S0-ANN-010

SURGICAL ONCOLOGY

SURGICAL

Springer
New York
Berlin
Heidelberg
Hong Kong
London
Milan
Paris
Tokyo

An Algorithmic Approach

ONCOLOGY

THEODORE J. SACLARIDES, M.D.
KEITH W. MILLIKAN, M.D.
CONSTANTINE V. GODELLAS, M.D.

Department of General Surgery
Rush Medical College
Chicago, IL

EDITORS

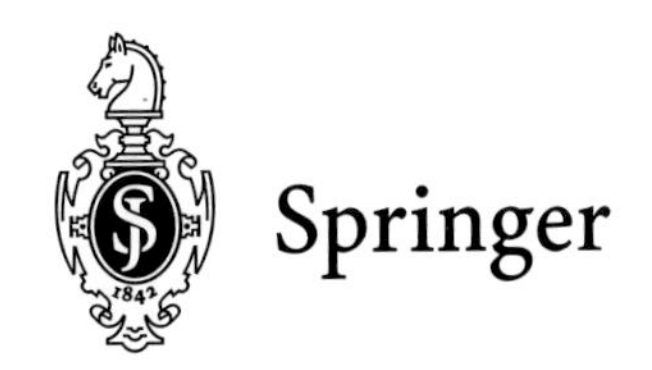

THEODORE J. SACLARIDES, M.D.
Professor of Surgery, Rush Medical College
Head, Section of Colon and Rectal Surgery
Department of General Surgery
Rush-Presbyterian-St. Luke's Medical Center
Chicago, IL 60612, USA

KEITH W. MILLIKAN, M.D.
Associate Professor of Surgery, Rush Medical College
Director of Undergraduate Surgical Education
Director, Nutrition Consultation Service
Department of General Surgery
Rush-Presbyterian-St. Luke's Medical Center
Chicago, IL 60612, USA

CONSTANTINE V. GODELLAS, M.D.
Assistant Professor of Surgery, Rush Medical College
Academic Program Coordinator
Department of General Surgery
Rush-Presbyterian-St. Luke's Medical Center
Chicago, IL 60612, USA

LIBRARY OF CONGRESS CATALOGING-IN-PUBLICATION DATA
Surgical oncology: an algorithmic approach / editors, Theodore J. Saclarides,
Keith W. Millikan, Constantine V. Godellas.
p. ; cm.
Includes bibliographical references and index.
ISBN 0-387-95201-2 (h/c : alk. paper)
1. Cancer—Surgery. 2. Oncology. 3. Algorithms. I. Saclarides, Theodore J., 1956–
II. Millikan, Keith W. III. Godellas, Constantine V.
[DNLM: 1. Neoplasms—surgery. 2. Surgical Procedures, Operative—methods. QZ 268
S961105 2001]
RD651 .S8833 2001
616.99'4059—dc21 2001032003

ISBN 0-387-95201-2 Printed on acid-free paper.

Text design by Steven Pisano.

Printed in the United States of America.

9 8 7 6 5 4 3 2 1 SPIN 10860606

www.springer-ny.com

Springer-Verlag New York Berlin Heidelberg
A member of BertelsmannSpringer Science+Business Media GmbH

My deepest gratitude to Frs. John Athas, George Scoulas (eternal be their memory) and Angelo Artemas for their inspiration and healing.

THEODORE J. SACLARIDES

I dedicate this work to my grandfather, Aunt Marge and Aunt Mary, who all suffered from lung cancer and, lastly, to Delores Deselich, who spent the majority of her shortened life nursing the sick, many of whom had the diseases described in the following pages.

KEITH W. MILLIKAN

In memory of my mother, Elaine, who was valiant in her fight against cancer, but ultimately lost the battle.

Also, for all the patients I have and will care for who fight the same battle, fortunately with better results.

I would also like to acknowledge my father, Dr. William Godellas, who practiced Internal Medicine for 40 years and taught me how to be a caring physician.

And finally, to my wife, Erin, who completes me.

CONSTANTINE V. GODELLAS

Foreword

It was not too many years ago that a hospital's daily surgical schedule included a number of "exploratory" operations. It was the era when the multipotential "general" surgeon was the star of the surgical amphitheater. While the need to make an incision to take a look inside the body might be compelling enough based on the presenting signs and symptoms, and often was lifesaving, beyond that what was found could be a total surprise, a thrilling adventure or a misguided exercise. That's why the "general" surgeon needed prolonged operating room exposure as an observer and then as an assistant, to gain the experience, confidence, and indeed the courage, to handle cases that today are commonly done by residents.

It was in just such a restricted, yet beckoning, climate that general surgery functioned until the great burst of progress that was triggered and fueled by the Second World War and its aftermath. The next several decades ushered in the establishment and maturation of the surgical specialties.

Inexorably from this fertile foundation the surgical subspecialties blossomed. It is now clear that surgery is in the midst of a multifaceted evolution, whose speed and breadth are truly impressive. While it also is true that some areas of surgery are not narrowly compartmentalized, so much new information of all sorts—technical and scientific—is being made available and is pertinent to good care, that to collect, analyze, and utilize it properly is a daunting challenge.

As just one example, it is no longer adequate for a physician to be defined as an "orthopedic" surgeon. By choice, or because of need, there are those orthopedic surgeons who confine their work just to neoplasms or to trauma; acquired or congenital disorders; only the foot and ankle; the hand, knee, hip, or spine and other areas. Many of these are legitimate subspecializations simply because of the considerable variety of available therapies for each anatomic area and the nuances that determine which therapeutic choice is most appropriate. As well, there is the need to perform enough of each of the applicable operations so as to both acquire the clinical judgment and develop the technical skills to confidently expect a high level of success. Multiply this by the robust growth of the other anatomic areas of surgical subspecialties and one can begin to understand the reasons why increasing numbers of surgeons have limited their repertoire of operations. At the same time, they improve their results and derive greater professional satisfaction.

Added to the specialization and subspecialization of surgery are the other two arms of the therapeutic trilogy, namely medicine and radiation therapy. Not surprisingly, they too have burgeoned to an extent unforeseen by most people who dispense health care. While all of the above developments have vastly expanded the choices of available treatments, they have also increased rather than lessened the challenges of deciding which therapy is most appropriate. Yet, in the final reckoning, it is from such a cornucopia of variable relevant choices that the clinician must select the therapy that will most likely lead to the desired result.

I applaud the book *Surgical Oncology: An Algorithmic Approach* by Drs. Theodore Saclarides, Keith Millikan and Constantine Godellas, because these young, but experienced, surgeons have wisely chosen to address an important, yet incompletely fulfilled, need in the current cancer textbooks—namely, to recognize the presence of an oncologic problem; to logically and methodically explore and treat it; and in an algorithmic fashion coordinate the efforts of the different disciplines necessary for treating the cancer patient.

I especially like the manner in which this book is arranged. The first part of each chapter is presented in a narrative exposition, offering the reader the choice of reading the material in a sweeping fashion or in a deliberate, studied way as the circumstances may require. The companion portion of each chapter is presented in the form of well-crafted algorithms that are logical and easy to follow. The concept of this book and the manner in which the contents are presented will make it an indispensable favorite of many physicians.

STEVEN G. ECONOMOU, M.D.

Professor of Surgery and Chairman Emeritus

Department of General Surgery

Rush-Presbyterian-St. Luke's Medical Center

Preface

The premise for this work is the realization that cancer cannot be adequately treated by a single specialty. The surgeon, medical oncologist, and radiation oncologist cannot and should not work or function in the secluded sphere of his/her own domain. Instead, successful management of the cancer patient must incorporate the best that each of these specialties has to offer. Added to the list of necessary healthcare professionals are genetic counselors, pain specialists, enterostomal therapists, and nutrition experts, just to name a few. Understanding the exact role of each of these entities can be a daunting challenge, thus the benefit of our work which has attempted to display in an algorithmic fashion how the various treatment and support modalities can be employed.

Treatment of the cancer patient must be individualized. One may incorrectly assume that an algorithmic approach advocates treatment of all patients with a particular cancer exactly the same or that a "cookbook" plan is being proposed. We firmly believe the contrary and comment throughout this work that controversy exists and that more that one approach may be taken depending on various institutional and geographic practices. Instead, our primary objective has been to display how many different specialties may interact and support one another with one goal in mind—to improve treatment and outcome. We hope that this work will accomplish our goal and organize care of the cancer patient in an easy to follow way.

THEODORE J. SACLARIDES, M.D.

KEITH W. MILLIKAN, M.D.

CONSTANTINE V. GODELLAS, M.D.

Contents

Section 2: Endocrine Malignancies

Section 3: Cancer of the Lung

Section 4: Breast Cancer

Section 5: Cutaneous Malignancies

Section 6: Gastrointestinal Malignancies

Section 12: Hematologic Malignancies

Section 13: Oncologic Emergencies

Contributors

Nadeem R. Abu-Rustum, M.D.
Department of Surgery, Gynecology Service, Memorial Sloan-Kettering Cancer Center, New York, NY 10021, USA

Roberto Angioli, M.D.
Department of Obstetrics and Gynecology, University of Rome Campus Biomedicó, Rome 00155, Italy

Hervy E. Averette, M.D.
Sylvester Comprehensive Breast Center, Miami, FL 33136, USA

Richard Barakat, M.D.
Department of Surgery, Memorial Sloan-Kettering Cancer Center, New York, NY 10021, USA

David Baldwin, Jr., M.D.
Department of Internal Medicine, Rush-Presbyterian-St. Luke's Medical Center, Chicago, IL 60612, USA

Roberto V. Barresi, M.D.
Department of Surgery, St. Alphonsus Regional Medical Center, Boise, ID 83705, USA

Steven D. Bines, M.D.
Department of General Surgery, Rush-Presbyterian-St. Luke's Medical Center, Chicago, IL 60612, USA

Philip Bonomi, M.D.
Department of Internal Medicine, Rush-Presbyterian-St. Luke's Medical Center, Chicago, IL 60612, USA

Marc I. Brand, M.D.
Department of General Surgery, Rush-Presbyterian-St. Luke's Medical Center, Chicago, IL 60612, USA

Murray F. Brennan, M.D.
Department of Surgery, Memorial Sloan-Kettering Cancer Center, New York, NY 10021, USA

Richard W. Byrne, M.D.
Department of Neurosurgery, Rush-Presbyterian-St. Luke's Medical Center, Chicago, IL 60612, USA

John R. Charters, M.D.
Department of Radiology, Rush-Presbyterian-St. Luke's Medical Center, Chicago, IL 60612, USA

James M. Church, B.Sc., M.B., Ch.B., M.Med.Sci.
Section of Colorectal Endoscopy, Department of Colorectal Surgery, The Cleveland Clinic Foundation, Cleveland, OH 44195, USA

Scott Cohen, M.D.
Sylvester Comprehensive Breast Center, Miami, FL 33136, USA

Christopher L. Coogan, M.D.
Department of Urology, Rush-Presbyterian-St. Luke's Medical Center, Chicago, IL 60612, USA

Domenico Coppola, M.D.
Division of Surgical Oncology, Moffit Cancer Center, Tampa, FL 33612-9497, USA

Marc L. Cullen, M.D.
Department of Pediatric Surgery, Children's Hospital of Michigan, Detroit, MI 48201-2196, USA

Andrew M. Davidoff, M.D.
Department of Pediatric Surgery, St. Jude Children's Hospital, Memphis, TN 38105, USA

Christopher J. DeWald, M.D.
Orthopedics and Scoliosis Ltd., Rush-Presbyterian-St. Luke's Medical Center, Chicago, IL 60612, USA

Daniel J. Deziel, M.D.
Department of General Surgery, Rush-Presbyterian-St. Luke's Medical Center, Chicago, IL 60612, USA

H. Drexel Dobson III, M.D.
Department of Colon and Rectal Surgery, Cook County Hospital, Chicago, IL 60612, USA

Philip E. Donahue, M.D., F.A.C.S
Department of Surgery, Cook County Hospital, Chicago, IL 60612, USA

Alexander Doolas, M.D.
Department of Surgery, Rush-Presbyterian-St Luke's Medical Center, Chicago, IL 60612, USA

Kambiz Dowlatshahi, M.D.
Department of Surgery, Rush-Presbyterian-St Luke's Medical Center, Chicago, IL 60612, USA

James S. Economou, M.D., Ph.D., F.A.C.S.
Division of Surgical Oncology, University of California, Los Angeles, School of Medicine, Los Angeles, CA 90024-1782, USA

Tasia S. Economou, M.D.
Southern California Permanente Medical Group: West Los Angeles, Los Angeles, CA 90034, USA

Lev Elterman, M.D.
Department of Urology, Rush-Presbyterian-St, Luke's Medical Center, Chicago, IL 60612, USA

David Esposito, M.D.
Department of Vascular and Cardiothoracic Surgery, Carolinas Medical Center, Charlotte, NC 28232, USA

Peter J. Fabri, M.D.
Surgical Service, James A. Haley Veteran's Administration Medical Center, Tampa, FL 33612, USA

Bejan Fakouri, M.D.
DuPage Urology Associates, Naperville, IL 60540, USA

Barry W. Feig, M.D.
Department of Surgical Oncology, University of Texas, M.D. Anderson Cancer Center, Houston, TX 77030-4095, USA

Carlos Fernandez-del Castillo, M.D.
Department of Surgery, Harvard Medical School, Massachusetts General Hospital, Boston, MA 02114, USA

Yuman Fong, M.D.
Department of Surgery, Memorial Sloan-Kettering Cancer Center, New York, NY 10021, USA

Gregory S. Foster, D.O.
Department of General Surgery, Rush-Presbyterian-St. Luke's Medical Center, Chicago, IL 60612, USA

Susan Galandiuk, M.D.
Department of Surgery, University of Louisville, Louisville, KY 40292, USA

G.E. Ghali, D.D.S., M.D.
Division of Surgical Oncology, Louisiana State University Medical Center, Shreveport, LA 71103, USA

Steven Gitelis, M.D.
Department of Orthopedic Surgery, Rush-Presbyterian-St. Luke's Medical Center, Chicago, IL 60612, USA

Constantine V. Godellas, M.D.
Department of General Surgery, Rush-Presbyterian-St. Luke's Medical Center, Chicago, IL 60612, USA

John A. Greager, M.D.
Department of Surgery, Cook County Hospital, Chicago, IL 60612, USA

Alexander A. Green, M.D.
Department of Pediatrics, Rush-Presbyterian-St. Luke's Medical Center, Chicago, IL 60612, USA

Seth P. Harlow, M.D.
Department of Surgery, University of Vermont, Burlington, VT 05405, USA

Jacqueline Harrison, M.D.
Department of Colon and Rectal Surgery, Cook County Hospital, Chicago, IL 60612, USA

Michael J. Hejna, M.D., Ph.D.
Department of Orthopedic Surgery, MacNeal Memorial Hospital, Berwyn, IL 60402, USA

Tina J. Hieken, M.D.
Department of General Surgery, Rush North Shore Medical Center, Skokie, IL 60076, USA

Jerome Hoeksema, M.D.
Department of Urology, Rush-Presbyterian-St. Luke's Medical Center, Chicago, IL 60612, USA

Edward F. Hollinger, M.D., Ph.D.
Department of General Surgery, Rush-Presbyterian-St. Luke's Medical Center, Chicago, IL 60612, USA

James R. Howe, M.D.
Department of Surgery, University of Iowa Hospitals and Clinics, Iowa City, IA 52442-1086, USA

William B. Inabnet III, M.D.
Division of Laparoscopic Surgery Department of Surgery, Mount Sinai Medical Center, New York, NY 10128, USA

Timothy W. James, M.D.
Elgin Cardiac Surgery, Elgin, IL 60120, USA

Richard Karl, M.D.
Division of Surgical Oncology, Moffit Cancer Center, Tampa, FL 33612-9497, USA

Nafeeza Khoka, M.D.
Department of Medical Oncology, Cook County Hospital, Chicago, IL 60612, USA

Edward H. Kolb, M.D.
Department of Surgery, Rush-Presbyterian-St. Luke's Medical Center, Chicago, IL 60612, USA

James M. Kozlowski, M.D. F.A.C.S.
Department of Urology, Northwestern University Medical School, Chicago, IL 60611-3009, USA

Daniel M. Labow, M.D.
Department of Surgery, Memorial Sloan-Kettering Cancer Center, New York, NY 10021, USA

Lily L. Lai, M.D.
Division of Surgery, City of Hope National Medical Center, Duarte, CA 91010-3000, USA

Benjamin D.L. Li, M.D.
Department of Surgical Oncology, Louisiana State University Medical Center, Shreveport, LA 71103, USA

Dennis T.H. Lim, M.D.
Head and Neck Service, Memorial Sloan-Kettering Cancer Center, New York, NY 10021, USA

Laurel A. Littrell, M.D.
Department of Radiology, Mayo Clinic, Rochester, MN 55901, USA

Ernst W. Lisek IV, M.D.
Department of Urology, DuPage Medical Group, Glen Ellyn, IL 60137, USA

James A. Madura II, M.D.
Department of General Surgery, Rush-Presbyterian-St. Luke's Medical Center, Chicago, IL 60612, USA

Sharmila Makhija, M.D.
Division of Gynecologic Oncology, University of Alabama at Birmingham, Birmingham, AL 35233, USA

Mark C. Mantooth, J.D.
American Medical Association, Washington, DC 20005, USA

Elizabeth Marcus, M.D.
Department of Surgery, Cook County Hospital, Chicago, IL 60612, USA

Thomas G. Matkov, M.D.
Department of Urology, All Saints-St. Mary Hospital, Racine, WI 53405, USA

Charles F. McKiel, Jr., M.D.
Department of Urology, Rush-Presbyterian-St. Luke's Medical Center, Chicago, IL 60612, USA

Arthur N.S. Mcunu, Jr., m.d.
Department of Surgery, Wayne State University, Harper Hospital, Detroit, MI 48201, USA

Janet Millikan, r.d., m.s., l.d.
Department of General Surgery, Rush-Presbyterian-St. Luke's Medical Center, Chicago, IL 60612, USA

Keith W. Millikan, m.d.
Department of General Surgery, Rush-Presbyterian-St. Luke's Medical Center, Chicago, IL 60612, USA

Emery A. Minnard, m.d.
Department of Surgery, Division of Surgical Oncology, Louisiana State University Medical Center, Shreveport, LA 71103, USA

Pinesh Monege, m.d.
Department of Medical Oncology, Cook County Hospital, Chicago, IL 60612, USA

J. Lawrence Munson, m.d.
Department of General Surgery, Lahey/Hitchcock Clinic, Burlington, MA 01805, USA

Peter Murphy, m.d.
Department of Anesthesiology, Rush-Presbyterian-St. Luke's Medical Center, Chicago, IL 60612, USA

Jonathan A. Myers, m.d.
Department of General Surgery, Rush-Presbyterian-St. Luke's Medical Center, Chicago, IL 60612, USA

Cam Nguyen, m.d., f.r.c.p. (c)
Department of Radiation Oncology, Rush-Presbyterian-St. Luke's Medical Center, Chicago, IL 60612, USA

Judith A. Paice, Ph.D., r.n., f.a.a.n.
Division of Hematology-Oncology, Northwestern University, Chicago, IL 60611, USA

William R. Panje, m.d., f.a.c.s.
Department of Otolaryngology and Bronchoesophagology, Rush-Presbyterian-St. Luke's Medical Center, Chicago, IL 60612, USA

Harvey I. Pass, m.d.
Departments of Surgery and Oncology, Thoracic Surgery, Karmanos Cancer Institute, Wayne State University, Detroit, MI 48201, USA

Geoffrey A. Porter, m.d.
Department of Surgical Oncology, University of Texas M.D. Anderson Cancer Center, Houston, TX 77030, USA

Paul Russo, M.D., F.A.C.S.
Urology Service, Department of Surgery, Memorial Sloan-Kettering Cancer Center, New York, NY 10021, USA

Richard A. Prinz, M.D.
Department of General Surgery, Rush-Presbyterian-St. Luke's Medical Center, Chicago, IL 60612, USA

Theodore J. Saclarides, M.D.
Department of General Surgery, Rush-Presbyterian-St. Luke's Medical Center, Chicago, IL 60612, USA

Nader Sadeghi, M.D., F.R.C.S.C.
Division of Otolaryngology, Head & Neck Surgery, George Washington University, Washington, DC 20037, USA

Nicholas C. Saenz, M.D.
Children's Specialists of San Diego, San Diego, CA 92123, USA

Pierre F. Saldinger, M.D.
Deparment of Surgery, Beth Israel Deaconess Medical Center, Boston, MA 02215, USA

Isaac Samuel, M.D., F.R.C.S.
Department of Surgery, University of Iowa Hospitals and Clinics, Iowa City, IA 52242, USA

V. Amod Saxena, M.D., F.R.C.R., F.A.C.R.
Department of Radiation Oncology, Rush-Presbyterian-St. Luke's Medical Center, Chicago, IL 60612, USA

Scott R. Schell, M.D., Ph.D.
Departments of Surgery and Molecular Genetics and Microbiology, University of Florida College of Medicine, Gainesville, FL 32610, USA

Robert Schreiber, M.D.
200 Winston Drive, Cliffside Park, NJ 07010, USA

Roderich E. Schwarz, M.D., Ph.D.
University of Medicine and Dentistry of New Jersey, Robert Wood Johnson Medical School, The Cancer Institute of New Jersey, New Brunswick, NJ 08901, USA

F. John Service, M.D., Ph.D.
Department of Medicine, Mayo Clinic, Rochester, MN 55905, USA

Ashok R. Shaha, M.D., F.A.C.S.
Head and Neck Service, Memorial Sloan-Kettering Cancer Center, New York, NY 10021, USA

Gail Shiomoto, m.d.
Department of Medical Oncology, Cook County Hospital, Chicago, IL 60612, USA

Norm Smith, m.d.
Department of Urology, Northwestern University Medical School, Chicago, IL 60611-3009, USA

Ronald H. Spiro, m.d.
Head and Neck Service, Memorial Sloan-Kettering Cancer Center, New York, NY 10021, USA

Mark S. Talamonti, m.d.
Department of Surgery, Northwestern University Medical School, Chicago, IL 60611-3009, USA

John V. Taylor, m.b., f.r.c.s.Ed.
Department of Surgery, University of Louisville, Louisville, KY 40292, USA

Geoffrey B. Thompson, m.d.
Department of General Surgery, Mayo Clinic, Rochester, MN 55905, USA

Theodore N. Tsangaris, m.d.
Department of Surgery, Breast Surgery, Division of Surgical Oncology, The Johns Hopkins Comprehensive Breast, Center, Sidney Kimmel Comprehensive Cancer Center at Johns Hopkins, Baltimore, MD 21287, USA

Robert Udelsman, m.d., m.b.a., f.a.c.s.
Department of Surgery, Yale University School of Medicine, New Haven, CT 06520-8062, USA

José M. Velasco, m.d.
Department of General Surgery, Rush North Shore Medical Center, Skokie, IL 60076, USA

T.K. Venkatesan, m.d.
Department of Otolaryngology, Illinois Masonic Medical Center, Rush-Presbyterian-St. Luke's Medical Center, Chicago, IL 60612, and Advocate, Illinois Masonic Medical Center, Chicago, IL 60657, USA

William H. Warren, m.d.
Department of Cardiovascular/Thoracic Surgery, Rush-Presbyterian-St. Luke's Medical Center, Chicago, IL 60612, USA

Marie Welshinger, m.d.
Women's Cancer Center at the Carol G. Simon Cancer Center, Morristown Memorial Hospital, Morristown, NJ 07962-1956, USA

David B. Wilson, m.d., major, usaf, mc
Division of General Surgery, Maxwell Clinic, Maxwell AFB, AL 36066, and Department of Surgery, University of Alabama at Birmingham, Birmingham, AL 35233, USA

Thomas R. Witt, m.d.
Department of General Surgery, Rush-Presbyterian-St. Luke's Medical Center, Chicago, IL 60612, USA

Peter Y. Wong, m.d.
Department of Vascular Surgery, Harper Hospital, Detroit Medical Center, Wayne State University Detroit, MI 48201, USA

Nader Yamin, m.d.
Department of General Surgery, Rush-Presbyterian-St. Luke's Medical Center, Chicago, IL 60612, USA

Section 1

Head and Neck

CHAPTER I

Cancer of the Lip

TINA J. HIEKEN

A. Epidemiology and Etiology

Carcinoma of the lip is estimated to occur in 3600 persons per year in the United States, an incidence of 1.8 persons per 100,000.[1] The incidence is slightly higher in Canada, at 2.7 cases per 100,000 per annum.[2] Ninety-five percent of cases occur in males.[3–5] Etiologic factors include ultraviolet (UV) light exposure, tobacco use of all types (cigarettes, pipes, cigars), and immunosuppression.[6–8] A causative role for poor oral hygiene, trauma, or exposure to topical carcinogens such as crude oils has not been substantiated.

The primary risk factor for carcinoma of the lip is actinic damage from ultraviolet light exposure. The decrease in the number of cases of carcinoma of the lip seen over the past 25 years may be attributable to the increased use of sunscreens. Almost all squamous cell carcinomas of the lip develop in areas of previous actinic cheilitis,[5,9] which manifests as blurring of the skin–vermilion junction, development of striations perpendicular to the skin–vermilion border, hyperkeratosis, and thickening of the skin below the lip. The proportion of cases of actinic cheilitis that develop into malignancy is unknown.

As the molecular level, as in other UV radiation-associated squamous cell carcinomas, mutations in the tumor suppressor gene *p53* have been demonstrated in up to 80% of squamous cell carcinomas of the lip.[10–12] Aberrant expression of p53 protein is also seen in a high proportion of precancerous lip lesions, suggesting that *p53* alterations are an early event in the pathogenesis of squamous cell lip cancers.[11] Mutations in the H-*ras* oncogene, detected in oral cavity squamous cell carcinomas due to chewing tobacco, have been observed in a large proportion of carcinomas of the lip.[13]

B. Histology

Most cancers of the lip are squamous cell carcinomas. Other tumors found in this location include basal cell carcinoma, malignant melanoma, and rarely minor salivary gland cancers. The three types of squamous cell carcinoma of the lip are exophytic, ulcerative, and verrucous (rare) types. Histologically,

Carcinoma of the Lip

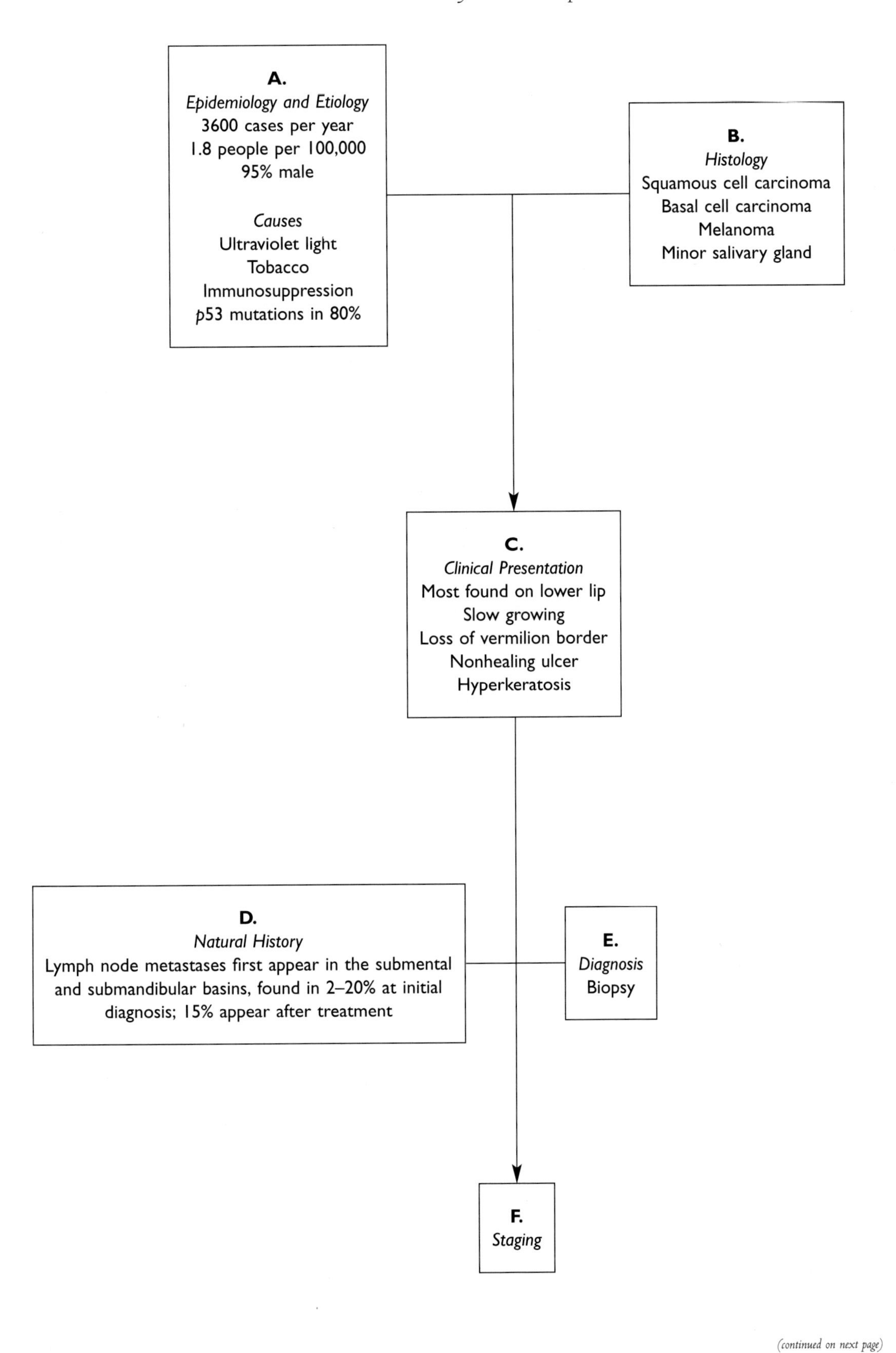

(continued on next page)

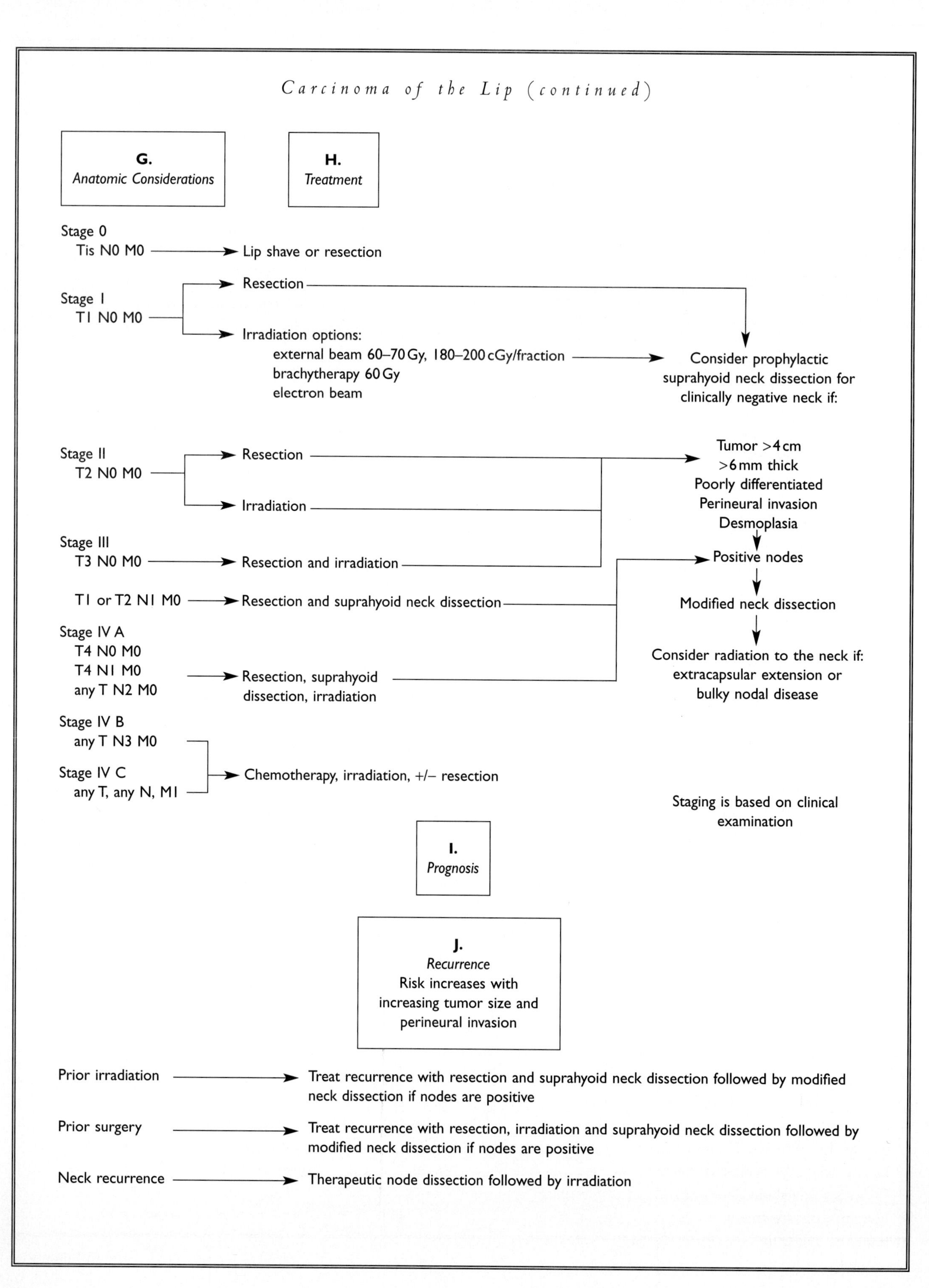

Carcinoma of the Lip (continued)
G.
Anatomic Considerations
H.
Treatment
Stage 0
Tis N0 M0
Lip shave or resection
Stage I
T1 N0 M0
Resection
Irradiation options:
external beam 60–70 Gy, 180–200 cGy/fraction
brachytherapy 60 Gy
electron beam
Consider prophylactic suprahyoid neck dissection for clinically negative neck if:
Stage II
T2 N0 M0
Resection
Irradiation
Tumor >4 cm
>6 mm thick
Poorly differentiated
Perineural invasion
Desmoplasia
Stage III
T3 N0 M0
Resection and irradiation
Positive nodes
T1 or T2 N1 M0
Resection and suprahyoid neck dissection
Modified neck dissection
Stage IV A
T4 N0 M0
T4 N1 M0
any T N2 M0
Resection, suprahyoid dissection, irradiation
Consider radiation to the neck if: extracapsular extension or bulky nodal disease
Stage IV B
any T N3 M0
Stage IV C
any T, any N, M1
Chemotherapy, irradiation, +/– resection
Staging is based on clinical examination
I.
Prognosis
J.
Recurrence
Risk increases with increasing tumor size and perineural invasion
Prior irradiation
Treat recurrence with resection and suprahyoid neck dissection followed by modified neck dissection if nodes are positive
Prior surgery
Treat recurrence with resection, irradiation and suprahyoid neck dissection followed by modified neck dissection if nodes are positive
Neck recurrence
Therapeutic node dissection followed by irradiation

lip carcinomas are graded from well differentiated (about 70% of lesions) to poorly differentiated (<5% of cases).

C. Clinical Presentation

Most carcinomas of the lip occur on the lower lip, with about 6% on the upper lip and 3% at the commissure.[4,5] Upper lip tumors are seen in a proportionally larger number of female patients.[5] Early carcinoma of the lip may be difficult to distinguish from actinic cheilitis. There may be loss of the sharply defined vermilion border or an area of induration. To detect early tumors, the lip must be palpated as well as inspected visually. Verrucous changes, erythema, nonhealing lesions, and hyperkeratosis may herald malignancy. Any of these lesions that persist for more than a few weeks should be biopsied. Advanced squamous cell carcinoma of the lip usually presents as a nonhealing chronic ulcer or an exophytic growth. Proper evaluation for suspected carcinoma of the lip includes not only inspection and palpation of the mucosal lip (both upper and lower lips, from the vermilion border to the commissures of the mouth) but careful examination of the neck as well. When present, cervical lymph node involvement from carcinoma of the lip usually first appears in the submental and submandibular lymph nodes, then the jugular nodes. Tumors of the upper lip may also metastasize to the preauricular lymph nodes.

D. Natural History

The biologic behavior of carcinoma of the lip is variable. Most tumors remain localized and grow slowly, spreading radially and peripherally rather than invading deeply into contiguous structures. Direct extension into adjacent bone and perineural invasion is exhibited by the occasionally aggressive form of this tumor. Regional lymph node metastases are present in 2–20% of cases (10% in most series) at the time of diagnosis.[4,5,14–17] An additional 5–30% of patients (15% on average) develop cervical lymph node metastases subsequent to treatment.[15,17,18]

E. Diagnosis

In general, all suspicious lesions should be biopsied prior to definitive treatment. Some surgeons, however, hold that small tumors of the lower lip should be treated without preliminary biopsy, claiming that an equivocal incisional or punch biopsy does not preclude the need for excision and that such biopsies may disseminate tumor cells into the circulation via disrupted blood vessels and lymphatics. In a small series of squamous cell carcinomas of the lip treated by primary resection without biopsy, the clinical diagnosis was correct in 87% of cases; prior biopsy would have altered the treatment of only one patient (3%).[19] Tissue should be obtained prior to initiating radiation therapy if this treatment modality is chosen. There is no role for toluidine blue staining in the evaluation of suspected carcinoma of the lip.

TABLE 1–1.
AJCC definition of TNM for carcinoma of the lip

Primary Tumor (T)	
TX	Primary tumor cannot be assessed
T0	No evidence of primary tumor
Tis	Carcinoma *in situ*
T1	Tumor 2 cm or less in greatest dimension
T2	Tumor more than 2 cm but not more than 4 cm in greatest dimension
T3	Tumor more than 4 cm in greatest dimension
T4 (lip)	Tumor invades adjacent structures (e.g., through cortical bone, inferior alveolar nerve, floor of mouth, skin of face)
Regional Lymph Nodes (N)	
NX	Regional lymph nodes cannot be assessed
N0	No regional lymph node metastasis
N1	Metastasis in a single ipsilateral lymph node, 3 cm or less in greatest dimension
N2	Metastasis in a single ipsilateral lymph node, more than 3 cm but not more than 6 cm in greatest dimension; or in multiple ipsilateral lymph nodes, none more than 6 cm in greatest dimension; or in bilateral or contralateral lymph nodes, none more than 6 cm in greatest dimension
N2a	Metastasis in single ipsilateral lymph node more than 3 cm but not more than 6 cm in greatest dimension
N2b	Metastasis in multiple ipsilateral lymph nodes, none more than 6 cm in greatest dimension
N2c	Metastasis in bilateral or contralateral lymph nodes, none more than 6 cm in greatest dimension
N3	Metastasis in a lymph node more than 6 cm in greatest dimension
Distant Metastasis (M)	
MX	Distant metastasis cannot be assessed
M0	No distant metastasis
M1	Distant metastasis

SOURCE: Used with permission of the American Joint Committee on Cancer (AJCC®), Chicago, IL. The original source for this material is the AJCC® Cancer Staging Manual, 5th edition (1997) published by Lippincott Williams & Wilkins Publishers, Philadelphia, PA.

F. Staging

The current TNM staging system for carcinoma of the lip is shown in Tables 1–1 and 1–2. To facilitate proper treatment and to compare treatment outcomes and prognostic factors, all cases should be staged according to these guidelines.

G. Anatomic Considerations

The lip is delineated by the junction of the vermilion border with the skin; it is well defined as an upper and lower lip joined at the commissures of the mouth. The arterial blood supply to the lip is by the superior and inferior labial arteries (branches of the facial artery), which create a circumoral vascular arcade at the level of the mucocutaneous ridge. Motor innervation comes from the buccal and mandibular branches

TABLE 1–2.
AJCC stage grouping for carcinoma of the lip

Stage	T	N	M
0	Tis	N0	M0
I	T1	N0	M0
II	T2	N0	M0
III	T3	N0	M0
	T1	N1	M0
	T2	N1	M0
	T3	N1	M0
IVA	T4	N0	M0
	T4	N1	M0
	Any T	N2	M0
IVB	Any T	N3	M0
IVC	Any T	Any N	M1

SOURCE: Used with permission of the American Joint Committee on Cancer (AJCC®), Chicago, IL. The original source for this material is the AJCC® Cancer Staging Manual, 5th edition (1997) published by Lippincott Williams & Wilkins Publishers, Philadelphia, PA.

of the facial nerve. Sensory nerve fibers travel via the infraorbital (upper) and mental (lower) nerves, both branches of the trigeminal (V) nerve. The primary lymph node drainage from the lower lip is to the submental and submaxillary lymph nodes. The upper lip may also drain to the parotid and preauricular lymph nodes.[21]

H. *Treatment*

It is important to remember that the foremost goal of treatment is retention of oral competence. Secondary goals include maintenance of articulation, deglutition, and cosmesis.

Carcinoma In Situ

Dysplasia and carcinoma in situ can be treated by vermilionectomy with advancement of a mucosal flap (lip shave). This approach is also effective for the treatment of carcinoma in situ with microinvasion.[22,23]

T1 and T2 Lesions

In the United States surgical resection is the most frequently used treatment for lesions involving less than 30% of the lip. Resection can be accomplished with a V-shaped excision and primary closure with excellent cosmesis and function.[4,24] Because of its technical ease and generally good results and the fact that resection can be done as a single ambulatory outpatient procedure, surgery is usually the preferred treatment for early invasive carcinomas of the lip. A V excision is performed under bilateral mental nerve blocks with additional local anesthetic infiltration as needed and intravenous sedation as required for patient comfort. The cutaneous–vermilion junction should be tattooed (using a 27-gauge needle dipped in methylene blue or a marking pen) to ensure proper realignment. Margins of 0.5 cm are marked; and a full-thickness wedge resection, including underlying orbicularis oris muscle, is performed. The inner mucosa is reapproximated with interrupted fine chromic sutures. The muscle layer is closed with 4-0 or 5-0 Vicryl; proper function of the oral sphincter requires careful reconstitution of the orbicularis oris muscle. The vermilion is everted with horizontal mattress sutures of 5-0 or 6-0 chromic material, taking meticulous care to realign the tattooed cutaneous–vermilion junction. The skin is then closed with 5-0 or 6-0 nylon sutures, which are removed 4–5 days postoperatively. A lip shave may be performed in conjunction with a V excision when there are extensive dysplastic changes of the adjacent vermilion.

Primary radiotherapy is also an effective treatment for T1 and T2 lesions. Brachytherapy or external beam radiation may be employed. Brachytherapy alone can be used for T1 and small T2 lesions and is usually delivered by iridium-192 (^{192}Ir) implantation at a dose of 60 Gy.[3,25] External beam radiation is customarily delivered as 60–70 Gy in 180- to 200-cGy fractions over 6–7 weeks. Other dose-fractionation schedules employed include a slightly lower dose in larger fractions (e.g., 51 Gy over 3 weeks in 300-cGy fractions).[26] Small carcinomas of the lip also may be treated with electron beam radiation.[27] The size and location of the primary tumor may govern the choice between surgery and radiation therapy. Iradiation should be avoided in young patients and when there are extensive premalignant changes of the remaining lip. Radiation therapy may be given postoperatively to improve local control after surgical excision with microscopically positive margins.

T3 Lesions

Surgery or radiotherapy may be used for T3 lesions (see above). Lesions that encompass more than 30% of the lip usually require flap reconstruction after resection for acceptable cosmesis and function. The Abbe-Estlander flap (Fig. 1–1), a transposition flap from the uninvolved opposite lip (lip-switch procedure or cross-lip flap), is satisfactory for defects of one-third to one-half of the lip.[24,28,29] The surgical treatment of tumors involving more than 50% of the lip represent a challenge to the surgeon. A variety of techniques, including nasolabial flaps (Fig. 1–2), the fan-type Gillies flap, and the Webster cheek advancement flap, may be employed.[24,30,31]

T4 and Large T3 Lesions

Defects of more than 80% of the lip resulting from resection of large tumors with or without chin invasion can be reconstructed with inferiorly based unilateral or bilateral nasolabial flaps. Total

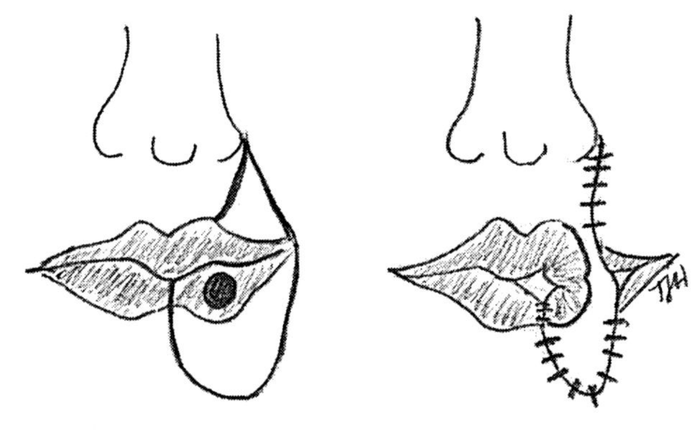

FIGURE 1–1
Abbe-Estlander flap.

lip resection with en bloc resection of the chin and mandible requires complex reconstruction with a distant flap such as a radial forearm flap.[24] Combined-modality treatment, consisting of resection and flap reconstruction followed by postoperative external beam radiation is the treatment of choice for advanced tumors. Complications of radiotherapy seen in this group of patients include soft tissue necrosis, necrosis of the mandible (rare), and moist desquamation (common).[26] The latter is usually self-limited and resolves within 6–8 weeks.

Management of Regional Lymph Nodes

Carcinoma of the lip has a much lower predilection for lymphatic spread than other squamous cell carcinomas of the oral cavity. Only 10–15% of patients present with positive lymph nodes.[4,5,14–17] An additional 10–15% of patients develop lymph node metastases after treatment.[15,17,18] Because of this low yield, routine prophylactic neck dissection for carcinoma of the lip usually is not performed. There are, however, some advocates of prophylactic suprahyoid lymph node dissection.[14] There is, as yet, no published data on the use of sentinel lymph node biopsy in the treatment of squamous cell carcinoma of the lip.

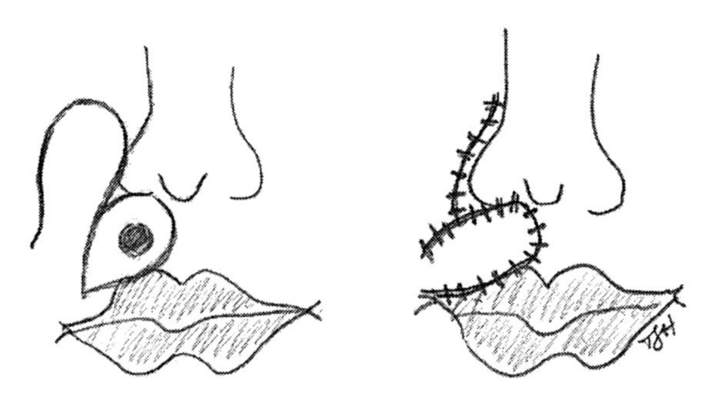

FIGURE 1–2
Nasolabial flap.

Risk factors for lymph node metastases include tumor size, histologic grade, tumor thickness, perineural invasion, and desmoplasia. Whereas only 5–7% of patients with T1 lesions have involved cervical lymph nodes at the time of diagnosis, more than twice as many patients with T2 and T3 lesions and more than 60% of patients with T4 lesions have cervical lymph node metastases at diagnosis.[5,24] Similarly, only a small percentage of patients with well differentiated carcinomas of the lip have concomitant lymph node metastases compared with more than 50% of those with poorly differentiated tumors.[15,17,24] Tumor thickness (depth of invasion) of ≥3–6 mm is associated with a 10-fold or greater increase in the likelihood of cervical lymph node metastases.[15,17] Perineural invasion is an uncommon finding but is associated with lymph node metastases at least 50% of the time.[15,17]

Desmoplastic squamous cell carcinomas (fewer than 5% of all such tumors) metastasize to regional lymph nodes six times more frequently than tumors lacking a significant stromal desmoplastic reaction.[17,32] Therefore it is reasonable to reserve prophylactic bilateral suprahyoid neck dissection for patients with a clinically negative neck to those with tumors >4 cm or >6 mm in vertical thickness, those with poorly differentiated tumors, and those exhibiting perineural invasion or significant desmoplasia. If any tumor-containing lymph nodes are found, a standard or modified radical neck dissection should then be performed on the affected side. More than one-third of these patients have additional metastatic disease in their jugular lymph nodes.[4,24]

Nearly half of the patients with *clinically* enlarged level I lymph nodes have only inflammatory or reactive changes on histologic examination.[4,5] Nevertheless, a suprahyoid neck dissection should be performed on patients with clinically enlarged submental or submandibular lymph nodes and converted to a standard or modified radical neck dissection if lymph node metastases are detected on frozen section. Postoperative adjuvant radiotherapy to the neck should be given to patients with extracapsular extension of tumor outside the lymph node and patients with massive, bulky nodal disease.

Stage IV Disease

Combined-modality treatment is usually employed for local control of the stage IV, advanced tumors. For metastatic disease, cisplatin-based chemotherapy, as used for other squamous cell carcinomas of the aerodigestive tract, may be given. There is no proven benefit of adjuvant chemotherapy for the treatment of patients with high risk tumors without distant disease.

I. *Prognosis*

Carcinoma of the lip has the most favorable prognosis of all squamous cell carcinomas of the oral cavity. Nonetheless,

10–15% of patients die of their disease.[5,17,24] Local control is achieved for more than 90% of T1 and T2 lesions but for only 45% of T4 lesions.[4,25,26] The 5-year survival for patients whose tumors are <2 cm and who are treated by surgery or radiotherapy alone generally exceeds 90%.[3–5,15] Patients with larger tumors or those who exhibit bony (usually mandibular) invasion generally have 5-year survival rates of less than 60%.[5] Other adverse prognostic factors include poor histologic grade, tumor thickness >6 mm, desmoplasia, stromal sclerosis, muscular invasion, and perineural invasion.[15,17,32,33] Growth of the tumor along perineural lymphatics into the point of exit from the mandible of the mental nerve (the mental foramen) can lead to extension along the inferior alveolar nerve and eventually toward the base of the skull. Angiogenesis has not been shown to have prognostic significance.[34] While *p53* mutations are found in about half of squamous cell carcinomas of the lip, the clinical significance of this observation is unknown.[35] Irrespective of tumor size, lymph node involvement further decreases survival. The average 5-year survival for all lymph node-positive patients is about 50%.[3,4,15]

There is also a significant incidence of metachronous lip neoplasia in the absence of total lip resurfacing. The risk of developing a second primary lip cancer is estimated to be approximately 20% by 10 years of follow-up.[36]

J. Recurrence

Local recurrence occurs infrequently. Not unexpectedly, recurrence rates increase in relation to the size of the primary tumor. The local recurrence rate is 10–15% for T1 lesions and more than 50% for T3 and T4 tumors.[24] Local recurrence is also more frequent for tumors exhibiting perineural invasion, even after apparently complete surgical resection.[17] Local recurrence after primary radiotherapy is best treated by resection. Local recurrence that occurs after surgical excision usually requires re-resection and adjuvant postoperative radiotherapy. Local recurrence is also associated with concomitant or subsequent lymph node metastasis.[15] A suprahyoid neck dissection (see above) should be performed for most patients with local recurrence despite a clinically negative neck.

Nodal recurrence is best treated by a therapeutic lymph node dissection. Most patients with recurrence in the neck, including those with extracapsular invasion of tumor cells or bulky nodal disease, should undergo postoperative radiation therapy.

References

1. Menck HR, Garfinkel L, Dodd GD. Preliminary report of the National Cancer Data Base. CA Cancer J Clin 1991;41:7.
2. Canadian Cancer Statistics. National Cancer Institute of Canada, Statistics Canada, 1995:80.
3. Jorgensen K, Elbrond O, Andersen AP. Carcinoma of the lip: a series of 869 cases. Acta Radiol 1973;12:177–190.
4. Heller KS, Shah JP. Carcinoma of the lip. Am J Surg 1979;138:600–603.
5. Zitsch RP, Park CW, Renner GJ, et al. Outcome analysis for lip carcinoma. Otolaryngol Head Neck Surg 1995;113:589–596.
6. Baker SR. Risk factors in multiple carcinoma of the lip. Otolaryngol Head Neck Surg 1980;88:248–260.
7. Berger HM, Goldman R, Gonick HC, et al. Epidermoid carcinoma of the lip after renal transplantation: report of two cases. Arch Intern Med 1971;128:609–612.
8. Pogoda JM, Preston-Martin S. Solar radiation, lip protection and lip cancer risk in Los Angeles County women. Cancer Causes Control 1996; 7:458–463.
9. Main JH, Pavone M. Actinic cheilitis and carcinoma of the lip. J Can Dent Assoc 1994;60:113–116.
10. Berner A, Holm R, Ane N, Hjortdal O. p53 Protein expression in squamocellular carcinomas of the lip. Anticancer Res 1993;13:2421–2424.
11. Crosthwaite N, Teale D, Franklin C, Foster GA, Stringer BMJ. p53 protein expression in malignant, pre-malignant and nonmalignant lesions of the lip. J Clin Pathol 1996;49:648–653.
12. Ibrahim SO, Johannessen AC, Vasstrand EN, et al. Immunohistochemical detection of p53 in archival formalin-fixed tissues of lip and intraoral squamous cell carcinomas from Norway. APMIS 1997;105: 757–764.
13. Milasin J, Pujic N, Dedovic N, Hikolic Z, Petrovic V, Dimitrijevic B. High incidence of H-ras oncogene mutations in squamous cell carcinoma of the lip vermilion. J Oral Pathol Med 1994;23:298–301.
14. Koc C, Akyol MU, Celikkanat S, et al. Role of suprahyoid neck dissection in the treatment of squamous cell carcinoma of the lower lip. Ann Otol Rhinol Laryngol 1997;106:787–789.
15. Frierson HF, Cooper PH. Prognostic factors in squamous cell carcinoma of the lower lip. Hum Pathol 1986;17:346–354.
16. McGregor GI, Davis NL, Hay JH. Impact of cervical lymph node metastases from squamous cell cancer of the lip. Am J Surg 1992;163:469–471.
17. Saywell MS, Weedon D. Histological correlates of metastasis in primary invasive squamous cell carcinoma of the lip. Australas J Pathol 1996; 36:193–195.
18. Marshall KA, Edgerton MT. Indications for neck dissection in carcinoma of the lip. Am J Surg 1977;133:216–218.
19. Hjortdal O, Naess A, Berner A. Squamous cell carcinomas of the lower lip. J Craniomaxillofac Surg 1995;23:34–37.
20. American Joint Committee on Cancer. Lip and oral cavity. In: AJCC Cancer Staging Manual, 5th ed. American Joint Committee on Cancer, Chicago, IL. 24–30.
21. Larson DL, Coers CR, Rodin AE, Parcansky GM, Corujo MB, Lewis SR. Lymphatics of the upper and lower lips. Am J Surg 1967;114:525–529.
22. Birt BD. The "lip shave" operation for pre-malignant conditions and microinvasive carcinomas of the lower lip. J Otolaryngol 1977;6:407–411.
23. Van der Wal JE, de Visscher JGAM, Baart JA, et al. Oncologic aspects of vermilionectomy in microinvasive squamous cell carcinoma of the lower lip. Int J Oral Maxillofac Surg 1996;25:446–448.
24. Luce EA, Goldberg DP. Oncologic and reconstructive considerations in nonmelanotic skin and lip cancers. Surg Oncol Clin N Am 1996; 5:751–784.
25. de Visscher JG, Grond AJ, Botke G, van der Waal I. Results of radiotherapy for squamous cell carcinomas of the vermilion border of the lower lip: a retrospective analysis of 108 patients. Radiother Oncol 1996;39:9–14.
26. Petrovich Z, Parker RG, Luxton G, et al. Carcinoma of the lip and selected sites of head and neck skin: a clinical study of 896 patients. Radiother Oncol 1987;8:11–17.

27. Sykes AJ, Allan E, Irwin C. Squamous cell carcinoma of the lip: the role of electron treatment. Clin Oncol 1996;8:384–386.
28. Abbe R. A new plastic operation for the relief of deformity due to double hairlip. Med Rec 1898;53:477–452.
29. Estlander JA. Eine methods aus der einen Lippe Sulstanzverluste der Andersen zu Ersetzen. Arch Klin Chir 1872;14:622–640.
30. Baker SR, Krause CJ. Pedicle flaps in reconstruction of the lip. Fac Plast Surg 1983;1:61–85.
31. MacGregor JA. Reconstruction of the lower lip. Br J Plast Surg 1983;36:40–59.
32. Breuninger H, Schaumburg-Lever G, Holzschuh J, et al. Desmoplastic squamous cell carcinoma of skin and vermilion surface: a highly malignant subtype of skin cancer. Cancer 1997;79:915–919.
33. Dos Santos LR, Cernea CR, Kowalski LP, et al. Squamous cell carcinoma of the lower lip: a retrospective study of 58 patients. Rev Paulista Med 1996;114:1117–1126.
34. Tahan SR, Stein AL. Angiogenesis in invasive squamous cell carcinoma of the lip: tumor vascularity is not an indicator of metastatic risk. J Cutan Pathol 1995;22:236–240.
35. Ostwald C, Gogacz P, Hillmann T, Schweder J, Gundlach K, Kundt G, Barten M. p53 Mutational spectra are different between squamous-cell carcinomas of the lip and the oral cavity. Int J Cancer 2000;88:82–86.
36. McCombe D, MacGill K, Ainslie J, Beresford J, Matthews J. Squamous cell carcinoma of the lip: A retrospective review of the Peter MacCallum Cancer Institute experience. ANZ J of Surg 2000;70:358–361.

Chapter 2

Cancer of the Floor of the Mouth

JOHN A. GREAGER

A. Epidemiology and Etiology

The floor of the mouth is one of the common sites for intraoral malignancies, although overall the annual incidence is quite low, with only about 0.6 cases occurring per 100,000 people in the United States. It is predominantly a disease of men (80%), with the median age being 55–65 years. Cigarette smoking, pipe smoking, tobacco or betel nut chewing, and heavy alcohol intake are believed to be etiologic factors. Poor oral hygiene and chronic trauma are also considered important associated factors.

B. Anatomy

The boundaries of the floor of the mouth include the surface mucosa from the mobile tongue to the alveolar process, extending from one tonsillar pillar to the other. The opening of the submandibular gland ducts, called Wharton's ducts, are located anteriorly and can become obstructed by tumor, leading to tenderness and enlargement of the submandibular gland. Sublingual glands and various minor salivary glands are also found in this location. The floor-of-mouth mucosa is nonkeratinizing stratified squamous epithelium; and the underlying musculature includes the genioglossus, geniohyoid, and mylohoid muscles. The blood and nerve supplies to the floor of the mouth are derived primarily from the paired lingual arteries and nerves.

C. Presentation

Premalignant lesions cause few if any symptoms, and the diagnosis depends on the awareness of the examining physician or dentist. White patches (leukoplakia) are known to become carcinoma if left untreated over time. Although less emphasized, red patches (erythroplasia) are commonly (90%) invasive cancers, carcinoma in situ, or severe epithelial dysplasia and must be seriously regarded for the correct diagnosis. Malignant lesions usually present as chronic, nonhealing ulcers; and although pain is rare with early lesions, its presence indicates advanced disease with deep invasion and perineural or

Cancer of the Floor of the Mouth

A.
Epidemiology and Etiology
Incidence: 0.6/100,000 in U.S.
Median age 55–65
80% Male
Risk factors: cigarette and pipe smoking, tobacco and betel nut chewing, alcohol

B.
Anatomy

C.
Presentation
Premalignant: leukoplakia, erythroplasia (usually asymptomatic)
Malignant: chronic nonhealing ulcers, pain with advanced lesions

D.
Diagnosis and Evaluation
Palpation of the mouth and neck
Biopsy, if negative, repeat if suspicion is high
Rule out synchronous upper aerodigestive cancers
Panorex mandibular radiographs to assess local extent
Chest radiograph or CT for distant disease

E.
Histology
Squamous cell carcinoma most common
Salivary gland tumors may be adenocarcinomas, adenoid cystic, mucoepidermoid

F.
Staging
(see Table 2–1)

G.
Treatment

Clinical stage	*Treatment of primary lesion*	*Treatment of clinical N0 neck*
T1 →	Surgery or irradiation →	Observation, irradiation, or neck dissection
T2 →	Surgery or irradiation →	Irradiation or neck dissection
T3,4 →	Negative-margin resection postoperative irradiation (6000–6300 cGy) →	Neck dissection and irradiation (see below)

H.
Prognosis
Risk of node metastases increases with T-stage: 12% for T1, 30% for T2, 50% for T3–4

Treatment of the clinically positive neck

Modified neck dissection →
- Negative → Observe
- Single, microscopic node → Observe
- Multiple nodes or extracapsular extension → 5000 cGy irradiation

bony involvement. Occasionally, an enlarged submandibular or digastric cervical lymph node initially causes the patient to seek medical assistance.

D. Diagnosis and Evaluation

To diagnose floor-of-mouth malignancies, careful inspection and palpation of the mouth and neck are essential. Suspicious lesions that are raised, are centrally ulcerated with indurated edges, and have an infiltrated base must be biopsied with forceps or by incisional or excisional biopsy. Negative biopsies should be repeated if the clinical index of suspicion is high. The upper aerodigestive tract must be evaluated endoscopically to help stage the disease properly and to check for synchronous malignancies. Extension and distal spread of disease is sought with panorex mandibular and chest radiography. If symptoms warrant chest tomograms or computed tomography (CT), bone or liver scans (or both) are obtained. Routine laboratory testing to help define the patient's general state of health is also mandatory.

E. Histology

Floor-of-mouth malignancies comprise approximately 10–15% of all intraoral cancers. Most of the lesions are classified histologically as squamous cell carcinomas, usually moderately to well differentiated varieties. Variant types include verrucous and sarcomatoid squamous cell carcinomas. The salivary glands may give rise to adenocarcinomas, adenoid cystic carcinomas, and mucoepidermoid carcinomas.

F. Staging

The American Joint Committee on Cancer (AJCC) (Table 2–1) has established an accepted staging system.

TABLE 2–1.
AJCC definition of TNM and stage grouping for carcinoma of the floor of the mouth

Primary Tumor (T)
TX Primary tumor cannot be assessed
T0 No evidence of primary tumor
Tis Carcinoma *in situ*
T1 Tumor 2 cm or less in greatest dimension
T2 Tumor more than 2 cm but not more than 4 cm in greatest dimension
T3 Tumor more than 4 cm in greatest dimension
T4 Tumor invades adjacent structures (e.g., through cortical bone, inferior alveolar nerve, floor of mouth, skin of face)

Regional Lymph Nodes (N)
NX Regional lymph nodes cannot be assessed
N0 No regional lymph node metastasis
N1 Metastasis in a single ipsilateral lymph node, 3 cm or less in greatest dimension
N2 Metastasis in a single ipsilateral lymph node, more than 3 cm but not more than 6 cm in greatest dimension; or in multiple ipsilateral lymph nodes, none more than 6 cm in greatest dimension; or in bilateral or contralateral lymph nodes, none more than 6 cm in greatest dimension
  N2a Metastasis in single ipsilateral lymph node more than 3 cm but not more than 6 cm in greatest dimension
  N2b Metastasis in multiple ipsilateral lymph nodes, none more than 6 cm in greatest dimension
  N2c Metastasis in bilateral or contralateral lymph nodes, none more than 6 cm in greatest dimension
N3 Metastasis in a lymph node more than 6 cm in greatest dimension

Distant Metastasis (M)
MX Distant metastasis cannot be assessed
M0 No distant metastasis
M1 Distant metastasis

Stage Grouping

Stage	*T*	*N*	M
0	Tis	N0	M0
I	T1	N0	M0
II	T2	N0	M0
III	T3	N0	M0
	T1	N1	M0
	T2	N1	M0
	T3	N1	M0
IVA	T4	N0	M0
	T4	N1	M0
	Any T	N2	M0
IVB	Any T	N3	M0
IVC	Any T	Any N	M1

SOURCE: Used with permission of the American Joint Committee on Cancer (AJCC®), Chicago, IL. The original source for this material is the AJCC® Cancer Staging Manual, 5th edition (1997) published by Lippincott Williams & Wilkins Publishers, Philadelphia, PA.

G. Treatment

Early floor-of-mouth cancer can be treated successfully with surgery or irradiation alone; these two approaches yield similar good results in selected patients. Malignancies that abut or lie in close proximity to mandibular periosteum, however, are generally not considered good candidates for radiotherapy (because of osteonecrosis), and such lesions are better treated surgically with en bloc mandibular resection. When radiotherapy is selected, external irradiation, interstitial implants, or implants combined with external irradiation are therapeutic options.

Treatment for palpable, suspicious cervical adenopathy is cervical lymph node dissection; postoperative irradiation may be necessary if multiple nodes are positive or if there is extracapsular extension of disease. For patients with clinically negative necks and small primary tumors, elective neck dissection, irradiation of the neck, or observation may be employed. For the latter patients who subsequently develop recurrence in the neck, neck dissection can be undertaken if the developing disease is detected promptly, but not all patients can be salvaged. In general, most clinicians advocate elective neck treatment for clinical N0 disease. Whether irradiation or neck dissection is chosen is determined by physician preference and the prescribed treatment for the primary tumor.

Advanced floor-of-mouth cancer (stage III or IV) is usually treated with a combination of surgery and postoperative radiation therapy; and the results are better than with surgery alone. Surgical resection of the primary cancer site can be extensive, including surrounding structures such as the tongue and mandible. Complete removal of the primary cancer should be confirmed by intraoperative frozen sections of the surgical margins. Full-thickness resection of the floor of the mouth, along with the tongue and mandible, may leave extensive, deforming surgical defects that necessitate complex reconstructive techniques. Use of myocutaneous flaps and osteomyocutaneous free flaps with microvasculature anastomoses has facilitated reconstruction and rehabilitation of these patients.

Ipsilateral neck dissection is necessary for all advanced floor-of-mouth cancers. When primary lesions approach or cross the midline of the mouth, bilateral cervical lymphadenectomy is indicated. Postoperative radiation therapy is usually administered to the primary site in total doses of 6000–6300 cGy. When positive surgical margins are identified, the area is treated with higher doses. During the first 5 weeks the primary site and upper neck are treated with a dose of 4500 cGy; after a spinal cord block is placed, the dose is increased to 5400 cGy. A boost to the primary lesion and any involved areas of the neck increase the total dose to 6000–6300 cGy.

H. *Prognosis*

The prognosis for patients with floor-of-mouth cancer is primarily determined by disease stage, patient performance status, and coexisting medical conditions. Floor-of-mouth cancer can be locally extensive without developing regional or distal spread. Early lesions (T1), however, can be associated with a 12% incidence of occult cervical nodal metastases; this rate increases progressively with increasing T stage: 30% for T2 lesions and aproximately 50% for T3 and T4 cancers. Common sites of lymph nodal metastases ae unusual. The overall 5-year survival rates vary according to stage: 90%, 80%, 66%, and 32% for stages I, II, III, and IV, respectively. Some consider poor tumor differentiation, perineural invasion, and deep primary tumor invasion as poor prognostic indicators for floor-of-mouth cancers.

Conclusions

Early floor-of-mouth tumors can be treated equally well with irradiation or surgery. Generally, surgery is preferred for lesions close to the mandible. Patients with palpable nodes in the neck should undergo a therapeutic neck dissection, with postoperative neck irradiation being reserved for patients with multiple positive nodes or extracapsular extension of the cancer. Treatment of clinically negative necks in patients with small lesions is controversial. Although observation may be considered, approximately 30% fail, and not all can be salvaged. Most physicians favor elective treatment of the clinically negative neck, using irradiation or surgery, the choice dictated by how the primary lesion is treated. Large lesions are treated with surgery followed by irradiation of the primary tumor site. The neck should be treated regardless of nodal status.

Suggested Reading

Arthur K, Farr HW. Prognostic significance of histologic grade in epideroid carcinoma of the mouth and pharynx. Am J Surg 1972;124:489–692.

Gilbert E, Goffinet D, Bradshaw M. Carcinoma of the oral tongue and floor of mouth: fifteen years experience with linear acceleration therapy. Cancer 1975;35:1517–1524.

Guillamondegui OM, Oliver B, Hayden R. Cancer of the anterior floor of mouth: selective choice of treatment and analysis of failures. Am J Surg 1980;140:560–562.

Lindbergh RD. Distribution of cervical lymph node metastasis from squamous cell carcinoma of the upper respiratory and digestive tracts. Cancer 1972;29:1446–1449.

Mazeron JJ, Grimard L, Raynal M, et al. Iridium-192 curietherapy for T1 and T2 epidermoid carcinomas of the floor of mouth. Int J Radiat Oncol Biol Phys 1990;18:1299–1306.

Mendenhall WM, Van Cise WJ, Bova FJ, Million RF. Analysis of time-dose factors in squamous cell carcinoma of the oral tongue and floor of mouth treated with radiation therapy alone. Int J Radiat Oncol Biol Phys 1981;7:1005–1011.

Shaha AR, Spiro RH, Shah JP, Strong EW. Squamous carcinoma of the floor of the mouth. Am J Surg 1984;148:455–459.

Soo KC, Carter RL, O'Brien CJ, et al. Prognostic implications of perineural spread in squamous carcinoma of the head and neck. Laryngoscope 1986;96:1145–1148.

Spiro RH, Huvos AG, Wong GY, et al. Predictive value of tumor thickness of squamous carcinoma confined to the tongue and floor of the mouth. Am J Surg 1986;152:345–350.

CHAPTER 3

Cancer of the Hard Palate

NADER SADEGHI
WILLIAM R. PANJE

A. Etiology

Squamous cell carcinoma (SCCA) accounts for one-half of hard palate cancers; minor salivary gland cancers, sarcomas, and melanomas account for the other half (Table 3–1).[1,2] A strong correlation between tobacco and alcohol consumption and SCCA of the oral cavity and soft palate is well established, but its relation to hard palate cancer is less convincing. A specific association between reverse smoking and hard palate SCCA has been noted in India.[3] In reverse smoking the lit end of the cigaret is placed in mouth. Less convincingly, ill-fitting dentures, mechanical irritation, poor oral hygiene, and chronic use of mouthwash have been implicated in oral cavity SCCA.[4–6]

B. Surgical Anatomy

The palate separates the oral cavity from the nasal cavity and the maxillary sinuses. The mucosa of the hard palate is a keratinizing, pseudostratified squamous epithelium; within the submucosa are numerous minor salivary glands. The periosteal covering of the palate is a relative barrier to the spread of cancer. The neurovascular supply to the palate comes through the palatine foramina located medial to the third molar teeth; these foramina provide a pathway of spread for tumor. Descending palatine arteries from the internal maxillary artery provide the blood supply and pass anteriorly through the nasopalatine foramen to the nose. Sensory and secretomotor fibers from the maxillary (V_2) branch of the trigeminal nerve and pterygopalatine ganglion travel to the hard palate via the greater and lesser palatine nerves (Fig. 3–1).

C. Presentation

Squamous cell carcinoma of the palate presents as an ulcerating surface lesion. It is often asymptomatic in its early stages but may become painful in advanced cases. The presence of a palatal mass, bleeding, foul odor, ill-fitting dentures in edentulous patients, or tooth loosening may be the presenting

Cancer of the Hard Palate

A.
Etiology
Possible causative role:
tobacco, alcohol, ill-fitting dentures, irritation, poor hygiene

B.
Anatomy

Differential Diagnosis
Squamous cell carcinoma
Minor salivary gland neoplasm
Pseudoepitheliomatosis hyperplasia
Necrotizing sialometaplasia
Bony hyperplasia

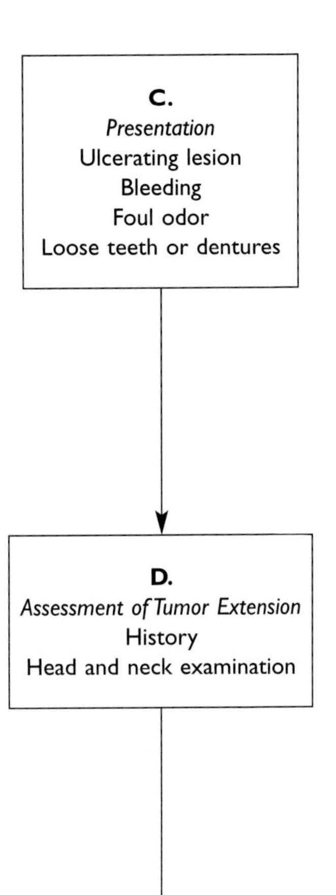

C.
Presentation
Ulcerating lesion
Bleeding
Foul odor
Loose teeth or dentures

D.
Assessment of Tumor Extension
History
Head and neck examination

E.
Radiographic Evaluation, Biopsy, and Staging

1. CT vs. MRI
   MRI is better for evaluating perineural invasion, paranasal sinus involvement, dural extension, associated inflammation
2. Biopsy
   Target periphery of ulcerating lesions, consider needle aspiration if cytologist is available
3. Rule out synchronous lesion in upper aerodigestive tract
   Panendoscopy vs. laryngoscopy, chest radiograph, barium swallow

(continued on next page)

Cancer of the Hard Palate (continued)

F.
Treatment of Squamous Cell Carcinoma

Primary lesion:

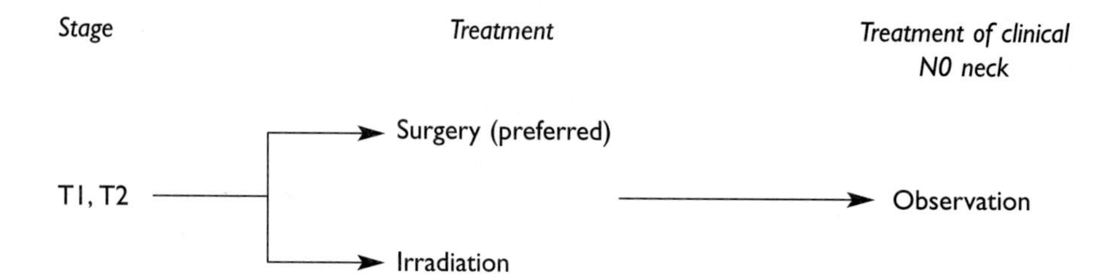

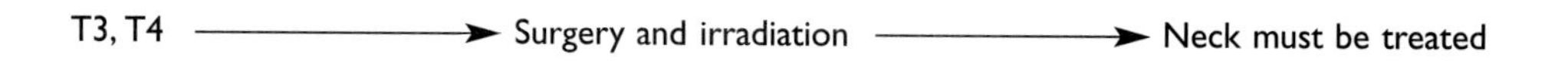

Neck:

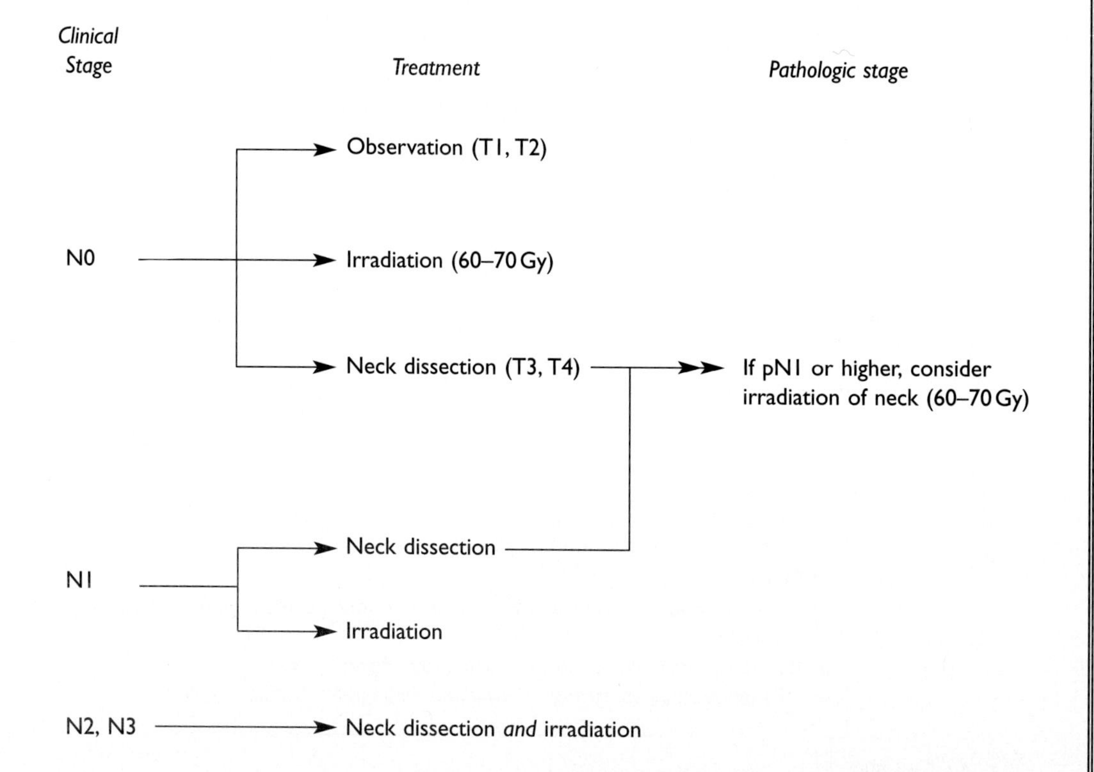

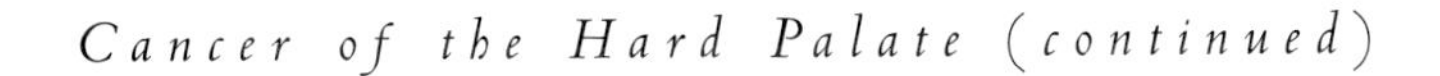

G.
Treatment of Minor Salivary Gland Tumors

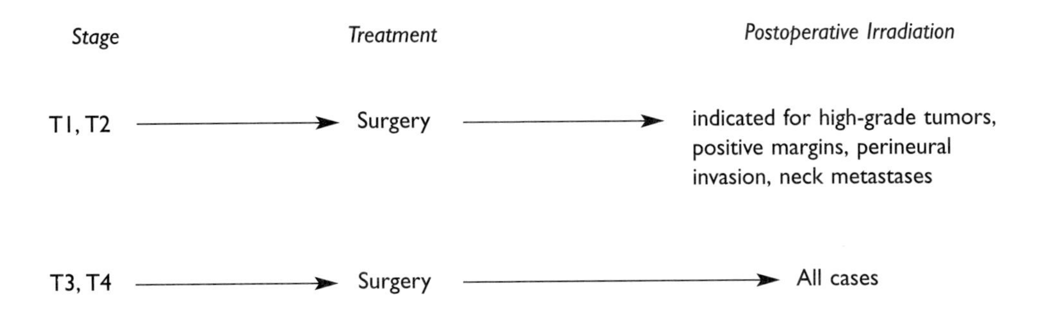

If adenoid cystic carcinoma is present, surgery followed by irradiation is the treatment of choice.

symptoms. Pseudoepitheliomatous hyperplasia and necrotizing sialometaplasia are benign self-limited lesions that may mimic SCCA and must be distinguished histologically. Minor salivary gland tumors, on the other hand, present as submucosal lesions with a smooth normal mucosal covering. Torus palatinus and bony hyperplasia of the palate are hard, asymptomatic, midline masses that should not be confused with tumors. Melanomas are usually smooth, black lesions but may be brown or brownish gray. Kaposi's sarcomas are bluish lesions commonly seen in patients with human immunodeficiency virus (HIV).

TABLE 3–1.
Distribution of hard palate malignant neoplasms

Histology	Frequency (%)
Squamous cell carcinoma	53
Adenoid cystic carcinomas	15
Mucoepidermoid carcinoma	10
Adenocarcinoma	4
Anaplastic carcinoma	4
Other	14

SOURCE: Petruzzelli and Myers.[2]

D. *Assessment of Tumor Extension*

A thorough history and physical examination help predict the extent of the tumor. One should assess not only the palate itself but possible extension of the tumor beyond the hard palate. Extension beyond the hard palate occurs with up to 70% of lesions.[1] Posterior extension into the soft palate may cause velopharyngeal insufficiency and hypernasal speech. Palatal hypesthesia indicates either trigeminal nerve involvement in the sphenopalatine foramen or pterygopalatine fossa extension. An absent corneal reflex is indicative of skull base extension through the foramen rotundum, foramen ovale, or inferior orbital fissure. Dental numbness may indicate perineural invasion. Middle ear effusion is suggestive of nasopharyngeal extension or invasion of the tensor veli palatini muscle. Involvement of the mandibular division of the trigeminal nerve may present as hypesthesia along the mandible or wasting of the temporalis or masseter muscle, indicative of infratemporal fossa involvement. Trismus, malocclusion, and pain are symptoms of invasion of the pterygoid muscles. Extension to the gingiva must be assessed. Dental sockets provide a pathway of invasion to the alveolar process of the maxillary bone and into the maxillary sinus. Nasal floor involvement may occur by direct extension through the palate.

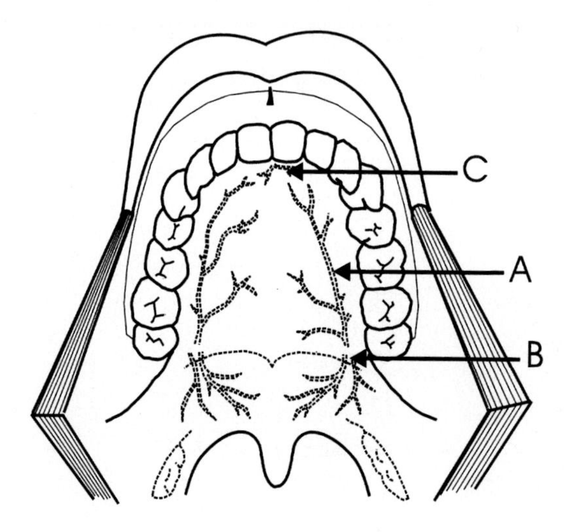

FIGURE 3–1
Anatomy of the palate and its blood supply. A, greater palatine artery; B, lesser palatine artery; C, nasopalatine artery.

Lymph node involvement is of special concern in SCCA and high-grade mucoepidermoid cancer. It is rare with other salivary gland carcinomas. About 30% of patients have cervical nodal metastasis at the time of presentation.[1] Submandibular nodes (level I) and upper deep jugular lymph nodes (level II) account for first-echelon nodal drainage.[7] In tumors with posterior soft palate extension, retropharyngeal nodes may be involved (Fig. 3–2).

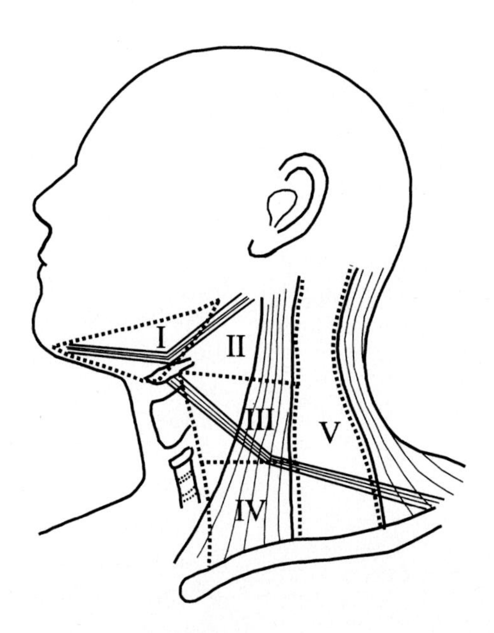

FIGURE 3–2
Classification of the nodal levels (I–V) of the neck. I, submental and submandibular area; II, upper internal jugular chain nodes down to the level of hyoid bone; III, middle internal jugular chain from the level of hyoid bone to cricoid cartilage; IV, lower jugular chain or supraclavicular nodes; V, posterior triangle nodes, including the spinal accessory chain.

E. Radiographic Evaluation, Biopsy, and Staging

Transoral biopsy of an ulcerative lesion may be easily performed in the office using local anesthesia. For ulcerating lesions it is important to biopsy near the edge of the tumor to avoid the necrotic central component. For large nonulcerated palatal lumps an incision through the intact mucosa may be required prior to biopsy. The surgeon should place the biopsy incision in such a manner that allows subsequent removal of the scar in continuity with the tumor. Alternatively, fine-needle aspiration cytologic studies may be performed if an experienced cytopathologist is available. Small submucosal lesions may be sampled with excisional biopsy. The tumor should be staged according to the American Joint Committee for Cancer Staging, as it is of critical importance for determining the prognosis (Table 3–2).

About 10% of patients with head and neck SCCA have a synchronous second primary cancer in the upper aerodigestive tract, lung, or esophagus.[8,9] Hence panendoscopy including esophagoscopy, bronchoscopy, and laryngopharyngoscopy should be performed in these patients. Alternatively, complete flexible nasopharyngolaryngoscopy, chest radiography, and barium esophagography may suffice for synchronous tumor assessment.

Radiologic evaluation helps increase the accuracy of the staging and is of utmost importance when planning treatment. Computed tomography (CT) scans should be performed in axial and coronal planes. Coronal images are best when assessing bony invasion of the palate and extension into the nasal fossa, maxillary sinus, and skull base. Enlargement of skull base foramina is indicative of tumor invasion. Axial images aid in assessing extension in horizontal planes into the soft palate, pterygoid plates and muscles, infratemporal fossa, and masticator space. CT scanning with intravenous contrast infusion should include the neck to assess for cervical nodal involvement. This is especially important for SCCA and high-grade mucoepidermoid carcinoma. Magnetic resonance imaging (MRI) is more accurate for assessing perineural extension along the foramina. This is especially important with adenoid cystic carcinoma, which has a propensity for perineural invasion. For advanced tumors with paranasal sinus involvement, MRI is superior to CT for distinguishing inflammatory changes from a neoplasm. For extensive lesions with intracranial involvement, MRI aids in assessing dural invasion. Chest radiography should be done to assess the possibility of a pulmonary metastasis or second primary (or both). A liver chemistry panel is adequate to assess for liver metastases. Abdominal and chest CT scans should be considered if distant metastases are suspected.

TABLE 3–2.
AJCC definition of TNM for cancer of the oral cavity

Primary Tumor (T)	
TX	Primary tumor cannot be assessed
T0	No evidence of primary tumor
Tis	Carcinoma *in situ*
T1	Tumor ≤2 cm in greatest dimension
T2	Tumor >2 cm but ≤4 cm in greatest dimension
T3	Tumor >4 cm in greatest dimension
T4 (oral cavity)	Tumor invades adjacent structures (e.g., through cortical bone, into deep [extrinsic] muscle of tongue, maxillary sinus, skin. Superficial erosion alone of bone/tooth socket by gingival primary is not sufficient to classify as T4)
Regional Lymph Nodes (N)	
NX	Regional lymph nodes cannot be assessed
N0	No regional lymph node metastasis
N1	Metastasis in a single ipsilateral lymph node, ≤3 cm in greatest dimension
N2	Metastasis in a single ipsilateral lymph node, >3 cm but ≤6 cm in greatest dimension; *or* in multiple ipsilateral lymph nodes, none >6 cm in greatest dimension; *or* in bilateral or contralateral lymph nodes, none >6 cm in greatest dimension
N2a	Metastasis in single ipsilateral lymph node >3 cm but ≤6 cm in greatest dimension
N2b	Metastasis in multiple ipsilateral lymph nodes, none >6 cm in greatest dimension
N2c	Metastasis in bilateral or contralateral lymph nodes, none >6 cm in greatest dimension
N3	Metastasis in a lymph node >6 cm in greatest dimension
Distant Metastasis (M)	
MX	Presence of distant metastasis cannot be assessed
M0	No distant metastasis
M1	Distant metastasis

SOURCE: Used with permission of the American Joint Committee on Cancer (AJCC®), Chicago, IL. The original source for this material is the AJCC® Cancer Staging Manual, 5th edition (1997) published by Lippincott Williams & Wilkins Publishers, Philadelphia, PA.

F. Treatment of Squamous Cell Carcinoma

T1, T2, and N0 Tumors

Surgery is the preferred treatment for SCCAs of the hard palate,[1,2,10] although radiation therapy is a viable alternative. Megavoltage radiation has also been utilized with some success in treating these tumors.[11,12] T1 and small T2 lesions can be managed with surgery or radiation therapy. With surgical management the 5-year survival is 75% for patients with stage I tumors and 50% for those with stage II tumors.[1] The proximity of the tumor to the bone and the potential complication of osteoradionecrosis (because the total radiation dose to the area is 60–70 Gy) make radiation therapy less desirable for treating these lesions. Moreover, surgery is simple and has little associated morbidity with no loss of function.

For tumors not involving the periosteum or bone, through-and-through excision of the palate and opening of the sinonasal fossa are not necessary; simple transoral excision into and including the periosteum suffices. A 1 cm margin is removed with the tumor. The periosteum serves as the superior margin. For extremely superficial lesions where the tumor is not close to the periosteum, the periosteum may be spared, a decision made intraoperatively. In most cases the surgical defect may be left open to heal by secondary intention and granulation. Skin grafting is discouraged. A palatal acrylic prosthesis (healing plate) should be fabricated by a dentist/prosthodontist prior to resection. It protects the palate wound during the healing process. In some cases palatal or buccal mucosal flaps (or both) are necessary to repair tissue defects, especially when radiation has been given preoperatively or if large defects are present.[13]

Clinical and radiologic N0 necks do not require elective treatment. However, if the neck is *clinically* positive, a staging modified radical neck dissection—sparing at minimum the spinal accessory nerve and potentially even the sternocleidomastoid muscle and internal jugular vein and including levels I, II, and III—is performed (Fig. 3–2). *Clinical* N1 disease may be treated with radiation as an alternative. If the pathologic stage of the neck is N2 or above after neck dissection, postoperative radiotherapy is applied to the neck.[1] Treatment of a patient with a *pathologic* N1 neck is controversial. Some physicians believe that these patients are adequately treated with neck dissection alone when there is no extracapsular extension. However, in many centers all patients with a pathologic N1 neck are treated with postoperative irradiation of the neck; this policy is recommended. When there is N1 disease with extracapsular extension, postoperative irradiation should always be undertaken.

T3 and T4 Tumors

Stage T3 and T4 lesions have a poor prognosis and require *combined treatment* with surgery and radiation therapy to the primary site; regardless of clinical stage, the neck must be treated as well. Clinical N1 disease in the neck may be treated with radiotherapy or neck dissection. Clinical N2 and above disease is treated with planned neck dissection followed by radiotherapy. A total dose of 60–70 Gy is given.

When planning surgery for lesions extending beyond the hard palate, it is important to determine the deficit that will result from resection. Resection of the soft palate poses significant risk of velopharyngeal insufficiency. Because the soft palate is a dynamic structure, reconstruction is difficult; hence primary radiation therapy may be considered for these lesions. Lesions invading the palatine bone require partial palatectomy with resulting oroantral and oronasal fistula. Invasion into the nasal cavity or the maxillary sinus requires inferior, partial, or total maxillectomy depending on the extent of the lesion. Prosthetic rehabilitation is highly effective in these patients.[14] Extension into the pterygopalatine and infratemporal fossa requires skull base approaches to extirpate the tumor effectively.

G. *Treatment of Minor Salivary Gland Tumors*

Eighty percent of minor salivary gland tumors are malignant (Table 3–3). The palate is the most common site for minor salivary gland carcinomas, and most of them occur in the hard palate.[15] Minor salivary gland malignancies are classified as high grade or low grade. High-grade tumors include adenoid cystic carcinoma, high-grade mucoepidermoid carcinoma, high-grade adenocarcinoma, malignant mixed tumor, and carcinoma ex-pleomorphic adenoma. Low-grade malignancies include low-grade mucoepidermoid carcinoma, polymorphous low-grade adenocarcinoma with its propensity to occur in the hard palate, acinic cell carcinoma, and other rare tumors.

For minor salivary gland tumors of the hard palate, surgery is the mainstay of treatment.[15–17] If perineural invasion is suspected, the greater palatine nerve should be identified and evaluated with frozen sections. If involved, it should be resected proximally until negative margins are attained. If negative margins cannot be attained at the foramen rotundum, postoperative radiation therapy should include the trigeminal ganglion. Radiotherapy, possibly combined with chemotherapy, is used as the primary treatment if the patient refuses surgery or is not a surgical candidate because of extensive unresectable disease. Postoperative radiotherapy with or without chemo-

TABLE 3–3.
Histologic types and frequencies of neoplasms of the minor salivary glands of the palate

Histologic type	%
Benign	26
Malignant	74
Adenoid cystic carcinoma	30
Mucoepidermoid carcinoma	16
Adenocarcinoma	18
Malignant mixed tumor	8
Other	2

SOURCE: King.[14]

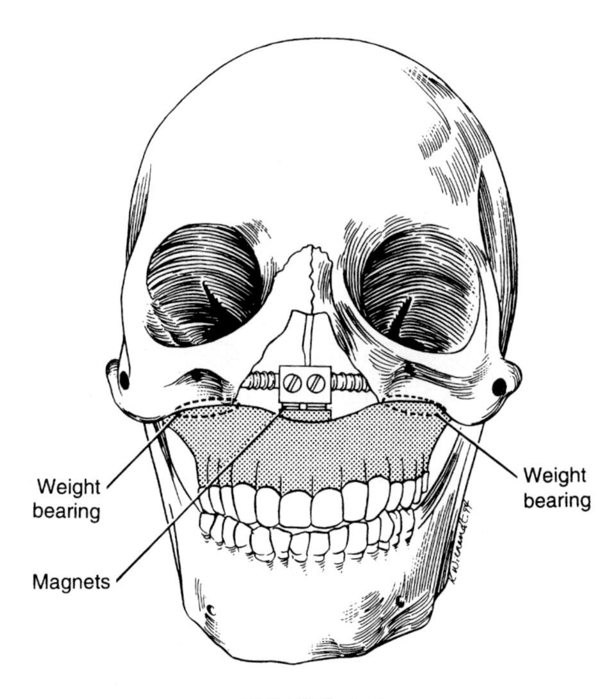

FIGURE 3–3
Prosthesis replacing total palate and bilateral maxillary defect. (From Panje and Hetherington, with permission.[22])

therapy is indicated for high-grade tumors, large T3 or T4 lesions, positive margins, tumors showing perineural invasion, and cervical lymph node metastasis.[16] The most important poor prognostic factors for malignant minor salivary gland tumors of the palate are grade 3 histology, tumor size >3 cm, and positive margins. Cervical nodal metastases are rarely seen, occurring in only 3% of cases.[16] Elective neck dissection is not indicated in the absence of clinical or radiologic signs of nodal metastases.

For adenoid cystic carcinoma, surgery followed by radiation therapy is the treatment of choice. Wide surgical margins are included, as this tumor is known for microscopic extension beyond the gross tumor margins. Propensity for perineural extension requires resection along the greater palatine nerves with frozen section control to achieve negative margins. Postoperative irradiation is preferred, as preoperative radiation therapy increases the surgical complications. There is some support for primary radiation therapy for small adenoid cystic carcinomas of the palate not involving the bone.[10]

Surgical Approaches

A transoral approach provides adequate exposure for superficial tumors of the hard palate that do not invade the bone (Table 3–4).[18] General anesthesia provides comfort for the patient and aids with exposure. The patient is placed in the supine position with head extended. A Dingman or Crochard mouth gag provides attachable cheek retractors to facilitate exposure. Alternatively, a hard rubber bite block or a Denhart gag may be used to open the mouth.

TABLE 3–4.
Surgical approaches to resection of hard palate tumors

Approach	Indication
Transoral	Small lesions with no or minimal bony invasion
Lateral rhinotomy	Infrastructure maxillectomy required
Nasal degloving	Infrastructure maxillectomy required
Weber-Ferguson incision	Total maxillectomy required
Infratemporal fossa approaches	Skull base invasion

Margins of 1 cm are mapped out surrounding the tumor, and the incision is made with electrocautery or a knife. Alternatively, a CO_2 laser may be used, as it provides adequate hemostasis and incurs less tissue damage.[19] The incision includes the periosteum if it is to be taken as the superior margin. Using a periosteal elevator the periosteum is elevated under direct vision, and the tumor is removed. In cases where the tumor involves the periosteum or bone, bone must be taken as the margin. This procedure can be performed using a cutting burr. The superior mucoperiosteal coverage should be preserved if

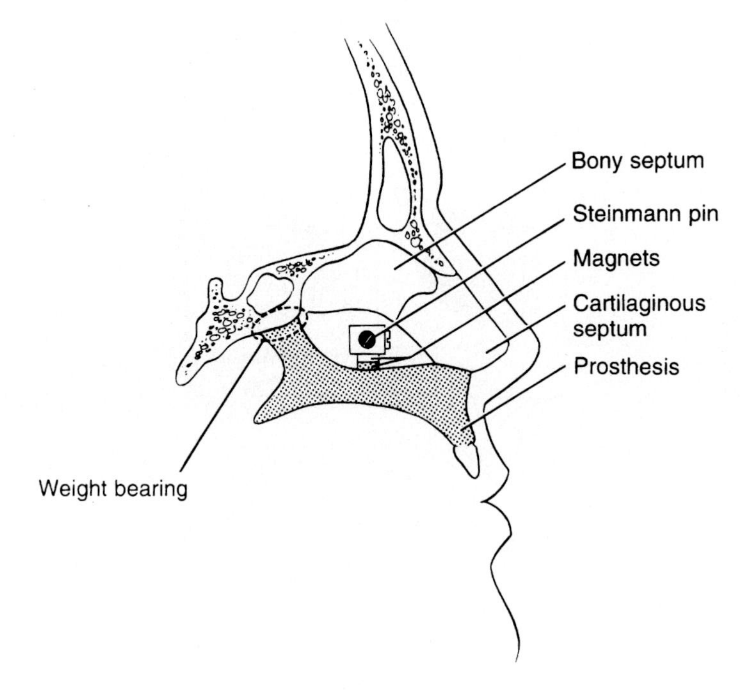

FIGURE 3–4
Sagittal view of the prosthesis in place. (From Panje and Hetherington, with permission.[22])

possible to prevent an oronasal fistula, although it may be difficult. A prosthetic device is highly effective for swallowing and speech rehabilitation.

In cases where the tumor is lateral and involves the alveolar ridge, a partial alveolectomy is included with the palate resection. To improve exposure, a buccogingival sulcus incision is made to the level of the anterior maxillary wall. A facial degloving approach is used to improve the exposure. The infraorbital nerve is preserved. An opening is made into the maxillary antrum to expose the superior surface of the palate. Following soft tissue incisions, bony cuts are made as needed using a Stryker saw, and the tumor is removed. Exposed soft tissue surfaces are covered with a split-thickness skin graft except for closed cavities. Immediate prosthetic rehabilitation is done with the aid of a prosthodontist who has prepared the temporary prosthetic device preoperatively.[20,21]

For extensive tumors of the hard palate that involve the hard palate bilaterally, total palatectomy and inferior bilateral maxillectomy is required. These resections leave the patient with extensive midfacial defects involving the palate, upper jaw, and sinuses (Fig. 3–3).

Flap and graft reconstruction of these defects is fraught with difficulty and often results in breakdown, with a consequent oroantral or oronasal fistula. Total midfacial prosthetic rehabilitation is highly effective in restoring deglutition and speech as well as the facial contour (Fig. 3–4).[22] It also allows easier postoperative examination of the surgical bed.

References

1. Evans JF, Shah JP. Epidermoid carcinoma of the palate. Am J Surg 1981;142:451–455.
2. Petruzzelli GJ, Myers EN. Malignant neoplasms of the hard palate and upper alveolar ridge. Oncology 1994;8:43–48.
3. Mahboubi E. The epidemiology of oral cavity, pharyngeal and esophageal cancer outside of North America and western Europe. Cancer 1977; 40:1879–1886.
4. Graham S, Dayal H, Rohrer T, et al. Dentition, diet, tobacco, and alcohol in the epidemiology of oral cancer. J Int Cancer Inst 1977;59:1611–1616.
5. Blot WJ, Winn DM, Fraumeni JF Jr. Oral cancer and mouthwash. J Natl Cancer Inst 1983;70:251–253.
6. Wynder EL, Kabat G, Rosenberg S, et al. Oral cancer and mouthwash use. J Natl Cancer Inst 1983;70:255–260.
7. Hollinshead WH. Anatomy for Surgeons. The Head and Neck, 3rd ed. Philadelphia: Lippincott, 1982: 331–345.
8. Gluckman JL. Synchronous multiple primary lesions of the upper aerodigestive system. Arch Otolaryngol 1979;105:597–598.
9. Leipzig B, Zellmer JE, Klug D, et al. The role of endoscopy in evaluating patients with head and neck cancer: a multiinstitutional prospective study. Arch Otolaryngol 1985;111:589–594.
10. Jaques DA. Epidermoid carcinoma of the palate. Otolaryngol Clin North Am 1978;12:125–128.
11. Chung CK, Rahman SM, Lim ML, et al. Squamous cell carcinoma of the hard palate. Int J Radiat Oncol Biol Phys 1979;5:191–196.
12. Chung CK, Johns ME, Cantrel RW, et al. Radiotherapy in the management of primary malignancies of the hard palate. Laryngoscope 1980;90:576–584.
13. Panje WR, Morris MR. Surgery of oral cavity, tongue, and oropharynx. In: Naumann HH, Helms J, Herberhold C, et al. (eds) Head and Neck Surgery, vol 1, part 2. New York: Thieme, 1995:739–753.

14. King GE. Rehabilitation of the nasal and paranasal sinus area: prosthetic rehabilitation. In: Thawly SE, Panje WR, Batsakis JG, Lindberg RD (eds) Comprehensive Management of Head and Neck Tumors, vol 1. Philadelphia: Saunders, 1987:408–433.
15. Spiro RH. Salivary neoplasms; overview of a 35-year experience with 2807 patients. Head Neck Surg 1986;8:177–184.
16. Beckhardt RN, Weber RS, Zane R, et al. Minor salivary gland tumors of the palate: clinical and pathologic correlates of outcome. Laryngoscope 1995; 105:1155–1160.
17. Spiro RH, Thaler HT, Hicks WF, et al. The importance of clinical staging of minor salivary gland carcinoma. Am J Surg 1991;162:330–336.
18. Panje WR, Morris MR. The oropharynx. In: Soutar DS, Tiwari R (eds) Excision and Reconstruction in Head and Neck Cancer. Edinburgh: Livingstone, 1994;141–157.
19. Panje WR, Scher N, Karnell M. Transoral carbon dioxide laser ablation for cancer, tumors and other lesions. Arch Otolaryngol Head Neck Surg 1989;115:681–688.
20. Aramany MA. Basic principles of obturator design for partially edentulous patients. Part I. Classification. J Prosthet Dent 1978;40:554–557.
21. Aramany MA. Basic principles of obturator design for partially edentulous patients. Part II. Design principles. J Prosthet Dent 1978;40:656–662.
22. Panje WR, Hetherington HE. Use of stainless steel implants in facial bone reconstruction. Otolaryngol Clin North Am 1995;28:341–349.

CHAPTER 4

Cancer of the Anterior (Oral) Tongue

BENJAMIN D.L. LI
G.E. GHALI
EMERY A. MINNARD

Introduction

An estimated 5500 new cases of tongue carcinoma are diagnosed each year in the United States. Of these patients, approximately 1900 die from their disease.[1] Carcinoma of the tongue is associated with alcohol and tobacco consumption. There is a 3 : 1 male/female preponderance, though with the increased use of tobacco by women this ratio is likely to change.[2,3] Carcinoma of the oral tongue (anterior two-thirds) behaves differently from carcinoma of the base of tongue (posterior one-third). The latter is more likely to be poorly differentiated and to have nodal metastases at presentation; and it is usually diagnosed at a later stage.[4] This chapter is devoted to the discussion of cancer of the anterior, or oral, tongue.

The oral tongue is the movable portion and extends from the circumvallate papillae to the junction at the anterior floor of the mouth. The oral tongue is divided into four regions: tip, lateral borders, and dorsal and ventral surfaces. Lymphatic drainage from the tongue is extensive; the anterior aspect drains into the submental nodes, and the lateral borders drain into the submandibular and upper deep jugular nodes. There is a rich lymphatic network in the neck, and communication across the midline can lead to contralateral neck drainage.[2,5]

Seventy-five percent of tongue cancers involve the oral tongue.[6] The cancer may begin as a painless ulcer that fails to heal spontaneously. Then, as it enlarges and compresses or infiltrates surrounding and adjacent structures, local pain, ipsilateral referred otalgia, and jaw pain can occur. Small cancers of the oral tongue may be asymptomatic. The intrinsic musculature (longitudinal, transverse, vertical) and the extrinsic musculature (genioglossus, hyoglossus, styloglossus, palatoglossus) of the tongue provide minimal hindrance to tumor growth. Thus the tumor may proliferate to considerable size before becoming symptomatic.

Initial Workup

The initial evaluation of a patient with tongue cancer begins with a complete history and physical examination. In addition to symptoms produced by the tumor, the age and general medical condition of the patient are vitally important when assessing his or her ability to tolerate the optimal therapeutic plan. Associated symptoms, such as hemoptysis or odynophagia, require careful evaluation; and a significant number of patients have a second malignancy of the aerodigestive tract.

Cancer of the Anterior (Oral) Tongue

5500 new cases per year
Risk factors: alcohol and tobacco
3 : 1 male to female ratio
Early lesions may be asymptomatic
Advanced lesions have jaw pain, referred otalgia

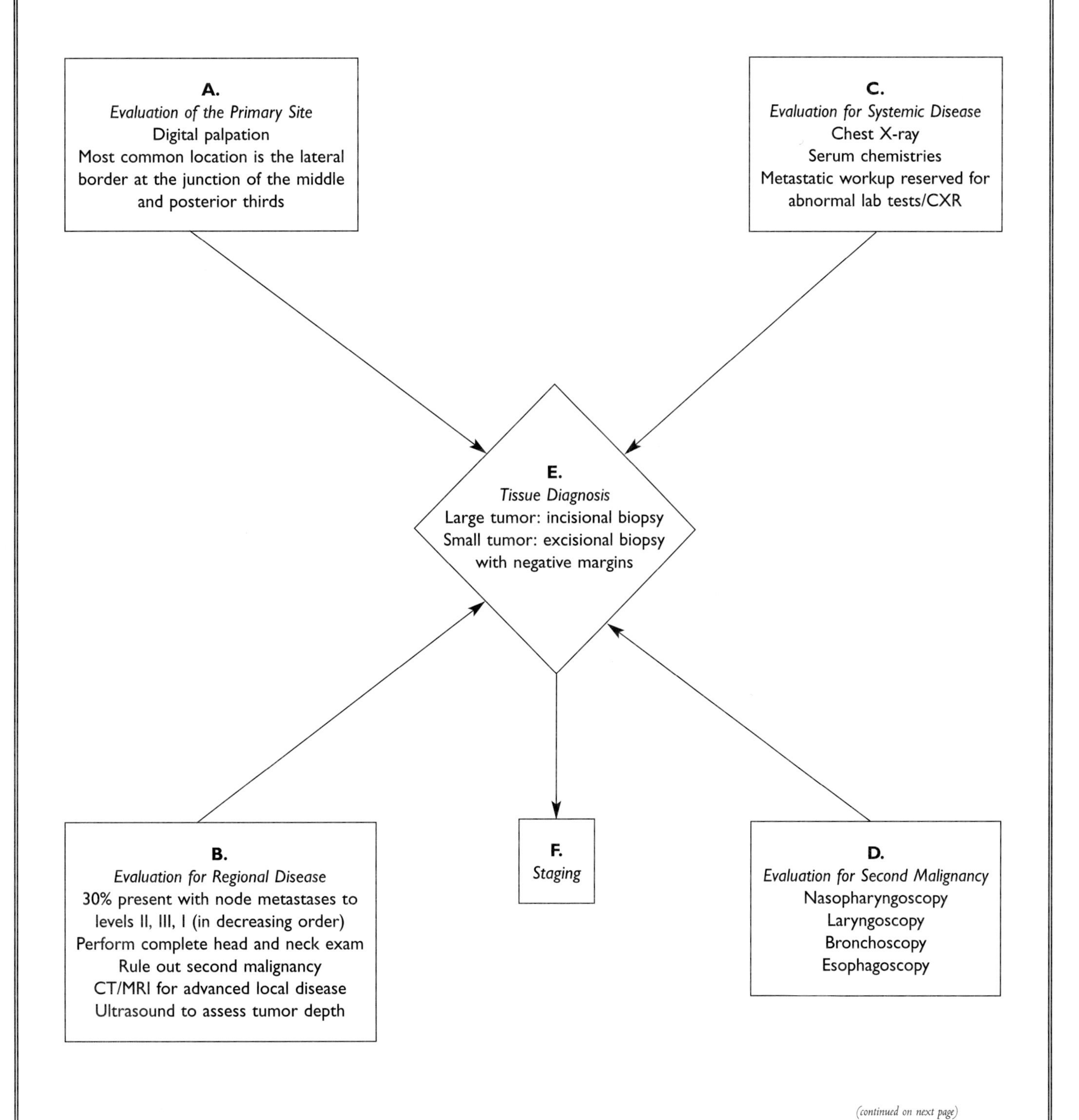

(continued on next page)

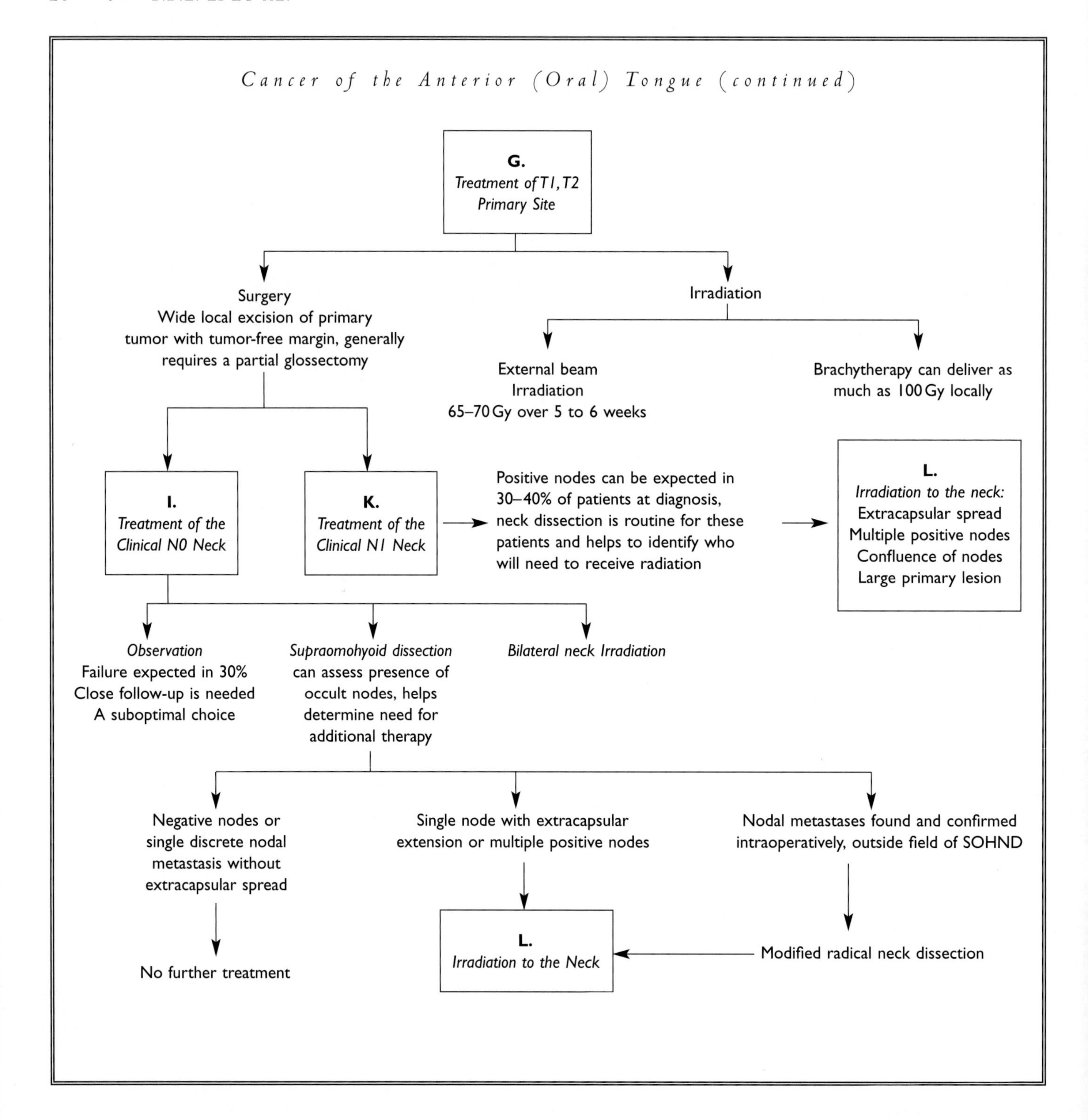

A. Evaluation of the Primary Site

The physical examination should be performed in a comfortable, relaxed setting. The primary tumor may be exophytic, endophytic, ulcerative, infiltrative, or occasionally occult. Careful visualization and digital palpation are necessary to assess the local extent of the disease. The most common primary site for oral tongue carcinoma is the lateral border, at the junction between the middle and posterior third of the tongue.[7] Oral tongue cancer can infiltrate adjacent structures, such as the floor of mouth (FOM), tongue base, and tonsillar pillars.

B. Evaluation for Regional Disease

In addition to the primary site, a complete head and neck examination entails careful evaluation of the scalp, skin of the face and neck, regional lymph nodes, thyroid gland, major salivary glands,

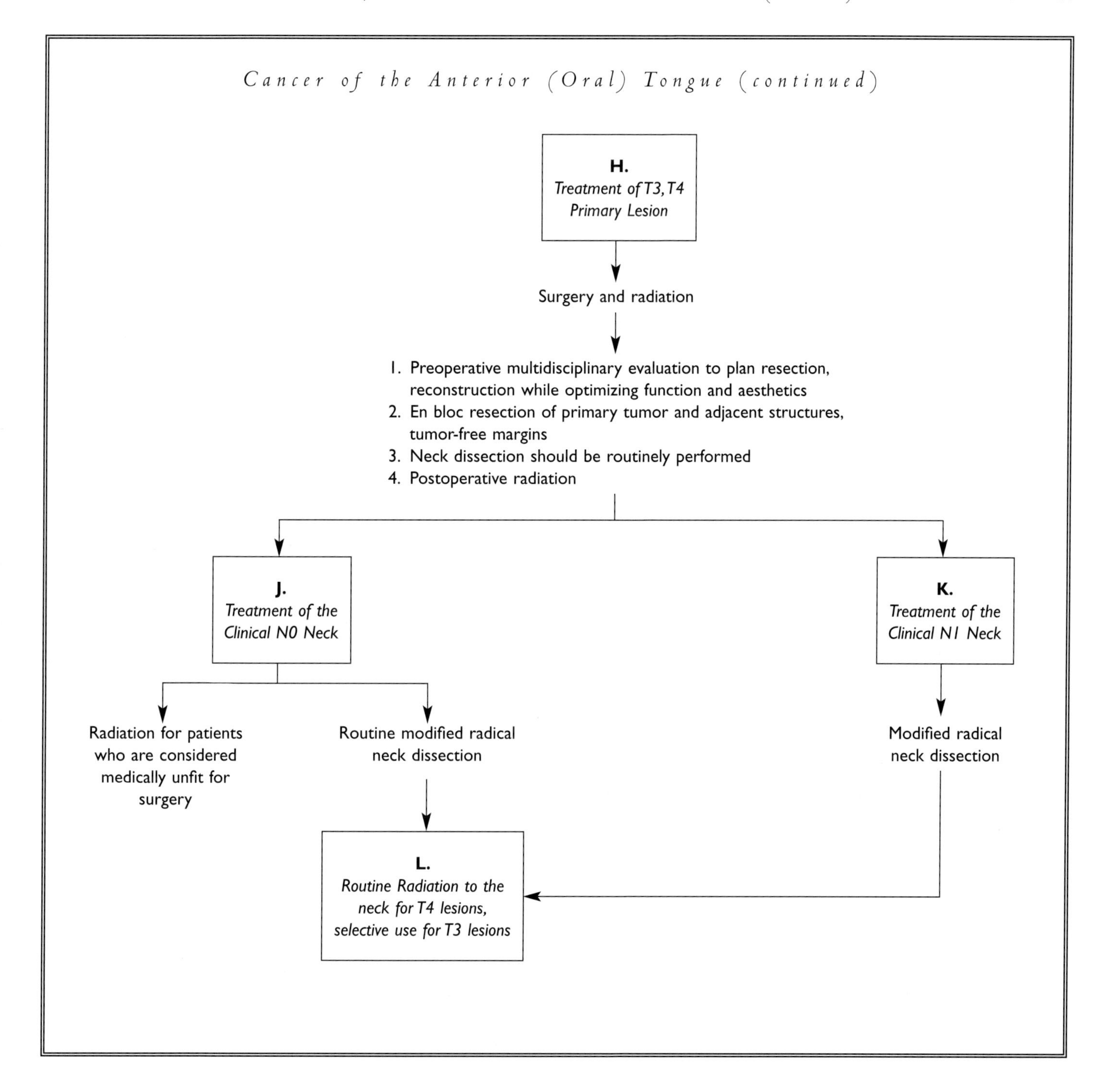

and cranial nerves. Additionally, the oral cavity, oropharynx, hypopharynx, larynx, nasopharynx, and nasal cavity require endoscopic or laryngeal mirror examination. Suspicious area(s) must be palpated if assessable and biopsied if appropriate.

Approximately 30% of oral tongue cancer patients present with clinical node metastases.[5,8,9] Lymphatic drainage of the oral tongue is principally to levels II, III, and I, in decreasing order (Fig. 4–1).[2,6] When the primary tumor is in the midline, bilateral neck metastases can occur. An adequate examination of the neck should assess for the presence or absence of palpable adenopathy (number, location, size) and any clinical manifestations of extracapsular extension (e.g., fixation of overlying skin or soft tissue, paralysis of cranial nerves).

Even with early lesions (T1 and T2), occult nodal metastases are present in 30–40% of patients.[2,5,8,11,12] In addition to tumor size, tumor thickness may independently predict nodal disease.[13] The use of ultrasonography to assess the thickness of the primary tumor has been advocated.[14] In our practice, computed tomography (CT) and magnetic resonance imaging (MRI) have been used in instances of locally advanced disease to ascertain muscular or mandibular invasion or major vessel involvement.[1,2,6]

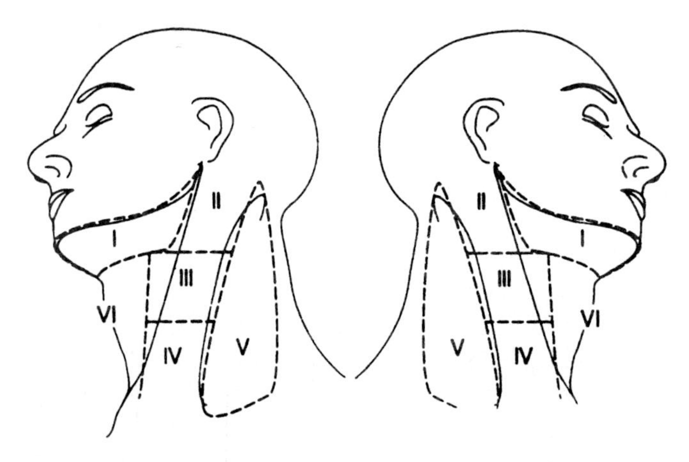

FIGURE 4–1
Lymphatic drainage of the oral tongue. (Used with permission of the American Joint Committee on Cancer (AJCC®), Chicago, IL. The original source for this material is the AJCC® Cancer Staging Manual, 5th edition (1997) published by Lippincott Williams & Wilkins Publishers, Philadelphia, PA.)

C. Evaluation for Systemic Disease

Extensive workup for distant metastatic disease is seldom indicated for primary carcinoma of the oral tongue unless the patient is symptomatic. The yield is low and usually not cost-effective.[15] A routine preoperative chest radiograph and blood chemistries, including liver function tests, are adequate in most instances. Further imaging studies are directed by abnormal laboratory and chest radiographic findings.[1,6]

D. Evaluation for Second Malignancy

The incidence of a second synchronous primary in the aerodigestive tract in patients with head and neck cancer has been estimated at 10–15%.[2,6] It is our practice therefore to perform panendoscopy (nasopharyngoscopy, laryngoscopy, bronchoscopy, and esophagoscopy) on all patients with head and neck cancer. It is performed under general anesthesia in an outpatient setting and permits a careful, detailed examination with minimal discomfort to the patient. It should be noted that there are those who employ a more selective approach, reserving panendoscopy for patients with locally advanced disease or clinically positive cervical node(s) or for those whose primary tumor is occult.[1,16]

E. Tissue Diagnosis

In the office setting, a small incisional biopsy may be performed with relative ease in selected patients. Excisional biopsy may achieve a tumor-free margin with early lesions. This situation is unusual, however, and partial glossectomy is generally necessary for complete tumor resection. Biopsies of deep lesions may be uncomfortable; therefore we prefer to perform the biopsy and careful local staging of suspicious areas concurrently with the panendoscopy in the operating room setting with the patient under general anesthesia.

Staging and Prognostic Factors

F. Staging

Table 4–1 is an adaptation of the most recent staging system for oral tongue cancer by the AJCC.[10] The two most important predictors of clinical outcome are the size of the primary tumor (T stage) and the presence of nodal metastases (N stage). The larger the primary lesion, the more likely it is that there is associated nodal disease (Table 4–2).[8,9]

Various investigators have reported that tumor thickness correlates with the likelihood of modal metastases and cancer recurrence.[13,17] Different depths of invasion (>2 mm vs. >4 mm) have been evaluated, but these studies tend to be retrospective in nature and involve subset analyses and small sample sizes. As such, although patients with thick lesions tend to do worse as a group, statistically significant data correlating tumor thickness and clinical outcome are unavailable.

Similarly, various histologic characteristics as predictors of poor clinical outcome have been reported, including poor histopathologic grade, nuclear grade, and perineural and perivascular invasion.[17–19] Unfortunately, due to interobserver variation, the subjective assessment of the histologic description, and the retrospective nature of most studies, histologic characteristics at present have not been demonstrated to be statistically significant independent prognostic markers.

Advances in molecular biology and diagnostics have affected certain aspects of clinical medicine. Various investigators have attempted to correlate molecular events and clinical outcome for cancer patients.[20–23] The most frequently altered oncogene in human cancers is the *p53* gene. This tumor suppressor gene has been found in conjunction with other head and neck squamous cell cancers, and its potential clinical implications have been reported, including its apparent association with a worse clinical outcome.[21,23] Similarly, overexpression of the eIF4E protein (a regulator of cellular protein synthesis) in tumor-free resection margins appears to be associated with local recurrence.[22] However, as exciting as these novel developments are, validation by large-scale prospective clinical trials is required before these molecular markers can be used reliably in the clinical setting.

Treatment of the Primary Site

G. Early Lesion (T1 and T2)

The mainstays of therapy for cancer of the oral tongue are surgery and radiation therapy. Irradiation may be curative for

TABLE 4–1.
AJCC definition of TNM and stage grouping for cancer of the anterior (oral) tongue

Primary Tumor (T)

TX	Primary tumor cannot be assessed
T0	No evidence of primary tumor
Tis	Carcinoma *in situ*
T1	Tumor ≤2 cm in greatest dimension
T2	Tumor >2 cm but ≤4 cm in greatest dimension
T3	Tumor >4 cm in greatest dimension
T4	Tumor invades adjacent structures (e.g., through cortical bone, into deep [extrinsic] muscle of tongue, maxillary sinus, skin. Superficial erosion alone of bone/tooth socket by gingirval primary is not sufficient to classify as T4)

Regional Lymph Nodes (N)

NX	Regional lymph nodes cannot be assessed
N0	No regional lymph node metastasis
N1	Metastasis in a single ipsilateral lymph node, ≤3 cm in greatest dimension
N2	Metastasis in a single ipsilateral lymph node, >3 cm but ≤6 cm in greatest dimension; or in multiple ipsilateral lymph nodes, none >6 cm in greatest dimension; or in bilateral or contralateral lymph nodes, none >6 cm in greatest dimension
N2a	Metastasis in single ipsilateral lymph nodes >3 cm but ≤6 cm in greatest dimension
N2b	Metastasis in multiple ipsilateral lymph nodes, none >6 cm in greatest dimension
N2c	Metastasis in bilateral or contralateral lymph nodes, none >6 cm in greatest dimension
N3	Metastasis in a lymph node >6 cm in greatest dimension

Distant Metastasis (M)

MX	Distant metastasis cannot be assessed
M0	No distant metastasis
M1	Distant metastasis

Stage Grouping

Stage	T	N	M
0	Tis	N0	M0
I	T1	N0	M0
II	T2	N0	M0
III	T3	N0	M0
	T1	N1	M0
	T2	N1	M0
	T3	N1	M0
IVA	T4	N0	M0
	T4	N1	M0
	Any T	N2	M0
IVB	Any T	N3	M0
IVC	Any T	Any N	M1

SOURCE: Used with permission of the American Joint Committee on Cancer (AJCC®), Chicago, IL. The original source for this material is the AJCC® Cancer Staging Manual, 5th edition (1997) published by Lippincott Williams & Wilkins Publishers, Philadelphia, PA.

early lesions (T1, T2) and preserves normal anatomy and tongue function in most cases.[11] Complications of treatment include significant edema of the tongue necessitating tracheotomy, xerostomia, loss of taste, and osteoradionecrosis.[24,25]

Irradiation can be administered as external beam radiation (EBRT) or brachytherapy (BCT). Conventional EBRT consists of 65–70 Gy over 5–6 weeks. BCT can deliver as much as 100 Gy locally to the oral tongue.[6,26] In a trial by Benk et al. comparing BCT alone versus EBRT plus a BCT boost in patients with stage II squamous cell carcinoma of the oral tongue, better local control rates were obtained with BCT alone.[26]

Prior to the initiation of irradiation, evaluation by an oral surgeon or dentist should be performed to assess the health of the patient's gingiva and dentition. Diseased teeth require extraction prior to irradiation to minimize the risk of osteoradionecrosis.

Surgical treatment of early oral tongue cancer consists of wide excision of the lesion with a tumor-free margin. It generally requires partial glossectomy, and functional results are usually good. The results of treatment by primary surgical resection compared to irradiation alone for early oral tongue cancer are equivalent.[25,27] Five-year local control rates of 85% for T1 lesions and 80% for T2 lesions can be expected.[27]

H. T3 and T4

Surgical resection is the mainstay of therapy for T3 and T4 lesions.[6,28] Locally advanced tumors may involve adjacent structures. The only potential for cure is complete en bloc resection of all tumor-associated tissue with microscopic tumor-free margins assessed at the time of surgery with frozen section. Additionally, neck dissection should be part of the treatment regimen, given the 50–70% probability of cervical node metastasis.[5] This may necessitate composite resection and reconstruction (traditional myocutaneous flap or vascular free flap) to preserve function and cosmesis.

Management of the Neck

I. N0 Neck and Early Lesions

Much has been written about the need for elective neck dissection (END) for clinically negative necks (N0) of patients with early lesions (T1 or T2). Franceschi and coworkers reported a 31% incidence of occult nodal metastasis in the clinically N0 neck for early oral tongue cancer.[29] Furthermore, for those who did not undergo END, 35% of patients with T1 or T2 lesions had developed cervical node metastases on follow-up.[8] Recent trends favor treatment of the N0 neck for early lesions with (1) selective

TABLE 4–2.
Incidence of regional metastases correlated with size of primary lesion (oral tongue)

Size	No. of patients	No. in whom positive nodes developed	%
T1	95	28	29
T2	77	33	43
T3	13	10	77

SOURCE: Data derived from Spiro and Strong.[8]

neck dissection: supraomohyoid neck dissection (SOHND); (2) modified radical neck dissection (MRND); or (3) irradiation.[3,6,12,19,30,31] This reflects an appreciation of the prevalence of occult neck disease even with early lesions. Data demonstrating survival benefit with this approach is not conclusive.

Supraomohyoid neck dissection refers to removal of lymph nodes from levels I, II, and III. The posterior limit of this dissection is marked by the cutaneous branches of the cervical plexus and the posterior border of the sternocleidomastoid muscle. The inferior limit is the superior belly of the omohyoid muscle where it crosses over the internal jugular vein. The superior limit is the inferior border of the mandible.

MRND refers to the removal of all lymph nodes at levels I, II, III, IV, and V while preserving one or more nonlymphatic structures (i.e., spinal accessory nerve, internal jugular vein, sternocleidomastoid muscle). The superior limit is the inferior border of the mandible; the inferior limit is the superior border of the clavicle. The medial limit is the lateral border of the sternohyoid muscle, hyoid bone, and contralateral anterior belly of the digastric muscle; the lateral limit is the anterior border of the trapezius muscle.

The only reported randomized prospective trial examining the use of END versus observation for oral tongue carcinoma was by Fakih et al.[12] These authors advocated the use of END in patients with early tongue cancer, specifically those with a tumor thickness of more than 4 mm. Unfortunately, the study involved only 70 patients, had a short median follow-up of 20 months, and did not reach statistical significance in survival benefit for END patients. Others, such as Cunningham et al.[32] and Byers et al.,[31] using retrospective data, suggested the efficacy of END over therapeutic neck dissection (when nodes are suspicious), as the salvage rate among patients who developed cervical metastasis after initial therapy is poor. In contrast, Franceschi et al. did not detect any survival benefit for patients who underwent END compared to those who were treated with therapeutic neck dissection when nodal disease became clinically evident.[29]

Elective irradiation is another option for treatment of the clinical N0 neck.[6,33,34] Northrop and coworkers compared the use of EBRT (50 Gy in 5 weeks) to the contralateral neck in conjunction with ipsilateral neck dissection versus ipsilateral neck dissection alone. The incidence of contralateral nodal disease at follow-up was 5% after contralateral irradiation and 34% after ipsilateral dissection alone.[33] Similarly, Mendenhall and coworkers reported lower neck recurrence in patients treated with elective irradiation.[34]

Until reliable prognostic factors are available to identify patients likely to have occult nodal metastases, or perhaps new technical applications such as the use of sentinel node biopsy prove efficacious, it appears that routine treatment of the neck is reasonable. Because the nodes that are at highest risk for metastases can be removed with a SOHND (levels I, II, and III), it is our philosophy that an elective SOHND should be performed to remove potential disease. If lymph nodes removed during SOHND are found to harbor metastatic disease, the following guidelines may apply: (1) For nodal metastases detected intraoperatively, one may proceed directly to MRND. Radiation is given to the neck if multiple nodes are involved or there is extracapsular extension. (2) If postoperative histology shows that only a single, discrete node is involved without extracapsular spread, no further treatment is needed. (3) If a single node is involved and the disease has spread extracapsularly, or if more than one node is positive at more than one level, postoperative irradiation of the neck is undertaken. Because of the lymphatic drainage of the tongue, patients whose lesions are midline can have bilateral neck disease; and thus bilateral END is necessary in selected patients.

J. N0 Neck and Advanced Lesions

Patients with N0 necks and advanced (T3 and T4) lesions should be considered for routine END.[1,6,35] The reported incidence of neck metastases in these instances is at least 50–70%.[13,36] Neck dissection not only provides potential cure, it identifies patients at high risk for regional recurrence, such as those with nodal disease and extracapsular spread, multiple node involvement, and confluence of nodal disease. The presence of these risk factors in patients with T3 lesions justifies the use of postoperative irradiation to both the neck and the primary site following neck dissection. Radiation applied to the primary site *and* the neck should be considered for all patients with T4 lesions after resection and node dissection irrespective of node status.

K. Treatment of the NI Neck

Patients with *clinically* involved necks require at least a modified radical neck dissection.[1,6,37] If these nodes are associated with a large primary lesion, adjacent organ involvement, or both, mandibulectomy (marginal versus segmental) may be necessary for resecting the primary lesion in addition to neck dissection. Depending on the size and site of the primary lesion, contralateral END (e.g., SOHND) may be indicated. Planning the reconstruction, preservation of critical function such as speech and swallowing, and rehabilitation must be kept in mind to optimize results. Patients with advanced lesions and nodal disease who are at high risk for cervical recurrence should be considered for postoperative irradiation.

Adjuvant Therapy

L. Role of Radiation Therapy

Numerous studies have reported that the combination of surgical resection and irradiation has a better outcome than surgery alone.[24,29] Indications for postoperative irradiation have included advanced disease (stage III and IV), positive surgical margins, multiple (more than three) positive lymph nodes, and extracapsular involvement.[1,6,37]

The role of chemotherapy in the adjuvant and neoadjuvant setting is in evolution. Though pilot studies have reported promising overall response rates and complete response rates with induction chemotherapy of head and neck cancers, the survival data are less promising using the most commonly prescribed regimen of cisplatin and 5-fluorouracil. Several large studies involving the usual active agents based on pilot studies failed to demonstrate survival benefits in the neoadjuvant or the adjuvant setting. The combination of chemotherapy and x-irradiation has shown some promise in organ preservation trials.[38]

References

1. Shah JP, Lydiatt W. Treatment of cancer of the head and neck. CA Cancer J Clin 1995;45:352–368.
2. Ghali GE, Li BDL, Minnard EA. Management of the neck relative to oral malignancy. Selected Readings in Oral Maxillofacial Surgery 1998;6(2):1–36.
3. Mendelson BC, Woods JE, Beahrs OH. Neck dissection in the treatment of carcinoma of the anterior two-thirds of the tongue. Surg Gynecol Obstet 1976;143:76–80.
4. Civantos FJ, Goodwin WJ. Cancer of the oropharynx. In: Myers EN, Suen JY (eds) Cancer of the Head and Neck, 3rd ed. Philadelphia: Saunders, 1996;361–380.
5. DiTroia JF. Nodal metastases and prognosis in carcinoma of the oral cavity. Otolaryngol Clin North Am 1972;5:333–342.
6. Alvi A, Myers EN, Johnson JT. Cancer of the oral cavity. In: Myers EN, Suen JY (eds) Cancer of the Head and Neck, 3rd ed. Philadelphia: Saunders, 1996;321–360.
7. Krupala JL, Gianol GJ. Carcinoma of the oral tongue. J La State Med Soc 1993;145:421–426.
8. Spiro RH, Strong EH. Epidermoid carcinoma of the mobile tongue treated by partial glossectomy alone. Am J Surg 1971;122:707.
9. Spiro RH, Alfonso AE, Farr HW, et al. Cervical node metastasis from epidermoid carcinoma of the oral cavity and oropharynx: a critical assessment of current staging. Am J Surg 1974;128:562.
10. American Joint Committee on Cancer Chicago, IL. American Joint Committee on Cancer. In: AJCC Cancer Staging Manual, 5th ed. American Joint Committee on Cancer, Chicago, IL. 1997:24–30.
11. Decroix Y, Ghossein NA. Experience of the Curie Institute in treatment of cancer of the mobile tongue. I. Treatment policies and results. CA Cancer J Clin 1981;47:496.
12. Fakih AR, Rao RS, Borges AM, et al. Elective versus therapeutic neck dissection in early carcinoma of the oral tongue. Am J Surg 1989;158:309–313.
13. Spiro RH, Huvos AG, Wong GY, et al. Predictive value of tumor thickness in squamous carcinoma confined to the tongue and floor of the mouth. Am J Surg 1986;152:345–350.
14. Shintani S, Nakayama B, Matsuura H, et al. Intraoral ultrasonography is useful to evaluate tumor thickness in tongue carcinoma. Am J Surg 1997;173:345–347.
15. Merino OR, Lindberg RD, Fletcher GH. An analysis of distant metastases from squamous cell carcinoma of the upper respiratory and digestive tracts. CA Cancer J Clin 1977;40:145–150.
16. McCombe A, Lund VJ, Howard DJ. Multiple synchronous carcinoma of the aerodigestive tract. J Laryngol Otol 1989;103:794–795.
17. Morton RP, Ferguson CM, Lambie NK, et al. Tumor thickness in early tongue cancer. Arch Otolaryngol Head Neck Surg 1994;120:717–720.
18. Woolgar JA, Scott J. Prediction of cervical lymph node metastasis in squamous cell carcinoma of the tongue/floor of mouth. Head Neck 1995;17:463–472.
19. Lydiatt DD, Robbins DT, Byers RM, et al. Treatment of stage I and II oral tongue cancer. Head Neck 1993;15:308–312.
20. Teixeira G, Antonangelo L, Kowalski L, et al. Argyrophilic nucleolar organizer regions staining is useful in predicting recurrence-free interval in oral tongue and floor of mouth squamous cell carcinoma. Am J Surg 1996; 172:684–688.
21. Brennan JA, Mao L, Hruban RH, et al. Molecular assessment of histopathological staging in squamous-cell carcinoma of the head and neck. N Engl J Med 1995;332:429–435.
22. Nathan CO, Li L, Li BDL, et al. Detection of the proto-oncogene eIF4E in surgical margins may predict recurrence in head and neck cancer. Oncogene 1997;15:579–584.
23. Shin DM, Kim J, Ro JY. Activation of p53 gene expression in premalignant lesions during head and neck tumorigenesis. Cancer Res 1994;54:321–326.
24. Amdur RJ, Parsons JT, Mendenhall WM, et al. Postoperative irradiation for squamous cell carcinoma of the head and neck: an analysis of treatment results and complications. Int J Radiat Oncol Biol Phys 1989;16:25–36.
25. Fein DA, Mendenhall WM, Parsons JT, et al. Carcinoma of the oral tongue: a comparison of results and complications of treatment with radiotherapy and/or surgery. Head Neck 1994;16:358–365.
26. Benk V, Mazeron JJ, Grimanrd L, et al. Comparison of curietherapy versus external irradiation combined with curietherapy in stage II squamous cell carcinomas of the mobile tongue. Radiother Oncol 1990;18:339–344.
27. Ridge JA, Hooks MA, Lee WR, et al. Head and neck tumors. In: Pazdur R, Coia LR, Hoskins WJ, Wagman LD (eds) Cancer Management: A Multidisciplinary Approach, 2nd ed. Huntington: PRR, 1998:468–471.
28. Magrin J, Kowalski LP, Saboia M, et al. Major glossectomy: end results of 106 cases. Oral Oncol Eur J Cancer 1996;32B:407–412.
29. Franceschi D, Gupta R, Spiro RH, et al. Improved survival in the treatment of squamous carcinoma of the oral tongue. Am J Surg 1993;166:360–365.
30. Ho CM, Lam KH, Wei WI, et al. Occult lymph node metastasis in small oral tongue cancers. Head & Neck 1992;14:359–363.
31. Byers RM, Weber RS, Andrews R, et al. Frequency and therapeutic implications of "skip metastases" in the neck from squamous carcinoma of the oral tongue. Head & Neck 1997;19:14–19.
32. Cunningham MJ, Johnson JT, Myers EN, et al. Cervical lymph node metastasis after local excision of early squamous cell carcinoma of the oral cavity. Am J Surg 1986;152:361–366.
33. Norhrop M, Flectcher GH, Jesse RH, et al. Evolution of neck disease in patients with primary squamous cell carcinoma of the oral tongue, floor of mouth, and palatine arch, and clinically positive neck nodes neither fixed nor bilateral. CA 1972;29(1):23–30.
34. Mendenhall WM, Million RR, Cassissi NJ. Elective neck irradiation in squamous cell carcinoma of the head and neck. Head Neck Surg 1980;3:15–20.
35. Silver CE, Moisa II. Elective treatment of the neck in cancer of the oral tongue. Semin Surg Oncol 1991;7:14.
36. Fujitani T, Ogasawara H, Hattori H, et al. Seventeen years experience in the treatment of carcinoma of the mobile tongue. Auris Nasus Larynx 1986;13:43.
37. Gujrathi D, Kerr P, Anderson B, et al. Treatment outcome of squamous cell carcinoma of the oral tongue. J of Otolaryn 1996;25(3):145–149.
38. Vokes EE. Combined-Modality therapy of head and neck cancer. Oncology 1997;11(9):27–30.

Chapter 5

Cancer of the Soft Palate

NADER SADEGHI
WILLIAM R. PANJE

A. Epidemiology and Etiology

Anatomically, the soft palate is part of the oropharynx. It consists of mucosa on both surfaces, connective tissue, muscle fibers, aponeurosis, numerous blood vessels, lymphatics, and minor salivary glands. Functionally, the soft palate serves to separate the oropharynx from the nasopharynx during swallowing and speech. The soft palate approximates the posterior pharyngeal wall during swallowing to prevent nasopharyngeal regurgitation and during speech to prevent air escaping into the nose.

Cancer of the soft palate accounts for fewer than 2% of head and neck mucosal malignancies. Among the hard and soft palate cancers, squamous cell carcinoma (SCCA) accounts for 75%.[1] In the soft palate, 80% of the lesions have squamous cell histology, with minor salivary tumors occurring less often. The incidence of oral cavity and oropharyngeal cancer varies geographically, with the highest incidence reported in India (accounting for 50% of all cancers).[2] SCCA of the soft palate, uvula, and anterior tonsillar pillar occurs much less frequently than cancers at other oropharyngeal sites, such as the tonsil and the base of the tongue.

Tobacco and alcohol are the major causes of oral cavity and oropharyngeal cancer including the soft palate. Reverse smoking is associated with a high incidence of palate cancer. The concept of field cancerization is particularly evident with soft palate cancer, where early neoplastic changes involve the mucosa beyond the visible tumor.

B. Presentation

Painful ulceration and odynophagia are the most common symptoms of SCCA of the soft palate. Minor salivary gland cancers, on the other hand, are usually asymptomatic submucosal masses. In advanced stages, velopharyngeal insufficiency, altered speech, difficulty swallowing, referred otalgia, trismus, or a neck mass may be present. Fortunately, tumors are often found incidentally in their early stages by the patient or the physician, as this area is easily visualized.

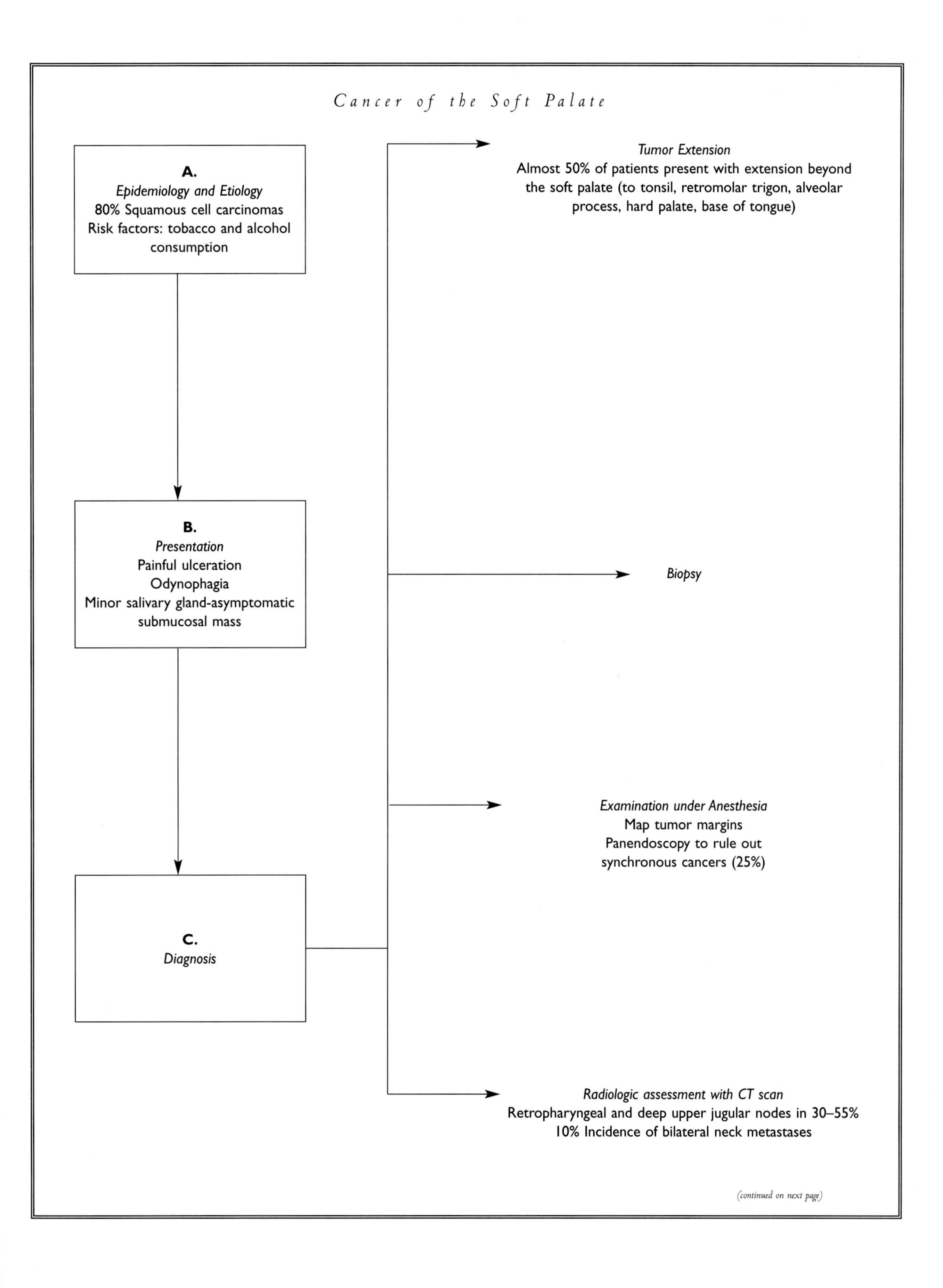
Cancer of the Soft Palate
A.
Epidemiology and Etiology
80% Squamous cell carcinomas
Risk factors: tobacco and alcohol consumption
B.
Presentation
Painful ulceration
Odynophagia
Minor salivary gland-asymptomatic submucosal mass
C.
Diagnosis
Tumor Extension
Almost 50% of patients present with extension beyond the soft palate (to tonsil, retromolar trigon, alveolar process, hard palate, base of tongue)
Biopsy
Examination under Anesthesia
Map tumor margins
Panendoscopy to rule out synchronous cancers (25%)
Radiologic assessment with CT scan
Retropharyngeal and deep upper jugular nodes in 30–55%
10% Incidence of bilateral neck metastases
(continued on next page)

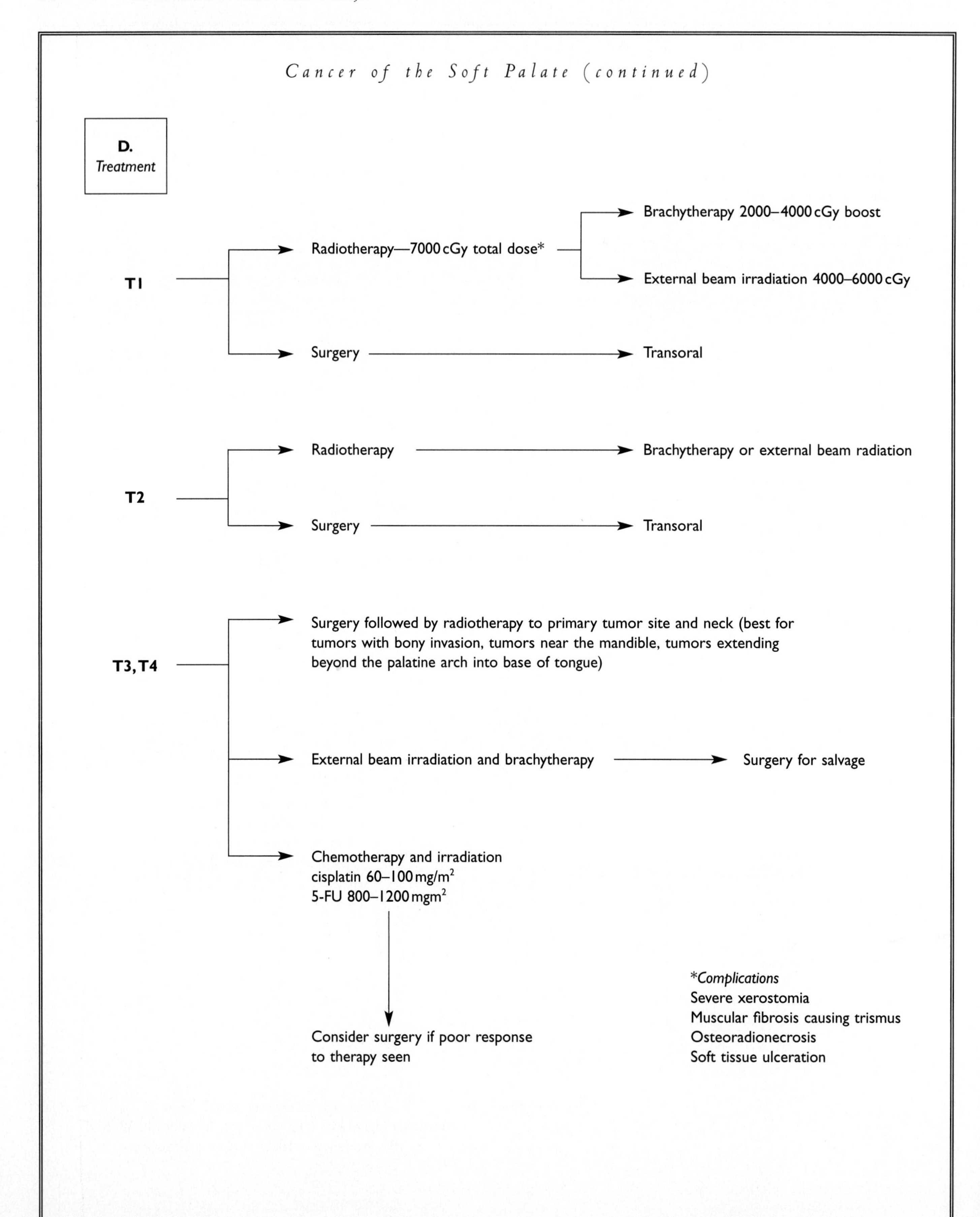
Cancer of the Soft Palate (continued)
D.
Treatment
T1
Radiotherapy—7000 cGy total dose*
Brachytherapy 2000–4000 cGy boost
External beam irradiation 4000–6000 cGy
Surgery
Transoral
T2
Radiotherapy
Brachytherapy or external beam radiation
Surgery
Transoral
T3, T4
Surgery followed by radiotherapy to primary tumor site and neck (best for tumors with bony invasion, tumors near the mandible, tumors extending beyond the palatine arch into base of tongue)
External beam irradiation and brachytherapy
Surgery for salvage
Chemotherapy and irradiation
cisplatin 60–100 mg/m2
5-FU 800–1200 mgm2
Consider surgery if poor response to therapy seen
*Complications
Severe xerostomia
Muscular fibrosis causing trismus
Osteoradionecrosis
Soft tissue ulceration

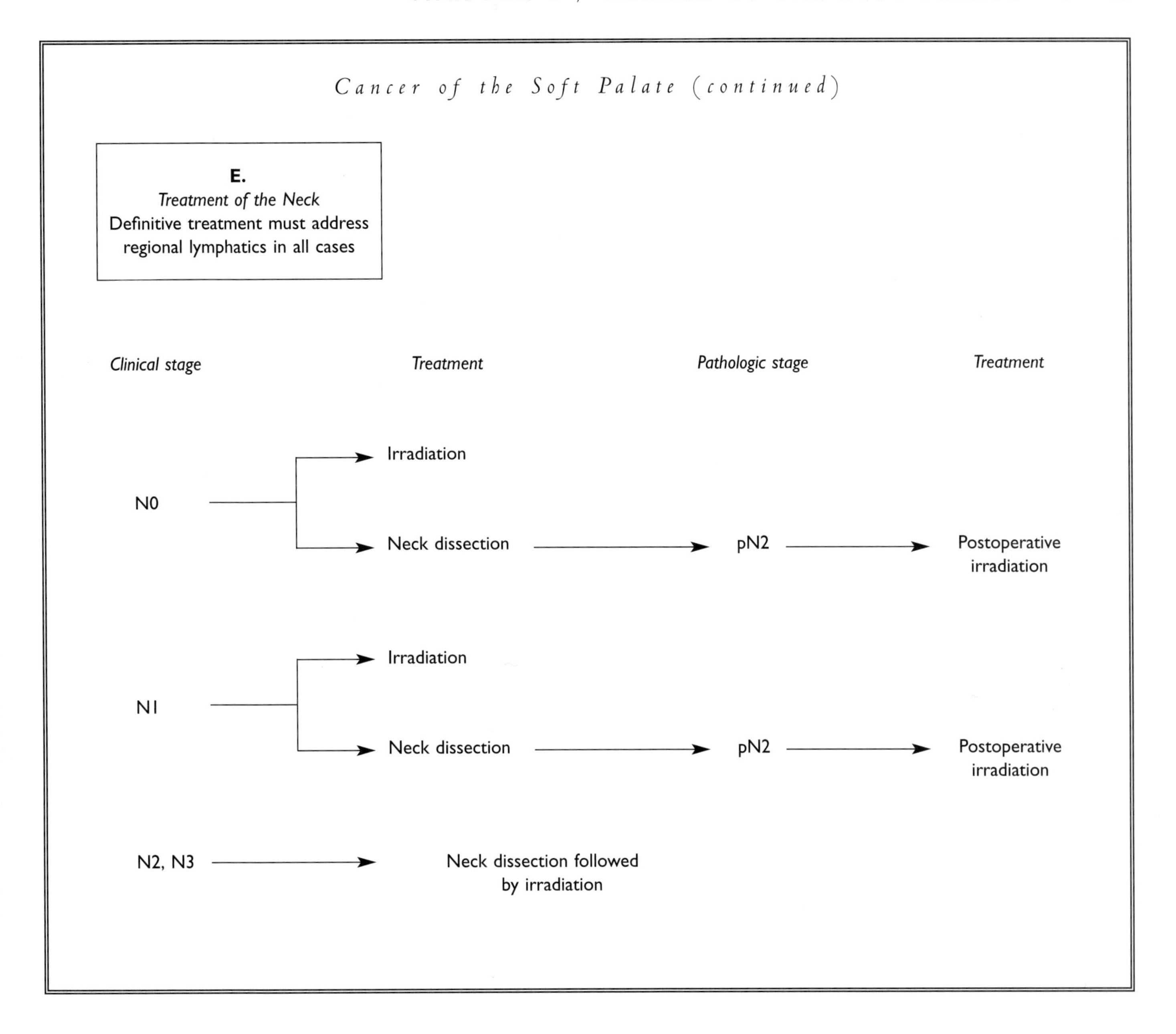

C. Diagnosis

Soft palate carcinomas are staged as oropharyngeal cancers according to the American Joint Committee for Cancer Staging (Table 5–1). Almost half of the patients present with *extension of the tumor* beyond the soft palate. Common sites of extension include tonsil, retromolar trigone, inferior or superior alveolar process, hard palate, and the base of the tongue.[3] Extension into the sphenopalatine foramen may result in palatal hypopsthesia. For extensive lesions invading the nasopharynx, there is often a middle ear effusion. The tumor may extend anterosuperiorly into the pterygomaxillary and infratemporal fossa.

Biopsy can often be performed in the office transorally with local anesthesia. For large nonulcerated lesions, an incision through the intact overlying mucosa may be required to perform the biopsy. The biopsy scar should be removed in continuity with the tumor during subsequent definitive excision. Alternatively, fine-needle aspiration cytologic studies may be performed if an experienced cytopathologist is available. Small submucosal lesions may be managed with an excisional biopsy.

Except for very small lesions, an *examination under anesthesia* is required for most squamous cell carcinomas of the soft palate to perform tumor mapping and margin assessment. Panendoscopy at the same time is performed to look for synchronous primary cancers of the upper aerodigestive tract or esophagus (10–15% incidence).[4] However, patients with soft palate cancer have an even higher incidence of synchronous and metachronous lesions, approaching 25%.[5] Alternatively, chest radio-

TABLE 5-1.
AJCC definition of TNM and stage grouping for cancer of the soft palate

Primary Tumor (T)

TX	Primary tumor cannot be assessed
T0	No evidence of primary tumor
Tis	Carcinoma *in situ*
T1	Tumor ≤2 cm in greatest dimension
T2	Tumor >2 cm but ≤4 cm in greatest dimension
T3	Tumor >4 cm in greatest dimension
T4	Tumor invades adjacent structures (e.g., pterygoid muscle[s], mandible, hard palate, deep muscle of tongue, larynx)

Regional Lymph Nodes (N)

NX	Regional lymph nodes cannot be assessed
N0	No regional lymph node metastasis
N1	Metastasis in a single ipsilateral lymph node, ≤3 cm
N2	Metastasis in a single ipsilateral lymph node, >3 cm but ≤6 cm
	N2a Single lymph node >3 cm but ≤6 cm
	N2b In multiple ipsilateral lymph nodes, none >6 cm
	N2c In bilateral or contralateral lymph nodes, none >6 cm
N3	Metastasis in a lymph node >6 cm

Distant Metastasis (M)

MX	Distant metastasis cannot be assessed
M0	No distant metastasis
M1	Distant metastasis

Stage Grouping

Stage	T	N	M
0	Tis	N0	M0
I	T1	N0	M0
II	T2	N0	M0
III	T3	N0	M0
	Any T1–3	N1	M0
IVA	T4	N0	M0
	T4	N1	M0
	T1–4	N2	M0
IVB	T1–4	N3	M0
IVC	Any T	Any N	M1

SOURCE: Used with permission of the American Joint Committee on Cancer (AJCC®), Chicago, IL. The original source for this material is the AJCC® Cancer Staging Manual, 5th edition (1997) published by Lippincott Williams & Wilkins Publishers, Philadelphia, PA.

graphy and barium esophagography may suffice for synchronous tumor assessment. Small tumors confined to the soft palate whose boundaries are visible do not require examination under anesthesia. In this situation, complete flexible nasopharyngolaryngoscopy and transoral inspection and palpation are adequate for tumor mapping.

Squamous cell carcinomas of the soft palate have a 30–55% incidence of metastasis to the retropharyngeal and upper deep jugular nodes.[3,6,7] There is a 10% incidence of bilateral neck metastases.[3] *Computed tomography* (CT) with infusion in both axial and coronal planes helps assess lymph node basins, particularly in the retropharyngeal space, and it helps identify extension of the primary tumor. *Magnetic resonance imaging* (MRI) is helpful if extension along nerves is suspected, particularly in cases of adenoid cystic carcinoma. MRI may be more sensitive than CT scans for assessing soft tissue extension by the tumor.

D. Treatment

Size, location, and contiguous spread by the primary tumor are important prognostic factors. Extension outside the palatine arch (especially to the base of the tongue), midline tumors, or tumors that extend across the palatine arch have a worse survival owing to a higher incidence of regional metastases. For small T1 lesions and superficial lesions with which no defect ensues after surgery, or for minimal defects that can be reconstructed with local flaps or left to close by secondary intention, surgery is acceptable therapy. Because resection of most other tumors of the soft palate cause velopharyngeal insufficiency, which affects both speech and swallowing, and because adequate reconstruction is technically difficult, radiation therapy has been the recommended treatment for most soft palate cancers.[5,8] Although advances in reconstructive techniques and prosthetic reconstruction has rendered surgical resection and subsequently rehabilitation of soft palate defects more effective, radiation therapy remains the primary treatment modality in most centers for T1, T2, and some T3 lesions. Most importantly, results are comparable to those achieved with surgery.[6,9–14]

Using radiotherapy as the primary treatment, tumor control is achieved in 80–90% of T1 lesions, 60–70% of T2 lesions, and 55–65% of T3 lesions.[6,9–14] For T4 lesions, where irradiation is routinely used as the primary treatment, this rate drops to less than 50%. Effective treatment of the primary lesion requires a dose approximating 7000 cGy.

The potential complications of radiotherapy include severe xerostomia, muscular fibrosis with resultant trismus, osteoradionecrosis of the mandible, and soft tissue ulceration. These complications are volume- and dose-dependent; and some centers use 2000–4000 cGy of interstitial brachytherapy with Ir^{192} to boost an initial external beam dose of 4000–6000 cGy. Brachytherapy is frequently added in patients with T3 tumors who are treated with external beam radiotherapy. Boosting the dose to the primary tumor site utilizing brachytherapy allows improved locoregional control of the tumor while reducing complications by avoiding wide-field high-dose irradiation.[9,13,14]

As mentioned, both radiotherapy and surgery are adequate for controlling early lesions (T1, T2, T3).[1,6] For advanced T4 lesions, traditional external beam radiotherapy alone has resulted in poor survival rates.[1] Consequently, for advanced stage III and IV tumors, combined treatment with surgical resection followed by radiation therapy to both the primary tumor and the neck is recommended.[1] An alternative regimen would be chemotherapy (cisplatin 60–100 mg/m^2 every 3 weeks and 5-fluorouracil 800–1200 mg/m^2 as an intravenous bolus or by infusion over 72–120 hours) combined with radiotherapy followed by surgical resection. Chemotherapy is given for two or three cycles, and the response to treatment is then assessed. Surgical resection is considered if the response to chemotherapy is poor.

If there has been a favorable response to chemotherapy, combined external beam radiation followed by brachytherapy is an alternative to surgery for management of these advanced lesions. The total dose given is 7000 cGy. Surgery is then reserved for salvage in these patients. Brachytherapy for tumors with bony invasion or those near the mandible results in a high incidence of osteoradionecrosis. These patients are best treated with planned surgical excision followed by external beam radiotherapy, as are patients with tumor extension beyond the palatine arch into the base of the tongue.

Adenoid cystic carcinoma and mucoepidermoid carcinoma are the two most common minor salivary gland tumors of the palate. Others include adenocarcinoma, malignant mixed tumor, and other rare tumors. Approximately 20–25% of minor salivary gland tumors found in the palate are benign. Adenocarcinomas and salivary gland cancers are best treated with surgery. Treatment strategies for minor salivary cancers of the palate are outlined elsewhere (see Chapter 3).

E. *Treatment of the Neck*

Squamous cell carcinoma of the soft palate and uvula is associated with occult regional metastasis in up to 20–30% of patients at presentation, even those with early primary tumors.[3,6,7] Therefore definitive treatment must address regional lymphatics in all cases. Midline lesions or those that cross the midline have a high incidence of bilateral metastasis; therefore treatment of both sides of the neck should be considered in these instances.[6,7] Tumor thickness is an excellent predictor of nodal metastasis with soft palate cancers. Baredes et al. found that all tumors thicker than 3.12 mm were associated with cervical metastasis, with the tumor thickness correlating more directly with nodal metastasis than the T stage.[15] Clinical regional metastases at presentation reduces the 5-year survival by half: from 80% in patients with N0 necks to 40% in those with clinically evident neck metastases.[6] For small tumors treated primarily with radiotherapy, clinical N0 and N1 disease can be adequately controlled with radiotherapy alone.[6] For clinical N2 and greater disease, 74% of patients have residual cancer following radiotherapy.[6] Hence these patients should be treated with planned combined therapy consisting of neck dissection followed by radiotherapy.

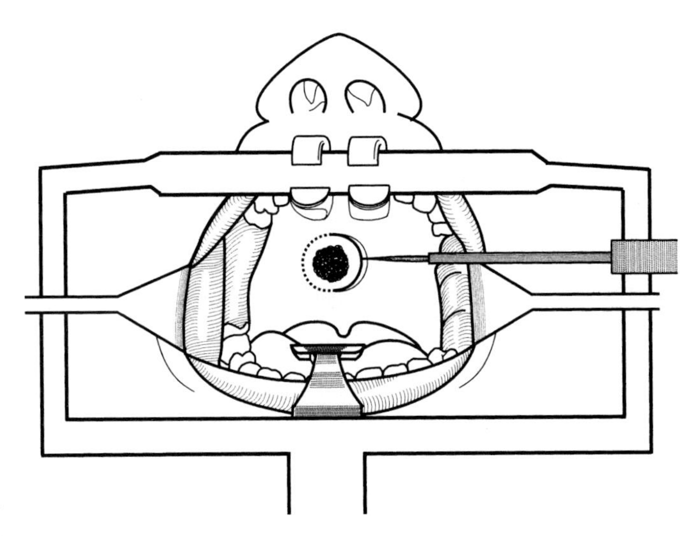

FIGURE 5–1
Transoral exposure for resection of small hard or soft palate cancers. Dingman mouth retractor provides excellent exposure.

Surgical Approaches

Transoral Approach

Transoral excision can be performed for most soft palate cancers when they are confined to the palatine arch without extension to the tonsils, lateral pharyngeal wall, or base of the tongue. A Dingman or Crochard mouth gag provides attachable cheek retractors to facilitate exposure (Figs. 5–1, 5–2). The tumor is mapped out with a margin of at least 1 cm. Electrocautery, cold knife, or CO_2 laser is used to perform the resection.[16] The margins are checked with frozen sections.

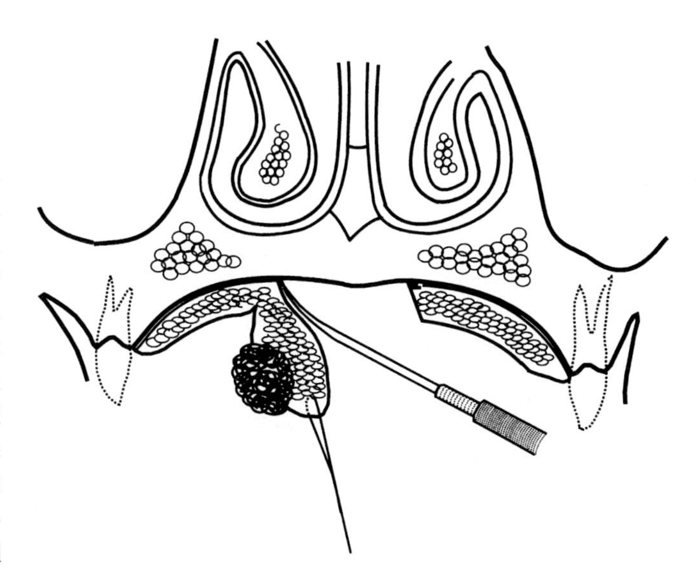

FIGURE 5–2
Coronal view of transoral resection of cancers of the palate.

Small mucosal lesions may be resected with preservation of the superior mucosa. If the defect is close to the hard palate, an advancement rotation flap from the hard palate may be used to close the defect. Small defects at the posterior margin of the soft palate may be closed by approximating the superior and inferior mucosa. The resulting velopharyngeal insufficiency corrects over time. A superiorly based pharyngeal flap may be used to close the defect. Submucosal resection may be done for small low-grade salivary gland tumors, preserving the mucosa for primary closure.

Pull-through Approach

For lesions that extend beyond the soft palate to involve the tonsil, base of the tongue, or lateral pharyngeal wall, a pull-through approach provides excellent exposure without mandibulotomy.[17,18] This technique allows en bloc resection of the primary tumor and neck dissection.

An upper transverse incision is made from the mastoid tip to the submentum. Following neck dissection including the submandibular triangle, a mucosal incision is made through the floor of the mouth. Mucosal incisions are made around the tumor with adequate margins. The mylohyoid muscle is cut from the neck, and the tongue is then delivered to the neck. Dissection is completed around the tumor, and the specimen is removed.[18]

Mandibulotomy Approach

A mandibulotomy approach provides wide exposure for resection of T4 soft palate cancers that extend to the hard palate, lateral pharynx, tonsil, base of the tongue, or the mandible. Visor flap or lip-splitting neck incisions may be used.

A horizontal incision is made from the mastoid tip to the submentum. The lip is split with a stair-step cut along the vermilion to prevent lip notching, and a Z incision is carried over the mentum to join the submental incision. Periosteum is raised on either side of the incision. A parasymphyseal stair-step osteotomy is made in such a fashion as to preserve the anterior muscular attachments of the mandible on the opposite side.[17] Once the position of the osteotomy is determined, mandibular miniplates are bent to adapt to the contour of the mandible for mandibular plating at the end of the procedure. An incision is made in the floor of the mouth in the labiogingival sulcus to the anterior resection margin. The mylohyoid muscle is then cut, which allows swinging the mandible open. Excellent exposure of the entire soft palate and oropharynx is thus provided. If, based on preoperative imaging, there is no mandibular bony invasion, the periosteum is raised as the margin. Relevant soft tissue cuts are made around the tumor, and it is removed. If there is invasion of the hard palate or the upper alveolus, osteotomies are made using a Stryker saw following adequate soft tissue cuts. This exposure allows an inferior maxillectomy. Attention should be given to assessing invasion of the medial pterygoid muscle; if invaded, adequate deep margins should be taken. In irradiated patients or whenever there is a chance for composite resection of the mandible, a lateral mandibulotomy is preferred.[18] The site of the cut varies depending on tumor extent. A visor flap can be used, obviating the need for lip splitting.

Reconstruction

A basic hard palate prosthesis can be designed that extends into the oropharynx.[19] When a posterior functioning band of soft palate is preserved, the obturator extension sits in the defect. During swallowing the posterior band is elevated against the obturator. For total soft palate defects, the posterior extension of the obturator sits in the oropharynx anterior to the pharyngeal constrictor. During swallowing the superior constrictor elevates against this static prosthesis to achieve velopharyngeal closure.

For extensive defects of the soft palate and lateral pharyngeal wall with exposed mandible, vascularized soft tissue reconstruction is mandatory. It is especially important in irradiated patients. The temporalis muscle or musculofascial flap is reliable and readily available for reconstruction.[17] It allows complete reconstruction of the soft palate and provides coverage for the lateral pharyngeal defect and exposed mandible. It may be combined with a superiorly based pharyngeal flap for double-layer closure of the palate. A dermal graft is used to cover the muscle if it is not covered by fascia. Microvascular radial forearm fasciocutaneous free flap reconstruction is another alternative for total soft palate reconstruction.

References

1. Evans JF, Shah JP. Epidermoid carcinoma of the palate. Am J Surg 1981;142:451–455.
2. Mahboubi E. The epidemiology of oral cavity, pharyngeal and esophageal cancer outside of North America and western Europe. Cancer 1977; 40:1879–1886.
3. Leemans CR, Engelbrecht WJ, Tiwari R, et al. Carcinoma of the soft palate and anterior tonsillar pillar. Laryngoscope 1994;104:1477–1481.
4. Gluckman JL. Synchronous multiple primary lesions of the upper aerodigestive system. Arch Otolaryngol 1979;105:597–598.
5. Russ JE, Applebaum EL, Sisson GA. Squamous cell carcinoma of the soft palate. Laryngoscope 1977;87:1151–1156.
6. Weber RS, Peters LJ, Wolf P, et al. Squamous cell carcinoma of the soft palate, uvula, and anterior faucial pillar. Otolaryngol Head Neck Surg 1988; 99:16–23.
7. Har-El G, Shaha A, Chaudry R, et al. Carcinoma of the uvula and midline soft palate: indications for neck treatment. Head Neck 1992;14:99–101.
8. Chung CK, Constable WC. Squamous cell carcinoma of the soft palate and uvula. Int J Radiat Oncol Biol Phys 1979;5:845–850.

9. Pernot M, Malissard L, Hoffstetter S, et al. Influence of tumoral, radiobiological, and general factors on local control and survival of a series of 361 tumors of the velotonsillar area treated by exclusive irradiation (external beam irradiation + brachytherapy or brachytherapy alone). Int J Radiat Oncol Biol Phys 1994;30:1051–1058.
10. Keus RB, Pontvert D, Brunin F, et al. Results of irradiation in squamous cell carcinoma of the soft palate and uvula. Radiat Oncol 1988;11:311–317.
11. Horton D, Tran L, Greenberg P, et al. Primary radiation therapy in the treatment of squamous cell carcinoma of the soft palate. Cancer 1989; 63:2442–2445.
12. Esche BA, Haie CM, Grebaulet AP, et al. Interstitial and external radiotherapy in carcinoma of the soft palate and uvula. Int J Radiat Oncol Biol Phys 1988;15:619–625.
13. Behar RA, Martin PJ, Fee WE, et al. Iridium-192 interstitial implant and external beam radiation therapy in the management of squamous cell carcinoma of the tonsil and soft palate. Int J Radiat Oncol Biol Phys 1993;28:221–227.
14. Levendag PC, Schmitz PIM, Jansen PP, et al. Fractionated high-dose-rate and pulsed-dose-rate brachytherapy: first clinical experience in squamous cell carcinoma of the tonsillar fossa and soft palate. Int J Radiat Oncol Biol Phys 1997;38:497–506.
15. Baredes S, Leeman DJ, Chen TS, et al. Significance of tumor thickness in soft palate carcinoma. Laryngoscope 1993;103:389–393.
16. Panje WR, Scher N, Karnell M. Transoral carbon dioxide laser ablation for cancer, tumors and other lesions. Arch Otolaryngol Head Neck Surg 1989;115:681–688.
17. Panje WR, Morris MR. Surgery of oral cavity, tongue, and oropharynx. In: Naumann HH, Helms J, Herberhold C, et al. (eds) Head and Neck Surgery, vol 1, part 2. New York: Thieme, 1995:739–753.
18. Panje WR, Morris MR. The oropharynx. In: Soutar DS, Tiwari R (eds) Excision and Reconstruction in Head and Neck Cancer. Edinburgh: Livingstone, 1994:141–157.
19. Johnson JT, Aramany MA, Myers EN. Palatal neoplasms: reconstructive considerations. Otolaryngol Clin North Am 1983;16:441–456.

Chapter 6

Tonsillar Cancer

ASHOK R. SHAHA

A. Etiology and Pathology

The oropharynx is anatomically divided into four areas: (1) tonsil and tonsillar pillar; (2) base of the tongue; (3) soft palate; and (4) pharyngeal wall. Although the oropharynx may be involved with systemic lymphoma as part of Waldeyer's ring, most tumors of this area are squamous cell cancers (95%). Sarcomas are rare. These tumors commonly extend from one anatomic site to another, and it may be difficult to pinpoint the exact location of the original lesion.

The overall incidence of tonsillar cancer is approximately 0.3% of all cancers and 6.7% of head and neck tumors. Tonsillar tumors fare better than the other lesions of the oropharynx and are more likely to be radiosensitive because of their lymphoepithelial nature. Even so, these lesions frequently present with clinically palpable lymph nodes and an advanced stage of disease. There is considerable debate as to the best way these tumors should be managed. This chapter attempts to enumerate the principles of treatment in a stepwise fashion.

The most common cause of tonsillar cancer is cigarette smoking and alcohol. Other causes, such as dietary deficiencies (vitamin A) and viruses such as the human papilloma virus (HPV), have been postulated. The human immunodeficiency virus (HIV) is probably related to the development of squamous cell carcinoma in high risk patients. Immunosuppression, especially after renal transplantation, may predispose to the evolution of cancers, as have *p53* mutation, overexpression of epidermal growth factor (EGF) receptor, and chromosome 18 tumor suppressor gene deletions.

B. Signs and Symptoms

Most of the tumors originating in the tonsil are relatively asymptomatic in their early stages. The patient may experience a mild sore throat, irritation in the back of the mouth, and occasionally pain referred to the ear. At locally advanced stages, the patient may present with odynophagia, dysphagia, slurred speech, and rarely trismus. The presence of trismus is a sign of advanced disease and is due to involvement of the pterygoid muscles.

Tonsillar Cancer

A.
Etiology and Pathology
Comprise 6.7% of head and neck cancers
Causes: smoking, alcohol, HPV and HIV infection, vitamin deficiencies
About 95% squamous cell cancers
Lymphomas occasionally seen

B.
Signs and Symptoms
Early: sore throat, ulceration in the tonsil
Advanced: neck mass, cervical metastasis with unknown primary, dysphagia, odynophagia, slurred speech, ear pain, trismus

C.
Diagnosis
Complete physical examination, detailed head and neck examination, palpation of the tumor
Biopsy of the lesion in the office or under anesthesia (assess pharyngeal wall)
Fiberoptic laryngoscopy to evaluate laryngopharynx
Chest radiography
Panoramic radiograph of the mandible
CT scan (local extension, presence of cervical adenopathy, mandibular invasion)
MRI (extent of soft tissue invasion, involvement of the base of the tongue)

(continued on next page)

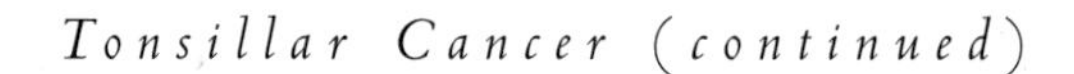

D.
Treatment

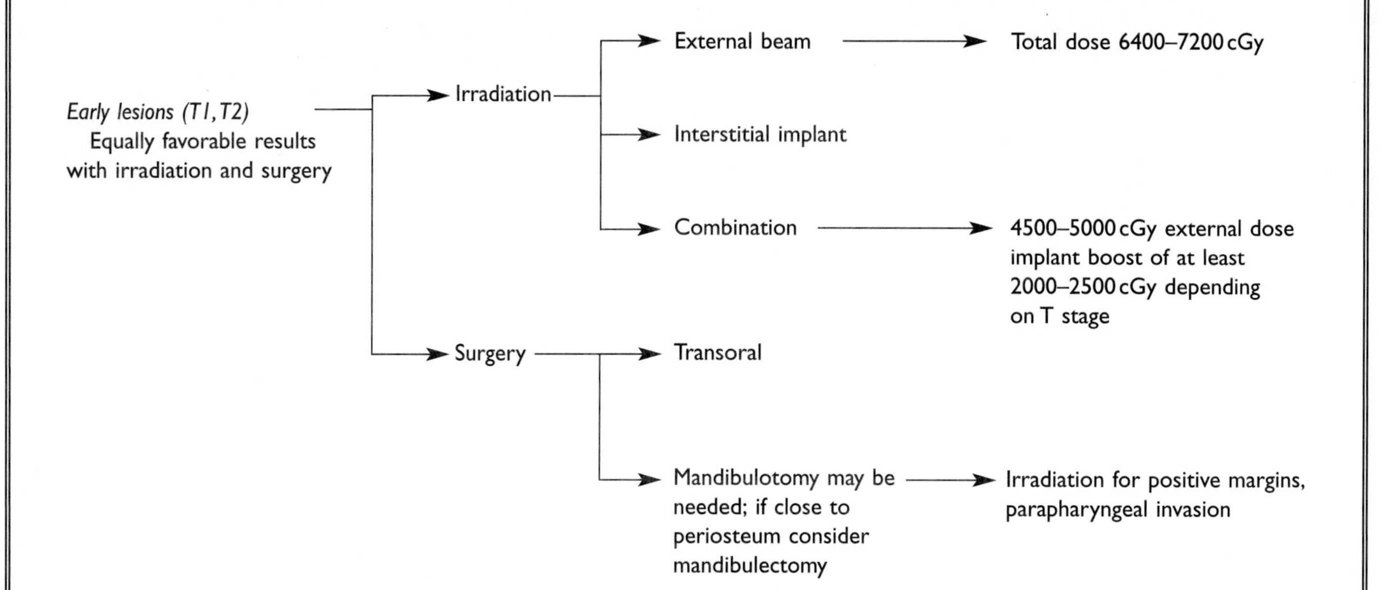

Advanced lesions (T3, T4)
Combined treatment with irradiation and surgery gives best results

→ Surgery followed by irradiation in 6 weeks
Primary closure of small defects
Large defects may require pectoralis myocutaneous or microvascular flaps
Tracheostomy may be needed
Gastrostomy may be required for long-term nutrition
Chemotherapy of uncertain benefit but may be used for patients with inoperable tumors

Treatment of the neck
Clinically negative neck: elective treatment, usually with irradiation
Clinically positive neck
Modified neck dissection, preserving XI nerve
Radical neck dissection for bulky nodal disease and for treatment failures after irradiation

→ Irradiation to the neck if multiple nodes positive or if there is extracapsular extension of disease

The incidence of clinically positive nodes is 65–75%. The most common areas of lymph node involvement are the level II, or jugulodigastric, nodes. The involvement of contralateral lymph nodes is rare, and approximately 10% of patients present with lymph node metastasis at level I (submandibular) or level V (posterior triangle) nodes. Occasionally, metastatic disease in the neck is the only clinical finding, and the primary tumor is found only after a diligent search.

The common clinical findings are an ulcerated exophytic irregular lesion involving the tonsil with surrounding erythema and raised margins. In the early stages the lesion may be small and difficult to appreciate clinically. In the advanced stages the primary lesion may extend into the surrounding areas, such as the pharyngeal wall or base of the tongue; or it may be adherent to the ascending ramus of the mandible.

C. *Diagnosis*

A complete, thorough examination of the head, neck, and oropharynx is essential. A mirror examination generally defines the extent of the disease; and flexible or rigid fiberoptic laryngoscopy is extremely helpful for evaluating posterior extension and extension to the pharyngeal wall or base of the tongue. Flexible laryngoscopy is also helpful for ruling out synchronous second primary tumors in the larynx or hypopharynx.

Biopsy of the suspected lesion can be performed easily in the office setting with topical anesthesia. Occasionally, the patient must be brought to the operating room and examined under general anesthesia for a detailed evaluation of the extent of the disease to the base of the tongue or the pharyngeal wall.

It is also important to evaluate the proximity of the disease to the mandible. Pretreatment computed tomography (CT) is helpful in this regard and for evaluating the presence of unsuspected lymph nodes in the neck. Chest radiography is performed routinely to rule out pulmonary metastases or second primary tumors, which are seen in approximately 5–7% of patients with tonsillar cancer. Magnetic resonance imaging (MRI) is rarely needed to determine the extent of disease, although it may give valuable information regarding involvement at the base of the tongue. Bronchoscopy is unnecessary if the chest radiograph is within normal limits. Esophagoscopy may be performed to rule out a second primary lesion in the esophagus. Following this evaluation, a clinical stage is assigned (Table 6–1).

D. *Treatment*

Early tonsillar squamous cell cancers can be treated with single-modality therapy (irradiation or surgery) with favorable results regardless of the treatment chosen. Because the surgical

TABLE 6–1.
AJCC definition of TNM and stage grouping for tonsillar cancers

Primary Tumor (T)

TX	Primary tumor cannot be assessed
T0	No existence of primary tumor
Tis	Carcinoma *in situ*
T1	Tumor ≤2 cm in greatest dimension
T2	Tumor >2 cm but ≤4 cm in greatest dimension
T3	Tumor >4 cm in greatest dimension
T4	Tumor invades adjacent structures [e.g., pterygoid muscle(s), mandible, hard palate, deep muscle of tongue, larynx]

Regional Lymph Nodes (N)

NX	Regional lymph nodes cannot be assessed
N0	No regional lymph node metastasis
N1	Metastasis in a single ipsilateral lymph node, ≤3 cm in greatest dimension
N2	Metastasis in a single ipsilateral lymph node, >3 cm but ≤6 cm in greatest dimension; or in multiple ipsilateral lymph nodes, none >6 cm in greatest dimension; or in bilateral or contralateral lymph nodes, none >6 cm in greatest dimension
N2a	Metastasis in a single ipsilateral lymph node >3 cm but ≤6 cm in greatest dimension
N2b	Metastasis in multiple ipsilateral lymph nodes, none >6 cm in greatest dimension
N2c	Metastasis in bilateral or contralateral lymph nodes, none >6 cm in greatest dimension
N3	Metastasis in a lymph node >6 cm in greatest dimension

Distant Metastasis (M)

MX	Distant metastasis cannot be assessed
M0	No distant metastasis
M1	Distant metastasis

Stage Grouping

Stage	T	N	M
0	Tis	N0	M0
I	T1	N0	M0
II	T2	N0	M0
III	T3	N0	M0
	T1	N1	M0
	T2	N1	M0
	T3	N1	M0
IVA	T4	N0	M0
	T4	N1	M0
	Any T	N2	M0
IVB	Any T	N3	M0
IVC	Any T	Any N	M1

SOURCE: Used with permission of the American Joint Committee on Cancer (AJCC®), Chicago, IL. The original source for this material is the AJCC® Cancer Staging Manual, 5th edition (1997) published by Lippincott Williams & Wilkins Publishers, Philadelphia, PA.

approaches are complex, current practice usually leans toward irradiation for early lesions. The ipsilateral neck should always be treated, even if it is clinically negative; contralateral failure in the neck is rare enough that routine treatment of the opposite side is not warranted. *Advanced* tonsillar tumors are treated with combination surgery and postoperative irradiation; the results are more favorable than those seen after irradiation alone. Generally, local control is jeopardized by disease extension to the lateral pharyngeal walls or to the base of the tongue.

Early Lesions

Small tonsillar cancers may be approached with a transoral operation, although exposure may be better with a lip-splitting incision and anterior midline or lateral mandibulotomy. Resection of part of the mandible may be needed if the disease extends to the periosteum. If necessary, resection of the primary tumor can be combined with neck dissection. The extent of lymphadenectomy in the neck varies among institutions and can be limited to a supraomohyoid dissection for the clinically negative neck, although this choice is controversial.

Irradiation is usually preferred over surgery for small cancers and can be given as external beam radiation, interstitial therapy, or a combination of the two. When external beam radiation is given, the contralateral neck should not be exposed; such careful application minimizes irradiation of the salivary glands, which can result in xerostomia. Furthermore, failure in the contralateral neck is uncommon.

The total dose of external beam radiation is 6400–7200 cGy. Local control is better than 90% for T1 lesions and is 80% for T2 lesions. Combining interstitial radiation with external beam radiation provides enhanced local control compared to that provided by external beam radiation alone, especially for lesions that extend to the base of the tongue. When used in this fashion, an external dose of 4500–5000 cGy is given with an implant dose of 2000–2500 cGy for T1 and T2 lesions and even higher doses for more advanced lesions. Complications of irradiation include xerostomia, necrosis of soft tissue, bone exposure, trismus, dysphagia, and osteoradionecrosis.

Advanced Lesions

Options for advanced tumors include irradiation alone or surgery followed by irradiation. Combined treatment yields better results. When large defects are created by an extensive resection, primary closure may be difficult. Reconstruction may then require use of a pectoralis myocutaneous flap or radial forearm free flap. A tracheostomy is usually required and may be needed for an extended length of time to protect the airways of patients who have difficulty swallowing. Irradiation is started approximately 6 weeks after surgery, when the surgical wound has healed satisfactorily.

Treatment of the Neck

The neck should be treated electively even if nodes are not clinically involved. Whether irradiation or lymphadenectomy is chosen depends on how the primary tumor is being treated. If the neck is clinically positive, a modified radical neck dissection is performed and radiation is given postoperatively to the neck if multiple nodes are involved, the node(s) are large and bulky, or there is extracapsular extension of disease.

Treatment Results

The local control of T1 and T2 cancer exceeds 80–85%, but the survival rate drops considerably for stage III and IV tumors. The 5-year survival is about 60% for patients with stage III tumors; for those with stage IV lesions, depending on the extent of the primary lesion and the nodal disease, the survival rate is 25–40%. Surgical salvage after initial radiation therapy is generally not satisfactory owing to local extension of the disease and frequent involvement of the mandible. Surgical intervention after a full course of radiation therapy is associated with a high incidence of complications related to soft tissue reconstruction and oropharyngeal dysfunction (e.g., dysphagia and aspiration).

Conclusions

Tonsillar cancers are the most common tumors of the oropharynx, and most have squamous cell histology. Cigarette smoking and alcohol consumption are the usual causative factors. Advanced lesions may involve more than one site in the oropharynx, and up to two-thirds of patients present with metastatic neck disease. Pretreatment evaluation includes a biopsy to establish the diagnosis, CT scan to evaluate regional extension and unsuspected disease in the neck, and endoscopy to rule out synchronous primaries. MRI scanning is indicated to inspect base-of-tongue involvement. Early tumors are treated equally well by irradiation and surgery. Advanced lesions are treated first with surgery (may require mandibulectomy) followed by irradiation in 6 weeks. The ipsilateral neck should be treated routinely; irradiation is chosen for the clinically negative neck. The clinically positive neck should be treated with neck dissection; postoperative irradiation to the neck is given if there are multiple positive nodes or extracapsular extension of disease.

Selected Reading

Dasmahapatra K, Mohit-Tabatabai M, Rush B, et al. Cancer of the tonsil: improved survival with combination therapy. Cancer 1986;57:451–455.

Givens CD, Johns ME, Cantrell RW. Carcinoma of the tonsil: analysis of 162 cases. Arch Otolaryngol 1981;107:730–734.

Mizono GS, Diaz RF, Fu KK, Boles R. Carcinoma of the tonsillar region. Laryngoscope 1986;96:240–244.

Perez CA, Purdy JA, Breaux SR, Ogura JH, von Essen S. Carcinoma of the tonsillar fossa: a non-randomized comparison of preoperative radiation and surgery and irradiation alone: long-term results. Cancer 1982;50:2314–2322.

Remmler D, Medina JE, Byers RM, Meoz R, Pfalzgraf K. Treatment of choice for squamous cell carcinoma of the tonsillar fossa. Head Neck Surg 1985;7:206–211.

Spiro J, Spiro R. Carcinoma of the tonsillar fossa: an update. Arch Otol Head Neck Surg 1989;115:1186–1189.

Chapter 7

Cancer of the Nasopharynx

V. Amod Saxena
Cam Nguyen

A. Epidemiology and Etiology

Cancer of the nasopharynx (NP) is rare in the United States and Europe,[1] but it is a common cancer in China, representing 18% of cancer cases in that population.[2] Chinese immigrants residing in the United States have a higher incidence of NP cancer than Americans, and California Caucasians born in Southeast Asia have a higher incidence of NP cancer than do American Caucasians.[3] The epidemiologic data suggest that genetic factors play an important role, as do environmental causes such as food containing preserved, salted fish. Other populations that show a high incidence of NP cancer, although less than the Chinese, are North Africans and Eskimos.

B. Anatomy

The NP is the superiormost portion of the pharynx (divided into the nasopharynx, oropharynx, and hypopharynx) located just below the sphenoid sinus. The NP is close to many critical structures. Superiorly, it is bounded by the pituitary gland, optic pathway, cavernous sinuses, and cerebrum. Anteriorly, it is bounded by the ethmoid sinus, maxillary sinus, and orbits. Laterally, it is surrounded by cranial nerves, carotid arteries, and jugular veins. Cranial nerves V and VI are the most commonly involved cranial nerves at presentation. Posterior to the eustachian tube opening is the fossa of Rosenmüller, which is probably the most frequent site of NP cancer (Fig. 7–1).

The NP has a rich network of lymphatics; consequently patients may present with a painless, enlarged lymph node in the posterior triangle of the neck. Frequently, an NP mass is discovered only after a diligent search for the primary tumor in such a patient. Because of its anatomic position, NP cancer, even in an early stage, can infiltrate many critical structures. Radiotherapy (RT) has been the treatment of choice for NP cancer, and chemotherapy has been used as an adjunct for advanced disease. Surgery has a limited role in the management of NP cancer and consists primarily of nasopharyngoscopy and biopsy; surgery is rarely performed as salvage therapy for persistent neck disease or for persistent primary site disease.

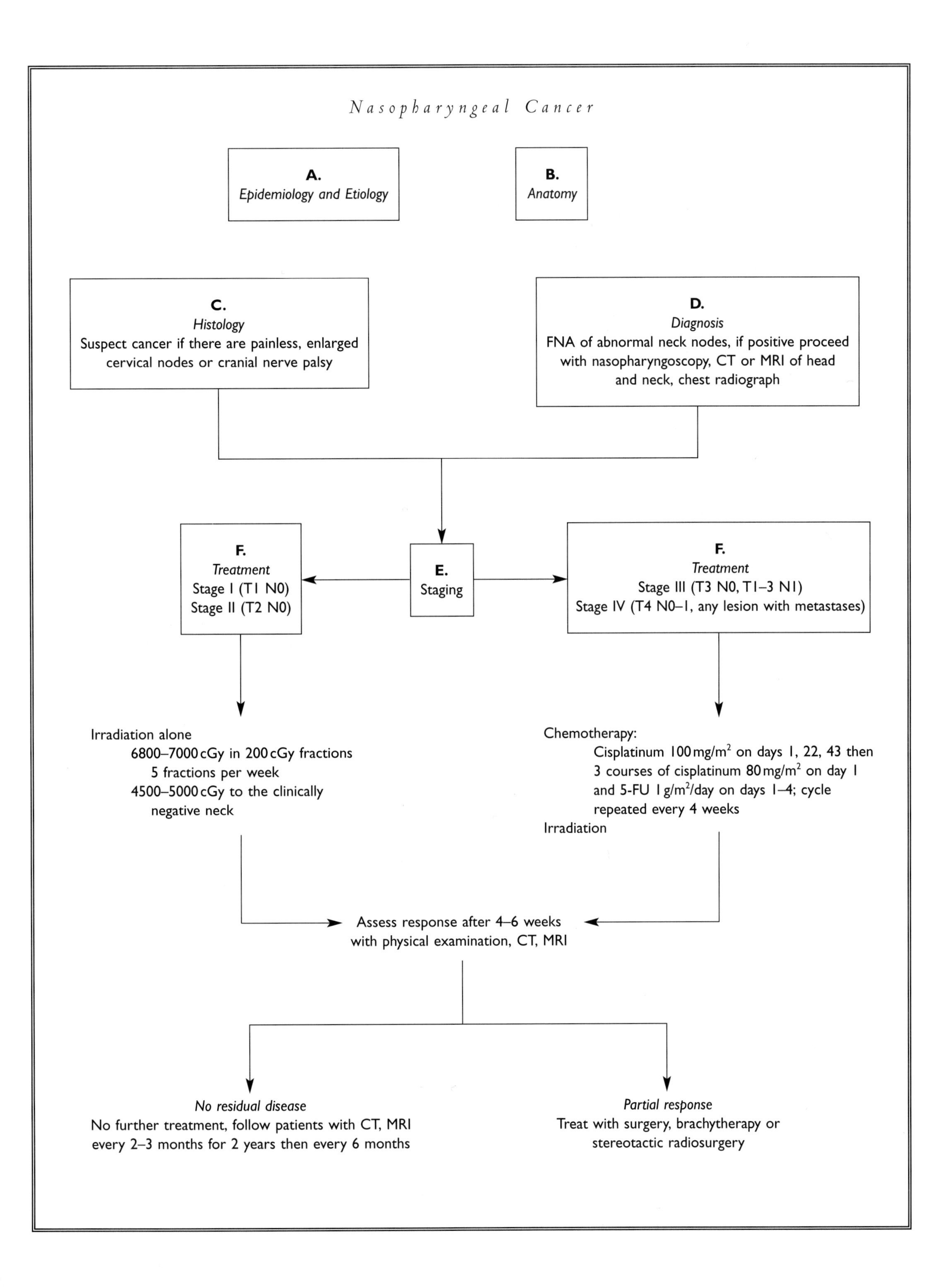
Nasopharyngeal Cancer
A.
Epidemiology and Etiology
B.
Anatomy
C.
Histology
Suspect cancer if there are painless, enlarged cervical nodes or cranial nerve palsy
D.
Diagnosis
FNA of abnormal neck nodes, if positive proceed with nasopharyngoscopy, CT or MRI of head and neck, chest radiograph
F.
Treatment
Stage I (T1 N0)
Stage II (T2 N0)
E.
Staging
F.
Treatment
Stage III (T3 N0, T1–3 N1)
Stage IV (T4 N0–1, any lesion with metastases)
Irradiation alone
6800–7000 cGy in 200 cGy fractions
5 fractions per week
4500–5000 cGy to the clinically negative neck
Chemotherapy:
Cisplatinum 100 mg/m2 on days 1, 22, 43 then 3 courses of cisplatinum 80 mg/m2 on day 1 and 5-FU 1 g/m2/day on days 1–4; cycle repeated every 4 weeks
Irradiation
Assess response after 4–6 weeks with physical examination, CT, MRI
No residual disease
No further treatment, follow patients with CT, MRI every 2–3 months for 2 years then every 6 months
Partial response
Treat with surgery, brachytherapy or stereotactic radiosurgery

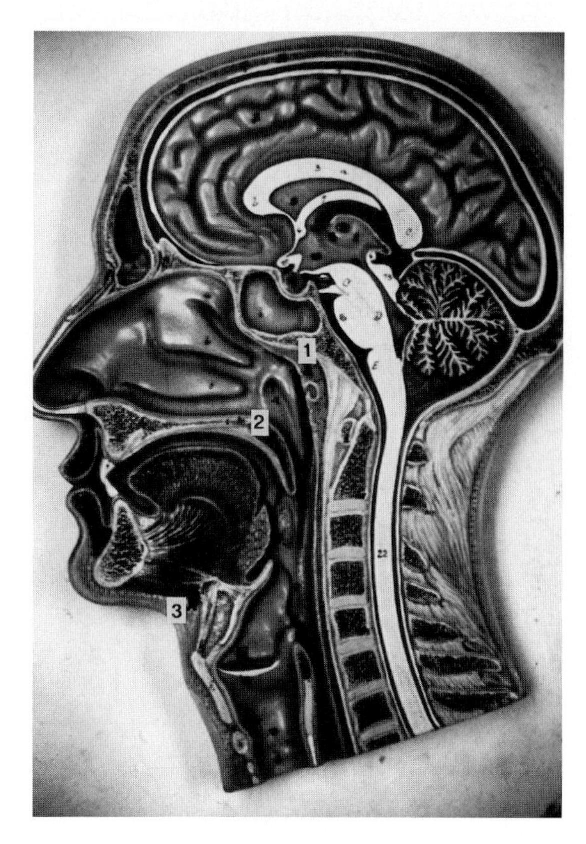

FIGURE 7–1
Boundaries and landmarks of the nasopharynx.

C. Histology

The most common histology of malignant NP tumors is squamous cell carcinoma; lymphoma and minor salivary gland cancers are less common. The World Health Organization (WHO) has classified NP squamous cell cancer[4] into three types.

Type 1: squamous cell carcinoma
Type 2: nonkeratinizing carcinoma with or without lymphoid stroma
Type 3: undifferentiated carcinoma with or without lymphoid stroma

Type 3 histology is common in the Chinese population; it is undifferentiated, is associated with a high incidence of metastatic disease, and responds well to local RT. In contrast, type 1 histology is more common in Americans, is well differentiated, and is associated with a lower incidence of metastatic disease; it responds to local RT less well than type 3.

D. Diagnosis

An NP mass is often discovered during a search for the cause of a cranial nerve palsy or because of painless cervical lymphadenopathy. Cranial nerves are often involved early because of their close proximity to the NP. Occasionally, the cavernous sinuses are invaded by tumor, which may cause cranial nerve palsy.

Most patients with NP cancer present with painless cervical lymphadenopathy, usually in the posterior triangle of the neck. Fine-needle aspiration (FNA) of the neck nodes should be done, as it can be performed safely and with minimal risk. Once the diagnosis of cancer is established by FNA, the next step is complete examination of the head and neck region to find a primary site. If an NP mass is seen by nasopharyngoscopy, it is biopsied to confirm the presence of cancer. Benign NP masses include lymphoid hypertrophy (requires no treatment) and juvenile angiofibroma, a benign childhood tumor that is managed with surgery or RT. The patient is then evaluated in a multidisciplinary clinic staffed by head and neck surgeons, medical oncologists, and radiation oncologists. Proper staging and treatment recommendations are thus determined.

The workup must include a complete history and physical examination and at least a computed tomographic (CT) scan or magnetic resonance image (MRI) of the head and neck regions. The CT scan is useful for identifying the NP mass and evaluating bone invasion (e.g., sphenoid or orbit invasion). MRI is better for determining soft tissue extension (e.g., parapharyngeal, cavernous sinus invasion). In addition, MRI provides a sagittal view of the tumor, which is extremely useful when planning definitive RT. A chest radiograph is obtained to rule out metastatic disease. A bone scan is not ordered routinely unless the patient has bone pain.

E. Staging

After the workup is complete, the tumor is staged to determine prognosis and appropriate therapy. Staging systems include Ho's classification[3,5] and the American Joint Commission on Cancer (AJCC) classification. The former is widely used in China and is considered to have better prognostic application. The latter is more commonly used in North America. Ho's staging system is outlined here for reference.

T1: tumor confined to the nasopharynx
T2: tumor extends to nasal fossa, oropharynx, or adjacent muscles/nerves below the base of skull
T3a: bone involvement below the base of skull
T3b: involvement of the base of the skull
T3c: involvement of cranial nerve(s)
T3d: involvement of the orbits/laryngopharynx/infratemporal fossa
N1: upper cervical node involvement
N2: midcervical node involvement
N3: lower cervical (supraclavicular) node involvement

TABLE 7–1.
Comparison of AJCC 1992 and 1998 staging systems for cancer of the nasopharynx

AJCC 1992		AJCC 1998	
T1	One NP subsite	T1	Confined to NP
T2	More than one NP subsite	T2	Extending to soft tissues of oropharynx and/or nasal fossa
		T2a	Without parapharyngeal extension
		T2b	With parapharyngeal extension
T3	Invading nasal cavity or oropharynx, or both	T3	Invading bony structures and/or paranasal sinuses
T4	Skull or cranial nerves, or both	T4	Intracranial extension and/or involvement of cranial nerves, infratemporal fossa, hypopharynx, or orbit
NX	Not assessed	NX	Not assessed
N0	No regional node metastasis	N0	No regional node metastasis
N1	Single lymph node <3 cm	N1	Unilateral lymph node(s) ≤ 6 cm in size; above supraclavicular fossa
N2	Multiple lymph nodes >3 cm but ≤ 6 cm	N2	Bilateral lymph node(s) ≤ 6 cm, above supraclavicular fossa
N2a	Single ipsilateral node		
N2b	Multiple ipsilateral nodes		
N2c	Multiple bilateral nodes		
N3	Lymph node(s) >6 cm	N3	Metastasis in a lymph node(s)
		N3a	Lymph node(s) >6 cm
		N3b	In the supraclavicular fossa

The AJCC modified its staging system in 1998[4] by taking into account the fact that lower cervical node involvement is associated with a worse prognosis.[6] The 1992 and 1998 staging systems are shown in Table 7–1 for comparison. The 1998 AJCC staging system is currently used to stage NP cancer and hopefully will prove to be of prognostic value with time. Here we use the AJCC 1992 staging system, as data from studies using combined chemotherapy and RT are based on this staging system.

F. *Treatment*

Because of the anatomic location of the nasopharynx in relation to other critical structures, the traditional treatment for NP cancer has been RT, which is effective for stages I and II but less so for stages III and IV, which requires combined chemotherapy and RT.

Stages I and II

For stage I (T1 N0) and stage II (T2 N0) RT alone is an effective treatment, but it must be individualized for each patient. The primary site requires an aggressive dose of RT (6800–7000 cGy, given in 200 cGy fractions, five fractions per week). The clinically N0 neck (i.e., no palpable disease and no nodes seen on CT scan) is treated with a "prophylactic" dose of 4500–5000 cGy, which effectively controls microscopic disease. However, if neck lymphadenopathy is present, the RT dose is given based on the extent of disease, with 6600 cGy given to nodes ≤ 2 cm and 7000 cGy to nodes >2 cm. Acute complications of RT include mucositis, loss of taste, fatigue, and xerostomia, but these problems are usually temporary. Late complications include xerostomia, loss of taste, fibrosis, and rarely osteoradionecrosis or radiation-induced myelitis (in $<1\%$).

With modern RT, CT-based treatment planning is used to outline the tumor volume accurately. This allows the RT to be focused on the tumor while restricting RT exposure of critical structures such as the optic chiasm, brainstem, and temporal lobes. One development in the field of radiation oncology is the use of three-dimensional treatment planning, which uses sophisticated computer software to focus multiple beams on the target as a booster, thereby maximizing the dose to the tumor while sparing the critical structures from radiation damage.[7] Figure 7–2 shows a CT scan of a patient with advanced NP cancer. Note the large mass occupying the NP and parapharyngeal extension. The air cavity of the NP one normally sees on a CT scan is now barely visible anterior to the mass.

A three-field technique is used most frequently for RT planning: Right and left lateral fields are used to cover the NP and upper neck nodes, and an anterior supraclavicular field (abutting the lateral fields) is used to treat the lower neck and supraclavicular nodes. Figure 7–3 shows a typical right lateral field for the same patient as in Figure 7–2. Note that the primary site (the NP), upper neck nodes, and posterior maxillary sinuses are treated. RT beams are typically rectangular, and any tissues not treated are blocked to individualize treatment for the patient. After the spinal cord tolerance dose is reached, usually 4400 cGy in 22 fractions, the field is reduced to cover the NP

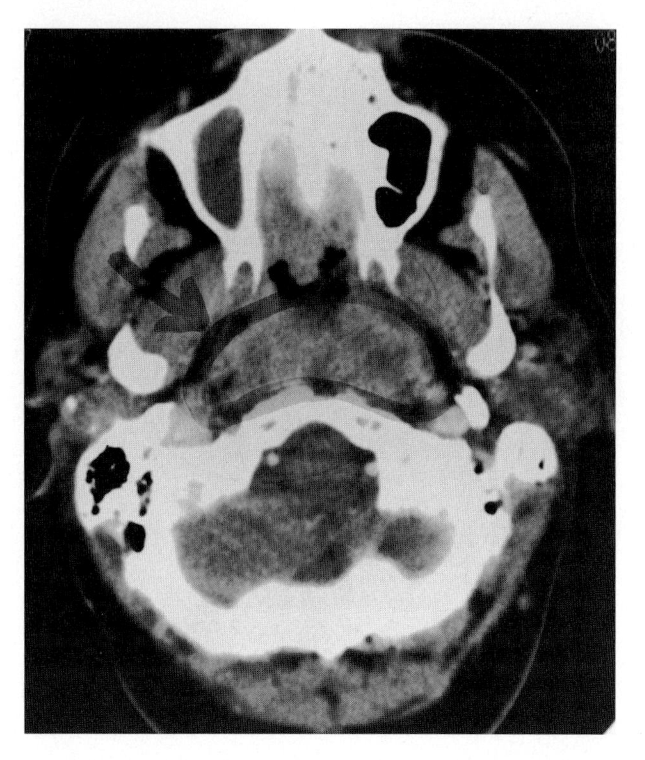

FIGURE 7–2
Computed tomography (CT) scan of a patient with advanced nasopharyngeal (NP) cancer. Note the large mass occupying the NP and parapharyngeal extension. The air cavity of the NP that one normally sees on a CT scan is now barely visible anterior to the mass, which itself is encircled.

and upper neck nodes. The involved posterior neck triangle, in this case the right side (area posterior to the broken line in Figure 7–3) is now treated with the electron beam, which has a limited depth of penetration (a few centimeters), to control the neck node that is not in the reduced photon portal to an adequate dose while sparing the spinal cord from excessive RT and potential radiation-induced myelitis.

Brachytherapy, the use of radioactive seeds implanted directly into the tumor, has been used by some investigators to boost the nasopharynx to a higher dose of RT. This practice is controversial, and most radiation oncologists treat early-stage NP cancer with the conventional technique of external RT.

Stages III and IV

For stage III (T3 N0 or T1–3 N1) and stage IV (T4 N0–1 or anyT anyN M1) lesions, RT alone does not provide effective local control of the disease. For this reason, chemotherapy has been used in combination with RT in many fashions: neoadjuvant (prior to RT), concurrent (at the same time as RT), and adjuvant (after RT). Data on the use of chemotherapy with RT have been conflicting, with many trials not randomized; however, the data from phase II trials[8,9] using this approach were promising.

The subsequent phase III intergroup study 0099[10] randomized patients with stages III and IV NP cancer to RT alone versus RT plus chemotherapy. In the experimental arm of this study, chemotherapy was used concurrently with RT. Chemotherapy included intravenous cisplatinum (100 mg/m^2) given on days 1, 22, and 43 of RT followed by three additional courses of cisplatinum (80 mg/m^2) on day 1 and 5-fluorouracil (5-FU) (1000 mg/m^2/day) on days 1–4 of each additional cycle, repeated every 4 weeks. This study showed a significant progression-free survival of 69% for the chemotherapy/RT group versus 24% for the RT-alone group. The 3-year survivals were 76% and 46%, respectively. Because of the encouraging results of this study, many investigators are now using combined chemotherapy/RT for advanced (stages III and IV) NP cancer. The RT techniques remain the same regardless whether chemotherapy is used. The rationale for using concurrent cisplatinum is that this drug has a radiosensitizing effect; that is, when combined with RT, the effect of the RT is greatly enhanced.

Approximately 4–6 weeks after completion of therapy, the patient is *assessed for response* to therapy by a repeat clinical examination and CT or MRI of the head and neck regions. Any suspicious areas (primary NP site or lymph nodes) should be biopsied to rule out residual malignancy.

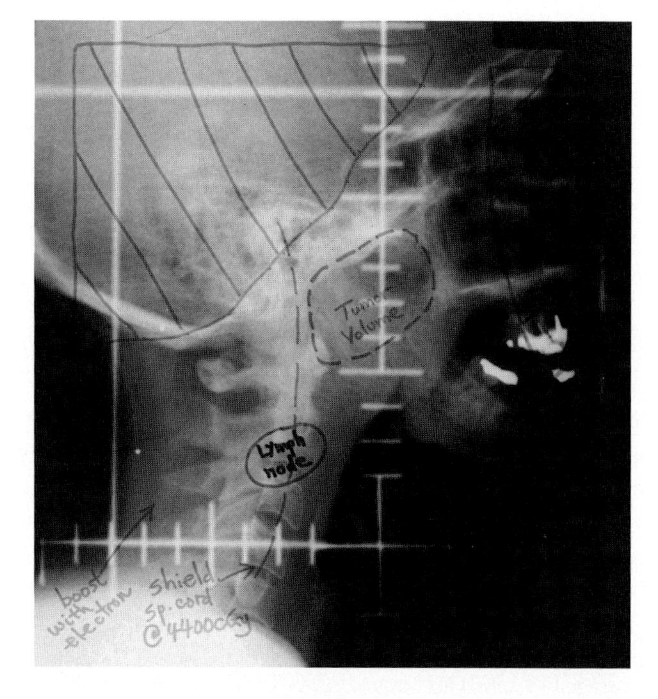

FIGURE 7–3
Planning film of a typical right lateral field for the same patient as in Figure 7–1. Note that the primary site (the NP), upper neck nodes, and posterior maxillary sinuses are treated. Radiotherapy (RT) beams are typically rectangular in shape, and any tissues not treated are blocked to individualize treatment. The shaded areas represent blocking of the RT beam; that is, the brainstem and posterior orbits are shielded from the photon beam. Dashed line, posterior edge of the photon beam. See text for more details.

If *no residual disease* is found, no further therapy is recommended. The patient is then followed with clinical examinations and CT or MRI every 2–3 months for the first 2 years and every 6 months thereafter.

If there is a *partial response* (it is rare to see no response), the patient should be assessed for possible surgery. Surgery of this region, especially after combined chemotherapy/RT, is a major undertaking and should be attempted only by those familiar with skull base surgery.

If the residual disease is confined to the nasopharynx, an alternative to surgery is brachytherapy. Brachytherapy techniques vary. One approach is to insert radioactive seeds (usually iodine-125) into the tumor; another approach is placement of afterloading plastic catheters in the NP to be loaded with radioactive sources (usually iridium-192). Brachytherapy allows delivery of high doses of radiation to the tumor while minimizing exposure to the surrounding critical structures. Erickson and Wilson reviewed this subject in detail, and the reader is encouraged to read their article for an in-depth review of brachytherapy.[11] Some centers have now used stereotactic radiosurgery, a sophisticated technique that allows multiple beams to converge on the same target. It can be carried out using a modified linear accelerator or a gamma knife instrument. Preliminary data from Stanford University showed encouraging results.[12] If there is residual disease in the neck, the patient is a possible candidate for salvage neck dissection or brachytherapy of the neck node(s). During the last 3 years, with new development of computer radiotherapy planning software and new design of linear accelerators with multi-leaf collimators, intensity-modulated radiotherapy (IMRT) has gained considerable popularity as a new tool for radiation oncologists to target the tumor with higher dose and greater precision, while limiting dose to critical organs, such as optic chiasm and brainstem, thus potentially improving the therapeutic index. In addition, F-18 Fluorodeoxyglucose Positron Emission Tomography (PET) appears to be a new promising tool to evaluate extent of disease for diagnosis and therapy.

Late Local Recurrence

Late local recurrence is a well known phenomenon. Some patients who are apparently cured of NP cancer may present with a recurrence in the NP many years later. Tumor staging should be repeated with CT or MRI. In the case of an isolated NP recurrence, this site can be retreated with RT. Many investigators use a combination of high-energy photon beams plus brachytherapy, with a cure rate of 35–40%.[11] Although data on the use of chemotherapy in this setting are limited, this modality should be considered in combination with RT to maximize the cure rate. Metastatic disease in the chest is treated with systemic chemotherapy; thoracotomy is generally not indicated, and the prognosis is extremely poor.

Conclusions

Nasopharyngeal cancer is a challenging disease for head and neck oncologists because of the advanced stage of the disease at diagnosis and the complex anatomy of this region. Radiation oncology has seen a major advance in technology with three-dimensional treatment planning and stereotactic radiosurgery. In addition, the encouraging results from the intergroup trial suggest that concurrent and adjuvant chemotherapy should be used for patients with advanced stages (III and IV) of the disease. Patients with advanced disease now have a higher cure rate with an acceptable rate of acute and late morbidity. This represents a significant step forward in the cure of this challenging cancer.

References

1. Sanguineti G, Geara FB, Garden AS, et al. Carcinoma of the nasopharynx treated by radiotherapy alone: determinants of local and regional control. Int J Radiat Oncol Biol Phys 1997;37:985–996.
2. Neel HB III. Nasopharyngeal carcinoma: clinical presentation, diagnosis, treatment and prognosis. Otolaryngol Clin North Am 1985;18:479–490.
3. Buell P. Race and place in the etiology of nasopharyngeal cancer: a study based on California death certificates. Int J Cancer 1973;11:268–272.
4. Fleming ID, Cooper JS, Henson DE, et al. American Joint Committee on Cancer: Manual for Staging of Cancer, 5th ed. Philadelphia: Lippincott-Raven, 1998.
5. Ho JHC. Stage classification of nasopharyngeal carcinoma: a review in nasopharyngeal carcinoma, etiology, and control. IARC Sci Publ 1978;20;99–113.
6. Beahrs OH, Henson DE, Hutter DE, Kennedy BJ. American Joint Committee on Cancer: Manual for Staging of Cancer, 4th ed. Philadelphia: Lippincott, 1992.
7. Liebel SA, Kutcher GJ, Harrison LB, et al. Improved dose distribution for 3-D conformal boost treatments in carcinoma of nasopharynx. Int J Radiat Oncol Biol Phys 1991;20:823–833.
8. Decker D, Drelichman A, Al-Sarraf M, et al. Chemotherapy for nasopharyngeal carcinoma. Cancer 1983;52:602–605.
9. Al-Sarraf M, Zundmanis M, Monciol V, et al. Concurrent cisplatin and radiotherapy in patients with locally advanced nasopharyngeal carcinoma: RTOG study [abstract]. Proc Am Soc Clin Oncol 1986;5:142.
10. Al-Sarraf M, Leblanc M, Giri S, et al. Chemoradiotherapy versus radiotherapy in patients with advanced nasopharyngeal cancer: phase III randomized intergroup study 0099. J Clin Oncol 1998;16:1310–1317.
11. Erickson BA, Wilson JF. Nasopharyngeal brachytherapy. Am J Clin Oncol 1993;16:424–443.
12. Cmelak AJ, Cox RS, Adler JR, et al. Radiosurgery for skull base malignancies and nasopharyngeal carcinoma. Int J Radiat Oncol Biol Phys 1997;37:997–1003.

Chapter 8

Laryngeal Cancer

Tasia S. Economou

A. Epidemiology and Etiology

The larynx is part of the respiratory system and is bounded superiorly by the pharynx and inferiorly by the trachea. The larynx is supported by muscle in the midneck area and the thyroid cartilage, which houses the larynx and forms the laryngeal prominence, or "Adam's apple." The larynx has a twofold purpose: It serves as (1) a sphincter or valve when protecting the lower respiratory airway during breathing and swallowing, and (2) the vibratory mechanism during human phonation.

Laryngeal cancer comprises about 1% of all newly diagnosed cancers each year. Most often, patients are male and close to 60 years of age. Several etiologic factors have been identified, of which tobacco use and excessive alcohol consumption are most often implicated; there appears to be a synergistic effect between the two. Laryngeal papillomatosis has been known to transform into squamous carcinoma in a small percentage of cases. It is also thought that acute and chronic inflammation of the cervical esophagus and posterior larynx secondary to persistent gastroesophageal reflux sometimes cause malignant changes. These risk factors affect all areas of the aerodigestive tract. Approximately 5–35% of patients with an aerodigestive tract cancer are found to have a synchronous or metachronous tumor.[1,2] Field cancerization, a term coined by Slaughter et al.,[3] describes the presence of multiple sites of squamous cell carcinoma.

B. Anatomy

The larynx is divided into three regions: the supraglottis, glottis, and subglottis.[4] A horizontal plane at the superior surface of the true vocal cords defines the inferior extent of the supraglottis. Also included in the supraglottis are the false vocal cords, epiglottis, aryepiglottic folds, and posterior portion of the arytenoid cartilage. The glottis contains the vocal cords back to and including the vocal process of the arytenoids. The subglottis begins 5 mm below the true vocal cords and extends to the inferior margin of the cricoid cartilage.

Laryngeal Cancer

A.
Epidemiology and Etiology
Male > female gender
sixth decade of life
Risk factors: tobacco, alcohol, laryngeal papillomatosis, GERD

B.
Anatomy
Supraglottis: false vocal cords, epiglottis aryepiglottic folds, posterior arytenoid cartilage
Glottis: vocal cords, vocal process of arytenoids
Subglottis: begins 5 mm below vocal cords, extends to inferior margin of cricoid cartilage

C.
Signs and Symptoms
Early: hoarseness, sore throat
Late: dysphagia, shortness of breath

D.
Diagnosis
History, head and neck examination
Indirect laryngoscopy
Flexible laryngoscopy
Direct laryngoscopy
CT scan (extension, nodes)
MRI (perineural spread, cartilage)

(continued on next page)

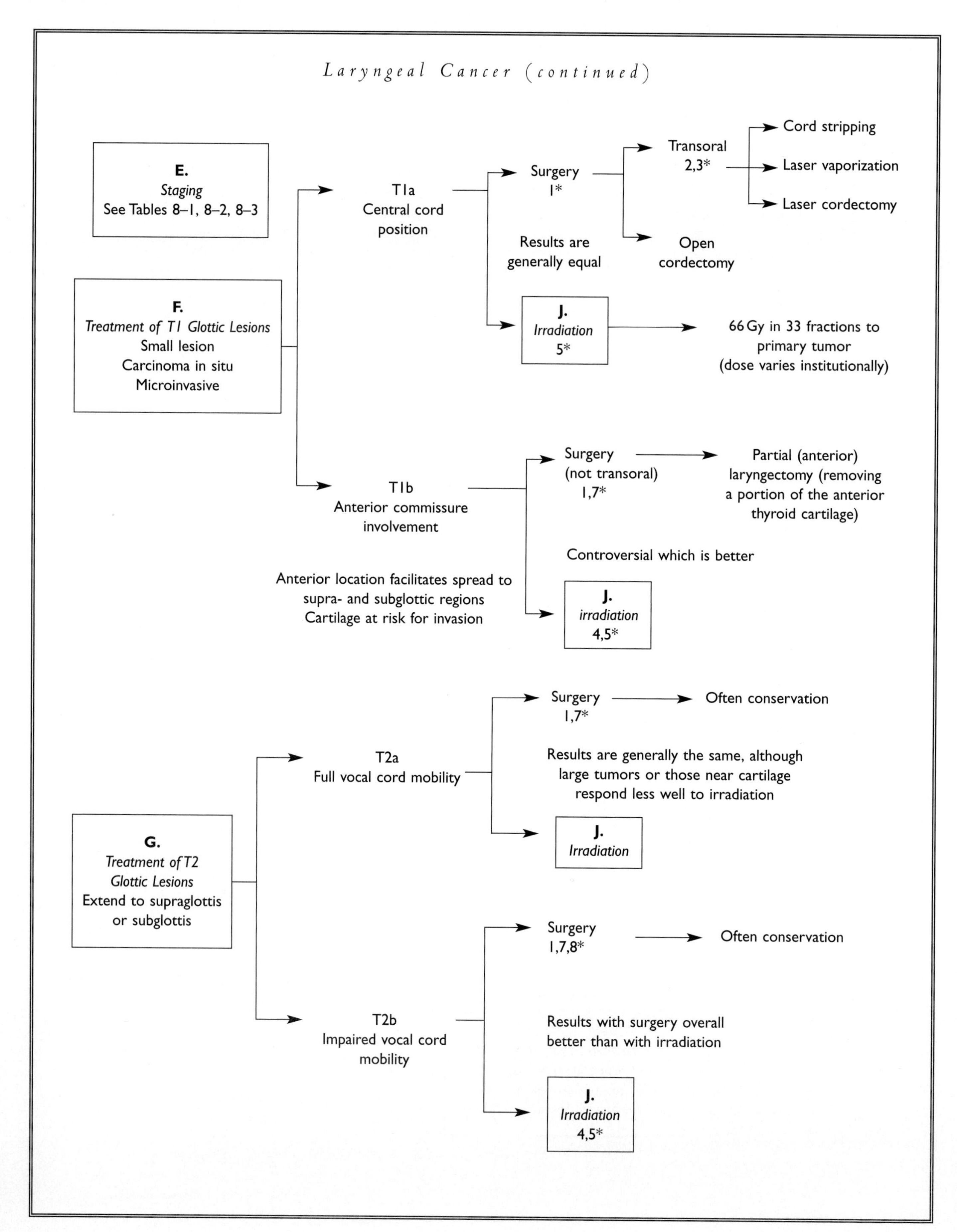

Laryngeal Cancer (continued)
E.
Staging
See Tables 8–1, 8–2, 8–3
F.
Treatment of T1 Glottic Lesions
Small lesion
Carcinoma in situ
Microinvasive
T1a
Central cord position
Surgery
1*
Transoral
2,3*
Cord stripping
Laser vaporization
Laser cordectomy
Open cordectomy
Results are generally equal
J.
Irradiation
5*
66 Gy in 33 fractions to primary tumor (dose varies institutionally)
T1b
Anterior commissure involvement
Surgery (not transoral)
1,7*
Partial (anterior) laryngectomy (removing a portion of the anterior thyroid cartilage)
Controversial which is better
Anterior location facilitates spread to supra- and subglottic regions
Cartilage at risk for invasion
J.
irradiation
4,5*
G.
Treatment of T2 Glottic Lesions
Extend to supraglottis or subglottis
T2a
Full vocal cord mobility
Surgery
1,7*
Often conservation
Results are generally the same, although large tumors or those near cartilage respond less well to irradiation
J.
Irradiation
T2b
Impaired vocal cord mobility
Surgery
1,7,8*
Often conservation
Results with surgery overall better than with irradiation
J.
Irradiation
4,5*

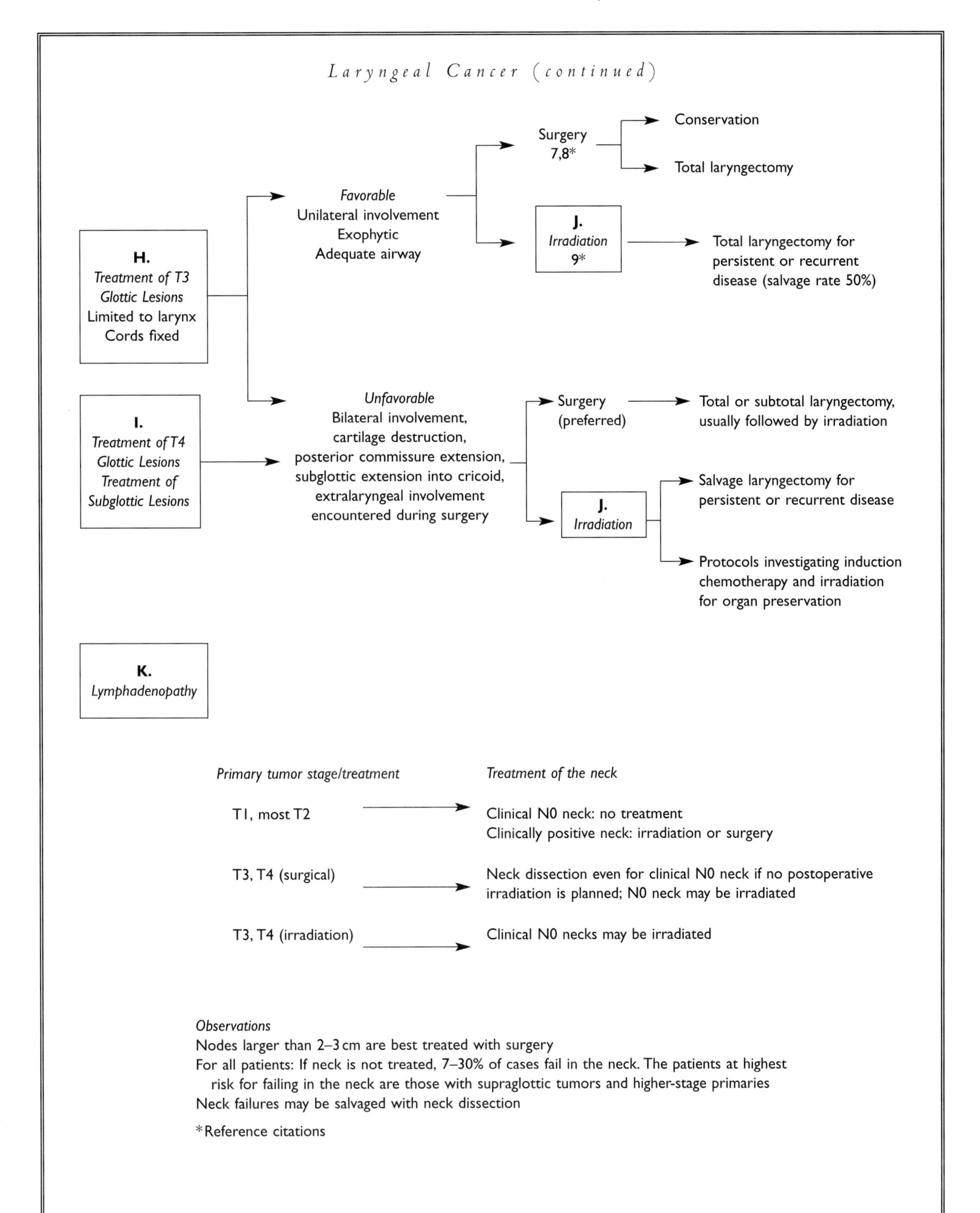
Laryngeal Cancer (continued)
H.
Treatment of T3
Glottic Lesions
Limited to larynx
Cords fixed
Favorable
Unilateral involvement
Exophytic
Adequate airway
Surgery
7,8*
Conservation
Total laryngectomy
J.
Irradiation
9*
Total laryngectomy for persistent or recurrent disease (salvage rate 50%)
I.
Treatment of T4
Glottic Lesions
Treatment of
Subglottic Lesions
Unfavorable
Bilateral involvement,
cartilage destruction,
posterior commissure extension,
subglottic extension into cricoid,
extralaryngeal involvement
encountered during surgery
Surgery
(preferred)
Total or subtotal laryngectomy, usually followed by irradiation
J.
Irradiation
Salvage laryngectomy for persistent or recurrent disease
Protocols investigating induction chemotherapy and irradiation for organ preservation
K.
Lymphadenopathy
Primary tumor stage/treatment
Treatment of the neck
T1, most T2
Clinical N0 neck: no treatment
Clinically positive neck: irradiation or surgery
T3, T4 (surgical)
Neck dissection even for clinical N0 neck if no postoperative irradiation is planned; N0 neck may be irradiated
T3, T4 (irradiation)
Clinical N0 necks may be irradiated
Observations
Nodes larger than 2–3 cm are best treated with surgery
For all patients: If neck is not treated, 7–30% of cases fail in the neck. The patients at highest risk for failing in the neck are those with supraglottic tumors and higher-stage primaries
Neck failures may be salvaged with neck dissection
*Reference citations

Two anatomic spaces of the larynx are important. The *paraglottic* space is that tissue lateral to the true and false vocal cords, the thyroid ala anterolaterally, and the conus elasticus. Penetration of tumor into this space often changes the stage of disease and requires more aggressive treatment. The *preepiglottic* space is located anterior to the epiglottis and posterior to the thyrohyoid membrane and the upper extent of the thyroid cartilage. Tumor extension into this space likewise precludes most conservation surgical techniques.

C. Signs and Symptoms

Signs and symptoms of a glottic tumor are often present during the early stages of the disease, with hoarseness and sore throat being the most common. As tumors enlarge, shortness of breath due to airway obstruction may become evident. Often the feeling of a "lump in the throat" or dysphagia is present with advancing disease. Tumors that begin subglottically more often present with dyspnea, as they can occlude the airway; they often do not cause hoarseness, as the true vocal cords are spared.

Supraglottic primary tumors may likewise present with dyspnea (owing to their size and location), some change in voice quality without true hoarseness, and dysphagia. Referred otalgia is common with all glottic cancers.

D. Diagnosis

Symptoms of hoarseness lasting more than 2 weeks, especially in a patient with a smoking history, requires a thorough head and neck examination. Indirect laryngoscopy with a mirror usually offers the best panoramic view of the glottic and supraglottic structures. When supplemented with a closer examination using a flexible nasopharyngoscope, indirect laryngoscopy often gives a reliable preliminary evaluation of a glottic lesion. Large, bulky lesions are occasionally biopsied at this time. More often direct laryngoscopy under general anesthesia is required, which permits palpation of the cords and the tumor and more thorough assessment of the mucosal extent and appearance of the lesion. One should remember to evaluate the esophagus and tracheobronchial tree, as there is an approximately 5% incidence of synchronous primary tumors in the aerodigestive tract.

Imaging studies are useful for staging the more advanced laryngeal tumors. The extent of most T1 and even some T2 lesions can be readily appreciated with endoscopy, and radiologic evaluation is not likely to add information in these early cases. An exception may be an anterior commissure or horseshoe lesion, in which case there may be exolaryngeal spread anteriorly.

Large lesions that extend into adjacent regions require further definition by computed tomography (CT) or magnetic resonance imaging (MRI). Submucosal extension and invasion of the preepiglottic or paraglottic spaces or the base of the tongue are usually well defined by CT imaging. Lymph node status is also well defined by CT; if nodes are larger than 1.0–1.5 cm in diameter or are of any size but have a low-density central area, they likely contain metastatic disease. Extranodal spread is suggested by an irregular border. MRI is the modality of choice for assessing perineural spread of tumor, cartilage invasion or destruction (or both), and tumor extent into surrounding tissue. Because of the multiplanar views afforded by MRI, subglottic and supraglottic extension by tumor are often better delineated by this modality.[5] CT and MRI are complementary modalities that not only enhance our knowledge of tumor extent but also facilitate patient preparation for treatment.

E. Staging

Accurate staging of a laryngeal tumor is imperative for discussing treatment alternatives, prognosis, and survival. The American Joint Committee of Cancer (AJCC) has devised a classification and staging system for primary tumors of the larynx.[6–8] (Tables 8–1, 8–2, 8–3). The T staging is divided into supraglottic, glottic, and subglottic categories. Nodal metastasis (N classification) denotes the number and size of involved nodes. Distant metastasis (M classification) recognizes disease beyond the neck and larynx. According to the AJCC guidelines, a T1 glottic tumor is limited to the true vocal cord(s). Many head and neck surgeons prefer to separate T1 lesions into two groups: T1a tumors are limited to one vocal cord, and T1b tumors involve both vocal cords, crossing the anterior commissure. Tumors may be small and on the central membranous cord; they may be large and bulky; or they may extend to the anterior or posterior commissure. All of these glottic lesions are classified as T1 by the AJCC so long as they are limited to the true vocal cords; it is no surprise, then, that there is broad variability in the reported cure rates.

T2 lesions are defined as tumors that extend to the subglottic or supraglottic regions with normal or impaired vocal cord mobility. T3 lesions are confined to the larynx, but there is vocal cord fixation (on one or both sides). T4 tumors extend through the thyroid cartilage or outside the larynx.

Treatment

The common triad of cancer therapies are surgery, irradiation, and chemotherapy, with the frequency of applicability heavily in favor of surgery or irradiation. Chemotherapy is reserved as an adjuvant modality to supplement the more traditional approaches especially when used in protocols. A host of factors decide a patient's treatment, including the following:

TABLE 8–1.
AJCC definition of TNM for laryngeal cancer

Primary Tumor (T)

TX	Primary tumor cannot be assessed
T0	No evidence of primary tumor
Tis	Carcinoma *in situ*
Supraglottis	
T1	Tumor limited to one subsite of supraglottis with normal vocal cord mobility
T2	Tumor invades mucosa of more than one adjacent subsite of supraglottis or glottis or region outside the supraglottis (e.g., mucosa of base of tongue, vallecula, medial wall of pyriform sinus) without fixation of the larynx
T3	Tumor limited to larynx with vocal cord fixation and/or invades any of the following: postcricoid area, preepiglottic tissues
T4	Tumor extends through the thyroid cartilage, and/or extends into soft tissues of the neck, thyroid, and/or esophagus
Glottis	
T1	Tumor limited to vocal cord(s) (may involve anterior or posterior commissures) with normal mobility
T1a	Tumor limited to one vocal cord
T1b	Tumor involves both vocal cords
T2	Tumor extends to supraglottis and/or subglottis, and/or with impaired vocal cord mobility
T3	Tumor limited to the larynx with vocal cord fixation
T4	Tumor invades through the thyroid cartilage and/or to other tissues beyond the larnyx (e.g., trachea, soft tissues of the neck, including thyroid, pharynx)
Subglottis	
T1	Tumor limited to the subglottis
T2	Tumor extends to vocal cord(s) with normal or impaired mobility
T3	Tumor limited to larynx with vocal cord fixation
T4	Tumor invades through cricoid or thyroid cartilage and/or extends to other tissues beyond the larynx (e.g., trachea, soft tissues of neck, including thyroid, esophagus)
Regional Lymph Node (N)	
NX	Regional lymph nodes cannot be assessed
N0	No regional lymph node metastasis
N1	Metastasis in a single ipsilateral lymph node, ≤3 cm in greatest dimension
N2	Metastasis in a single ipsilateral lymph node, >3 cm but ≤6 cm in greatest dimension, or in multiple ipsilateral lymph nodes, none >6 cm in greatest dimension, or in bilateral or contralateral lymph nodes, none >6 cm in greatest dimension
N2a	Metastasis in a single ipsilateral lymph node >3 cm but ≤6 cm in greatest dimension
N2b	Metastasis in multiple ipsilateral lymph nodes, none >6 cm in greatest dimension
N2c	Metastasis in bilateral or contralateral lymph nodes, none >6 cm in greatest dimension
N3	Metastasis in a lymph node >6 cm in greatest dimension
Distant Metastasis (M)	
MX	Distant metastasis cannot be assessed
M0	No distant metastasis
M1	Distant metastasis

SOURCE: Used with permission of the American Joint Committee on Cancer (AJCC®), Chicago, IL. The original source for this material is the AJCC® Cancer Staging Manual, 5th edition (1997) published by Lippincott Williams & Wilkins Publishers, Philadelphia, PA.

1. Precise location of the tumor
2. Stage of the cancer
3. Histologic type and grade
4. Expected cure rate
5. Therapeutic and posttherapeutic morbidity and mortality
6. Age and general health of the patient
7. Desires and expectations of the patient and family after they have been informed of all the qualifying conditions
8. Ability or likelihood of the patient to comply
9. Proximity and availability of an appropriate therapeutic facility
10. Experience and preference of the physician

TABLE 8–2.
AJCC stage grouping for laryngeal cancer

Stage	*T*	*N*	M
0	Tis	N0	M0
I	T1	N0	M0
II	T2	N0	M0
III	T3	N0	M0
	T1	N1	M0
	T2	N1	M0
	T3	N1	M0
IVA	T4	N0	M0
	T4	N1	M0
	Any T	N2	M0
IVB	Any T	N3	M0
IVC	Any T	Any N	M1

SOURCE: Used with permission of the American Joint Committee on Cancer (AJCC®), Chicago, IL. The original source for this material is the AJCC® Cancer Staging Manual, 5th edition (1997) published by Lippincott Williams & Wilkins Publishers, Philadelphia, PA.

F. T1 Lesions

Surgery (Transoral) The management of T1 laryngeal cancer is controversial given the wide range of lesions that fit the T1 definition. A small carcinoma in situ or early microinvasive carcinoma on the central part of the cord can often be managed endoscopically with vocal cord stripping and close observation, repeating the procedure if necessary. Laser cordectomy may be considered for membranous T1 lesions that can be fully visualized during endoscopy. The CO_2 or KTP laser with its excellent hemostatic ability can be used effectively to excise a local lesion with little damage to adjacent tissues. Although the margins of the excised specimen may be difficult to assess, biopsy specimen from of the underlying muscle bed can be obtained to determine tumor clearance using frozen sections. Vocal cord stripping, laser vaporization, and laser resection of vocal cord lesions impose little morbidity and require only brief if any hospitalization. Voice quality remains good, and these modalities offer excellent cure rates of 87–100%.[9–11]

The basis of conservation surgery involves removal of disease with adequate margins while preserving as much normal muscle and cartilage as possible to maintain optimal laryngeal function. Consideration for conservation surgery should include factors such as the patient's general health, age, and occupation. Continuity of care, patient compliance, and proximity to the hospital or radiation therapy center are strong factors as well. Histologic factors play a role: Certain tumors, such as verrucous cancers and chondromas, are relatively radioresistant, so surgery is the preferred form of management. The surgeon's experience with conservation surgery and the radiotherapists' results with such treatment are also considerations. Finally, a patient's inclination toward surgery or irradiation plays a major role. With these early-stage tumors there is no clear advantage for surgical or radiation treatment of squamous cell carcinoma.

Glottic lymphatics are limited; therefore nodal metastases from T1 lesions are seen infrequently. Lesions involving the anterior commissure can spread more easily to the supraglottic and subglottic larynx owing to tumor abutting cartilage. The cartilage itself can be easily invaded in such instances. This anterior involvement is not considered conducive to transoral or laser treatment. Tumors of the anterior commissure may, in fact, be understaged because of undetected penetration of the thyroid cartilage at this location. Irradiating such a lesion would clearly result in decreased local control. An open procedure, including removal of a vertical strut of anterior thyroid cartilage, is considered by many to be an oncologically appropriate operation.[12–14] External conservation procedures such as these yield 5-year control rates of 85–91%, thus strongly supporting their use.

Irradiation There is an abundance of literature to support the treatment of T1 lesions with radiation therapy. Large series describe initial and ultimate local control rates ranging from 91% to more than 97%.[15–17] Voice preservation was accomplished with good to excellent voice quality in 80–90% of such patients.

There is support for irradiation or surgical treatment for early glottic squamous cell carcinoma. T1a lesions treated by either modality have cure rates of 88–100%,[18,19] although there is considerable controversy regarding the appropriate treatment modality for T1b lesions. According to some authors, T1b tumors that have anterior commissure involvement and close abutment of the anterior thyroid cartilage generally respond less favorably to irradiation (73–96%) than to an external surgical approach (85–91%).[20,21] Other series have not shown that anterior commissure involvement alone adversely affects outcome following radiotherapy.[22,23] My opinion is that, as a group, T1b lesions are better treated by an open surgical conservation technique for more accurate tumor staging and optimal control.

The benefits of organ preservation and maintaining function of the larynx cannot be overstated. Preservation of a useful voice while achieving acceptable control rates is a strong factor for considering radiotherapy as a primary treatment modality. The health, occupation, compliance, and bias of the patient are also important factors.

G. T2 Lesions

The T2 tumors can extend to the supraglottis or subglottis with or without impaired vocal cord mobility. As with T1 lesions, the T2 definition encompasses a wide range of tumors, and some authors prefer to subdivide these lesions further.[24] T2a lesions have full vocal cord mobility, whereas T2b tumors have limited vocal cord mobility and the cords are not fixed. Decreased cord mobility is often due to tumor invasion of the underlying vocalis muscle. Invasion of the cricoarytenoid joint or the recurrent laryngeal nerve or tumor bulk alone may hinder full motion of the cord. The controversy continues among surgeons as to when a cord with impaired mobility (T2b) becomes a fixed cord (T3). This subjective decision may affect treatment bias among surgeons and radiotherapists.

The T2a lesions fare the same whether treated by radiation therapy (67–87%) or surgery (80–91%). However, with increasing tumor size or proximity to cartilage, external beam radiation becomes less effective. For this reason T2b lesions, with their impaired vocal cord mobility, do not respond as well to irradiation, with cure rates of 64–76%. External surgical treatment, often conservative, offers an improved rate of control (73–90%).[20,22,25]

H. T3 Lesions

The T3 carcinomas are limited to the larynx, but there is vocal cord(s) fixation. The rigidity of the AJCC staging system makes it necessary to accommodate numerous exceptions. For example, a relatively small but penetrating true vocal cord lesion that is invading the vocalis muscle or the inner perichondrium of the thyroid cartilage may cause vocal cord fixation (T3). A large transglottic lesion covering far more mucosa may only impair (T2b) the affected cord rather than cause fixation. The same management for these two lesions may therefore result in different outcomes.

Traditionally, total laryngectomy was the recommended treatment for T3 cancer. Yuen et al. reported a 5-year survival rate of 80% in patients with T3 glottic carcinomas undergoing total laryngectomy with or without postoperative irradiation.[26] The following, however, have been presented as favorable indications for *conservation surgery* of the larynx for T3 lesions: unilateral disease, exophytic tumors, and an adequate airway at presentation. Unfavorable factors include extensive bilateral disease, subglottic extension down to the cricoid, cartilage destruction, posterior commissure extension, or extralaryngeal disease found during surgery (T4).[27]

As previously discussed, T3 glottic tumors are a heterogeneous group of tumors with a wide range of size and growth patterns. With proper selection, a small group of patients with T3 lesions may be amenable to conservation surgery with acceptable cure rates. These same favorable lesions tend to be more suitable for radiotherapy, with control rates of approximately 40–70% in most studies.[28–30] If there is residual or recurrent tumor, up to 50% of patients can be salvaged with surgery, usually total laryngectomy. The less favorable large, bulky, bilateral transglottic carcinomas do not respond as well to radiation treatment; they are best treated with laryngectomy and irradiation, which gives them the best chance of survival.

Vertical partial laryngectomy techniques performed on selected groups of patients with T3 tumors produced 2-year disease control rates of 60–85%.[31–33] Important in that selection process is information garnered from direct laryngoscopy, CT or MRI (or both), and frozen section assessment of mucosal margins at the time of surgery. The surgeon's familiarity with conservation techniques and the patient's acceptance of limiting factors and consent for possible total laryngectomy also play important roles.

I. T4 Lesions

There is little controversy that total laryngectomy is the "standard" treatment for most T3, T4, and subglottic lesions. Residual or recurrent tumor after radiation therapy is usually treated with total laryngectomy rather than something less radical because the original tumor size and location is often difficult to ascertain. For selected patients, extended conservation surgery, including "near total" laryngectomy, has yielded favorable results. As surgeons, we remain challenged when trying to devise ways to decrease the morbidity associated with the treatment of these lesions.

A total laryngectomy involves removal of the hyoid bone, epiglottis, thyroid cartilage, larynx, and cricoid cartilage. The inferior extent of the resection depends somewhat on the subglottic extent of the tumor; but for most glottic lesions, removing the second tracheal ring is sufficient. Supraglottic lesions that extend into the base of the tongue or the hypopharynx require extended resection in these areas. Most often the pharyngeal defect can be closed primarily. For more extensive defects, pectoralis myocutaneous or microvascular free flaps may be used for closure. The trachea is sewn directly to the skin, creating a permanent laryngostome. A cricopharyngeal myotomy performed easily at the time of surgery aids in postoperative swallowing and in the acquisition of voice during rehabilitation.

Patients play a crucial role in their treatment plan, as many are unwilling to lose their larynx. The issue of quality of life often is more important to the patient than our opinion of the treatment that offers the best chance of cure.

J. Radiotherapy Techniques

There is some variation in the radiation technique for T1 and T2 glottic squamous cell carcinomas. Most institutions use opposed lateral wedged portals with $4 \times 4\,cm^2$ to $5 \times 5\,cm^2$ field sizes. Large T2 lesions may require a field size of $6 \times 6\,cm^2$. Total doses used are most commonly 66 Gy in 33 daily fractions of 200 cGy or 63 Gy in 28 daily fractions of 225 cGy. There is some variability in total dose and number of days of treatment. Given the paucity of true vocal cord lymphatics, metastasis from T1 and most T2 lesions remains less than 5%; this does not justify prophylactic radiation therapy of the neck.

Several factors are known to affect the outcome of radiation therapy. Previously mentioned was anterior commissure involvement by some tumors; extension of tumor this close to cartilage is probably reason enough to choose surgery over irradiation. Variable irradiation results may be due to inadequate dosing at this anterior extent of the tumor. When anterior tumor location is taken into account, meticulous planning and dosing to this area for a tumor whose stage has been accurately determined should not yield significantly poorer results according to some authors.[22,23,34] Indeed, tumor at the anterior commissure that has already penetrated cartilage is no longer stage T1 but has advanced to stage T4. This may account for some of the poor results reported with irradiation for "T1b" tumors, as cartilage involvement mandates surgical treatment.

Impaired vocal cord mobility, as seen with T2b and T3 lesions, makes it less likely that radiotherapy can cure the patient. Small tumor volume, tumors that are unilateral, and patients not requiring tracheostomy tend to have better local control. It is not surprising that in selected subgroups of patients with T2 and T3 tumors improved outcomes can be realized with radiation treatment.

The duration of the irradiation has been shown to affect the overall response rate. Comparison of various radiotherapeutic schedules has shown a 10–15% lower control rate for patients whose fractionation schedule exceeded 35 days.[35] Another study likewise showed a decrease in local control (by 18%) in T2 and T3 patients whose treatment protocols were prolonged.[36] A dose of more than 200 cGy per fraction was as efficacious as lower doses when patients were treated to the same endpoint. Unplanned breaks during treatment may therefore compromise the end result, and a higher total dose may be needed to regain adequate control of the tumor, at the expense of increased morbidity. Noncompliant patients whose tumor stage would fit well into the group favorable for irradiation might instead be better treated with surgery for fear they might never receive a full, uninterrupted course of radiotherapy.

Minor complications of radiotherapy include a localized sore throat, some erythema, and a globus sensation. Severe complications, such as laryngeal swelling requiring tracheostomy, laryngeal necrosis, or chondritis, occur in fewer than 1% of cases.

Advantages of radiotherapy include voice preservation and improved voice quality compared with partial laryngectomy in most cases. Irradiation is performed on an outpatient basis and is associated with a low rate of severe complications. The 6–7 weeks needed to complete a full course of radiation may make this a less desirable option for some patients. Lesions that are borderline amenable to conservation surgery are less likely to be salvageable by the same conservation technique after failing a full course of radiation. Residual or recurrent disease following irradiation is often not evident early owing to mucosal changes or swelling and must be treated in a much more aggressive surgical fashion. What might have been treated primarily by a conservation surgical technique may now require more radical surgery to obtain negative margins.

K. *Lymphadenopathy*

Glottic lymphatics are unique owing to the embryologic origin of these tissues. The supraglottis arises from tongue base analogues, and the subglottis arises from tracheobronchial analogues. Both of these regions have a rich lymphatic supply; and in a high percentage of these cancers adenopathy is present at the time of the initial examination. The glottis is the point of fusion of these two planes, and there is a paucity of lymphatics. Cancers limited to the cord rarely metastasize; and if they do, it is usually to the ipsilateral neck. The exception occurs with T1b lesions, which abut the thyroid cartilage anteriorly where there is a richer supply of lymphatics and blood vessels. This accounts for a nodal metastasis rate of up to 8% for T1b tumors. Only if a vocal cord tumor invades superiorly or inferiorly into the areas abundant with lymphatics does one see a significant incidence of nodal metastases.

For the above reasons, T1 and most T2 lesions do not require specific treatment for the clinically N0 neck. T3 and T4 lesions, even with clinically N0 necks, have a high enough incidence of occult nodes that treatment is warranted. If treatment of the primary tumor is surgical, a conservative neck dissection may be performed concurrently. If radiation therapy is used for primary T3 or T4 disease, N0 necks may be irradiated. Generally, nodes >2–3 cm are best treated surgically. Occasionally, for cases in which the primary tumor might be treated equally well with surgery or radiation therapy, extensive nodal disease that would require surgical intervention may sway one toward surgical treatment for the primary tumor as well.[37,38]

There is some question regarding the need for elective treatment of the N0 neck in patients with laryngeal cancer. One study reviewed cases in which the primary lesion was surgically resected and the necks were left untreated; 7–30% of patients later developed neck metastases. In this and other series, patients who had undergone elective neck dissection were found to have a 3–30% rate of occult positive nodes demonstrated histologically. The highest number of occult positive neck nodes were found in patients with supraglottic primaries and a high-stage tumor. The authors could find no substantial influence on survival outcomes for these two groups of patients, as the patients in whom neck disease eventually developed were salvaged with a neck dissection.[39] It is perhaps prudent to consider an elective neck dissection in the patient population who may be noncompliant for follow-up or radiation therapy appointments.

Chemotherapy has no role in the treatment of early T1 or T2 lesions of the larynx. Surgical and irradiation modalities offer excellent cure rates. More advanced lesions (stages III and IV) are most often treated with combined therapy to include conservation or total laryngectomy and irradiation. Trials have been used to randomize patients to induction chemotherapy followed by irradiation in an attempt to preserve laryngeal function. Multiple trials have not yet demonstrated an increase in survival using this technique, although the ability to preserve laryngeal function in some cases makes this an appealing area for intense future study.[40–42]

Management of laryngeal cancer requires a multidisciplinary approach among the surgeon, radiation oncologist, and medical colleagues. Close, frequent follow-up of patients and thorough examinations are necessary to detect any recurrence early. Speech therapists, social workers, and family members offer continued support to these patients during their posttreatment course.

References

1. Mansel RN, Vermeersch H. Panendoscopy for second primaries in head and neck cancer. Ann Otol Rhinol Laryngol 1981 Sep–Oct;90 (5 Pt1):460–464.
2. McGuint WF, Matthews B, Koufman JA. Multiple simultaneous tumors in patients with head and neck cancer. Cancer 1982;50:1195–1199.
3. Slaughter DL, Southwick HW, Smejkal W. Field cancerization in oral stratified squamous epithelium: clinical implications of multicentric origin. Cancer 1953;6:963–968.

4. Silver CE. Surgical management of neoplasms of the larynx, hypopharynx, and cervical esophagus. Curr Probl Surg 1977;14:2–69.
5. Williams DW, 3rd. Imaging of laryngeal cancer. Otolaryngol Clin North Am 1997;30:35–58.
6. AJCC. Staging of primary tumor (T) in laryngeal cancer. American Joint Committee for Cancer Staging and End-Results Reporting: Manual for Staging of Cancer, 1997.
7. AJCC. Staging of metastasis (N,M) in laryngeal cancer. American Joint Committee for Cancer Staging and End-Results Reporting: Manual for Staging of Cancer, 1997.
8. AJCC. Stage grouping for laryngeal cancer. American Joint Committee for Cancer Staging and End-Results Reporting: Manual for Staging of Cancer, 1997.
9. Blakeslee D, Vaughan CW, Shapshay SM, et al. Excisional biopsy in the selected management of T1 glottic cancer: a three-year follow-up study. Laryngoscope 1984;94:488–494.
10. Davis RK, Kelly SM, Parkin JL, et al. Selective management of early glottic cancer. Laryngoscope 1990;100:1306–1309.
11. McGuint WF, Koufman JA. Endoscopic laser surgery. Arch Otolaryngol Head Neck Surg 1987;113:501–505.
12. Neel BH III, Devine KD, DeSanto LW. Laryngofissure and cordectomy for early cordal carcinoma: outcome in 182 patients. Otolaryngol Head Neck Surg 1980;88:79–84.
13. Thomas JV, Olson KD, Neel HB, et al. Early glottic carcinoma treated with open laryngeal procedures. Arch Otolaryngol Head Neck Surg 1994;120: 264–268.
14. Olson KD, DeSanto LW. Partial vertical laryngectomy: indications and surgical technique. Am J Otolaryngol 1990;11:153–160.
15. Mendenhall WM, Parsons JT, Million RR, et al. T1–T2 squamous cell carcinoma of the glottic larynx treated with radiation therapy: relationship of dose-fractionation factors to local control and complications. Int J Radiat Oncol Biol Phys 1988;15:1267.
16. Wang CC. Carcinomas of the larynx. In: Radiation Therapy for Head and Neck Neoplasms: Indications, Techniques, and Results, 2nd ed., Chicago: Year Book, 1990.
17. Terhaard CHJ, Snippe K, Ravasz LA, et al. Radiotherapy in T1 laryngeal cancer: prognostic factors for locoregional control and survival; uni- and multivariate analysis. Int J Radiat Oncol Biol Phys 1991;21:1179.
18. Rucci L, Gallo O, Fini-Storchi D. Glottic cancer involving anterior commissure and surgery vs. radiotherapy. Head Neck 1991;13:403.
19. Ton-Van J, Lafebure SL, Stern JC, et al. Comparison of surgery and radiotherapy in T1 and T2 glottic carcinomas. Am J Surg 1991;162:337.
20. Johnson J, Myers E, Hao S, et al. Outcome of open surgical therapy for glottic carcinoma. Ann Otol Rhinol Laryngol 1993;102:752.
21. Olson K, Thanas J, DeSanto L, et al. Indications and results of cordectomy for early glottic carcinoma. Otolaryngol Head Neck Surg 1993;108:277.
22. Fein DA, Mendenhall WM, Parsons TJ, et al. T1–T2 squamous cell carcinoma of the glottic larynx treated with radiotherapy: a multivariate analysis of variables potentially influencing local control. Int J Radiat Oncol Biol Phys 1993;25:605.
23. Pellittori PK, Kennedy TL, Vrabec DP, et al. Radiotherapy: the mainstay in the treatment of early glottic carcinoma. Arch Otolaryngol Head Neck Surg 1991;117:297.
24. Kaplan M, John M, McLean W, et al. Stage II glottic carcinoma: prognostic factors and management. Laryngoscope 1983;93:725.
25. Howell-Burke D, Peters L, Goepfert H, et al. T2 glottic carcinoma. Arch Otolaryngol Head Neck Surg 1990;116:830.
26. Yuen A, Medina JE, Goepfert H, et al. Management of stage T3 and T4 glottic carcinomas. Arch Otolaryngol Head Neck Surg 1984;148:467–472.
27. Osguthorpe J, Putney F. Open surgical management of early glottic carcinoma. Otolaryngol Clin North Am 1997;30:87–99.
28. Bryant GP, Poulson MG, Tripcony L, et al. Treatment decisions in T3N0M0 glottic carcinoma. Int J Radiat Oncol Biol Phys 1995;31:285.
29. Harwood AR, Hawkins NV, Beale FA, et al. Management of advanced glottic cancer: a 10-year review of the Toronto experience. Int J Radiat Oncol Biol Phys 1979;5:899.
30. Wang CC. Radiation therapy of laryngeal tumors. In: Thawley SE, Panje WR (eds) Comprehensive Management of Head and Neck Tumors. Philadelphia: Saunders, 1987.
31. Kirchner JA, Som ML. Clinical significance of fixed vocal cord. Laryngoscope 1971;81:1029–1044.
32. Kessler DJ, Trapp TK, Cacaterra TC. The treatment of T3 glottic carcinoma with vertical partial laryngectomy. Arch Otolaryngol Head Neck Surg 1987;113:1196–1199.
33. Biller HF, Lawson W. Partial laryngectomy for vocal cord cancer with marked limitation or fixation of the vocal cord. Laryngoscope 1986; 96:61–64.
34. Rudoltz MS, Benammar A, Mohiuddin M. Prognostic factors for local control and survival in T2 squamous cell carcinoma of the glottis. Int J Radiat Oncol Biol Phys 1993;26:767.
35. Robertson AG, Robertson C, Boyle RP, et al. The effect of differing radiotherapeutic schedules on the response of glottic carcinomas of the larynx. Eur J Cancer 1993;29A:501.
36. Wang CC, Efind JT. Does prolonged treatment course adversely affect local control of carcinoma of the larynx? Int J Radiat Oncol Biol Phys 1994; 29:652.
37. Byer RM, Wolf PF, Ballantyne AJ. Rationale for elective modified neck dissection. Head Neck Surg 1988;10:160.
38. Million RR, Cassisi NJ, Mancuso AA. Larynx. In: Million RR, Cassisi NJ (eds) Management of Head and Neck Cancer: A Multidisciplinary Approach, 2nd ed. Philadelphia: Lippincott, 1994.
39. Calhoun KH, Stiennberg CM, Hokanson JA, et al. Laryngeal cancer without spread to the node: treatment options and outcome. South Med J 1988;81:1369–1374.
40. Adjuvant chemotherapy for advanced head and neck squamous carcinoma: final report of the Head and Neck Contacts Program. Cancer 1987; 60:301–311.
41. Schuller DE, Metch B, Stein DW, Mattox D, McCracken JD. Preoperative chemotherapy in advanced resectable head and neck cancer: final report of the Southwest Oncology Group. Laryngoscope 1988;98:1205–1211.
42. The Department of Veterans Affairs Laryngeal Cancer Study Group. Induction chemotherapy plus radiation compared with surgery plus radiation with advanced laryngeal cancer. N Engl J Medicine 1991;324:1685–1690.

Chapter 9

Malignant Tumors of Salivary Glands

RONALD H. SPIRO
DENNIS T.H. LIM

Salivary Gland Tumors

A. Epidemiology and Etiology

Salivary gland tumors comprise fewer than 3% of head and neck neoplasms and are especially challenging to the clinician because of their remarkable variation in presentation and clinical behavior. Most arise in the major or paired salivary glands: 75–85% occur in the parotid gland and fewer than 10% in the submandibular gland. The sublingual gland, a most uncommon site for salivary gland neoplasms, accounts for only 0.05% of salivary neoplasms. In our experience, about 20% of salivary gland tumors originate from the unpaired or minor salivary glands. These tiny, predominantly mucus-secreting glands are found everywhere underneath the mucous membrane of the upper aerodigestive tract but are clustered most densely on the palate.[1]

The probability of cancer is less than 25% in patients with parotid gland tumors, about 50% in those with submandibular gland tumors, more than 80% in our experience with minor salivary lesions, and virtually 100% in those few who present with sublingual gland lesions. It is important to remember that statistics on the distributions of salivary gland tumors and the proportion that are malignant usually derive from tumor registries of large tertiary care centers, where there is an obvious referral bias. In the community setting, salivary tumor experience is mostly limited to the parotid gland; minor salivary gland tumors are uncommon, and the proportion that proves to be malignant is certainly much lower than we have reported.

B. Histology

The histologic classification now used in most centers is basically a modification of that proposed years ago by Foote and Frazell (Table 9–1).[2] In 1978 Batsakis and Regezi offered a more detailed classification of salivary gland cancers (Table 9–2),[3] and the second edition of the World Health Organization's classification of salivary gland cancers gives an even more complex histologic breakdown (Table 9–3).[4]

Salivary Gland Tumors

A.
Epidemiology and Etiology
Salivary gland tumors constitute <3% of head/neck tumors
Parotid tumors 75–80%: 25% are malignant, most common mucoepidermoid
Submandibular tumors <10%: 50% are malignant, most common adenoid cystic
Sublingual tumors <1%: 100% are malignant
Minor salivary gland tumors: 80% are malignant (most common adenoid cystic)

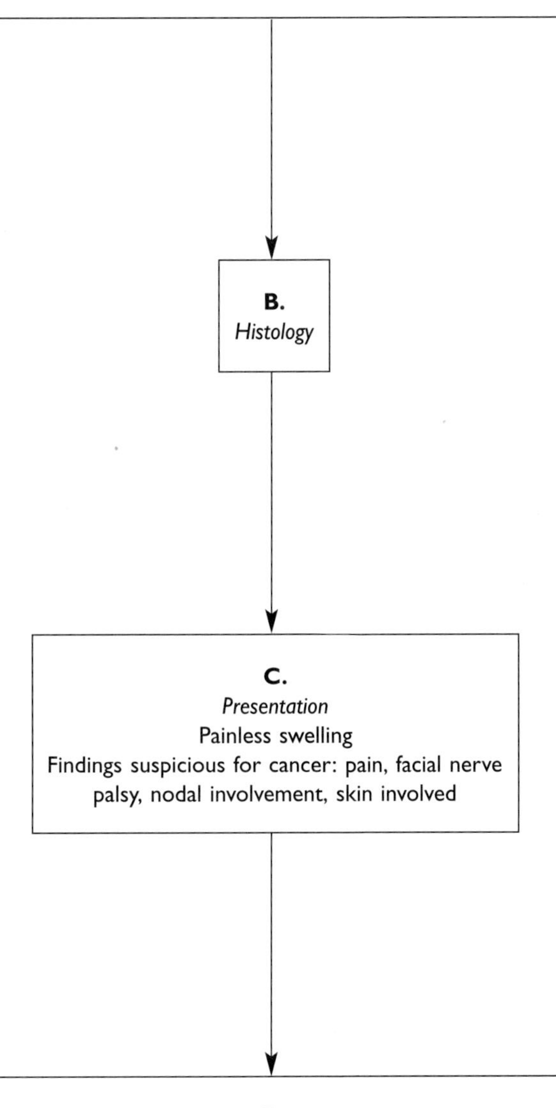

B.
Histology

C.
Presentation
Painless swelling
Findings suspicious for cancer: pain, facial nerve palsy, nodal involvement, skin involved

D.
Diagnosis
Fine-needle aspiration: not routinely advised for small, mobile lesions in a parotid gland; is indicated for larger parotid lesions, submandibular tumors
Imaging: not necessary for small, mobile parotid tumors but is indicated for deep lobe tumors, high grade lesions, and minor salivary gland tumors

TABLE 9–1.
Classification and incidence of malignant salivary gland tumors at Memorial Hospital

Tumor type	No. of patients 1939–1973	1988–1993
Mucoepidermoid carcinoma	439 (34%)	119 (34%)
Adenoid cystic carcinoma	281 (22%)	72 (21%)
Adenocarcinoma	225 (17%)	73 (21%)
Malignant mixed tumor	161 (13%)	22 (6%)
Acinic cell carcinoma	84 (7%)	25 (7%)
Epidermoid carcinoma	53 (4%)	19 (6%)
Anaplastic and others	33 (3%)	16 (5%)
Total	1278 (100%)	346 (100%)

SOURCE: Foote and Frazell.[2]

Although unique subtypes of malignant tumors are better defined by this classification, it is unwieldy and rather confusing to clinicians.

In the Memorial Hospital experience, more than 80% of benign tumors are pleomorphic adenomas; and in patients with malignant neoplasms, mucoepidermoid carcinoma is the most common diagnosis (34%). The latter is followed by adenoid cystic carcinoma (23%), adenocarcinoma (19%), and malignant mixed tumor (13%). Less frequently diagnosed malignant tumors are acinic cell carcinoma (7%), epidermoid carcinoma (4%), and other anaplastic variants (4%).

The incidence of malignant tumors varies by site. For example, mucoepidermoid carcinoma is the most common cancer diagnosis in the parotid gland, whereas adenoid cystic carcinoma is the most commonly encountered malignant tumor in the submandibular and minor salivary glands.

GRADING Stewart and colleagues first described the concept of grading in a study of mucoepidermoid carcinomas of salivary gland origin reported in 1945.[5] Since then, the importance of salivary tumor grading has become widely accepted. Significant differences in clinical behavior are apparent among histologic grades. Low-grade mucoepidermoid carcinomas, for example, almost never metastasize and typically behave in a relatively benign fashion. Similarly, less aggressive growth patterns are evident in certain patients with low-grade acinic cell carcinomas or adenocarcinomas.

Adenoid cystic carcinoma (ACC) accounts for 4–15% of all salivary gland cancers and is the most common cancer arising in minor salivary glands. It is characterized by aggressive but indolent behavior with a strong propensity for local recurrence, a significant incidence of distant metastasis, and minimal likelihood of nodal involvement. Tubular, cribriform, and solid tumor patterns occur in varying proportions. High-grade tumors showing more than a 30% solid pattern seem to behave more aggressively, but our experience suggests that significant survival

TABLE 9–2.
Classification of malignant salivary gland tumors

Carcinoma ex pleomorphic adenoma (carcinoma arising in a mixed tumor)
Malignant mixed tumor (biphasic malignancy)
Mucoepidermoid carcinoma
Low grade
Intermediate grade
High grade
Adenoid cystic carcinoma
Acinous (acinic) cell carcinoma
Adenocarcinoma
Mucus-producing adenopapillary and nonpapillary
Salivary duct carcinoma (ductal carcinoma)
Other adenocarcinoma
Oncocytic cell carcinoma (malignant oncocytoma)
Clear cell carcinoma (nonmucinous and glycogen-containing or non-glycogen-containing
Primary squamous cell carcinoma
Undifferentiated carcinoma
Epithelial-myoepithelial carcinoma
Metastatic
Unclassified

SOURCE: Batsakis and Regezi.[3]

TABLE 9–3.
World Health Organization classification of malignant salivary gland tumors

Acinic cell carcinoma
Mucoepidermoid carcinoma
Adenoid cystic carcinoma
Polymorphous low-grade adenocarcinoma
Epithelial myoepithelial carcinoma
Basal cell adenocarcinoma
Sebaceous carcinoma
Papillary cystadenocarcinoma
Mucinous adenocarcinoma
Oncocytic carcinoma
Salivary duct carcinoma
Adenocarcinoma
Malignant myoepithelioma
Carcinoma in pleomorphic adenoma
Squamous cell carcinoma
Small-cell carcinoma
Undifferentiated carcinoma
Incidence, in decreasing frequency
Mucoepidermoid (34%)
Adenoid cystic (23%)
Adenocarcinoma (19%)
Malignant mixed (13%)
Acinic cell (7%)

SOURCE: Seifert and Sobin.[4]

differences based only on adenoid cystic tumor grade tend to disappear when patients are followed for more than 10 years.[6]

STAGING Included in our 1975 report on 288 previously untreated patients with parotid carcinoma was a proposal for a simple staging system that accurately predicted the probability of survival.[7] With modification, this system was adopted by the American Joint Committee on Cancer (AJCC) in 1978 (Table 9–4).[8] Clearly, the staging of salivary gland tumors is important for treatment planning and is essential for meaningful comparison of end results. Although there is no AJCC staging system for minor salivary tumors, they can be staged using criteria identical to those described for squamous carcinoma in similar sites.[9] Multivariate analyses have indicated that clinical stage is clearly the most important predictor of survival. Our data showed 10-year overall survivals of 83%, 53%, 35%, and 24% for patients with stage I, II, III, and IV disease, respectively.[6]

C. PRESENTATION

Painless swelling is the most common presenting symptom of salivary gland tumors, regardless of the site of origin or the histology. Pain usually suggests that a tumor is malignant but does not exclude the possibility of a benign diagnosis. The duration of symptoms may range from months to years but tends to be shorter in patients with malignant tumors.

Clinical findings are determined by the location of the tumor. Most parotid gland tumors present as a preauricular mass near the angle of the mandible. In our experience, about 10% of parotid tumors arise below the plane of the facial nerve in the deep lobe. Most are indistinguishable from their counterparts that arise lateral to the nerve. About 1% of parotid tumors arise from the small piece of accessory parotid tissue at the anterior border of the gland, near Stenson's duct. Retromandibular origin of a deep lobe parotid tumor is uncommon and is characterized by soft palate or pharyngeal swelling alone or in combination with an external mass. Computed tomography (CT) or magnetic resonance imaging (MRI) can help distinguish deep parotid tumors from other parapharyngeal neoplasms. Small benign and malignant parotid gland tumors are clinically indistinguishable, but a diagnosis of malignancy is obvious when there is facial nerve palsy, nodal involvement, or skin involvement. Minor salivary gland tumors typically present as swellings underneath intact mucosa, but ulceration is not unusual.

Nodal metastasis was confirmed, initially or subsequent to initial treatment, in 26% of our patients with major salivary gland cancers and in 21% of those with minor salivary lesions, most of which were clinically apparent at presentation. This occurs most often in patients with high-grade tumors and is unusual in those with low-grade tumors or adenoid cystic carcinoma.

D. DIAGNOSIS

Any swelling near the ear is considered a parotid tumor until proven otherwise. Open biopsy of a parotid or submandibular gland is ill-advised, as it risks tumor seeding and may complicate

TABLE 9–4.
AJCC definition of TNM and stage grouping for salivary gland tumors

Primary Tumor (T)

TX	Primary tumor cannot be assessed
T0	No evidence of primary tumor
T1	Tumor 2 cm or less in greatest dimension without extraparenchymal extension
T2	Tumor more than 2 cm but not more than 4 cm in greatest dimension without extraparenchymal extension
T3	Tumor having extraparenchymal extension without seventh nerve involvement and/or more than 4 cm but not more than 6 cm in greatest dimension
T4	Tumor invades base of skull, seventh nerve, and/or exceeds 6 cm in greatest dimension

Regional Lymph Nodes (N)

NX	Regional lymph nodes cannot be assessed
N0	No regional lymph node metastasis
N1	Metastasis in a single ipsilateral lymph node, 3 cm or less in greatest dimension
N2	Metastasis to a single ipsilateral lymph node, more than 3 cm but not more than 6 cm in greatest dimension, or in multiple ipsilateral lymph nodes, none more than 6 cm in greatest dimension, or in bilateral or contralateral lymph nodes, none more than 6 cm in greatest dimension
N2a	Metastasis in a single ipsilateral lymph node more than 3 cm but not more than 6 cm in greatest dimension
N2b	Metastasis in multiple ipsilateral lymph nodes, none more than 6 cm in greatest dimension
N2c	Metastasis in bilateral or contralateral lymph nodes, none more than 6 cm in greatest dimension
N3	Metastasis in a lymph node more than 6 cm in greatest dimension

Distant Metastasis (M)

MX	Distant metastasis cannot be assessed
M0	No distant metastasis
M1	Distant metastasis

Stage Grouping

Stage	*T*	*N*	*M*
I	T1	N0	M0
	T2	N0	M0
II	T3	N0	M0
III	T1	N1	M0
	T2	N1	M0
IV	T4	N0	M0
	T3	N1	M0
	T4	N1	M0
	Any T	N2	M0
	Any T	N3	M0
	Any T	Any N	M1

SOURCE: Used with permission of the American Joint Committee on Cancer (AJCC®), Chicago, IL. The original source for this material is the AJCC® Cancer Staging Manual, 5th edition (1997) published by Lippincott Williams & Wilkins Publishers, Philadelphia, PA.

the indicated surgery. When a minor salivary gland tumor is suspected, on the other hand, biopsy is important as the differential diagnosis includes sarcoma, lymphoma, or melanoma. Treatment varies accordingly.

Fine-needle aspiration biopsy (FNAB) is not recommended for all parotid tumors, as a tissue diagnosis is not essential for treatment planning in the patient who presents with a small, mobile mass that is obviously within the substance of the gland. Clearly, FNAB is appropriate when parotid gland origin is uncertain or when the size and location of the tumor suggest that the facial nerve dissection is likely to be tedious.

The argument for FNAB of a mass in the submandibular triangle is much more compelling, as relatively few such "lumps" turn out to be primary neoplasms of the submandibular gland.[10] Many of these patients have inflammation or a neoplasm involving adjacent lymph nodes, and knowledge of the histology is likely to influence treatment.

Although some centers claim that FNAB for salivary gland tumors is highly accurate, we and others have noted significant errors in interpretation even when a frozen section technique is used on adequate tissue fragments or surgical specimens. FNAB certainly has an important role in selected patients, but it is no substitute for careful clinical assessment.

Another area of controversy in the management of salivary gland tumors is the role of imaging (i.e., CT and MRI). Few question the importance of imaging a patient with a deep lobe parotid tumor, a high-stage tumor that has invaded adjacent structures, or a high-grade tumor that is likely to be associated with occult cervical metastases. Conversely, CT should not be routine for all patients with parotid tumors because it is not likely to change the management of small to moderate-size, freely mobile tumors that are obviously confined to the gland.

Imaging assumes more importance in the evaluation of the patient with a minor salivary gland tumor, particularly those that arise in inaccessible sites. Better assessment of tumor extent has greatly enhanced treatment planning in some patients with salivary gland tumors, particularly those with lesions arising in the palate or sinuses. Although MRI offers some advantage because of its multiplanar capability and the ability to distinguish tumor from secretion in the sinuses, it is our impression that high quality CT with contrast often provides adequate information.

Parotid Tumors

E. Diagnosis and Treatment

Benign-Appearing Parotid Mass A mass < 3 cm arising from the parotid gland that is discrete and confined to the gland, with no skin involvement or associated adenopathy, can be safely treated with subtotal parotidectomy that preserves the facial nerve. FNAB is often unnecessary, as it seldom changes the treatment approach. Imaging in this setting seldom adds more information than can be derived from a careful clinical examination. When the facial nerve is found to be densely adherent to, or involved by the tumor, it is wiser to sacrifice it and perform a cable graft, rather than risk piecemeal excision of the lesion in an overly zealous attempt to preserve the nerve. It is important to remember that adjunctive radiation therapy is no substitute for a complete en bloc resection.

When the diagnosis of malignancy is confirmed, postoperative radiation therapy may be indicated if: (1) there has been obvious tumor spillage; (2) the surgeon is concerned about the excision margins; or (3) the pathology report suggests ominous histologic features, such as unsuspected margin involvement, perineural extension, or vascular invasion. In our experience, adjunctive radiation therapy failed to yield survival benefit in patients who had adequately excised malignant tumors that were < 4 cm in size.[11]

Possibly Malignant Parotid Mass When the origin and extent of a large (> 3 cm) mass in the parotid region is not clear, or there is suspicion clinically that adjacent structures or the retromandibular space are involved, FNAB can provide useful information. A diagnosis of malignancy allows the surgeon and patient to prepare for the possibility of a more radical procedure. Imaging with CT scans and intravenous contrast or MRI with gadolinium can help define the deep extent of the disease, involvement of the great vessels, or encroachment of the retromandibular space. Treatment may involve subtotal or total parotidectomy, often with facial nerve sparing. For those with retromandibular deep lobe tumors, transcervical resection is usually possible, but a mandibulotomy is occasionally required (Fig. 9–1).

Adjuvant external radiotherapy (ERT) is indicated for malignant tumors when the lesion is of high grade, there are concerns about the adequacy of the resection, or there are ominous histologic features such as perineural invasion or vascular infiltration. Practically speaking, ERT is indicated for all patients after resection of a malignant retropharyngeal tumor because margins are invariably close. The dose given to the parotid bed is 60 Gy.

Because there is no evidence to support elective lymphadenectomy (for the N0 neck), the ipsilateral neck should be included in the portal when postoperative ERT is given, particularly when dealing with a high-grade tumor. When performed for a clinically positive neck, the lymphadenectomy consists of a modified radical neck dissection that preserves the spinal accessory nerve; a supraomohyoid dissection (SOH) may suffice in selected patients with a single positive node in the upper neck (level 2).

Obviously Malignant Parotid Mass A parotid tumor associated with facial paralysis, nodal metastasis,

Parotid Tumors

E.
Diagnosis and Treatment

Benign-Appearing Lesion → Subtotal parotidectomy with preservation of facial nerve VII unless densely adherent to or grossly involved with tumor → If malignant, consider irradiation if: (1) there has been tumor spillage; (2) margins are positive; (3) there is perineural extension or vascular invasion

Lesion < 3 cm
Confined to parotid,
No sign of malignancy

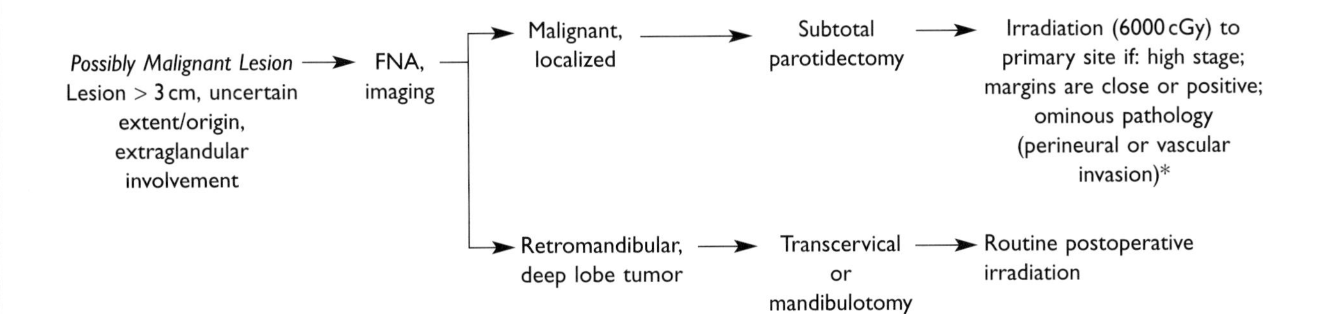

Obviously Malignant Mass → FNA, imaging → Extended parotidectomy with sacrifice of cranial nerve VII, skin excision, possible composite resection and reconstruction as required → *Additional treatment:* Irradiation to the primary site. If neck clinically positive, perform modified neck dissection. For the negative neck, consider irradiation or supraomohyoid neck dissection for high-grade lesion in the parotid tail

Facial nerve palsy
suspicous nodes
skin ulceration

Unresectable tumor or Distant Metastasis → FNA, imaging → Palliative radiotherapy; multiagent chemotherapy: cisplatin, doxorubicin, fluorouracil

**Treatment of the neck:*
Neck clinically positive: perform neck disseaction

Neck clinically negative: include neck in irradiation field

Large Mass Suspicious for Carcinoma An asymptomatic mass > 3 cm in the submandibular triangle with reduced mobility should raise concerns about the possibility of carcinoma arising in the gland. Again, FNAB and an imaging study should confirm the diagnosis and define the extent of the tumor. The procedure of choice in the clinically node-negative setting is an extended SOH dissection with in-continuity removal of the muscles adjacent to the gland. On occasion, the hypoglossal or lingual nerves (or both) may have to be sacrificed. Lymphadenectomy facilitates exposure of the deeper plane of the dissection in the submandibular triangle, but a radical neck dissection is unnecessary unless there are obvious nodal metastases. It should be noted that occult nodal metastasis is uncommon in patients with adenoid cystic carcinoma, which is the most common tumor encountered at this site. ERT to a full therapeutic dose (at least 60 Gy) is advisable for any patient who has a sizable malignant tumor that extends beyond the capsule of the gland. The radiation dose to the lower part of the neck can be less provided the lymph nodes in this area are uninvolved.

Obvious Cancer The patient with a large, ill-defined submandibular mass associated with lower facial nerve, hypoglossal, or lingual nerve dysfunction, cervical lymphadenopathy, fixation to the mandible, or skin involvement should undergo FNAB and an imaging study to confirm the presence of an advanced submandibular gland carcinoma. An open or core biopsy occasionally is necessary to resolve a conflict between the clinical impression of cancer and a benign or nondiagnostic FNAB. The precise extent of the resection required obviously depends on the extent of the tumor as defined clinically and radiographically. If there is adherence to or infiltration of the adjacent muscles, the muscles should be resected, including the hypoglossal nerve when necessary. When the tumor arises high in the submandibular triangle, it may be necessary to include the lingual nerve, the marginal branch of the facial nerve, and the adjacent floor of the mouth in the resection.

Direct invasion of bone is unusual even in patients with advanced disease, but encroachment or envelopment by tumor may necessitate a lower marginal or even a segmental mandibulectomy. In the worst case scenario, advanced submandibular gland cancer may be clinically indistinguishable from similar locally advanced lesions arising in sublingual or floor-of-mouth sites, and a composite resection with hemimandibulectomy and jaw reconstruction is required.

Radical or modified neck dissection is indicated to remove clinically obvious nodal metastases. In the N0 setting, elective en bloc resection of level II and III lymph nodes is appropriate because it facilitates access to the plane of dissection deep to the digastric tendon and removes the nodes most likely to harbor occult metastases. All of these patients require adjuvant radiation therapy, as described above.

Oral or Oropharyngeal Minor Salivary Tumors

Neoplasms arising in minor salivary glands in these sites usually present as a submucosal mass, but occasionally they are ulcerated and mimic squamous carcinoma. Typically, this swelling is asymptomatic. The palate is the most common site, and radiographic studies are essential in these patients lest the inferior extension of an occult antral tumor be mistaken for a palate primary.

Although there are no reliable clinical features predictive of a malignant diagnosis, pain, rapid growth, and ulceration suggest this possibility. When the lesion is small (< 1 cm), the histologic diagnosis is best established with an excisional biopsy that is adequate therapy even if the tumor proves malignant. When an incomplete excision is performed for biopsy purposes, the patient often requires a wider definitive excision than was originally necessary. In patients with larger tumors, FNAB or core biopsy with a dermatologic punch is less disruptive than partial excision and is usually adequate for at least a "benign" versus "malignant" diagnosis. Treatment can then be planned accordingly.

The detailed management of these clinically and histologically diverse tumors is beyond the scope of this chapter. Suffice it to say that they are treated surgically with procedures virtually identical to those employed for squamous cell carcinomas in similar sites. Margins must be generous in patients with adenoid cystic carcinoma because this tumor infiltrates well beyond what can be appreciated clinically or radiologically. The indications for lymphadenectomy and adjunctive irradiation are similar to those described above.

References

1. Spiro RH. Salivary neoplasm: overview of a 35-year experience with 2807 patients. Head Neck Surg 1986;8:177–184.
2. Foote FW, Frazell EL. Tumors of the major salivary glands. Cancer 1953; 6:1065–1153.
3. Batsakis JG, Regezi JA. The pathology of head and neck tumors: salivary glands. Part 1. Head Neck Surg 1978;1:59–68.
4. Seifert G, Sobin LH. The World Health Organization's classification of salivary gland tumors. Cancer 1992;70:379–385.
5. Stewart FW, Foote FW Jr, Becker WF. Mucoepidermoid tumors of salivary glands. Am Surg 1945;122:820–844.
6. Spiro RH, Huvos AG. Stage means more than grade in adenoid cystic carcinoma. Am J Surg 1992;164:623–628.
7. Spiro RH, Huvos AG, Strong EW. Cancer of the parotid gland: a clinicopathological study of 288 primary cases. Am J Surg 1975;130:452–459.
8. AJCC. American Joint Committee for Cancer Staging and End Results Reporting. Manual for Staging of Cancer. Chicago: American Joint Committee, 1978.
9. Spiro RH, Thaler HT, Hicks WF, et al. The importance of clinical staging of minor salivary gland carcinoma. Am J Surg 1991;162:330–336.

10. Spiro RH, Hajdu SI, Strong EW. Tumors of the submaxillary gland. Am J Surg 1976;132:463–468.
11. Armstrong JG, Harrison LB, Spiro RH, Fass DE, Strong EW, Fuks ZY. Malignant tumors of major salivary gland: a match pair analysis of the role of combined surgery and postoperative radiotherapy. Arch Otolaryngol Head Neck Surg 1990;116:290–293.
12. Laramore GE, Krall JM, Griffin TW. Neutron versus photon irradiation for unresectable salivary gland tumors: final report of an RTOG-MRC randomized clinical trial. Int J Radiat Oncol Biol Phys 1993;27:235–240.
13. Kaplan MJ, Johns ME, Cantrell RW. Chemotherapy for salivary gland cancer. Otolaryngol Head Neck Surg 1986;95:165–170.

Section 2

Endocrine Malignancies

CHAPTER 10

Thyroid Neoplasms

PETER Y. WONG
RICHARD A. PRINZ

Thyroid Nodules

A. Epidemiology and Etiology

The presence of a single or multiple nodule(s) in an otherwise apparently normal thyroid gland is termed nodular thyroid disease. Even though most thyroid nodules are benign, both physicians and patients are concerned about cancer. According to epidemiologic studies in North America, the prevalence of a palpable thyroid nodule in adults is 4–7%, with new nodules developing at a rate of 0.1% per year.[1] Thyroid nodules are more common in women than in men.[2] They are also more common in older persons, people who live in endemic areas of iodine deficiency,[3] and people with previous exposure to ionizing radiation.[4] Infants and children who received 200–500 cGy of ionizing radiation develop new nodules at a rate of 2% per year, reaching a peak incidence in 15–25 years.[5]

In the United States approximately 12,000 new thyroid cancers are diagnosed annually, and about 1000 patients die from the disease.[2] Fifteen percent of clinically solitary thyroid nodules are malignant.[6] During the 1980s fine-needle aspiration biopsy (FNAB) became the diagnostic tool of choice for thyroid nodules, and its use increased the yield of thyroid cancer at operation and decreased the number of unnecessary thyroidectomies. This chapter discusses the evaluation of thyroid nodules and the management of patients with papillary, follicular, Hurthle cell, and medullary cancer, lymphoma, and anaplastic cancer of the thyroid gland.

B. Diagnosis

History and Physical Examination The initial evaluation of a thyroid nodule is no different from that for any other disease: No diagnostic test can replace the history and physical examination. The history should determine whether there has been prior external irradiation of the head and neck area, as these patients have a 40% chance of harboring a malignancy in a palpable thyroid nodule. The possibility of malignancy increases if a thyroid nodule has grown rapidly or caused symptoms of local compression (i.e., difficulty speaking, breathing, or swallowing).

Thyroid Nodules

A.

Epidemiology and Etiology

Thyroid nodules

≤10% Malignant

Risk factors
- Previous irradiation
- Extremes of age
- Male gender
- Rapid growth
- Local compression

High risk conditions
- Family history of medullary cancer
- MEN 2
- Familial polyposis
- Cowden's disease

B.

Diagnosis

History and physical examination
Fine-needle aspiration biopsy (FNAB)
Consider ultrasonography directed for a small nodule or previously negative FNAB

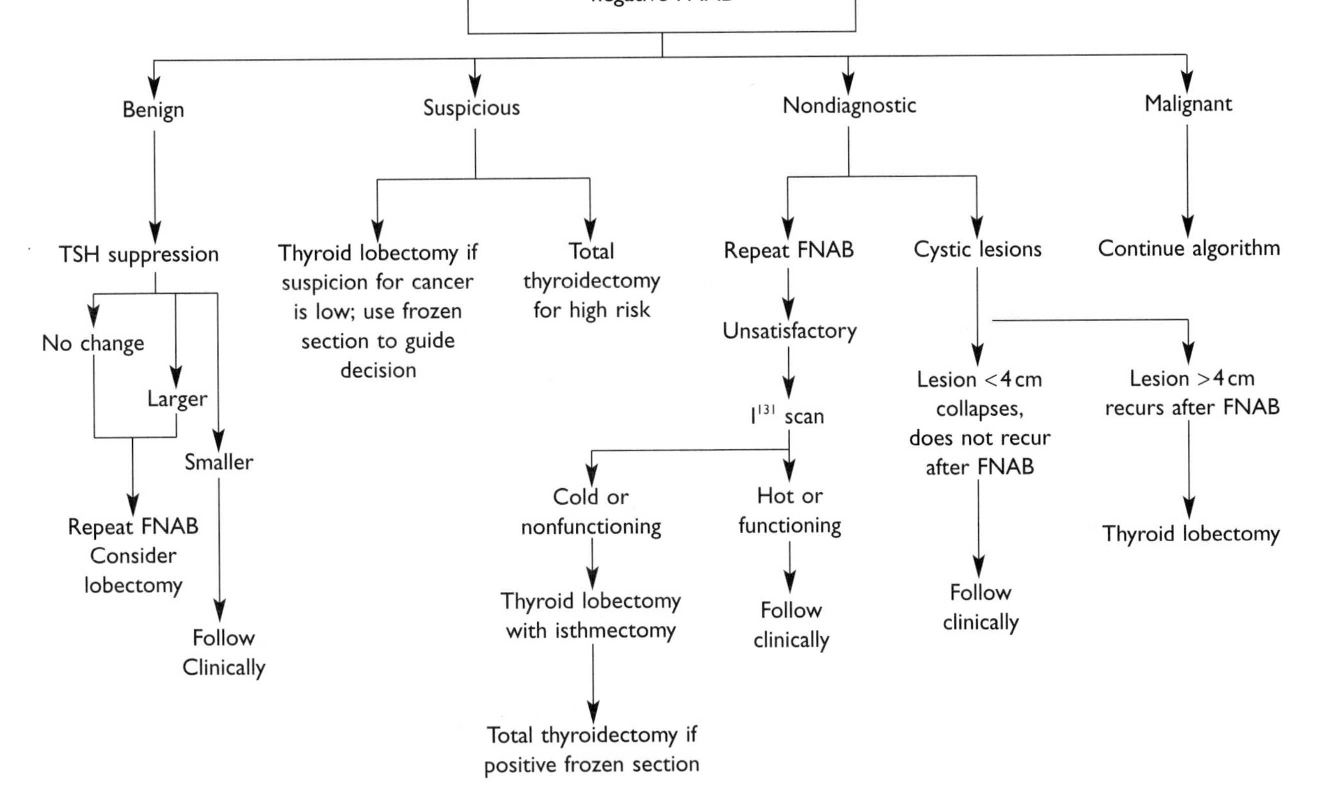

Nodules found in men and in patients at the extremes of age are more likely to be cancerous. A family history of thyroid malignancy, particularly medullary carcinoma [a feature of multiple endocrine neoplasia (MEN)] increases the chance of a thyroid nodule being malignant. *MEN 2A syndrome* consists of parathyroid hyperplasia, pheochromocytoma, and medullary carcinoma of the thyroid; *MEN 2B* consists of ganglioneuromas, pheochromocytoma, and medullary carcinoma of the thyroid (see Chapter 17) *Familial adenomatous polyposis coli* carries a high risk of developing carcinomas of the colon, stomach, duodenum, periampullary region, and thyroid. The incidence of papillary carcinoma in patients with familial polyposis can be as high as 86%.[7] Patients with *Cowden's disease*, which consists of trichilemmomas of the adnexa, adenomas and carcinomas of the breast, and polyposis of the intestinal tract are at risk of developing a differentiated thyroid cancer.[8] On physical examination, a thyroid nodule is suspicious for malignancy if it is fixed to the adjacent tissue, if there is lymphadenopathy, and if there is ipsilateral vocal cord paralysis on indirect laryngoscopy.[1,2,9]

FINE-NEEDLE ASPIRATION BIOPSY The initial diagnostic test should be FNAB because it is accurate, inexpensive, and safe. FNAB has an overall sensitivity of 80–85%, specificity of 90–95%, false-negative rate of less than 5%, false-positive rate of 1–3%, and diagnostic accuracy of more than 95%.[10]

The results of cytodiagnosis can be divided into four categories: benign (70–75%), suspicious or indeterminate (10–15%), malignant (5%), unsatisfactory or nondiagnostic (5%). Nondiagnostic results may be due to inadequate samples, lack of sufficient cells to evaluate, or sampling error due to improper needle placement. Suspicious or indeterminate results are usually due to difficulty differentiating benign Hurthle cell and follicular cell neoplasms from their malignant counterparts. A complete evaluation of the capsule is needed for this differentiation.

There is an increased risk of sampling error in large nodules (>4 cm) because acellular, cystic, or necrotic tissue may be obtained. Conversely, small nodules (<1 cm) may be missed altogether.[11] Ultrasound-guided FNAB is recommended if a thyroid nodule is smaller than 1 cm or cannot be palpated or if the FNAB is repeatedly nondiagnostic based on palpation-guided biopsies.

Benign Nodules Patients with benign nodules are given synthroid to suppress thyroid-stimulating hormone (TSH) and are reevaluated regularly during the course of the ensuing year by physical examination to assess nodule size. A repeat FNAB is performed if the size of the nodule does not decrease. If the nodule size increases, FNAB is repeated sooner or the nodule removed via thyroid lobectomy.[10]

Suspicious or Indeterminate Results We and others[1,2,10] recommend thyroidectomy if suspicious or indeterminate cytology is obtained following FNAB, as up to 30% of such nodules harbor cancer. At especially high risk are nodules with FNAB findings that show a predominance of follicular cells, as they have a 60% chance of being a neoplasm.[12] Near-total or total thyroidectomy is recommended when the likelihood of cancer is high (i.e., patients with a family history of thyroid cancer, especially medullary carcinoma or MEN 2, a rapidly growing tumor, hard nodules, fixation to adjacent structures, vocal cord paralysis, enlarged lymph nodes, or distant metastases). Lobectomy with isthmectomy is recommended when the clinical suspicion of malignancy is low.[13]

Unsatisfactory or Nondiagnostic Results Cytology studies are unsatisfactory or nondiagnostic for fewer than 5% of nodules. In such cases we recommend repeat FNAB, as satisfactory results can be obtained in more than 50%.[2] Ultrasound-guided FNAB may be helpful in this situation, especially if the nodule is intrathyroid, <1 cm, or a mixed cystic lesion. Clinical correlation and iodine-123 (I^{123}) or technetium-99m (Tc^{99m}) thyroid scintigraphy should be used if repeated aspirates still yield unsatisfactory results. About 10–15% of cold nodules, <5% of warm nodules, and <1–2% of hot nodules are malignant.[1] We recommend surgical excision (total lobectomy with isthmectomy) for cold nodules when FNAB cytology has been indeterminate; if a frozen section shows malignancy, total thyroidectomy is performed. Warm and hot nodules can be observed clinically if there are no other clinical features suggesting cancer.[1,9,10]

Cystic Lesions Cystic lesions account for as many as 30% of all thyroid nodules. Most are benign, but about 10–15% of cystic lesions are malignant. If cystic lesions are >4 cm, recur after three aspirations, or do not decompress completely after aspiration, they should be surgically excised. Conversely, if a cyst is <4 cm, totally collapses, and does not recur after aspiration, the patient can simply be followed.

Malignant Thyroid Lesions

Thyroid carcinomas comprise fewer than 1% of all human cancers.[14] The incidence ranges from 0.5 to 10.0 cases per 100,000 population per year in different parts of the world.[15] Thyroid malignancies are two to four times more common in women than in men, with the median age at diagnosis 45–50 years. Investigators have discovered that as many as one-third of papillary carcinomas have *RET* gene rearrangements, which increases to 60–80% if the patient has a history of external irradiation.[16–22] Other evidence suggests that *RAS* gene mutation is an early event in thyroid tumorigenesis; a similar frequency of *RAS* gene mutations is found in follicular adenomas and carcinomas.[23,24] In some follicular carcinomas, mutations are found in the genes encoding the thyrotropin receptor and the α-subunit

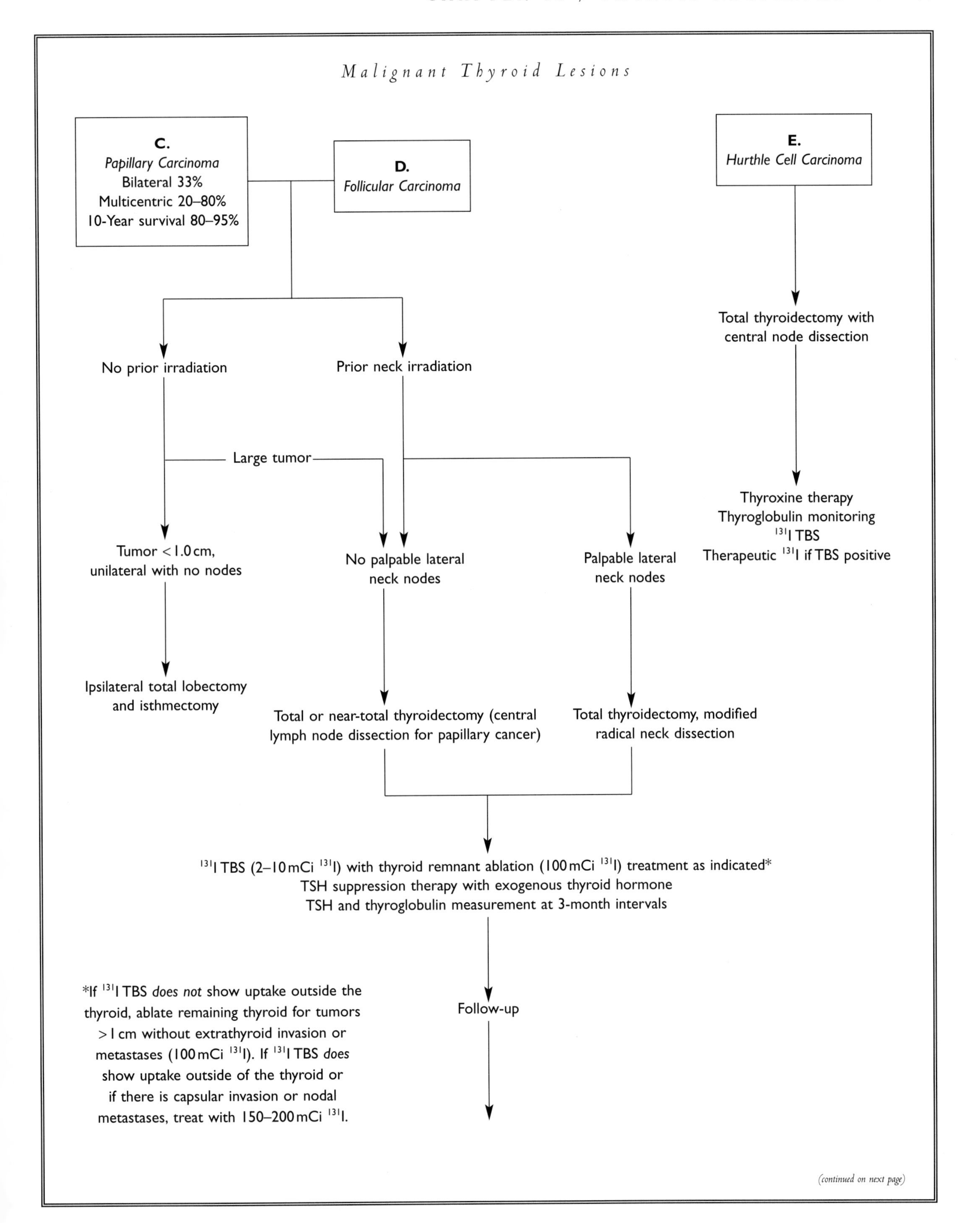
Malignant Thyroid Lesions
C.
Papillary Carcinoma
Bilateral 33%
Multicentric 20–80%
10-Year survival 80–95%
D.
Follicular Carcinoma
E.
Hurthle Cell Carcinoma
No prior irradiation
Prior neck irradiation
Large tumor
Tumor < 1.0 cm, unilateral with no nodes
No palpable lateral neck nodes
Palpable lateral neck nodes
Ipsilateral total lobectomy and isthmectomy
Total or near-total thyroidectomy (central lymph node dissection for papillary cancer)
Total thyroidectomy, modified radical neck dissection
Total thyroidectomy with central node dissection
Thyroxine therapy
Thyroglobulin monitoring
131I TBS
Therapeutic 131I if TBS positive
131I TBS (2–10 mCi 131I) with thyroid remnant ablation (100 mCi 131I) treatment as indicated*
TSH suppression therapy with exogenous thyroid hormone
TSH and thyroglobulin measurement at 3-month intervals
Follow-up
*If 131I TBS does not show uptake outside the thyroid, ablate remaining thyroid for tumors > 1 cm without extrathyroid invasion or metastases (100 mCi 131I). If 131I TBS does show uptake outside of the thyroid or if there is capsular invasion or nodal metastases, treat with 150–200 mCi 131I.
(continued on next page)

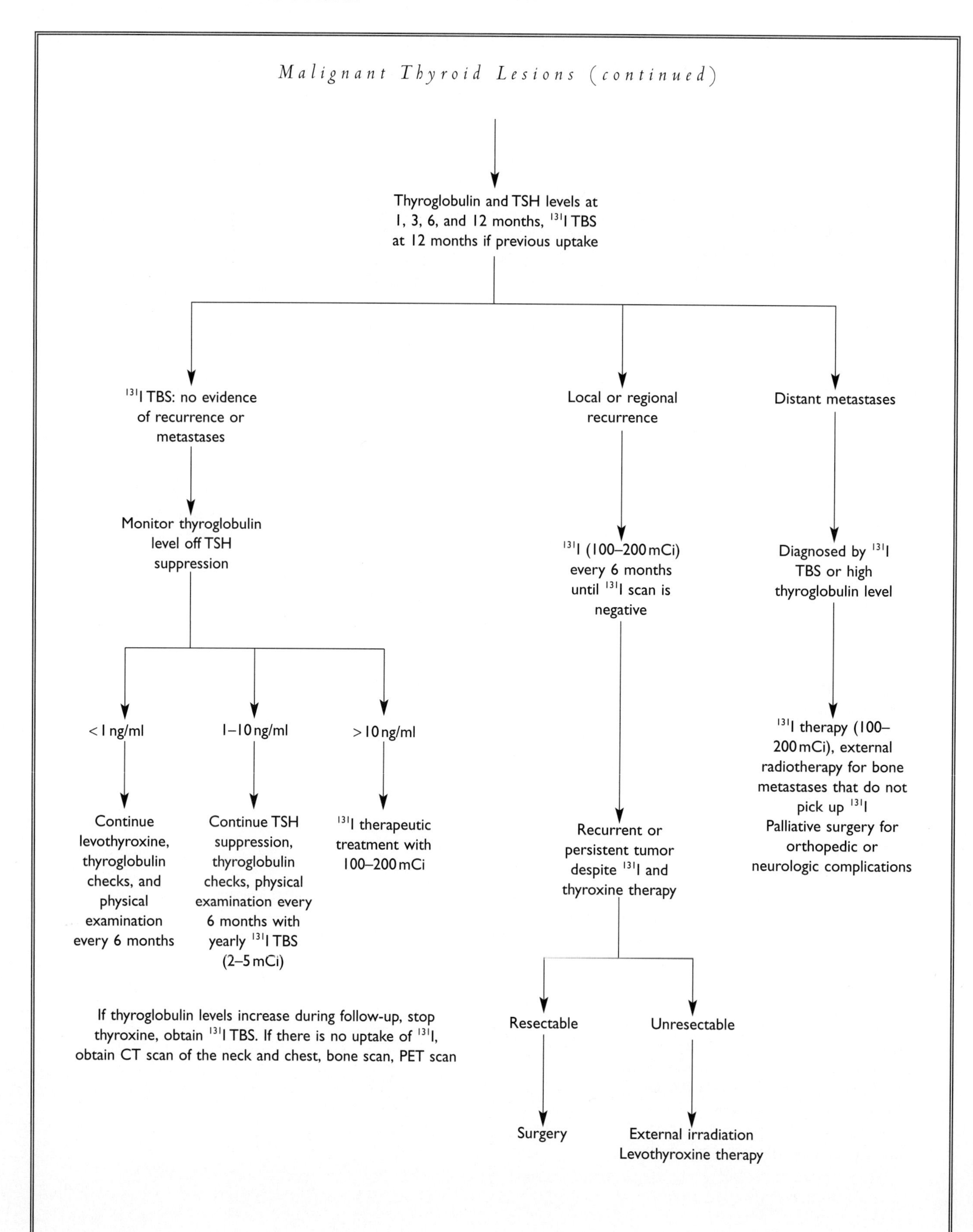
Malignant Thyroid Lesions (continued)
Thyroglobulin and TSH levels at 1, 3, 6, and 12 months, 131I TBS at 12 months if previous uptake
131I TBS: no evidence of recurrence or metastases
Local or regional recurrence
Distant metastases
Monitor thyroglobulin level off TSH suppression
131I (100–200 mCi) every 6 months until 131I scan is negative
Diagnosed by 131I TBS or high thyroglobulin level
< 1 ng/ml
1–10 ng/ml
> 10 ng/ml
131I therapy (100–200 mCi), external radiotherapy for bone metastases that do not pick up 131I
Palliative surgery for orthopedic or neurologic complications
Continue levothyroxine, thyroglobulin checks, and physical examination every 6 months
Continue TSH suppression, thyroglobulin checks, physical examination every 6 months with yearly 131I TBS (2–5 mCi)
131I therapeutic treatment with 100–200 mCi
Recurrent or persistent tumor despite 131I and thyroxine therapy
If thyroglobulin levels increase during follow-up, stop thyroxine, obtain 131I TBS. If there is no uptake of 131I, obtain CT scan of the neck and chest, bone scan, PET scan
Resectable
Unresectable
Surgery
External irradiation
Levothyroxine therapy

of the stimulatory G (G_s) protein.[24,25] Moreover, inactivating mutations of *p53* are common in anaplastic thyroid carcinomas.[26,27]

Radiation exposure before the age of 15 is a major risk factor. Most thyroid carcinomas caused by external radiation to the neck during childhood are papillary carcinomas.[28–30] The risk of thyroid carcinoma is increased by a factor of 7.7 in a child exposed to a dose of 1 Gy.[29] The risk is increased with a dose as low as 10 cGy. At doses >1.5 Gy, the risk decreases because of cell killing. The latent period between radiation exposure and diagnosis is at least 5 years, and the risk continues to increase for 20–30 or even more years after exposure. Patients receiving I^{131} for diagnostic or therapeutic purposes do not have an increased risk of thyroid cancer.[28–30] However, intense environmental radiation exposure due to isotopes of iodine increases the incidence of thyroid cancer, as evidenced by the rise in papillary thyroid carcinoma in the Marshall Islands after atomic bomb testing and in Belarus and Ukraine after the Chernobyl nuclear accident.[31,32]

Management of a thyroid malignancy depends on the type of cancer, its etiology, the patient's family history, the symptoms, and the physical findings. Thyroid carcinomas are classified as follows.

- Differentiated tumors
  - Papillary
  - Follicular
  - Hurthle cell
- Medullary
- Anaplastic
- Other
  - Lymphoma
  - Metastatic carcinoma
  - Squamous cell carcinoma

C. Papillary Carcinoma

Papillary carcinoma comprises approximately 80% of primary thyroid cancers. It is a heterogeneous group of malignancies that originate from the follicular epithelial cells.[33] Papillary carcinoma is often bilateral (33%) and multicentric (20–80%). It typically spreads through the lymphatics in the thyroid to the regional lymph nodes and less commonly to lungs, bone, and brain.[14] The overall 10-year survival rate is approximately 80–95% for middle-age and younger adults. According to Schlumberger,[14] 5–20% of patients have local or regional recurrences and 10–15% have distant metastasis. There are three prognostic indicators for recurrent disease or death.

1. Age is important. Patients younger than 15 or older than 50 are at greater risk.[34,35]

2. Certain histologic subtypes, such as tall cell, columnar cell, and diffuse sclerosing variants of papillary carcinoma carry a less favorable prognosis.[36,37]

3. Tumors >4 cm, invade beyond the thyroid capsule, or metastasize to lymph nodes and distant organs are more likely to recur or cause death.

These prognostic factors should guide the initial and follow-up treatment.

No Prior Radiation Exposure When papillary carcinoma is diagnosed by FNAB, surgical resection is indicated. If the thyroid nodule is ≤1 cm in diameter, unifocal, intrathyroid, and nonmetastatic with a clinically normal contralateral lobe, it may be treated by ipsilateral total lobectomy and isthmectomy.[33]

Prior Irradiation to the Head and Neck and Other Factors For patients with a history of irradiation to the neck, bilateral disease, tumor size >1.5 cm in diameter, or cervical metastases, a total or near-total thyroidectomy by an experienced surgeon is the best treatment. The rationale for total thyroidectomy is as follows.

1. Tumor is present in the contralateral lobe in 30–85% of patients with papillary carcinoma.[38]

2. Tumor recurrence appears in the contralateral lobe in 5–10% of patients.[39]

3. Fifty percent of patients with central neck recurrence die because of recurrent disease.[40]

4. The recurrence rate is lower and the long-term survival rate is better with initial aggressive therapy.[40,41]

5. Total thyroidectomy facilitates detection and treatment of recurrent or metastatic carcinoma by I^{131} scanning.[33]

6. Serum thyroglobulin determinations for persistent, recurrent, or metastatic tumor are more sensitive and accurate if there is no remaining normal thyroid tissue.[42]

7. The small chance of a differentiated tumor degenerating into an anaplastic carcinoma is eliminated.[43]

The operation can and should be performed with negligible mortality and a complication rate of less than 2–3%.[44–48] In addition to total or near-total thyroidectomy, the lymph nodes in the central compartment (paratracheal and tracheoesophageal areas), in the lower third of the jugulocarotid chain, and in the ipsilateral supraclavicular area should be evaluated.[14] In approximately two-thirds of the patients who have lymph node metastasis, more than 80% of the positive lymph nodes are found in

Distant Metastases Distant metastases to the lungs and bones are most common and occur in 10–15% of patients. Distant metastasis can be diagnosed in two-thirds of the patients using ^{131}I TBS. Almost all patients with distant metastasis have high serum thyroglobulin levels.[14] Patients should be treated with ^{131}I using 100–150 mCi if the metastatic tumor picks up ^{131}I. Surgery is palliative and is done mostly for orthopedic or neurologic complications.[58,59,60] External radiotherapy is given to patients with bony metastases that do not pick up ^{131}I.[61]

D. Follicular Carcinoma

Follicular carcinoma constitutes approximately 10% of primary thyroid cancers. Follicular carcinomas are encapsulated tumors that invade through their capsule and into blood vessels. They tend to metastasize hematogenously to distant sites, mainly lung and bone. Follicular carcinoma can be distinguished from a follicular adenoma only by examining the capsule or blood vessels for invasion. Therefore it is difficult if not impossible to diagnose follicular carcinoma by FNAB. Lymph node involvement is uncommon with follicular carcinoma compared to papillary carcinoma (25–35% vs. 10–15%). However, as many as 33% of patients with follicular carcinoma have distant metastases at initial presentation.[9,39]

Follicular carcinoma, like papillary carcinoma, is classified as a differentiated thyroid cancer. Treatment is similar for both follicular and papillary carcinoma. Ipsilateral total lobectomy and isthmectomy are recommended for patients without prior radiation exposure who have unilateral tumors <1 cm in size. Patients with prior radiation exposure require total or near-total thyroidectomy. Lymph node dissection is performed only if palpable nodes are found during surgery. Thyroxine therapy and clinical follow-up with serum thyroglobulin levels and ^{131}I TBS are similar to that discussed for papillary carcinoma (see above).[14]

E. Hurthle Cell Carcinoma

Hurthle cell carcinomas constitute about 3–5% of all thyroid malignancies. Hurthle cells are derived from the follicular epithelium; therefore they produce thyroglobulin and have TSH receptors, as do papillary and follicular carcinomas. Like follicular cancer, Hurthle cell carcinoma is difficult to diagnose by FNAB and is distinguished from a Hurthle cell adenoma by examining for capsular or vascular invasion.[9] Benign lesions such as Hashimoto's thyroiditis and multinodular goiter can be confused with a Hurthle cell neoplasm on FNAB. Hurthle cell carcinomas invade the regional lymph nodes more often than follicular carcinomas and are frequently multifocal and bilateral. Only 10% of Hurthle cell carcinomas take up radioactive iodine.[62]

Hurthle cell carcinomas are treated by total thyroidectomy with central compartment lymph node dissection. If the central neck nodes are involved or there are clinically palpable nodes in the lateral neck, a modified radical neck dissection is warranted.[62] Because Hurthle cell carcinomas produce thyroglobulin and have TSH receptors, postoperative TSH suppression therapy and thyroglobulin monitoring for recurrence and metastases are warranted. Even though 90% of Hurthle cell carcinomas do not pick up ^{131}I, an initial ^{131}I TBS should be performed and ^{131}I radioiodine therapy given if the ^{131}I TBS is positive.[9,62]

Other Thyroid Carcinomas

F. Medullary Carcinoma

Medullary thyroid carcinomas (MTCs) constitute about 5% of all thyroid cancers[63] and are derived from the thyroid parafollicular cells (C-cells). These neuroendocrine cells secrete calcitonin; and plasma calcitonin levels can be used as a marker for diagnosing and monitoring the course and treatment of MTCs. It was once the best marker for screening family members for hereditary forms of the disease, but this can now be accomplished by genetic screening for the *RET* proto-oncogene abnormality on chromosome 10. MTC occurs as a sporadic or hereditary tumor with an incidence of approximately 60% or 40%, respectively. In its sporadic form the tumor is usually single and unilateral. In its hereditary form the tumor is usually multifocal, bilateral, and inherited in an autosomal dominant pattern. The sporadic and hereditary tumors are typically more aggressive than the differentiated thyroid cancers (papillary and follicular), and lymph node metastases are often present at the initial presentation. The hereditary forms occur in MEN 2A, MEN 2B and familial MTC (FMTC). The MTC in patients with MEN 2B is more aggressive than in those with MEN 2A; FMTC is the most indolent type.[9,64]

Preoperative Evaluation The preoperative evaluation of patients with known MTC includes the following measures.

1. Carcinoembryonic antigen (CEA) level (elevated CEA levels are associated with metastatic disease)[65]
2. Basal or stimulated calcitonin levels (or both)
3. Screening for hyperparathyroidism (serum calcium and intact parathyroid hormone)
4. Screening for pheochromocytoma (24 hour urine collection for catecholamines, vanillylmandelic acid, and metanephrines)

Treatment Total thyroidectomy with central compartment lymph node dissection is the primary treatment for patients with MTC. For those with palpable jugular or paratracheal lymph nodes or a tumor >2 cm, ipsilateral modified radical neck dissection is warranted. Patients are followed by physical examination and plasma calcitonin levels. Elevated calcitonin levels indicate residual or recurrent disease. One should attempt to localize an occult recurrence using ultrasonography, CT scans, a nuclear imaging study with ^{131}I metaiodobenzylguanidine (MIBG), or selective venous catheterization. Surgical neck exploration and lymph node dissection should be performed for localized recurrences.[9,64]

FAMILY SCREENING The precursor of MTC, C-cell hyperplasia is found in the hereditary form of the disease. Investigators have found that defects in the *RET* proto-oncogene are responsible for FMTC, MEN 2A, and MEN 2B.[66–69] Family screening should be done for MTC; individuals are at 50% risk for the disease if they have an affected parent or sibling. First degree relatives of patients with MTC should be screened for the *RET* mutation on chromosome 10; if the *RET* mutation test is negative, the tested individual will not develop MTC and no further testing or treatment is needed. On the other hand, if the *RET* mutation is present, prophylactic total thyroidectomy is recommended for affected individuals starting at age 5.[9,64]

G. Lymphoma

Primary thyroid lymphoma accounts for 1% of all thyroid cancers.[70] Non-Hodgkin's lymphoma is the predominant type and usually occurs in older women with Hashimoto's thyroiditis.[71–73] The diagnosis can be established by FNAB or open biopsy. If a lymphoma is confined within the thyroid, total thyroidectomy with radiotherapy achieves favorable results. The 5-year survival rate for patients with resectable intrathyroid lymphoma is 75–85%.[9,74–76] Thyroid lymphoma that has invaded adjacent tissue is unresectable. FNAB or open biopsy is used to obtain the diagnosis. Irradiation and chemotherapy comprise the treatment of choice. The 5-year survival rate for patients with extrathyroid lymphoma is 35–40%.[9,74–76]

H. Anaplastic Carcinoma

Anaplastic thyroid carcinoma occurs more often in endemic goiter areas. It should be suspected in any elderly patient with a rapidly growing thyroid nodule. Well differentiated thyroid carcinomas (papillary and follicular) can dedifferentiate into anaplastic thyroid cancer. In fact, differentiated thyroid cancer is found in approximately 80% of patients with anaplastic cancer.[9] Fifty percent of patients with anaplastic cancers have a long history of thyroid nodules. Even though anaplastic carcinoma accounts for only 1% of all primary thyroid carcinomas, it is the most lethal form of thyroid malignancy.[77] Five-year survival is rare, and the median survival averages only 6 months.[78] Open biopsy and tracheostomy are the most common surgical procedures, reflecting the advanced stage of the disease at presentation.

The latest treatment is multimodality therapy. Described by Tennvall et al.,[79] it involves preoperative high-voltage irradiation with a target dose of 30 Gy and a postoperative total dose of 46 Gy. Chemotherapy consists of 20 mg doxorubicin given intravenously each week for 7–9 weeks. The first dose is begun 1–2 hours before the first radiation treatment up to a dose of 400–750 mg/m^2. In Tennvall et al.'s study debulking was possible in 70% of patients so treated; almost 50% of patients had no recurrence, but approximately 25% of treated patients died because of local failure.

References

1. Rojeski MT, Gharib H. Nodular thyroid disease. N Engl J Med 1985; 313:428–436.
2. Mazzaferri JF. Management of thyroid neoplasms. N Engl J Med 1993; 328:553–559.
3. Vigneri R. Studies on the goiter endemia in Sicily. J Endocrinol Invest 1988;11:831–843.
4. Hanson GA, Komorowski RA, Cerletty JM, et al. Thyroid gland morphology in young adults: normal subjects versus those with prior low-dose neck irradiation in childhood. Surgery 1983;94:984–988.
5. DeGroot LJ. Clinical review. 2. Diagnostic approach and management of patients exposed to irradiation to the thyroid. J Clin Endocrinol Metab 1989;69:925–928.
6. Staunton MD, Greening WP. Clinical diagnosis of thyroid cancer. BMJ 1973;4:532–535.
7. Bell B, Mazzaferri EL. Familial adenomatous polyposis (Gardner's syndrome) and thyroid carcinoma: a case report and review of the literature. Dig Dis Sci 1993;38:185–190.
8. Sogol PB, Sugawara M, Gordon HE, et al. Cowden's disease: familial goiter and skin hamartomas; a report of three cases. West J Med 1983;139: 324–328.
9. Soh EY, Clark OH. Surgical considerations and approach to thyroid cancer. Endocrinol Metab Clin North Am 1996;25:115–139.
10. Gharib H, Goellner JR. Fine-needle aspiration biopsy of the thyroid: an appraisal. Ann Intern Med 1993;118:282–289.
11. Caruso D, Mazzaferri EL. Fine needle aspiration biopsy in the management of thyroid nodules. Endocrinologist 1991;1:194–202.
12. De Jong SA, Demeter JG, Castelli M, et al. Follicular cell predominance in the cytologic examination of dominant thyroid nodules indicates a sixty percent incidence of neoplasia. Surgery 1990;108:794–800.
13. Hamming JF, Goslings BM, Van Steenis GJ, et al. The value of fine-needle aspiration biopsy in patients with nodular thyroid disease divided into groups of suspicion of malignant neoplasms on clinical grounds. Arch Intern Med 1990;150:113–116.
14. Schlumberger MJ. Papillary and follicular thyroid carcinoma. N Engl J Med 1998;338:297–306.
15. Parkin DM, Muir CS, Whelan SL, et al. Cancer Incidence in five continents. IARC Sci Publ 6(120–145).
16. Santoro M, Carlomagno F, Hay ID, et al. RET oncogene activation in human thyroid neoplasms is restricted to the papillary cancer subtype. J Clin Invest 1992;89:1517–1522.
17. Bongarzone I, Fugazzola L, Vigneri P, et al. Age related activation of the tyrosine kinase receptor protooncogenes RET and NTRK1 in papillary thyroid carcinoma. J Clin Endocrinol Metab 1996;81:2006–2009.

18. Zou M, Shi Y, Farid NR. Low rate of ret proto-oncogene activation (PTC/RET^{TPC}) in papillary thyroid carcinomas from Saudi Arabia. Cancer 1994;73:176–180.
19. Fugazzola L, Pilotti S, Pinchera A, et al. Oncogenic rearrangements of the RET proto-oncogene in papillary thyroid carcinomas from children exposed to the Chernobyl nuclear accident. Cancer Res 1995;55:5617–5620.
20. Klugbauer S, Lengfelder E, Demidchik EP, et al. High prevalence of RET rearrangement in thyroid tumors of children from Belarus after the Chernobyl reactor accident. Oncogene 1995;11:2459–2467.
21. Nikiforov YE, Rowland JM, Bove KE, et al. Distinct pattern of ret oncogene rearrangements in morphological variants of radiation-induced and sporadic thyroid papillary carcinomas in children. Cancer Res 1997;57: 1690–1694.
22. Bounacer A, Wicker R, Caillou B, et al. High prevalence of activating RET proto-oncogene rearrangements in thyroid tumors from patients who had received external radiation. Oncogene 1997;15:1263–1273.
23. Fagin JA. Molecular pathogenesis. In: Braverman LE, Utiger RD (eds) Werner and Ingbar's The Thyroid: A Fundamental and Clinical Text, 7th ed. Philadelphia: Lippincott-Raven, 1996;909–916.
24. Challeton C, Bounacer A, Du Villard JA, et al. Pattern of ras and gsp oncogene mutations in radiation-associated human thyroid tumors. Oncogene 1995;11:601–603.
25. Russo D, Arturi F, Schlumberger M, et al. Activating mutations of the TSH receptor in differentiated thyroid carcinomas. Oncogene 1995;11: 1907–1911.
26. Fagin JA, Matsuo K, Karmakar A, et al. High prevalence of mutations of the p53 gene in poorly differentiated human thyroid carcinomas. J Clin Invest 1993;91:179–184.
27. Ito T, Seyama T, Mizuno T, et al. Unique association of p53 mutations with undifferentiated but not with differentiated carcinomas of the thyroid gland. Cancer Res 1992;52:1369–1371.
28. Shore RE. Issues and epidemiological evidence regarding radiation-induced thyroid cancer. Radiat Res 1992;131:98–111.
29. Ron E, Lubin JH, Shore RE, et al. Thyroid cancer after exposure to external radiation: a pooled analysis of seven studies. Radiat Res 1995;141: 259–277.
30. Schneider AB, Ron E. Pathogenesis. In: Braverman LE, Utiger RD (eds) Werner and Ingbar's The Thyroid: A Fundamental and Clinical Text, 7th ed. Philadelphia: Lippincott-Raven, 1996;902–909.
31. Dobyns BM, Hyrmer BA. The surgical management of benign and malignant thyroid neoplasms in Marshall Islanders exposed to hydrogen bomb fallout. World J Surg 1992;16:126–140.
32. Kazakov VS, Demidchik EP, Astakhova LN. Thyroid cancer after Chernobyl. Nature 1992;359:21.
33. LiVolsi VA. Surgical Pathology of the Thyroid. Philadelphia: Saunders, 1990.
34. Brander A, Viikinikoski P, Nickels J, et al. Thyroid gland: ultrasound screening in middle-aged women with no previous thyroid disease. Radiology 1989;173:507.
35. Brander A, Viikinikoski P, Nickels J, et al. Thyroid gland: ultrasound screening in a random adult population. Radiology 1991;181:683.
36. Bottger IG. Minimal thyroid cancer: clinical consequences. Recent Results Cancer Res 1988;106:139.
37. Bronner MP, LiVolsi VA. Spindle cell squamous carcinoma of the thyroid: an unusual anaplastic tumor associated with tall cell papillary cancer. Mod Pathol 1991;4:637.
38. Russel WO, Ibanez ML, Clark RL, et al. Thyroid carcinoma: classification, intraglandular dissemination, and clinicopathological study based upon whole organ section of 80 glands. Cancer 1963;16:1425.
39. Hirabayashi RN, Lindsay S. Carcinoma of the thyroid gland: a statistical study of 390 patients. J Clin Endocrinol Metab 1961;21:1596–1610.
40. Mazzaferri EL, Young RL. Papillary thyroid carcinoma: a 10 year follow-up report of the impact of therapy in 576 patients. Am J Med 1981;70:511–518.
41. Mazzaferri EL, Jhiany SM. Long-term impact of initial surgical and medical therapy on papillary and follicular thyroid cancer. Am J Med 1994; 97:418–428.
42. Pineda JD, Lee T, Ain KB, et al. ^{131}I therapy for thyroid cancer patients with elevated thyroglobulin and negative diagnostic scan. J Clin Endocrinol Metab 1995;80:1488.
43. Massin JP, Savoie JC, Garnier H, et al. Pulmonary metastases in differentiated thyroid carcinoma: study of 58 cases with implications for the primary tumor treatment. Cancer 1984;53:982–992.
44. Attie JN, Moskowitz GW, Marfouleff D, et al. Feasibility of total thyroidectomy in the treatment of thyroid carcinoma. Am J Surg 1979;138: 555–560.
45. Beierwaltes WH, Nishiyama RH, Thompson NW, et al. Survival time and cure in papillary and follicular thyroid carcinoma with distant metastases: statistics following University of Michigan therapy. J Nucl Med 1982; 23:561.
46. Clark OH. Total thyroidectomy: the treatment of choice for patients with differentiated thyroid cancer. Ann Surg 1982;196:361–370.
47. Lennquist S. Surgical strategy in thyroid carcinoma: a clinical review. Acta Chir Scand 1986;152:321–338.
48. Thompson NW, Nishiyama RH, Harness JK. Thyroid carcinoma: current controversies. Curr Probl Surg 1978;15:1–67.
49. DeGroot LJ, Kaplan EL, McCormick M, et al. Natural history, treatment, and course of papillary carcinoma. J Clin Endocrinol Metab 1990;71: 414–424.
50. Mazzaferri EL, Jhiang SM. Long term impact of initial surgical and medical therapy on papillary and follicular thyroid cancer. Am J Med 1994;97: 418–428.
51. Lakshmanan M, Schaffer A, Robbins J, et al. A simplified low iodine diet in ^{131}I scanning and therapy of thyroid cancer. Clin Nucl Med 1988;13:866.
52. Benua RS, Leeper RD. A method and rationale for treating metastatic thyroid carcinoma with the largest safe dose of ^{131}I. In: Medeiros-Neto G, Gaitan E (eds) Frontiers in Thyroidology. New York: Plenum, 1986;1317.
53. Bartalena L, Martino E, Pacchiarotti A, et al. Factors affecting suppression of endogenous thyrotropin secretion by thyroxine treatment: retrospective analysis in athyreotic and goitrous patients. J Clin Endocrinol Metab 1987;64:849–855.
54. Marcocci C, Golia F, Bruno-Bossio G, et al. Carefully monitored levothyroxine suppressive therapy is not associated with bone loss in premenopausal women. J Clin Endocrinol Metab 1994;78:818–823.
55. Hoefnagel CA, Delprat CC, Marcuse HR, et al. Role of thallium-201 total-body scintigraphy in follow-up of thyroid carcinoma. J Nucl Med 1986; 27:1854–1857.
56. Lind P, Gallowitsch HJ, Langsteger W, et al. Technetium-99m-tetrofosmin whole-body scintigraphy in the follow-up of differentiated thyroid carcinoma. J Nucl Med 1997;38:348–352.
57. Feine U, Lietzenmayer R, Hanke JP, et al. Fluorine-18-FDG and iodine-131-iodide uptake in thyroid cancer. J Nucl Med 1996;37:1468–1472.
58. Hoie J, Stenwig AE, Kullmann G, et al. Distant metastases in papillary thyroid cancer: a review of 91 patients. Cancer 1988;61:1–6.
59. Marcocci C, Pacini F, Eliser R, et al. Clinical and biological behavior of bone metastases from differentiated thyroid carcinoma. Surgery 1989;106: 960–966.
60. Niederle B, Roka R, Schemper M, et al. Surgical treatment of distant metastases in differentiated thyroid cancer: indication and results. Surgery 1986;100:1088–1097.
61. Schlumberger M, Challeton C, De Vathaire F, et al. Radioactive iodine treatment and external radiotherapy for lung and bone metastases from thyroid carcinoma. J Nucl Med 1996;37:598–605.

62. Azadian A, Irving RB, Walfish PG, et al. Management considerations in Hurthle cell carcinoma. Surgery 1995;118:711–715.
63. Block MA. Surgical treatment of medullary carcinoma of the thyroid. Otolaryngol Clin North Am 1990;23:453–473.
64. Moley JF. Medullary thyroid cancer. Surg Clin North Am 1995;75:405–420.
65. Busnardo B, Girelli M, Sinioni N, et al. Nonparallel patterns of calcitonin and carcinoembryonic antigen levels in the follow-up of medullary thyroid carcinoma. Cancer 1984;53:278.
66. Carlson K, Dou S, Chi D, et al. Single missense mutation in the tyrosine kinase catalytic domain of the RET protooncogene is associated with multiple endocrine neoplasia type 2B. Proc Natl Acad Sci USA 1994;91: 1579.
67. Donis-Keller H, Dou S, Chi D. Mutations in the RET proto-oncogene are associated with MEN 2A and FMTC. Hum Mol Genet 1993;2:851.
68. Goodfellow P. Inherited cancers associated with the RET proto-oncogene. Curr Opin Genet Dev 1994;4:446.
69. Mulligan L, Kwok J, Healy C. Germ-line mutations of the RET protooncogene in multiple endocrine neoplasia type 2A. Nature 1993;363: 458.
70. Samaan NA, Ordonez NG. Uncommon types of thyroid cancer. Endocrinol Metab Clin North Am 1990;19:637–648.
71. Compagno J, Oertel JE. Malignant lymphoma and other lymphoproliferative disorders of the thyroid gland: a clinicopathologic study of 245 cases. Am J Clin Pathol 1980;74:1–11.
72. Russel WO, Ibanez ML, Clark RL. Thyroid carcinoma: classification, intraglandular dissemination, and clinicopathological study based upon whole organ section of 80 glands. Cancer 1963;16:1425.
73. Sirota DK, Segal RL. Primary lymphomas of the thyroid gland. JAMA 1979;242:1743–1746.
74. Rosen IB, Sutcliffe SB, Gospodarowicz MK, et al. The role of surgery in the management of thyroid lymphoma. Surgery 1988;104:1095–1099.
75. Devine RM, Edis AJ, Banks PM. Primary lymphoma of the thyroid: a review of the Mayo Clinic experience through 1978. World J Surg 1981;5:33–38.
76. Pyke CM, Grant CS, Habermann TM, et al. Non-Hodgkin's lymphoma of the thyroid: is more than biopsy necessary? World J Surg 1992;16:604–610.
77. Aldinger KA, Samaan NA, Ibanez M, et al. Anaplastic carcinoma of the thyroid: a review of 84 cases of spindle and giant cell carcinoma of the thyroid. Cancer 1978;41:2267–2275.
78. Demeter JG, De Jong SA, Lawrence AM, et al. Anaplastic thyroid carcinoma: risk factors and outcome. Surgery 1991;110:956–967.
79. Tennvall J, Lundell G, Hallquist A, et al. Combined doxorubicin, hyperfractionated radiotherapy and surgery in anaplastic thyroid carcinoma. Cancer 1994;74:1348–1354.

CHAPTER 11

Parathyroid Cancer

CONSTANTINE V. GODELLAS

Cancer of the parathyroid glands is rare. It was first described by de Quervain in 1909. His patient presented with a large, locally invasive neck mass and subsequently developed lung metastases. de Quervain did not mention hypercalcemia in his report, but we know that most patients with parathyroid cancer also present with *marked* hypercalcemia.

It may be difficult to differentiate a parathyroid cancer from a parathyroid adenoma intraoperatively or even histologically; frequently the diagnosis is made only when there is local recurrence or when metastases arise. This chapter focuses on the epidemiology, diagnosis, treatment, and follow-up of the patient with suspected or documented parathyroid cancer.

A. Epidemiology and Staging

Parathyroid cancer occurs in 0.14–2.30% of patients with hyperparathyroidism. Cancer of the parathyroid gland accounts for fewer than 1% of all cases of hypercalcemia. The incidence in the general population is less than 1%. Reported studies are usually from tertiary referral centers that specialize in endocrine diseases; therefore these reports probably overestimate what the true incidence is nationally.

Although there is a marked female preponderance noted for benign parathyroid adenoma, there is only a slight increase in the incidence of parathyroid cancer in females. Most series report the median age at diagnosis to be in the fifth decade.

There is no clear causative factor. Some have postulated that exposure to radiation may lead to an increased incidence of this disease. There is also a belief that there may be a genetic predilection. A single factor, however, has not been definitively associated with the development of parathyroid cancer.

There is no standardized staging system for parathyroid cancer probably because of the rarity of the disease and the difficulty making the diagnosis. Because there are no clear histologic criteria that establish a diagnosis of cancer when the tumor is not invasive and has not metastasized, it stands to reason that establishing a staging system would be difficult.

B. Diagnosis

As with most things in medicine, a thorough history and physical examination are important for the diagnosis. Parathyroid cancers are almost always functional, unlike many other malignancies of the endocrine glands. The tumors secrete large amounts of parathyroid hormone (PTH), which causes a

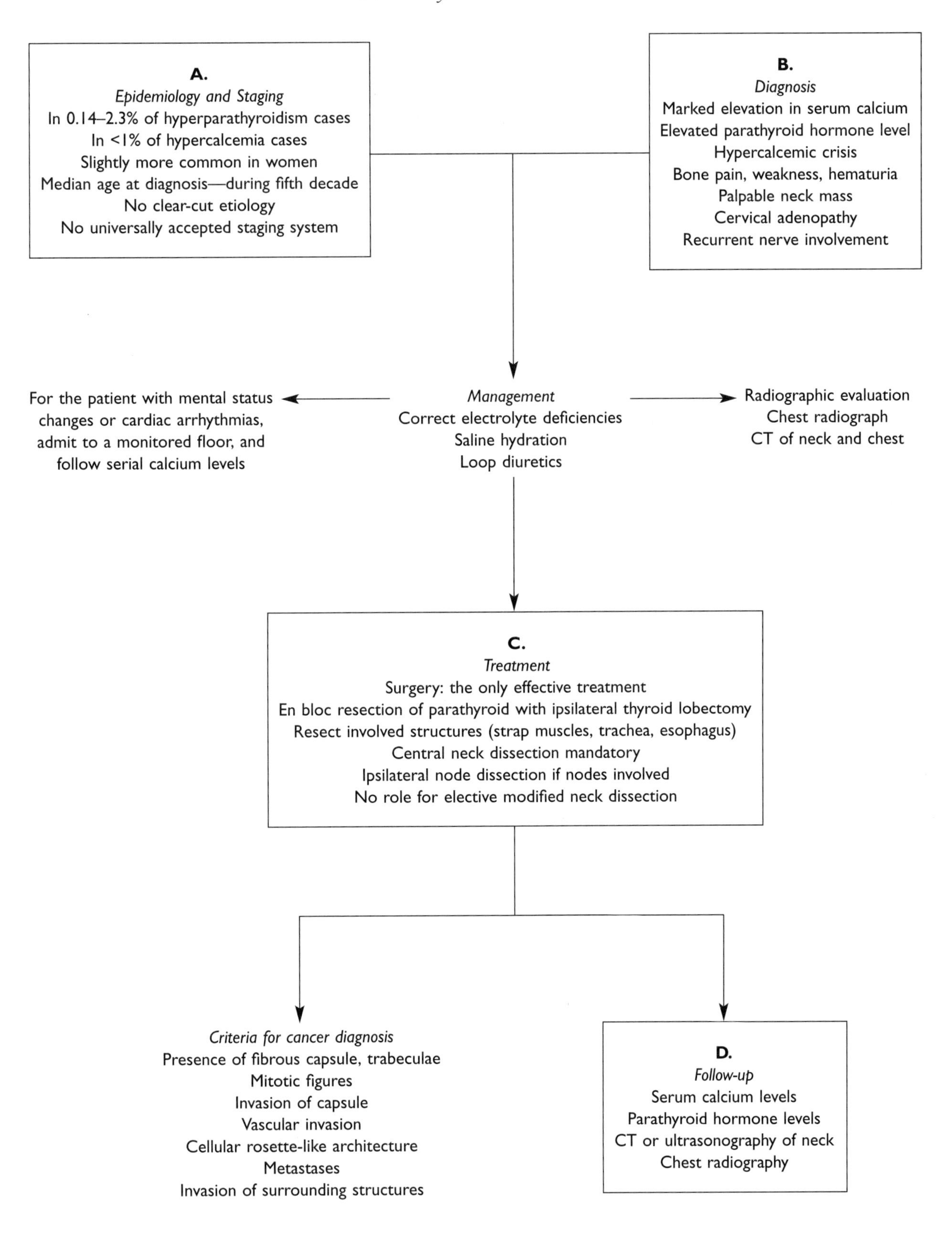
Parathyroid Cancer
A.
Epidemiology and Staging
In 0.14–2.3% of hyperparathyroidism cases
In <1% of hypercalcemia cases
Slightly more common in women
Median age at diagnosis—during fifth decade
No clear-cut etiology
No universally accepted staging system
B.
Diagnosis
Marked elevation in serum calcium
Elevated parathyroid hormone level
Hypercalcemic crisis
Bone pain, weakness, hematuria
Palpable neck mass
Cervical adenopathy
Recurrent nerve involvement
For the patient with mental status changes or cardiac arrhythmias, admit to a monitored floor, and follow serial calcium levels
Management
Correct electrolyte deficiencies
Saline hydration
Loop diuretics
Radiographic evaluation
Chest radiograph
CT of neck and chest
C.
Treatment
Surgery: the only effective treatment
En bloc resection of parathyroid with ipsilateral thyroid lobectomy
Resect involved structures (strap muscles, trachea, esophagus)
Central neck dissection mandatory
Ipsilateral node dissection if nodes involved
No role for elective modified neck dissection
Criteria for cancer diagnosis
Presence of fibrous capsule, trabeculae
Mitotic figures
Invasion of capsule
Vascular invasion
Cellular rosette-like architecture
Metastases
Invasion of surrounding structures
D.
Follow-up
Serum calcium levels
Parathyroid hormone levels
CT or ultrasonography of neck
Chest radiography

marked elevation of serum calcium levels. It is not uncommon to find serum calcium levels above 14–15 mg/dl; levels this high are usually not seen in patients with benign parathyroid adenomas. For this reason, patients with parathyroid cancer present much more commonly with symptoms related to renal and skeletal complaints than do patients with benign hyperparathyroidism. The most common complaints are bone pain, proximal muscle weakness, hematuria, and renal colic. Patients who present in hypercalcemic crisis, also known as parathyroid storm, are more likely to have a parathyroid cancer than a benign adenoma as the cause of their hyperparathyroidism.

Patients should be asked in depth about a history of a prior malignancy or signs or symptoms that may lead one to suspect metastatic disease from a primary lesion other than parathyroid cancer as the reason for the hypercalcemia. Familial endocrinopathies also suggest that the hypercalcemia is secondary to parathyroid adenoma or hyperplasia as a result of the multiple endocrine neoplasia (MEN) syndrome.

Patients with parathyroid carcinoma are much more likely to have a palpable neck mass on physical examination than are patients with benign parathyroid pathology. In fact, a benign parathyroid adenoma or hyperplastic gland is almost never palpable. Furthermore, any patient with hypercalcemia and cervical lymphadenopathy should be suspected of having a malignancy. The malignancy does not have to be parathyroid cancer, as clearly lung cancer and lymphoma (as well as other cancers) may cause cervical adenopathy and hypercalcemia. However, a patient with an elevated PTH level, hypercalcemia, and cervical adenopathy should be suspected of having a parathyroid cancer. Hoarseness should also lead one to suspect parathyroid cancer or other malignancy invading or compressing the recurrent laryngeal nerve. This is rarely seen secondary to benign parathyroid pathology.

The laboratory evaluation of hypercalcemia must include assessment of the fluid and electrolyte status. This is especially important for patients with *marked* hypercalcemia, which is usually accompanied by severe deficits in extracellular fluid. Abnormalities in fluid and electrolytes are likely secondary to gastrointestinal dysfunction, renal insufficiency, and abnormalities in calcium homeostasis. Intact PTH is measured by radioimmunometric techniques to confirm that the parathyroid gland is the cause of the hypercalcemia. PTH levels in patients with parathyroid cancer are usually severalfold higher than in patients with benign parathyroid disease.

Radiologic evaluation should include, at minimum, a chest radiograph. The presence of multiple nodules suggests metastatic disease, whereas a solitary nodule may herald the presence of a primary lung cancer. If there is a high degree of suspicion for parathyroid cancer, a computed tomography (CT) scan of the neck and even the chest can determine the extent of the cervical disease (including substernal extension, local invasion, or lymphadenopathy) and the need to look for pulmonary metastases. As yet, there is no clear role for magnetic resonance imaging (MRI) or positron emission tomography (PET) scanning; however, advances in these techniques may make them more sensitive for establishing the diagnosis of malignancy preoperatively at some later date. For the patient who has a history of cancer that preferentially metastasizes to bone (breast, prostate, lung cancer), a bone scan is performed to determine the presence, extent, and location of metastases.

As already mentioned, other nonparathyroid entities in the differential diagnosis of hypercalcemia should be entertained. An elevated PTH level frequently rules out most of these other causes. If metastasis or an invasive cancer is not identified preoperatively, the diagnosis of parathyroid cancer cannot be made with certainty. Although parathyroid cancer may still be suspected, adenoma or hyperplasia should be considered the most likely diagnosis because of the rarity of parathyroid malignancy. For the patient with a palpable neck mass and marked hypercalcemia secondary to hyperparathyroidism, parathyroid cancer should be strongly considered, even without other evidence for malignancy (metastasis, local invasiveness, hoarseness).

C. *Treatment*

Surgery is the only effective treatment for parathyroid cancer. Preoperative preparation must address the severe hypercalcemia and the associated metabolic abnormalities. The confused, obtunded patient with marked hypercalcemia should be promptly admitted to the hospital, preferably to a patient care unit equipped with cardiac monitors. Arrhythmias must be promptly recognized and treated. Vigorous hydration with saline must be instituted; and once urine output is established, loop diuretics are given to promote calcium elimination. The medical management for hypercalcemic crisis is further described in Chapter 63. If medical therapy fails to lower serum calcium promptly or if the patient's mental status or cardiac rhythm worsens, the patient should be prepared for neck exploration.

If an elective operation is planned and the patient is considered an acceptable surgical candidate, a high index of suspicion of malignancy must be maintained to expect a reasonable chance for cure. In other words, preoperatively one should suspect cancer if a patient has an extremely high serum calcium level, a markedly elevated PTH level, and a palpable neck mass. Likewise, any patient with clear evidence of metastases or recurrent laryngeal nerve involvement should be approached with the understanding that there is likely a cancer present. Intraoperatively, a markedly enlarged gland in association with extreme hypercalcemia, a grayish white, firm, fibrotic gland, or a gland that is locally invasive into surrounding structures should all be considered malignant.

The procedure of choice for a patient with a parathyroid cancer is radical or en bloc resection of the parathyroid gland including the ipsilateral thyroid lobe and any associated structures that appear to be invaded. It is frequently necessary to resect ipsilateral strap muscles because of local invasion or to allow better exposure during resection. Resection of the recurrent laryngeal nerve should be undertaken if in so doing it allows complete removal of the cancer. If the nerve is involved, the patient has already lost function of the cord; therefore sacrificing the nerve to obtain clearance of all tumor is advisable. In rare instances the cancer is extremely aggressive and invades the trachea and esophagus. This situation is usually identified preoperatively from symptoms of dysphagia or respiratory difficulties or by CT scan or other imaging modalities; appropriate preparations should be made for tracheal or esophageal resection if complete tumor clearance can be obtained.

Along with en bloc resection of the parathyroid gland, all patients with documented or suspected parathyroid cancer should undergo dissection of the central or pretracheal lymph nodes. Ipsilateral modified radical neck dissection is performed only if there is evidence of adenopathy on the affected side. There is currently no role for elective modified radical neck dissection in patients with parathyroid carcinoma.

Frequently, parathyroid cancer is not diagnosed even after pathologic examination. The histopathologic features of parathyroid cancer can be similar to those of a benign adenoma. Criteria have been suggested to facilitate establishing the diagnosis, the most common being those of Schantz and Castleman: Their criteria include the presence of (1) a fibrous capsule or trabeculae; (2) mitotic figures; (3) invasion of the capsule or surrounding vessels; and (4) cellular architecture with a trabecular or rosette-like appearance. Cytologic criteria include nuclear pleomorphism and enlargement. Taken alone, none of these microscopic features is specific for parathyroid carcinoma. The gross features of the tumor comprise the most important factors for diagnosing cancer. Intraoperatively, if there is obvious invasion of the thyroid tissue or surrounding muscles, or metastases to lymph nodes, the diagnosis can be made with certainty. There are some patients in whom parathyroid cancer cannot be conclusively diagnosed until the patient develops local recurrence or nodal or distant metastases.

Anecdotal evidence suggests that postoperative radiation therapy may be beneficial to the surgical bed; but because of the small number of treated patients and long disease latency periods prior to recurrence, there has been no conclusive proof to indicate this is true. There is no good evidence to suggest that postoperative chemotherapy is of benefit, even for the patient with metastatic disease. Isolated metastases should be aggressively resected in hopes of both enhancing survival and controlling hypercalcemia.

D. Follow-up

Serum calcium and PTH levels should be followed because they are sensitive markers for recurrence of parathyroid cancer. Physical examination of the neck is also useful for identifying a locally recurrent tumor or nodal metastasis. In some patients whose neck examination is difficult because of excessive scar tissue from a previous operation or body habitus, it may be difficult to identify a small recurrence. Serial ultrasonography or CT scans can be useful in these patients for identifying a recurrence.

It is important to realize that long-term follow-up is necessary in the patient with documented or suspected parathyroid cancer because this is usually a slow-growing malignancy marked by late local recurrence, metastases to lung and bone, or both. The 5-year survival rate is on the order of 50%, although it is higher for patients who have undergone a curative resection.

The major sequelae of recurrent or metastatic disease is similar to that for other endocrine cancers in that patients have symptoms related to excess hormone production and to the local effects of the tumor. Patients with recurrent or metastatic disease usually have elevated serum PTH levels and resultant hypercalcemia. Tumor progression and marked hypercalcemia may cause problems, but tracheal and esophageal obstruction can also occur. Because there is no evidence to suggest that chemotherapy or radiation therapy has a role in recurrent or metastatic disease, resection of recurrent and metastatic tumors should be considered if technically possible. Other pharmacologic means directed at controlling hypercalcemia may be necessary in the patient who is not a surgical candidate, including drugs such as mithramycin, calcitonin, pamidronate, and biphosphonates. A more complete discussion of the control of hypercalcemia is found in Chapter 63.

Conclusions

A patient presenting with extreme hypercalcemia secondary to markedly elevated levels of parathyroid hormone and a palpable neck mass should be suspected of having a parathyroid carcinoma. Surgical excision can be curative if the surgeon's index of suspicion is high and a complete resection is performed. Locally recurrent or metastatic disease is not a contraindication to surgery, and an operation may be the only means available to control the resultant hypercalcemia.

Suggested Reading

DeVita VT Jr, Hellman S, Rosenberg SA (eds). Cancer: Principles and Practice of Oncology, 5th ed. Philadelphia: Lippincott, 1997.

Hakaim G, Esselstyn CB Jr. Parathyroid carcinoma: 50-year experience of the Cleveland Clinic Foundation. Cleve Clin J Med 1993;60:331–335.

Obara T, Fujimoto Y. Diagnosis and treatment of patients with parathyroid carcinoma: an update and review. World J Surg 1991;15:738–744.

Sandelin K, Thompson NW, Bondeson L. Metastatic parathyroid carcinoma: dilemmas in management. Surgery 1991;110:978–988.

Schantz A, Castleman B. Parathyroid carcinoma: a study of 70 cases. Cancer 1973;31:600–605.

Van Heerden JA, Weiland LH, Re Mine WH, Walls JT, Purnell DC. Cancer of the parathyroid glands. Arch Surg 1979;114:475–480.

Vetto JT, Brennan MF, Woodruff J, Burt M. Parathyroid carcinoma: diagnosis and clinical history. Surgery 1993;114:882–892.

Wang CA, Gaz RD. Natural history of parathyroid carcinoma: diagnosis, treatment, and results. Am J Surg 1985;149:522–527.

Wynne AG, van Heerden J, Carney JA, Fitzpatrick LA. Parathyroid carcinoma: clinical and pathologic features in 43 patients. Medicine 1992;71:197–205.

Chapter 12

Adrenal Cancer

SCOTT R. SCHELL
ROBERT UDELSMAN

A. Epidemiology

Adrenal cancer is an extremely rare neoplasm, accounting for 0.05–0.20% of all cancers. This risk translates to approximately two cases per million population worldwide and approximately 200 new cases each year in the United States.[1,2]

There is a gender bias for adrenal cancer, with women developing functioning adrenal cortical carcinomas more commonly than men; nonfunctioning adrenal cancers are more frequently seen in men and older patients. These cancers are found in patients of all ages, with a median age at presentation of 40 years. There are no reported etiologic factors associated with adrenal cancer, nor does there appear to be a geographic or climatic predisposition. Previous reports have described adrenal cancer in combination with a complex hereditary syndrome of breast, lung, and soft tissue cancers.[3]

B. Clinical Behavior

Adrenal cancers typically present with local extension, displacement, obstruction or destruction of adjacent structures, or as a large abdominal mass. The tumor may rupture into the abdominal cavity, presenting with the clinical picture of an acute abdomen. Adrenal masses may directly involve the kidney, causing hematuria or pain. Similar to renal cancer, they can directly invade the left renal vein or vena cava, causing tumor embolism, venous thrombosis, and occlusion.[1] Lower extremity edema is seen in approximately 10% of patients. Fever, anorexia, and weight loss are common associated symptoms.

Adrenal cancer most frequently spreads to the lungs and liver, with most patients ultimately developing disease in these organs. Widespread metastases can be seen in any location or organ system. These metastases can be symptomatic or silent and should be considered for biopsy if the diagnosis is not certain. Metastases to bone, although uncommon, may be radiographically blastic or lytic.

A.
Epidemiology
Functioning tumors more common in women
Nonfunctioning tumors more common in men
Median age at presentation 40 years
Represents 0.05–0.2% of all cancers
200 New cases per year in U.S.

B.
Clinical Behavior
Large mass
Compression of surrounding structures
Hematuria
Lower extremity edema (10%)
Metastatic disease to lungs, liver

C.
Hormonal Function (Table 12–1)
Nonfunctioning
Functioning without syndrome
Syndrome producing
Medullary

D.
Imaging, Localization, and Laboratory Studies (Table 12–2)
Remove all functioning tumors regardless of size or whether producing syndrome
Nonfunctioning tumors <4.5 cm should be imaged again in 3–4 months

(continued on next page)

Adrenal Cancer (continued)

E.
Preoperative Considerations
Surgery considered for all fuctioning tumors and lesions <4.5 cm
For pheochromocytomas, provide alpha-adrenergic blockade with phenoxybenzamine, start with 10–20 mg bid and increase dose until patient develops orthostatic hypotension
Beta blockade not routine
Correct electrolytes
Replace steroids
Vaccinate if splenectomy likely
Bowel preparation if colectomy contemplated

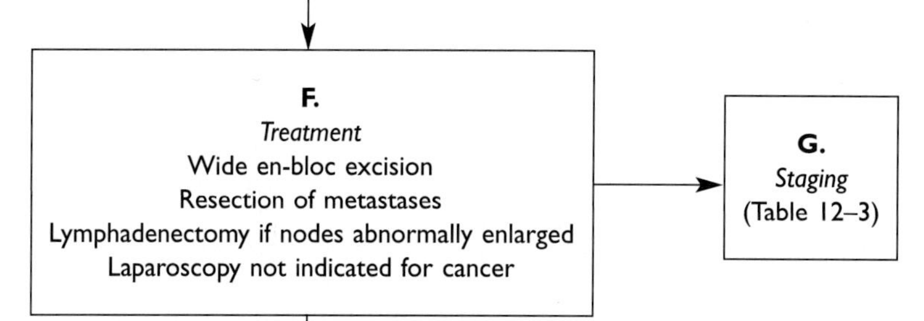

H.
Postoperative Treatment
Irradiation to palliate bony metastases
Chemotherapy is generally not helpful
Mitotane is given for adrenal suppression (inhibits corticosteroid synthesis, 1–6 g/day, dose titrated)
Follow-up with serial CT, MRI, biochemistry
Resect recurrent disease if possible

I.
Prognosis
(Table 12–4)

Mitotane caveats
Dose-dependent side effects develop in 90%
Used for patients with residual or recurrent disease and virtually all following curative resection (duration of therapy not clear)

TABLE 12–1.
Hormonal function in adrenal cancer

Hormonal Status	Comments
Nonfunctioning	Steroid production and excretion are normal or low.
Functioning	Steroid production is increased without evidence of clinical syndrome.
Syndrome-producing (approx. 50% of cases)	
Cushing syndrome	It is most commonly seen in females and represents approximately 20% of syndrome-producing cancers. It is typically present as an advanced clinical picture.
Virilization	Amenorrhea, hair and skin changes, and voice deepening in females are seen.
Feminization	Gynecomastia, impotence, loss of libido, and testicular atrophy are seen in males.
Hypertension	It results from glucocorticoid binding to mineralocorticoid receptors. Rarely it is due to elevated renin levels caused by renal artery compression (or rarely aldosterone production).
Polypeptide production	Although rare, cortical cancers can produce catecholamines, gonadotropins, insulin-like factors, and antidiuretic-type hormone.
Medullary tumors	
Pheochromocytoma	Hypertension that ranges from clinically inapparent to obviously symptomatic is present.

C. Hormonal Function

Previous reports of functioning adrenal cortical cancers may be misleading because excessive production of 17-hydroxycorticoids (17-HOC) or 17-ketosteroids (17-KS), without clinical evidence of steroid overproduction, has been described.[4,5] Currently, there are four recognized categories of hormone function, which are summarized in Table 12–1. Adrenal cortex cancers may be nonfunctioning, produce steroids but fail to create a hormonal syndrome, or develop into a specific syndrome depending on the particular hormone overproduced. Pheochromocytomas arising in the adrenal medulla produce catecholamines, with resultant hypertension and vasoactive symptoms.

D. Imaging, Localization, and Laboratory Studies

Many asymptomatic adrenal tumors are detected during routine computed tomographic (CT) scanning for other reasons. These "incidentalomas" should be selectively evaluated for occult hormone production and possible malignancy. In a review of 171 incidental adrenal masses, 25.7% were cortical adenomas, 4.1% were metastases from other primary tumors, 4.7% were adrenocortical carcinomas, and 0.06% were pheochromocytomas. The remainder were not specified.[6] All patients with incidental adrenal masses should have 24-hour urine specimens collected for catecholamine, metanephrine, and vanillylmandelic acid (VMA) assays. Hypertensive patients with hypokalemia should undergo testing for an aldosterone-producing tumor. Routine screening for hypercortisolism and hyperandrogenism in patients with adrenal incidentalomas is not indicated but should be considered for patients with clinical features suggestive of these disorders.

Cancer in adrenal tumors directly correlates with size; tumors <5 cm are rarely malignant. CT remains the single most effective imaging modality for screening the adrenal gland, providing high-resolution imaging of the adrenal glands, kidney, and liver. A multicenter retrospective study of 210 patients demonstrated that a 5 cm cutoff discriminated between benign and malignant adrenal cortical lesions with a sensitivity of 93% and a specificity of 64%. In many series, however, cancers have been reported in smaller lesions.[7,8] Retroperitoneal structures are well visualized with CT scanning, and the relation of the tumor to adjacent structures and vasculature can be delineated. Masses >1 cm are reliably detected by CT scan whether they are primary adrenal tumors, suspicious regional lymph nodes, or distant metastases.[6] Figure 12–1 demonstrates a sizeable left-sided pheochromocytoma.

We recommend the following: (1) All *functioning* adrenal masses should be removed even if they are not causing a clinical syndrome, regardless of size; and (2) all tumors >4.5 cm in diameter should be removed. For *nonfunctioning* lesions <4.5 cm, a follow-up imaging study is obtained in 3–4 months; if serial growth is detected, the tumor is excised.

More recently, magnetic resonance imaging (MRI) has gained favor because of better quality imaging of adrenal neoplasms and retroperitoneal structures. T2-weighted MRI images provide bright enhancement of adrenal masses and metastases; and image intensity greater than that seen in the liver is

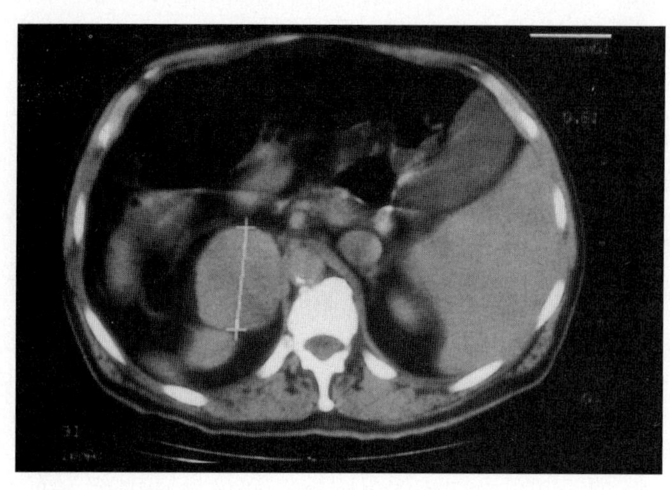

FIGURE 12–1
Computed tomography scan showing a large left pheochromocytoma.

suggestive of cancer and the need for surgery. Application of magnetic resonance angiography (MRA) provides more accurate assessment of vascular involvement than CT and often eliminates the need for invasive angiographic procedures.[7] Some centers utilize ultrasonographic imaging of adrenal masses. However, its accuracy is examiner-dependent and is significantly lessened by the patient's fat, thereby decreasing its usefulness for patients who are severely cushingoid.[8] Ultrasonography is useful for serial examination of adrenal tumors. Nuclear medicine imaging using iodocholesterol or I^{131}-6-β-iodomethyl-19-norcholesterol (NP-59) can be used as a physiologic assay of corticosteroid production or adrenal function inhibition by unilateral tumor obliteration. This scan is most useful in patients with small aldosteronomas or ACTH-independent Cushing syndrome who have a normal CT scan.[9]

Computed tomography and ultrasound imaging can be used to guide fine-needle aspiration biopsy (FNAB) of suspicious adrenal masses. Needle biopsy cannot distinguish an adrenal adenoma from a primary adrenal carcinoma and is therefore rarely indicated for this purpose. It can be useful, however, for diagnosing metastatic tumors. Patients under consideration for needle biopsy should undergo urine catecholamine metabolite screening to rule out pheochromocytoma prior to biopsy.

Laboratory studies primarily assess the urinary presence of excreted steroids. Normal or decreased steroid levels can be seen in patients who have nonfunctioning tumors. Some cancers

TABLE 12–2.
Imaging and laboratory diagnostic procedures for adrenal cancers

Procedure	Comments
Computed tomography	Accurate for adrenal masses, lymph nodes, and metastases >1 cm; good visualization of retroperitoneum, kidney, and liver
Magnetic resonance imaging, magnetic resonance angiography (MRA)	High resolution images of mass; T2 enhancement of adrenal lesions. MRA demonstrates vascular involvement, often obviating need for invasive angiography
Ultrasonography	Accurate for assessing adrenal masses; requires skilled operator and radiologist; decreased accuracy in patients with large amounts of body fat (cushingoid patients)
Nuclear medicine studies	Iodocholesterol and NP-59 are useful physiologic tests; "hot" adrenal shows active steroid production; "cold" adrenal shows obliteration of functional tissue by tumor or suppressed contralateral gland; useful in patients with small functional adrenal adenomas that are not well visualized by other techniques
Fine-needle biopsy	Rarely indicated; cannot discriminate between adrenal adenoma and carcinoma; can be used to diagnose metastatic lesions in the adrenal gland; patients must be screened for pheochromocytoma prior to biopsy, as biopsy can precipitate a hypertensive crisis
Urinary screening	1. Normal or decreased steroid levels in patients with nonfunctioning tumors 2. Elevated 17-KS or 17-HOC levels in patients without clinically apparent syndrome 3. Elevated 17-KS most common; elevated DHEA suggestive of cancer 4. Elevated 17-HOC less common; no suppression following 72-hour dexamethasone suppression suggests ACTH-independent process 5. Some cancers lack β-hydroxylation; elevated precursor accumulation, including DHEA, androstenedione, deoxycortisosterone, androgens, estrogens, and aldosterone, are observed 6. Pheochromocytomas commonly demonstrate elevated VMA and metanephrines

17-KS, 17-ketosteroids; 17-HOC, 17-hydroxycorticoids; DHEA, dihydroepiandrosterone; VMA, vanillylmandelic acid.

produce 17-KS or 17-HOC in excess without clinical manifestations. Functional cancers most commonly produce 17-KS, which is commonly associated with an increase in the androgen dihydroepiandrosterone (DHEA). Increased 17-HOC production is less common than 17-KS production, and failure of suppression following 72 hours of dexamethasone suggests an ACTH-independent process (adrenal adenoma or adrenal carcinoma). Some adrenal cancers lack adequate β-hydroxylation of steroid biosynthesis, resulting in increased intermediate production, and these substances may be the principal steroid products detected in urine. Urinary screening positive for VMA and metanephrines is diagnostic for pheochromocytoma. Table 12–2 summarizes the imaging and diagnostic procedures for adrenal cancers.

E. Preoperative Considerations

Patients with pheochromocytomas are treated with selective α-adrenergic receptor blockade using phenoxybenzamine for several weeks prior to surgery. The starting dose is 10–20 mg PO twice a day, which is escalated preoperatively until the patient develops symptoms of orthostatic hypotension and nasal congestion. After adequate α-blockage is achieved, β-blockade is occasionally added to control tachycardia; propranolol is frequently used for this purpose. Fluid repletion is required prior to surgery.

Electrolyte abnormalities should be corrected prior to surgery. Perioperative steroid replacement can be considered, as contralateral adrenal suppression is common, and inadequate steroid levels following resection may result in an addisonian crisis.

Patients with a large tumor should undergo preoperative mechanical and antibiotic bowel preparation in anticipation of possible bowel resection. Patients who may require splenectomy should receive preoperative vaccinations against encapsulated organisms, including *Hemophilus influenzae*, pneumococcus, and meningococcus. At operation, patients receive prophylactic antibiotic coverage against gram-negative and anaerobic bacteria in the event the operation dictates manipulation or resection of portions of the gastrointestinal or genitourinary tract.

F. Treatment

Surgical resection is the only potential curative treatment for adrenal carcinoma. A variety of approaches can be employed depending on the location and extent of the tumor. In general, when operating for a primary adrenal carcinoma, an anterior, flank, or thoracoabdominal approach may be employed. Posterior or laparoscopic approaches are not indicated when attempting a curative resection of a known or suspected cancer. Kocherization of the duodenum and opening the lesser sac provide access to the retroperitoneum; excision of enlarged periaortic lymph nodes may be included in the retroperitoneal exploration.

Patients with tumor extending into the mediastinum should be prepared for a median sternotomy. If preoperative imaging studies reveal tumor extension into the vena cava or left atrium, bypass or circulatory arrest may be used to allow access to, and resection of, tumor from these involved areas.

En bloc resection of the primary tumor and involved adjacent structures is the goal. Resection of hepatic or pulmonary metastases aids in improving long-term survival. Noncurative debulking is helpful for reducing symptoms and prolonging the time to symptomatic recurrence.[10–12]

G. Staging

Adrenal cancers are staged based on the size of the primary tumor, completeness of the resection, and histologic tumor grade. Table 12–3 reviews the staging system proposed by Bradley.[13] Sixty to seventy percent of patients are found to have stage III or IV disease at operation. Only 50% of patients are eligible for curative resection.

TABLE 12–3.
Proposed clinical staging system for adrenal cancers

Parameter	Stage	Criteria
Primary tumor extent	1	<5 cm; confined to adrenal gland
	2	>5 cm and <10 cm; *or* adherent to kidney
	3	>10 cm; *or* invading surrounding structures or renal vein
Metastases	0	No metastases
	1	Regional lymphatics
	2	Distant metastases (lung, liver, bone)
Tissue remaining after resection	0	Tumor completely excised
	1	Tumor capsule violated at surgery
	2	Tumor remaining after resection
Histologic differentiation	1	Differentiated, without capsular or vascular invasion
	2	Moderately undifferentiated, with capsular or vascular invasion
	3	Anaplastic; both capsular and vascular invasion
Stage	1	≤3
	2	4–5
	3	6–7
	4	≥8

H. Postoperative Treatment

Radiation therapy is not helpful for preoperative or postoperative cytoreduction, but it may relieve pain in patients with bony metastases.[14] Single-agent chemotherapy using alkylating agents, cisplatinum, or doxorubicin and combination therapies based on 5-fluorouracil (5-FU) and methotrexate have shown some antitumor activity in a limited number of patients. Because of the low incidence of these tumors, randomized, multiinstitution trials are required to determine efficacy.

Mitotane (*o,p′*-DDD) was introduced during the 1960s and remains the mainstay of adjuvant therapy for adrenal cancer. Occasional long-term remissions and regression of metastases have been noted (25%). Tumor response tends to be partial and transient. Mitotane inhibits corticosteroid biosynthesis, causing atrophy of adrenal tissue and palliation of symptoms in up to 75% of treated patients. Patients are given 1–6 g/day, titrating the dosage to suppression of plasma cortisol levels. Patients should be expected to experience complete adrenal suppression and so require mineralocorticoid and glucocorticoid replacement. As many at 90% of patients on mitotane therapy develop significant gastrointestinal, neuromuscular, dermatologic, and depression side effects. Because the toxicity is dose-dependent, these side effects can be reversed by decreasing the mitotane dose.[13,15] The goal of therapy is 6 g per day (divided doses), but side effects may keep one from reaching this goal. The duration of therapy is lifelong.[16–18]

Mitotane was initially intended to treat residual or recurrent disease following surgery. There has been a progressive trend to use it for virtually all patients as adjuvant chemotherapy following even "curative" resections. Despite the absence of randomized, prospective, placebo-controlled trials, its use has been adopted by most centers as standard adjuvant therapy.[19] The duration of this therapy has not been determined.

Patients should be followed with serial CT or MRI scans and the appropriate biochemical profiles to assess possible tumor recurrence and metastatic disease. Metastases to regional lymph nodes occur in 68% of patients, to lung in 71%, to liver in 42%, and to bone in 26%. Reoperation and resection of metastases can prolong survival and alleviate symptoms. The Italian National Registry for Adrenal Carcinoma reported a mean survival of 16 ± 15 months in 20 reoperated patients, which was significantly higher than for patients in whom resection was not performed (survival of 3 ± 3 months).[20]

I. Prognosis

The prognosis for patients with adrenal cancer is poor, with a median survival of 22–47 months. Patients with anaplastic tumors have the worst survival (5 months, median) compared to those with differentiated tumors (40 months, median). Patients with weight loss, vascular invasion, tumor cell necrosis, and a diffuse growth pattern have a worse prognosis and earlier metastasis.[21] Table 12–4 summarizes the survival by clinical stage.

TABLE 12–4.
Survival by stage of adrenal cancer

Stage	Mean survival
I/II	5 Years
III	2.3 Years
IV	12 Months
Anaplastic	5 Months

References

1. Lipsett MB, Hertz R, Ross GT. Clinical and pathophysiological aspects of adrenal cortical carcinoma. Am J Med 1963;35:374.
2. Hajjar RA, Hickey RC, Samaan NA. Adrenal cortical carcinoma: a study of 32 patients. Cancer 1975;35:549.
3. Lynch HT, Katz DA, Bogard PJ, Lynch JF. The sarcoma, breast cancer, lung cancer, and adrenocortical carcinoma syndrome revisited. Am J Dis Child 1985;139:134.
4. Fukushima DK, Bradlow HL, Hellman L, Gallagher TF. Origin of prenanetriol in a patient with adrenal carcinoma. J Clin Endocrinol 1962;22:765.
5. Fukushima DK, Gallagher TF. Steroid production in "nonfunctioning" adrenal cortical tumor. J Clin Endocrinol 1963;23:923.
6. Gajraj H, Young AE. Adrenal incidentaloma. Br J Surg 1993;80:422.
7. Terzolo M, Ali A, Oscella G, et al. Prevalence of adrenal carcinoma among incidentally discovered adrenal masses. Arch Surg 1997;132: 914–919.
8. Linos DA, Stylopoulos N, Raptis SA. Adrenaloma: a call for more aggressive management. World J Surg 1996;20:788–793.
9. Javadpour N, Woltering EA, Brennan MF. Adrenal neoplasms. Curr Probl Surg 1980;17:16.
10. Doppman JL, Reinig JW, Dwyer AJ, et al. Differentiation of adrenal masses by magnetic resonance imaging. Surgery 1987;102:1018.
11. Ghorashi B, Holmes JH. Gray scale sonographic appearance of an adrenal mass: a case report. J Clin Ultrasound 1976;4:121.
12. Watanabe K, Kamoi I, Nakayama C, et al. Scintigraphic detection of a hepatic metastasis with iodine-131-labelled steroid in recurrent adrenal carcinoma: case report. J Nucl Med 1976;17:904.
13. Bradley EL. Primary and adjunctive therapy in carcinoma of the adrenal cortex. Surg Gynecol Obstet 1975;141:507.
14. Cohn K, Gottesman L, Brennan M. Adrenocortical carcinoma. Surgery 1986;100:1170.
15. Schteinbart DE, Mtazedi A, Noonan RA, et al. Treatment of adrenal carcinomas. Arch Surg 1982;117:1142.
16. King DR, Lock EE. Adrenal cortical carcinoma: a clinical and pathological study of 49 cases. Cancer 1979;44:239.

17. Hutter AM, Kayhoe DE. Adrenal cortica carcinoma: clinical features of 128 patients. Am J Med 1966;41:572.
18. Lubitz JA, Freeman L, Okun R. Mitotane use in inoperable cortical carcinoma. JAMA 1973;223:1109.
19. Luton JP, Cerdas S, Billaud L, et al. Clinical features of adrenocortical carcinoma prognostic factors, and the effect of mitotane therapy. N Engl J Med 1990;322:1195–2001.
20. Bellantone R, Ferrante A, Boscherini M, et al. Role of reoperation in recurrence of adrenal cortical carcinoma: results from 188 cases collected in the Italian National Registry for adrenal cortical carcinoma. Surgery 1997; 122:1212–1218.
21. Hough AJ, Hollifield JW, Page DL, et al. Prognostic factors in adrenal cortical tumor: a mathematical analysis of clinical and morphological data. Am J Clin Pathol 1979;73:390.

Chapter 13

Hypergastrinemia, Gastrinoma, and Multiple Endocrine Neoplasia 1

PETER J. FABRI

A. Epidemiology

Gastrinoma [Zollinger-Ellison (ZE) syndrome] is an uncommon tumor. Because reports come from institutions where cases are clustered, the surgical literature gives the impression that the tumor is more common than it actually is. Multiple endocrine meoplasia type 1 (MEN 1), which includes gastrinoma, hyperparathyroidism, and pituitary adenomas, has been widely described and small series reported.[1,2] It appears true that "more papers have been written about the ZE syndrome than there are patients with the disease."

Hypergastrinemia, an elevation of the serum gastrin level (normal 100–200 pg/ml), is commonly identified because of the widespread availability of the assay. A fasting gastrin over 1000 pg/ml is generally diagnostic of gastrinoma when it occurs in the presence of peptic ulcer disease or hyperchlorhydria. Intermediate values (200–1000 pg/ml) may be found in patients with gastrinoma, but other potential causes for hypergastrinemia must be sought. The challenge for the clinician is to distinguish between elevated gastrin levels due to gastrinoma and those due to other diseases, as the incidence of true gastrinoma is perhaps one patient per million.

B. Differential Diagnosis

Hypergastrinemia may be due to decreased clearance, increased production secondary to a physiologic or pharmacologic process, or increased production due to gastrinoma. Decreased clearance is seen in renal failure and with short bowel syndrome. *Increased production* can be due to hypercalcemia of all causes (parathyroid adenomas rarely also produce gastrin) and to decreased gastric acid production, which may be caused by achlorhydria or pharmacologic suppression of acid production by histamine receptor antagonists or proton pump inhibitors.

Gastrinoma

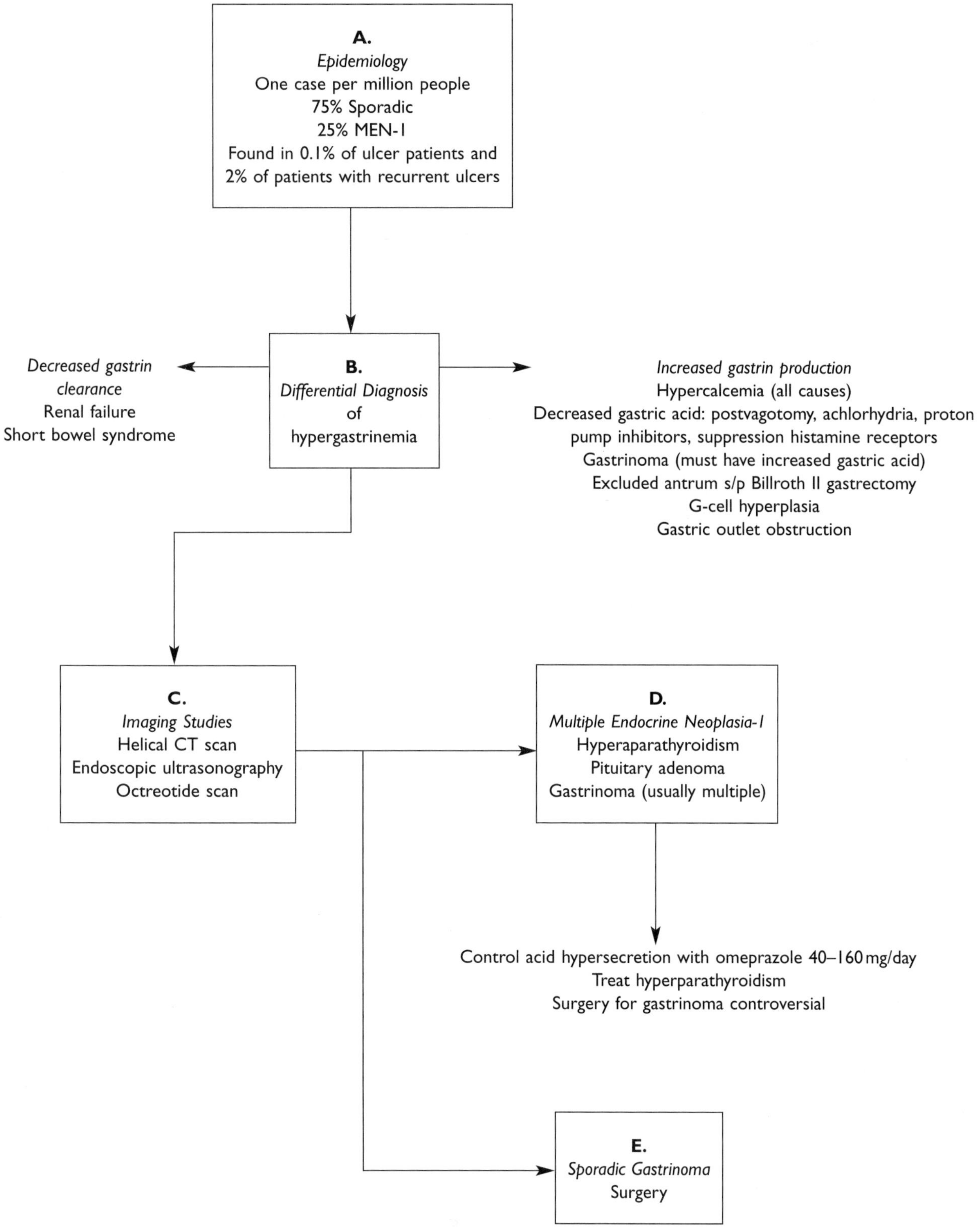

A.
Epidemiology
One case per million people
75% Sporadic
25% MEN-1
Found in 0.1% of ulcer patients and
2% of patients with recurrent ulcers

B.
Differential Diagnosis
of
hypergastrinemia

Decreased gastrin clearance
Renal failure
Short bowel syndrome

Increased gastrin production
Hypercalcemia (all causes)
Decreased gastric acid: postvagotomy, achlorhydria, proton pump inhibitors, suppression histamine receptors
Gastrinoma (must have increased gastric acid)
Excluded antrum s/p Billroth II gastrectomy
G-cell hyperplasia
Gastric outlet obstruction

C.
Imaging Studies
Helical CT scan
Endoscopic ultrasonography
Octreotide scan

D.
Multiple Endocrine Neoplasia-1
Hyperaparathyroidism
Pituitary adenoma
Gastrinoma (usually multiple)

Control acid hypersecretion with omeprazole 40–160 mg/day
Treat hyperparathyroidism
Surgery for gastrinoma controversial

E.
Sporadic Gastrinoma
Surgery

(continued on next page)

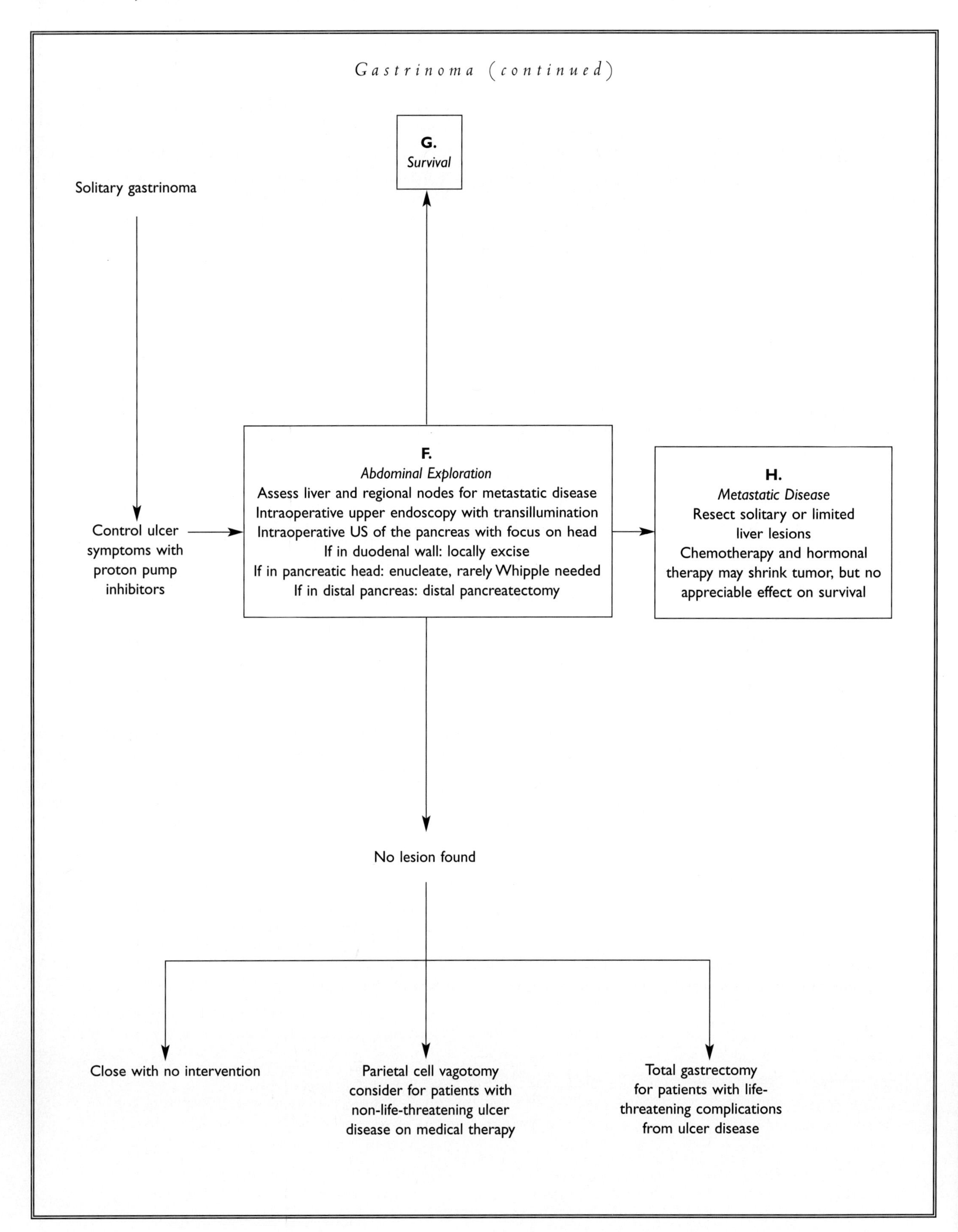
Gastrinoma (continued)
G.
Survival
Solitary gastrinoma
Control ulcer symptoms with proton pump inhibitors
F.
Abdominal Exploration
Assess liver and regional nodes for metastatic disease
Intraoperative upper endoscopy with transillumination
Intraoperative US of the pancreas with focus on head
If in duodenal wall: locally excise
If in pancreatic head: enucleate, rarely Whipple needed
If in distal pancreas: distal pancreatectomy
H.
Metastatic Disease
Resect solitary or limited liver lesions
Chemotherapy and hormonal therapy may shrink tumor, but no appreciable effect on survival
No lesion found
Close with no intervention
Parietal cell vagotomy consider for patients with non-life-threatening ulcer disease on medical therapy
Total gastrectomy for patients with life-threatening complications from ulcer disease

An elevated serum gastrin level can be confirmed by repeating the assay; and the patient's history, drug list, and family history are reviewed. If the repeat gastrin level is increased, the patient's serum blood urea nitrogen (BUN), creatinine, and calcium level are checked. If these parameters are normal, it is imperative that one be certain the patient has not been ingesting gastric acid antagonists, which are in widespread use.

Hypergastrinemia without acid production is clearly *Not due to gastrinoma*. Gastric acid analysis is performed after stopping all antisecretory medications, and the basal acid output and maximal acid output are then measured. A basal acid output of >15 mEq/hr (or >5 mEq/hr in previously operated patients) suggests the diagnosis of gastrinoma.

When hypergastrinemia occurs in the presence of increased acid production, it may still be due to a physiologic rather than a neoplastic process. Short bowel syndrome should be easy to identify by history, as should the possibility of excluded gastric antrum in patients who have had a previous gastrectomy with Billroth II reconstruction. With the marked decrease in peptic ulcer surgery, this should be a rare diagnosis. Gastrin (G)-cell hyperplasia, a diffuse increase in the number of gastrin cells in the antrum, may occur as a distinct syndrome and may require provocative testing with secretin. Intravenous administration of secretin (2 units/kg IV) helps distinguish G-cell hyperplasia from gastrinoma: With G-cell hyperplasia, gastrin levels fall in response to secretin; and with gastrinoma, gastrin rises significantly and paradoxically. The increase in gastrin level after secretin administration is diagnostic for gastrinoma.[3,4]

A clinical diagnosis of gastrinoma historically (before the availability of the gastrin radioimmunoassay) was based on the presence of fulminant and atypical peptic ulcer disease, marked gastric acid hypersecretion, and a non-beta islet cell tumor of the pancreas. It is now recognized that gastrinoma, although usually malignant and often metastatic, is a slow-growing, indolent tumor with a natural history measured in decades.[5] Patients identified by these clinical manifestations presumably have had the disease for 20–30 years before diagnosis. Today this rare tumor is usually identified biochemically in a patient without a particularly unusual ulcer history or perhaps even with diarrhea as the only symptom. Even sophisticated imaging studies often fail to demonstrate a tumor, and surgical exploration may be negative.

It is estimated that 0.1% of patients with primary duodenal ulcer disease and 2.0% of those with recurrent ulcers after standard therapy have a gastrinoma. Indeed ulceration, abdominal pain, and diarrhea are common symptoms, the latter occurring in up to 50% of patients. Formerly, patients died from the complications of acid oversecretion; and the most reliable way to treat the disease was total gastrectomy. With the advanced pharmacologic therapy available today, emphasis has shifted to approaching ZE syndrome for its oncologic potential rather than its ulcerogenic potential.

C. Imaging Studies

Imaging in patients with biochemical evidence of gastrinoma should include helical computed tomography (CT) scanning, endoscopic ultrasonography, and octreotide scanning.[6–8] Currently, helical CT scanning has the highest accuracy among the radiographic procedures, superior to standard CT or magnetic resonance imaging (MRI). Nevertheless, fewer than 50% of studies are positive. Endoscopic ultrasonography has the ability to identify small lesions in the pancreas or duodenal wall.[9] Reported data are sparse, however, and the accuracy is unknown. Octreotide scanning does not improve the identification of primary tumors but can identify multiple or metastatic lesions, usually precluding surgical intervention.[10,11] If all imaging studies are negative, arteriographic injection of secretin selectively into pancreatic and duodenal arteries with sampling for gastrin levels in the left hepatic vein may identify the site of an occult lesion.[12]

D. Multiple Endocrine Neoplasia Type 1

Multiple endocrine neoplasia type 1 is a familial syndrome characterized by hyperparathyroidism (often precedes the diagnosis of gastrinoma by several years) and *pancreatic tumors*. Pituitary adenomas occur less frequently and, when present, usually are diagnosed later in the course of the syndrome.

About 25% of gastrinomas are associated with MEN 1. The remaining 75% occur sporadically and are less likely to be multiple; they generally have a more favorable prognosis. Although MEN 1 is widely recognized, the number of kindreds is small, and most patients are aware of their family history. Data suggest that the long-term outlook for "cure" of MEN 1-associated gastrinoma is small because of multicentric disease and the likelihood of recurrence.[1,13] Although previous series have documented excellent clinical results after surgical excision,[14] similar results can be obtained with medical management (proton pump inhibition).

Benzimidazoles (omeprazole and lansoprazole) selectively inhibit the H^+-K^+-adenosine triphosphatase on the luminal surface of the gastric parietal cell. These drugs are preferred over the histamine H_2-receptor antagonists for patients with gastrinoma when treating primary disease before surgery or unresectable or metastatic disease. Omeprazole doses vary from 40 to 160 mg/day.

Investigators with experience in managing MEN 1 families currently do not recommend surgical exploration for most. Careful attention should be paid to identifying initial or recurrent hyperparathyroidism (always caused by hyperplasia), which can produce hypergastrinemia through hypercalcemia and is substantially alleviated by treating the hyperparathyroidism.

E. Sporadic Gastrinoma

The diagnosis of sporadic gastrinoma is reached when all of the above causes of hypergastrinemia have been excluded. Sporadic gastrinoma, although indolent, must be considered a malignant neoplasm; and surgical excision is currently the only treatment with a potential for clinical and biochemical cure.[14]

F. Abdominal Exploration

Surgical exploration for gastrinoma should be performed electively, with the intention of long-term cure. Ulcer disease is initially managed medically with proton pump inhibition. Preoperative preparation includes evaluation of cardiac and pulmonary function. Occasionally (10%), pheochromocytoma occurs in the setting of MEN 1.[14] Surgical exploration should exclude metastasis to the liver or regional lymph nodes. The duodenum should be examined by intraoperative endoscopy with transillumination of the duodenal wall, which frequently identifies small (1–2 mm) lesions that may be multiple.[15,16] Intraoperative ultrasonography is performed on the entire head of the pancreas, within which 80% of gastrinomas are found. The entire distal pancreas is mobilized from the retroperitoneum, taking care to avoid injuring the spleen. The mobilized pancreatic tail should be palpated bimanually and examined with ultrasonography. A lesion or lesions are found in most patients and should be removed. Duodenal lesions are removed through a duodenotomy. Pancreatic head lesions are enucleated; pancreaticoduodenectomy (Whipple's procedure) is rarely required. Lesions in the body or tail of the paucreas are included in a distal pancreatectomy. In cases where no lesion is identified, options include closure without intervention, parietal cell vagotomy, or total gastrectomy. A highly selective vagotomy facilitates postoperative medical management for patients who have not experienced serious ulcerogenic complications such as hemorrhage. Gastrectomy is reserved for patients who have had life-threatening complications from their ulcer disease while on appropriate medical management. Radiolabeled octreotide with an intraoperative handheld gamma probe has been used to localize lesions.[17]

G. Survival

For patients without gross tumor identified at surgery the 10-year survival is 100%. For patients without liver metastasis the 10-year survival is >90%, whereas for those with liver involvement survival at 10 years is only 30%.[14,18,19]

H. Metastatic Disease

Metastatic disease may preclude surgical treatment, although solitary liver metastases may be resected and patients cured "biochemically." Limited metastatic disease identified at the time of surgery should be resected if all disease can be removed. Metastases identified during long-term follow-up may benefit from resection if they are solitary or limited and easily resectable. Although earlier studies showed a beneficial effect after surgical debulking, medical management probably produces a comparable long-term outcome. Long-term survival is possible for patients with metastatic disease treated with adequate acid control alone. Previous studies using chemotherapy (streptozotocin) occasionally have shown a reduction in tumor volume, as does treatment with somatostatin or its analogue octreotide. Whether such treatment improves survival over that seen with omeprazole treatment alone is questionable.[20]

Conclusions

Gastrinomas occur sporadically in most instances, although 25% are associated with MEN 1. Complications of acid hypersecretion can be ameliorated with proton pump inhibitors, and gastrectomy is rarely necessary for hemorrhage. Most contend that surgery for MEN 1-associated gastrinomas should not be proposed routinely because of multicentric disease, high recurrence rates, and long-term survival regardless of treatment. Sporadic gastrinomas, however, should be considered for resection if imaging studies do not show a large volume or distant disease. Most gastrinomas can be localized. If operative maneuvers fail to identify the lesion, choices include closing without intervention, parietal cell vagotomy (if no ulcer-related complications have occurred) or total gastrectomy (for life-threatening ulcer-related complications).

References

1. Jenson RT. Management of the Zollinger-Ellison syndrome in patients with multiple endocrine neoplasia type 1. J Intern Med 1998;243:477–488.
2. Migon M, Cadiot G. Diagnostic and therapeutic criteria in patients with Zollinger-Ellison syndrome and multiple endocrine neoplasia type 1. J Intern Med 1998;243:489–494.
3. Hirschowitz BI. Zollinger-Ellison syndrome: pathogenesis, diagnosis, and management. Am J Gastroenterol 1997;92:44S–48S.
4. Jensen RT. Gastrin-producing tumors. Cancer Treat Res 1997;89:293–334.
5. Botnman PC, Radebold K. Changing therapy for gastrinoma. HPB Surg 1998;10:411–413.
6. Kisker O, Bastian D, Bartsch D, et al. Localization, malignant potential, and surgical management of gastrinomas. World J Surg 1998;22:651–657.
7. Norton JA. Gastrinoma: advances in localization and treatment. Surg Oncol Clin North Am 1998;7:845–861.
8. Prinz RA. Localization of gastrinomas. Int J Pancreatol 1996;19:79–91.

9. Ruzniewski P, Amouyal P, Amouyal G, et al. Localization of gastrinomas by endoscopic ultrasonography in patients with Zollinger-Ellison syndrome. Surgery 1995;117:629–635.
10. Alexander HR, Fraker DL, Norton JA, et al. Prospective study of somatostatin receptor scintigraphy and its effect on operative outcome in patients with Zollinger-Ellison syndrome. Ann Surg 1998;228:228–238.
11. Zimr T, Stolzel U, Bader M, et al. Endoscopic ultrasonography and somatostatin receptor scintigraphy in the preoperative localization of insulinomas and gastrinomas. Gut 1996;39:562–568.
12. Cohen MS, Picus D, Lairmore TC, et al. Prospective study of provocative angiograms to localize functional islet cell tumors on the pancreas. Surgery 1997;122:1091–1100.
13. Thompson NW. Current concepts in the surgical management of multiple endocrine neoplasia type 1 pancreatic-duodenal disease: results in the treatment of 40 patients with Zollinger-Ellison syndrome, hypoglycemia, or both. J Intern Med 1998;243:495–500.
14. Ellison EC. Forty-year appraisal of gastrinoma: back to the future. Ann Surg 1995;222:511–521.
15. Bhutani MS, Dexter D, McKellar DP, et al. Intraoperative endoscopic ultrasonography in Zollinger-Ellison syndrome. Endoscopy 1997;29:754–756.
16. Sugg S, Norton JA, Fraker DL, et al. A prospective study of intraoperative methods to diagnose and resect duodenal gastrinomas. Ann Surg 1993; 218:138–144.
17. Benevento A, Dominioni L, Carcano G, et al. Intraoperative localization of gut endocrine tumors with radiolabeled somatostatin analogs and a gamma-detecting probe. Semin Surg Oncol 1998;15:239–244.
18. Soga J, Yakuwa Y. The gastrinoma/Zollinger-Ellison syndrome: statistical evaluation of a Japanese series of 359 cases. J Hepatobiliary Pancreat Surg 1998;5:77–85.
19. Weber HC, Venzon DJ, Lin JT, et al. Determinants of metastatic rate and survival in patients with Zollinger-Ellison syndrome: a prospective long-term study. Gastroenterology 1995;108:1637–1649.
20. Qureshi W, Rashid S. Zollinger-Ellison syndrome: improved treatment options for this complex disorder. Postgrad Med J 1998;104:155–164.

Chapter 14

Insulinoma

GEOFFREY B. THOMPSON
F. JOHN SERVICE

A. Epidemiology and Etiology

Insulinomas arise from the beta cells of the islets of Langerhans. Although the most common islet cell tumor, they are rare, with an incidence of four cases per one million patient-years in persons of northern European descent.[1] Sixty percent of patients are female, with a median age at presentation of 47 years (range 8–82 years). Insulinomas are all intrapancreatic and are equally distributed among the head, uncinate, body, and tail of the pancreas. More than 90% of the tumors are solitary, and more than 80% are <2 cm. Among these lesions, 10% are multiple, 6% are malignant, and 8% occur in patients from multiple endocrine neoplasia type 1 (MEN 1) kindreds. More than 90% of patients are cured by initial surgery, with long-term survival no different from that of age- and gender-matched controls.[1] Recurrence rates of 7% and 21% have been reported in sporadic and familial cases, respectively.

B. Neuroglycopenic Symptoms

A variety of nonspecific symptoms are frequently attributed to hypoglycemia, but true hypoglycemic symptoms rarely occur at plasma glucose levels >55 mg/dl. If normal plasma glucose levels are repeatedly obtained at the time of such symptoms, the diagnosis of a hypoglycemic disorder is eliminated, and other potential causes for the patient's symptoms must be sought. Generally, central nervous system function is not impaired until plasma glucose levels fall below 50 mg/dl. Although symptoms are classically associated with fasting and exercise, patients with insulinomas may have postprandial hypoglycemia as well.

The classic symptoms of *neuroglycopenia* are confusion, tiredness, dizziness, visual blurring, headache, difficulty thinking and speaking, and inability to concentrate. *Autonomic symptoms*, including sweating, trembling, nausea, anxiety, hunger, and palpitations, may occur in combination with neuroglycopenic symptoms. More than 80% of patients describe a history of various combinations of diplopia, blurred vision, palpitations, sweating, weakness, confusion, or abnormal behavior. More than half of the patients experience amnestic episodes or coma, and approximately 10% have generalized seizures. Whipple's

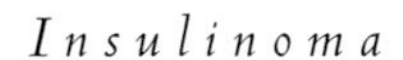

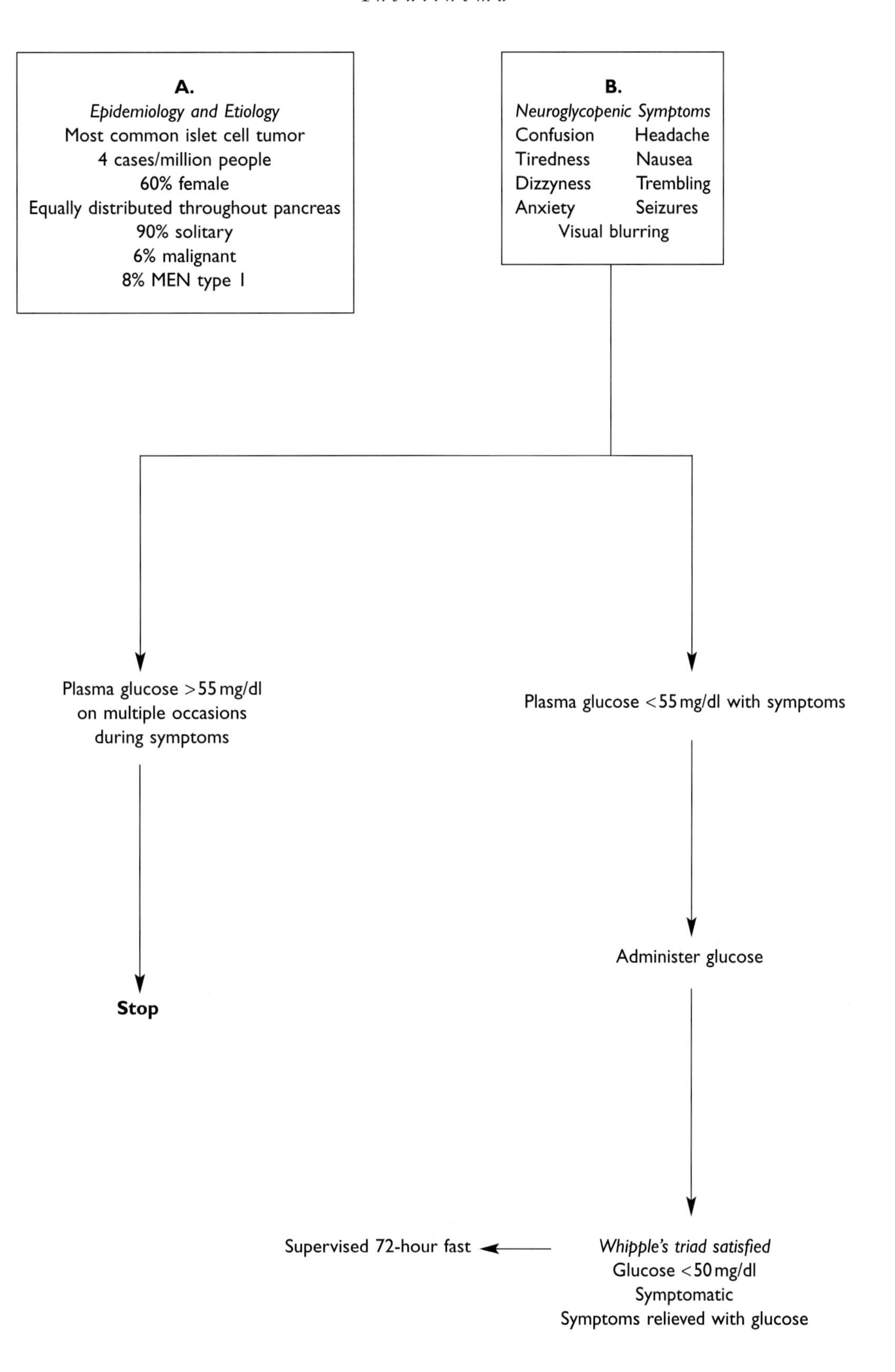

(continued on next page)

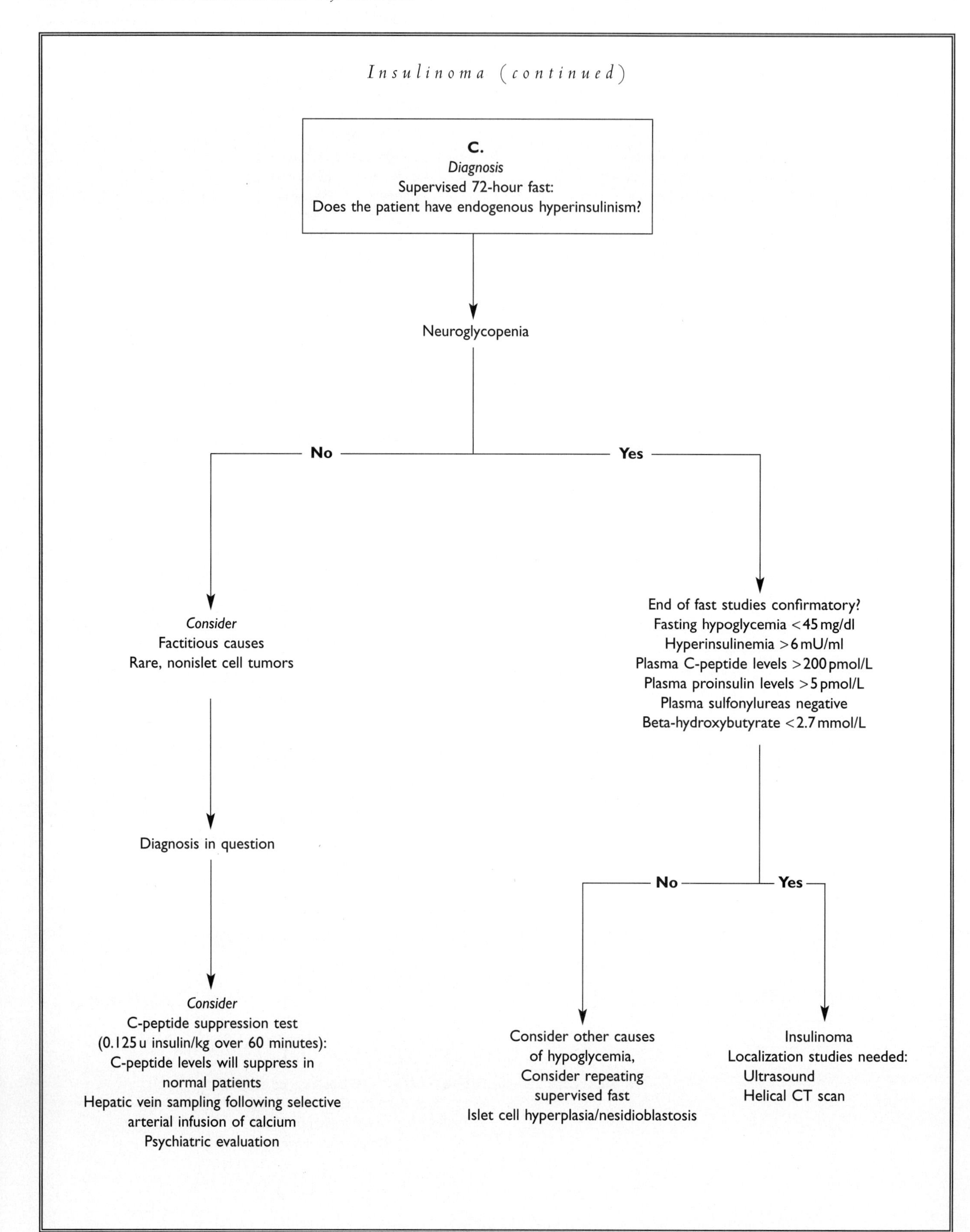
Insulinoma (continued)
C.
Diagnosis
Supervised 72-hour fast:
Does the patient have endogenous hyperinsulinism?
Neuroglycopenia
No
Yes
Consider
Factitious causes
Rare, nonislet cell tumors
Diagnosis in question
Consider
C-peptide suppression test
(0.125 u insulin/kg over 60 minutes):
C-peptide levels will suppress in
normal patients
Hepatic vein sampling following selective
arterial infusion of calcium
Psychiatric evaluation
End of fast studies confirmatory?
Fasting hypoglycemia <45 mg/dl
Hyperinsulinemia >6 mU/ml
Plasma C-peptide levels >200 pmol/L
Plasma proinsulin levels >5 pmol/L
Plasma sulfonylureas negative
Beta-hydroxybutyrate <2.7 mmol/L
No
Yes
Consider other causes
of hypoglycemia,
Consider repeating
supervised fast
Islet cell hyperplasia/nesidioblastosis
Insulinoma
Localization studies needed:
Ultrasound
Helical CT scan

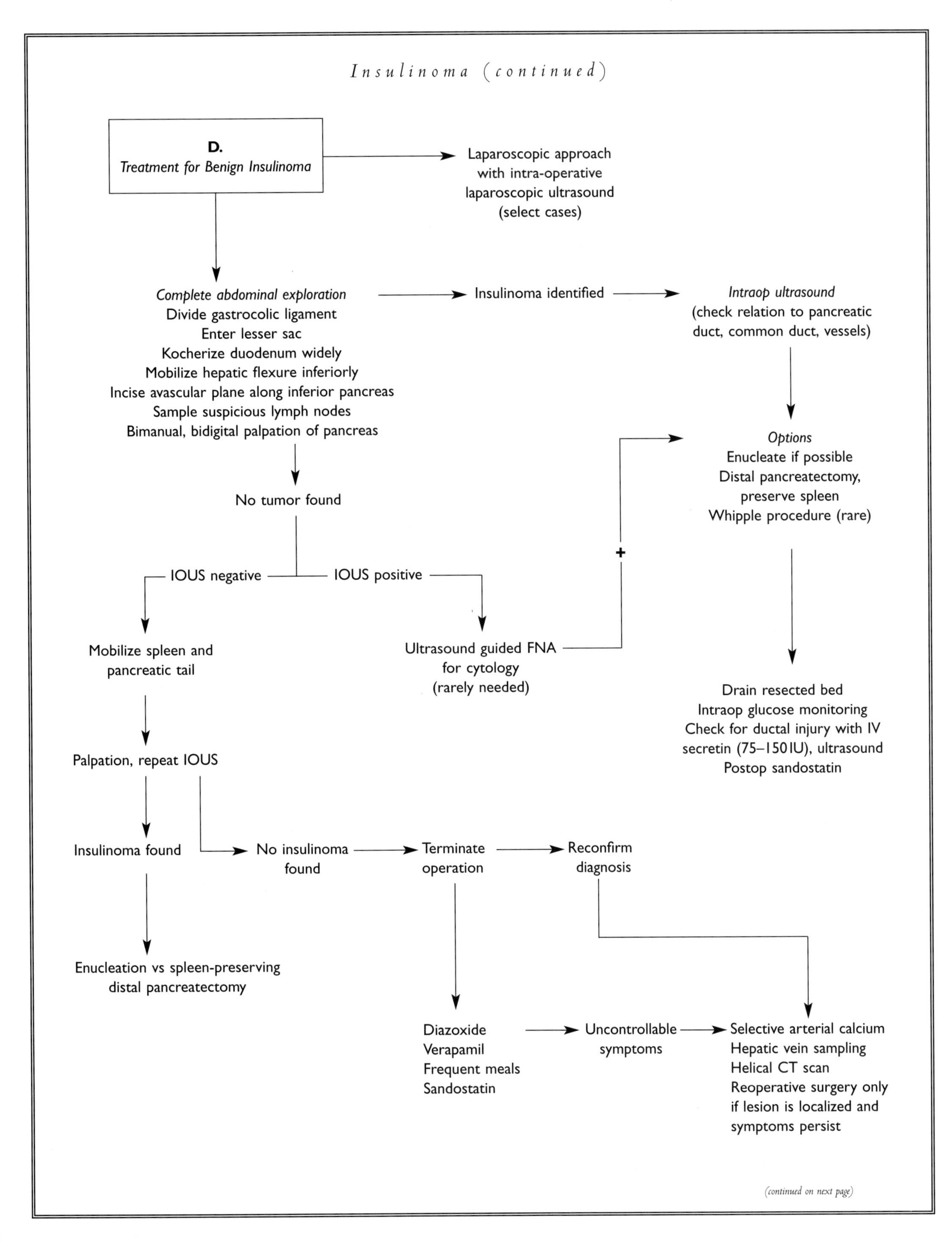

(continued on next page)

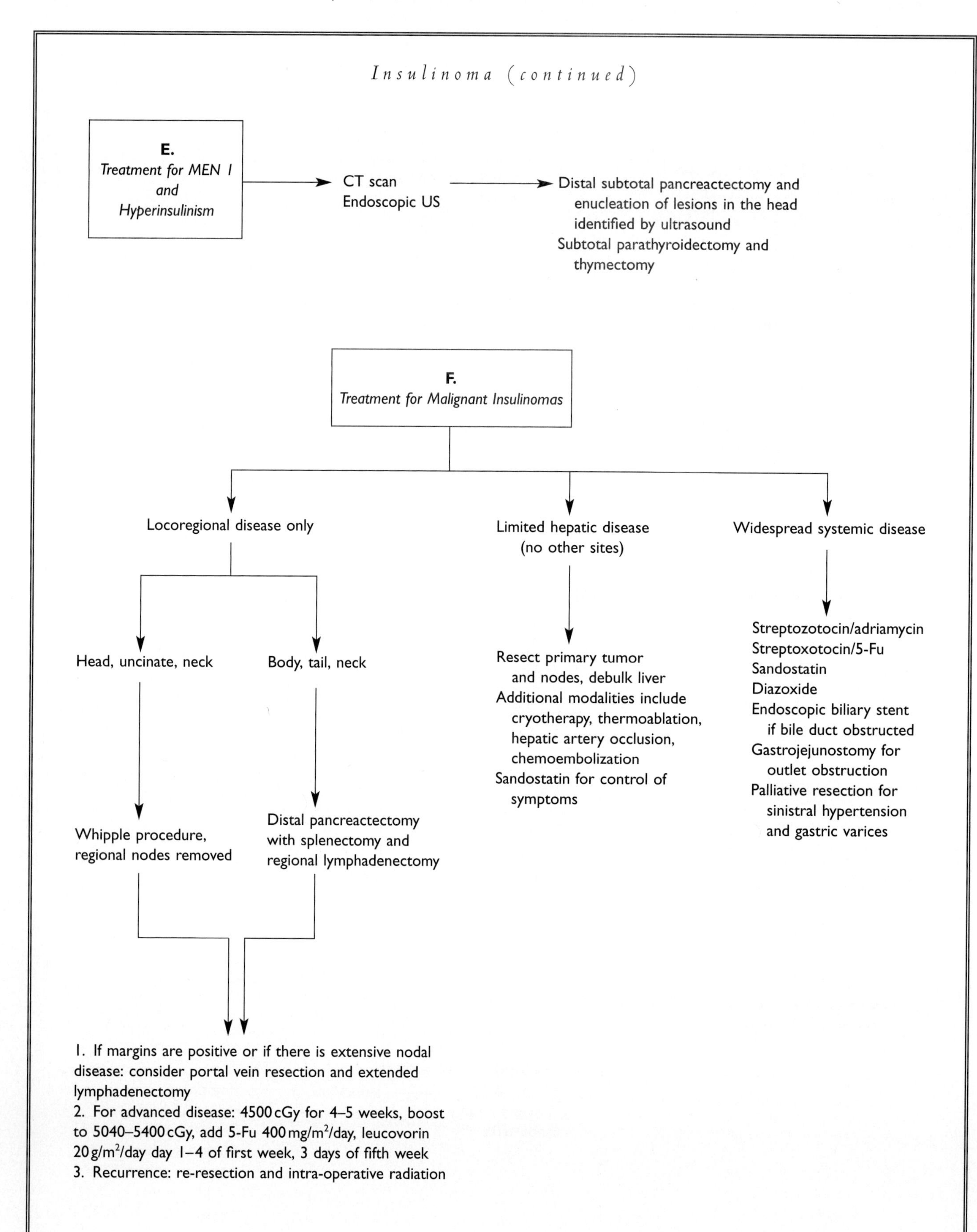
Insulinoma (continued)
E.
Treatment for MEN I and Hyperinsulinism
CT scan
Endoscopic US
Distal subtotal pancreactectomy and enucleation of lesions in the head identified by ultrasound
Subtotal parathyroidectomy and thymectomy
F.
Treatment for Malignant Insulinomas
Locoregional disease only
Limited hepatic disease (no other sites)
Widespread systemic disease
Head, uncinate, neck
Body, tail, neck
Whipple procedure, regional nodes removed
Distal pancreactectomy with splenectomy and regional lymphadenectomy
Resect primary tumor and nodes, debulk liver
Additional modalities include cryotherapy, thermoablation, hepatic artery occlusion, chemoembolization
Sandostatin for control of symptoms
Streptozotocin/adriamycin
Streptoxotocin/5-Fu
Sandostatin
Diazoxide
Endoscopic biliary stent if bile duct obstructed
Gastrojejunostomy for outlet obstruction
Palliative resection for sinistral hypertension and gastric varices
1. If margins are positive or if there is extensive nodal disease: consider portal vein resection and extended lymphadenectomy
2. For advanced disease: 4500 cGy for 4–5 weeks, boost to 5040–5400 cGy, add 5-Fu 400 mg/m²/day, leucovorin 20 g/m²/day day 1–4 of first week, 3 days of fifth week
3. Recurrence: re-resection and intra-operative radiation

TABLE 14–1.
Insulinoma: diagnostic criteria after 72-hour fast

Neuroglycopenia: present
Plasma glucose: ≤ 45 mg/dl
Plasma insulin (RIA): ≥ 6 μU/ml
Plasma C-peptide (ICMA): ≥ 200 pmol/L
Plasma proinsulin (ICMA): ≥ 5 pmol/L
Plasma sulfonylureas (first and second generation): negative
β-Hydroxybutyrate: < 2.7 mmol/L
Δ Glucose with 1 mg IV glucagon: 25 mg/dl within 30 minutes

RIA, radioimmunoassay; ICMA, immunochemilumineatric assay.

triad, characterized by plasma glucose levels <50 mg/dl, symptoms of hypoglycemia, and symptoms relieved by the administration of glucose, confirm the diagnosis of hypoglycemia. Evaluation with a supervised 72-hour fast would be the next step.[1]

C. Diagnosis

The *supervised 72-hour fast*[2] is necessary to determine which patients truly have endogenous (nonfactitious) hyperinsulinism; 35% of these patients have a positive test within 12 hours, 75% within 48 hours, and 92% within 48 hours. It is a rarity for a patient with endogenous (nonfactitious) hyperinsulinism to have a negative 72-hour fasting test. If both symptoms and hypoglycemia (plasma ≤45 mg/dl) are demonstrated at any time during the 72-hour fast, the fast can be terminated and end-of-fast studies obtained (Table 14–1). A positive fast consists of fasting hypoglycemia (plasma ≤45 mg/dl) with concomitant hyperinsulinemia (plasma insulin ≥6 mU/ml by radioimmunoassay). Plasma C-peptide levels measured by immunochemilumimetric (ICMA) assay of ≥200 pmol/L and plasma proinsulin levels (ICMA) ≥5 pmol/L confirm that the hyperinsulinemic state is due to endogenous rather than factitious causes.[3]

Patients with factitious hypoglycemia undergoing a 72-hour supervised fast may not have symptoms during the fast because they may have lost their access to insulin, oral agents, or both. Patients with hyperplasia or nesidioblastosis may experience neuroglycopenia only postprandially and often have a negative 72-hour fast.

To rule out a factitious cause in patients with elevated plasma insulin and C-peptide levels, assays for both first- and second-generation sulfonylureas must be performed using plasma obtained at completion of the fast; Typically, insulin, C-peptide, and proinsulin levels are not available for 24–48 hours. Insulin surrogates[4] can be measured rapidly at the end of the fast; if positive, they strongly suggest a hyperinsulinemic state warranting localization studies.[2] Plasma β-hydroxybutrate levels tend to be especially low in insulinoma patients because of the antiketogenic effect of insulin (<2.7 mmol/L). The administration of glucagon 1 mg IV raises the glucose level by ≥25 mg/dl within 30 minutes of fast completion. This is due to the glycogenic and antiglycogenolytic effects of insulin that maintain a supply of glucose in the liver.

If a witnessed hypoglycemic event occurs prior to a supervised 72-hour fast, the end-of-fast laboratory studies can be performed immediately. If confirmatory, the prolonged supervised fast can be avoided. If the end-of-fast criteria are not met or if there is evidence of exogenous insulin or sulfonylurea administration, no radiographic studies should be obtained nor should exploratory surgery be performed. The use of exogenous agents should be suspected when patients are in the health care field, care for diabetic family members, or seek medical evaluation without the support of family members and friends. Another possible cause for such a clinical presentation is adult nesidioblastosis,[5] which is generally a diffuse pancreatic process characterized histologically by beta cells budding off exocrine pancreatic ducts. Although this can be a histologic variant of normal, it has been associated with hyperinsulinemic hypoglycemia in children and in rare adults.

If the diagnosis is still in question, if further investigation is desired, and if factitious causes have been ruled out as best as they can be, consideration should be given to performing angiographic selective arterial calcium injection with hepatic vein sampling (SACI/HVS) for insulin.[6] This test is best performed in reoperative situations, when the diagnosis is still suspected but prior surgery has not identified a lesion. It should also be used in patients suspected of having nesidioblastosis based on the typical negative 72-hour fast. SACI/HVS is useful because of the territorial distribution of the pancreatic blood supply. Typically, the splenic artery perfuses the body and tail of the pancreas. The gastroduodenal artery supplies the head of the gland and the superior mesenteric artery, the uncinate process. Although there is overlap between these arterial territories, selective calcium injection, a known insulin secretagogue, stimulates abnormal beta cells to produce insulin in concentrations two- to threefold higher than normal beta cells. Patients who do not have an insulinoma or nesidioblastosis do not exhibit this response when the selected pancreatic arteries are injected with calcium. Patients with a discrete insulinoma generally regionalize to the area supplied by the vessel injected. Patients with nesidioblastosis often demonstrate a step-up in all three arterial distributions. In one report, there was a 94% accuracy rate.[6] In addition to regionalizing the insulinoma, an angiographic blush helps specifically localize the site of the tumor approximately 50% of time.

On rare occasion the C-peptide suppression test is helpful. In normal individuals administration of insulin 0.125 U/kg over 60 minutes results in defined suppression of plasma C-peptide levels. In patients with autonomous secretion of insulin and C-peptide, administration of exogenous insulin generally does not suppress C-peptide levels to the same degree as is seen in normal individuals. Normal responses are based on patient age and body mass index.[7]

Once endogenous nonfactitious hyperinsulinism has been confirmed, localizing studies are performed. Localizing studies should never be done just to diagnose an insulinoma, as false-positive and false-negative studies occur. Preoperative localization helps plan the operation, educate the patient, and relieve surgeon and patient anxiety.

All insulinomas are intrapancreatic, and 90% are solitary. Nearly all insulinomas can be found intraoperatively by an experienced endocrine surgeon aided by an experienced ultrasonographer utilizing intraoperative real-time ultrasonography (IOUS).[8–10] Several localizing studies have been utilized with varying degrees of success.[11] At the present time, we favor the use of transabdominal real-time ultrasonography, although it is, at best, only 60% accurate.[8] Should it show a well defined insulinoma, no other tests are necessary, and more invasive preoperative imaging studies can be avoided. If ultrasonography is negative, we use helical or spiral computed tomography (CT) scanning; triple-phase contrast methods scan the patient prior to injection of intravenous contrast and during the arterial and parenchymal phases. Although we believe this method is more accurate than conventional CT, supportive data are not yet available. Some centers almost exclusively use preoperative endoscopic ultrasonography (EUS), which has reported accuracy rates of 60–90%.[12] Lesions in the tail may be missed, although they are generally easily detected in the operating room.[13]

With a firm biochemical diagnosis of endogenous hyperinsulinism, the next step is to proceed to the operating room whether preoperative localizing studies are positive or negative. The basis for this philosophy is as follows: Although a positive preoperative localizing study has value, the highest degree of success is achieved by an experienced endocrine surgeon working in conjunction with an experienced ultrasonographer utilizing IOUS. IOUS has an accuracy of 92%.[10] Among our last 119 patients who underwent surgery for hyperinsulinism with the aid of IOUS, there were only three failures (unpublished data). Two of these patients had diffuse disease, and in only one was there a suspected missed adenoma, for an overall success rate of 98%. These results would not justify the routine use of SACI/HVS in patients with negative preoperative localization studies.

D. *Treatment for Benign Insulinoma*

Laparoscopic Approach

Anecdotal reports describe enucleation and distal pancreatic resections for insulinomas utilizing a transabdominal/retroperitoneal laparoscopic approach. This has been facilitated by the availability of laparoscopic IOUS instrumentation. The efficacy and safety of this approach has yet to be proven, and such an approach should be reserved for tumors that are pedunculated within the distal body and tail of the gland. A few surgeons worldwide have limited experience with these techniques.[14] Reported fistula rates have been higher than conventional surgery.

Standard Approach

The peritoneal cavity is explored through a transverse epigastric or long midline incision. After ruling out obvious metastatic disease, primarily on the surface of the liver, peritoneum, and regional lymph nodes, the gastrocolic ligament is divided just outside the gastroepiploic arcade; alternatively, the greater omentum can be taken down off the transverse colon from left to right entering the lesser sac, which exposes the body and proximal tail of the pancreas. The duodenum is widely kocherized up to and including the ligament of Treitz. In many instances, mobilization of the hepatic flexure facilitates exposure of the uncinate process. The avascular plane along the inferior border of the body of the pancreas is then incised, allowing bimanual and bidigital palpation of the body and proximal tail of the gland as well as the head, neck, and uncinate process of the pancreas. If an insulinoma is identified by this point, IOUS is performed for confirmation, to rule out additional occult lesions in the pancreas and liver, and to demonstrate the proximity of the islet cell tumor to the pancreatic and bile ducts and the major blood vessels.

Most insulinomas, because of their benign and well encapsulated nature, are amenable to enucleation after incising the overlying pancreatic capsule and exposing the underlying insulinoma. It is most helpful to perform the enucleation utilizing a carotid endarterectomy spatula. Small vessels are coapted with bipolar cautery. Sutures and clips are best avoided if possible. Once the superficial portion of the insulinoma is free, placing a stay suture in a figure-of-eight fashion through the adenoma often facilitates completion of the enucleation by providing slight countertraction. When the insulinoma is right on the main pancreatic duct within the body and tail of the gland, a spleen-preserving distal pancreatectomy is advisable rather than risk major ductal injury. For tumors in the head of the gland in close proximity to the bile and pancreatic ducts, a Whipple procedure, although generally frowned upon and rarely indicated, can be performed safely rather than taking the chance of missing a major bile or pancreatic ductal injury. Helpful hints for doing a pancreaticojejunostomy in the setting of a soft, normal pancreas include using as few absorbable sutures as possible, thereby minimizing necrosis, covering the anastomosis with fibrin glue, and maintaining the patient on continuous intravenous Sandostatin at 600–800 μg/24 hr until the patient is eating well without signs of a pancreatic leak.

Whether enucleation or resection is undertaken, closed suction drainage is imperative and should be maintained until the patient is eating without signs of a pancreatic leak. Following enucleation procedures, we always administer 75–150 IU secretin intravenously to check for major ductal disruption. IOUS can also be beneficial at this point, as secretin causes dilation of the pancreatic duct, making it possible to visualize its entire course with the ultrasound probe.

Intraoperative glucose monitoring is utilized routinely at our institution. Patients are brought to the operating room off all glucose-containing fluids for a few hours prior to surgery. Frequent plasma glucose levels are determined, and patients are maintained at levels >60 mg/dl utilizing incremental doses of 50% dextrose administered intravenously. Following removal of the tumor, plasma glucose levels are checked at 5-minute intervals with the aid of a radial arterial line until rebound hyperglycemia is demonstrated. Typically, after successful removal of an insulinoma, blood glucose levels rebound by 20 mg or more over the first 20 minutes. However, false-negative and false-positive results do occur. Surgical judgment should be the final determinant, not the plasma glucose level, for determining the completeness of resection. Patients generally develop rebound hyperglycemia within a few hours following surgery, if not sooner. Depending on the extent of pancreatic resection, glucose levels >300 mg/dl may occur within the first 24–48 hours. Typically, plasma glucose levels return to normal levels within 7–10 days. Approximately 5–7% of patients develop diabetes mellitus long term.[1]

Apparent ductal injuries following enucleation can be managed in various ways. Minor side branch injuries can be treated with simple ligation with absorbable suture and closed suction drainage. Major pancreatic ductal injury involving the body and tail of the pancreas is best treated with distal pancreatectomy. Major ductal injury in the head of the gland can be treated with closure of the side hole with fine interrupted absorbable sutures and closed suction drainage, although others close this type of injury over a small Silastic stent brought out through the papilla. Another option is to drain the injury site into a defunctionalized Roux limb. Finally, if all else fails, a Whipple procedure can be considered, but in general it should be a procedure of last resort.

If palpation and IOUS of the head, neck, body, and proximal tail of the gland is inconclusive, the next step is to mobilize the spleen and pancreatic tail. If repeat palpation/IOUS is positive, one should then continue with the procedures previously outlined.

If no tumor is found at the time of operation, the abdomen should be closed and the operation terminated. Blind distal resections should be condemned[15] for the following reasons: (1) most missed insulinomas are ultimately found in the head and uncinate, where they are most difficult to localize; (2) only 50% of insulinomas occur in the body and tail; (3) reoperations following blind distal resection are associated with a much higher incidence of pancreatic complications (fistula, abscess, pseudocyst formation, diabetes mellitus). Patients undergoing completion pancreatectomy for endogenous hyperinsulinism trade one life-threatening problem for another. Although many of these patients live several decades, life expectancy is clearly shortened as a result of the apancreatic state.[15]

Patients who have undergone unsuccessful surgery can be treated with frequent meals, calcium channel blockers, diazoxide, and Sandostatin injections, with varying degrees of success.[2] In patients with significant symptomatology, none of these palliative measures offers complete symptom relief, and all are associated with side effects. In patients with uncontrolled symptoms, selective arterial calcium injection with hepatic vein insulin sampling should be the next step after reconfirming the diagnosis of endogenous hyperinsulinism. If SACI/HVS is negative along with repeat standard localizing studies, one should not reoperate unless symptoms are truly unmanageable. In patients with a positive gradient on hepatic vein sampling, reoperative surgery can be performed once the initial perioperative inflammation has subsided (usually 6–12 months). At that time, palpation and IOUS are repeated; if negative, a gradient-guided resection is performed. In patients with a gradient in the splenic artery distribution, a distal pancreatectomy just to the left of the superior mesenteric vein is undertaken, preferably with splenic preservation. If the gradient is confined to the gastroduodenal artery or superior mesenteric artery distribution (or both) and no tumor is visualized by IOUS, a Whipple procedure can be performed. If a step-up is noted throughout the gland, an extended distal resection to the right of the superior mesenteric vein can render selected patients euglycemic.

E. MEN 1 and Hyperinsulinism

Twenty percent of patients with the MEN 1 syndrome have hyperisulinism. These glands are characterized by diffuse adenomatosis, hyperplasia, and nesidioblastosis. Once the diagnosis is confirmed, CT scanning and endoscopic US are all that is required preoperatively to rule out metastatic disease and to demonstrate the existence of large tumors in the pancreatic head. Surgical management involves a distal subtotal pancreatic resection with enucleation of additional tumors in the head of the gland using IOUS as a guide.[16,17] Subtotal parathyroidectomy and transcervical thymectomy with cryopreservation can be performed in the same setting for patients with concomitant hyperparathyroidism. Most of the pituitary tumors seen in these patients are microprolactinomas and are most often treated nonoperatively. Transsphenoidal surgery is reserved for patients with refractory hyperprolactinemia, enlarging prolactinomas, and pressure-related symptoms.

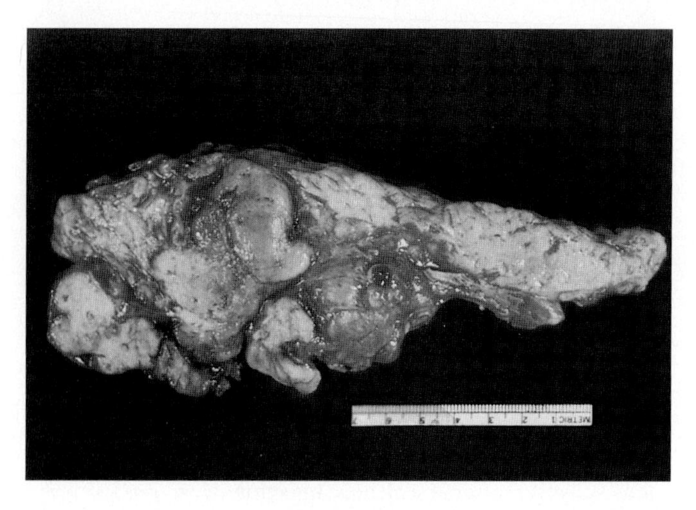

FIGURE 14–1
Distal pancreatectomy specimen containing malignant insulinoma with regional lymph node metastases.

F. *Treatment for Malignant Insulinomas*

Locoregional Disease Only

Fewer than 10% of insulinomas are malignant[1] (Fig. 14–1), the diagnosis of which is established by demonstrating distant or nodal metastases or invasion of surrounding structures. Malignant insulinomas tend to be larger than their benign counterparts, are more infiltrative in nature, and are easily localized by conventional CT scanning. Magnetic resonance imaging (MRI) is most helpful for delineating the extent of hepatic metastases. Disease localized to the primary site or surrounding regional lymph nodes is best treated by resection. Tumors located in the body, tail, and neck can generally be treated by distal pancreatectomy with splenectomy, along with regional lymphadenectomy. Malignant tumors confined to the head, uncinate, or distal neck are best treated by a Whipple procedure with extended regional lymph node dissection. If margins are histologically positive or there is extensive nodal disease, one can consider concomitant superior mesenteric vein/portal vein (SMV/PV) resection along with extended lymphadenectomy for gross total resection.

Postoperatively, such patients can be treated with external beam radiation, 5-fluorouracil (5-FU), and leucovorin. There are, however, no strong data to support this particular regimen. This approach has been extrapolated from the Gastrointestinal Study Group data for pancreatic ductal adenocarcinoma.[18,19] Radiation therapy is given as follows: large field, 4500 cGy for 4–5 weeks (25 fractions) with a boost to 5040–5400 cGy given in three to five additional fractions. Chemotherapy is as follows: 5-FU 400 mg/m^2/day plus leucovorin 20 g/m^2/day rapid IV push daily within 2 hours of irradiation for 4 days of the first week and 3 days of the fifth week.

In the setting of local recurrence, re-resection utilizing intraoperative radiation therapy can be considered, once again without well defined studies to support its use.

Limited Metastatic Disease Confined to the Liver

For patients with limited metastatic disease confined to the liver, an aggressive multimodality approach has been shown to provide effective palliation from hormonal sequelae and occasionally to improve survival.[20] This multimodality approach includes resection of the primary tumor and regional lymph nodes and hepatic debulking,[21] preferably with removal of more than 90% of the tumor burden, leaving behind at least two well vascularized hepatic segments. Additional modalities[20,22] incorporating cryotherapy or thermoablation as well as hepatic artery occlusion techniques and chemoembolization have also provided effective symptomatic palliation in select patients. The long-acting somatostatin analogue octreotide[23] can also be utilized for hormonal suppression therapy. The use longer-acting analogues may effectively reduce the need for multiple daily injections.

Widespread Systemic Disease

In the instance of widespread systemic disease, therapy is primarily offered to symptomatic patients who suffer from hormonal sequelae, obstruction, pain, or bleeding. Occasionally, palliative distal pancreatectomy and splenectomy are necessary for patients with sinistral hypertension due to splenic vein occlusion and bleeding gastric varices. Patients with gastric outlet obstruction can be managed with gastrojejunostomy, performed as an open or a laparoscopic procedure. In most cases biliary obstruction can be managed by placing an endoscopic biliary stent. The combination of streptozotocin (STZ) and adriamycin has been shown to provide a 69% response rate in patients with metastatic islet cell carcinoma,[24] an improvement over the standard regimen of streptozotocin and 5-FU (45% response rate). STZ is given by intravenous injection at a dose of 500 mg/m^2/day for 5 days and repeated every 6 weeks. Doxorubicin (adriamycin) is given along with STZ by intravenous injection at a dose of 50 mg/m^2 on days 1 and 22 of each 6-week treatment cycle, with a maximal total dose of 500 mg/m^2. Diazoxide, a nondiuretic benzothiadiazine that acts directly on beta cells to reduce insulin secretion, has been utilized in patients with widespread metastatic disease and symptoms. Side effects, particularly gastrointestinal, hypotension, edema, and hirsutism, have made its use unpleasant for most patients.[25]

References

1. Service FJ, McMahon MM, O'Brien PC, Ballard DJ. Functioning insulinoma: incidence, recurrence, and long-term survival of patients; a 60-year study. Mayo Clin Proc 1991;66:711–719.
2. Service FJ. Hypoglycemic disorders. N Engl J Med 1995;332:1144–1152.
3. Service FJ, O'Brien PC, McMahon MM, Kao PI. C-peptide during the prolonged fast in insulinoma. J Clin Endocrinol Metab 1993;76:655–659.
4. O'Brien T, O'Brien PC, Service FJ. Insulin surrogates in insulinoma. J Clin Endocrinol Metab 1993;77:448–451.
5. Harness JK, Geelhoed GW, Thompson NW, et al. Nesidioblastosis in adults. Arch Surg 1981;116:575.
6. Brown CK, Bartlett DL, Doppman JL, et al. Intra-arterial calcium stimulation and intraoperative ultrasonography in the localization and resection of insulinomas. Surgery 1997;122:1189–1193.
7. Service FJ, O'Brien PC, Kao PC, Young WF. C-peptide suppression test: effects of gender, age, and body mass index; implications for the diagnosis of insulinoma. J Clin Endocrinol Metab 1992;74:204–210.
8. Gorman B, Charboneau JW, James EM, et al. Benign pancreatic insulinoma: preoperative and intraoperative monographic localization. AJR Am J Roentgenol 1986;147:929–934.
9. Grant CS. Gastrointestinal endocrine tumors: insulinoma. Baillieres Clin Gastroenterol 1996;10:645–671.
10. Grant CS, van Heerden JA, Charboneau JW, James EM, Reading CC. Insulinoma: the value of intraoperative ultrasonography. Arch Surg 1988;123:843–848.
11. Pasieka JL, McLeod MK, Thompson NW, Burney RE. Surgical approach to insulinomas: assessing the need for preoperative localization. Arch Surg 1992;127:442.
12. Schumacher B, Lubke HJ, Frieling T, Strohmeyer G, Starke AA. Prospective study on the detection of insulinomas by endoscopic ultrasonography. Endoscopy 1996;28:273–276.
13. Rösch T, Lightdale J, Botet JF, et al. Localization of pancreatic endocrine tumors by endoscopic ultrasonography. N Engl J Med 1992;326:1721.
14. Gagner M, Pomp A, Herrera MF. Early experience with laparoscopic resections of islet cell tumors. Surgery 1996;120:1051–1054.
15. Thompson GB, Service FJ, van Heerden JA, et al. Reoperative insulinomas, 1927 to 1992: an institutional experience. Surgery 1993;114:1196–1206.
16. Thompson NW. Multiple endocrine neoplasia type. I. Surgical therapy. Cancer Treat Res 1997;89:407–419.
17. Rasbach DA, van Heerden JA, Telander RL, et al. Surgical management of hyperinsulinism in the multiple endocrine neoplasia type 1 syndrome. Arch Surg 1985;120:584.
18. Kalser MH, Ellenberg SS, Gastrointestinal Tumor Study Group. Pancreatic cancer: adjuvant combined radiation and chemotherapy following curative resection. Arch Surg 1985;120:899–903.
19. Gastrointestinal Tumor Study Group. Further evidence of effective adjuvant combined radiation and chemotherapy following curative resection of pancreatic cancer. Cancer 1987;59:2006–2010.
20. Que FG, Nagorney DM. Cytoreductive hepatic surgery for metastatic gastrointestinal neuroendocrine tumors. Front Gastrointest Res 1995; 23:416–430.
21. McEntee GP, Nagorney DM, Kvols LK, Moertel CG, Grant CS. Cytoreductive hepatic surgery for neuroendocrine tumors. Surgery 1990; 108:1091–1096.
22. Siperstein AE, Rogers SJ, Hansen PD, Gitomirsky A. Laparoscopic thermal ablation of hepatic neuroendocrine tumor metastases. Surgery 1997; 122:1147–1155.
23. Maton PN. Use of octreotide acetate for the control of symptoms in patients with islet cell tumors. World J Surg 1993;17:504.
24. Moertel CG, Lefkopoulo M, Lipsitz S, Hahn RG, Klaassen D. Streptozocin-doxorubicin, streptozocin-fluorouracil, or chlorozotocin in the treatment of advanced islet cell carcinoma. N Engl J Med 1992;326:519–523.
25. Goode PN, Farndon JR, Anderson J. Diazoxide in the management of patients with insulinoma. World J Surg 1986;10:586.

Chapter 15

Glucagonoma

MARK S. TALAMONTI

A. Epidemiology and Etiology

Glucagonomas are rare pancreatic islet cell tumors that produce a distinct clinical syndrome because of excess production of glucagon by the alpha cells of the pancreatic islets. Glucagon-producing tumors occur less frequently than gastrinomas and insulinomas, but they produce a clinical syndrome that is just as distinctive. Becker et al. first described the features of this syndrome in 1942,[1] and McGavran et al. reported the first well documented case of hyperglucagonemia in 1966.[2] Mallinson et al. reported nine cases in 1974, detailing the characteristic features of the syndrome.[3] The most notable features of the glucagonoma syndrome are diabetes or abnormal glucose tolerance, a unique rash known as necrotizing migratory erythema, and thromboembolic problems.[4] Women appear to outnumber men, with a frequency of 3:1. The mean age at diagnosis is 52 years (range 20–73 years). Although glucagonomas have been associated with the multiple endocrine neoplasia type 1 (MEN 1) syndrome, this is a rare occurrence. Other common findings in patients with glucagonomas include weight loss and anemia. Less frequently associated symptoms are gastrointestinal and neurologic disorders.[5]

B. Physiology and Pathology

Glucagon from pancreatic alpha cells plays an important role in modulating serum glucose concentrations. Glucagon is a catabolic hormone that antagonizes the effects of insulin. Its principal physiologic function is to increase blood glucose levels. It is the exaggeration of these effects that leads to the biochemical and clinical features of the glucagonoma syndrome. Glucagon is stored and released by the pancreas in response to hypoglycemia or stress. It is a *potent stimulator* of gluconeogenesis, glycogenolysis, and ketogenesis. It also *inhibits* glycolysis and lipogenesis. Other physiologic roles of glucagon are hepatic ketogenesis and mild hepatic proteolysis. With the glucagonoma syndrome there is a marked increase in hepatic proteolysis with conversion of amino acid nitrogen to urea nitrogen. This leads to decreased blood amino acid levels, particularly the glycogenic molecules such as alanine, glycine, and

Glucagonoma

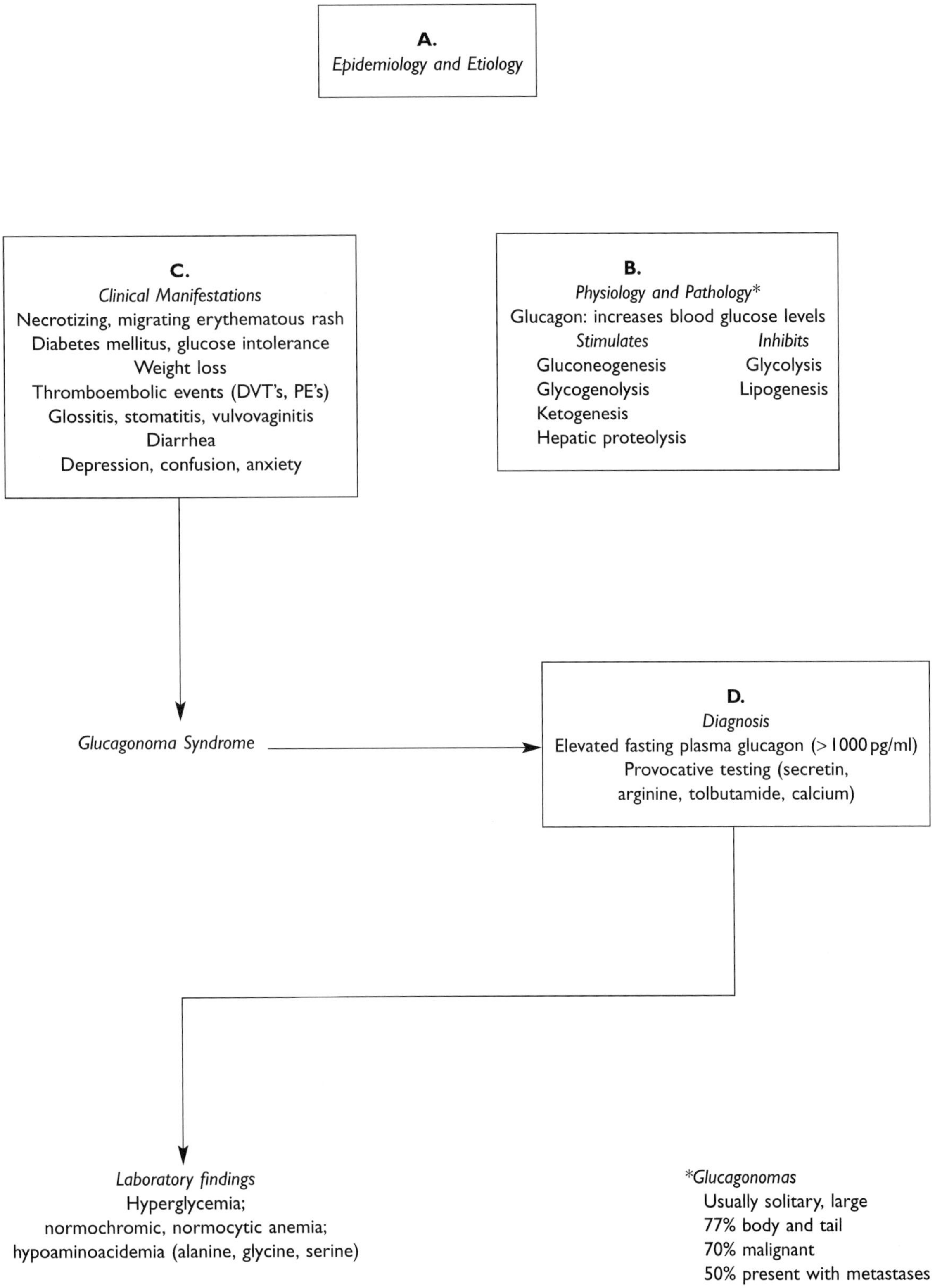

A.
Epidemiology and Etiology

B.
*Physiology and Pathology**
Glucagon: increases blood glucose levels

Stimulates	*Inhibits*
Gluconeogenesis	Glycolysis
Glycogenolysis	Lipogenesis
Ketogenesis	
Hepatic proteolysis	

C.
Clinical Manifestations
Necrotizing, migrating erythematous rash
Diabetes mellitus, glucose intolerance
Weight loss
Thromboembolic events (DVT's, PE's)
Glossitis, stomatitis, vulvovaginitis
Diarrhea
Depression, confusion, anxiety

↓

Glucagonoma Syndrome →

D.
Diagnosis
Elevated fasting plasma glucagon (>1000 pg/ml)
Provocative testing (secretin, arginine, tolbutamide, calcium)

↓

Laboratory findings
Hyperglycemia;
normochromic, normocytic anemia;
hypoaminoacidemia (alanine, glycine, serine)

**Glucagonomas*
- Usually solitary, large
- 77% body and tail
- 70% malignant
- 50% present with metastases

(continued on next page)

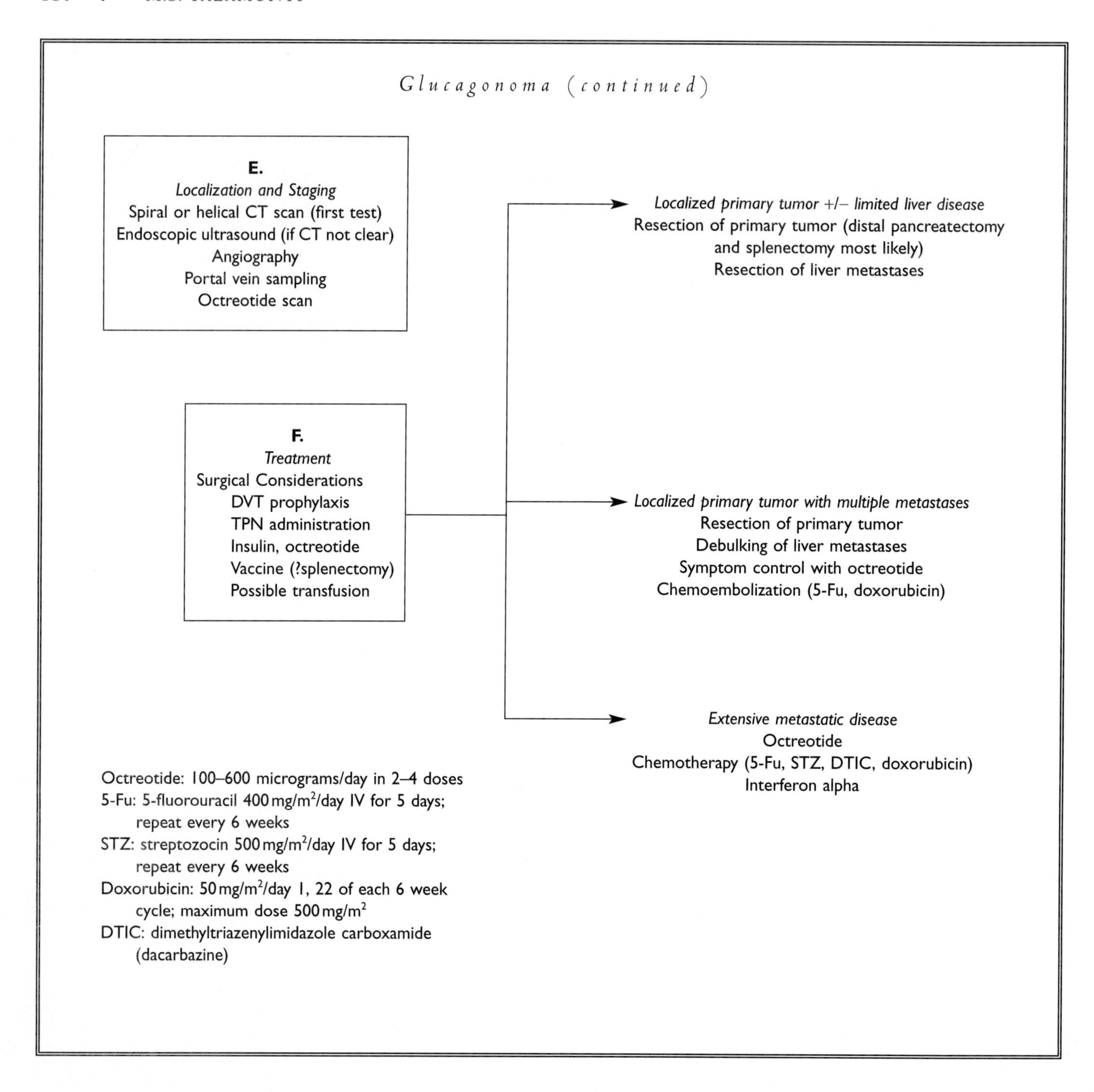

serine, which are also required for increased gluconeogenesis. Circulating levels often fall to less than 25% of normal, resulting in organ protein catabolism and hence decreased lean body mass. This is probably a major factor in the weight loss associated with the syndrome.[6]

Glucagonomas are usually solitary tumors; they tend to be large (>5 cm) and occur most often (77%) in the body and tail of the pancreas.[7] The tumors are usually solid, but they can undergo central necrosis with hemorrhage.

Approximately 70% of glucagonomas are malignant, but, malignancy can be diagnosed only by finding local invasion or distant metastases.[8] Because of the frequent delay in diagnosis, many of these tumors (at least 50%) present with metastatic disease. The liver is the most common site of distant metastases followed by the peripancreatic lymph nodes. The tumors may become quite large before detection and show signs of local invasion, including portal vein thrombosis, mesenteric artery encasement, and retroperitoneal extension.

C. Clinical Manifestations

The most striking clinical feature of the glucagonoma syndrome is its characteristic rash, known as necrolytic migratory erythema (NME),[9] which occurs in approximately two-thirds of patients.

The rash usually starts in the groins and migrates to the distal extremities, thighs, buttocks, and perineum. Erythematous blotches are the first manifestation, followed by scaling. The lesions become raised, with vesicopustules and bullae; then erosion and crusting occurs. The lesions may become confluent, and clearing begins centrally. Healing leaves indurated pigmented areas. The process is chronic, relapsing, and migratory.[10] The rash is attributed to the hypoaminoacidemia that results from the profound, catabolic effects of glucagon.[11] The diagnosis of NME is suggested by the clinical presentation of the rash and can be confirmed by characteristic findings on biopsy.

The most common clinical feature of the glucagonoma syndrome is diabetes mellitus. This is nearly a universal finding in patients with glucagonoma,[6,9] although patients often go undiagnosed for many years until the effects of metastatic disease become apparent or the characteristic necrotizing skin rash develops. The diabetes associated with glucagonomas differs from the usual insulin-dependent disease. It is generally milder, and patients are less prone to ketoacidosis or microvascular complications. Natural insulin production may vary during the course of the disease. Replacement of the normal beta cells by an enlarging tumor may exacerbate the diabetes.[5]

Weight loss without anorexia is also common in this syndrome. The weight loss may be severe and may be explained by excessive lipolysis and gluconeogenesis. Deep venous thrombosis (DVT) and thromboembolism are frequent in patients with glucagonomas,[6,9] occurring in 30–50% of patients. Because thromboembolic complications are fatal in a significant proportion of these patients, those undergoing surgery must receive appropriate DVT prophylaxis. Long-term anticoagulation therapy is considered for patients with incurable or advanced disease. Other common but less characteristic findings with this syndrome are diarrhea, stomatitis, glossitis, and chronic vulvovaginitis. Alterations in mental status, although nonspecific, are frequent in patients with glucagonoma. These alterations include depression, disorientation, and a general sense of nervousness.[6,9]

A normochromic, normocytic anemia occurs in about 85% of patients with glucagonomas. The exact etiology of the anemia is unclear, but glucagon does have the ability to suppress erythropoiesis.[12] Hypoaminoacidemia is another unique clinical characteristic of this syndrome. Concentrations of most amino acids are usually depressed to less than 25% of normal. The depressed plasma amino acid levels are though possibly to play a role in the development of the characteristic skin rash. Correction of the hypoaminoacidemia by surgical removal of the tumor or amino acid supplementation is associated with resolution of the characteristic rash.[11]

D. Diagnosis

The diagnosis is suggested by the characteristic clinical presentation and is confirmed by demonstrating a plasma glucagon concentration that is inappropriately elevated relative to the plasma glucose level. Normal glucagon values range from 25 to 250 pg/ml. Although glucagon levels can be elevated in patients with hepatic insufficiency, renal failure, severe stress, hypoglycemia, diabetic ketoacidosis, and starvation, the level rarely exceeds 500 pg/ml in the presence of these conditions. Almost all patients with glucagonomas have plasma glucagon levels above 250 pg/ml; levels exceeding 1000 pg/ml are diagnostic. The diagnosis is further suggested by failure of glucose to suppress glucagon. Provocative testing with secretin, arginine, tolbutamide, or calcium may be helpful but is usually not necessary.[4,5]

E. Localization and Staging

Glucagonomas are less difficult to localize preoperatively than other endocrine tumors of the pancreas because of their large size at presentation. Most are >3–5 cm in diameter, and most are located in the body and tail of the pancreas.[7,8] Dynamic, sequential computed tomography (CT) scanning with thin cuts through the region of the pancreas can usually localize these tumors. Additional information regarding the local extent of the tumor can also be obtained from a CT scan. The absence of portal vein thrombosis and the lack of encasement of the hepatic artery or superior mesenteric artery suggest a localized primary tumor amenable to surgical resection. CT scans can also identify intraabdominal metastases especially in the liver and peripancreatic lymph nodes. Angiography and percutaneous transhepatic venous sampling can be helpful for localizing small tumors that were difficult to identify on CT scan.[13–15] Endoscopic ultrasonography (EUS) of the pancreas is a relatively new modality. It has demonstrated enhanced sensitivity in terms of localizing pancreatic endocrine tumors and may be useful when CT images suggest the presence of a small but not well visualized tumor. It is less invasive than angiography and selective venous sampling and should be considered the second test to use after CT scanning in ambiguous situations.[16]

Somatostatin receptor scintigraphy is a new imaging method for localizing and determining the extent of gastrointestinal neuroendocrine tumors. An indium-labeled somatostatin analogue is injected, which then binds to tumor cells with somatostatin receptors; localization is accomplished then through nuclear medicine imaging. The advantages of this technique are that it may provide biochemical evidence that somatostatin receptors are present in the tumor, and it may be able to identify small or occult disease in the liver that has escaped detection with CT scanning.[17] The treatment implications of a somatostatin receptor-positive tumor are discussed below.

F. Treatment

Localized Primary Tumor with or without Limited Liver Disease

Surgery offers the only chance of cure for neuroendocrine tumors. Approximately 25% of glucagonomas are benign and are therefore cured by surgery. For patients with malignant tumors confined to the pancreas, resection results in an estimated cure rate on approximately 30%. Most of these cancers recur, with the most frequent site of recurrence being the liver. Approximately 50–60% of patients with malignant glucagonomas have metastases at the time of diagnosis. Aggressive surgical resection, including excision of the primary tumor and debulking of liver metastases, should be considered, as tumor volume reduction may significantly reverse the debilitating effects of excess glucagon secretion.[6] A number of reports have documented rapid reversal of the clinical syndrome after removing the primary tumor and liver-directed therapy for the metastases.[6,8] Limited liver resections of peripherally based metastases are indicated when feasible. Formal hepatic resections should be undertaken if all gross disease can be removed in this fashion. Alternative forms of liver surgery, including cryosurgical ablation and radiofrequency ablation, have been applied to treat metastatic neuroendocrine tumors; and preliminary reports suggest favorable response rates.[18] It is the general recommendation that aggressive removal of as much tumor as possible be undertaken if curative resection is not possible.

Surgery may be complicated by the tendency to form deep venous thrombi, the catabolic effects of hyperglucagonemia, and anemia. Administration of total parenteral nutrition (TPN) containing insulin and simultaneous administration of octreotide may help minimize the operative risks associated with these adverse consequences. For severely debilitated patients, some recommend several weeks of TPN to help reverse the catabolic effects of glucagon and to raise serum amino acid levels. Perioperative heparin administration is indicated, as 30% of these patients have thromboembolic phenomena. In preparation for a likely splenectomy with distal pancreatic resection, pneumococcal vaccine administration is indicated. Transfusions should be considered if profound anemia exists prior to surgical exploration.[8]

At the time of surgical exploration, the pancreas, peripancreatic lymph nodes, and liver are thoroughly evaluated. For the few patients in whom clinical, radiographic, and operative findings suggest the presence of a benign tumor, enucleation may be indicated. For patients with malignant lesions in the body and tail of the pancreas, aggressive resection of the primary tumor, including the spleen and peripancreatic lymph nodes, should be considered. Occasionally, patients with tumors in the head of the pancreas require a Whipple resection. Usually patients with liver metastases have bulky, diffuse disease that precludes complete removal of all metastases. Even so, an aggressive attempt at resection of peripherally based nodules should be made. Tumor debulking can provide dramatic, rapid alleviation of many of the characteristic symptoms.[4,5] In addition, removal of a significant volume of metastatic tumor may improve the response to systemic therapy with octreotide.[19] In addition to relief from the debilitating effects of the disease, survival may also be prolonged in these patients. In some reports, approximately 50% of patients survived 5 years following a combination of aggressive surgical resection and systemic therapy consisting of chemotherapy or octreotide administration.[20,21] Octreotide is administered subcutaneously every 8–12 hours. The initial dose is 100–600 μg/day in two to four divided doses. The effective dose varies among patients and must be titrated to the individual's symptoms.

Localized Primary Tumor with Multiple Metastases

Patients who succumb to malignant glucagonoma usually do so because of progressive disease in the liver. Thus therapy directed at controlling symptoms and progression of the liver metastases appears warranted. Liver metastases from glucagonomas are particularly hypervascular; consequently, these tumors are potential targets for hepatic artery embolization, which has been combined with simultaneous intraarterial chemotherapy. Theoretic advantages of hepatic artery chemoembolization include delivery of high doses of concentrated chemotherapy to the tumor deposits and interruption of the arterial blood supply to these hypervascular lesions. Chemotherapeutic agents delivered at the time of chemoembolization have included 5-fluorouracil (5-FU) and doxorubicin. Significant radiographic responses can be expected in approximately 50% of patients, and nearly all patients have some alleviation of their clinical symptoms. In addition, patients who have undergone hepatic artery chemoembolization may have improved symptom control with octreotide subsequent to the liver-directed therapy.[22–25] Orthotopic liver transplantation has also been used occasionally in patients with malignant glucagonomas.

Extensive Metastatic Disease

Octreotide Therapy Somatostatin is a naturally occurring peptide hormone thought to be a potent inhibitor of peptide release. The clinical usefulness of somatostatin has been limited by its short half-life of less than 4 minutes. A long-acting analogue of somatostatin, octreotide has become a mainstay in controlling the hormonal manifestations of neuroendocrine tumors. Usually administered by subcutaneous injection, it has been used effectively in patients with glucagonomas. The dose is 100–600 μg/day in two to four divided doses.

Somatostatin receptor scintigraphy, as noted, has been used to help identify subclinical disease and may also identify tumors that express significant levels of somatostatin receptor. It is these tumors that are most likely to be palliated with octreotide.

Several studies have documented clinical responses in addition to decreased levels of circulating glucagon after administration of octreotide. Octreotide can be administered preoperatively in an attempt to diminish the debilitating effects of hyperglucagonemia. In addition, following surgical resection or liver-directed therapy, octreotide may have enhanced effectiveness in reducing the clinical manifestations of the disease and is particularly effective against the rash (necrolytic migratory erythema). Octreotide is less consistently effective in reversing the weight loss, diabetes, and anemia seen in these patients.[8,21,26]

CHEMOTHERAPY Cytotoxic chemotherapy with 5-FU and streptozocin (STZ) provides reasonably successful palliation of metastatic disease. Response rates of 70–80% have been reported.[27,28] For the combination regimens, STZ is given by intravenous injection at a dose of $500\,mg/m^2$/day for 5 consecutive days, repeated every 6 weeks. 5-FU is given by intravenous injection at a dose of $400\,mg/m^2$/day for 5 days, concurrently with the streptozocin. Doxorubicin has also been used with streptozocin, at a dose of $50\,mg/m^2$ IV on days 1 and 22 of each 6-week treatment cycle, with a maximal total dose of $500\,mg/m^2$. The most active therapeutic agent is probably dimethyltriazenyl imidazole carboxamide (DTIC), which is active against many of the islet cell tumors but has been shown to be particularly successful for treating glucagonomas.[29] Interferon-α (IFNα) has been used with some success to treat malignant endocrine tumors including glucagonomas; and if combined with 5-FU, it produces response rates approaching 40–50%.[30] Recombinant INFα 2a is given at a daily dose of 3×106 IU for the first 3 days. The dose is then increased to 6×106 IU, administered daily for the first 8 weeks and three times per week thereafter. It is given intramuscularly into one of the gluteal muscles. The most active and effective combination of therapeutic agents (5-FU/streptozotocin/DTIC) and biologic therapy (IFNα) is currently being addressed by ongoing clinical trials.

References

1. Becker SW, Kahn D, Rothman S. Cutaneous manifestations of internal malignant tumors. Arch Dermatol Syphilol 1942;45:1069–1080.
2. McGavran MH, Unger RH, Recant L, Polk HC, Kilo C, Levin ME. A glucagon-secreting alpha cell carcinoma of the pancreas. N Engl J Med 1966;274:1408–1413.
3. Mallinson GN, Bloom SR, Warin AP, Salmon PR, Cox B. A glucagonoma syndrome. Lancet 1974;2:1–5.
4. Sabel MS, Prinz RA. Glucagonoma. Surg Dis Pancreas 1998;79:745–756.
5. Van Heerden FA, Thompson GB. Islet cell tumours of the pancreas. Surg Pancreas 1993;49:545–561.
6. Joyce CD, Prinz RA. The glucagonoma syndrome. Probl Gen Surg 1994; 11:1–16.
7. Howard JH, Stabile BE, Zinner MJ, Chang S, Belur BS, Passero E. Anatomic distribution of pancreatic endocrine tumors. Am J Surg 1990;159:258–264.
8. Prinz RA, Badrinath K, Banerji M, Sparagana M, Dorsch TR, Lawrence AM. Operative and chemotherapeutic management of malignant glucagon-producing tumors. Surgery 1981;90:713–719.
9. Bloom SR, Polak JM. Glucagonoma syndrome. Am J Med 1987;82(suppl): 25–36.
10. Fujita J, Seino Y, Ishida H, et al. A functional study of a case of glucagonoma exhibiting typical glucagonoma syndrome. Cancer 1986;57:860–865.
11. Norton JA, Hahn CR, Schiebinger R, et al. Amino acid deficiency and the skin rash associated with glucagonoma. Ann Intern Med 1979;91:213–215.
12. Naets JP, Guns M. Inhibitory effect of glucagon on erythropoiesis. Blood 1980;55:997–1002.
13. Wawrukiewicz AS, Rosch J, Keller FS, Lieberman DA. Glucagonoma and its angiographic diagnosis. Cardiovasc Intervent Radiol 1982;5:318–324.
14. Cho KJ, Wilcox CW, Reuter SR. Glucagon producing islet cell tumor of the pancreas. AJR Am J Roentgenol 1977;145:509–516.
15. Ingemansson S, Holst J, Larsson LI, et al. Localization of glucagonomas by catheterization of the pancreatic veins and with glucagon assay. Surg Gynecol Obstet 1977;145:509–516.
16. Rosch T, Lightdale CJ, Botet JF. Localization of pancreatic endocrine tumors by endoscopic ultrasonography. N Engl J Med 1992;326:1721–1726.
17. Krenning EP, Kwekkeboom DJ, Oei HY, et al. Somatostatin-receptor scintigraphy in gastroenteropancreatic tumors. Ann NY Acad Sci 1994; 773:416–424.
18. Bilchik AJ, Sarantou T, Foshag L, Giuliano AE, Ramming KP. Cryosurgical palliation of metastatic neuroendocrine tumors resistant to conventional therapy. Surgery 1997;122:1040–1048.
19. Modlin JM, Lewis JJ, Ahlman H, Bilchik AJ, Jumar RR. Management of unresectable malignant endocrine tumors of the pancreas. Surg Gynecol Obstet 1993;176:507–518.
20. Moertel CG. An Odyssey in the land of small tumors. J Clin Oncol 1987;5:1503–1522.
21. Altimari AF, Bhoopalam N, Prinz RA, et al. Use of a somatostatin analog (SMS201-995) in the glucagonoma syndrome. Surgery 1986;100:989–996.
22. Carrasco D, Jackson NA, Samaan R, et al. The carcinoid syndrome: palliation by hepatic arterial embolization. Am J Radiol 1986;147:149–154.
23. Hajarizadeh H, Ivancev K, Mueller CR, et al. Effective palliative treatment of metastatic carcinoid tumors with intra-arterial chemotherapy/chemoembolization combined with octreotide acetate. Am J Surg 1992;163:479–483.
24. Perry JL, Stuart K, Stokes KR, Clouse ME. Hepatic arterial chemoembolization for metastatic neuroendocrine tumors. Surgery 1994;116:1116–1117.
25. Urszniewski P, Rougier P, Roche A, et al. Hepatic arterial chemoembolization in patients with liver metastases of endocrine tumors: a prospective phase II study in 24 patients. Cancer 1993;71:2624–2630.
26. Jockenhovel F, Lederbogen S, Olbricht T, et al. The long-acting somatostatin analogue octreotide alleviates symptoms by reducing post-translational conversion of preproglucagon to glucagon in a patient with malignant glucagonoma, but does not prevent tumor growth. Clin Invest 1994; 72:127–133.
27. Moertel C, Hauley J, Johnson L. Streptozotocin alone compared with streptozotocin plus fluorouracil in the treatment of advanced islet cell carcinoma. N Engl J Med 1980;303:1189–1194.
28. Broder LE, Carter SK. Pancreatic islet cell carcinoma: results of therapy with streptozotocin in 52 patients. Ann Intern Med 1973;79:101–107.
29. Kessinger A, Floley JF, Lemon HM. Therapy of malignant APUD cell tumors: effectiveness of DTIC. Cancer 1983;51:790–794.
30. Jones DV Jr, Samaan NA, Sellin RV, et al. Metastatic glucagonoma: clinical response to a combination of 5-FU and alpha-interferon. Am J Med 1992;93:348–349.

CHAPTER 16

Carcinoid Tumors

KEITH W. MILLIKAN
EDWARD F. HOLLINGER

Oberndorfer first used the term *kazenoide* to describe a class of intestinal tumors that have a more homogeneous histologic appearance and slower rate of growth than intestinal adenocarcinomas.[1] It was later suggested that these tumors might arise from enterochromaffin cells of the glands of Lieberkühn, indicating that they were of endocrine origin.[2]

Currently, "carcinoid" is used to describe a spectrum of neoplasms that originate from neuroendocrine cells and may produce biologically active agents. These tumors may show benign or malignant behavior and may be clinically functional or nonfunctional in regard to producing biologically active amines or peptides. In general, carcinoids derive from cells of the diffuse endocrine system and have the capacity for *a*mine *p*recursor *u*ptake and *d*ecarboxylation; thus these tumors can be classified as a subset of APUDomas.[3] Because these lesions are often found incidentally, the measured incidence rate varies significantly; in the United States the incidence is approximately 7–15 per 1 million population per year. In approximately 45% of reported cases metastases are already evident at the time of diagnosis, and an overall 5-year survival rate of approximately 50% for all carcinoid tumors has been reported.[4]

Carcinoid tumors can cause symptoms as a result of direct local organ effects (e.g., pulmonary or gastrointestinal tract obstruction) or as the result of hormones released into the systemic circulation. In particular, expression of serotonin by carcinoids outside anatomic areas subserved by the portal circulation can result in a "carcinoid syndrome" consisting of cutaneous flushing, diarrhea, right-sided valvular heart disease, and bronchoconstriction.

Characteristics and Classification

Several classifications have been developed for characterizing carcinoid tumors, anticipating their patterns of spread, and predicting patient survival. Characteristics used include the anatomic location of the primary tumor; its embryonic origin, which is closely related to the tumor's histochemical and biochemical properties; tumor size and stage; and the histologic appearance of the tumor.

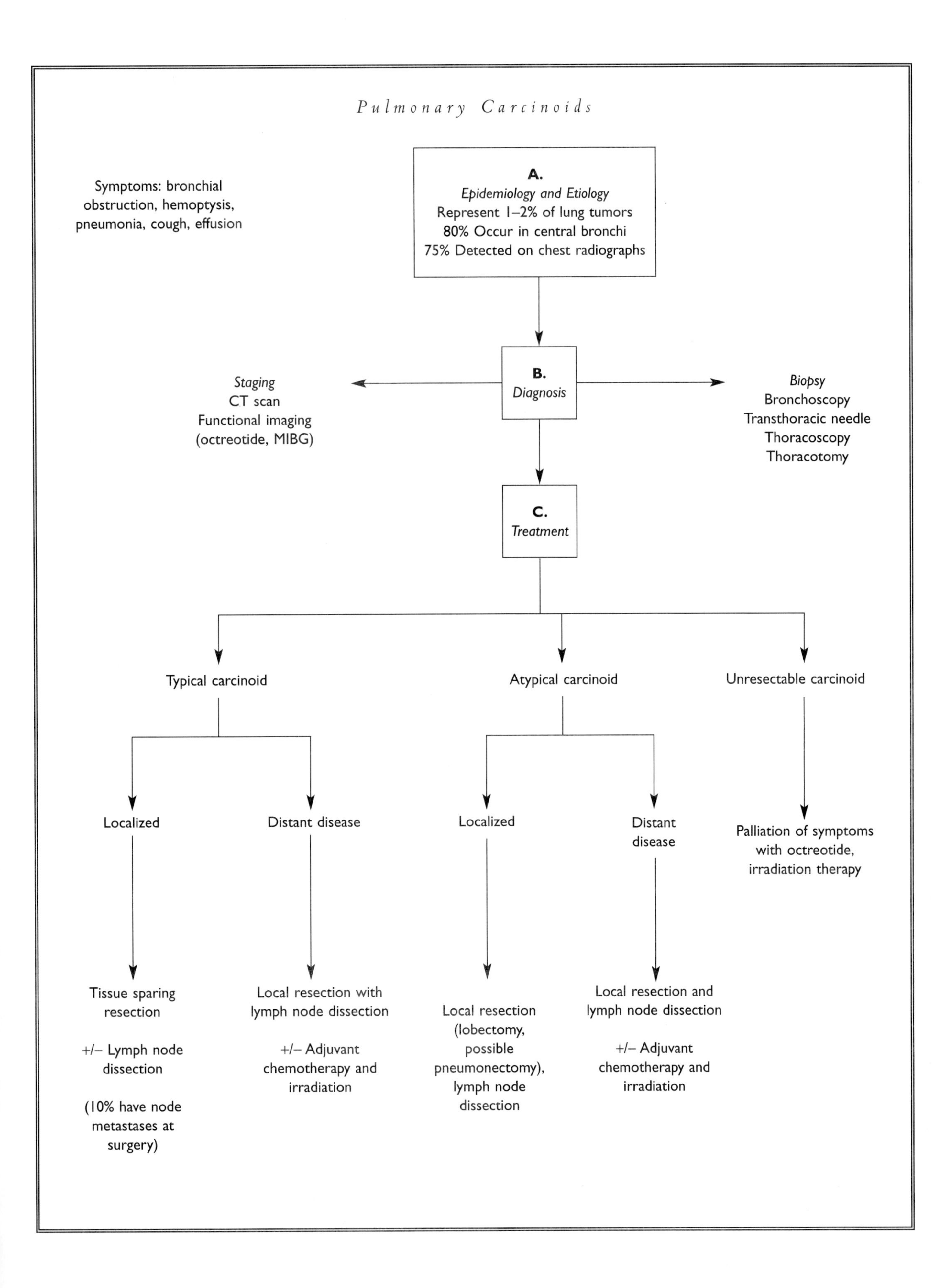

Pulmonary Carcinoids
Symptoms: bronchial obstruction, hemoptysis, pneumonia, cough, effusion
A.
Epidemiology and Etiology
Represent 1–2% of lung tumors
80% Occur in central bronchi
75% Detected on chest radiographs
B.
Diagnosis
Staging
CT scan
Functional imaging
(octreotide, MIBG)
Biopsy
Bronchoscopy
Transthoracic needle
Thoracoscopy
Thoracotomy
C.
Treatment
Typical carcinoid
Atypical carcinoid
Unresectable carcinoid
Localized
Distant disease
Localized
Distant disease
Palliation of symptoms with octreotide, irradiation therapy
Tissue sparing resection
+/– Lymph node dissection
(10% have node metastases at surgery)
Local resection with lymph node dissection
+/– Adjuvant chemotherapy and irradiation
Local resection (lobectomy, possible pneumonectomy), lymph node dissection
Local resection and lymph node dissection
+/– Adjuvant chemotherapy and irradiation

Anatomic Location

The most common location for carcinoid tumors is the gastrointestinal (GI) tract (74–85%), but tumors also may develop as bronchial carcinoids in the lungs (10–25%) or in other organs such as skin, ovary, prostate, and kidney (1–5%).[4,5] A large retrospective review of carcinoid tumor epidemiology showed that the most frequent locations in the GI tract are the appendix (about 20% of all carcinoid tumors), ileum (about 15%), and rectum (about 12%).[4]

Embryonic Origin

The most common system for classifying carcinoid tumors divides them according to their site of origin in the embryonic foregut, midgut, or hindgut,[6] although revisions of this classification scheme have been proposed.[7] This scheme is particularly helpful for predicting the hormone products various carcinoid tumors produce. Carcinoid tumors of the respiratory tract, stomach, duodenum, and pancreas arise from foregut derivatives. These tumors typically produce serotonin and its immediate precursor 5-hydroxytryptophan (5-HTP). Respiratory (bronchial) carcinoids may also secrete pituitary hormones such as adrenocorticotropic hormone (ACTH) or neuropeptides; and those of the proximal GI tract (stomach and duodenum) may also secrete GI peptides and histamine. Foregut tumors usually show argyrophilic staining when subjected to silver impregnation. Carcinoid tumors of the midgut (jejunum, ileum, right colon) may produce high levels of serotonin and peptides of the tachykinin group but rarely produce 5-HTP. Midgut carcinoids usually show argentaffin staining. Hindgut carcinoids (left colon, rectum) may produce gut peptides but rarely produce significant amounts of serotonin or 5-HTP. Carcinoid tumors of the hindgut usually do not react with silver stains.[8,9]

Tumor Size and Staging

As is the case with many neoplasms, survival rates of patients with carcinoid tumors usually depend on the size of the primary tumor and the presence of metastases. Several studies have demonstrated that survival at 5 years is significantly better for patients with midgut and hindgut carcinoids <2 cm in diameter than for those with larger tumors.[10,11] Additionally, the tendency to metastasize correlates well with primary tumor size. In one series of 307 rectal carcinoids, 1.7% of tumors <1 cm in largest diameter metastasized, and 10% of tumors 1–2 cm and 82% of tumors >2 cm showed metastatic spread.[12] As with most "rules" associated with carcinoid tumors, however, there are exceptions. For example, the survival rate for patients with (rare) carcinoid tumors of the ampulla of Vater does not appear to correlate well with tumor size.[13] The presence of regional and distant metastases is associated with a worse prognosis. Godwin reported relative survival rates of 94% for patients with localized disease, 64% for patients with only regional metastases, and 18% for patients with disseminated disease.[5] A review by Modlin and Sandor reported 5-year survival rates for all types of carcinoid tumors of 79.7%, 50.6%, and 21.8% for patients with localized disease, regional metastases, and distant metastasis, respectively.[4]

Histologic Appearance

On light microscopy, carcinoid tumors typically show uniform round cells arranged in one of five typical growth patterns: insular, trabecular, glandular, undifferentiated, or mixed. Johnson et al. assessed the frequency and survival associated with each of these growth patterns for carcinoid tumors >1 cm in diameter.[14] They showed that an insular pattern, where carcinoid cells form solid nests with clearly defined boundaries, occurs most frequently (33%) and is associated with a relatively favorable prognosis (median survival 3 years). A trabecular growth pattern, where carcinoid cells form anastomosing bands and loops with a prominent vascular network, occurs in approximately 18% of tumors and also is associated with a more favorable prognosis (median survival 2.5 years). Carcinoids with a glandular pattern show cells arranged to form small acinar structures, whereas those with an undifferentiated pattern show none of the three pure differentiated growth patterns. Glandular and undifferentiated patterns were relatively uncommon (2% and 4%, respectively) and were associated with median survival times of less than 1 year. The most common growth pattern is a mix of two or more of the above pure patterns; a mixed pattern is observed in approximately 43% of carcinoid tumors and is associated with median survivals of 1.4 years (mixed undifferentiated and trabecular) to 4.4 years (mixed insular and glandular). The growth pattern also appears to correlate with the anatomic location of the tumor. A trabecular pattern is most common in foregut carcinoids, an insular pattern predominates in midgut tumors, and a mixed pattern is the most common growth pattern in hindgut tumors.[15]

Pathogenesis

Because most carcinoid tumors occur in the GI tract, much of the research into understanding the pathogenesis of carcinoids tumors has focused on those occurring in this area. Carcinoid tumors account for just over one-half of all GI endocrine tumors. Within the gut, enterochromaffin (EC) cells are the most common endocrine cells and occur with the greatest frequency in the duodenum, ileum, and appendix; they are less common in the large bowel and are usually absent in the esophagus. The mechanism that induces the proliferation of EC cells to form a carcinoid tumor is not well understood. In some cases overproduction of stimulatory hormones has been shown to increase the incidence of endocrine cell hyperplasia and carcinoids; for example, a significant increase in the incidence of gastric carcinoids has been shown in patients with long-standing hypergastrinemia.[16–18] However, the incidence of other carcinoids, especially those that develop sporadically or in connection with multiple endocrine neoplasia type 1 (MEN 1) is independent of gastrin levels. Carcinoid tumors of this type often behave in a more malignant fashion than those associated with hypergastrinemia.[19]

Carcinoid tumors may show changes in DNA content, and some studies suggest that DNA aneuploid tumors have a significantly worse prognosis than near-diploid tumors.[20] Other studies, however, appear to refute this correlation.[21] Early studies also indicated that carcinoid tumors may overexpress oncogenes such as *p53*,[10] but more recent investigations suggest that this may not be necessary for the development of carcinoids.[22,23] Finally, the activation of nuclear oncogenes such as N-*myc* and c-*jun*[24] or c-*myc* and *bcl-2*[25] may be important in carcinoid tumorigenesis. Such observations may offer assistance in predicting the outcomes of various classes of carcinoid tumors and indicate underlying mechanisms of the development of these lesions. However, much of the pathogenesis of carcinoids remains unclear.

Carcinoid Syndrome

In addition to local symptoms, carcinoid tumors may cause systemic manifestations because of ectopic hormone production. Classic acute symptoms of carcinoid syndrome include cutaneous flushing (94%), diarrhea (78%), bronchoconstriction (19%), and peripheral edema (19%).[9] Fibrosis of the pulmonic and tricuspid valves may also cause cardiac symptoms in as many as 40% of patients with long-standing disease.[26] Although carcinoid syndrome was classically associated with tumors producing serotonin, evidence suggests that histamine, dopamine, substance P, and other tachykinins may play significant roles. For example, serotonin antagonists effectively treat the diarrhea associated with carcinoid syndrome but do not reduce the cutaneous flushing. Tumors of the midgut characteristically produce serotonin, and carcinoids in other locations may as well. Carcinoid tumors localized to the GI tract usually do not cause carcinoid syndrome because the liver inactivates any hormones released by the tumor. However, hepatic metastasis of GI carcinoids or extraportal primary tumors can release hormones directly into the systemic circulation, causing the syndrome.

Elevated levels (>10 mg/24 hr) of the serotonin metabolite 5-hydroxyindoleacetic acid (5-HIAA) in the urine confirm the diagnosis of carcinoid syndrome. Diarrhea associated with carcinoid syndrome can be treated with serotonin antagonists such as methysergide, cyproheptadine, and ondansetron.[27] These drugs have largely been replaced by long-acting somatostatin analogues such as octreotide, which reduce both flushing and diarrhea.[28] Somatostatin analogues can be used for both prophylactic and acute therapy of carcinoid syndrome. They have relatively few significant side effects, the one exception being the formation of gallstones with prolonged administration. If extended therapy is planned, cholecystectomy should be performed when the primary tumor is resected. Studies have tested long-acting somatostatin analogues such as lanreotide (biweekly injections) for their ability to reduce the inconvenience of the twice-daily subcutaneous injections required for octreotide.[29]

Pulmonary Carcinoids

A. Epidemiology and Etiology

Neuroendocrine bronchopulmonary tumors comprise a spectrum of tumors from the low-grade malignancy of typical carcinoids to atypical carcinoids to the high-grade malignancy of small-cell carcinomas. Pulmonary carcinoid tumors arise from the neuroendocrine (Kulchitsky) cells at the basal aspect of the bronchial mucosa. They account for 1–2% of all lung neoplasms and occur at a mean age of 35–60 years. The gender distribution differs among studies but generally shows an approximately equal incidence in males and females.[30,31] Approximately 80% of carcinoid tumors occur in central bronchi, most commonly on the right side; the remaining tumors occur peripheral to the segmental bronchi. Pulmonary carcinoids can be classified as typical (less malignant) or atypical (more malignant) based on histopathology.

B. Diagnosis

Pulmonary carcinoids may be diagnosed because of symptoms or be discovered as an incidental finding on chest imaging. Clinical symptoms include bronchial obstruction, hemoptysis, pneumonia, pleural effusions, and cough, although a significant number of cases are asymptomatic.[32] Peripheral lesions most frequently present as asymptomatic solitary nodules on chest radiographs. Endocrine symptoms are most common with atypical carcinoids, especially after metastasis to the liver.[33] More than 75% of pulmonary carcinoids are detected using conventional posteroanterior chest radiography.[34]

Computed tomography (CT) may be helpful for localizing small tumors that are occult on conventional roentgenography and for staging.[34] Positron emission tomography (PET) using ^{18}F-fluorodeoxyglucose (FDG) is finding increasing use as a noninvasive means for determining the malignant potential of pulmonary lesions, although carcinoid tumors frequently show relatively low FDG uptake compared to other malignancies.[31] Other functional imaging agents, such as ^{111}In-octreotide (a somatostatin analogue) and ^{131}I-meta-iodobenzylguanidine (MIBG) have been used with greater success in evaluating bronchial carcinoids.[35,36]

Definitive diagnosis requires biopsy by bronchoscopy, transthoracic needle aspiration, thoracoscopy, or open thoracotomy. The sensitivity of bronchoscopy depends on tumor location, as peripheral tumors may not be accessible using this technique. Reported sensitivities range from 37% to 92%.[37,38] Endoscopically, bronchial carcinoids have a regular mucosa with a smooth, glistening, blue-red "mulberry" appearance.[30] The tumors are well vascularized and may bleed easily; excessive hemorrhage or necrosis suggests an atypical carcinoid. Because of the risk of hemorrhage, some clinicians prefer to avoid endoscopic biopsy.[39] Others suggest that for lesions that do not appear extensively vascular application of a dilute epinephrine solution (1:10,000) followed by flexible bronchoscopy can provide adequate tissue for diagnosis with minimal risk to the patient. These authors reserve rigid bronchoscopy for vascular tumors and those requiring deeper biopsy sections for definitive diagnosis. If hemorrhage is encountered, it can be controlled by topical application of a dilute solution of epinephrine, cautery, Nd:YAG laser, or in extreme cases emergent thoracotomy.[32]

Pulmonary resection is the treatment of choice for bronchial carcinoids, but such choice depends on the histology of the tumor. Complete tumor excision is of paramount importance in all cases; hence thoracotomy is usually necessary. Because many tumors have extrabronchial components, endoscopic tumor resection is generally limited to establishing airway patency prior to definitive tumor resection or for palliation in patients who are poor operative candidates and who have a limited life expectancy.[37]

C. Treatment

Typical Carcinoids Typical pulmonary carcinoids show a regular arrangement of small polygonal cells with clear to eosinophilic cytoplasm but without significant pleomorphism. They rarely spread beyond the thorax. Because of the limited malignant potential, a conservative operative approach (segmentectomy, wedge resection, sleeve resection) may be appropriate for typical carcinoids, especially when clinical considerations such as a lack of pulmonary reserve or increased patient age suggest procedures that spare lung parenchyma.[40,41] However, intraoperative lymph node examination is recommended because approximately 10% of typical carcinoids show nodal involvement at the time of surgery. If distant disease is present, more aggressive resection and adjuvant chemotherapy or irradiation may be indicated. Typical carcinoids rarely recur after complete resection and generally have little influence on life expectancy.[32]

Atypical Carcinoids Atypical carcinoids are usually large and demonstrate a less regular architecture, nuclear pleomorphism with irregular nuclear chromatin, necrosis, mitotic figures, and lymphatic or vascular invasion.[34,42] They often metastasize to regional lymph nodes (66%), lung, liver, or bone.[43] Additionally, atypical carcinoids more frequently show paraneoplastic effects, such as carcinoid or Cushing syndrome.[34] There is general agreement that aggressive surgical intervention is indicated for these tumors. At minimum this consists of lobectomy and mediastinal lymph node dissection, and sometimes total pneumonectomy is required.[40,44] Adjuvant irradiation or chemotherapy may also be indicated, especially for patients with distant metastasis. Patients with atypical carcinoids show average 5- and 10-year survivals of 60% and 40%, respectively.[32]

Unresectable Carcinoids For patients with unresectable tumors, symptomatic palliation may be possible using radiation therapy.[45] Somatostatin analogues (e.g., octreotide) can be used to control symptoms of the carcinoid syndrome, which may be significant with unresectable primary or metastatic disease. Octreotide administration can also prevent carcinoid storm during anesthesia or surgery.[46,47]

With treatment, the overall 5- and 10-year survival rates for patients with pulmonary carcinoids are approximately 93% and 82%, respectively.[41] The 10-year survival rates are significantly worse for patients with atypical carcinoids (18–60%) than for those with typical carcinoids (85–100%).[32]

Gastric Carcinoids

Gastric carcinoids are relatively rare tumors, accounting for fewer than 0.3–0.5% of all gastric malignancies, although they may represent as many as 10–30% of all GI carcinoids. They are associated with other malignant neoplasms in about 8% of cases.[48] Gastric carcinoids are generally subtyped into three groups. Type I and type II are associated with hypergastrinemia; type III occurs sporadically.

D. Presentation and Diagnosis

Gastric carcinoids may mimic ulcers, polyps, or carcinoma, presenting with symptoms that include abdominal pain, hematemesis, diarrhea, and gastric outlet obstruction.[49] Alternatively, they may be discovered incidentally during gastroscopy for conditions such as atrophic gastritis. Gastroscopy with biopsy is generally the most useful test for evaluating gastric carcinoids, which may present with the classic finding of an irregularly shaped erythematous depression in the center of a rounded submucosal mass.[50] Grossly, lesions may appear as multiple small, yellowish fundic polyps. CT and endoscopic ultrasonog-

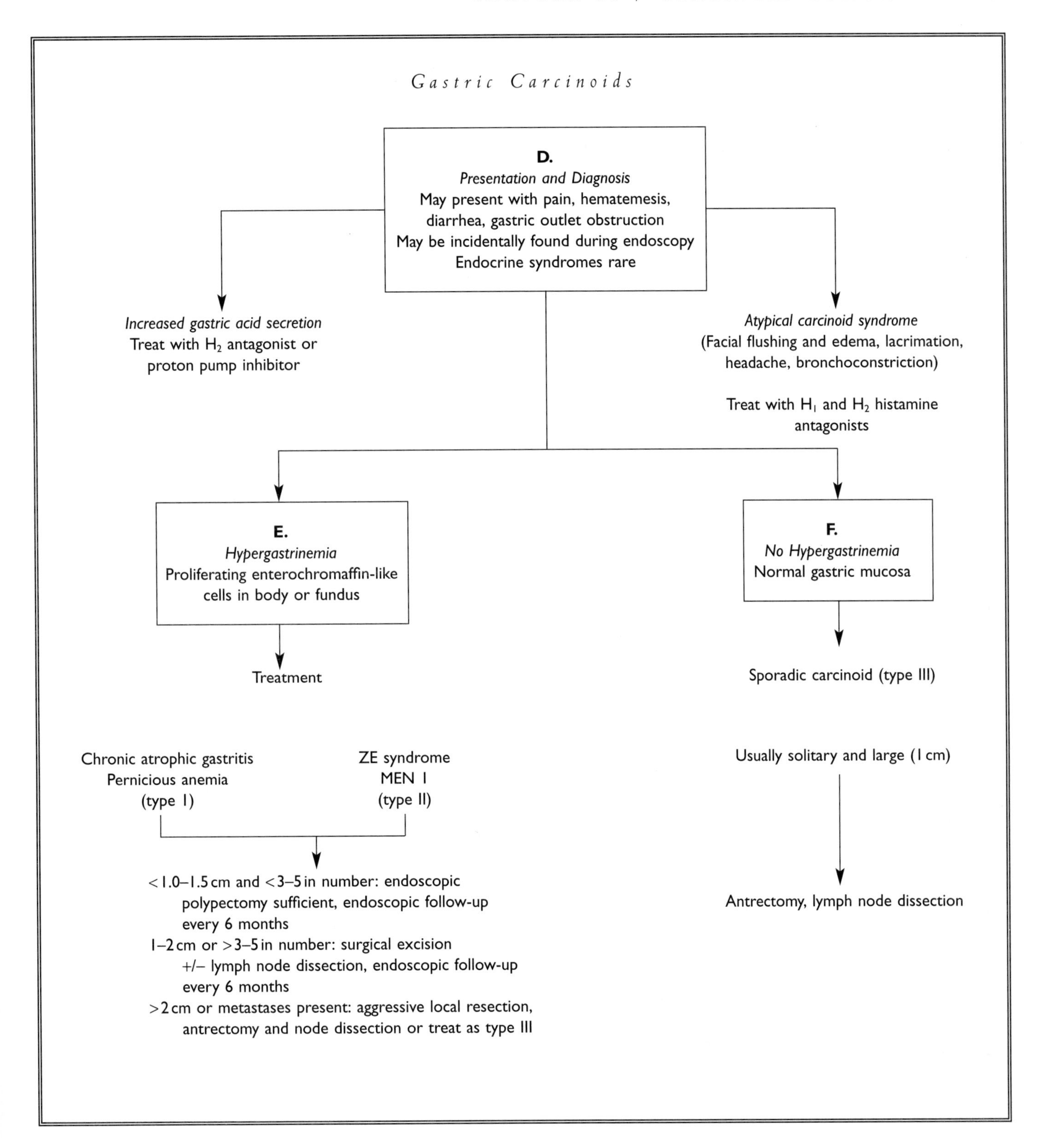

raphy (EUS) are of limited value for initial detection but may assist in staging submucosal lesions. Functional imaging with octreotide or MIBG may also assist in assessing lesion number and stage.[35,51]

Endocrine syndromes rarely result from gastric carcinoids.[52] The symptoms may be those of a typical carcinoid syndrome; but more frequently an atypical carcinoid syndrome characterized by prolonged, patchy, bright red flushing, facial edema, lacrimation, headache, and bronchoconstriction occurs. Atypical carcinoid syndrome can be treated with H_1- and H_2-histamine antagonists; and excessive gastric acid secretion can be controlled by H_2-receptor and proton pump antagonists.

E. Hypergastrinemia

Type I gastric carcinoids are the most common and occur secondary to hypergastrinemia in patients with chronic atrophic gastritis and pernicious anemia. These tumors are generally small (<1 cm) and multiple, exhibit relatively slow growth, and rarely metastasize. The tumors are usually composed of proliferating enterochromaffin-like (ECL) cells and occur concomitantly with ECL hyperplasia in the gastric body or fundus. Type II gastric carcinoids occur less frequently and are associated with hypergastrinemia attributable to Zollinger-Ellison syndrome or MEN 1. These tumors are also generally small (<1.5 cm), multiple, and slow growing; but they metastasize more frequently than type I gastric carcinoids. Like type I carcinoids, they are usually composed of ECL cells and are associated with ECL hyperplasia in the gastric body or fundus.

Management of type I and type II gastric carcinoids differs depending on the tumor size, number, and presence of metastasis. Fewer than three to five small (<1.0–1.5 cm) type I or II carcinoids without evidence of metastasis are unlikely to exhibit highly malignant behavior and so may be removed by endoscopic polypectomy with follow-up by endoscopic surveillance. Type I and II lesions 1–2 cm in diameter should be surgically excised with consideration give to local lymph node dissection. Tumors >2 cm in the presence of hypergastrinemia increase the suspicion of a type III (sporadic) carcinoid and should be treated with aggressive local resection, antrectomy (to remove all gastrin producing G-cells in the antrum), and lymph node dissection; alternatively, they are treated as type III gastric carcinoids. The presence of metastases also suggests the need for aggressive local resection, lymph node dissection, and possible antrectomy. For patients with treated gastrin-dependent carcinoids, studies reveal little alteration in life expectancy.[53]

F. No Hypergastrinemia

Type III gastric carcinoids occur sporadically, independent of hypergastrinemia. They are most often solitary and large (>1 cm) and consist of multiple gastric endocrine cells (EC, ECL, and X cells). Tumors show rapid, aggressive progression with local invasion and often metastasize to regional lymph nodes (55%) and the liver (24%).[52,54,55] Because of their aggressive behavior, gastric resection (including antrectomy) with lymph node dissection is the treatment of choice for sporadic gastric carcinoids. Neuroendocrine carcinomas, which were previously known as "atypical" gastric carcinoids, are aggressive lesions that resemble type III gastric carcinoids and carry a poor prognosis. For patients with treated sporadic carcinoid tumors, an age-corrected survival rate of 79% has been reported.[53]

Duodenal and Pancreatic Carcinoids

Carcinoid tumors of the duodenum and pancreas represent fewer than 2% of all GI neuroendocrine tumors and are much less common than adenomas and adenocarcinomas. True pancreatic carcinoids are rare. Duodenal neuroendocrine tumors are further classified into five subtypes: gastrinomas, somatostatinomas, gangliocytic paragangliomas, serotonin/calcitonin/pancreatic polypeptide (PP)-producing tumors, and poorly differentiated carcinomas. Surgical excision is the therapy of choice for all duodenal and pancreatic carcinoid tumors, in part because most tumors respond poorly to cytotoxic chemotherapy. With the exception of poorly differentiated neuroendocrine carcinomas, most are associated with a favorable outcome.

G. Diagnosis

Duodenal and pancreatic carcinoids may be suggested by clinical symptoms or associated syndromes, or they may be discovered incidentally. The diagnosis can usually be narrowed to a specific type of duodenal carcinoid based on clinical symptoms and the anatomic location of the primary tumor. Magnetic resonance imaging (MRI) has been shown to have a higher sensitivity than CT or abdominal ultrasonography for detecting pancreatic carcinoids.[56] EUS can also be used to locate duodenal and pancreatic tumors but is dependent on operator experience and expertise.[57]

H. Duodenal Carcinoids

Gastrinomas Gastrin-producing tumors are the most common, accounting for approximately 60% of duodenal carcinoids. Gastrinomas are most commonly located in the first or second portions of the duodenum, are small (<1 cm), and metastasize to regional lymph nodes in 30–70% of cases but rarely metastasize further without significant delay. Approximately 30% of gastrinomas are associated with Zollinger-Ellison syndrome (ZES) or MEN 1. In patients with ZES secondary to MEN 1, the incidence of duodenal gastrinomas may be 70–90%.[58] Gastrinomas associated with ZES are usually small (<1 cm) submucosal lesions,[59] whereas those associated with MEN 1 are usually multicentric.[60]

Because of the small size of gastrinomas, they are rarely identified by endoscopy or preoperative CT, MRI, or ultrasonography. Intraoperative ultrasonography (IOUS) and endoscopic transillumination have been shown to aid in identifying primary duodenal gastrinomas;[61] and somatostatin receptor scintigraphy using ^{111}In-octreotide has been shown to have good accuracy (92%) in identifying both primary and metastatic lesions.[62] However, duodenotomy remains the gold standard for localizing these lesions.[63] Achieving biochemical cures for hypergastrinemia in patients with ZES and MEN 1 can be difficult because many patients with duodenal gastrinomas have lymph node

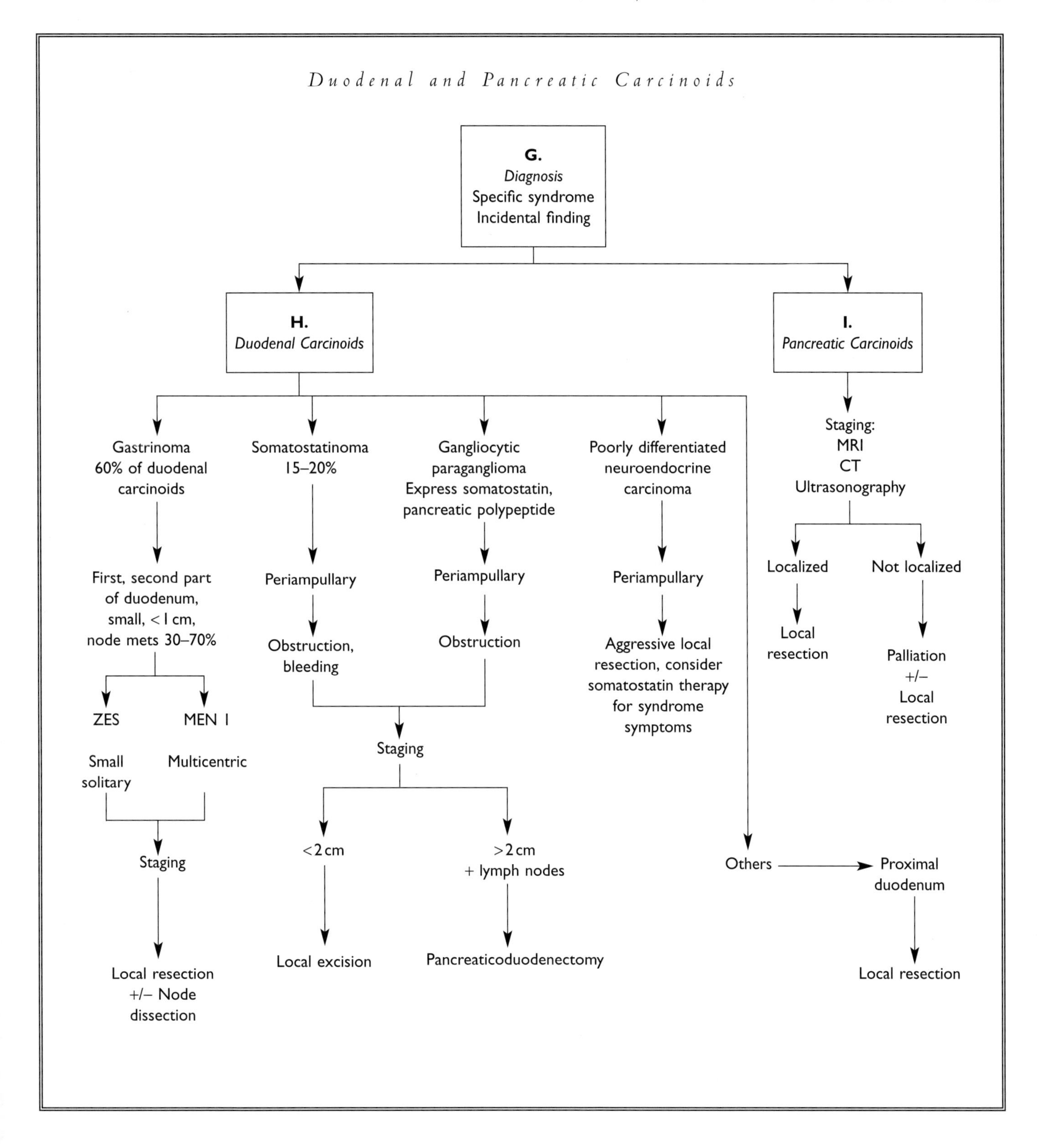

metastases (86%) or multiple tumors (43%) at diagnosis.[58] Intraoperative measurement of gastrin levels can help determine whether complete tumor resection has been achieved.[64] Because these tumors generally do not metastasize beyond the lymph nodes, the 10-year survival following local resection approaches 85%.[65]

Somatostatinomas Somatostatin-producing tumors account for 15–20% of duodenal carcinoids. About one-fourth occur in patients with type I neurofibromatosis (von Recklinghausen's disease).[66,67] Somatostatinomas usually appear at the ampulla of Vater and are identified once ampullary obstruction, pancreatitis, or bleeding occurs. They present as 1- to 2-cm homogeneous nodules that rarely ulcerate. On biopsy they show a characteristic glandular growth pattern and contain concentrically laminated psammoma bodies.

GANGLIOCYTIC PARAGANGLIOMAS Gangliocytic paragangliomas contain identifiable gangliocytic elements and typically occur in the periampullary portion of the duodenum. These tumors most frequently express somatostatin and PP, are large (>2 cm), and may invade the muscularis propria. They are usually encountered incidentally or following hemorrhage. Biopsy of the lesion shows a combination of paraganglioma, ganglioneuroma, and carcinoid tissues that stain for somatostatin and PP.[68]

Tumor size and the presence of lymph node involvement determine the therapy for somatostatinomas, gangliocytic paragangliomas, and other periampullary tumors. Local excision is recommended for small tumors (<2 cm); larger tumors or those with lymph node involvement should be treated with pancreaticoduodenectomy. Periampullary carcinoid tumors of these types generally have a good prognosis, with 5-year survivals of 90% reported in some series.[69]

POORLY DIFFERENTIATED NEUROENDOCRINE CARCINOMAS Poorly differentiated neuroendocrine carcinomas, which are identified by positive staining for neuroendocrine markers, are rare. They usually occur in the periampullary region and exhibit highly malignant behavior.[68] Patients typically present with symptoms of ampullary obstruction. Pancreatic carcinoids may also produce an atypical carcinoid syndrome of pain, diarrhea, and weight loss without skin flushing. The diagnosis is based on typical carcinoid histologic features together with increased serotonin metabolism.[70] Symptoms associated with carcinoid syndrome may respond to somatostatin analogues. Poorly differentiated neuroendocrine carcinoma may also be aggressively resected, but outcomes remain poor because of the aggressive nature of these tumors.

OTHERS Duodenal carcinoids producing calcitonin or PP are rare. They infrequently produce clinically significant amounts of hormones and generally exhibit low-grade malignant behavior. They usually appear as small (<2 cm), gray polyps in the proximal duodenum.[68] Local resection is generally curative.

I. Pancreatic Carcinoids

Pancreatic carcinoids are rare. They stain for serotonin (and sometimes other biogenic amines) and exhibit classic carcinoid morphology on microscopy. These carcinoids are usually detected late but may be locally resected if adjacent organs have not been invaded. A high frequency of distant metastases and a poor response to chemotherapy precludes long-term survival in many patients.[70,71] Pancreatic islet cell tumors (e.g., insulinoma, gastrinoma) are characterized with respect to their predominant hormone expression and are not considered carcinoids.

Jejunoileal Carcinoids

In the GI tract most carcinoids occur in the small bowel. Because appendiceal carcinoids behave differently than other midgut carcinoids, they are considered separately. Carcinoids of the jejunum and ileum, which behave in a similar fashion, are considered together.

J. Epidemiology and Etiology

Up to one-third of malignant small bowel tumors are carcinoids. Incidental small (<1 cm) localized midgut carcinoids are frequently found at autopsy. The tumors are relatively slow growing, but the lack of overt symptoms from the primary tumor means that a large number of patients (>70%) have large tumors (>1 cm) and often disseminated disease at the time of diagnosis. The tumor may invade the mesentery, distorting the architecture of the bowel wall by inducing desmoplastic tissue growth. Up to 40% of these patients have multiple tumors.[68] Midgut carcinoids most commonly metastasize to regional lymph nodes and then to the liver; they may rarely metastasize to bone. They are also associated with synchronous or metachronous tumors, most commonly adenocarcinomas of the colon, in a significant number (17%) of cases.[4,72] Most of the tumors in the ileum are composed of EC cells arranged in an insular pattern and show argentaffin staining. The most common biochemical products are serotonin and substance P.[73] Approximately 20% of malignant carcinoids are associated with the classic carcinoid syndrome, almost always because of hepatic metastases. Related carcinoid tumors can also occur in the jejunum or in association with Meckel's diverticulum,[74] but these lesions are much less common, more commonly show a trabecular growth pattern, and produce gastrin or somatostatin rather than serotonin.[68]

K. Diagnosis

Small localized midgut carcinoids generally remain asymptomatic and are discovered incidentally or at autopsy. Large tumors are associated with a higher incidence of metastases. Patients may present with localized symptoms caused by the primary tumor or systemic symptoms due to ectopic hormone production. Local effects include mucosal ulceration, abdominal pain, and GI bleeding.[75] Bioactive carcinoid tumors also may produce significant intraabdominal and retroperitoneal fibrosis, as well as distortion of the bowel wall by tumor-induced extracelluar matrix production. These changes may cause symptomatic bowel obstruction, although total bowel obstruction is relatively uncommon. Mesenteric and retroperitoneal fibrosis can also result in intestinal ischemia or infarction or in ureteral obstruction.[76] Tumor metastasis to the retroperitoneum or liver can

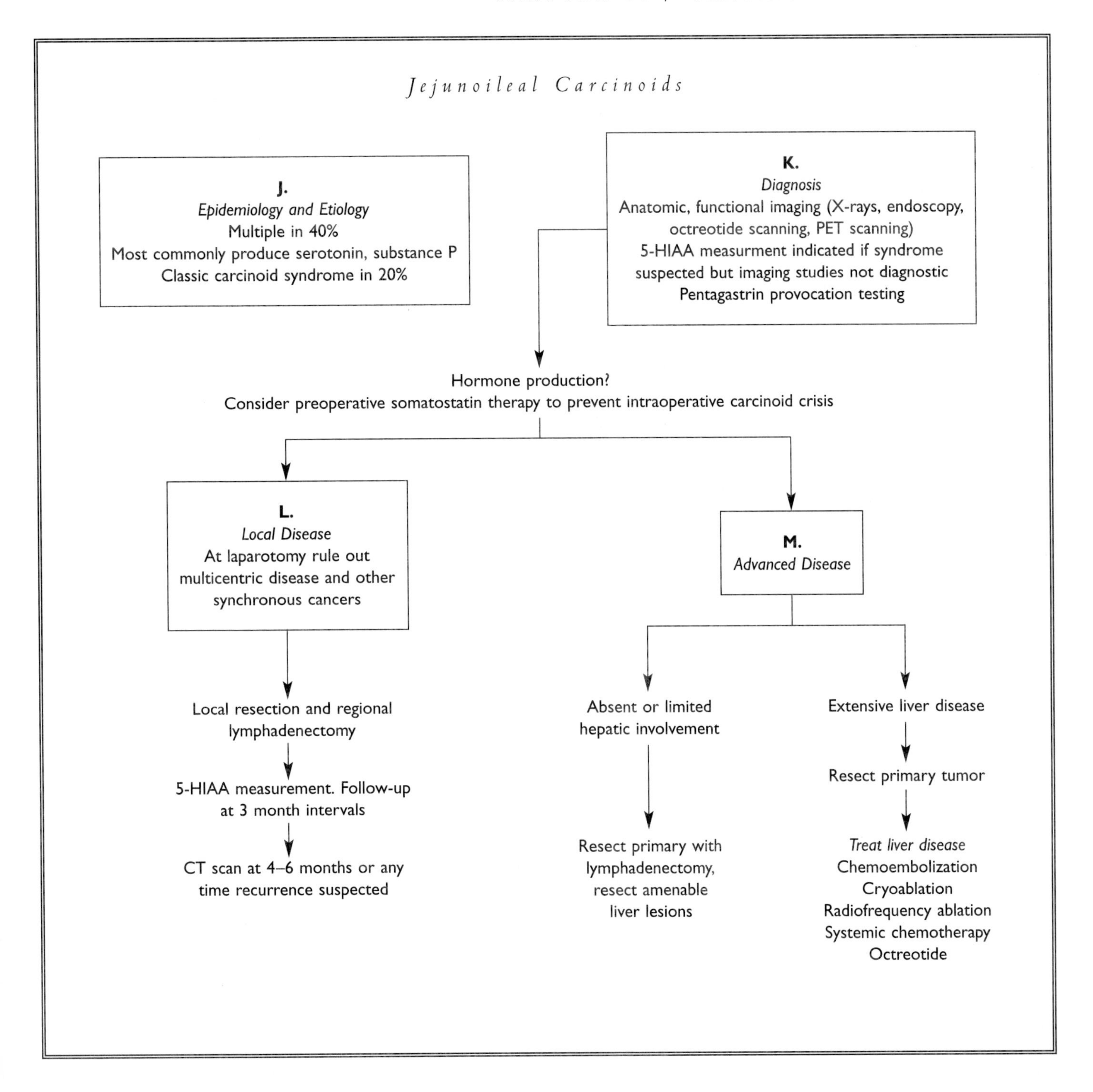

result in the classic carcinoid syndrome. Both anatomic techniques (upper and lower bowel contrast roentgenography, enteroclysis, endoscopy, CT) and functional imaging (somatostatin scintigraphy, serotonin positron emission tomography) may assist in localizing tumors.[77–80] Biochemical characterization by quantitative 5-HIAA measurement may be useful when anatomic imaging is equivocal.[76] Finally, provocation testing with pentagastrin can be used where clinical suspicion of carcinoid tumor persists in the presence of negative imaging and biochemical studies.[81]

L. Local Disease

Primary carcinoid tumors of the midgut that have not metastasized should be resected together with the corresponding regional mesenteric lymph nodes. Intraoperative examination for multicentric carcinoid disease or other simultaneous malignancy should be undertaken, and tumor localization may be aided by use of intraoperative somatostatin scintigraphy.[82] Patients with tumors that express ectopic hormones may be treated with octreotide preoperatively to prevent intraoperative carcinoid crisis.[46,47] Follow-up should include physical examination, assessment of symptoms, and urinary 5-HIAA measurements approximately every 3 months; abdominal CT scans are performed less frequently, although if symptoms warrant, imaging is performed promptly.[83]

M. Advanced Disease

Therapy for advanced lesions is more controversial. Invasive disease with no or limited hepatic metastasis should be treated by aggressive local resection of the primary tumor with the associated mesentery. Debulking of involved local and retroperitoneal lymph nodes is advised even if all disease cannot be removed. Superficial solitary hepatic lesions can be treated by wedge resection at the time of primary surgery. For hormone-producing tumors, preoperative prophylaxis with octreotide may prevent carcinoid crisis. Octreotide prophylaxis is especially important if hepatic metastases are present. When octreotide therapy is to be used for a significant length of time, the initial surgical procedure should include cholecystectomy to avoid cholecystitis secondary to octreotide-induced gallstones. If hepatic embolization is to be used to control hepatic metastases, cholecystectomy should be performed to preclude gallbladder gangrene during embolization, and collateral blood vessels to the liver may be ligated to decrease the accessory blood supply to the tumor.[84] For patients with more advanced disease, the initial surgery should focus on removing the primary tumor and associated local metastases; it reduces the tumor burden and decreases the incidence of local symptoms such as bowel obstruction.[83,85,86] Surgical or medical therapy (or both) for hepatic metastasis can follow. The 5-year survival for patients with localized small intestine carcinoids has been reported as 65%; survival decreases to 35% when distant disease is present.[4]

Appendiceal Carcinoids

Carcinoid tumors of the appendix occur relatively frequently compared to other carcinoids and fortuitously are associated with the most favorable prognosis. They present at a relatively early age (42 years) compared to other carcinoid tumors (62 years) and have a 0.47 : 1 male/female ratio.[87] In contrast to other midgut carcinoids, appendiceal carcinoids usually follow a benign course. The reason for their less malignant clinical presentation is not known. Concurrent adenocarcinoma at another site in the GI tract occurs with 10–15% of appendiceal carcinoids.[4,87]

N. Diagnosis

Appendiceal carcinoids are most commonly diagnosed during appendectomy (about 50%) or incidentally during other surgical procedures. The incidence of appendicitis may be increased with appendiceal carcinoids because the tumor contributes to obstruction of the appendiceal lumen; this clinical presentation may explain the relatively early diagnosis of this type of carcinoid. Most appendiceal carcinoids occur near the tip of the appendix.[88] Most (70–90%) of the tumors are < 1 cm at the time of discovery; tumors of this size are not associated with metastasis. Tumors of intermediate size (1–2 cm) are rarely (0.5–0.7%) associated with metastases, whereas metastases are more common (average 30%) with rare large (> 2 cm) appendiceal carcinoids.[89]

O. Treatment

Distal Appendiceal Carcinoids For carcinoids < 1 cm in largest diameter in any location in the appendix, simple appendectomy is curative. With tumors of 1–2 cm the incidence of metastasis is low, so simple appendectomy is curative in most cases.[89] More extensive resection can be undertaken if evidence of aggressive behavior (e.g., invasion of the mesoappendix or subserosal lymphatics) is observed. In particular, more extensive resection may be advised for young patients, whereas the risk of operative complications may outweigh the benefit of an extended surgical procedure in older patients. Right hemicolectomy should be performed for large tumors (> 2 cm).[89]

Proximal Appendiceal or Cecal Carcinoids Therapy for carcinoids at the base of the appendix remains controversial. Because appendiceal carcinoids almost always metastasize first to regional lymph nodes, accurate intraoperative assessment of tumor spread should be undertaken. Patients without metastases or evidence of tumor invasion are probably best treated by appendectomy alone. As with distal carcinoids, more aggressive procedures may be warranted in younger patients with intermediate-size tumors. Right hemicolectomy is indicated for tumors that have extensive local invasion or lymph node involvement.[88]

Prognosis

The prognosis for patients with appendiceal carcinoids is quite favorable. The 5-year survivals are 94% for localized lesions, 85% for regional disease, and 34% for patients with distant metastases.[87]

Colon Carcinoids

P. Epidemiology

Carcinoid tumors of the colon comprise about 8% of all carcinoids and occur most frequently in the cecum (about 50%) and right colon.[90] The male/female ratio differs among studies, but a small female predominance (60%) has been noted. The peak

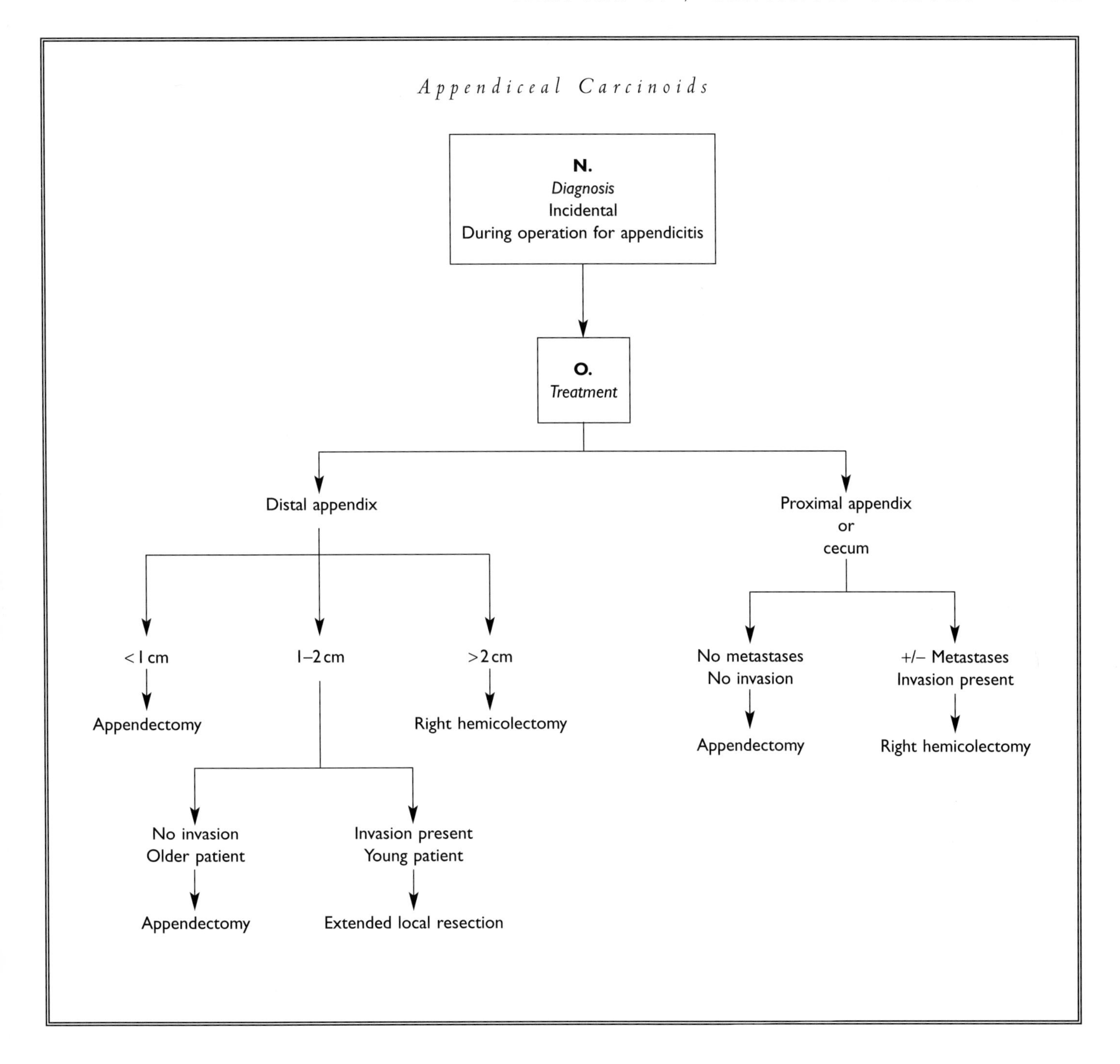

incidence of colonic carcinoids occurs during the seventh decade of life. A large proportion (60–70%) of colon carcinoids have metastases at the time of diagnosis, which contributes to a relatively poor 5-year survival for all colon carcinoids (42%) despite the relatively good survival (71%) for patients with localized disease.[4] Colon carcinoids are associated with a high frequency (25–40%) of other concomitant neoplasms, most commonly adenocarcinomas.[5,90]

Q. Diagnosis and Staging

Most patients with colon carcinoids are diagnosed after complaining of pain, anorexia, and weight loss of an extended duration. Some patients are identified prior to the onset of significant symptoms during routine colonoscopy; others may present with signs of bowel obstruction. Hemoccult-positive stools are unusual unless the lesion is located in the left colon, and carcinoid syndrome is rare unless significant liver metastases are present. Some patients have elevated carcinoembryonic antigen (CEA) levels, although this is not universal.[91]

Direct visualization during colonoscopy allows identification of some colonic carcinoids, and others are first identified radiographically. Barium enema usually demonstrates symptomatic tumors; the most common appearances are a large polypoid mass or a circumferential "apple core" lesion similar to that observed with adenocarcinoma.[90] Carcinoids of the colon may

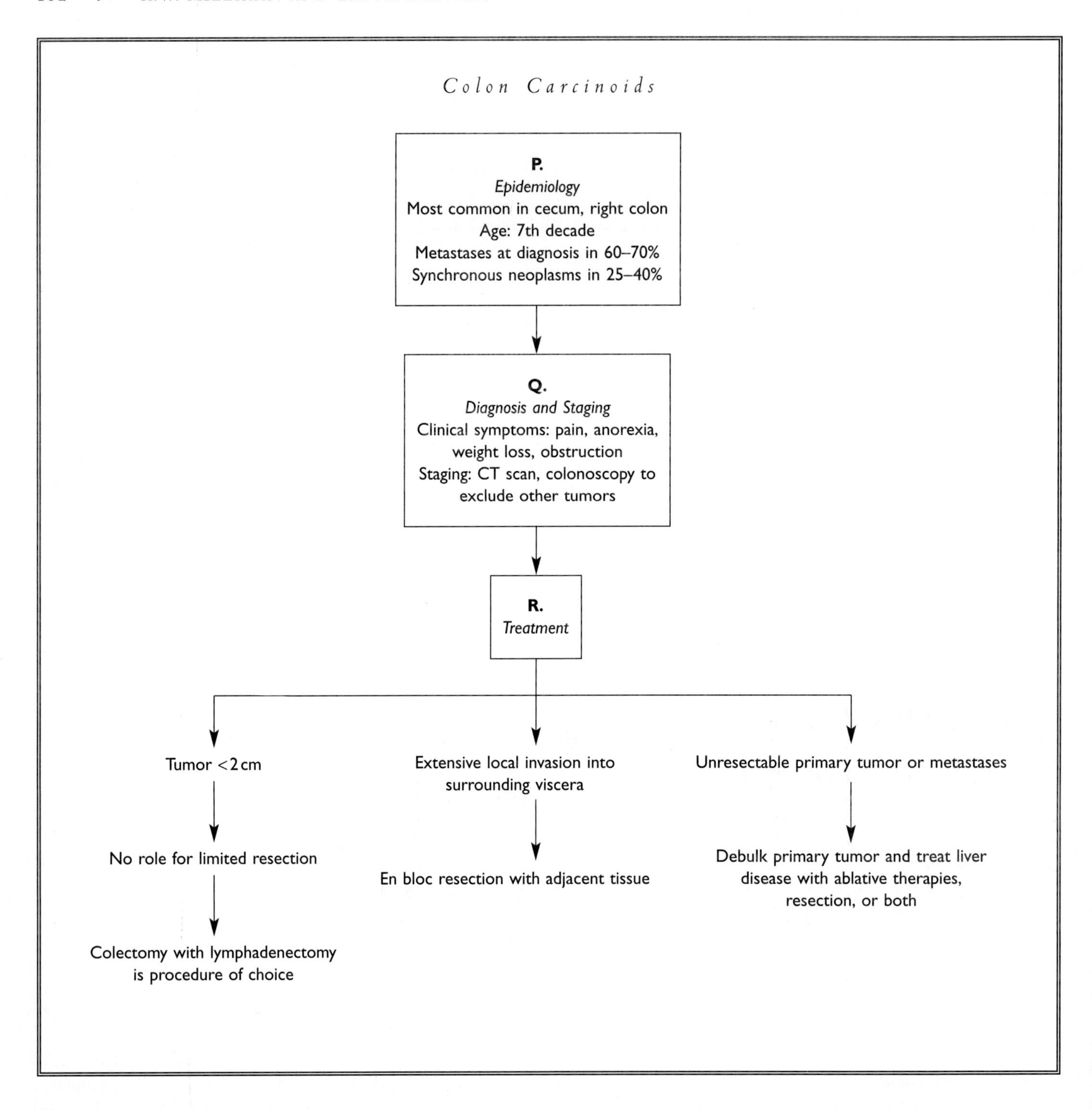

metastasize to distant sites without significant involvement of regional lymph nodes. Therefore preoperative evaluation for metastatic disease should be performed in a manner similar to that described for other GI carcinoids.[4]

R. Treatment

It has been suggested that, like other GI carcinoids, colon *carcinoids* <2 cm should be treated by limited resection, with radical colectomy reserved for larger lesions or those with evidence of invasion. However, the appreciable risk of lymph node invasion and relatively comparable operative risks for limited resection and standard colon resection suggest that resection of the colon and associated lymphatic drainage should be standard therapy for all colonic carcinoids regardless of size.[89,90]

If *local invasion* into contiguous organs has occurred, colectomy should be supplemented with en bloc resection of all affected tissues. If isolated hepatic metastases are present, they should also be resected. Colon carcinoids generally respond

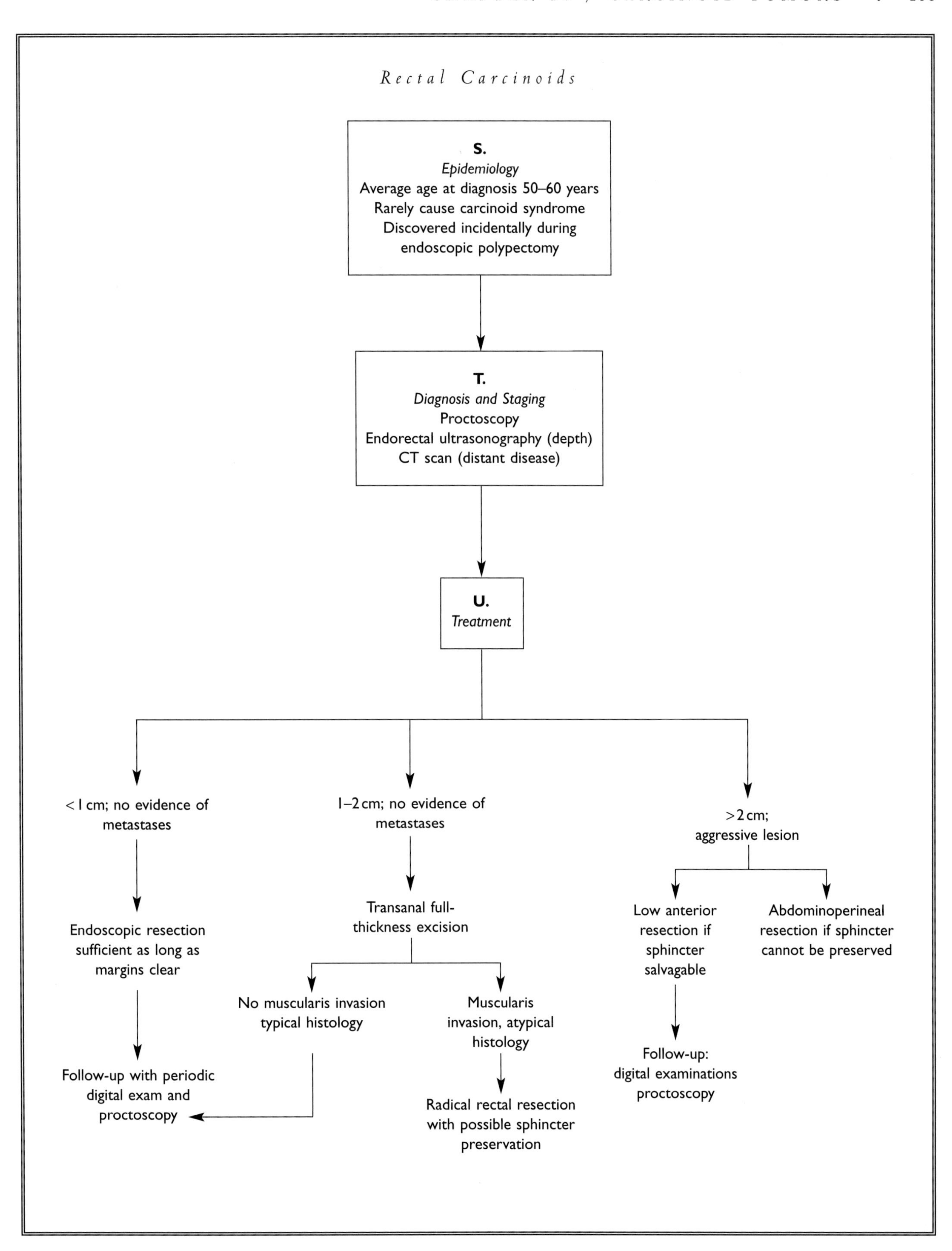
Rectal Carcinoids
S.
Epidemiology
Average age at diagnosis 50–60 years
Rarely cause carcinoid syndrome
Discovered incidentally during endoscopic polypectomy
T.
Diagnosis and Staging
Proctoscopy
Endorectal ultrasonography (depth)
CT scan (distant disease)
U.
Treatment
<1 cm; no evidence of metastases
Endoscopic resection sufficient as long as margins clear
Follow-up with periodic digital exam and proctoscopy
1–2 cm; no evidence of metastases
Transanal full-thickness excision
No muscularis invasion typical histology
Muscularis invasion, atypical histology
Radical rectal resection with possible sphincter preservation
>2 cm; aggressive lesion
Low anterior resection if sphincter salvagable
Follow-up: digital examinations proctoscopy
Abdominoperineal resection if sphincter cannot be preserved

poorly to chemotherapy or irradiation, so adjuvant therapy appears to be of little value in prolonging survival.[90]

Unresectable tumors should be debulked and isolated hepatic metastases resected if possible. Aggressive surgical debulking of liver involvement is especially important for reducing or eliminating symptoms of carcinoid syndrome, if present; repeated procedures may also prolong life.[90]

Rectal Carcinoids

S. Epidemiology

The rectum is the most common site for large bowel carcinoid tumors and the third most frequent site in the GI tract. The average age at diagnosis is 50–60 years, and no gender predominance has been shown. The age-adjusted incidence has been noted to be three- to fourfold higher in the Africa-American population. Rectal tumors are frequently discovered early in their course and show a low propensity for metastasis. Rectal carcinoids may express a variety of hormones, including serotonin, PP, and less frequently glucagon, gastrin, or somatostatin. Frequently more than one hormone is expressed. They may be argyrophil-positive (55%) or argentaffin-positive (28%).[92] They are not often associated with carcinoid syndrome.[93] Finally, rectal carcinoids are associated with noncarcinoid tumors in approximately 10% of cases.[4]

T. Diagnosis and Staging

Rectal carcinoids are usually detected earlier in the course of the disease than other GI carcinoids because many are detectable during routine digital rectal examination or proctoscopy. Rectal carcinoids typically are firm, yellow, submucosal lesions that have a firm or hard, discrete, mobile feel on digital examination. Only about 50% of tumors cause symptoms, such as bleeding per rectum, constipation, rectal pain, or pruritus ani.[89] Benign anorectal conditions such as hemorrhoids may be responsible for the observed symptoms in many patients with small rectal carcinoids.[94] The presence of symptoms attributable to the carcinoid tumor itself may indicate a poorer prognosis.[95] Elevated prostatic acid phosphatase and CEA levels have been observed in 80% and 25% of cases, respectively.[89]

Staging for rectal carcinoids consists of evaluating the remaining colon with colonoscopy, ruling out metastatic disease, and determining the depth of invasion. The latter is best determined with rectal ultrasomography; distant disease is assessed with CT scanning.

U. Treatment

Most (>60%) rectal carcinoids are *<1 cm* in diameter at the time of diagnosis; tumors of this size are associated with metastases in fewer than 2% of cases. Endoscopic excision is usually curative for these localized lesions.[96]

Carcinoid tumors *1–2 cm in largest diameter* were associated with nonlocalized disease in approximately 15% of cases in a study by Mani et al.,[97] although Koura et al. indicated that 47% of patients with 1- to 2-cm rectal carcinoids had or later developed metastases.[11] Localized invasion of the muscularis propria is also associated with significantly higher rates of metastases, most commonly to the liver, lungs, and bone. Tumors of 1–2 cm should be treated by transmural resection with adequate margins to evaluate invasion of the muscularis. Appropriate additional therapy is then determined based on pathology.

Transmural resection is usually curative for typical rectal carcinoids that show no evidence of invasion of the muscularis. Typical carcinoids have uniform cells, no or rare mitotic figures, are arranged in nests or strands in the submucosa, and show no mucin production or invasion.

Atypical carcinoids show invasion of vessels, lymphatics, perineurium, or muscularis propria, an anaplastic appearance, mitoses, cellular pleomorphism, or mucin production. Atypical tumors are more frequently associated with metastatic spread, regardless of tumor size.[11] Therefore lesions that have invaded the muscularis or have histology suggesting an atypical carcinoid should be treated further by radical excision of the rectum with potential sphincter preservation if located in the mid or upper rectum. For the poor risk patient, local reexcision may be considered, but this approach does not address possible extraluminal spread in the mesorectum.

Rectal carcinoids *>2 cm in diameter* are frequently (60–80%) associated with metastases.[97] Therapy for large or metastatic rectal carcinoids remains controversial. Chemotherapy and irradiation have not been shown to have significant benefit; therefore surgery remains the treatment of choice. Several studies have suggested that extensive surgical resection does not improve disease-free survival in patients with tumors >2 cm.[11,95] Others continue to advocate major resection for rectal carcinoids with features indicating an aggressive lesion (size >2 cm, mucosal ulceration or umbilication, symptomatic tumors, or fixation seen by digital rectal examination) if no evidence of distant disease is present.[94] Tumors that can be resected without compromising sphincter function should be treated with low anterior resection; if complete resection cannot be undertaken without compromising sphincter function, abdominoperineal resection may be required. The decreased quality of life incurred by patients undergoing abdominoperitoneal resection must be considered in light of the high risk of disease recurrence.[11]

For any patient undergoing surgical therapy, follow-up by digital examination and proctoscopy should be undertaken to detect any subsequent tumors while they are still at a treatable stage. Five-year survival rates of 81% for localized lesions have been reported, with significantly poorer survival rates of 47%

and 18% for regional or distant lymph node involvement, respectively.[4]

Hepatic Manifestations of Carcinoid Disease

Hepatic metastases of carcinoid tumors may present with significant symptoms, especially the carcinoid syndrome. Therapy for advanced carcinoid disease should begin with a procedure aimed at resecting the primary tumor, resecting or debulking regional metastases, and if indicated cholecystectomy prior to octreotide therapy or hepatic embolization. Prior to any intervention, 1–2 weeks of octreotide pretreatment has been suggested to prevent carcinoid storm.[83] Optimal therapy for liver disease consists, whenever possible, of complete tumor resection.[98] Patients with isolated unilobar lesions can be treated by lobar or segmental resection with the intent of removing all of the disease.

Patients with multilobar liver metastases can be treated in several ways. The most common method is to induce tumor ischemia by percutaneous selective hepatic artery embolization. The relative efficacy of repeated temporary occlusion compared to relatively more permanent embolization remains unclear.[99] Contraindications to hepatic embolization include a tumor burden exceeding 50% of the liver volume, occlusion of the portal vein, hyperbilirubinemia, or persistently elevated liver enzyme levels. Relative contraindications include contrast allergy, coagulopathies, significant extrahepatic tumor, or poor performance status.[100] Side effects of hepatic embolization include abdominal pain, fever, nausea, and vomiting. More serious complications include gallbladder ischemia or necrosis, pancreatitis, lives abscess, hepatorenal syndrome, and carcinoid crisis.[85,101] Laparoscopic thermal ablation[102] and cryosurgery[103] have also been proposed for treating hepatic metastases of carcinoid tumors.

Chemotherapy and interferon-alpha therapy can be useful for palliation of local symptoms and carcinoid syndrome but appear to have little effect on tumor progression. Therapy with ^{131}I-MIBG has also been used to achieve temporary relief of symptoms.[104] Finally, combined therapy with octreotide, sequential intraarterial 5-fluorouracil (5-FU) infusions, and hepatic tumor chemoembolization has been reported to retard tumor progression and decrease symptoms.[105] The long-term benefit of concurrent or sequential chemotherapy with embolization remains to be determined. Percutaneous intrahepatic injection of alcohol has also been used for palliation of symptoms in elderly patients with carcinoid syndrome, and cytotoxic drugs delivered by regional hyperthermic liver perfusion have been used to treat carcinoid syndrome in patients whose disease is sufficiently advanced to preclude hepatic embolization.[85]

Finally, orthotopic liver transplantation (OLT) can be considered for patients with severe symptoms after the extrahepatic disease has been controlled.[106] Even patients who had no demonstrable extrahepatic disease at the time of transplant have tumor recurrence rates approaching 50%.[107] This may be caused, in part, by accelerated tumor growth following immunosuppression. The best candidates for OLT appear to be patients who have undergone aggressive surgical resection of both local and hepatic carcinoid disease and who fail to respond to adjuvant therapy. In such cases, liver transplantation remains a high risk procedure, but it can provide long-term palliation of symptoms and increased patient survival.[108]

References

1. Oberndorfer S. Karzinoide Tumoren des Dunndarms. Frankfurt Z Pathol 1907;1:426–430.
2. Gosset A, Masson P. Tumeurs endocrine de l'appendice. Presse Med 1914;22:237.
3. Pearse AG, Polak JM. Endocrine tumours of neural crest origin: neurolymphomas, apudomas and the APUD concept. Med Biol 1974;52:3–18.
4. Modlin IM, Sandor A. An analysis of 8305 cases of carcinoid tumors. Cancer 1997;79:813–829.
5. Godwin JD. Carcinoid tumors: an analysis of 2837 cases. Cancer 1975; 36:560–569.
6. Williams ED, Sandler M. The classification of carcinoid tumors. Lancet 1963;1:238–239.
7. Capella C, Heitz PU, Hofler H, Solcia E, Kloppel G. Revised classification of neuroendocrine tumors of the lung, pancreas and gut. Digestion 1994;55:11–23.
8. Neary PC, Redmond PH, Houghton T, Watson GR, Bouchier-Hayes D. Carcinoid disease: review of the literature. Dis Colon Rectum 1997; 40:349–362.
9. Creutzfeldt W. Carcinoid tumors: development of our knowledge. World J Surg 1996;20:126–131.
10. Cheng JY, Sheu LF, Meng CL, Lin JC. Expression of p53 protein in colorectal carcinoids. Arch Surg 1996;131:67–70.
11. Koura AN, Giacco GG, Curley SA, Skibber JM, Feig BW, Ellis LM. Carcinoid tumors of the rectum: effect of size, histopathology, and surgical treatment on metastasis free survival. Cancer 1997;79:1294–1298.
12. Bates HR Jr. Carcinoid tumors of the rectum: a statistical review. Dis Colon Rectum 1996;9:90.
13. Walton GF, Gibbs ER, Spencer GO, Laws HL. Carcinoid tumors of the ampulla of Vater. Am Surg 1997;63:302–304.
14. Johnson LA, Lavin P, Moertel CG, et al. Carcinoids: the association of histologic growth pattern and survival. Cancer 1983;51:882–889.
15. Soga J, Tazawa K. Pathologic analysis of carcinoids: histologic reevaluation of 62 cases. Cancer 1971;28:990–998.
16. Modlin IM, Zhu Z, Tang LH, et al. Evidence for a regulatory role for histamine in gastric enterochromaffin-like cell proliferation induced by hypergastrinemia. Digestion 1996;57:310–321.
17. Bordi C, D'Adda T, Azzoni C, Pilato FP, Caruana P. Hypergastrinemia and gastric enterochromaffin-like cells. Am J Surg Pathol 1995;19:S8–19.
18. Modlin IM, Lawton GP, Miu K, et al. Pathophysiology of the fundic enterochromaffin-like (ECL) cell and gastric carcinoid tumours. Ann R Coll Surg Engl 1996;78:133–138.
19. Rindi G, Luinetti O, Cornaggia M, Capella C, Solcia E. Three subtypes of gastric argyrophil carcinoid and the gastric neuroendocrine carcinoma: a clinicopathologic study. Gastroenterology 1993;104:994–1006.

20. Cheng JY, Lin JC, Yu DS, Lee WH, Meng CL. Flow cytometric DNA analysis of colorectal carcinoid. Am J Surg 1994;168:29–32.
21. Fitzgerald SD, Meagher AP, Moniz-Pereira P, Farrow GM, Witzig TE, Wolff BG. Carcinoid tumor of the rectum: DNA ploidy is not a prognostic factor. Dis Colon Rectum 1996;39:643–648.
22. O'Dowd G, Gosney JR. Absence of overexpression of p53 protein by intestinal carcinoid tumours. J Pathol 1995;175:403–404.
23. Wang DG, Johnston CF, Anderson N, Sloan JM, Buchanan KD. Overexpression of the tumour suppressor gene p53 is not implicated in neuroendocrine tumour carcinogenesis. J Pathol 1995;175:397–401.
24. Dietrich WF, Radany EH, Smith JS, Bishop JM, Hanahan D, Lander ES. Genome-wide search for loss of heterozygosity in transgenic mouse tumors reveals candidate tumor suppressor genes on chromosomes 9 and 16. Proc Natl Acad Sci USA 1994;91:9451–9455.
25. Wang DG, Johnston CF, Buchanan KD. Oncogene expression in gastroenteropancreatic neuroendocrine tumors: implications for pathogenesis. Cancer 1997;80:668–675.
26. Connolly HM, Nishimura RA, Smith HC, Pellikka PA, Mullany CJ, Kvols LK. Outcome of cardiac surgery for carcinoid heart disease. J Am Coll Cardiol 1995;25:410–416.
27. Wilde MI, Markham A. Ondansetron: a review of its pharmacology and preliminary clinical findings in novel applications. Drugs 1996;52:773–794.
28. Melnyk DL. Update on carcinoid syndrome. AANA J 1997;65:265–270.
29. Ruszniewski P, Ducreux M, Chayvialle JA, et al. Treatment of the carcinoid syndrome with the longacting somatostatin analogue lanreotide: a prospective study in 39 patients. Gut 1996;39:279–283.
30. Froudarakis M, Fournel P, Burgard G, et al. Bronchial carcinoids: a review of 22 cases. Oncology 1996;53:153–158.
31. Erasmus JJ, McAdams HP, Patz EF Jr, Coleman RE, Ahuja V, Goodman PC. Evaluation of primary pulmonary carcinoid tumors using FDG PET. AJR Am J Roentgenol 1998;170:1369–1373.
32. Dusmet ME, McKneally MF. Pulmonary and thymic carcinoid tumors. World J Surg 1996;20:189–195.
33. Rea F, Binda R, Spreafico G, et al. Bronchial carcinoids: a review of 60 patients. Ann Thorac Surg 1989;47:412–414.
34. Davila DG, Dunn WF, Tazelaar HD, Pairolero PC. Bronchial carcinoid tumors. Mayo Clin Proc 1993;68:795–803.
35. Hoefnagel CA, Den Hartog Jager FC, Van Gennip AH, Marcuse HR, Taal BG. Diagnosis and treatment of a carcinoid tumor using iodine-131 meta-iodobenzylguanidine. Clin Nucl Med 1986;111:150–152.
36. Christin-Maitre S, Chabbert-Buffet N, Mure A, Boukhris R, Bouchard P. Use of somatostatin analog for localization and treatment of ACTH secreting bronchial carcinoid tumor. Chest 1996;109:845–846.
37. McCaughan BC, Martini N, Bains MS. Bronchial carcinoids: review of 124 cases. J Thorac Cardiovasc Surg 1985;89:8–17.
38. Torre M, Barberis M, Barbieri B, Bonacina E, Belloni P. Typical and atypical bronchial carcinoids. Respir Med 1989;83:305–308.
39. Okike N, Bernatz PE, Payne WS, Woolner LB, Leonard PF. Bronchoplastic procedures in the treatment of carcinoid tumors of the tracheobronchial tree. J Thorac Cardiovasc Surg 1978;76:281–291.
40. Shah R, Sabanathan S, Mearns J, Richardson J, Goulden C. Carcinoid tumour of the lung. J Cardiovasc Surg 1997;38:187–189.
41. Chughtai TS, Morin JE, Sheiner NM, Wilson JA, Mulder DS. Bronchial carcinoid—twenty years' experience defines a selective surgical approach. Surgery 1997;122:801–808.
42. Arrigoni MG, Woolner LB, Bernatz PE. Atypical carcinoid tumors of the lung. J Thorac Cardiovasc Surg 1972;64:413–421.
43. Kayser K, Kayser C, Rahn W, Bovin NV, Gabius HJ. Carcinoid tumors of the lung: immuno- and ligandohistochemistry, analysis of integrated optical density, syntactic structure analysis, clinical data, and prognosis of patients treated surgically. J Surg Oncol 1996;63:99–106.
44. Marty-Ane CH, Costes V, Pujol JL, Alauzen M, Baldet P, Mary H. Carcinoid tumors of the lung: do atypical features require aggressive management? Ann Thorac Surg 1995;59:78–83.
45. Chakravarthy A, Abrams RA. Radiation therapy in the management of patients with malignant carcinoid tumors. Cancer 1995;75:1386–1390.
46. Karmy-Jones R, Vallieres E. Carcinoid crisis after biopsy of a bronchial carcinoid. Ann Thorac Surg 1993;56:1403–1405.
47. Vaughan DJ, Brunner MD. Anesthesia for patients with carcinoid syndrome. Int Anesthesiol Clin 1997;35:129–142.
48. Modlin IM, Sandor A, Tang LH, Kidd M, Zelterman D. A 40-year analysis of 265 gastric carcinoids. Am J Gastroenterol 1997;92:633–638.
49. Roncoroni L, Costi R, Canavese G, Violi V, Bordi C. Carcinoid tumor associated with vascular malformation as a cause of massive gastric bleeding. Am J Gastroenterol 1997;92:2119–2121.
50. Nakamura S, Iida M, Yao T, Fujishima M. Endoscopic features of gastric carcinoids. Gastrointest Endosc 1991;37:535–538.
51. Fruauff A, Irwin GA, Williams HC, Gold B. CT demonstration of gastric carcinoid. AJR Am J Roentgenol 1987;148:1276–1277.
52. Gilligan CJ, Lawton GP, Tang LH, West AB, Modlin IM. Gastric carcinoid tumors: the biology and therapy of an enigmatic and controversial lesion. Am J Gastroenterol 1995;90:338–352.
53. Rappel S, Altendorf-Hofmann A, Stolte M. Prognosis of gastric carcinoid tumours. Digestion 1995;56:455–462.
54. Kokkola A, Sjoblom SM, Haapiainen R, Sipponen P, Puolakkainen P, Jarvinen H. The risk of gastric carcinoma and carcinoid tumours in patients with pernicious anaemia: a prospective follow-up study. Scand J Gastroenterol 1998;33:88–92.
55. Rindi G, Bordi C, Rappel S, La Rosa S, Stolte M, Solcia E. Gastric carcinoids and neuroendocrine carcinomas: pathogenesis, pathology, and behavior. World J Surg 1996;20:168–172.
56. Moore NR, Rogers CE, Britton BJ. Magnetic resonance imaging of endocrine tumours of the pancreas. Bri J Radiol 1995;68:341–347.
57. Pelley RJ, Bukowski RM. Recent advances in diagnosis and therapy of neuroendocrine tumors of the gastrointestinal tract. Curr Opin Oncol 1997;9:68–74.
58. MacFarlane MP, Fraker DL, Alexander HR, Norton JA, Lubensky I, Jensen RT. Prospective study of surgical resection of duodenal and pancreatic gastrinomas in multiple endocrine neoplasia type 1. Surgery 1995;118:973–979.
59. Thom AK, Norton JA, Axiotis CA, Jensen RT. Location, incidence, and malignant potential of duodenal gastrinomas. Surgery 1991;110:1086–1091.
60. Donow C, Pipeleers-Marichal M, Schroder S, Stamm B, Heitz PU, Kloppel G. Surgical pathology of gastrinoma: site, size, multicentricity, association with multiple endocrine neoplasia type 1, and malignancy. Cancer 1991;68:1329–1334.
61. Frucht H, Norton JA, London JF, et al. Detection of duodenal gastrinomas by operative endoscopic transillumination: a prospective study. Gastroenterology 1990;99:1622–1627.
62. Schirmer WJ, Melvin WS, Rush RM, et al. Indium-111-pentetreotide scanning versus conventional imaging techniques for the localization of gastrinoma. Surgery 1995;118:1105–1113.
63. Sugg SL, Norton JA, Fraker DL, et al. A prospective study of intraoperative methods to diagnose and resect duodenal gastrinomas. Ann Surg 1993;218:138–144.
64. Proye C, Pattou F, Carnaille B, Paris JC, d'Herbomez M, Marchandise X. Intraoperative gastrin measurements during surgical management of

patients with gastrinomas: experience with 20 cases. World J Surg 1998;22:643–649.

65. Akerstrom G. Management of carcinoid tumors of the stomach, duodenum, and pancreas. World J Surg 1996;20:173–182.
66. Wheeler MH, Curley IR, Williams ED. The association of neurofibromatosis, pheochromocytoma, and somatostatin-rich duodenal carcinoid tumor. Surgery 1986;100:1163–1169.
67. Fuller CE, Williams GT. Gastrointestinal manifestations of type 1 neurofibromatosis (von Recklinghausen's disease). Histopathology 1991;19: 1–11.
68. Kloppel G, Heitz PU, Capella C, Solcia E. Pathology and nomenclature of human gastrointestinal neuroendocrine (carcinoid) tumors and related lesions. World J Surg 1996;20:132–141.
69. Neoptolemos JR, Talbot IC, Shaw DC, Carr-Locke DL. Long-term survival after resection of ampullary carcinoma is associated independently with tumor grade and a new staging classification that assesses local invasiveness. Cancer 1988;61:1403–1407.
70. Maurer CA, Baer HU, Dyong TH, et al. Carcinoid of the pancreas: clinical characteristics and morphological features. Eur J Cancer 1996;32A: 1109–1116.
71. Moertel CG, Hanley JA. Combination chemotherapy trials in metastatic carcinoid tumor and the malignant carcinoid syndrome. Cancer Clin Trials 1979;2:327–334.
72. Feldman JM. Carcinoid tumors and the carcinoid syndrome. Curr Probl Surg 1989;26:835–885.
73. Burke AP, Thomas RM, Elsayed AM, Sobin LH. Carcinoids of the jejunum and ileum: an immunohistochemical and clinicopathologic study of 167 cases. Cancer 1997;79:1086–1093.
74. Weber JD, McFadden DW. Carcinoid tumors in Meckel's diverticula. J Clin Gastroenterol 1989;11:682–686.
75. Makridis C, Rastad J, Oberg K, Akerstrom G. Progression of metastases and symptom improvement from laparotomy in midgut carcinoid tumors. World J Surg 1996;20:900–906.
76. Basson MD, Ahlman H, Wangberg B, Modlin IM. Biology and management of the midgut carcinoid. Am J Surg 1993;165:288–297.
77. Orlefors H, Sundin A, Ahlstrom H, et al. Positron emission tomography with 5-hydroxytryptophan in neuroendocrine tumors. J Clin Oncol 1998; 16:2534–2541.
78. Woodard PK, Feldman JM, Paine SS, Baker ME. Midgut carcinoid tumors: CT findings and biochemical profiles. J Comput Assist Tomogr 1995; 19:400–405.
79. Wallace S, Ajani JA, Charnsangavej C, et al. Carcinoid tumors: imaging procedures and interventional radiology. World J Surg 1996;20:147–156.
80. Sugimoto E, Lorelius LE, Eriksson B, Oberg K. Midgut carcinoid tumours: CT appearance. Acta Radiol 1995;36:367–371.
81. Ahlman H, Nilsson O, Wangberg B, Dahlstrom A. Neuroendocrine insights from the laboratory to the clinic. Am J Surg 1996;172:61–67.
82. Ohrvall U, Westlin JE, Nilsson S, et al. Intraoperative gamma detection reveals abdominal endocrine tumors more efficiently than somatostatin receptor scintigraphy. Cancer 1997;80:2490–2494.
83. Wangberg B, Westberg G, Tylen U, et al. Survival of patients with disseminated midgut carcinoid tumors after aggressive tumor reduction. World J Surg 1996;20:892–899.
84. Persson BG, Nobin A, Ahren B, Jeppsson B, Mansson B, Bengmark S. Repeated hepatic ischemia as a treatment for carcinoid liver metastases. World J Surg 1989;13:307–311.
85. Ahlman H, Westberg G, Wangberg B, et al. Treatment of liver metastases of carcinoid tumors. World J Surg 1996;20:196–202.
86. Box JC, Watne AL, Lucas GW. Small bowel carcinoid: review of a single institution experience and review of the literature. Am Surg 1996;62: 280–286.
87. Sandor A, Modlin IM. A retrospective analysis of 1570 appendiceal carcinoids. Am J Gastroenterol 1998;93:422–428.
88. Roggo A, Wood WC, Ottinger LW. Carcinoid tumors of the appendix. Ann Surg 1993;217:385–390.
89. Stinner B, Kisker O, Zielke A, Rothmund M. Surgical management for carcinoid tumors of small bowel, appendix, colon, and rectum. World J Surg 1996;20:183–188.
90. Rosenberg JM, Welch JP. Carcinoid tumors of the colon: a study of 72 patients. Am J Surg 1985;149:775–779.
91. Tobi M, Darmon E, Rozen P, et al. Shared tumor antigens in colorectal carcinoma and neuroendocrine tumors. Cancer Detect Prev 1998; 22:147–152.
92. Federspiel BH, Burke AP, Sobin LH, Shekitka KM. Rectal and colonic carcinoids: a clinicopathologic study of 84 cases. Cancer 1990;65:135–140.
93. Soga J. Carcinoids of the rectum: an evaluation of 1271 reported cases. Surg Today 1997;27:112–119.
94. Jetmore AB, Ray JE, Gathright JB Jr, McMullen KM, Hicks TC, Timmcke AE. Rectal carcinoids: the most frequent carcinoid tumor. Dis Colon Rectum 1992;35:717–725.
95. Sauven P, Ridge JA, Quan SH, Sigurdson ER. Anorectal carcinoid tumors: is aggressive surgery warranted? Ann Surg 1990;211:67–71.
96. Higaki S, Nishiaki M, Mitani N, Yanai H, Tada M, Okita K. Effectiveness of local endoscopic resection of rectal carcinoid tumors. Endoscopy 1997;29:171–175.
97. Mani S, Modlin IM, Ballantyne G, Ahlman H, West B. Carcinoids of the rectum. J Am Coll Surg 1994;179:231–248.
98. Chen H, Hardacre JM, Uzar A, Cameron JL, Choti MA. Isolated liver metastases from neuroendocrine tumors: does resection prolong survival? J Am Coll Surg 1998;187:88–92.
99. Winkelbauer FW, Niederle B, Pietschmann F, et al. Hepatic artery embolotherapy of hepatic metastases from carcinoid tumors: value of using a mixture of cyanoacrylate and ethiodized oil. AJR Am J Roentgenol 1995;165:323–327.
100. Ajani JA, Carrasco CH, Wallace S. Neuroendocrine tumors metastatic to the liver: vascular occlusion therapy. Ann NY Acad Sci 1994;733: 479–487.
101. de Baere T, Roche A, Amenabar JM, et al. Liver abscess formation after local treatment of liver tumors. Hepatology 1996;23:1436–1440.
102. Siperstein AE, Rogers SJ, Hansen PD, Gitomirsky A. Laparoscopic thermal ablation of hepatic neuroendocrine tumor metastases. Surgery 1997;122: 1147–1154.
103. Bilchik AJ, Sarantou T, Foshag LJ, Giuliano AE, Ramming KP. Cryosurgical palliation of metastatic neuroendocrine tumors resistant to conventional therapy. Surgery 1997;122:1040–1047.
104. Bongers V, de Klerk JM, Zonnenberg BA, de Kort G, Lips CJ, van Rijk PP. Acute liver necrosis induced by iodine-131-MIBG in the treatment of metastatic carcinoid tumors. J Nucl Med 1997;38:1024–1026.
105. Diaco DS, Hajarizadeh H, Mueller CR, Fletcher WS, Pommier RF, Woltering EA. Treatment of metastatic carcinoid tumors using multimodality therapy of octreotide acetate, intra-arterial chemotherapy, and hepatic arterial chemoembolization. Am J Surg 1995;169;523–528.
106. Ramage JK, Catnach SM, Williams R. Overview: the management of metastatic carcinoid tumors. Liver Transpl Surg 1995;1:107–110.
107. Routley D, Ramage JK, McPeake J, Tan KC, Williams R. Orthotopic liver transplantation in the treatment of metastatic neuroendocrine tumors of the liver. Liver Transpl Surg 1995;1:118–121.
108. Dousset B, Houssin D, Soubrane O, Boillot O, Baudin F, Chapuis Y. Metastatic endocrine tumors: is there a place for liver transplantation? Liver Transpl Surg 1995;1:111–117.

Chapter 17

Multiple Endocrine Neoplasia Syndromes

JAMES R. HOWE

The multiple endocrine neoplasia (MEN) syndromes are divided into two broad categories, designated MEN 1 and MEN 2. MEN 1, also known as Wermer syndrome, is an autosomal dominant condition in which patients develop hyperparathyroidism, pituitary tumors, and pancreatic islet cell tumors. MEN 2 is further divided into three autosomal dominant subtypes, known as MEN 2A, MEN 2B, and familial medullary thyroid carcinoma (FMTC). MEN 2A, also known as Sipple syndrome, is characterized by medullary thyroid carcinoma, pheochromocytoma, and hyperparathyroidism. Patients with MEN 2B share the first two components with MEN 2A, but in place of hyperparathyroidism they have a marfanoid body habitus, mucosal neuromas of the lips and tongue, and ganglioneuromas of the gastrointestinal tract. Patients with FMTC do not develop pheochromocytomas or hyperparathyroidism.

MEN 1

Hyperparathyroidism	95%
Pituitary tumors	30%
Pancreatic islet cell tumors	40%

The first description of MEN 1 was in 1903 by Erdheim, who described a patient with acromegaly and parathyroid hyperplasia.[1] Cushing and Davidoff were the first to describe a patient with tumors of the pituitary (acromegaly), parathyroids, and pancreatic islet cells in 1927.[2] Underahl et al. reported eight cases in which patients had developed tumors involving at least two of these three endocrine glands in 1953,[3] and Wermer coined the term "adenomatosis of endocrine glands" when describing five members of a family with MEN 1 in 1954.[4] A follow-up study of this family reported 20 affected individuals spanning four generations, 19 of whom had severe peptic ulcer disease and 10 who had documented tumors of the parathyroids, pituitary, pancreatic islet cells, thyroid, or adrenal cortex.[5] This report helped confirm the importance of the new syndrome reported by Zollinger and Ellison in 1955, in which severe ulcer disease was associated with pancreatic islet cell tumors.[6] We now know that the most common feature of MEN 1 is hyperplasia of the parathyroid glands, which is seen in 95% of these

MEN 1 Syndrome

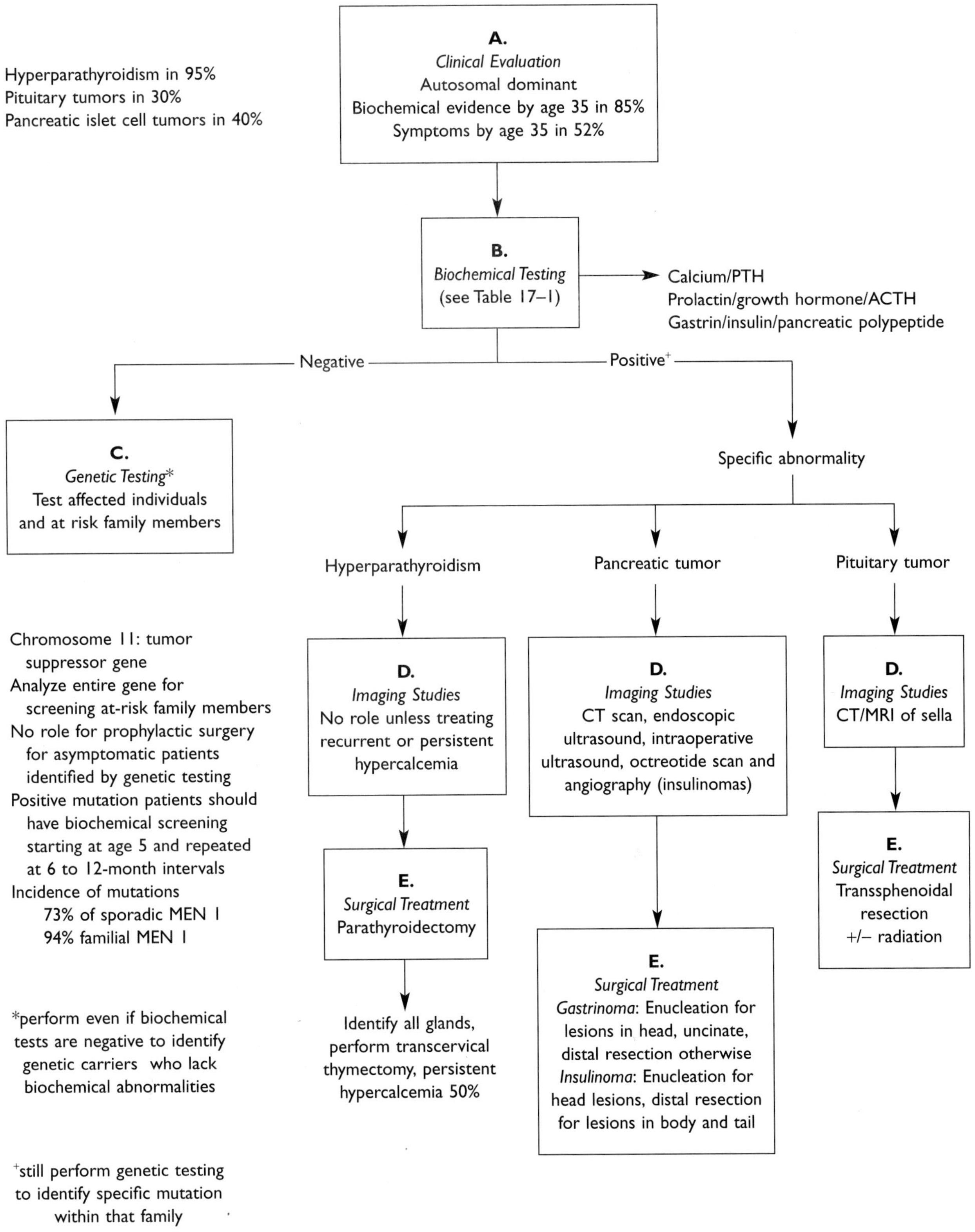

Hyperparathyroidism in 95%
Pituitary tumors in 30%
Pancreatic islet cell tumors in 40%

A.
Clinical Evaluation
Autosomal dominant
Biochemical evidence by age 35 in 85%
Symptoms by age 35 in 52%

B.
Biochemical Testing
(see Table 17–1)

→ Calcium/PTH
Prolactin/growth hormone/ACTH
Gastrin/insulin/pancreatic polypeptide

Negative →

C.
*Genetic Testing**
Test affected individuals
and at risk family members

Chromosome 11: tumor suppressor gene
Analyze entire gene for screening at-risk family members
No role for prophylactic surgery for asymptomatic patients identified by genetic testing
Positive mutation patients should have biochemical screening starting at age 5 and repeated at 6 to 12-month intervals
Incidence of mutations
73% of sporadic MEN 1
94% familial MEN 1

*perform even if biochemical tests are negative to identify genetic carriers who lack biochemical abnormalities

+still perform genetic testing to identify specific mutation within that family

Positive+ →

Specific abnormality

Hyperparathyroidism

D.
Imaging Studies
No role unless treating recurrent or persistent hypercalcemia

E.
Surgical Treatment
Parathyroidectomy

Identify all glands, perform transcervical thymectomy, persistent hypercalcemia 50%

Pancreatic tumor

D.
Imaging Studies
CT scan, endoscopic ultrasound, intraoperative ultrasound, octreotide scan and angiography (insulinomas)

E.
Surgical Treatment
Gastrinoma: Enucleation for lesions in head, uncinate, distal resection otherwise
Insulinoma: Enucleation for head lesions, distal resection for lesions in body and tail

Pituitary tumor

D.
Imaging Studies
CT/MRI of sella

E.
Surgical Treatment
Transsphenoidal resection
+/– radiation

patients; approximately 40% have pancreatic islet cell tumors, and 30% have adenomas of the pituitary. Family members less commonly manifest adrenal cortical tumors, follicular neoplasms of the thyroid, multiple lipomas, and bronchial or intestinal carcinoids.

A. Clinical Evaluation

The presentation of MEN 1 depends on which components of the disease are involved. Typically, the age of onset is 20–40 years. Patients with *hyperparathyroidism*, may have nephrolithiasis or osteitis fibrosa cystica, but most are asymptomatic. Symptoms related to *pancreatic islet cell tumors* vary according to which hormone is being produced: primarily gastrin or insulin and less commonly glucagon, somatostatin, and vasoactive intestinal peptide (VIP). MEN 1 patients with gastrinomas have severe peptic ulcer disease and account for 25% of patients with Zollinger-Ellison syndrome[7,8]; these patients are likely to present with complications of ulcer disease, such as perforation, obstruction, or bleeding. Epigastric pain is common, as is diarrhea due to acid hypersecretion and steatorrhea due to precipitation of bile salts and the acidic denaturation of lipase. Patients with insulinomas typically have fasting hypoglycemia, which stimulates the release of epinephrine; patients may be confused or comatose and commonly manifest palpitations, tachycardia, and sweating. Many patients have significant weight gain, as they eat frequently to avoid these events. Patients with VIPomas have profuse *w*atery *d*iarrhea, *h*ypokalemia, *a*chlorhydria (collectively known as the WDHA syndrome), and flushing. No clear-cut syndrome is recognized for pancreatic polypeptide (PP)-producing tumors; and plasma levels of PP may be elevated with other islet cell neoplasms. Glucagonomas produce a syndrome of diabetes, weight loss, anemia, psychiatric symptoms, and a distinctive rash called necrolytic migratory erythema. Somatostatinomas are more likely to cause symptoms related to a peripancreatic mass than excess hormone production; mild diabetes, gallstones, and steatorrhea may be seen.

Pituitary tumors are usually prolactinomas, which present with amenorrhea, galactorrhea, and infertility in females; males are more likely to present with symptoms related to a mass lesion in the sella turcica. Pituitary adenomas may also produce growth hormone (GH), causing acromegaly, increased sellar volume, hyperhidrosis, weakness, arthralgia, and abnormal glucose tolerance tests. Less commonly, pituitary adenomas produce adrenocorticotropic hormone (ACTH), leading to the adrenal hyperplasia of Cushing's disease. Some tumors are nonsecretory, and others produce more than one hormone.[9] Pituitary tumors may also cause visual disturbances such as diplopia, headaches, or symptoms secondary to loss of other pituitary hormones caused by tumor compression.

There is usually a strong family history of parathyroid, pancreatic, or pituitary neoplasms, as MEN 1 is inherited as an autosomal dominant trait. There is no predilection for either gender. Among 220 affected patients reported by Trump et al., 30% were asymptomatic and diagnosed only by biochemical screening. The age at diagnosis ranged from 8 to 79 years, 52% developed symptoms by the age of 35 years, and 85% had biochemical evidence of disease by age 35.[10]

B. Biochemical Testing

Table 17–1 summarizes the components of MEN 1 syndrome and the biochemical testing needed for diagnosis. The measurement of fasting PP in MEN 1 patients may also be useful as a screening test for islet cell neoplasms; when PP levels are elevated to more than three times the normal values (which vary with age from approximately 150 to 325 pg/ml), the sensitivity for detecting these tumors is 95% with 88% specificity.[11]

C. Genetic Testing

The gene for MEN 1 was mapped to the long arm of chromosome 11 in 1988 by Larsson and associates, who also demonstrated that allelic losses were present in tumor tissues, consistent with a tumor suppressor function.[12] Over the following 9 years the interval containing the MEN 1 gene was progressively narrowed, and deletions of this region were reported in MEN 1-related tumors as well as sporadic parathyroid tumors and gastrinomas.[13,14] In 1997 the gene for MEN 1 (named *MENIN*) was identified; it was found to be 2.8 kb in size, contain 10 exons, and encode for a 610-amino-acid protein. Mutations were found in 14 of 15 MEN 1 families studied and were consistent with loss of function, confirming earlier hypotheses of a tumor suppressor role. The gene is expressed in all tissues and shares little similarity with other known sequences.[15] It appears that the MENIN protein is located in the cell nucleus, but its function remains unclear.[16]

Another group of investigators confirmed these finding by also identifying this gene, finding nine mutations in 10 MEN 1 families.[17] The mutations seen in different families are widely distributed across the gene, with few families sharing the same mutation, in contrast to the MEN 2 syndromes. Further studies have revealed *MENIN* mutations in 8 of 11 (73%) sporadic MEN 1 cases and 47 of 50 (94%) familial MEN 1 cases, with a total of 40 different mutations. No *MENIN* mutations were seen in five families with familial hyperparathyroidism, suggesting a different mechanism for the development of this syndrome.[18] Analysis of 63 unrelated MEN 1 kindreds by another group demonstrated 47 different mutations scattered throughout the coding region; approximately 10% of them appeared to arise de novo in patients without a family history and were inherited by the next generation. This study allowed determination of the age-related penetrance of MEN 1, which was 7% by age 10, 52% by age 20, 87% by age 30, and 98% by age 40. Among 201 family

TABLE 17–1.
MEN 1 biochemical testing

Condition	Laboratory findings	Provocative testing
Hyperparathyroidism	High normal, elevated serum calcium Elevated PTH Hypophosphatemia, hyperchloremia Chloride/phosphate ratio > 33 Elevated 24-hour urine calcium	
Gastrinoma	Elevated fasting serum gastrin (> 500 pg/ml) Gastrin level 100–500 pg/ml → provocative tests	Secretin (2 U/kg IV); check gastrin levels at 0, 2, 5, 10, 15 minutes; expect > 50% increase with gastrinoma
Insulinoma	Hypoglycemia and elevated insulin (normal < 30/U/ml) C-peptide level (normal < 1.2 ng/ml) (rules out exogenous insulin)	After 72-hour fast, measure glucose, insulin, and C-peptide levels when symptoms develop Tolbutamide test, calcium infusion
VIPoma	Stool volume exceeding 3 L/day Elevated fasting VIP level	
Glucagonoma	Serum glucagon levels > 150 pg/ml	
Pituitary adenoma	Prolactin level (normal: women < 23 ng/ml, men < 20 ng/ml) Growth hormone level (normal < 5 ng/ml) ACTH level (normal < 60 mg/ml) Ectopic ACTH tumor > 500 pg/ml Pituitary ACTH tumor 75–200 pg/ml	Give 75–100 g glucose PO; measure growth hormone at 1 and 2 hours; if pituitary tumor, no suppression of growth hormone and insulin levels stay elevated

PTH, parathyroid hormone; VIP, vasoactive intestinal peptide; ACTH, adrenocorticotrophic hormone.
The fasting pancreatic polypeptide (PP) assay may be useful as a screening test for islet cell neoplasms; when PP levels are elevated to more than three times normal (150–325 pg/ml), the sensitivity for detecting these tumors is 95% with 88% specificity.[11]

members found to carry a mutant *MENIN* allele, 50% had already presented with symptoms, 27% were asymptomatic but were positive by biochemical screening, and 23% were asymptomatic and negative by biochemical screening.[19] The diversity of the mutations throughout the *MENIN* gene requires analysis of the entire coding region for screening new families. Owing to the location of the tumors associated with MEN 1 and their generally benign nature (except for gastrinomas), there seems to be little need for prophylactic surgery in asymptomatic patients based on genetic testing. Bassett and colleagues recommended that those identified with *MENIN* mutations undergo standard biochemical screening beginning at age 5 and repeated at 6- to 12-month intervals. This approach would allow early detection and treatment of MEN 1-associated neoplasms.[19]

All MEN 1 patients should undergo genetic testing. Mutations have been detected in more than 90% of the families studied; and once the mutation is known in a family, testing of at-risk family members is a relatively simple matter. All affected members of the same family have the same mutation; identification of asymptomatic gene carriers allows more rigorous biochemical and radiologic screening. This type of testing is performed using DNA extracted from *peripheral* blood. Patients with sporadic MEN 1 should also undergo testing if they have or are planning to have children. These germline defects presumably result from a mutation in an egg or sperm cell of an otherwise normal parent and are passed on to his or her offspring. The success at finding mutations in sporadic MEN 1 cases has also been good (about 70%).

A study of 33 sporadic parathyroid tumors for mutations of the *MENIN* gene revealed somatic mutations in 7 (21%); the normal gene was found to be deleted in all tumors with *MENIN* mutations. These results suggested that mutations in the *MENIN* gene also contribute to the development of sporadic tumors.[20] A similar study of 27 sporadic gastrinomas and 12 sporadic insulinomas found *MENIN* mutations in 33% and 17% of these tumors, respectively, and deletion of one copy of the gene in 93% and 50% of the tumors with mutations, respectively. This suggests a role for *MENIN* in the development of both sporadic gastrinomas and insulinomas.[21] A study of sporadic pituitary adenomas in 38 patients revealed deletion of the normal copy in 3 (8%) and *MENIN* mutations in two of these three tumors. Although these mutations were less common than those seen in other sporadic MEN 1-associated neoplasms, they may be involved in the development of a subset of these tumors, although this was not demonstrated by this study.[22]

D. Imaging Studies

There is currently little role for parathyroid imaging in patients with MEN 1 who have not previously undergone neck exploration. In patients in whom fewer than four glands were identified at their initial operation and who later had persistent or recurrent hyperparathyroidism, imaging may be helpful. Similarly, if four glands were identified during subtotal or total parathyroidectomy and the patient has persistent hyperparathyroidism, imaging may help identify an ectopic gland. High-resolution ultrasonography (US), computed tomography (CT), and sestamibi pertechnetate scanning are currently the non-invasive tests of choice.

Islet cell tumors in MEN 1 patients are usually multicentric and may be benign or malignant. Approximately 80% of *gastrinomas* are found within the duodenal wall, are small, and are not reliably identified by preoperative imaging. Most of these tumors are malignant, and up to 50% of MEN 1 patients have lymph node metastases at the time of diagnosis. Although CT or US may not detect small duodenal gastrinomas, it may show liver metastases and thereby select patients for medical management. In those without signs of metastatic disease by these imaging tests, the combination of intraoperative ultrasonography (IOUS), intraoperative endoscopic transillumination of the duodenum, and duodenotomy with palpation yield the highest success rates for finding these neoplasms.[23]

Insulinomas occur almost exclusively in the pancreas, with equal distribution throughout the gland. Approximately 85–90% of these tumors are benign; when malignant, metastases most often are to the regional nodes and liver. Up to 90% of these tumors are <2 cm in size, 40% are <1 cm, and 90% are multicentric in MEN 1 patients. CT with 5 mm cuts through the pancreas identifies about 60% of these tumors, with octreotide scanning yielding similar results. Angiography may demonstrate a tumor blush and allows identification of up to 60–80% of these tumors.[24] A more sensitive technique for diagnosing insulinoma is the measurement of hepatic venous insulin levels after intra-arterial injection of calcium into the hepatic, gastroduodenal, splenic, and superior mesenteric arteries; calcium causes secretion of insulin from these tumors, and the levels measured in a hepatic vein after injection into these arteries allows regionalization of the tumor(s). However, owing to the multicentricity of these tumors in MEN 1 patients, this method is less valuable in these patients than in sporadic cases where 90% of the tumors are solitary. IOUS may be the most sensitive localization procedure; and coupled with palpation of the pancreas it allows localization of more than 90% of these tumors.[25] Thompson currently recommends endoscopic ultrasonography (EUS) as the only preoperative imaging test for insulinoma.[26] Thorough mobilization and manual palpation of the pancreas should be performed at operation, and IOUS can enhance the detection of additional lesions. The data on the optimal approach for other pancreatic islet cell tumors in MEN 1 patients are limited by their small numbers. Thin-cut, helical CT is a reasonable approach to these patients as it identifies tumors >1 cm and demonstrates the presence of liver metastases; octreotide scanning may also be a useful adjunct in these patients.

Approximately 60% of MEN 1 patients with *pituitary tumors* have microadenomas (<1 cm), and about 40% have macroadenomas (>1 cm). The incidence of macroadenomas is higher in males than in females.[9] The hormone being produced by a pituitary adenoma is generally not evident from imaging tests unless they also show bony features characteristic of acromegaly or Cushing's disease. Currently, magnetic resonance imaging (MRI) has become the diagnostic test of choice for imaging these tumors. Thin-cut coronal and axial CT with intravenous contrast is also useful for identifying micro- and macroadenomas.

E. Surgical Treatment

Hyperparathyroidism Most patients with MEN 1 present with hyperparathyroidism, and neck exploration through a low collar incision is undertaken in those meeting the biochemical criteria. The primary objective is to identify all parathyroid glands. To achieve this objective, transcervical thymectomy is recommended because of the high incidence of ectopic or supernumerary glands in MEN patients. The surgical options are total parathyroidectomy and autotransplantation versus subtotal parathyroidectomy.

With total parathyroidectomy all four glands are removed, and a 25- to 50-mg portion of one parathyroid gland is cut into 1 × 3 mm pieces, which are placed in iced saline; approximately 15–20 pieces are implanted into the nondominant brachioradialis muscle. Each pocket containing several fragments is marked with a nonabsorbable suture so it can be identified in the future should the patient develop recurrent hyperparathyroidism.[27]

With subtotal parathyroidectomy, the three largest glands are removed. If the fourth gland is also enlarged, a clip is placed across the gland, and the distal portion is removed, leaving an approximately 50 mg remnant attached to the blood supply; if this gland is of normal size, a clip is placed to mark the end of the gland, which is also marked with a long nonabsorbable suture to facilitate future identification should the patient develop recurrent hyperparathyroidism. It is essential that there is no compromise to the blood supply of this remaining gland; one way to do this is to select the gland to be preserved first and attempt to obtain a well vascularized 50 mg remnant prior to removing the other glands. In this way, the other glands can potentially be used should the viability of the first remnant appear to be in question.

The biggest risk of both procedures is permanent hypoparathyroidism, which may be reduced by cryopreservation of parathyroid tissue at the initial procedure. Recurrent hyperparathyroidism is more problematic with subtotal parathyroidectomy patients in that it requires a repeat neck exploration. With autotransplantation, some of the implanted parathyroid tissue can be removed under local anesthesia. Graft function can be followed by measuring parathyroid hormone (PTH) levels from the ipsilateral antecubital vein.

The result of surgical treatment for hyperparathyroidism in MEN 1 patients is not nearly as favorable as that seen in patients with sporadic disease. In one study with long-term follow-up after surgery for hyperparathyroidism in 61 MEN 1 patients, the rate of persistent or recurrent hyperparathyroidism was 54%. In patients rendered normocalcemic after the original neck exploration, the rate of recurrent hyperparathyroidism was 21% at 5 years and 41% at 10 years of follow-up. Ten percent of these patients were chronically hypocalcemic.[28] In centers with particular expertise in this area, the rate of persistent or recurrent hyperparathyroidism can be reduced to less than 20%,[26] but long-term follow-up is essential to monitor for recurrence of this component of the disease.

PANCREATIC TUMORS The surgical treatment of *islet cell neoplasms* in MEN 1 has changed significantly over the past few decades, especially for gastrinomas. Early surgical experience with gastrinomas in MEN 1 suggested that few patients were cured by surgery[29] but that total gastrectomy provided good palliation. With the advent of H_2-blockers, many patients could be managed medically without surgery. Later it became appreciated that a large proportion of these tumors were extrapancreatic, and that gastrinomas were often malignant and could progress and metastasize when managed medically. Furthermore, many tumors removed from the pancreas in these patients were immunohistochemically negative for gastrin. It is now known that most gastrinomas (80–90%) are located in the gastrinoma triangle, which is defined by the cystic and common bile duct confluence superiorly, the second and third portions of the duodenum inferiorly, and the region of the neck and body of the pancreas medially.[30] Current recommendations are that all patients with Zollinger-Ellison syndrome (ZES) without signs of metastatic disease should undergo exploration. During exploration the duodenum is extensively kocherized, and the peritoneal attachments of the spleen are taken down to mobilize the body and tail of the pancreas. The pancreas and duodenum are palpated to identify small tumors. At this time IOUS should be carried out to identify small tumors in the pancreas. Tumors in the head or uncinate process are enucleated, and distal pancreatectomy is performed to remove tumors in the neck, body, or tail of the gland. To identify duodenal tumors, intraoperative endoscopy is performed to transilluminate the wall of the duodenum, which aids in identifying small gastrinomas; the duodenal wall should be palpated. Next, a longitudinal duodenotomy is performed in the second portion of the duodenum, encompassing any tumors that may have been identified. Additional tumors found upon opening the duodenum are locally excised with full-thickness margins of normal tissue. The duodenotomy is then closed transversely in two layers. Lymph nodes in the porta hepatis along the common hepatic artery, celiac axis, and peripancreatic region are also removed at exploration because they may be sites of metastases.[23]

In Thompson's[26] experience with 17 MEN 1 ZES patients, 76% of patients had tumors in the duodenum, 59% in the pancreas (24% in pancreas only), and 35% in the duodenum and pancreas. All of their patients also had neuroendocrine tumors identified in the body or tail of the pancreas, but they were not necessarily gastrinomas. Approximately half of the patients had nodal metastases. Of these 17 patients, 29% had negative postoperative secretin tests (implying cure of disease), 35% of others had negative basal gastrin levels and were asymptomatic, and 35% had increased basal gastrin levels.

A prospective study from the National Institutes of Health in 10 MEN 1 patients with ZES found duodenal gastrinomas in seven patients (two also had pancreatic tumors), isolated pancreatic tumors in two, and gastrinoma in a lymph node in one other. Eighty percent of these patients had lymph node metastases, but one of the criteria for inclusion in the study was the presence of a lesion >3 cm in diameter seen by preoperative imaging. Although all 10 patients had significant reductions in serum gastrin levels, none of these patients was cured (as defined by normal gastrin levels). This may have been influenced by selecting only patients with large tumors for exploration.[31]

Survival of patients with MEN 1-related and sporadic gastrinomas was evaluated by Ellison, who also proposed a staging system for gastrinoma based on a 40 year experience with 74 patients. Stage I tumors are those <2 cm without liver metastases; stage II lesions are >2 cm without liver metastases; and stage III is defined by the presence of liver metastases. The status of the regional nodes is not a factor in this staging system. The 10-year survival rates for patients with resected stage I tumors were 94–96% and 68–82% for those with lesions not resected (depending on tumor size). For those with resected stage II tumors the 10-year survival was 86–91%, and that for patients with unresected lesions, 40–55%. Among patients with stage III tumors it was 65–90% for those with resected tumors and 7–50% for those with unresected tumors.[32]

About 99% of insulinomas occur in the pancreas, and approximately 85% are benign. Attention is directed at the pancreas and determining if metastatic disease is present. A Kocher maneuver is performed, as is division of the omental attachments to the colon to visualize the lesser sac. This allows for thorough palpation of the head and uncinate process of the pancreas. Next, the peritoneum overlying the inferior edge of the pancreas is divided, and the peritoneal attachments to the spleen are taken down to mobilize the body and tail of the gland. These portions of the pancreas are carefully palpated, and IOUS is performed. Tumors in the body or tail are treated by distal pancreatectomy, and those in the head or uncinate process are enucleated. If no tumor is found, surgical options include blind distal pancreatectomy or cessation of operation and further diagnostic workup. Most of the less common islet cell tumors, such as vasoactive intestinal protein tumors (VIPomas), glucagonomas, and pancreatic polypeptide tumors (PPomas), have significant malignant potential and usually are found in the pancreas. The surgical approach to these lesions is similar to that used for insulinoma, except they have higher malignant potential and therefore are more likely to have regional nodal involvement or liver metastases. For somatostatinomas, which are usually in the head of the pancreas or duodenum, pancreaticoduodenectomy must be considered.

There is no clear benefit of chemotherapy for patients with gastrinoma metastatic to regional lymph nodes who have postoperative hypergastrinemia. In contrast, if there is distant disease in the liver or elsewhere, chemotherapy may be of benefit. Combination streptozocin (500 mg/m^2/day for 5 days every 6 weeks) and doxorubicin (50 mg/m^2 on days 1 and 22 of each cycle) is superior to streptozocin and 5-fluorouracil (400 mg/m^2/day for 5 days every 6 weeks), with response rates of 69% and a median survival of 2.2 years for those with advanced islet cell tumors.[33] Liver metastases may be treated by debulking, hepatic artery ligation, or chemoembolization. Treatment of unresectable insulinoma is similar, except palliation may be achieved with diazoxide or octreotide. Metastatic glucagonoma or VIPoma may also be palliated with octreotide.

Pituitary Tumors The treatment of MEN 1 patients with documented pituitary tumors depends on the tumor size and the hormones being produced. Virtually all patients with growth hormone (GH)- or adrenocorticotropic hormone (ACTH)-producing tumors should have surgery because of the deleterious metabolic effects associated with these tumors. The approach of choice for most tumors is transsphenoidal resection with preservation of normal pituitary tissue adjacent to the adenoma. Large tumors are more likely to require craniotomy. Long-term remission rates are best in patients with GH-producing tumors, ranging from 60% to 90%; they depend on tumor size, the presence of extrasellar extension, and preoperative GH levels. The remission rate associated with Cushing's disease is approximately 75–90% in patients with intrasellar tumors but is less than 50% in patients with extrasellar tumors. No tumor is found in 10–15% of patients thought to have Cushing's disease; these patients may have ectopic ACTH-producing tumors or pituitary hyperplasia. They may benefit from total hypophysectomy, which results in panhypopituitarism. In children or young adults, radiation therapy may be preferable in this situation as it is more likely to allow continued growth and the chance for procreation.

There is effective medical therapy for prolactin (PRL)-producing tumors in the form of the dopamine agonist bromocriptine. Side effects include primarily nausea, vomiting, dizziness, and orthostatic hypotension. The results of surgery for large tumors (>2 cm) and those with PRL levels >600 ng/ml are poor, with cure rates of approximately 10%. Therefore these patients are commonly treated with bromocriptine, which may normalize the PRL levels and provide good long-term control. Exceptions include patients with visual compromise and those planning to have children in the future, as rapid growth of the tumor may occur during pregnancy. There is a higher recurrence rate (15–50%) for PRL-producing microadenomas after transsphenoidal surgery, which is influenced by tumor size, extrasellar extension, and preoperative PRL levels. Patients with small, localized tumors and PRL levels <100 ng/ml have the highest remission rates. If patients treated with bromocriptine have continued growth of their tumor, or if the PRL levels are not effectively lowered, surgery should be considered.[34] The results of surgical treatment for pituitary disease in MEN 1 patients is similar to that observed in non-MEN 1 patients.[9]

Adjuvant therapy should be considered in patients with incompletely excised pituitary adenomas, tumors with unfavorable characteristics (large tumors or those with extrasellar extension), or recurrent tumors. Radiation therapy may be useful in this situation, and medical management with bromocriptine is helpful for most patients with PRL-secreting tumors and to a lesser extent those with GH-secreting tumors. In patients with recurrent ACTH-producing tumors or in those in whom no tumor was found after pituitary surgery, pituitary irradiation or bilateral adrenalectomy should be considered.

MEN 2

MEN 2A
- Medullary thyroid cancer in 100%
- Pheochromocytoma in 6–100%
- Hyperparathyroidism in 0–53%

MEN 2B
- Medullary thyroid cancer
- Pheochromocytoma
- Marfanoid body habitus
- Mucosal neuromas

The feature common to all subtypes of the MEN 2 syndromes is medullary thyroid cancer (MTC). This was first reported as a distinct entity in 1959 by Hazard, Hawk, and Crile. In 1961 Sipple estimated that the incidence of thyroid carcinoma was 14 times higher in patients with pheochromocytoma relative to the normal population.[35] It was not until 1965 that Williams reported that MTC was the thyroid cancer associated with pheochromocytoma,[36] and he later suggested that the parafollicular cells (C-cells) might produce the hormone calcitonin.[37] Then in 1968 the term "multiple endocrine neoplasia type 2" was coined by Steiner et al.[38] Tashjian et al. made early

MEN 2 Syndrome

MEN 2A
- Medullary thyroid cancer in 100%
- Pheochromocytoma in 6–100%
- Hyperparathyroidism in 0–53%

F.
Clinical Evaluation
History
Physical examination
Family history

MEN 2B
- Medullary thyroid cancer
- Pheochromocytoma
- Marfinoid habitus
- Neuromas

↓

G.
Biochemical Testing
Stimulated calcitonin levels: calcium gluconate 2 mg/kg/min followed by pentagastrin (0.5 micrograms/kg/5 sec); then measure serum calcitonin at 1, 3, 5 minutes
24 hour urine for catecholamines, metanephrine, VMA
Serum calcium

↓

H.
Genetic Testing
Advised for MEN 2 family members
Family members at risk may be carriers even if biochemical testing is negative and therefore genetic testing advised
Gene identified on chromosome 10(RET)
Mutation present in 98% of MEN 2A
Mutation present in 95% MEN 2B

(continued on next page)

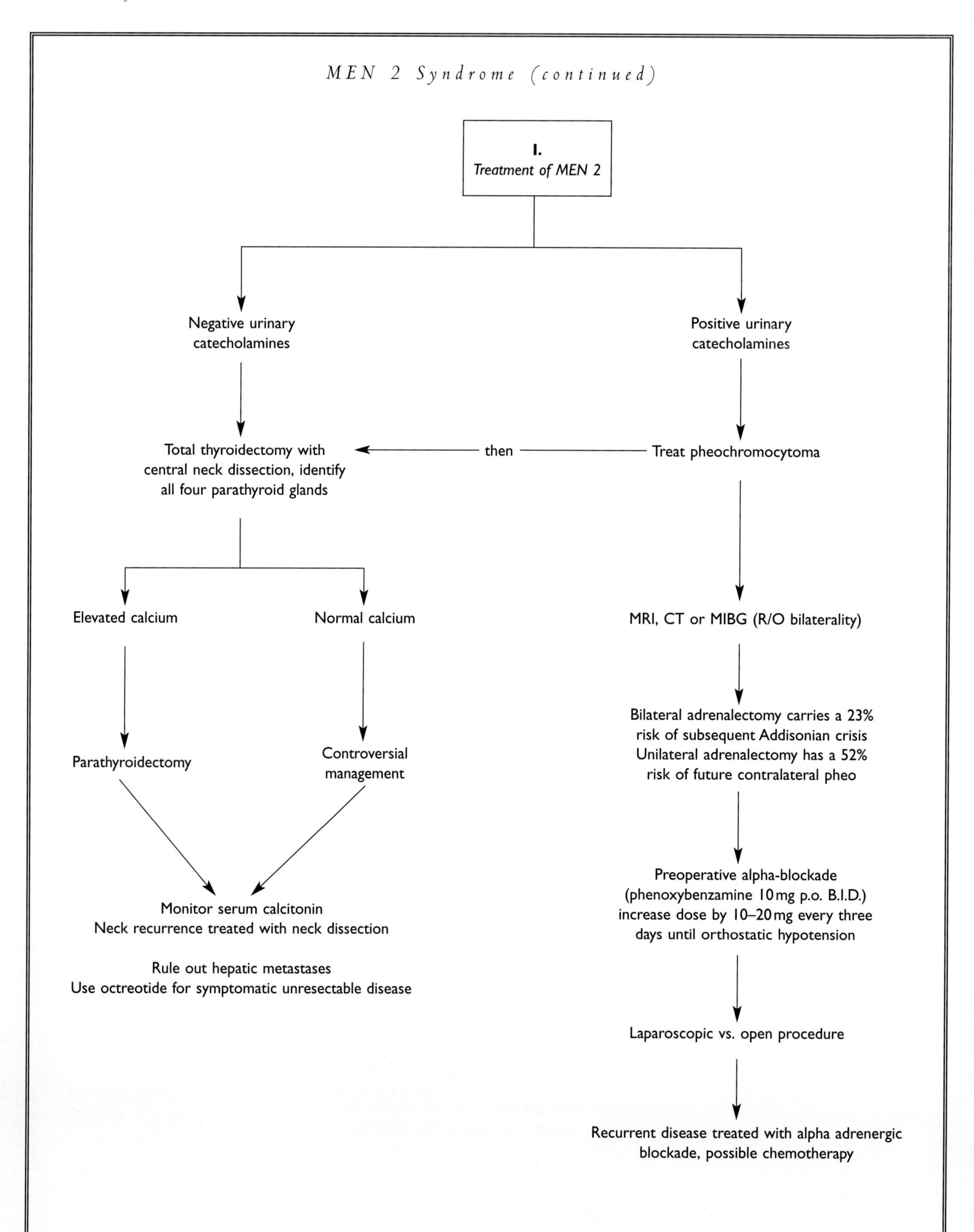
MEN 2 Syndrome (continued)
I.
Treatment of MEN 2
Negative urinary catecholamines
Positive urinary catecholamines
Total thyroidectomy with central neck dissection, identify all four parathyroid glands
then
Treat pheochromocytoma
Elevated calcium
Normal calcium
MRI, CT or MIBG (R/O bilaterality)
Parathyroidectomy
Controversial management
Bilateral adrenalectomy carries a 23% risk of subsequent Addisonian crisis
Unilateral adrenalectomy has a 52% risk of future contralateral pheo
Monitor serum calcitonin
Neck recurrence treated with neck dissection
Rule out hepatic metastases
Use octreotide for symptomatic unresectable disease
Preoperative alpha-blockade (phenoxybenzamine 10 mg p.o. B.I.D.) increase dose by 10–20 mg every three days until orthostatic hypotension
Laparoscopic vs. open procedure
Recurrent disease treated with alpha adrenergic blockade, possible chemotherapy

diagnosis of MTC possible in 1970 by developing the immunoassay for calcitonin.[39] MEN 2B was defined as a separate entity in 1968,[40,41] and the first report of FMTC as a distinct syndrome appeared in 1986.[42]

F. Clinical Evaluation

Most patients with the MEN 2 syndromes who are not screened biochemically for its various components present with a neck mass. Some patients may also complain of dysphagia, hoarseness, or cervical lymphadenopathy; patients with large tumors or metastatic disease may develop diarrhea as a side effect of high calcitonin levels. In a review of 86 MEN 2A patients with a minimum 10-year follow-up, the mean age at which MTC was diagnosed was 29 years, hyperparathyroidism at 36 years, and pheochromocytoma at 37 years of age; only 10% of patients with pheochromocytoma or hyperparathyroidism were diagnosed with this component of MEN 2A prior to the MTC diagnosis.[43] The most common symptoms seen in 49 MEN 2A and 9 MEN 2B patients with pheochromocytoma were headaches (69%), palpitations (62%), hypertension (57%), sweating (50%), nausea (26%), flushing (21%), tremulousness/anxiety (21%), and syncope (17%); 7% were asymptomatic.[44] Most MEN 2A patients with hyperparathyrodism are asymptomatic and are usually identified by screening laboratory tests (hypercalcemia). Patients with MEN 2B are recognizable early in life by their unusual physical appearance, which includes multiple mucosal neuromas (especially on the lips and tongue), thickened eyelids, soft tissue prognathism, a broad base to the nose, a marfanoid body habitus (characterized by an elongated, gracile build), skeletal abnormalities (kyphosis, pectus excavatum, pes cavus, scoliosis, lordosis, valgus deformities), and visible corneal nerves.[45] These patients also have ganglioneuromatosis of the gastrointestinal tract, which leads to poor peristalsis; patients often develop constipation during early childhood.

Because the MEN 2 syndromes are autosomal dominant disorders, there is usually a strong family history of thyroid cancer, although 5–10% of cases appear de novo without a family history.[46] The latter presentation is relatively common in MEN 2B. Virtually all patients with MEN 2A develop MTC; 93% are diagnosed biochemically by age 31, and 59% present with symptoms by age 70.[47] The prevalence of pheochromocytoma and hyperparathyroidism is highly variable among kindreds. In one large study of 12 kindreds the prevalence of pheochromocytoma was 42% but varied between 6% and 100% among kindreds; the prevalence of hyperparathyroidism was 35% and ranged from 0 to 53% among these kindreds.[43]

G. Biochemical Testing

Medullary carcinomas develop in the parafollicular cells, or C-cells, which are derived from the neural crest and are found predominantly in the superior poles of the thyroid gland. The neuroendocrine C-cells secrete calcitonin (CTN), a 32-amino-acid peptide whose exact function remains unclear in humans. One of the effects of CTN is to inhibit osteoclast function, which causes diminished bone resorption.[48] In many animals CTN causes hypocalcemia and hypophosphatemia owing to diminished bone resorption; but in humans the effect of CTN on calcium homeostasis is less critical, as patients are not hypercalcemic after total thyroidectomy and patients with sporadic MTC (producing high levels of CTN) are not hypocalcemic. Patients with small tumors may have normal basal levels of CTN, whereas most patients with MTC and its precursor C-cell hyperplasia (CCH) have elevated stimulated CTN levels. Stimulation testing involves collecting blood samples immediately before and at several-minute intervals (typically 1, 3, and 5 minutes) after administration of CTN secretagogues. Sequential administration of calcium gluconate (2 mg/kg/min) followed by pentagastrin (0.5 μg/kg/5 sec) produces high CTN levels in patients with MTC[49]; testing may also be performed using either agent alone. Normal CTN values vary depending on the radioimmunoassay used; levels may be as high as 100 pg/ml in females and 350 pg/ml in males after calcium/pentagastrin stimulation testing. Unfortunately, pentagastrin has recently been removed from the market by the manufacturer, and no good replacement secretagogue is currently available. The biochemical diagnosis of hyperparathyroidism is the same as that discussed for MEN 1.

It is important to test patients for the presence of a pheochromocytoma prior to operation for other components of MEN 2A or MEN 2B. Patients with pheochromocytomas are at high risk for intraoperative complications, such as labile hypertension and significant hypotension once the tumor is removed. Pheochromocytoma is diagnosed by measuring a 24-hour urine sample (in a container with 20 ml of 6N HCl), for catecholamines, metanephrines, and vanillylmandelic acid (VMA). Fractionation of the urine catecholamines for the individual measurement of epinephrine, norepinephrine, dopamine, normetanephrine, metanephrine, and VMA is useful; an elevated epinephrine level is the most consistent abnormality in MEN 2 patients.[50] Screening using norepinephrine and epinephrine (100% sensitivity, 97% specificity) or normetanephrine and metanephrine (100% sensitivity, 98% specificity) was highly reliable for the diagnosis of pheochromocytoma in 20 patients with proven pheochromocytoma and more than 1000 controls.[51] A variety of medications can interfere with the assay; therefore this collection is best done off-medication. The antihypertensive drugs that cause the least interference with urinary catecholamine measurement are calcium channel blockers, vasodilators (e.g., hydralazine), angiotensin-converting enzyme inhibitors, and diuretics.

H. Genetic Testing

In 1987 genetic linkage studies demonstrated that the locus for MEN 2A mapped to the pericentromeric region of chromosome

10.[52,53] The genes for MEN 2B and FMTC were found to map to the same region in 1991,[54] and in 1993 the predisposing gene for both MEN 2A and FMTC was found to be the *RET* proto-oncogene.[55,56] Mutations in *RET* were subsequently found in individuals with MEN 2B[57] and Hirschsprung's disease.[58,59] Soon after these discoveries Wells et al. performed prophylactic thyroidectomy on children from MEN 2A families with *RET* mutations and demonstrated foci of MTC and C-cell hyperplasia in patients with negative provocative CTN tests.[60]

The *RET* proto-oncogene consists of twenty exons and encodes for a cell surface receptor with tyrosine kinase activity. Transgenic knockout mice lacking a functional *RET* gene display renal agenesis and lack of enteric neurons in the gastrointestinal tract; they die shortly after birth.[61] Most of the germline mutations in MEN 2A and FMTC have been found in cysteine residues from exons 10 and 11 of the gene in the extracellular domain of this receptor. *RET* mutations have been found in approximately 98% of MEN 2A families, 85% (169/199 families) of which are at codon 634 of exon 11 and the remainder in codons 609, 611, 618, and 620 of exon 10.[62] The presence of codon 634 mutations appear to be significantly correlated with the presence of pheochromocytoma or hyperparathyroidism in MEN 2A families.[63] Approximately 88% of FMTC families have been found to have *RET* mutations, with approximately one-third at codon 618, one-third at codon 634, and the others in codons 609, 611, 620, and 768.[62,64] It is believed that changes seen in *RET* from MEN 2A and FMTC patients at highly conserved cysteine results in the formation of stable RET homodimers, which causes constitutive activation of the RET kinase.[65]

Among 79 MEN 2B families, 75 (95%) were found with *RET* mutations, all of which occurred at codon 918 of exon 16[62]; this changes a highly conserved methionine to threonine in the substrate recognition site of the tyrosine kinase domain of the intracellular portion of the RET protein. Mutation at codon 918, as seen in MEN 2B, is believed to result in phosphorylation of improper substrates.[65] Interestingly, 66% of patients with sporadic MTC have somatic codon 918 mutations.[66] In contrast, patients with Hirschsprung's disease have deletions, missense, nonsense, or frame-shift mutations throughout the gene.[58,59] These changes appear to result in loss of RET kinase activity.[67]

Prior to identification of the MEN 2 gene, family members at risk for MEN 2 were screened annually by provocative testing for CTN, 24-hour urine collection, and serum calcium levels. If these parameters are negative through the age of 35, the risk of being a gene carrier is reduced to approximately 5%.[68] The problem with biochemical screening is the inconvenience of the tests and the fact that administration of pentagastrin is usually followed by a several-minute period of nausea or substernal pressure; compliance with this type of screening has been problematic. Baseline biochemical screening should be performed in new patients suspected of having one of the MEN 2 syndromes; the same is true for family members at risk, as even if genetic testing is to be performed it is important to know whether there is biochemical evidence of MTC or pheochromocytoma at this point in time. Genetic testing should be performed in MEN 2 family members and is simplified once the specific mutation in a family has been identified. Family members who lack the *RET* mutation can be spared further biochemical testing and are not at risk for the disease. In some families, however, *RET* mutations are not present, even in affected individuals; in such families biochemical screening tests are needed. The lack of a mutation in a family may be due to a laboratory error, incomplete testing to identify new mutations, mutations at sites not identified by standard assays, or genetic heterogeneity. In those who carry an MEN 2A or MEN 2B mutation, prophylactic thyroidectomy is recommended and may be performed as early as age 5.[60] Management of the parathyroid glands at the time of prophylactic thyroidectomy is more controversial, with some advocating routine total parathyroidectomy and autotransplantation[69] and others leaving the glands in situ in patients with normal preoperative calcium levels.[70] Gene carriers should be followed by CTN tests to monitor for recurrence and by 24-hour urine testing for diagnosis of pheochromocytoma.

I. Treatment

The surgical treatment of MTC in MEN 2 patients is total thyroidectomy with a central neck dissection. Both recurrent laryngeal nerves are carefully identified and protected. All four parathyroid glands are identified; if they appear normal in size and the preoperative calcium level is normal, they should be carefully marked with nonabsorbable sutures and not disturbed. In contrast, others believe that total parathyroidectomy and autotransplantation should be performed in MEN 2 patients for two reasons: a 35% incidence of future hyperparathyroidism and possible injury to the parathyroids if they are left in place during central neck dissection.[69] The management of normal parathyroid glands in normocalcemic MEN 2 patients with MCT, however, is controversial; most surgeons favor leaving the glands alone in this situation. The incidence of permanent hypoparathyroidism after total thyroidectomy is approximately 5% when the glands are left in situ versus 1% when parathyroid tissue is autotransplanted.[71] When autotransplantation is performed in patients without hyperparathyroidism, it is preferable to transplant one and a half to two glands (rather than a 25–50 mg portion of one gland as performed for hyperplasia) in the nondominant forearm in the fashion described under the surgical treatment of MEN 1. The borders of the central neck dissection are the carotid sheath laterally, the tracheoesophageal groove medially, the innominate artery inferiorly, and the hyoid bone superiorly. If grossly involved nodes are present lateral to the central compartment, a modified radical neck dissection should be performed on that side.

Screening for pheochromocytoma is performed by 24-hour urinary measurement for catecholamines, as discussed above. If this test is positive, the patient should undergo MRI or CT to confirm the presence of an enlarged adrenal and to determine the status of the contralateral gland. With MRI, pheochromocytomas characteristically have high signal intensity in T2-weighted images, which allows them to be distinguished from other adrenal neoplasms.[72] Metaiodobenzylguanidine (MIBG) scintigraphy is a useful technique for localizing paragangliomas, pheochromocytomas, and their metastases. MIBG is especially useful for identifying lateral or ectopic pheochromocytomas.[73] The disadvantages are that MIBG is expensive, requires that patients take iodine to avoid thyroid ablation, takes several days to perform, and still requires correlation with other anatomic studies such as MRI or CT.

Bilateral Pheochromocytoma

Patients with MEN 2A or MEN 2B are at risk for bilateral pheochromocytoma. The surgical approach to patients with these adrenal neoplasms has been controversial. Some advocate bilateral adrenalectomy because of the high incidence of bilateral involvement,[74] but permanent corticosteroid and mineralocorticoid replacement is required, and patients are at risk for addisonian crisis. A more selective strategy is to perform (1) bilateral adrenalectomy when bilateral adrenal enlargement is seen on preoperative imaging tests or (2) unilateral adrenalectomy with contralateral exploration in patients with unilateral enlargement. Among 23 MEN 2A and MEN 2B patients managed in this fashion, 52% developed pheochromocytoma of the contralateral adrenal at a mean follow-up of 11.9 years (range 0.4–21.2 years) after treatment of the first pheochromocytoma. Among patients who had undergone bilateral adrenalectomy, 23% (10 of 43) had experienced at least one episode of adrenal insufficiency.[44] Although Carney and associates found that 3 of 19 MEN 2 patients had malignant pheochromocytomas and suggested it as another reason to perform bilateral adrenalectomy,[74] none of 58 patients described by Lairmore and colleagues had a malignant pheochromocytoma.[44]

Exploration has traditionally been via a transabdominal route, which allows access to both adrenal glands and examination of extraadrenal regions, such as the organ of Zuckerhkandl. Laparoscopic adrenalectomy has raised questions regarding the need for routine laparotomy in all patients. Gagner et al. suggested that unilateral or bilateral laparoscopic adrenalectomy can be performed for pheochromocytoma safely but incurs longer operative times than open procedures and with a higher complication rate than for other adrenal lesions removed laparoscopically.[75] All patients must undergo preoperative α-blockade to restore their plasma volume; we generally begin with phenoxybenzamine 10 mg PO bid, which is increased by 10 mg every 3 days until orthostatic hypotension is achieved. This process takes approximately 2 weeks, at the end of which the patients become extremely fatigued. Intraoperatively, patients are monitored with an arterial line and central venous line. An experienced anesthesiologist is required for these cases, as there may be significant swings of hypertension and hypotension that require rapid treatment with sodium nitroprusside or neosynephrine and volume, respectively.

Patients with a history of MTC are followed with CTN levels to monitor for tumor recurrence; when the levels are elevated, venous sampling from both sides of the neck and from the hepatic veins is indicated. Unilateral recurrence in the neck can be treated by neck dissection with meticulous clearing of nonessential tissue in the neck; bilateral recurrence is treated by staged neck dissections. This approach can result in cure rates of up to 38% in patients without evidence of distant metastases.[76] Hepatic metastases should be ruled out by laparoscopy prior to neck exploration. Patients with metastatic MTC and CTN levels exceeding several thousand picograms per milliliter may become symptomatic with diarrhea (presumably as a result of high hormone levels) treatment with octreotide may provide good palliation. Currently, there is no role for adjuvant therapy in patients with advanced or metastatic MTC. A variety of chemotherapeutic regimens have been attempted without significant benefit, and these tumors are relatively radioresistant.[77] The role of adjuvant or therapeutic chemotherapy in malignant pheochromocytoma is also limited; and when possible, recurrent or metastatic pheochromocytoma should be removed surgically. When this is not possible, symptoms may be controlled with α-adrenergic blockade. Although initially ^{131}I-MIBG appeared to hold promise for the treatment of malignant pheochromocytoma, the results thus far have been disappointing, with no complete responses, partial response rates of approximately 30%, and biochemical response rates of approximately 45%.[78,79] The chemotherapeutic regimen of cyclophosphamide (750 mg/m^2 on day 1, q21days), vincristine (1.4 mg/m^2 on day 1, q21days), and dacarbazine (600 mg/m^2 on days 1 and 2, q21days), used primarily in patients with metastatic neuroblastoma, has been used with some success in those with malignant pheochromocytoma. This regimen resulted in a complete/partial response rate of 57% (median duration 21 months) and a complete/partial biochemical response rate of 79%.[80] Symptomatic bone metastases may be palliated by radiation therapy.

References

1. Erdheim J. Zur normalen und pathologischen histologie der glandula thyroidea, parathyroidea und hypophysis. Beitr Pathol Anat 1903;33:158.
2. Cushing H, Davidoff LM. The pathologic findings in four autopsied cases of acromegaly with a discussion of their significance Monograph 22. New York: Rockefeller Institute for Medical Research, 1927.

3. Underahl LO, Wollner LB, Black BM. Report of eight cases in which the pituitary, parathyroid, and pancreatic islets were involved. J Clin Endocrinol Metab 1953;13:20–47.
4. Wermer P. Genetic aspects of adenomatosis of endocrine glands. Am J Med 1954;16:363–371.
5. Wermer P. Endocrine adenomatosis and peptic ulcer complex in a large kindred: inherited multiple tumors and mosaic pleiotropism in man. Am J Med 1963;35:205–212.
6. Zollinger RM, Ellison EH. Primary peptic ulceration of the jejunum associated with islet cell tumors of the pancreas. Am J Surg 1955;142:709–728.
7. Zollinger RM, Ellison EC, O'Dorisio TM, et al. Thirty years' experience with gastrinoma. World J Surg 1984;8:427–435.
8. Wolfe MM, Jensen RT. Zollinger-Ellison syndrome: current concepts in diagnosis and management. N Engl J Med 1987;317:1200–1209.
9. O'Brien T, O'Riordan DS, Gharib H, et al. Results of treatment of pituitary disease in multiple endocrine neoplasia, type I. Neurosurgery 1996; 39:273–278.
10. Trump D, Farren B, Wooding C, et al. Clinical studies of multiple endocrine neoplasia type 1 (MEN1) Q J Med 1996;89:653–669. Erratum. Q J Med 1996;89:957–958.
11. Mutch MG, Frisella MM, DeBenedetti MK, et al. Pancreatic polypeptide is a useful plasma marker for radiographically evident pancreatic islet cell tumors in patients with multiple endocrine neoplasia type 1. Surgery 1997;122:1012–1019.
12. Larsson C, Skogseid B, Oberg K, et al. Multiple endocrine neoplasia type 1 gene maps to chromosome 11 and is lost in insulinoma. Nature 1988; 332:85–87.
13. Bale AE, Norton JA, Wong EL, et al. Allelic loss on chromosome 11 in hereditary and sporadic tumors related to familial multiple endocrine neoplasia type 1. Cancer Res 1991;51:1154–1157.
14. Sawicki MP, Wan YJ, Johnson CL, et al. Loss of heterozygosity on chromosome 11 in sporadic gastrinomas. Hum Genet 1992;89:445–449.
15. Chandrasekharappa SC, Guru SC, Manickam P, et al. Positional cloning of the gene for multiple endocrine neoplasia-type 1. Science 1997;276: 404–407.
16. Guru SC, Goldsmith PK, Burns AL, et al. Menin, the product of the MEN1 gene, is a nuclear protein. Proc Natl Acad Sci USA 1998;95:1630–1634.
17. Lemmens I, Van de Ven WJ, Kas K, et al. Identification of the multiple endocrine neoplasia type 1 (MEN1) gene: the European Consortium on MEN1. Hum Mol Genet 1997;6:1177–1183.
18. Agarwal SK, Kester MB, Debelenko LV, et al. Germline mutations of the MEN1 gene in familial multiple endocrine neoplasia type 1 and related states. Hum Mol Genet 1997;6:1169–1175.
19. Bassett JH, Forbes SA, Pannett AA, et al. Characterization of mutations in patients with multiple endocrine neoplasia type 1. Am J Hum Genet 1998;62:232–244.
20. Heppner C, Kester MB, Agarwal SK, et al. Somatic mutation of the MEN1 gene in parathyroid tumours. Nat Genet 1997;16:375–378.
21. Zhuang Z, Vortmeyer AO, Pack S, et al. Somatic mutations of the MEN1 tumor suppressor gene in sporadic gastrinomas and insulinomas. Cancer Res 1997;57:4682–4686.
22. Zhuang Z, Ezzat SZ, Vortmeyer AO, et al. Mutations of the MEN1 tumor suppressor gene in pituitary tumors. Cancer Res 1997;57:5446–5451.
23. Sugg SL, Norton JA, Fraker DL, et al. A prospective study of intraoperative methods to diagnose and resect duodenal gastrinomas. Ann Surg 1993; 218:138–144.
24. Bottger TC, Junginger T. Is preoperative radiographic localization of islet cell tumors in patients with insulinoma necessary? World J Surg 1993; 17:427–432.
25. Zeiger MA, Shawker TH, Norton JA. Use of intraoperative ultrasonography to localize islet cell tumors. World J Surg 1993;17:448–454.
26. Thompson NW. The surgical management of hyperparathyroidism and endocrine disease of the pancreas in the multiple endocrine neoplasia type 1 patient. J Intern Med 1995;238:269–280.
27. Wells SA Jr, Farndon JR, Dale JK, et al. Long term evaluation of patients with primary parathyroid hyperplasia managed by total parathyroidectomy and heterotopic autotransplantation. Ann Surg 1980;192: 451–458.
28. Rizzoli R, Green JD, Marx SJ. Primary hyperparathyroidism in familial multiple endocrine neoplasia type I: long-term follow-up of serum calcium levels after parathyroidectomy. Am J Med 1985;78:467–474.
29. van Heerden JA, Smith SL, Miller LJ. Management of the Zollinger-Ellison syndrome in patients with multiple endocrine neoplasia type I. Surgery 1986;100:971–977.
30. Stabile BE, Morrow DJ, Passaro E Jr. The gastrinoma triangle: operative implications. Am J Surg 1984;147:25–31.
31. MacFarlane MP, Fraker DL, Alexander HR, et al. Prospective study of surgical resection of duodenal and pancreatic gastrinomas in multiple endocrine neoplasia type 1. Surgery 1995;118:973–979.
32. Ellison EC. Forty-year appraisal of gastrinoma: back to the future. Ann Surg 1995;222;511–521.
33. Moertel CG, Lefkopoulo M, Lipsitz S, et al. Streptozocin-doxorubicin, streptozocin-fluorouracil or chlorozotocin in the treatment of advanced islet-cell carcinoma. N Engl J Med 1992;326:519–523.
34. Baskin DS. Neurosurgical management of pituitary-hypothalamic neoplasms. In: Becker KL (ed) Principles and Practice of Endocrinology and Metabolism. Philadelphia: Lippincott, 1995;238–247.
35. Sipple JH. The association of pheochromocytoma with carcinoma of the thyroid gland. Am J Med 1961;31:163–166.
36. Williams ED. A review of 17 cases of carcinoma of the thyroid and pheochromocytoma. J Clin Pathol 1965;18:288–292.
37. Williams ED. Histogenesis of medullary carcinoma of the thyroid. J Clin Pathol 1966;19:114–118.
38. Steiner AL, Goodman AD, Powers SR. Study of a kindred with pheochromocytoma, medullary thyroid carcinoma, hyperparathyroidism and Cushing's disease: multiple endocrine neoplasia type 2. Medicine 1968;47: 371–409.
39. Tashjian AH Jr, Howland BG, Melvin KEW, et al. Immunoassay of human calcitonin: clinical measurement, relation to serum calcium and studies in patients with medullary carinoma. N Engl J Med 1970;283:890–895.
40. Gorlin RJ, Sedano HO, Vickers RA, et al. Multiple mucosal neuromas, pheochromocytoma and medullary carcinoma of the thyroid—a syndrome. Cancer 1968;22:293–299.
41. Schimke RN, Hartmann WH, Prout TE, et al. Syndrome of bilateral pheochromocytoma, medullary thyroid carcinoma and multiple neuromas. N Engl J Med 1968;279:1–7.
42. Farndon JR, Leight GS, Dilley WG, et al. Familial medullary thyroid carcinoma without associated endocrinopathies: a distinct clinical entity. Br J Surg 1986;73:278–281.
43. Howe JR, Norton JA, Wells SA. Prevalence of pheochromocytoma and hyperparathyroidism in multiple endocrine neoplasia type 2A: results of long-term follow-up. Surgery 1993;114:1070–1077.
44. Lairmore TC, Ball DB, Baylin SB, et al. Management of pheochromocytomas in patients with the multiple endocrine neoplasia type 2 syndromes. Ann Surg 1993;217:596–601.
45. Norton JA, Froome LC, Farrell RE, et al. Multiple endocrine neoplasia type IIb. Surg Clin North Am 1979;59:109–118.
46. Schuffenecker I, Ginet N, Goldgar D, et al. Prevalence and parental origin of de novo RET mutations in multiple endocrine neoplasia type 2A and familial medullary thyroid carcinoma: le Groupe d'Etude des Tumeurs a Calcitonine. Am J Hum Genet 1997;60:233–237.

47. Easton DF, Ponder MA, Cummings T, et al. The clinical and screening age-at-onset distribution for the MEN-2 syndrome. Am J Hum Genet 1989;44:208–215.
48. Chambers TJ, Chambers JC, Symonds J, et al. The effect of calcitonin on the cytoplasmic spreading of rat osteoclasts. J Clin Endocrinol Metab 1986; 63:1080–1085.
49. Wells SA Jr, Baylin SB, Linehan WM, et al. Provocative agents and the diagnosis of medullary carcinoma of the thyroid gland. Ann Surg 1978; 188:139–141.
50. Hamilton BP, Landsberg L, Levine RJ. Measurement of urinary epinephrine in screening for pheochromocytoma in multiple endocrine type II. Am J Med 1978;65:1027–1032.
51. Graham PE, Smythe GA, Edwards GA, et al. Laboratory diagnosis of pheochromocytoma: which analytes should we measure? Ann Clin Biochem 1993;30:129–134.
52. Simpson NE, Kidd KK, Goodfellow PJ, et al. Assignment of multiple endocrine neoplasia type 2A to chromosome 10 by genetic linkage. Nature 1987;328:528–530.
53. Mathew CGP, Chin KS, Easton DF, et al. A linked genetic marker for multiple endocrine neoplasia type 2A on chromosome 10. Nature 1987;328:527–528.
54. Lairmore TC, Howe JR, Korte JA, et al. Familial medullary thyroid carcinoma and multiple endocrine neoplasia type 2B map to the same region of chromosome 10 as multiple endocrine neoplasia type 2A. Genomics 1991;9:181–192.
55. Donis-Keller H, Dou S, Chi D, et al. Mutations in the RET proto-oncogene are associated with MEN2A and FMTC. Hum Mol Genet 1993;2:851–856.
56. Mulligan LM, Kwok JBJ, Healey CS, et al. Germline mutations of the RET proto-oncogene in multiple endocrine neoplasia type 2A. Nature 1993; 363:458–460.
57. Carlson KM, Dou S, Chi D, et al. Single missense mutation in the tyrosine kinase catalytic domain of the RET proto-oncogene is associated with multiple endocrine neoplasia type 2B. Proc Natl Acad Sci USA 1994;91:1579–1583.
58. Romeo G, Ronchetto P, Luo Y, et al. Point mutations affecting the tyrosine kinase domain of the RET proto-oncogene in Hirschsprung's disease. Nature 1994;367:377–378.
59. Edery P, Lyonnet S, Mulligan LM, et al. Mutations of the RET proto-oncogene in Hirschsprung's disease. Nature 1994;367:378–380.
60. Wells SA Jr, Chi DD, Toshima K, et al. Predictive DNA testing and prophylactic thyroidectomy in patients at risk for multiple endocrine neoplasia type 2A. Ann Surg 1994;220:237–247.
61. Schuchardt A, D'Agati V, Larsson-Bloomberg L, et al. Defects in the kidney and enteric nervous system of mice lacking the tyrosine kinase receptor RET. Nature 1994;367:380–383.
62. Eng C, Clayton D, Schuffenecker I, et al. The relationship between specific RET proto-oncogene mutations and disease phenotype in multiple endocrine neoplasia type 2: international RET mutation consortium analysis. JAMA 1996;276:1575–1579.
63. Marsh DJ, Mulligan LM, Eng C. RET proto-oncogene mutations in multiple endocrine neoplasia type 2 and medullary thyroid carcinoma. Horm Res 1997;47:168–178.
64. Boccia LM, Green JS, Joyce C, et al. Mutation of RET codon 768 is associated with the FMTC phenotype. Clin Genet 1997;51:81–85.
65. Santoro M, Carlomagno F, Romano A, et al. Activation of RET as a dominant transforming gene by germline mutations of MEN2A and MEN2B. Science 1995;267:381–383.
66. Marsh DJ, Learoyd DL, Andrew SD, et al. Somatic mutations in the RET proto-oncogene in sporadic medullary thyroid carcinoma. Clin Endocrinol (Oxf) 1996;44:249–257.
67. Pasini B, Borrello MG, Greco A, et al. Loss of function effect of RET mutations causing Hirschsprung disease. Nat Genet 1995;10:35–40.
68. Ponder BA, Ponder MA, Coffey R, et al. Risk estimation and screening in families of patients with medullary thyroid carcinoma. Lancet 1988;1:397–401.
69. Skinner MA, Norton JA, Moley JF, et al. Heterotopic autotransplantation of parathyroid tissue in children undergoing total thyroidectomy. J Pediatr Surg 1997;32:510–513.
70. Decker RA, Geiger JD, Cox CE, et al. Prophylactic surgery for multiple endocrine neoplasia type IIa after genetic diagnosis: is parathyroid transplantation indicated? World J Surg 1996;20:814–820.
71. Olson JA Jr, DeBenedetti MK, Baumann DS, et al. Parathyroid autotransplantation during thyroidectomy: results of long-term follow-up. Ann Surg 1996;223:472–478.
72. Doppman JL, Reinig JW, Dwyer AJ, et al. Differentiation of adrenal masses by magnetic resonance imaging. Surgery 1987;102:1018–1026.
73. Shapiro B, Copp JE, Sisson JC, et al. Iodine-131 metaiodobenzylguanidine for the locating of suspected pheochromocytoma: experience in 400 cases. J Nucl Med 1985;26:576–585.
74. Carney JA, Sizemore GW, Sheps SG. Adrenal medullary disease in multiple endocrine neoplasia, type 2: pheochromocytoma and its precursors. Am J Clin Pathol 1976;66:279–290.
75. Gagner M, Breton G, Pharand D, et al. Is laparoscopic adrenalectomy indicated for pheochromocytomas? Surgery 1996;120:1076–1079.
76. Moley JF, Dilley WG, DeBenedetti MK. Improved results of cervical reoperation for medullary thyroid carcinoma. Ann Surg 1997;225:734–740.
77. Norton JA, Levin B, Jensen RT. Cancer of the endocrine system. In: DeVita VT, Hellman S, Rosenberg SA (eds) Cancer: Principles and Practice of Oncology. Philadelphia: Lippincott, 1993;1333–1435.
78. Shapiro B, Sisson JC, Wieland DM, et al. Radiopharmaceutical therapy of malignant pheochromocytoma with [^{131}I]metaiodobenzylguanidine: results from ten years of experience. J Nucl Biol Med 1991;35:269–276.
79. Krempf M, Lumbroso J, Mornex R, et al. Use of m-[^{131}I]iodobenzylguanidine in the treatment of malignant pheochromocytoma. J Clin Endocrinol Metab 1991;72:455–461.
80. Averbuch SD, Steakley CS, Young RC, et al. Malignant pheochromocytoma: effective treatment with a combination of cyclophosphamide, vincristine, and dacarbazine. Ann Intern Med 1988;109:267–273.

Section 3

Cancer of the Lung

Chapter 18

Small Cell Cancer of the Lung

PHILIP BONOMI

A. Epidemiology and Etiology

Lung cancer is the leading cause of cancer deaths in both men and women in the United States. Although most of the patients have non-small cell lung cancer, the number of patients with small cell tumors is still relatively large, with approximately 30,000 cases having been diagnosed in 1999. Although the absolute number of patients who have small cell lung cancer has increased, the percentage relative to those with non-small cell tumors appears to have decreased. Prior to 1990 approximately 20% of patients had small cell histology, and more recent studies have shown that small cell lung cancer constitutes approximately 16–17% of all cases.[1,2] The reasons for the changes in the histologic patterns is not clear. Despite the decrease in the percentage of small cell tumors, this neoplasm continues to be a major problem. Only breast cancer, prostate cancer, colon cancer, and non-small lung cancer occur more frequently in the United States.

Lung cancer is strongly related to cigarette smoking; patients who have smoked a large number of cigarettes have a high risk of developing small cell lung cancer. It is encouraging to see that there has been a significant decline in the incidence of cigarette smoking among adult American men, although there has been no decrease among American women. It is distressing to see that the frequency of smoking among teenagers of all socioeconomic groups is increasing. The current smoking trends suggest that small cell lung cancer will continue to be a major health problem for many decades.

B. Presentation

Most of the patients present with relatively large central tumors and extensive bulky mediastinal lymphadenopathy. Patients frequently have a cough and dyspnea because of the central location of their tumors. In addition, the tumor tends to compress or invade mediastinal structures, which may cause superior vena cava syndrome, esophageal obstruction, or pericardial effusion. Small cell lung cancer has a strong tendency to disseminate early and widely. The most common metastatic sites are the brain, liver, bone, bone marrow, and adrenals. Patients frequently have metastases in multiple sites, and they

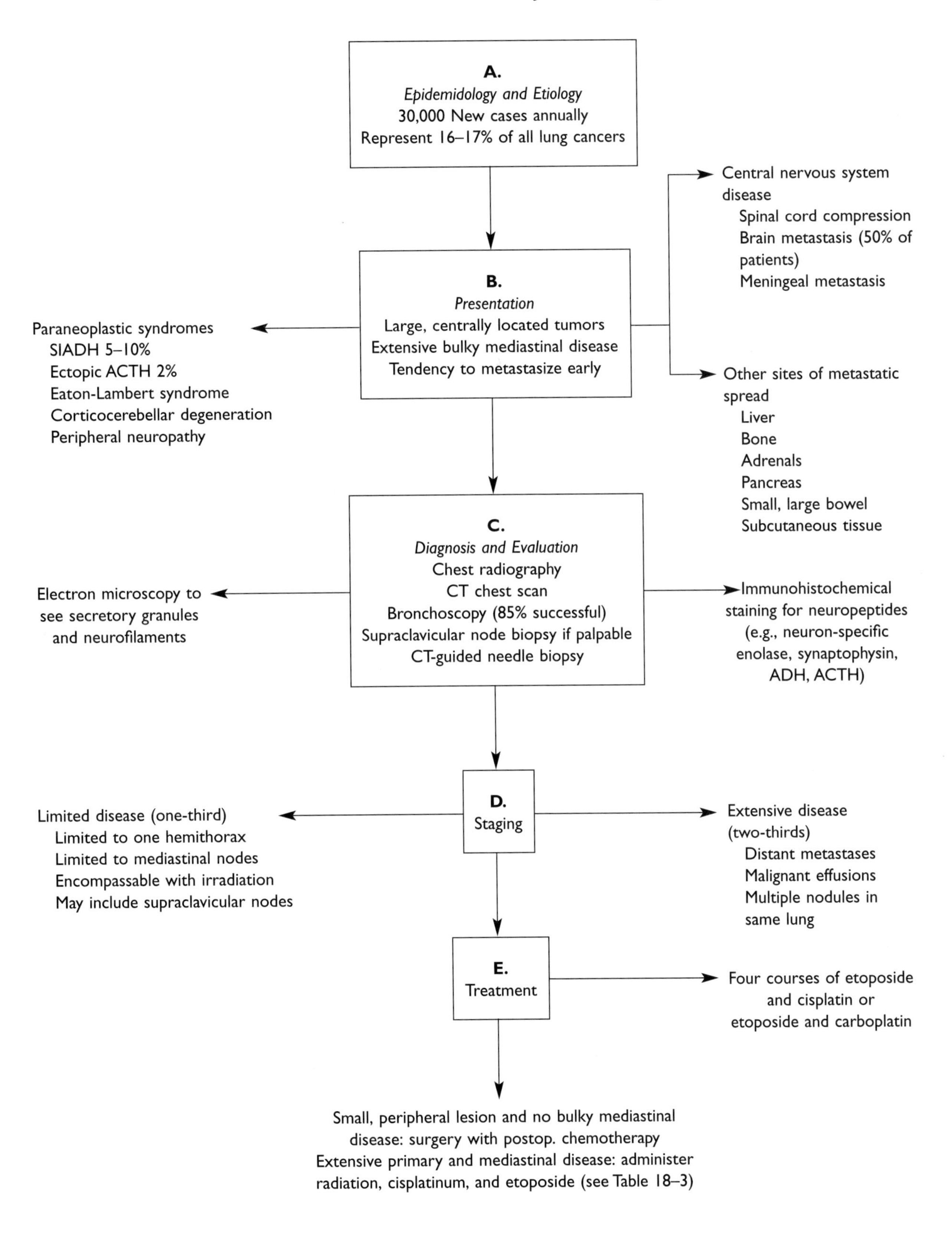
Small Cell Cancer of the Lung
A.
Epidemiology and Etiology
30,000 New cases annually
Represent 16–17% of all lung cancers
B.
Presentation
Large, centrally located tumors
Extensive bulky mediastinal disease
Tendency to metastasize early
Central nervous system disease
Spinal cord compression
Brain metastasis (50% of patients)
Meningeal metastasis
Other sites of metastatic spread
Liver
Bone
Adrenals
Pancreas
Small, large bowel
Subcutaneous tissue
Paraneoplastic syndromes
SIADH 5–10%
Ectopic ACTH 2%
Eaton-Lambert syndrome
Corticocerebellar degeneration
Peripheral neuropathy
C.
Diagnosis and Evaluation
Chest radiography
CT chest scan
Bronchoscopy (85% successful)
Supraclavicular node biopsy if palpable
CT-guided needle biopsy
Electron microscopy to see secretory granules and neurofilaments
Immunohistochemical staining for neuropeptides (e.g., neuron-specific enolase, synaptophysin, ADH, ACTH)
D.
Staging
Limited disease (one-third)
Limited to one hemithorax
Limited to mediastinal nodes
Encompassable with irradiation
May include supraclavicular nodes
Extensive disease (two-thirds)
Distant metastases
Malignant effusions
Multiple nodules in same lung
E.
Treatment
Four courses of etoposide and cisplatin or etoposide and carboplatin
Small, peripheral lesion and no bulky mediastinal disease: surgery with postop. chemotherapy
Extensive primary and mediastinal disease: administer radiation, cisplatinum, and etoposide (see Table 18–3)

TABLE 18–1.
Evaluation of patients with mass lesions seen on chest radiographs

Complete history
- Present illness
- Review of systems
  - Information regarding extent of local disease
  - Information regarding distant metastases
  - Information regarding functional status

Physical examination
- Careful evaluation of supraclavicular areas may provide site to obtain tissue for biopsy
- Chest examination: extent of local disease

Chest CT scan
- Extent of primary tumor and evaluation of regional lymph nodes.
- Evaluate for distant disease: lungs, pleura, liver, adrenals, upper abdominal nodes, pancreas

Bronchoscopy
- For central lesions

Mediastinoscopy
- Considered for patients in whom bronchoscopy has failed to indicate the diagnosis

CT guided needle biopsy
- Considered for patients in whom bronchoscopy and mediastinoscopy have failed to indicate the diagnosis

often lose significant weight and have severely impaired functional capacity. The suggested evaluation of patients with respiratory complaints or abnormal chest radiographs (or both) is outlined in Table 18–1. Staging for patients with established small cell lung cancer is described in Table 18–2.

Central Nervous System Metastases

Small cell lung cancer frequently metastasizes to the spine, which may cause spinal cord compression. Patients with spinal metastases frequently present with neck or back pain that is exacerbated by coughing and sneezing. Cervical spine involvement may cause pain radiating down the arms. Lumbosacral spine involvement frequently causes pain radiating down the lower extremities, and involvement of the thoracic spine may cause a band-like pain that encircles one or both sides of the hemithorax.

It is important to recognize spinal cord compression promptly, as early treatment with steroids and radiation therapy can reverse the neurologic deficits in a significant percentage of patients. This has profound implications for the patient's quality of life. Brain metastases develop in as many as 50% of patients,

TABLE 18–2.
Staging for distant metastases in patients with small cell lung cancer

CT chest
- Examine for pulmonary metastases and pleural effusion

CT brain scan with infusion/MRI brain scan
- Either study can be done to evaluate for brain metastases
- Infusion must be used with CT scan because noninfusion scans miss some lesions
- If meningeal metastases are suspected, MRI scan with infusion should be used

CT scan of the liver and adrenal glands
- Routinely performed with the CT chest scan in patients with possible lung tumors

Bone scan
- Evaluation for osseous metastases

Bone marrow biopsy and aspirate
- Done in patients with abnormal CBC, LDH, or both and no evidence of distant metastases
- Provides no significant useful information in patients who have evidence of distant metastases in other sites

who experience headaches, neurologic deficits, or both. Meningeal metastases are also relatively common and may cause cranial nerve palsies and widespread, disparate neurologic signs and symptoms. The diagnosis of meningeal carcinomatosis can be established by spinal fluid cytology, which shows malignant cells, and by spinal fluid chemistry, which frequently reveals elevated protein and decreased glucose levels.

Paraneoplastic Syndromes

Mental status changes are frequently caused by brain metastases, but it is important to remember that such changes may also accompany inappropriate antidiuretic hormone (ADH) secretion, which produces symptomatic hyponatremia in 5–10% of patients with small cell lung cancer. Significant hyponatremia may lead to coma, seizures, and death. Symptoms due to excessive production of adrenocorticotropic hormone (ACTH) occur in approximately 2% of small cell lung cancer patients. Other paraneoplastic syndromes are the Eaton-Lambert syndrome (a variant of myasthenia gravis), corticocerebellar degeneration, and peripheral neuropathy.

Miscellaneous Sites of Metastases

Other sites of metastasis include the pancreas (which is sometimes associated with pancreatitis), the small and large bowel (which may cause obstruction), and subcutaneous tissue. Extensive involvement of the mediastinal lymph nodes may cause retrograde lymphatic flow resulting in metastases to supraclavicular nodes and to upper abdominal lymph nodes.

C. Diagnosis and Evaluation

The diagnosis of small cell lung cancer can be established by bronchoscopic biopsy or brushings in approximately 85% of patients because of the central location of most of these tumors. If bronchoscopy does not provide a diagnosis, careful examination of the supraclavicular areas may identify lymph nodes that are accessible for biopsy. Computed tomography (CT)-directed needle biopsy of thoracic masses and mediastinoscopy are other ways to obtain tissue.

Previously, small cell lung cancer was classified as an oat cell or an intermediate subtype. More recently, pathologists have recommended that the terms "oat cell" and "intermediate" be discarded.[3] They recommended that the lymphocyte type (previously called oat cell) and the intermediate type, which was subdivided into fusiform and polygonal subtypes, be grouped together and called "*small cell lung cancer*." Ninety percent of the tumors fall into this classification. A smaller group of patients have tumors classified as small cell/large cell variant, which contains small cells and a subpopulation of cells that resemble large cell carcinoma. A third group of small cell tumors consists of small cells and a subpopulation of squamous or adenocarcinoma cells; these tumors are called mixed small cell and squamous carcinoma or mixed small cell and adenocarcinoma.

Small cell lung cancer has characteristic ultrastructural features, including the presence of neurosecretory granules and neurofilaments, giving rise to the name "neuroendocrine cancer." In addition, these tumors may secrete some or all of the following peptides: neuron-specific enolase, synaptophysin, ACTH, ADH, amine decarboxylase enzymes, and biologic amines. Electron microscopy and immunohistochemical staining for these peptides help establish the diagnosis of small cell carcinoma.

Within the family of neuroendocrine carcinomas, there is a wide variation in biologic behavior. With its tendency for rapid proliferation and widespread dissemination, small cell carcinoma is the most aggressive member of the neuroendocrine family. At the opposite end of the spectrum is bronchial carcinoid, which has been described as a tumor growing in slow motion. Bronchial carcinoid virtually never metastasizes to distant sites.

There is a small group of neuroendocrine lung tumors whose behavior is intermediate between small cell carcinoma and bronchial carcinoid. These tumors grow more slowly than small cell lung cancer, but unlike bronchial carcinoid they tend to spread to distant sites. This neoplasm has been called anaplastic carcinoid or well differentiated neuroendocrine pulmonary carcinoma.

D. Staging

Although the TNM classification for staging can be applied to small cell lung cancer, most investigators do not use this system and prefer to classify tumors according to whether they are associated with limited or extensive disease. Patients whose disease is confined to one hemithorax and mediastinal lymph nodes and is encompassable in an irradiation portal are classified as having *limited disease*. Patient who have metastases to supraclavicular lymph nodes without evidence of distant metastases are also included in the limited disease category. The *extensive disease* category includes all patients with distant metastases and those with malignant pleural effusions. Patients with multiple lung nodules within the same lung are classified as having extensive disease. Approximately two-thirds of small cell lung cancer patients present with extensive disease.

E. Treatment

Limited Disease

Surgery Tumor resection has a relatively limited role in the treatment of small cell lung cancer. Prior to the introduction of chemotherapy, surgery was used relatively frequently, although the median survival was measured in months and virtually no patients achieved long-term survival. The reason for these disappointing results was that most patients experienced early, rapid development of distant metastases.

During the 1960s a trial was conducted in Great Britain in which surgery was compared to thoracic irradiation. This study showed that patients who received radiation therapy survived slightly longer.[4] During the 1970s it became apparent that combination chemotherapy could produce a relatively high rate of tumor regression of small cell lung cancer; more importantly, survival was prolonged by treatment with chemotherapy. At this point, chemotherapy became the primary treatment for small cell lung cancer, and the use of surgery was greatly curtailed. It soon became apparent, however, that chemotherapy-resistant disease developed in virtually all patients with small cell lung cancer. Tumor regrowth at the primary site and in the regional lymph nodes was common. These observations led to renewed interest in surgery following treatment with chemotherapy. A large randomized study was conducted in which patients received five courses of chemotherapy. Patients whose tumors responded favorably to chemotherapy were randomly assigned to undergo thoracic irradiation or surgery. This study failed to show a survival advantage for the patients who underwent surgery for bulky primary tumors and extensive mediastinal lymph node metastases.[5]

At the present time, therefore, surgery is primarily limited to the small subset of patients (fewer than 5% of all patients) who present with a peripheral lesion and no evidence of mediastinal lymph node involvement. In most of these cases the peripheral location of the tumor precludes obtaining tissue for diagnosis, and thoracotomy is undertaken to obtain tissue for histologic assessment.

Some critics argue that fine-needle aspiration in these instances is preferable to surgery so an unnecessary thoracotomy could be avoided when small cell histology is present. The following considerations seem to refute this argument. First, in the absence of distant disease, suspicious peripheral nodules should be resected even if fine needle aspirate was unsuccessful in obtaining tissue. Second, there is considerable evidence supporting the fact that chemotherapy alone rarely results in long-term survival of patients with limited-stage disease and that local therapy combined with chemotherapy results in a better chance of long-term survival. Tumor resection in the absence of mediastinal lymph node involvement is reasonable local therapy for patients with peripheral nodules, and the procedure provides adequate tissue to firmly establish the diagnosis. Once the diagnosis of small cell carcinoma is established, it is essential that the patient receive postoperative chemotherapy.[6]

Radiation During the 1980s there was considerable controversy regarding the role of thoracic radiation therapy for limited-stage small cell lung cancer. This arose from the fact that there were conflicting results from randomized trials in which chemotherapy alone was compared to irradiation and chemotherapy. A meta-analysis of multiple trials showed that the addition of thoracic irradiation was associated with prolongation of the median survival and improvement in the 2- and 5-year survival rates.[7] A variety of chemotherapy regimens and radiation therapy schedules and doses were used, but no "standard" regimen was identified based on these trials. More recently a regimen consisting of cisplatin/etoposide and concurrent thoracic radiation therapy has established a new standard of care for limited-stage small cell lung cancer patients despite the fact that this regimen has not been tested in a phase III trial comparing it to other chemoradiotherapy regimens. Multiple phase II and phase III trials testing etoposide/cisplatin and concurrent radiation therapy have produced median survival rates of approximately 20 months. The 2-year survival is 40%; and the 5-year survival is approximately 20%.[8] This represents a significant improvement over previous results obtained with irradiation or surgery alone, which produced a median survival of approximately 3–4 months with virtually no survivors at 2 years.

Results with cisplatin/etoposide and concurrent radiation therapy are also superior to those observed with previous chemotherapy regimens. Critics might argue that some of these improvements are the result of more accurate identification and selection of patients with limited disease. In the earlier trials, staging was suboptimal because CT scan evaluation of the brain, chest, and abdomen was not done routinely. It is likely that improved staging has identified a number of patients with distant metastases whose stage would have been classified as limited disease in earlier trials. It is also possible that inclusion of patients with an inherently more favorable prognosis (a phenomenon called stage migration) may be at least partially responsible for the superior results observed in recent studies. In all likelihood, however, treatment with etoposide/cisplatin and simultaneous thoracic irradiation represents a significant advance for patients with limited-stage small cell lung cancer.

Chemotherapy regimens using medications other than etoposide/cisplatin may have improved effectiveness, but extensive disease trials have not identified a regimen clearly superior to etoposide/cisplatin. Etoposide and cisplatin can be given in full doses concurrently with thoracic irradiation; other regimens, such as cyclophosphamide/doxorubicin/vincristine (CAV), cause excessive toxicity when given concurrently with thoracic irradiation. Trials testing newer chemotherapy regimens given concurrently with irradiation for non-small cell lung cancer have shown that the newer drugs cannot be given in full doses because of excessive esophageal or pulmonary toxicity.

TABLE 18–3.
Treatment of limited-stage small cell lung cancer

Chemotherapy	
Cisplatin	$60\,mg/m^2$ IV on day 1
Etoposide	$100\,mg/m^2$ on days 1,2,3
Schedule:	every 21 days
Treatments for irradiation regimen	
Chemotherapy	
Cisplatin $60\,mg/m^2$ IV on day 1	
Etoposide $100\,mg/m^2$ IV on days 1, 2, 3	
Schedule: every 21 days	
Total of four courses	
Irradiation	
1.8 Gy daily, 25 fractions, 5 weeks	
1.5 Gy bid, 30 fractions, 3 weeks	

The question of the optimum sequence for etoposide/cisplatin and thoracic irradiation has been addressed in several randomized trials. In a study of sequential versus simultaneous etoposide/cisplatin and irradiation, Gotak et al. observed acceptable toxicity with both regimens and longer survival in patients who underwent simultaneous etoposide/cisplatin chemotherapy and thoracic irradiation.[9] Another trial compared treatment with concurrent etoposide/cisplatin and thoracic irradiation during the second course versus the sixth course of chemotherapy. Longer survival was noted in patients who underwent early concurrent chemotherapy and irradiation.[10] Two studies have addressed the question of radiation dose and schedule. In each trial all patients received the same dose and schedule of etoposide/cisplatin, but they were randomly assigned to undergo irradiation given as single daily fractions (conventional dose schedule) or courses of twice-daily fractions (accelerated dose schedule). Conflicting results were observed in these studies, with one of the trials showing no difference in survival[11] and the other reporting a 26% five-year survival rate for patients who received radiation on a twice-daily basis compared to 16% for patients who received single daily fractions of radiation.[8] Investigators are proposing a new trial in which patients are randomized to twice-daily irradiation or to a higher total dose of radiation given in a single daily fraction.

In view of the easier application of single daily fractions, if a higher dose given in a single daily fraction provides comparable results, it would have important, practical implications for limited disease. Etoposide/cisplatin plus thoracic irradiation regimens are described in Table 18–3.

PROPHYLACTIC CRANIAL IRRADIATION Brain metastases are identified in 10–15% of small cell lung cancer patients at the time of diagnosis, and they occur in as many as 50% of patients who survive for 2 years. Numerous randomized trials have shown that prophylactic irradiation reduces the incidence of brain metastases, but individual trials have failed to show an overall survival advantage for patients who have undergone prophylactic cranial irradiation. A meta-analysis that evaluated multiple randomized trials has shown that prophylactic cranial irradiation increases the 3-year survival rate by 5% for patients whose disease is in complete remission after treatment with chemotherapy alone or chemotherapy combined with thoracic irradiation.[12] Based on the results of the meta-analysis, it is reasonable to recommend prophylactic cranial irradiation for patients who are in complete remission following treatment.

EXTENSIVE DISEASE

During the mid-1970s it became apparent that small cell lung cancer was relatively sensitive to chemotherapy. A variety of combination chemotherapy regimens have produced remissions in 50–60% of small cell lung cancer patients with extensive disease. More importantly, the median survival for patients treated with chemotherapy is 8–10 months compared to a median survival of 8 weeks for patients who received supportive care only.[13]

Initial enthusiasm for chemotherapy and the large number of trials attesting to the interest in various drug combinations were tempered by the realization that there were virtually no long-term survivors among those with extensive disease and that drug resistance was common. Despite the fact that many regimens have been tested, none has emerged as clearly superior. The most commonly used regimens are etoposide/carboplatin and cyclophosphamide/doxorubicin/vincristine.[13] Multiple drug regimens, some consisting of as many as eight drugs, have been tested; but none has proven superior to the etoposide/cisplatin regimen.[14] One possible exception is a combination consisting of ifosfamide (an alkylating agent), etoposide, and cisplatin (the ICE regimen). In a relatively small trial, superior survival was observed with the ICE regimen compared to etoposide/cisplatin. The 2-year survival rate for patients treated with ICE was 12% compared to 5% for those given etoposide/cisplatin.[15] If additional trials testing this regimen show similar results, it would represent a modest improvement for patients with *extensive* small cell lung cancer.

During the mid-1980s as it became more apparent that the development of drug resistance following initial tumor regression was a major problem, investigators tested a variety of treatment strategies designed to overcome drug resistance. Increasing total dose and increasing dose intensity have been tested in multiple randomized trials. Unfortunately, these trials have shown no improvement in survival, and worse toxicity was observed with the more intensive treatments.[14]

TABLE 18–4.
New chemotherapy drugs for small cell lung cancer

Taxanes
Paclitaxel
Docetaxel
Antimetabolites
Gemcitabine
Topoisomerase Inhibitors
Topotecan
Irinotecan

One of the more promising strategies to overcome drug resistance involves the use of alternating chemotherapy regimens. This approach is based on a mathematic model that suggested alternating regimens might overcome drug resistance and on assumptions that regimens that were truly cross resistant were available and complete remission was highly possible. In fact, none of the tested regimens in these trials fulfilled these criteria, and significant improvements in survival were not observed with alternating chemotherapy regimens.[14]

Another variation of this approach involved giving different chemotherapy drugs on a weekly basis with the hope that the rapid, sequential administration of drugs with different mechanisms of action would overcome resistance. This approach also failed to produce significantly improved survival.[14]

Some investigators have proposed maintenance chemotherapy as a means to suppress the emergence of drug resistance. Unfortunately, these randomized trials have failed to show a benefit from prolonged treatment; and based on the results of the studies, most investigators recommend stopping chemotherapy for extensive disease after a total of four to six courses.[14]

Conclusions

Approximately 25 years after the discovery that small cell lung cancer is relatively sensitive to chemotherapy, we remain at a plateau for extensive disease, which carries a median survival of 8–10 months and 2-year survival rates of less than 5%. This situation has focused the attention of investigators on the development of newer and hopefully more effective drugs.

During the late 1980s and early 1990s five new drugs[16] active against small cell lung cancer were identified (Table 18–4). Whether these agents are more effective remains to be seen. One of these, topotecan, has been tested in a recently completed phase III trial, which showed no advantage for giving topotecan after etoposide/cisplatin. Another of the new agents, paclitaxel, is currently being tested in a nationwide phase III trial. In both of these studies the new agent has been added to the etoposide/cisplatin regimen.

In contrast to *extensive* disease, significant progress has been made in the treatment of *limited* disease, with the 5-year survival rate increasing from less than 1% to approximately 20% as a result of treatment with etoposide/cisplatin and concurrent thoracic irradiation. Investigators are currently discussing new treatment strategies for limited disease. At this point the leading issues are the addition of one of the newer drugs to the etoposide/cisplatin plus irradiation regimen. Alternatively, some investigators have suggested testing the following irradiation options: giving a higher total dose of radiation with single daily fractions or reducing the size of the radiation field.

Perhaps the use of biologic treatment is the most promising idea to be tested on small cell lung cancer. A variety of agents are being developed, and some are already being tested. Such therapeutic approaches include inhibition of growth factors, inhibition of signal transduction, inhibition of matrix metalloproteinase inhibitors, antiangiogenesis agents, and tumor vaccines.

References

1. Travis WD, Travis LB, Devesa SS. Lung cancer. Cancer 1999;75:101–102.
2. EL-Torky M, EL-Zeky F, Hall JC. Significant changes in the distributor of histologic types of lung cancer. Cancer 1990;65:2361–2367.
3. Hirsch FR, Matthews MJ, Aisner S, et al. Histopathologic classification of small cell lung cancer: changing concepts and terminology. Cancer 1988;62:973–978.
4. Working Party on the Evaluation of Different Methods of Therapy in Carcinoma of the Bronchus. Comparative trial of surgery and radiotherapy for the primary treatment of small-celled or oat-celled carcinoma of the bronchus. Lancet 1966;2:979–983.
5. Lad T, Piantadosi S, Thomas P, et al. A prospective randomized trial to determine the benefit of surgical resection of residual disease following response of small cell lung cancer to combination chemotherapy. Chest 1994;106(suppl 6):320–323.
6. Shepherd FA, Evans WK, Feld R, et al. Adjuvant chemotherapy following surgical resection for small cell lung carcinoma of the lung. J Clin Oncol 1988;6:832–837.
7. Pignon JP, Arriagada R, Ihde DC, et al. A meta-analysis of thoracic radiotherapy for small-cell lung cancer. N Engl J Med 1992;327:1618–1624.
8. Turrisi AT, Kim K, Blum R, et al. Twice daily compared with one daily thoracic radiotherapy in limited small-cell lung cancer treated concurrently with cisplatin and etoposide. N Engl J Med 1999;340:265–271.
9. Gotak NY, Takada M, et al. Final results of a phase III study of concurrent versus sequential thoracic radiotherapy in combination with cisplatin and etoposide for limited-stage small cell lung cancer: the Japan Clinical Oncology Group study. Proc Am Soc Clin Oncol 1999;18:468a.
10. Murray N, Coy D, Pater JL, et al. Importance of timing for thoracic irradiation in the combined modality treatment of limited-stage small-cell lung cancer. J Clin Oncol 1993;11:336–344.
11. Bonner JA, Sloan JA, Hillman SH, et al. A quality adjusted re-analysis of a phase III trial comparing once-daily thoracic radiation therapy versus twice-daily thoracic radiation therapy in patients with limited stage small cell lung cancer. Proc Am Soc Clin Oncol 1999;18:466a.

12. Auperin A, Arriagad A, Pignon JPP, et al. Prophylactic cranial irradiation for patients with small-cell lung cancer in complete remission: prophylactic cranial irradiation overview collaborative group. N Engl J Med 1999;341:476–484.
13. Ihde DC. Current perspectives in the treatment of small cell lung cancer: educational symposium of the VII World Congress on Lung Cancer. Lung Cancer 1997;12(suppl 3):S1–S3.
14. Bonomi P. Review of selected randomized trials in small cell lung cancer. Semin Oncol 1998;25(suppl 9):70–78.
15. Loehrer PJ, Ansari R, Conin R, et al. Cisplatin plus etoposide with or without ifosfamide in extensive small cell lung cancer: a Vassier Oncology Group study. J Clin Oncol 1995;13:2594–2599.
16. Murray N. New drugs for small cell lung cancer. Oncology 1997;11(suppl 9):38–42.

CHAPTER 19

Non-Small Cell Cancer of the Lung

WILLIAM H. WARREN
TIMOTHY W. JAMES

A. Epidemiology and Etiology

Carcinoma of the lung is the leading cause of cancer deaths in men and women in the United States. The leading risk factor for its development is tobacco consumption, which is estimated to be responsible for more than 90% of this malignancy in men and at least 80% in women. Lung cancer is aggressive with respect to both local invasion and dissemination. Once spread has occurred, as with all cancers the chance for cure declines precipitously.

To understand the staging of lung carcinoma, one must be familiar with the pulmonary and mediastinal lymph node mapping proposed by Naruke et al.[1] All current literature discusses the staging of lung cancer according to the TNM international staging system described by Mountain in 1997.[2] The definitions for T, N and M descriptors are provided in Table 19–1. The TNM staging system is as follows: stage I is T1–2 N0 M0; stage II is T1–2 N1 M0; stage IIIA is T1–3 N2 M0 *or* T3 N0–1 M0; stage IIIB is any T N3 M0 or T4 any N, M0; stage IV is any T any N M1 (Tables 19–2 and 19–3). The 5-year survival for patients with a completely resected non-small cell stage I lung carcinoma approaches 80%, especially when the tumor is ≤2 cm. However, when considering all patients presenting with lung cancer, only 25% are found to have tumors deemed surgically resectable (stage I, II, or IIIA). Of the remainder, 25% have IIIB disease and 50% stage IV. The 5-year survival statistics for the various stages of non-small cell carcinoma are provided in Figure 19–1. The 5-year survival for stage I is 60–80%, for stage IIA 30–40%, for stage IIB 25–40%, for stage IIIA 10–45%, for stage IIIB 5%, and for stage IV <5%.[3] Therefore for most patients with lung cancer the outlook is poor. Accurate staging is thus of paramount importance when selecting patients for curative resection.

B. Initial Evaluation

The evaluation and treatment of the lung cancer patient requires careful clinical assessment and interpretation of special studies. A diagnosis of lung cancer is usually clinically suspected based on radiographic criteria. Subsequently, clinical staging is performed to determine if local structures are involved

Non-Small Cell Carcinoma of the Lung

A.
Epidemiology and Etiology
Leading cause of cancer deaths
Leading risk factor: tobacco use
Only 25% are resectable

B.
Initial Evaluation
Historical points: prior tobacco use, prior treatment for cancer, cough, hemoptysis, shortness of breath, exposure to asbestos
Physical signs of advanced disease: palpable supraclavicular node, Horner's syndrome, hoarseness, SVC obstruction

C.
Diagnosis
Attempt FNA of suspicious cervical adenopathy; if not possible, perform excisional node biopsy
Chest radiography: look for solitary pulmonary nodule, R/O pleural effusion, R/O multiple nodules (implies metastatic disease), compare with old films
CT of chest and abdomen to evaluate mediastinum and R/O metastatic disease in the liver or adrenal gland; consider FNA of suspicious lesions
PET scan: efficacy still in question
MRI to evaluate involvement of vascular structures and brachial plexus
Mediastinoscopy

D.
Indications for Endoscopy

Mediastinal nodes (N2, N3) < 1.5 cm:
Bronchoscopy indicated if central lesion or peripheral lesion > 3 cm
Mediastinoscopy not needed

Peripheral lesion < 3 cm:
consider percutaneous needle aspirate vs. excisional biopsy

Mediastinal nodes (N2, N3) > 1.5 cm:
Bronchoscopy indicated if central lesion or peripheral lesion > 3 cm
Mediastinoscopy indicated

(continued on next page)

Non-Small Cell Carcinoma of the Lung (continued)

E.
Staging

F.
Treatment

For a good risk patient with a stage I, II, IIIA lesion, lobectomy with mediastinal node dissection is the procedure of choice. Wedge resections are associated with a higher recurrence rate.
For a poor risk patient who could not tolerate loss of substantial lung volume, wedge or segmental resection is preferred.

Stage		*Treatment*
I		→ Lobectomy with hilar and mediastinal lymph node dissection; postop. chemotherapy and irradiation (RT) not indicated
II		→ Lobectomy with hilar and mediastinal lymph node dissection; postop. chemotherapy/RT does not prolong survival
IIIA	T3N0–1 T1–3N2	→ If clinically IIIA, preop. chemotherapy (VP-16, cisplatin, taxol) and RT followed by surgery*
	T1–3, bulky N2	→ Preop. chemotherapy/RT; then surgery if there has been a favorable response to therapy
IIIB	T4N0	→ Chemotherapy/RT (+surgery in highly selected cases)
	T4N1–2	→ Chemotherapy/RT
	Any T, N3	→ Chemotherapy/RT
IV	Resectable brain metastasis	→ Surgery followed by chemotherapy/RT
	All other M+	→ Chemotherapy/RT

Special cases

Pancoast tumor	→ Preop. chemotherapy/RT followed by surgery
T3 chest wall, non-Pancoast	→ If large resection anticipated, preop. chemotherapy/RT followed by surgery If limited chest wall involvement, surgery alone
T4, invading trachea, aorta, or great vessels	→ Preop. chemotherapy/RT (see stage IIIB) followed by surgery

*If IIIA disease is diagnosed only after surgery, postoperative irradiation and chemotherapy are given; the combination yields significantly longer disease-free survival than irradiation alone. Postoperative irradiation alone improves local control but has no appreciable effect on survival.

Non-Small Cell Carcinoma of the Lung (continued)

G.
Assessment of Operative Risk
Cardiovascular history
- Age
- Prior MI, CHF, DM
- History of angina
- Exercise tolerance
- Murmur

Pulmonary history
- History and physical examination
- Chest radiography

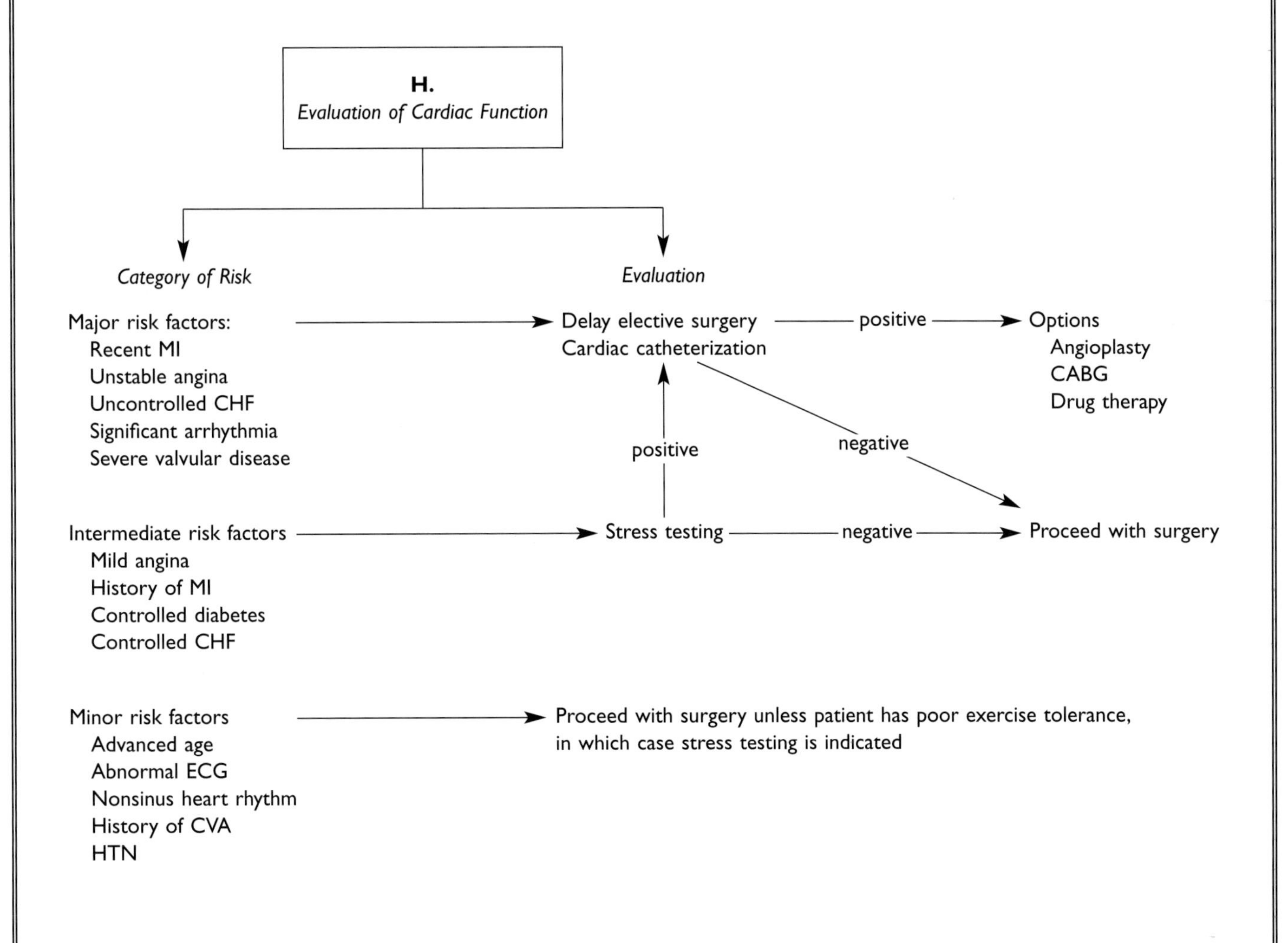

MI, myocardial infarction; CHF, congestive heart failure; DM, diabetes mellitus; CABG, coronary artery bypass graft; ECG, electrocardiogram; CVA, cerebral vascular accident; HTN, hypertension

(continued on next page)

Non-Small Cell Carcinoma of the Lung (continued)

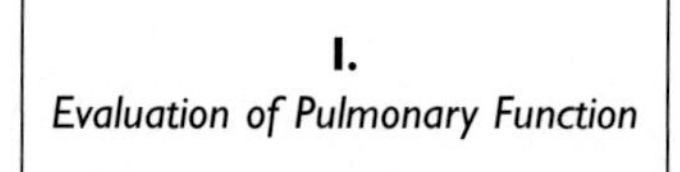

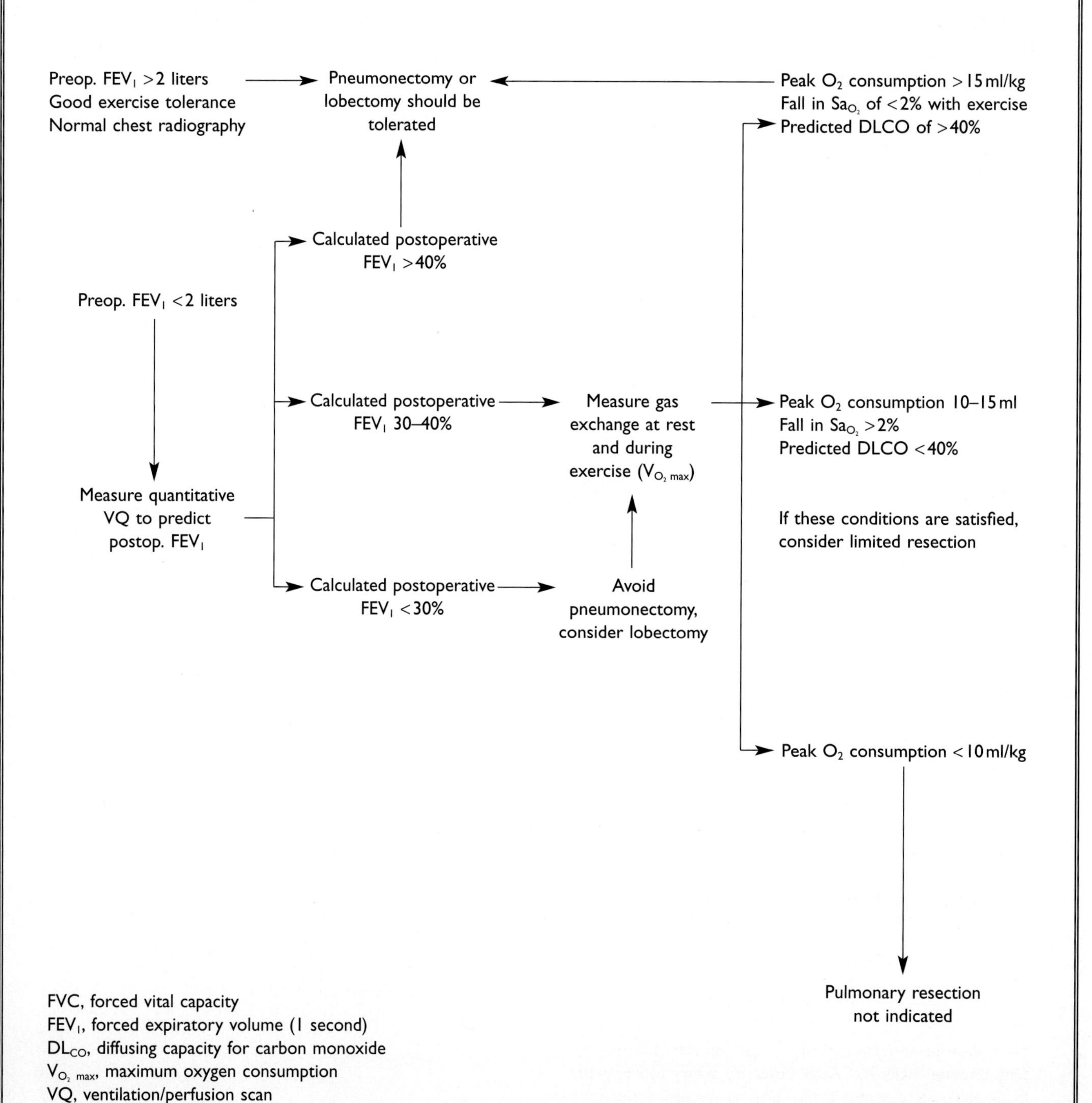

TABLE 19–1.
AJCC definition of TNM for lung cancer

Primary Tumor (T)

TX Primary tumor cannot be assessed, or tumor proven by the presence of malignant cells in sputum or bronchial washings but not visualized by imaging or bronchoscopy

T0 No evidence of primary tumor

Tis Carcinoma *in situ*

T1 Tumor 3 cm or less in greatest dimension, surrounded by lung or visceral pleura, without bronchoscopic evidence of invasion more proximal than the lobar bronchus* (i.e., not in the main bronchus)

T2 Tumor with any of the following features of size or extent:
More than 3 cm in greatest dimension
Involves main bronchus, 2 cm or more distal to the carina
Invades the visceral pleura
Associated with atelectasis or obstructive pneumonitis that extends to the hilar region but does not involve the entire lung

T3 Tumor of any size that directly invades any of the following: chest wall (including superior sulcus tumors), diaphragm, mediastinal pleura, parietal pericardium; or tumor in the main bronchus less than 2 cm distal to the carina but without involvement of the carina; or associated atelectasis or obstructive pneumonitis of the entire lung

T4 Tumor of any size that invades any of the following: mediastinum, heart, great vessels, trachea, esophagus, vertebral body, carina; separate tumor nodule(s) in the same lobe; or tumor with a malignant pleural effusion**

* The uncommon superficial tumor of any size with its invasive component limited to the bronchial wall, which may extend proximal to the main bronchus, is also classified T1.

** Most pleural effusions associated with lung cancer are due to tumor. However, there are a few patients in whom multiple cytopathologic examinations of pleural fluid are negative for tumor. In these cases, fluid is nonbloody and is not an exudate. When these elements and clinical judgment dictate that the effusion is not related to the tumor, the effusion should be excluded as a staging element and the patient should be staged T1, T2, or T3.

Regional Lymph Nodes (N)

NX Regional lymph nodes cannot be assessed

N0 No regional lymph node metastasis

N1 Metastasis to ipsilateral peribronchial and/or ipsilateral hilar lymph nodes, and intrapulmonary nodes involved by direct extension of the primary tumor

N2 Metastasis to ipsilateral mediastinal and/or subcarinal lymph node(s)

N3 Metastasis to contralateral mediastinal, contralateral hilar, ipsilateral or contralateral scalene, or supraclavicular lymph node(s)

Distant Metastasis (M)

MX Distant metastasis cannot be assessed

M0 No distant metastasis

M1 Distant metastasis present
Note: M1 includes separate tumor nodule(s) in a different lobe (ipsilateral or contralateral).

SOURCE: Used with permission of the American Joint Committee on Cancer (AJCC®), Chicago, IL. The original source for this material is the AJCC® Cancer Staging Manual, 5th edition (1997) published by Lippincott Williams & Wilkins Publishers, Philadelphia, PA.

TABLE 19–2.
AJCC stage grouping for lung cancer

Occult carcinoma	TX	N0	M0
0	Tis	N0	M0
IA	T1	N0	M0
IB	T2	N0	M0
IIA	T1	N1	M0
IIB	T2	N1	M0
	T3	N0	M0
IIIA	T1	N2	M0
	T2	N2	M0
	T3	N1	M0
	T3	N2	M0
IIIB	Any T	N3	M0
	T4	Any N	M0
IV	Any T	Any N	M1

SOURCE: Used with permission of the American Joint Committee on Cancer (AJCC®), Chicago, IL. The original source for this material is the AJCC® Cancer Staging Manual, 5th edition (1997) published by Lippincott Williams & Wilkins Publishers, Philadelphia, PA.

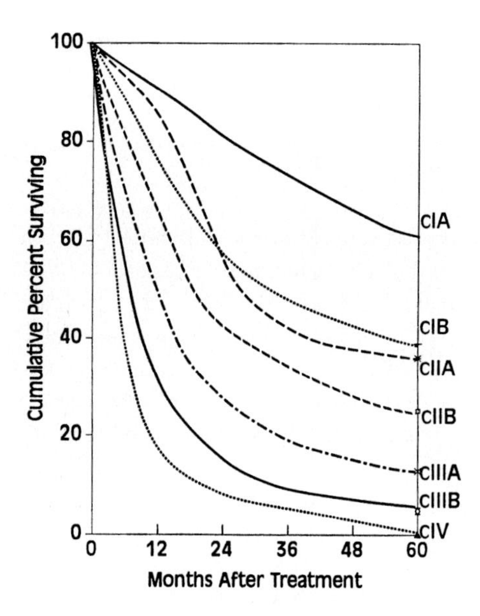

FIGURE 19–1
Survival rates for clinical stage lung cancer.

and if there is evidence of spread to regional nodes or distant sites. Finally, treatment must be proposed based on histologic and cytologic assessment of the tumor, clinical staging (i.e., resectability), and the ability of the patient to tolerate a planned procedure (i.e., operability).[4]

C. *Diagnosis*

The suspicion that a given lesion represents a carcinoma is usually based on finding a solitary pulmonary nodule, mass, or localized infiltrate on a chest radiograph. The solitary pulmonary nodule (SPN) is defined as a single, well demarcated opacity <3 cm in diameter and completely within the pleural boundaries.[5] Among the general population, the incidence of cancer in patients with an SPN is 3–6%.[6] Nodules must be >9 mm before they are reliably detected by a chest roentgenogram.[7] Upon reaching this size, a tumor has already undergone 30 of the 40 cell doublings that are estimated to occur before the death of a patient.[8] Although it follows that early detection should confer a benefit to patients, three large trials of routine chest radiographs and sputum screening of male smokers failed to show a sufficient survival benefit to recommend routine screening of the smoking public.

A careful history and physical examination must accompany the initial evaluation. Particular attention must be paid to a history of any prior malignancy, tobacco use, exposure to asbestos, and respiratory symptoms including cough, hemoptysis, wheezing, and shortness of breath. Weight loss, malaise, and loss of energy are also worrisome complaints. On examination, the findings of a palpable supraclavicular node, Horner's syndrome, hoarseness (recurrent nerve palsy), physical signs of consolidated lung or pleural effusion, localized wheezing, or findings of SVC obstruction all suggest advanced disease. Old chest films should be diligently sought, as they may establish that a nodule has been unchanged for years and no further workup is warranted.

If a pleural effusion is of significant size and can be safely tapped, thoracentesis should be done early in the workup of the patient as a low risk way to establish the diagnosis and palliate the patient. Furthermore, an effusion should be drained *prior* to computed tomography (CT) imaging, as most findings are better assessed in an optimally reexpanded lung. Cytologic analysis should be performed on the pleural fluid. Likewise, a palpable supraclavicular lymph node should be biopsied by fine-needle aspiration or an excisional biopsy. The presence of a malignant pleural effusion (T4) or positive supraclavicular node (N3) renders the patient stage IIIB and thus not a candidate for resection. CT scanning is still indicated to plan therapy and assess future response to treatment. In selected cases, a nuclear bone scan and CT of the brain with and without contrast may be indicated (see below).

The radiographic features of a nodule or infiltrate on a plain chest radiograph can suggest not only the diagnosis of a primary malignancy but also its histologic type.[9] Squamous cell tumors are located centrally two-thirds of the time and have a tendency to cavitate (Fig. 19–2). Occasionally, a patient is found to have positive sputum cytology but no visible tumor radiographically. In these instances most are squamous carcinomas. Adenocarcinomas tend to be peripheral or subpleural nodules or masses (Fig. 19–3). The notable exception is bronchoalveolar carcinoma, which tends to present initially as a parenchymal infiltrate. Large cell carcinomas tend to be peripheral, and two-thirds are >4 cm in diameter at presentation. Small cell neuroendrocine lung cancer tends to present with bulky lobar and mediastinal adenopathy, which can overshadow the underlying pulmonary nodule or infiltrate (Figs. 19–4 and 19–5).

To further define the anatomy of the lesion, CT scans of the chest and upper abdomen with and without contrast are performed. Several important features of the plain radiograph and the CT scan aid in determining the differential diagnosis. Pulmonary granulomatous disease is suspected when the lesion is found to have a lamellar pattern of calcification. Pulmonary hamartomas have a characteristic "popcorn" pattern of calcification. The size of the lesion and its shape are important features; large lesions and those with spiculated, irregular borders tend to be malignant.[10] Spherical lesions with smooth margins tend to be benign unless there is a history of malignancy. In clinical practice, the chest radiograph and CT scan usually cannot be used to rule out malignancy definitively once the question has been raised. There are three exceptions to this statement: (1) a pulmonary nodule that has remained unchanged for 2 years or more, (2) a nodule with a "popcorn" calcification pattern indicative of hamartoma, and (3) a nodule that is heavily calcified.

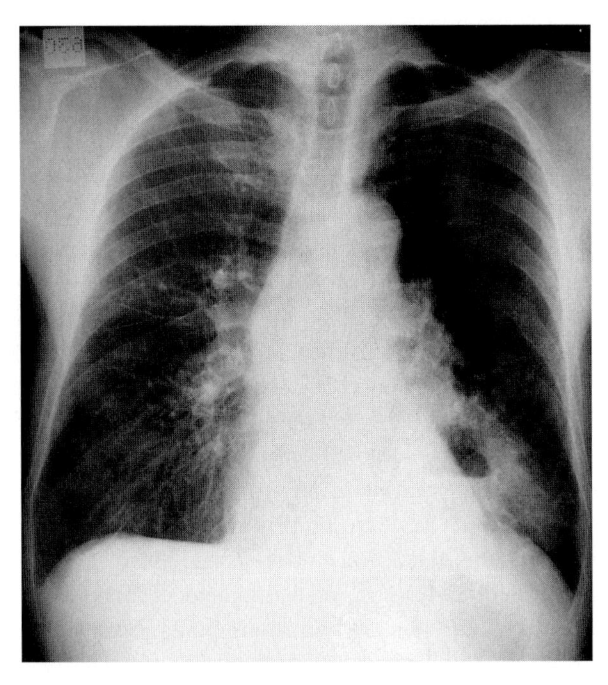

FIGURE 19–2
Posteroanterior chest radiograph of a 56-year-old man presenting with hemoptysis. Note the cavitating mass in the left lower lobe with an air-fluid level. On bronchoscopy the patient was found to have a squamous carcinoma.

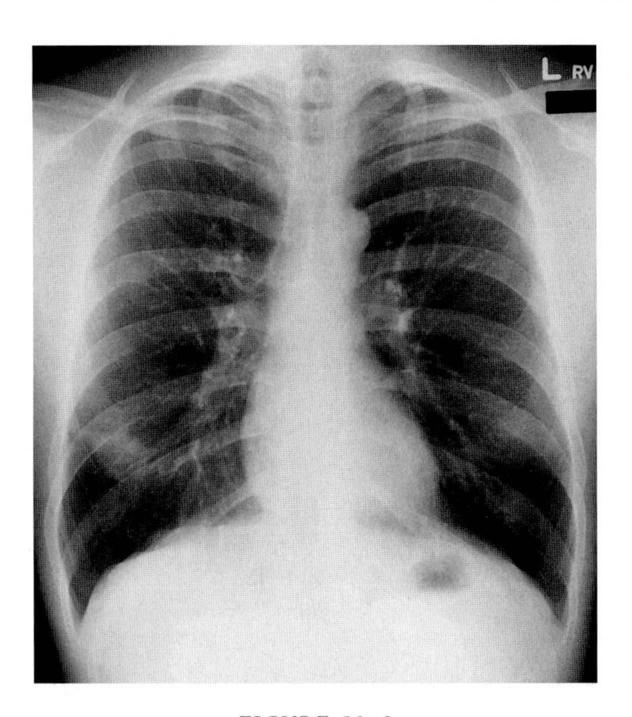

FIGURE 19–3
Posteroanterior chest radiograph of a 42-year-old nonsmoker presenting asymptomatically. A nodule was found in the right lobe. On bronchoscopy the nodule proved to be adenocarcinoma. No extrapulmonary primary tumor could be found.

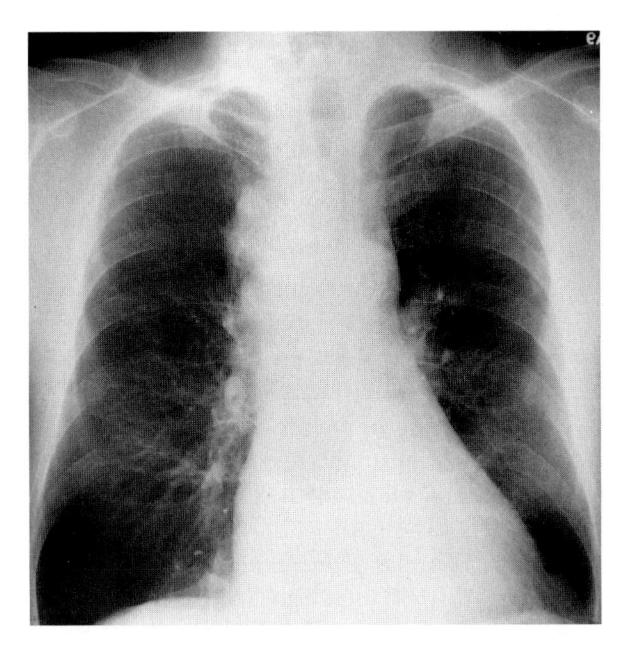

FIGURE 19–4
Posteroanterior chest radiograph of a 62-year-old patient presenting with a 4-month history of cough and sudden onset of facial swelling. Extensive mediastinal adenopathy was suspected. On mediastinoscopy the patient was found to have small cell neuroendocrine carcinoma causing SVC obstruction.

In addition to assessing the features of the lesion, CT is used to assess the relation of the lesion to surrounding structures (evidence of local invasion), the size and location of regional and mediastinal lymph nodes (evidence of lymph node involvement), and the presence or absence of adrenal and hepatic lesions (evidence of distant metastases).

There is considerable controversy regarding the assessment of mediastinal nodes. Reported series note that the sensitivity and specificity for detecting nodal metastases by CT ranges from 50% to 85%.[11] Of nodes ≥1 cm in diameter, 7–15% contain metastatic cancer.[12] Among nodes ≥2 cm in diameter, about two-thirds contain cancer,[13] and those >3 cm nearly always contain tumor in this setting. Overall, the incidence of metastatic adenocarcinoma in patients with non-small cell lung cancer and 1.5 cm mediastinal lymph nodes is much greater than in similar-size mediastinal nodes in patients with squamous cell carcinoma.[14,15]

Among stage IIIA patients, those with "minimal N2 disease" (i.e., a single positive node, no extracapsular spread) have a much better 5-year survival with surgery and radiotherapy (30% five-year survival) than those with either multilevel "nonbulky" or "bulky" N2 disease. For the latter groups, survivals are about 20% and 5%, respectively. For these patients, surgical resection alone is unlikely to be curative. Instead, several cycles of chemoradiotherapy are given to down-

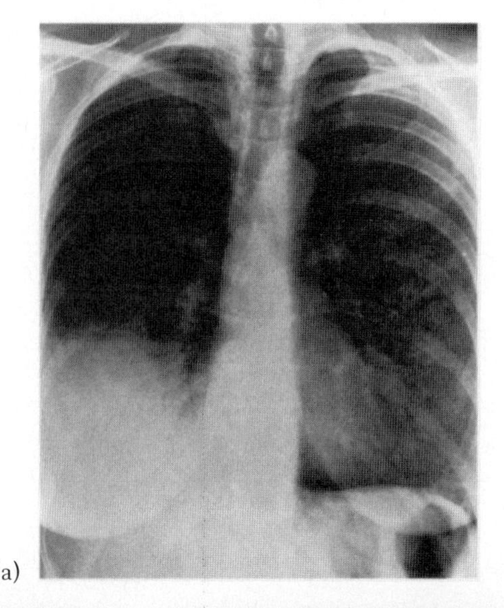

(a)

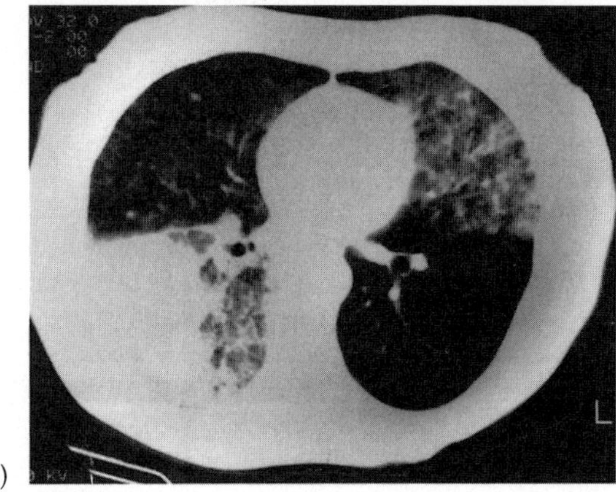

(b)

FIGURE 19–5
(a) Posterioranterior chest radiograph showing bronchioalveolar carcinoma with nearly complete consolidation of the right lower lobe and extensive consolidation of the lingular segment, (Contralateral disease is designated M1). (b) Computed tomographic scan of the chest (lung windows) shows the above findings to greater advantage.

stage the tumor and treat clinically occult distant metastases. Surgery may be reconsidered if there has been a favorable response to therapy. In patients with stage IIIA disease with minimal or no N2 involvement, preoperative chemoradiotherapy with subsequent complete resection is considered to be the treatment of choice.[16]

It should be noted that position emission tomography (PET) is being used increasingly to stage lung cancer. Although PET scans are not widely available, preliminary data suggest improved staging sensitivity and specificity compared to CT scans.[17–19] Ultimately, unequivocal findings of mediastinal lymph node metastases on PET scan may obviate the need for mediastinoscopy, but for the present mediastinoscopy should be performed to confirm PET scan findings.

D. Indications for Endoscopy

There are a variety of possible outcomes in the diagnostic algorithm following CT/PET scans. If mediastinal nodes are <1.5 cm, mediastinoscopy is not needed. Bronchoscopy is performed for central lesions or large (>3 cm) peripheral lesions. Resection is then recommended unless the lesion is highly likely to be benign or the patient represents a prohibitive operative risk (see below). On occasion, a *small cell neuroendocrine carcinoma* is diagnosed (bronchoscopic biopsy) or suspected, even when the only finding is a coin lesion and mediastinal nodes are not enlarged. In the setting of clinical stage I disease, this diagnosis should not be accepted without considerable skepticism, as true small cell carcinomas only rarely are discovered in stage I. In general, if surgical resection is contemplated this diagnosis warrants, at the very least, further staging procedures such as mediastinoscopy, even if the mediastinal nodes are not enlarged. CT of the brain and nuclear bone scans should also be performed on the basis of this histologic diagnosis alone. If after this workup there appears to be no evidence of a more advanced tumor, resection should be considered for the peripheral nodule, the rationale being that the diagnosis of small cell cancer is mistaken.[20,21] If, as is usually the case with small cell carcinoma, the tumor presents as a central mass or more extensive disease is present, including stage IIIA disease, there is no survival advantage offered even to patients undergoing an apparently complete surgical resection after chemoradiotherapy when compared to those undergoing chemoradiotherapy alone.[22]

If the CT scan demonstrates that the nodes are ≥1.5 cm or the PET scan suggests the presence of positive mediastinal nodes, bronchoscopy *and* mediastinoscopy should be performed In the absence of histologically proven mediastinal nodal involvement, subsequent resection is usually undertaken. If mediastinal nodes are involved but there is no distant metastatic disease, preoperative chemoradiotherapy is usually administered. If a significant amount of pleural fluid is discovered by CT scan that was not suspected by plain chest radiographs, thoracentesis should be performed to rule out cancer. In the case of multiple lung nodules, the patient requires a complete workup to assess for a primary extrathoracic tumor (i.e., the pulmonary nodules are metastases from another primary lesion).

An unsuspected adrenal mass >2 cm may require biopsy, especially if the diagnosis of the primary lesion is in question.[23] Chemical shift magnetic resonance imaging (MRI)[24] may accurately distinguish between an adrenal metastasis and an adrenal "adenoma," obviating the need for biopsy in a significant number of patients. Likewise, hepatic lesions thought to be cystic should undergo ultrasonographic assessment; well demarcated and solitary cystic lesions are usually benign. Solid hepatic lesions with or without necrotic centers may be malignant and require percutaneous needle biopsy to establish the diagnosis. In some superior sulcus tumors the CT scan may not adequately delineate the relation of the tumor to the brachial plexus and, in particular, the subclavian vessels. In this setting, MRI is indicated and has proved to be a valuable tool.[25] Needle biopsy is usually required to establish the diagnosis in superior sulcus tumors, as they are difficult to diagnose by bronchoscopy owing to the apical and peripheral location of the tumor. A diagnosis must be established prior to initiating preoperative radiation therapy (either alone or in conjunction with chemotherapy). If a percutaneous needle aspirate fails to establish the diagnosis, a core biopsy using a cutting needle is sometimes necessary.

Generally speaking, T4 tumors (malignant pleural effusion or invasion of mediastinal structures) are unresectable. However, there have been good risk patients who have survived beyond 5 years after complete resection of select T4 N0 or T4 N1 tumors, including patients whose tumors invaded the carina, superior vena cava, subclavian vessels, and aorta. Those patients considered for surgical resection must be carefully staged to rule out distant disease and to determine suitability for surgery. In general, these patients are best treated utilizing preoperative neoadjuvant chemoradiotherapy and then are restaged radiographically prior to resection. As is always the case with these locally advanced tumors, a diagnosis must be established prior to embarking on a course of aggressive therapy.

E. *Staging*

In many cases staging is complete after following the steps outlined above. In particular, CT and PET evaluation of the mediastinum and upper abdomen has become an integral part of staging. Although there is some controversy, most believe that additional studies to search for bone and brain metastases are not warranted routinely. CT of the brain or nuclear bone scans (or both) may be indicated based on the patient's history, physical examination, and biochemical profile. The history of recent and unexplained weight loss or fall in performance status, new neurologic complaints or deficits, focal bone pain, or any evidence of locally advanced disease in the chest justifies further studies to assess for distant metastatic disease. Prior imaging studies that showed mediastinal nodal enlargement or suspicious liver or adrenal masses also are indications for brain and bone imaging studies. In addition, patients with clinical or biochemical evidence of syndromes of ectopic hormonal production (e.g., hyponatremia) or biochemical evidence of metastatic disease (e.g., hypercalcemia) should also be worked up for distant metastases owing to a high incidence of metastatic disease in this group.

F. *Treatment*

A tissue diagnosis should be made prior to making treatment decisions. This is usually accomplished with bronchoscopy or, on occasion, with percutaneous needle aspiration. When the diagnosis of carcinoma is established and the stage determined, therapeutic options can be considered. If by clinical impression the lesion is judged to be highly suspicious for carcinoma but the diagnosis cannot be established by bronchoscopy, especially in a patient who has a low operative risk, thoracotomy is warranted to establish a diagnosis. The surgeon may then proceed with the appropriate curative resection. With the preoperative imaging studies and the diagnostic tools currently available, thoracotomy is rarely performed simply to establish a diagnosis for an unresectable lung cancer.

Stages I and II

Surgical resection is the standard treatment for patients with stage I or stage II disease. Systemic dissection of hilar and mediastinal lymph nodes is performed at thoracotomy. Long-term survival with lung cancer predictably exceeds 70% only in patients with T1 N0 stage I disease undergoing complete resection. With regard to extent of resection, the role of limited resection (i.e., wedge or segmental resection) for stage I lung carcinoma has undergone recent reevaluation. Patients undergoing a wedge resection or segmentectomy for stage I disease have a survival similar to that of patients treated with lobectomy, but the incidence of local recurrence is increased.[26–28] Most surgeons agree, therefore, that limited lung resections should be reserved for patients with severely compromised pulmonary function whose stage I carcinomas are located peripheral enough in the lung to permit limited resection. For the patient able to tolerate a lobectomy with low perioperative mortality, lobectomy with mediastinal node dissection is the procedure of choice.[29,30] Other options for complete resection include sleeve lobectomy, pneumonectomy, and sleeve pneumonectomy. The scope of the resection is obviously dictated by the location and extent of the tumor and must be anticipated before embarking on a thoracotomy. The mere presence of positive, but resectable, hilar or mediastinal nodes (or both) does not mandate a pneumonectomy.[31]

Perioperative morbidity and mortality are functions of the extent of the resection and the medical status of the patient. Overall, lobectomy is associated with 2% operative mortality, whereas the operative mortality associated with pneumonectomy may reach 10–15%. The 5-year survival is a function primarily of TNM status and the overall medical status of the patient. Survival after an incomplete resection approximates that of patients not undergoing resection; hence there is no role for "debulking" in the management of carcinoma of the lung.[32] In the unusual circumstance where a complete resection cannot be accomplished, some have advocated addition of intraoperative brachytherapy,[33] but the long-term results have been predictably poor. Generally, neither irradiation nor chemotherapy is advised postoperatively for completely resected stage I lung cancer. For pathologic stage II disease, postoperative irradiation alone may lower the local recurrence rate, but it has no appreciable effect on overall survival.

Stage IIIA

Stage IIIA includes T3 tumors, N2 nodal disease, or both. Surgical resection of T3 N0 tumors produces better survival rates than resection of N2 cancers. In either case, the goal of surgery is complete resection. T3 tumors invade the chest wall, diaphragm, mediastinal pleura, or pericardium or are within 2 cm of the carina. If completely resected, approximately half of the patients with T3 N0 tumors survive 5 years; in contrast, those with node-positive, completely resected T3 tumors have less than a 10% five-year survival. If resection is not complete, there are no long-term survivors. Postoperative irradiation alone improves local control but does not enhance survival.

Tumors within 2 cm of the carina can be resected with a pneumonectomy. Conservation of lung tissue is paramount, however; and if complete resection can be accomplished with a sleeve resection, this approach is preferable. The cure rates for patients with T3 N0 tumors undergoing pneumonectomy and sleeve resection are comparable. Sleeve lobectomy and pulmonectomy provide comparable 5-year survivals for appropriately selected patients with T3 N0 carcinomas.

Minimal N2 disease is defined as single-station lymph node involvement with microscopic disease. For such patients, the mediastinum may appear radiographically normal and nodal involvement is not discovered until after surgery. Resection of the primary tumor and complete mediastinal lymph node dissection is warranted provided all disease can be resected. Postoperatively, irradiation and chemotherapy are undertaken for N2 disease or in instances where the surgical margins are positive; combined adjuvant therapy administered in this fashion reduces recurrence rates and prolongs disease-free survival. If preoperatively there is strong evidence that a patient has clinical stage IIIA disease based on radiographic tests, preoperative chemoradiation is applied. The regimen includes VP-16, cisplatin, and taxol. Bulky N2 disease is defined as multiple levels of nodal metastases, multiple nodes at one level, or extranodal spread of disease. Most surgeons believe such cases to be unresectable, and these patients are treated with radiotherapy with or without chemotherapy. Surgery may then be considered, depending on tumor response to treatment.

Stage IIIB

Based on the "traditional" definition of resectability (T4 or advanced nodal spread N3) surgery is generally contraindicated for stage IIIB disease. However, selected T4 N0 tumors, such as those involving the carina, superior vena cava, left atrium, or aorta, occasionally can be completely resected. Most of these patients undergo preoperative combination chemoradiotherapy to downstage the tumor and increase the likelihood of obtaining negative resection margins. Preoperative combined chemotherapy and irradiation may render tumors resectable with a 2-year survival of approximately 40%. Tumors staged T4 because of cytologically positive malignant effusions do not fall into this category.

Stage IV

Surgery is contraindicated for stage IV disease with few exceptions. There has been evidence demonstrating a 5-year survival advantage for patients with a resectable lung cancer and a solitary brain metastasis who undergo staged resections of both. This is especially true if the lung resection is less than a pneumonectomy and there has been an interval of 6 months or more before discovery of the brain lesion.[34,35] There are also occasional case reports suggesting that patients with a solitary adrenal metastasis may also undergo resection of both, with a survival advantage over patients denied surgical resections. However, resection of liver or bone metastases from a primary lung carcinoma—even those that appear solitary and can be apparently "completely" resected—have not been shown to confer a survival advantage to the patient.[36]

G. *Assessment of Operative Risk*

H. Evaluation of Cardiac Function

Patients considered to be in the high risk category for resection, based on poor cardiac reserve or poor pulmonary reserve, may be treated with radiation therapy. The 5-year survival in these instances is less than 10%.

Coincident with assessment of the patient's tumor and planning of the surgical resection, there must also be careful assessment of the patient's overall physical status and suitability for the planned procedure. Preexisting cardiac and pulmonary disease are the primary determinants of postoperative morbidity and mortality, and each must be carefully assessed.[37,38]

Patients who have undergone coronary revascularization within 5 years and lack recurrent symptoms, those with a negative workup for cardiac ischemia, and those who have had a negative coronary angiogram within 2 years require no further investigation. Patients with recurrent cardiac symptoms may be stratified for further testing based on the presence of certain clinical variables. These variables fall into three categories (major, intermediate, minor risk) according to the cardiac risk.

Major predictors of bad outcome include the presence of unstable angina, recent myocardial infarction, uncontrolled congestive heart failure, significant arrhythmia, or severe valvular disease. Patients who have had a recent myocardial infarction are at risk for reinfarction and death. This risk is greatest if they undergo elective noncardiac surgery within 6 months.

These patients usually require cardiac catheterization prior to major noncardiac surgery.[39,40]

Those with intermediate variables (mild but stable angina, history of myocardial infarction or congestive heart failure well controlled medically, well managed diabetes mellitus) should undergo stress testing. If a patient is unable to undergo exercise stress testing, a dipyridamole (Persantine IV) stress test can be performed. Those with a negative stress test may proceed with surgery. Those with a positive or borderline stress test merit further testing or cardiac catheterization.

Minor risk factors are advanced age, abnormal electrocardiogram (ECG), nonsinus heart rhythms, history of stroke, and hypertension. Surgery may be undertaken in these patients without extensive preoperative testing unless the operation is high risk or the patient has poor exercise tolerance, in which case stress testing is indicated.

Noninvasive testing for ischemia is done with the stress ECG, dobutamine echocardiography, or Persantine-thallium. Criteria for a positive test include the following.

1. Stress ECG showing evidence of ischemia with a drop in systolic blood pressure ≥10 mm Hg
2. Stress perfusion scan with reversibility in half or more of 10 (single photon emission) CT slices
3. Stress echocardiographic ischemia in more than five segments, two or more coronary zones, or four left anterior descending artery zones

Management options for patients demonstrated to have ischemic changes can be classified as a revascularization strategy (coronary angioplasty, coronary artery bypass surgery) or a nonrevascularization strategy. A detailed discussion of these options is beyond the scope of this chapter. Management for patients with ischemia who do not require revascularization includes appropriate perioperative monitoring and the use of perioperative β-blockers or calcium channel blockers. The medical management of coronary or valvular heart disease is determined by the pathophysiologic findings of the individual patient. A more detailed discussion of preoperative cardiac assessment is available in the guidelines for perioperative cardiovascular evaluation for noncardiac surgery.[41,42]

I. Evaluation of Pulmonary Function

The pulmonary assessment begins with the history, physical examination, and chest radiograph. A history of smoking, asthma, exercise intolerance, dyspnea, or tachypnea; a occupational history (including exposure to coal, asbestos, or fumes); a history of serious pulmonary infection including tuberculosis, prior lung surgery, chest wall trauma; and a diagnosis of chronic obstructive pulmonary disease or systemic disease involving the lung alert the surgeon to a potentially significant loss of lung reserve. Stair climbing provides a measure of the patient's cardiovascular and pulmonary reserve, with studies now reported that support its value.[43,44] Surgical patients require objective measurement of lung function with spirometry and measurement of arterial blood gases preoperatively.

Patients under age 45 with an unremarkable history and physical examination require no further physiologic workup prior to resection. However, for patients older than 45 years or those with a history of significant underlying pulmonary disease, pulmonary function testing is appropriate. Patients with maximum oxygen consumption ($V_{O_2\ max}$) >20 ml/kg/min, forced vital capacity (FVC) >2 liters, diffusing capacity for carbon monoxide (DL_{CO}) >60%, and P_{CO_2} <45 mm Hg are candidates for surgery so long as there is no reason to think that the postoperative forced expiratory volume at 1 second (FEV_1) will be <1200 ml. This determination is of paramount importance when one considers the patient's ability to tolerate a pneumonectomy. Ideally, the patient has a calculated postoperative FEV_1 of 800 ml. Currently, the best single estimate of the postoperative FEV_1 is calculated by multiplying the preoperative FEV_1 by the percent perfusion of the remaining lung, as determined by a quantitative ventilation/perfusion lung scan.

Patients with a preoperative FEV_1 >2 liters, good exercise tolerance, and a normal chest radiograph (apart from the known tumor) can safely undergo lobectomy or pneumonectomy. However, if one of these conditions is not met, a quantitative ventilation/perfusion scan is done to predict the postoperative FEV_1. A postoperative FEV_1 that is more than 40% of the predicted value in an asymptomatic patient implies that pneumonectomy or lobectomy would be tolerated. Patients whose predicted postoperative FEV_1 is 30–40% of normal or those with dyspnea are at high risk of developing postoperative pulmonary insufficiency after a major thoracic resection. For these patients, $V_{O_2\ max}$ studies have been used to define further their risk as surgical candidates. A peak O_2 consumption of >15 ml/kg/min, a fall in Sa_{O_2} of 2% or less with exercise, and a predicted DL_{CO} of >40% imply that a formal lobectomy or pneumonectomy should be tolerated. A $V_{O_2\ max}$ of 10–15 ml/kg/min, a fall in Sa_{O_2} of >2% with exercise, or a predicted DL_{CO} of <40% place the patient at much higher risk for postoperative pulmonary insufficiency. In this patient population, only limited pulmonary resections should be entertained. A $V_{O_2\ max}$ of <10 ml/kg/min places the patient at prohibitive risk, and pulmonary resection should not be considered.[45] It must be emphasized that these are only guidelines for patient selection and that individual assessment and the surgeon's experience are of paramount importance.

Conclusions

Resection is the accepted treatment for patients with stage I or II lung cancer; unfortunately, only 25% of patients fall into this category. Following resection, adjuvant therapy has no proven benefit for stage I or II patients. If stage IIIA (N2) disease is suspected on clinical grounds (CT scan, PET scan) and is confirmed histologically (needle biopsy or mediastinoscopy), initial surgery is generally contraindicated. Instead, chemotherapy and radiation are administered to downstage the lesion and potentially render it resectable. If unsuspected, pathologic stage IIIA (N2) disease is discovered following thoracotomy and lobectomy, postoperative irradiation and chemotherapy have proven benefit in terms of prolonging disease-free survival. Stage IIIB disease without N3 involvement may be treated first with chemotherapy and radiation followed by surgery, depending on tumor response. Most surgeons consider N3 disease a sign of inoperability.

References

1. Naruke T, Suemasu K, Ishikawa S. Lymph node mapping and curability at various levels of metastasis in resected lung cancer. J Thorac Cardiovasc Surg 1978;76:832–839.
2. Mountain CF. Revisions in the international system for staging lung cancer. Chest 1997;111:1710–1717.
3. Naruke T, Goya T, Tsuchiya R, et al. Prognosis and survival in resected lung carcinoma based on the new international staging system. J Thorac Cardiovasc Surg 1988;96:440–447.
4. Ginsberg RJ. Preoperative assessment of the thoracic surgical patient: a surgeon's viewpoint. In: Pearson FG, Deslauriers J, Hiebert CA, McNeally MF, Ginsberg RJ, Urschel HC (eds) Thoracic Surgery. New York: Churchill Livingstone, 1995:29–36.
5. O'Donovan PB. The radiologic appearance of lung cancer. Oncology 1997;11:1387–1424.
6. Steele JD. The solitary pulmonary nodule. J Thorac Cardiovasc Surg 1963;46:21–39.
7. Kundel HL. Predictive values and threshold detectability of lung tumors. Radiology 1981;139:25–29.
8. Geddes DM. The natural history of lung cancer: a review based on rates of tumor growth. Br J Dis Chest 1979;73:1–17.
9. Byrd RB, Carr DT, Miller WE, et al. Radiographic abnormalities in carcinoma of the lung as related to histologic cell type. Thorax 1969;24:573–575.
10. Zwirewich CV, Vedal S, Miller RR, et al. Solitary pulmonary nodule: high-resolution CT and radiologic-pathologic correlation. Radiology 1991;179:469–476.
11. Primack SL, Lee KS, Logan PM, et al. Bronchogenic carcinoma: utility of CT in the evaluation of patients with suspected lesions. Radiology 1994;193:795–800.
12. Gross BH, Glazer GM, Orringer MB, et al. Bronchogenic carcinoma metastatic to normal-sized lymph nodes: frequency and significance. Radiology 1988;166:71–74.
13. McLoud TC, Bourgouin PM, Greenberg RW, et al. Bronchogenic carcinoma: analysis of staging in the mediastinum with CT by correlative lymph node mapping and sampling. Radiology 1992;182:319–323.
14. Maddeus M, Ginsberg RJ. Cancer: diagnosis and staging. In: Pearson FG, Deslauriers J, Hiebert CA, McNeally MF, Ginsberg RJ, Urschel HC (eds) Thoracic Surgery. New York: Churchill Livingstone, 1995:671–690.
15. Shields TW. Diagnosis and staging of lung cancer. In: Baue AE, Geha AS, Hammond GL, et al. (eds) Glenn's Thoracic and Cardiovascular Surgery. Stamford, CT: Appleton & Lange, 1996;391–419.
16. Greco FA, Hainsworth JD. Multidisciplinary approach to potentially curable non-small cell carcinoma of the lung. Oncology 1997;11:27–36.
17. Wahl RL, Quint LE, Greenough RL. Staging of mediastinal non-small cell lung cancer with FDG, PET, CT and fusion images: preliminary prospective evaluation. Radiology 1994;191:371–377.
18. Minn H, Zasadny KR, Quint LE, et al. Lung cancer: reproducibility of quantitative measurements for evaluating 2-[F-18]-fluoro-2-deoxy-D-glucose uptake at PET. Radiology 1995;196:167–173.
19. Schiepers C. Role of position emission tomography in the staging of lung cancer. Lung Cancer 1997;17(suppl 1):S29–S35.
20. Warren WH, Gould VE. Differential diagnosis of small cell neuroendocrine carcinoma of the lung. Chest Surg Clin N Am 1997;7:49–63.
21. Urschel J. Surgical treatment of peripheral small cell lung cancer. Chest Surg Clin N Am 1997;7:95–103.
22. Kohman LJ. Is there a place for surgery in central small cell lung cancer? Chest Surg Clin N Am 1997;7:105–112.
23. Burt M, Heelan RT, Coit D, et al. Prospective evaluation of unilateral adrenal masses in patients with operable non-small-cell lung cancer: impact of magnetic resonance imaging. J Thorac Cardiovasc Surg 1994;107:584–589.
24. Schwartz LH, Ginsberg MS, Burt ME, et al. MRI as an alternative to CT guided biopsy of adrenal masses in patients with lung cancer. Ann Thorac Surg 1998;65:193–197.
25. Gamsu G. Magnetic resonance imaging in lung cancer. Chest 1986;89:242s–244s.
26. Martini N, Bains MS, Burt ME, et al. Incidence of local recurrence and second primary tumors in resected stage I lung cancer. J Thorac Cardiovasc Surg 1995;109:120–129.
27. Warren WH, Faber LP. Segmentectomy versus lobectomy in patients with stage I pulmonary carcinoma: five year survival and patterns of recurrence. J Thorac Cardiovasc Surg 1994;107:1087–1094.
28. Ginsburg RJ. The role of limited resection in the treatment of early stage lung cancer. Lung Cancer 1994;11(suppl 2):S35–S36.
29. Martini N, Flehinger BJ. The role of surgery in N2 lung cancer. Surg Clin North Am 1987;67:1037–1049.
30. Thomas PH, Piantadosi S, Mountain CF. Should subcarinal lymph nodes be routinely examined in patients with non-small cell lung cancer? J Thorac Cardiovasc Surg 1988;95:883–887.
31. Shields TW. Presentation, diagnosis and staging of bronchial carcinoma and of the asymptomatic solitary pulmonary nodule. In: Shields TW (ed) General Thoracic Surgery, 4th ed. Philadelphia: Williams & Wilkins, 1994:1122–1154.
32. Hara N, Ohta M, Tanaka K, et al. Assessment of the role of surgery for stage III bronchogenic carcinoma. J Surg Oncol 1984;25:153–158.
33. Burt ME, Pomerantz AH, Bains MS, et al. Results of surgical treatment of stage III lung cancer invading the mediastinum. Surg Clin North Am 1987;67:987–1000.
34. Raviv G, Klein E, Yellin A, et al. Surgical treatment of solitary adrenal metastases from lung carcinoma. J Surg Oncol 1990;43:123–124.
35. Reyes L, Parvez Z, Nemoto T, et al. Adrenalectomy for adrenal metastasis from lung carcinoma. J Surg Oncol 1990;44:32–34.
36. Luketich JD, Martini N, Ginsberg RJ, et al. Successful treatment of solitary extracranial metastases from non-small cell lung cancer. Ann Thorac Surg 1995;60:1609–1611.
37. Wernly JA, DeMeester TR. Preoperative assessment of patients undergoing lung resection for cancer. In: Roth JA, Ruchdeschel JC, Weisenburger TH (eds) Thoracic Oncology. Philadelphia: Saunders, 1989:156–176.
38. Martinez FJ, Paine R. Medical evaluation of the patient with potentially resectable lung cancer. In: Pass HI, Mitchell JB, Johnson DH, Turisi AT (eds) Lung Cancer: Principles and Practice. Philadelphia: Lippincott-Raven, 1995:511–534.

39. Cohen MC, Eagle KA. Expert opinion regarding indications for coronary angiography before non-coronary cardiac surgery. Am Heart J 1997; 134:321–329.
40. Goldman L. Cardiac risks and complications of non-cardiac surgery. Ann Surg 1983;198:780–791.
41. Eagle KA. Surgical patients with heart disease: summary of the ACC/AHA guidelines. Am Fam Physician 1997;56:811–818.
42. Eagle KA, Brundage BH, Chaitman BR, et al. Guidelines for perioperative cardiovascular evaluation for non-cardiac surgery. J Am Coll Cardiol 1996;27:910–948.
43. Olsen GN, Bolton JWR, Weiman DS, et al. Stair climbing as an exercise test to predict the postoperative complications of lung resection: two years experience. Chest 1991;99:587–590.
44. Morice RC, Peters EJ, Ryan MB, et al. Exercise testing in the evaluation of patients at high risk for complications from lung resection. Chest 1992;101:356–361.
45. Bechard D, Wetstein L. Assessment of exercise consumption as a pre-operative criterion for lung resection. Ann Thorac Surg 1987;44:344–349.

CHAPTER 20

Metastatic Cancer to the Lung

ARTHUR N.S. MCUNU, JR.
HARVEY I. PASS

A. Epidemiology and Etiology

The lungs are the second most common site of metastatic disease.[1] A review of autopsy studies of patients dying from extrathoracic malignancies yields an incidence of metastatic disease to the lungs of 20–54%.[2–4] Among these patients, 10–15% had metastatic disease confined to the lungs.[4] Improved survival has been seen following surgical treatment of patients with certain histologies. This chapter presents an approach to the care of patients with pulmonary metastases from extrathoracic sources.

The first resection of pulmonary metastases occurred in 1882 and is credited to Weinlechner.[5] In 1883 Kronlein removed a metastatic nodule from a young woman during resection of a chest wall sarcoma.[6] The first isolated pulmonary metastasectomy was performed by Divis in 1927.[7] In 1930 Torek performed the first resection of pulmonary metastases in the United States.[8] Resection of metastatic pulmonary nodules was further supported by the improved survival benefit noted by Barney and Churchill in 1939[9] and by Alexander and Haight in 1947.[10] The approach has been expanded to include resection of multiple lesions, and an extended survival has been seen for certain tumor types.

The most common mechanism for the development of pulmonary metastases is hematogenous tumor embolization.[3,4,11] Tumor cells are released from the primary lesion by enzymatic degradation of the basement membrane.[12] Tumor emboli are then released into the circulation and filtered into the pulmonary capillary bed,[3,4,13–15] where they interact with endothelial cells, thrombocytes, and fibrin, becoming attached to the vascular endothelium.[3,14,16] Metastatic growth is subsequently determined by tumor and local factors.[14,16]

Another mode of metastasis to the lungs involves lymphatic spread from the primary site to regional lymph nodes and subsequent progressive spread along lymphatic chains.[3,4,11,14,17–19] Retrograde extension from pulmonary and hilar lymphatics has also been demonstrated.[19,20] Direct bronchial invasion from an involved node or transbronchial dissemination via aspiration can cause endobronchial metastases.[20,21]

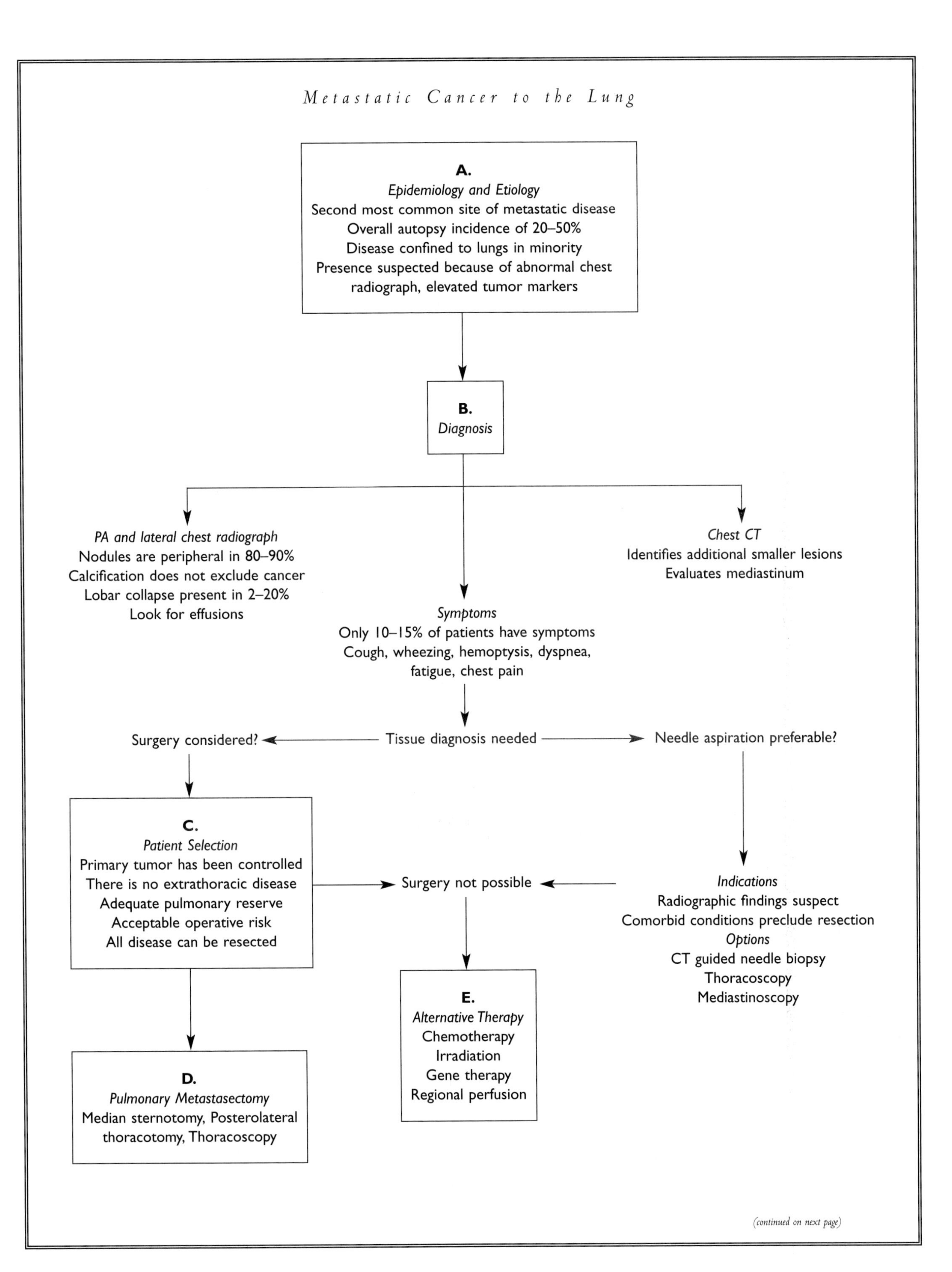

(continued on next page)

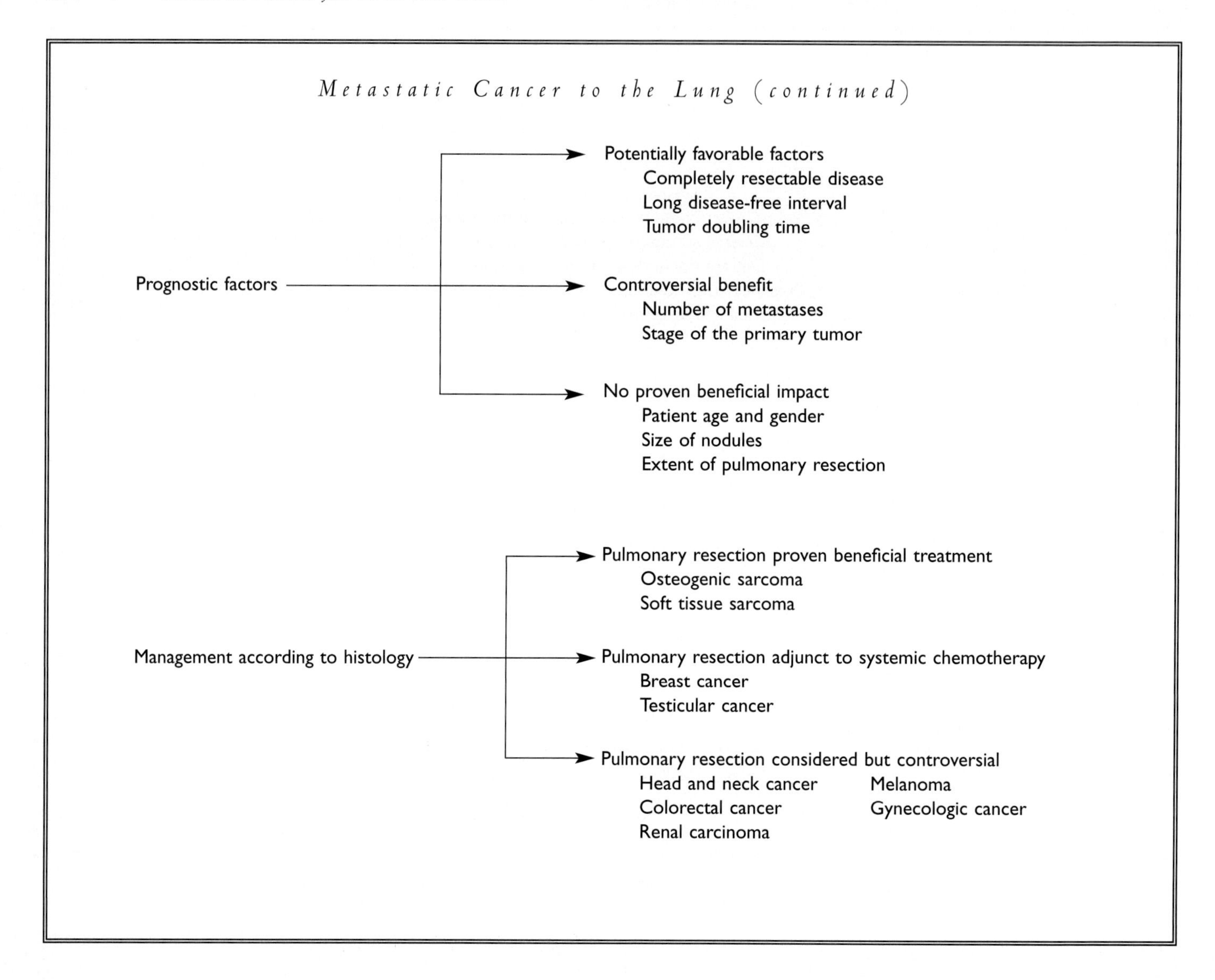

B. *Diagnosis*

About 80–90% of pulmonary metastases are found in the peripheral or outer one-third, subpleural location.[22–24] These lesions present radiographically as spherical nodules with clearly defined borders without linear densities.[3,4,11,24,25] The nodules may be single or multiple. In general, multiple nodules are highly suggestive of metastatic disease but are certainly not pathognomic.[25] Lung tumors such as bronchoalveolar carcinoma and multiple synchronous primary lung carcinomas may present with multiple nodules on roentgenograms.[11,16,25]

Calcification of a malignant nodule may occur[26] and can be seen following chemotherapy and with certain primary tumors such as osteosarcoma, chondrosarcoma, synovial sarcoma, and carcinomas of the breast, gastrointestinal tract, thyroid gland, and ovaries.[11,16,26,27] Approximately 2–20% of patients present with at least one lobar collapse from endobronchial metastases.[28–30] These metastases frequently arise from breast, colon, and kidney carcinomas.[31] Predilection of metastatic lesions to the left or right has not been demonstrated.[32] The location of the metastases is most often at the bases because of circulatory physiology.[33] Patients are usually asymptomatic; only 5–15% develop symptoms because of the location and size of the tumors.[34–36] Symptoms include cough, wheezing, hemoptysis, dyspnea, fatigue, and chest pain.

The posteroanterior and lateral roentgenograms are excellent screening tools that can detect changes from previous examinations.[3,4,11] Computed tomography (CT) has become the standard method used to evaluate pulmonary metastases[33] and is capable of detecting lesions as small as 3 mm. In the clinical setting of a known malignancy, the presence of multiple nodules on CT usually indicates metastatic disease.[8] Even without a known extrathoracic malignancy, 73% of 114 patients with multiple pulmonary nodules detected on CT had metastatic disease in one series.[8] The disadvantage of the CT scan is its low specificity; myriad disease entities, such as infectious and noninfectious granulomatous disease, pneumoconiosis, collagen vascular disease, drug reactions, septic emboli, and multifocal primary bronchogenic carcinoma, may present with multiple nodules on the CT scan. The definitive diagnosis of pulmonary metastases therefore should rest with tissue diagnosis.[8,11,21]

Certain clinical scenarios warrant obtaining a tissue diagnosis without thoracotomy, including cases where there is uncertainty regarding the radiographic appearance of the lesion and doubt about the ability of the patient to tolerate a major resection. For high risk patients, fine-needle aspiration may provide a histologic diagnosis with sensitivities of approximately 88% for metastatic lesions.[37,38] The peripheral disposition of pulmonary metastases renders this approach ideal in patients with prohibitive co-morbid conditions.

Thoracoscopy is another diagnostic technique but necessitates general anesthesia. It is suitable for obtaining tissue from peripheral parenchymal lesions.[39–41] Mediastinoscopy or mediastinotomy has a limited role in the diagnosis of pulmonary metastases,[42] but it has been proposed as part of the evaluation of patients with large proximal tumors or for breast cancer.

C. *Patient Selection*

There are no consistently reliable predictors of survival after surgical resection of pulmonary metastases.[43] Only a small percentage of patients are cured, and only a small cohort of other patients experience any survival benefit. The approach to each patient therefore must be individualized. The essential requirements when selecting patients to undergo resection are whether the primary tumor is locally controlled and if there is evidence of extrathoracic disease. Radiographic, radionuclide, and endoscopic examinations may assist in ruling out disease outside the chest. Additionally, the pulmonary disease must be completely resectable with preservation of adequate postoperative lung function. Finally, there should be no other effective therapeutic options, and the patient should be free of co-morbid medical conditions that would render the surgery too risky. Unfortunately, only one-third of patients with pulmonary metastases meet these criteria.[30]

As mentioned above, no established factors reliably predict survival following pulmonary metastasectomy.[43] The problem stems from the fact that available data on prognostic factors derive from retrospective analyses of various tumor histologies from different primary sites. In addition, treatment has varied; patients may have received adjuvant chemotherapy, radiation therapy, or immunotherapy in addition to surgery. Certain factors have been studied and serve as guidelines, including resectability, disease-free interval, number of metastases, tumor doubling time, and others.

Resectability

For all histologies, complete resection of pulmonary metastatic disease results in improved survival.[34,35,44–47] Resectability is determined by intraoperative findings; anatomic features that should be assessed include discontinuous involvement of the pericardium or diaphragm, metastatic lymph nodes, associated malignant pleural effusion, or pleural metastases, each of which precludes resectability. In highly selected patients, aggressive surgical resection via pneumonectomy or en bloc pulmonary resections may lead to long-term survival.[48]

Disease-free Interval

Disease-free interval (DFI) refers to the time from treatment of the primary tumor to detection of pulmonary metastases.[49,50] It might be inferred that a shorter DFI portends diminished survival of the patient, but the data on the impact of the DFI on patient survival is controversial.[51–54] It appears that DFI duration has prognostic significance for breast and head and neck cancers, but its prognostic significance has not been clearly established for other histologies.[55–65]

Number of Metastases

Preoperative radiologic examinations can underestimate the number of nodules by a factor of two.[33] The prognostic impact of the number of metastases and the implications regarding surgery depends on tumor histology.[45] For instance, one study demonstrated a resection benefit for patients with metastatic soft tissue sarcomas in whom up to 15 nodules were resected. Other reports, however, offer contrary conclusions.[35,44,47,53,55,58–62,64,66–71] Overall the data on the prognostic impact of the number of metastases varies widely, but most authors report no significant correlation with patient survival.

Tumor Doubling Time

Tumor doubling time (TDT) has been quantitated as a means of correlating growth rate with prognosis. Several authors have demonstrated decreased patient survival in association with tumors with shorter TDTs.[51,72,73] Therapeutic agents such as chemotherapy can alter the TDT, which may potentially improve survival.[74]

Other Possible Prognostic Indicators

Other prognostic indicators have been studied, albeit in a nonrandomized fashion, and no significant impact on patient survival has been demonstrated. They include the laterality of the lesions, patient age and gender, symptoms, nodal status, size of the nodules, use of adjuvant chemotherapy, and the extent of resection.[34,35,45,57,59,75–79]

D. Treatment: Pulmonary Metastasectomy

There are four surgical approaches for resecting pulmonary metastases: median sternotomy, posterolateral thoracotomy, clamshell incision, and video-assisted thoracoscopy. Regardless of the approach selected, every effort should be made to conserve lung tissue while ensuring satisfactory margins of resection. Because most metastatic nodules are found peripherally, wedge resections can usually be accomplished. Larger resections may be necessary (e.g., lobectomy, segmentectomy, en bloc resections) to effect complete resection.

For bilateral disease, the preferred initial approach is through a median sternotomy, which allows exploration of both thoracic cavities[45–47,80] and visualization of the mediastinum, pulmonary parenchyma, hilar lymph nodes, chest wall, and diaphragm to determine resectability. The mortality rate approaches 0%,[45] and the recovery of postoperative pulmonary function is more rapid than that after posterolateral thoracotomy.[81] The major drawback with this approach is the difficult access to posteromedial lesions, nodules in the left lower lobe, and the narrow retrosternal spaces. This approach should be avoided when a sleeve resection is anticipated, there is central staple line recurrence, or in the presence of a history of sternal irradiation.[82,83]

Posterolateral thoracotomy offers an excellent view of the entire hemithorax and is ideal for posteromedially placed lesions.[82,83] Bilateral thoracotomy can be performed in one or two stages. Bilateral anterior thoracotomy, the "clam-shell" incision, can be used without significant morbidity.[84] Video-assisted thoracic surgery (VATS) has been applied to the management of pulmonary metastases.[39–41,84] Proponents of this technique cite excellent visualization of the lung surface, less patient discomfort, and a shorter hospital stay as the greatest advantages. VATS offers excellent exposure for biopsy and is helpful for determining resectability. Its major disadvantages are the inability to feel, detect, and resect all metastases, particularly when they are deep-seated.[84] The ultimate affect on survival using VATS remains to be established.

Specific Histologies

Osteogenic Sarcoma

Osteogenic sarcoma most frequently metastasizes to the lungs. Prior to the use of chemotherapy, 80% of patients with osteogenic sarcoma died during the first year following amputation alone, and 95% died within 3 years.[85] Survival has been improved by the use of multidrug chemotherapy combined with radical resection of the primary tumor.[86]

Although hampered by a lack of randomization, all reported series advocate aggressive resection of pulmonary metastases for these patients.[34,52–54,68,74,87] The 5-year survival rates range from 25% to 58% in the literature.[87] Once the primary tumor has been controlled with multimodality therapy, the preferred approach is aggressive pulmonary metastasectomy,[88–90] even in cases where multiple thoracotomies are required.[89]

Soft Tissue Sarcoma

The lung is frequently the sole site of metastases in patients with soft tissue sarcoma (STS). The metastases are most commonly encountered within the first 2 years after diagnosis of the primary tumor. Surgical resection alone can remove isolated and resectable metastases. Following pulmonary metastasectomy the 5-year survival rate is approximately 33%, according to several series.[35,36,45,46,67,76,78,90–93] Factors associated with an increased risk of pulmonary metastases include higher primary tumor grade, tumor size >3 cm, lower extremity site, and histologic type.[76] Favorable predictors of survival following thoracotomy have been retrospectively identified for the various soft tissue sarcomas and include complete resection, long DFI between the first and second metastasectomies, and completely resected disease. The actual number of nodules removed has no influence on survival.

Urinary Tract Cancer

Fifty percent of patients with isolated renal cell carcinoma who undergo nephrectomy and 75% of those with stage IV disease develop pulmonary metastases.[94] Review of the literature reveals 5-year survival rates ranging from 13% to 50% with a median survival of 23–33 months following pulmonary metastasectomy.[36,44,75,94–97] The indications for and benefits of resection remain variable and inconclusive.

Testicular Cancer

Testicular cancer is considered a curable tumor with more than 90% overall long-term survival. Many patients can achieve a complete response with chemotherapy despite the presence of widespread metastases.[98] First-line therapy in the management of patients with pulmonary metastases is cisplatin-based combination chemotherapy. With this regimen, 75% of patients achieve a complete response.[99–101] Pulmonary metastasectomy renders an additional 10–15% of patients disease-free. Surgery for this disease therefore is reserved for patients who do not have a favorable response to chemotherapy. Adverse prognostic factors include prechemotherapy human chorionic gonodotropin (hCG) levels of at least 10,000 IU, incomplete resection, and the extent of the disease.[102] The most significant predictor for relapse is incomplete resection.

Head and Neck Cancer

When primary tumors of the lip, tonsil, and adenoid are excluded, the first site of metastases from head and neck cancer is to the lung. These patients also have a high incidence of primary lung cancer because of tobacco exposure. Pulmonary metastasectomy yields 5-year survival rates of up to 44%.[36,44,66,103] With locoregional control of the primary tumor, the most significant prognostic factor is complete resection.[66] A DFI of 1–2 years has favorably influenced survival in some studies.[66,104]

Colorectal Cancer

An estimated 10% of patients with colorectal carcinoma develop pulmonary metastases. Among these patients only 10% have disease confined to the lungs.[105] Distal rectal primary tumors have a greater predilection for *isolated* pulmonary metastases than do colon cancers owing to their systemic, rather than portal, venous drainage.[106,107] The 5-year survival rates after pulmonary metastasectomy range from 9% to 58%.[36,58–60,75,95,108–115] The best survival rates have been reported in the patients with a solitary metastasis and a normal postresection carcinoembryonic antigen (CEA) level.[60,115] Simultaneous resection of pulmonary and hepatic metastases has been conducted with actuarial 1-, 3-, and 5-year survival rates of 89%, 78%, and 52%, respectively.[114]

Gynecologic Cancer

The resection of pulmonary metastases resulting from uterine-cervical cancer has been reported, with 5-year survival rates of 8–52%.[36,55,56,95] A heterogeneous group of patients with primary tumors involving the cervix, endometrium, ovary, uterine sarcoma, and choriocarcinoma has been reported with 5-year survival of 36% after resection of metastases.[55] In that series patients with lesions <4cm in diameter had the most favorable prognosis.

Breast Cancer

Pulmonary metastases accounts for 25% of the deaths related to breast cancer.[116] The 5-year survival rates following pulmonary metastasectomy range between 27% and 50%.[36,66,71,104,117–119] A DFI of more than 12 months and an estrogen receptor (ER)-positive status predict longer survival.[86] Systemic therapy should be considered first, reserving thoracotomy for patients whose lung disease is the sole site of metastasis.

Melanoma

The incidence of pulmonary metastases from melanoma varies widely among reports. In one study of 200 melanoma patients, a pulmonary nodule was the first sign of dissemination in 38% of the patients.[120] Another study revealed a 50% incidence of pulmonary metastases as the initial site of recurrence.[61] The 5-year survival rates range from 5% to 33%. Complete resection is a consistent predictor of survival.[62]

Other Tumors

In addition to osteogenic sarcoma and STS, children can develop pulmonary metastases from Wilms' tumor, hepatoma, hepatoblastoma, and, rarely, neuroblastoma.[121] Multiple thoracotomies may be necessary.

E. *Alternative Treatment*

Chemotherapy

As noted previously, only one-third of all patients with isolated pulmonary metastases benefit from complete resection with prolonged survival. The development of more effective chemotherapeutic agents has increased interest in applying this treatment modality to pulmonary metastases. Thus far the available data have failed to demonstrate a survival benefit of chemotherapy alone for all histologies except testicular cancer. The role of metastasectomy and chemotherapy as combined therapy awaits further clarification.

In general, with the exception of osteogenic sarcoma, chemotherapy for metastatic sarcomas continues to yield unsatisfactory results, with response rates around 30%.[122,123] For metastatic breast carcinoma, systemic treatment is given first, reserving surgery for patients with persistent, resectable disease. Effective chemotherapy has not yet been developed for metastatic colon cancer, renal cell carcinoma, or melanoma; therefore resection of metastatic disease should be considered, provided the patient is an acceptable candidate for surgery.

Radiation Therapy

Radiation therapy has little or no role in the management of patients with pulmonary metastases. It is currently reserved for palliation of patients with symptoms of advanced metastases such as bone invasion.

Gene Therapy

The overall poor survival of patients with pulmonary metastases treated with available measures has sparked an interest in more novel therapeutic approaches. Some of this interest has naturally focused on molecular biology to predict events that account for the aggressive behavior of some tumors. Alterations in the *p53* gene have been associated with the uncontrolled cell growth of soft tissue sarcoma. An in vitro study has been reported in which transduction of wild-type *p53* into soft tissue sarcomas with the mutated gene altered the malignant potential of the tumor, as demonstrated by decreased proliferation.[124] Others have reported on the correlation of the early development of pulmonary metastases, poor survival, and the expression of *ErbB-2* in patients with osteogenic sarcoma.[125] The use of these and other specific genetic markers may improve the selection of patients and their stratification to determine who can benefit from surgery, chemotherapy, or other therapies.

Regional Lung Perfusion

The optimal delivery of systemic chemotherapy is frequently limited by toxicity. The theoretic advantage of regional delivery of antineoplastic agents is that larger doses can be administered with minimal systemic "spillover" and thus reduced likelihood of toxicity. Several experimental models have been designed to evaluate isolated lung perfusion.[126–130] The feasibility of delivering higher doses of chemotherapy than can be achieved through the systemic route has been established. Currently, phase I trials are being conducted in patients with unresectable pulmonary metastases from STS at the University of Texas M.D. Anderson Cancer Center.

Conclusions

Once extrathoracic disease has been excluded and operative suitability determined, patients with isolated pulmonary metastases may be considered for thoracotomy. Complete surgical resection consistently correlates with improved survival. The results of multimodality therapy have been unsatisfactory, prompting a search for innovative therapies such as gene therapy and isolated lung perfusion. Clinical trials are necessary to define the optimal treatment approach to patients with pulmonary metastases.

References

1. Willis RA. The Spread of Tumors in the Human Body. London: Butterworth, 1973;167–174.
2. Crow J, Slavin G, Kreel L. Pulmonary metastasis: a pathologic and radiologic study. Cancer 1981;47:2595–2602.
3. Spencer H. Pathology of the Lung (Excluding Pulmonary Tuberculosis). Oxford: Pergamon, 1985.
4. Cahan WG, Shaw JP, Castro EL. Benign solitary lung lesions in patients with cancer. Ann Surg 1977;187:241–244.
5. van Dongen JA, van Slooten EA. The surgical treatment of pulmonary metastases. Cancer Treat Rev 1978;5:29–48.
6. Meade RH. A History of Thoracic Surgery. Springfield, IL: Charles C Thomas, 1961;1194–1197.
7. Divis G. Ein Beitraq Zur Operafiven Behandfung der Lungeschwulste. Acta Chir Scand 1927;62:329–341.
8. Torek F. Removal of metastatic carcinoma of the lung and mediastinum. Arch Surg 1930;21:1416–1424.
9. Barney JD, Churchill EJ. Adenocarcinoma of the kidney with metastasis to the lung cured by nephrectomy and lobectomy. Urology 1939; 42:269–276.
10. Alexander J, Haight C. Pulmonary resection for solitary metastatic sarcomas and carcinomas. Surg Gynecol Obstet 1947;85:129–146.
11. Libshitz HL, Jing B-S, Wallace S, et al. Sterilized metastases: a diagnostic and therapeutic dilemma. AJR Am J Roentgenol 1983;140:15–19.
12. Muller KM, Respondek M. Pulmonary metastases: pathological anatomy. Lung 1990;168:1137–1144.
13. Hirakata K, Nakata H, Harakate J. Appearance of pulmonary metastases on high resolution CT scans: comparison with histopathological findings from autopsy specimen. AJR Am J Roentgenol 1993;161:7–43.
14. Weiss L, Gilbert HA. Pulmonary Metastasis. Boston: GK Hall, 1978.
15. Hirata K, Nakata H, Naganawa T. CT of pulmonary metastases with pathological correlation. Semin Ultrasound CT MR 1995;16:379–394.
16. Zwirenwich CV, Vedal S, Miller RR. Solitary pulmonary nodule: high resolution CT and radiologic-pathologic correlation. Radiology 1991; 179:469–476.
17. Coppage L, Shaw C, McBride-Curtis A. Metastatic disease to the chest in patients with extrathoracic malignancy. J Thorac Imaging 1987;2:24–37.
18. Davis S. CT evaluation for pulmonary metastases in patients with extrathoracic malignancy. Radiology 1991;180:1–12.
19. Janower ML, Blennerhassett JB. Lymphangitic spread of metastatic cancer to the lung. Radiology 1971;101:267–273.
20. Marchevsky AM. Metastatic tumors of the lungs. Lung Biol Health Dis 1990;44:231–245.
21. Sadoff F, Grossman J, Weiner N. Lymphangitic pulmonary metastases secondary to breast cancer with normal chest x-rays and abnormal perfusion lung scans. Oncology 1975;31:164–171.
22. Morton DL, Joseph WL, Ketcham AS, Geelhoed GW, Adkins PC. Surgical resection and adjunctive immunotherapy for selected patients with multiple pulmonary metastases. Ann Surg 1973;178:360–365.
23. McCormack PM, Ginsberg KB, Bains MJ, et al. Accuracy of lung imaging in metastases with implications for the role of thoracoscopy. Ann Thorac Surg 1993;56:863–866.
24. Fuerstein IM, Jicha DL, Pass HI, et al. Pulmonary metastases: MR imaging with surgical correlation; a prospective study. Radiology 1992;182:123–129.
25. Rosenfield AT, Sanders RC, Custer LE. Widespread calcified metastases from adenocarcinoma of the jejunum. Am J Dig Dis 1975;20:990–993.
26. Panella J, Mintzer RA. Multiple calcified pulmonary nodules in an elderly man. JAMA 1980;244:2559–2560.
27. Gerle R, Felson B. Metastatic endobronchial hypernephroma. Chest 1963;44:225–233.
28. King DS, Castleman B. Bronchial involvement in metastatic pulmonary malignancy. J Thorac Surg 1943;12:305–315.
29. Braman SS, Whitcomb ME. Endobronchial metastases. Arch Intern Med 1975;135:543–547.
30. Sheperd MP. Endobronchial metastatic disease. Thorax 1982;37:362–370.
31. Dwyer AJ, Reichert CM, Woltering EA, Flye MW. Diffuse pulmonary metastasis in melanoma: radiologic pathologic correlation. AJR Am J Roentgenol 1984;143:983–984.
32. Roth JA, Pass HI, Wesley MN, White D, Putman JB, Seipp C. Comparison of median sternotomy and thoracotomy for resection of pulmonary metastases in patients with adult soft tissue sarcomas. Ann Thorac Surg 1986;42:134–138.

33. Pass HI, Dwyer MA, Makuchi R, Roth JA. Detection of pulmonary metastases in patients with osteogenic and soft tissue sarcoma: the superiority of CT scan compared with conventional linear tomograms using dynamic analyses. J Clin Oncol 1985;3:1261–1265.
34. Putman JB, Roth JA, Wesley MN, Johnston MR, Rosenberg SA. Survival aggressive resection of pulmonary metastases from osteogenic sarcoma analysis of prognostic factors. Ann Thorac Surg 1983;36:516–523.
35. Putman JB, Roth JA, Wesley MN, Johnston MR, Rosenberg SA. Analysis of prognostic factors in patients undergoing resection of pulmonary metastases for soft tissue sarcomas. J Thorac Cardiovasc Surg 1984; 87:260–268.
36. Mountain CF, McMurtrey MJ, Hermes KE. Surgery for pulmonary metastases: a 20-year experience. Ann Thorac Surg 1984;38:323–329.
37. Johnston WW. Percutaneous needle aspiration biopsy of 1015 patients. Acta Cytol 1984;28:218–224.
38. Nordenstrom BEW. Technical aspects of obtaining cellular material from lesions deep in the lung. Acta Cytol 1984;28:233–242.
39. Page RD, Jeffrey RR, Donnelly RJ. Thoracoscopy: a review of 121 consecutive surgical procedures. Ann Thorac Surg 1989;48:66–68.
40. Bonniot JP, Homasson JF, Roden SL, Angelbault ML, Renault PC. Pleural and lung cryobiopsies during thoracoscopy. Chest 1989;95:492–493.
41. Lewis RJ, Caccavale RJ, Sisler GE. Special report: video-endoscopic thoracic surgery. N J Med 1991;88:473–475.
42. Todd TR. Pulmonary metastasectomy: current indications for lung metastases. Chest 1993;103:4015–4035.
43. Matthay RA, Arroliga AC. Resection of pulmonary metastases. Am Rev Respir Dis 1993;148:1691–1696.
44. Vogt-Moykopf I, Bulzebruck H, Merkle NM, Probst G. Results of surgical treatment of pulmonary metastases. Eur J Cardiothorac Surg 1988;2: 224–232.
45. Jablons D, Steinberg SM, Roth J, Pittaluga S, Rosenberg SA, Pass HI. Metastasectomy for soft tissue sarcoma. J Thorac Cardiovasc Surg 1989; 97:695–705.
46. Pastrorino U, Valente M, Gasparini M, et al. Median sternotomy and multiple lung resections for metastatic sarcomas. Eur J Cardiothorac Surg 1990;4:477–481.
47. Lanza LA, Miser JS, Pass HI, Roth JA. The role of resection in the treatment of pulmonary metastases from Ewing's sarcoma. J Thorac Cardiovasc Surg 1987;94:181–187.
48. Putman JB, Suell DM, Natarajan G, Roth JA. Extended resection of pulmonary metastasectomy: is the risk justified? Ann Thorac Surg 1993; 55:1440–1446.
49. Telander RL, Pairolero PC, Pritchard DJ, Sim FH, Gilchrist GS. Resection of pulmonary metastatic osteogenic sarcoma in children. Surgery 1978; 84:335–341.
50. Lienard D, Rocman P, Lejeune FJ. Resection of lung metastases from sarcomas. Eur J Surg Oncol 1989;15:530–534.
51. Roth A, Putman JB, Wesley MN, Rosenberg SA. Differing determinants of prognosis following resection of pulmonary metastases from osteogenic and soft tissue sarcoma patients. Cancer 1985;55:1361–1366.
52. Meyer WH, Schell MJ, Jumar EP, et al. Thoracotomy for pulmonary metastatic osteosarcoma: an analysis of prognostic indicators of survival. Cancer 1987;59:374–379.
53. Goorin AM, Delorey MJ, Lack EE, et al. Prognostic significance of complete surgical resection of pulmonary metastases in patients with osteogenic sarcoma: analysis of 32 patients. J Clin Oncol 1984;2:425–431.
54. Carter SR, Grimer RJ, Sneath RS, Matthews H. Results of thoracotomy in osteogenic sarcoma with pulmonary metastases. Thorax 1991;46:727–731.
55. Fuller AF, Scannell JG, Wilkins EW. Pulmonary resection for metastases from gynecologic cancers, Massachusetts General Hospital experience; 1943–1982. Gynecol Oncol 1985;22:174–180.
56. Seki M, Nakagawa K, Tsuchiya S, et al. Surgical treatment of pulmonary metastases from uterine cervical cancer. J Thorac Cardiovasc Surg 1992; 104:876–881.
57. Levenback C, Rubin SC, McCormack PM, Haskins WJ, Atkinson EN, Lewis JL. Resection of pulmonary metastases from uterine sarcoma. Gynecol Oncol 1992;45:202–205.
58. Goya T, Miyazawa N, Kondo H, Tsuchiya R, Naruke T, Suesmasu K. Surgical resection of pulmonary metastases from colorectal cancer. Cancer 1989;64:1418–1421.
59. Mori M, Tomodo H, Ishida T, et al. Surgical resection of pulmonary metastases from colorectal adenocarcinoma. Arch Surg 1991;126:1297–1301.
60. McAbe MK, Aken MS, Trastek VF, Ilstrup DM, Deschamp PC, Pairolero PL. Colorectal lung metastases: results of surgical excision. Ann Thorac Surg 1992;53:780–786.
61. Saclarides TJ, Krueger BL, Szeluga DS, Warren WH, Faber LP, Economou SG. Thoracotomy for colon and rectal cancer metastases. Dis Colon Rectum 1993;36:425–429.
62. Pogrebriak HW, Stovroff M, Roth JA, Pass HI. Resection of pulmonary metastases from malignant melanoma: results of a 16-year experience. Ann Thorac Surg 1988;46:20–23.
63. Karp NS, Boyd A, De Pan HJ, et al. Thoracotomy for metastatic malignant melanoma. Surgery 1990;107:256–261.
64. Harpole DH, Johnson LM, Wolfe WG, et al. Analysis of 945 cases of pulmonary metastatic melanoma. J Thorac Cardiovasc Surg 1992;103: 743–750.
65. Gorenstein LA, Putman JB, Natarajan G, et al. Improved survival after resection of pulmonary metastases from malignant melanoma. Ann Thorac Surg 1991;52:204–210.
66. Flye MN, Woltering G, Rosenberg JA. Aggressive pulmonary resection for metastatic osteogenic and soft tissue sarcomas. Ann Thorac Surg 1984; 37:123–127.
67. Casson AG, Putman JB, Natarajan G, et al. Five-year survival after pulmonary metastasectomy for adult soft tissue sarcoma. Cancer 1992; 69:662–668.
68. Spanos PK, Payne WS, Ivins JC, Pritchard DJ. Pulmonary resection for metastatic osteogenic sarcoma. J Bone Joint Surg (Am) 1976;58:624–628.
69. Stewart JR, Carey JA, Merrill WH, Frist WH, Hamond JW, Bender HW. Twenty years experience with pulmonary metastasectomy. Am Surg 1992; 58:100–103.
70. Venn GE, Sarin S, Goldstraw P. Survival following pulmonary metastasectomy. Eur J Cardiothorac Surg 1989;3:105–110.
71. Ishida T, Kaneko S, Yokoyama H, et al. Metastatic lung tumors and extended indications for surgery. Int Surg 1992;77:173–177.
72. Joseph WI, Morton DL, Adkins PC. Prognostic significance of tumor doubling time in evaluating operability in pulmonary metastatic disease. J Thorac Cardiovasc Surg 1971;61:23–32.
73. Takita H, Edgerton F, Karakousis C, Douglass HO, Vincent RG, Beckey S. Surgical management of metastases to the lung. Surg Gynecol Obstet 1981;152:191–194.
74. Giritsky AS, Etcubanas E, Mark JBD. Pulmonary resection in children with osteogenic sarcoma: improved survival with surgery chemotherapy and irradiation. J Thorac Cardiovasc Surg 1978;75:354–361.
75. Roberts DG, Lepore V, Cardillo G, et al. Long-term follow-up of operative treatment for pulmonary metastases. Eur J Cardiothorac Surg 1989;3: 292–296.
76. Gadd MA, Casper ES, Woodruff JM, McCormack PM, Brennan MF. Development and treatment of pulmonary metastases in adult patients with extremity soft tissue sarcoma. Ann Surg 1993;218;705–712.

77. Huth JF, Holmes EC, Vernon SE, Callery CD, Ramming KP, Morton DL. Pulmonary resection for metastatic sarcoma. Am J Surg 1980;140:9–16.
78. Lanza LA, Putman JB Jr, Benjamin RS, Roth JA. Response to chemotherapy does not predict survival after resection of sarcomatous pulmonary metastases. Ann Thorac Surg 1991;51:219–224.
79. Carsky S, Ondrus D, Schnorrer M, Majek M. Germ cell testicular tumours with lung metastases: chemotherapy and surgical treatment. Int Urol Nephrol 1992;24:305–311.
80. Regal A-M, Reese P, Antkowiak J, Hart T, Takita H. Median sternotomy for metastatic lung lesions in 131 patients. Cancer 1985;55:1334–1339.
81. Cooper JD, Nelems JM, Pearson FG. Extended indications for median sternotomy in patients requiring pulmonary resection. Ann Thorac Surg 1978;26:413–419.
82. Pogrebniak HW, Pass HI. Initial and reoperative pulmonary metastasectomy: indications, technique, and results. Semin Surg Oncol 1993;9:142–149.
83. Pass HI. Treatment of metastatic cancer to the lung. In: De Vita VT, Hellman S, Rosenberg SA (eds) Principles and Practice of Oncology. Philadelphia: Lippincott, 1993;2186.
84. Bains MS, Ginsberg RJ, Jones WG II, et al. The clamshell incision: an improved approach to bilateral pulmonary and mediastinal tumors [abstract]. Ann Thorac Surg 1994;58:30–33.
85. Marcove RC, Mike V, Hajek JV, Levin AG, Hutter RVP. Osteogenic sarcoma under the age of twenty-one. Am J Bone Joint Surg 1970;52:411–423.
86. Guiliano AE, Feig S, Eilber FR. Changing metastatic patterns of osteosarcoma. Cancer 1984;54:2160–2164.
87. Pastorino U, Casparini M, Valente M, et al. Primary childhood osteosarcoma: the role of salvage surgery. Ann Oncol 1992;3:543–546.
88. Bacci G, Avella M, Picci P, Briccoli A, Dallari D, Campandacci M. Metastatic patterns in osteosarcoma. Tumori 1988;74:421–427.
89. Goorin AM, Shuster JJ, Baker A, Horowitz ME, Meyer WH, Link MP. Changing pattern of pulmonary metastases with adjuvant chemotherapy in patients with osteosarcoma: results from the multi-institutional osteosarcoma study. J Clin Oncol 1991;9:600–605.
90. Yamaguchi H, Nojima T, Yagi T, et al. The alteration in the pattern of pulmonary metastases with adjuvant chemotherapy in osteosarcoma. Int Orthop 1988;12:305–308.
91. Eckersberger F, Moritz E, Wolner E. Results and prognostic factors after resection of pulmonary metastases. Eur J Cardiothorac Surg 1988;2:433–437.
92. Martini N, McCormack PM, Bains MS, Beattie ES Jr. Surgery for solitary and multiple pulmonary metastases. NY State J Med 1978;78:1711–1713.
93. Creagen ET, Fleming TR, Edmonson JH, Pairolero PC. Pulmonary resection for metastatic nonosteogenic sarcoma. Cancer 1979;44:1908–1912.
94. Pogrebniak HW, Hass G, Linehan M, Rosenberg SA, Pass HI. Renal cell carcinoma: resection of solitary and multiple metastases. Ann Thorac Surg 1992;54:33–38.
95. Morrow CE, Vassilopoulos PP, Grace TB. Surgical resection of metastatic neoplasms of the lung: experience at the University of Minnesota Hospitals. Cancer 1980;45:2981–2985.
96. di Silverio F, Facciolo F, D'Eramo G, Lauretti S, Ricci C. Surgery of pulmonary metastases from renal and bladder carcinoma. Scand J Urol Nephrol 1991;138:215–218.
97. Cerfolio RJ, Allen MS, Deschamps C, et al. Pulmonary resection of metastatic renal cell carcinoma. Ann Thorac Surg 1994;57:339–344.
98. Li MC, Whitmore WF, Colbey R, Grabstald H. Effects of combined drug therapy on metastatic cancer of the testes. JAMA 1960;174:145–153.
99. Einhorn LH, Donohue J. Cis-diamine dichloroplatinum, vinblastine, and bleomycin combination chemotherapy in disseminated testicular cancer. Ann Intern Med 1977;87:293–298.
100. Einhorn LH, Williams SD, Mandelbaum I, Donohue JP. Surgical resection in disseminated testicular cancer following chemotherapeutic cytoreduction. Cancer 1981;48:904–908.
101. Mandelbaum I, Yaw PB, Einhorn LH, Williams SD, Rowland RG, Donohue JP. The importance of one-stage median sternotomy and retroperitoneal node dissection in disseminated testicular cancer. Ann Thorac Surg 1983;36:524–528.
102. Steyerberg EW, Keizer HJ, Zwartendijk J, et al. Prognosis of residual masses following chemotherapy for metastatic nonseminomatous testicular cancer: a multivariate analysis. Br J Cancer 1993;68:195–200.
103. McCormack PM, Martini N. The changing role of surgery for pulmonary metastases. Ann Thorac Surg 1979;41:833–840.
104. Mazer TM, Robbins KT, McMurtrey MJ, Byers RM. Resection of pulmonary metastases from squamous carcinoma of the head and neck. Am J Surg 1988;156:238–242.
105. McCormack PM, Attiyeh FF. Resected pulmonary metastases from colorectal cancer. Dis Colon Rectum 1979;22:553–556.
106. Gallandiuk S, Wieand HS, Moertel CG, et al. Patterns of recurrence after curative resection of carcinoma of the colon and rectum. Surg Gynecol Obstet 1992;174:27–32.
107. Turk PS, Wanebo HJ. Results of surgical treatment of nonhepatic recurrence of colorectal carcinoma. Cancer 1993;711:4267–4277.
108. Vincent RG, Choksi LB, Takita H, Guiterrez AL. Surgical resection of the solitary pulmonary metastasis. In: Weiss L, Gilbert HA (eds) Pulmonary Metastases. Boston: GK Hall, 1978;224.
109. Cahan WG, Castro EB, Hajou SI. The significance of a solitary lung shadow in patients with colon carcinoma. Cancer 1974;33:414–421.
110. Wilking N, Petrelli NJ, Herrera L, Regal AM, Mittelman A. Surgical resection of pulmonary metastases from colorectal adenocarcinoma. Dis Colon Rectum 1985;28:562–564.
111. Mansel JK, Zinsmeister AR, Pairolero PC, Jett JR. Pulmonary resection of metastatic colorectal adenocarcinoma: a 10-year experience. Chest 1986;89:109–112.
112. Brister SJ, Devarennes B, Gordon PH, Sheiner NM, Pym J. Contemporary operative management of pulmonary metastases of colorectal origin. Dis Colon Rectum 1988;31:786–792.
113. Pihl E, Hughes ES, McDermott FT, Johnson WR, Katrivessish H. Lung recurrence after curative surgery for colorectal cancer. Dis Colon Rectum 1987;30:417–419.
114. Smith JW, Fortner JG, Burt M. Resection of hepatic and pulmonary metastases from colorectal cancer. Surg Oncol 1992;1:399–404.
115. Yano T, Hara N, Ichinose Y, Yokoyama H, Miuro T, Ohta M. Results of pulmonary resection of metastatic colorectal cancer and its application. J Thorac Cardiovasc Surg 1993;106:875–879.
116. Ramming KP. Surgery for pulmonary metastases. Surg Clin North Am 1980;60:815–824.
117. Wright JO, Brandt B, Ehrenhaft JL. Results of pulmonary resection for metastatic lesions. J Thorac Cardiovasc Surg 1982;83:94–99.
118. Staren ED, Salerno C, Rongione A, Witt TR, Faber LP. Pulmonary resection for metastatic breast cancer. Arch Surg 1992;127:1282–1284.
119. McDonald ML, Deschamps C, Ilstrup DM, Allen MJ, Trastek VF, Pairolero PC. Pulmonary resection for metastatic breast cancer [poster]. Presented at the 30th Annual Meeting of the Society of Thoracic Surgeons, New Orleans, 1994.
120. Balch CM, Soong S, Murad TM, Smith JW, Maddox WA, Durant JR. A multifactorial analysis of melanoma. IV. Prognostic factors in 200 melanoma patients with distant metastases (stage III). J Clin Oncol 1983;1:126–134.

121. Winkler K. Surgical treatment of pulmonary metastases in childhood. J Thorac Cardiovasc Surg 1986;34:133–136.
122. Bacci G, Picci P, Briccoli A, et al. Osteosarcoma of the extremity metastatic at presentation: results achieved in 26 patients treated with combined therapy (primary chemotherapy followed by simultaneous resection of the primary and metastatic lesion). Tumori 1992;78:200–206.
123. Weh HJ, Zugel M, Wingberg D, et al. Chemotherapy of metastatic soft tissue sarcoma with a combination of adriamycin and DTIC or adriamycin and ifosfamide. Onkologie 1990;13:448–452.
124. Scotlandi K, Serra M, Nicoletti G, et al. Multidrug resistance and malignancy in human osteosarcoma. Cancer Res 1996;10:2434–2439.
125. Onda M, Matsuda S, Higaki S, et al. ErbB-2 expression is correlated with poor prognosis for patients with osteosarcoma. Cancer 1996;77:71–78.
126. Johnston MR, Michen RF, Dawson CA. Lung perfusion with chemotherapy in patients with unresectable metastatic sarcoma to the lung or diffuse bronchoalveolar carcinoma. J Thorac Cardiovasc Surg 1995;110:368–373.
127. Pass HI, Mew DJ, Kranda KC, et al. Isolated lung perfusion with tumor necrosis factor for pulmonary metastases. Ann Thorac Surg 1996; 61:1609–1617.
128. Weksler B, Ng B, Lenert JT, Burt ME. Isolated single-lung perfusion with doxorubicin is pharmacokinetically superior to intravenous injection. Ann Thorac Surg 1993;56:209–214.
129. Weksler B, Schneider A, Ng B, Burt ME. Isolated single lung perfusion in the rat: an experimental model. J Appl Physiol 1993;74:2736–2739.
130. Weksler B, Lenert JT, Ng B, Burt M. Isolated single lung perfusion with doxorubicin is effective in eradicating soft tissue sarcoma lung metastases in a rat model. J Thorac Cardiovasc Surg 1994;107:50–54.

Section 4

Breast Cancer

CHAPTER 21

Abnormal Mammography

KAMBIZ DOWLATSHAHI

A. Screening Mammography

Screening mammography for the early detection of breast cancer became the Papanicolaou smear of the 1990s. Sixty-five percent of women age 40–50 years and 55% over age 50 years undergo annual mammography in the United States.[1] The general acceptance of screening is based on long-term follow-up studies showing that patients whose cancer was detected solely with mammograms have a 30% reduction in mortality.[2,3] The disadvantage of screening mammography is its low positive predictive value (20–25%),[4,5] which means that when the indication for biopsy is an abnormal mammogram 75–80% of women undergo unnecessary surgical biopsy, a significant physical, emotional, and financial disincentive.

Image-guided breast biopsy techniques (principally stereotactic and ultrasonographic) in conjunction with various needle-like devices have been instrumental in introducing minimally invasive procedures. This approach enables the surgeon or radiologist to obtain highly accurate information regarding the nonpalpable breast lesion at much less discomfort to the patient and cost to the payer.

Despite these advances, the primary question concerning the patient and the physician alike is unchanged: Is the mammographic abnormality cancer? A secondary question concerns in situ versus invasive histology, a subject that has gained significance in terms of subsequent surgical management. For example, if the mammographic abnormality proves to be an in situ carcinoma, the patient is likely to undergo wire localization and excisional biopsy. On the other hand, if the lesion is invasive cancer, lumpectomy and sentinel node biopsy as a one-step operation is considered.

B. Abnormal Mammogram

An abnormal mammogram is defined as a breast image containing a mass or microcalcifications, parenchymal distortion, dilated ducts, or skin thickening. Any of these findings may be noted on the screening mammogram of an asymptomatic woman or they may be associated with pain, nipple discharge, or a palpable mass.

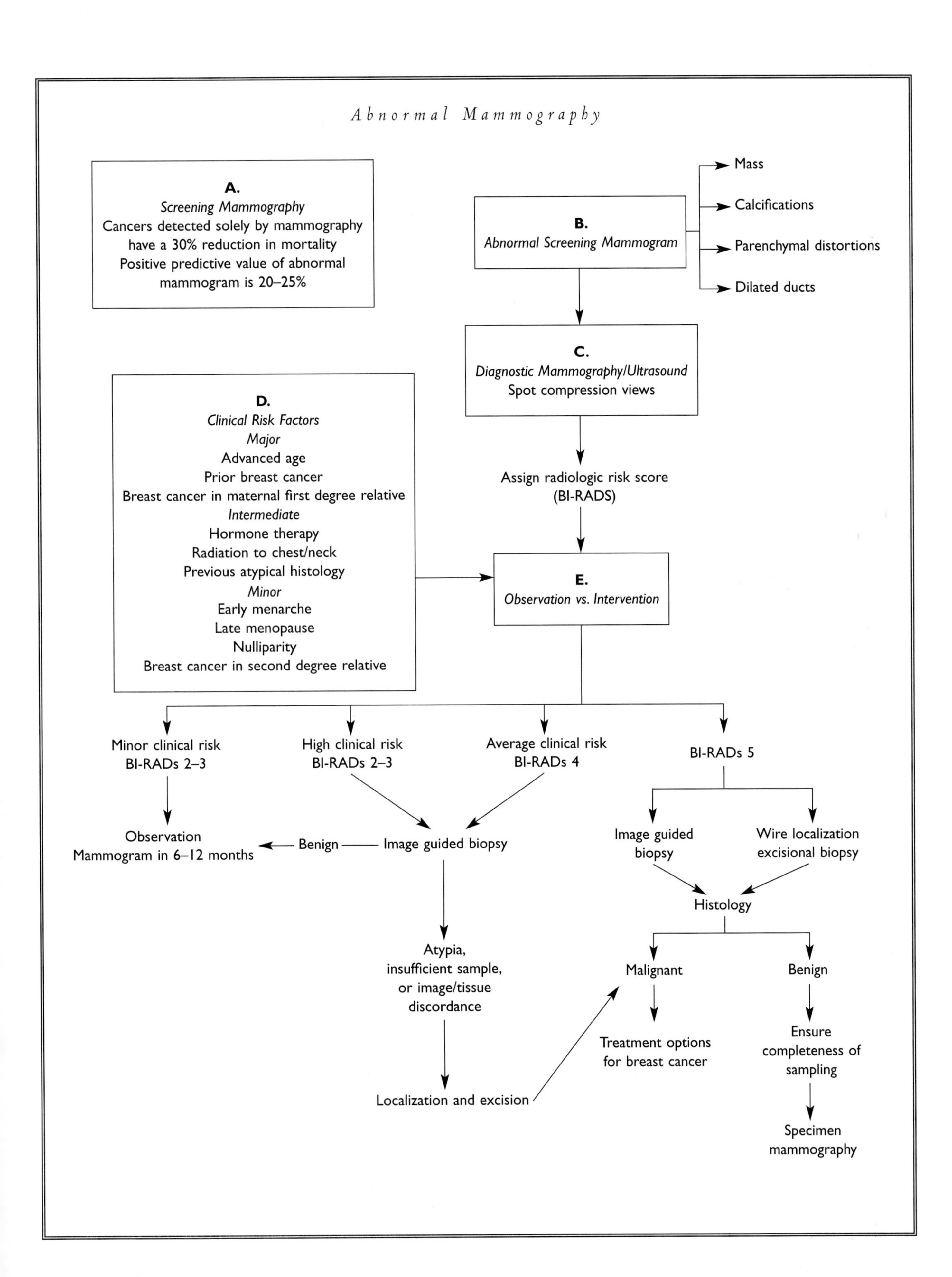

Abnormal Mammography
A.
Screening Mammography
Cancers detected solely by mammography have a 30% reduction in mortality
Positive predictive value of abnormal mammogram is 20–25%
B.
Abnormal Screening Mammogram
Mass
Calcifications
Parenchymal distortions
Dilated ducts
C.
Diagnostic Mammography/Ultrasound
Spot compression views
D.
Clinical Risk Factors
Major
Advanced age
Prior breast cancer
Breast cancer in maternal first degree relative
Intermediate
Hormone therapy
Radiation to chest/neck
Previous atypical histology
Minor
Early menarche
Late menopause
Nulliparity
Breast cancer in second degree relative
Assign radiologic risk score (BI-RADS)
E.
Observation vs. Intervention
Minor clinical risk BI-RADs 2–3
High clinical risk BI-RADs 2–3
Average clinical risk BI-RADs 4
BI-RADs 5
Observation Mammogram in 6–12 months
Benign
Image guided biopsy
Image guided biopsy
Wire localization excisional biopsy
Histology
Atypia, insufficient sample, or image/tissue discordance
Malignant
Benign
Treatment options for breast cancer
Ensure completeness of sampling
Localization and excision
Specimen mammography

Mass Lesions

The following features of a mass lesion should be noted and recorded in a consistent fashion.

Location: consider the breast as the face of a clock when describing it
Size: measured in millimeters
Shape: round or oval, for example
Borders: lobular, ill-defined, jagged
Density: hyperdense, for example

Calcifications

Calcifications represent a common mammographic abnormality. The following features should be noted.

Location: quadrant of the breast, for example
Size: micro, macro
Shape: round, linear, branching
Distribution: focal, segmental, uni- or bilateral (Fig. 21–1)

Parenchymal Densities

Soft tissue densities may be characterized as diffuse (e.g., in young women with dense fibroglandular parenchyma or in postmenopausal women receiving hormone therapy). Unilateral density is seen in patients with edema due to irradiation, infection, or inflammatory carcinoma. Segmental/asymmetric density is seen in a normal involutional breast.

Tissue Distortions/Dilated Ducts

Tissue distortions and dilated ducts are seen in previously operated breasts, early breast cancer, or fibrocystic changes such as radial scar. Figure 21–1 illustrates common mammographic abnormalities and associated risk factors for cancer.

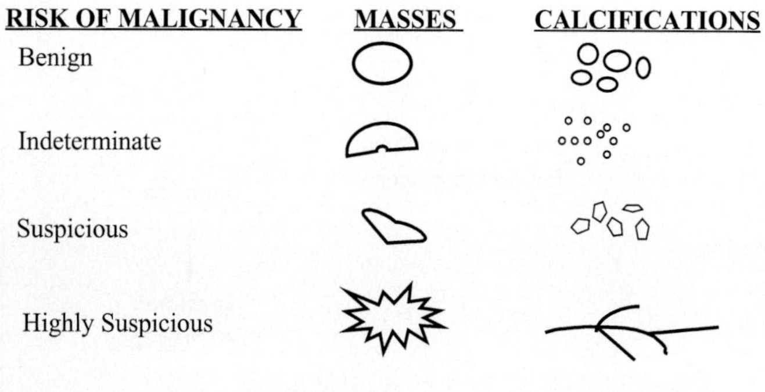

RISK OF MALIGNANCY — MASSES — CALCIFICATIONS
Benign
Indeterminate
Suspicious
Highly Suspicious

FIGURE 21–1
Mammographic masses and calcifications as related to the risk of malignancy.

NOTE: When evaluating a mammographic abnormality to determine its risk for malignancy, it is important to compare the current films with previous images to detect change or stability.

C. Diagnostic Mammography Workup

Additional imaging procedures are needed to determine whether a *screening* mammographic abnormality is benign or malignant. *Diagnostic* mammography and ultrasonography are the imaging modalities used for this purpose, and the following steps are taken.

1. Spot compression of ill-defined masses
2. Spot compression magnification of calcifications
3. Open field magnification of segmentally distributed calcifications
4. Ultrasound examination to differentiate between solid and cystic lesions and to characterize solid lesions further
5. Ninety-degree views to identify milk of calcium in small breast cysts

Magnetic resonance imaging (MRI) and mammoscintigraphy are other diagnostic modalities increasingly employed for a patient with a dense fibroglandular pattern. MRI requires a breast coil and is useful in the following instances: detecting tumor recurrence in a breast previously treated with surgery and irradiation, demonstrating multicentricity, or searching for an occult primary lesion in a patient with metastatic adenocarcinoma in an axillary node.[6,7] Mammoscintigraphy is a relatively new procedure: Technetium-99m sestamibi, a nonspecific radiolabeled colloid solution, is injected intravenously prior to scanning the breast. This procedure has low sensitivity for tumors <1 cm in diameter.[8]

Having completed the diagnostic workup, one may assign a risk score to the lesion for its probability of malignancy. In 1996 the American College of Radiology proposed a system known as BI-RADS (Breast Imaging Reporting and Data Systems), shown in Table 21–1.

D. Clinical Risk Factors

Personal and family history, careful physical examination, and the psychological makeup of the patient are important components for determining whether the patient with a mammographic abnormality should be kept under surveillance or undergo biopsy. *Major risk factors* are advanced age, previous history of breast cancer or carcinoma in situ, and a history of premenopausal breast cancer in a first-degree maternal relative. *Intermediate risk factors* include age 50–60, hormone replacement

TABLE 21–1.
Breast Imaging Reporting and Data System (BI-RADS) of the American College of Radiology

Category	Assessment	Description and management recommendation
0	Incomplete	Needs additional workup (e.g., spot compression or ultrasonography) prior to assigning final assessment.
1	Negative	There is nothing on which to comment. Routine screening.
2	Benign finding: negative	Definitely benign finding described. Routine screening.
3	Probably benign finding	High probability of being benign. *Short-term follow-up (usually 6 months) to establish stability.*
4	Suspicious abnormality	Not characteristic but has reasonable probability of being malignant. *Biopsy is urged.*
5	Highly suggestive of malignancy	High probability of being cancer. *Appropriate action should be taken.*

SOURCE: Adapted from the American College of Radiology Breast Imaging Reporting and Data System (BI-RADS).

therapy, prior irradiation of the chest and neck, and a previous breast biopsy with atypia. *Minor risk factors* consist of early menarche, late menopause, nulliparity, and breast cancer in a second-degree family member (Table 21–2).

E. *Observation Versus Intervention*

At this point in the overall assessment of the patient for breast cancer, one must combine the imaging risk score with the clinical risks for malignancy and arrive at a decision.

Observation

As a general rule, patients with slight clinical risk factors and mammographic lesions of BI-RADS scores of 2 and 3 may be followed with mammography every 6–12 months. Examples of probably benign mammographic lesions are well defined, round or oval masses (especially if the abnormality is noted for the first time), mass-like lesions proven to be simple cysts by ultrasonography, and nonclustered round microcalcifications. The author's personal series of 1250 cases and those in other reports[9] indicate that the incidence of malignancy in probably benign mammographic lesions is 1–2%. Approximately 20% of all abnormal mammograms fall into this category (i.e., definitely or probably benign) (Table 21–2).

Intervention

Patients with a BI-RADS score of 2 or 3 and high risk clinical factors and patients with BI-RADS 4 lesions of all clinical risk backgrounds should undergo image-guided breast biopsy to rule out malignancy (Table 21–2). This intermediate group accounts for approximately 50% of all abnormal mammograms.

Patients with mammographic abnormalities of BI-RADS 5 regardless of clinical risk background, should undergo (1) image-guided breast biopsy to rule in malignancy prior to definitive treatment or (2) wire localization and excisional biopsy. This high suspicion group accounts for 30% of all mammographic abnormalities (Fig. 21–2).

There are two common imaging technologies—stereotactic and ultrasonographic—used with various biopsy devices to obtain tissue samples from suspicious, nonpalpable breast lesions. Wire localization/excisional biopsy is the conventional technique against which stereotactic or ultrasound-guided needle biopsies are judged.

Stereotactic Breast Biopsy

The concept of breast stereotactic biopsy was developed in Sweden and was introduced to the United States in 1986.[10–13] Briefly, the stereotactic device consists of a table top on which the patient lies in a prone position, with the breast suspended through an opening and immobilized by a compression plate against an image receptor. The breast position is adjusted so the suspicious lesion is seen through a 5 × 5 cm window on the compression plate. Two images of the lesion at 30° angles are obtained (Fig. 21–3). Using the triangulation principle, the location of the lesion in the breast is calculated by a computer, which determines the direction and depth of the sampling needle.

TABLE 21–2.
Clinical risk factors for breast cancer in asymptomatic women

Low risk
Age < 50 years
Nulliparous
Family history: second-degree maternal relative with breast cancer
Intermediate risk
Age 50–60 years
Hormone therapy
Prior radiation to the chest/neck
Prior atypical breast pathology
High risk
Age > 60 years
Prior breast cancer or in situ lesion
First-degree relative with breast cancer

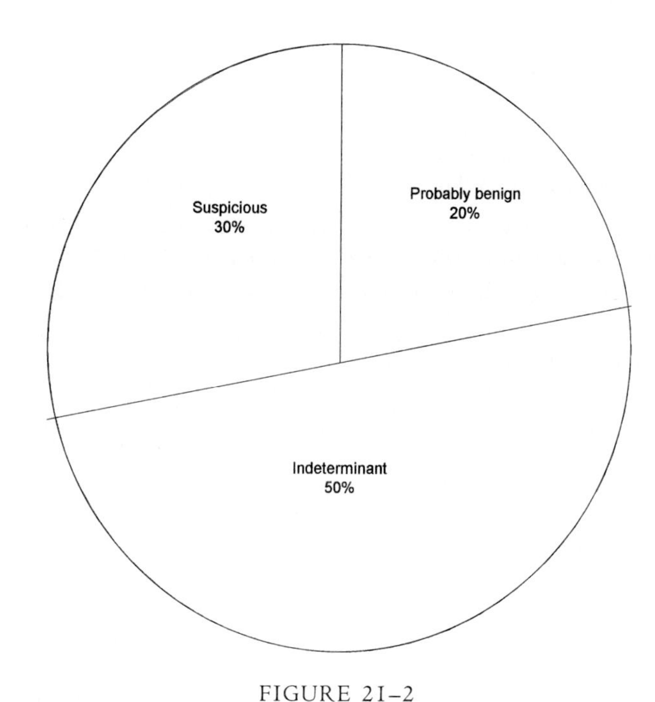

FIGURE 21–2
Distribution of mammographic abnormalities according to histologic findings in 1250 cases.

Since the introduction of digital mammography in 1993, image acquisition is faster than with the film screening technique. Additionally, the image may be processed to obtain optimal visualization of the lesion. Under local anesthesia the sampling needle is introduced into the breast with stereotactic guidance. Multiple samples are obtained with radiographic confirmation of the needle traversing the lesion. If the suspected lesion has calcifications, specimen mammograms are obtained by the device to confirm the presence of calcifications in the core samples. Stereotactic breast biopsy is a minimally morbid outpatient procedure that usually takes 30–45 minutes to perform.

Ultrasonography

The application of breast ultrasonography by surgeons and radiologists has rapidly increased. Ultrasonography is employed diagnostically to detect cystic breast lesions and therapeutically to guide needles for core biopsies and to drain cysts. It is also utilized for wire localization prior to excisional breast biopsy. Ultrasound devices are less expensive than stereotactic instruments and are easier to use. However, if the indication for tissue sampling is the presence of abnormal calcifications, the procedure is best performed by stereotactic means.

Fine-Needle Aspiration Cytology

Stereotactic fine-needle aspiration (FNA) is not widely used in the United States because it provides insufficient tissue for diagnosis in 10–20% of cases and because experienced cytopathologists are not present at all medical centers. FNA is a simple technique, easy to learn, and inexpensive. It is employed in conjunction with ultrasonography to sample complex cysts and small nonpalpable, ultrasonographically visible solid tumors such as intramammary lymph nodes.

Core-Needle Biopsy

Automated spring-loaded core-needle biopsy is a widely used device for obtaining tissue samples from patients with an abnormal mammogram. Fourteen-gauge needles are inserted under stereotactic or ultrasound guidance. Several reports indicate the diagnostic accuracy to be comparable to wire localization/excisional biopsy.[14–17] The associated complications are a less than 1% incidence of hematoma and infection.

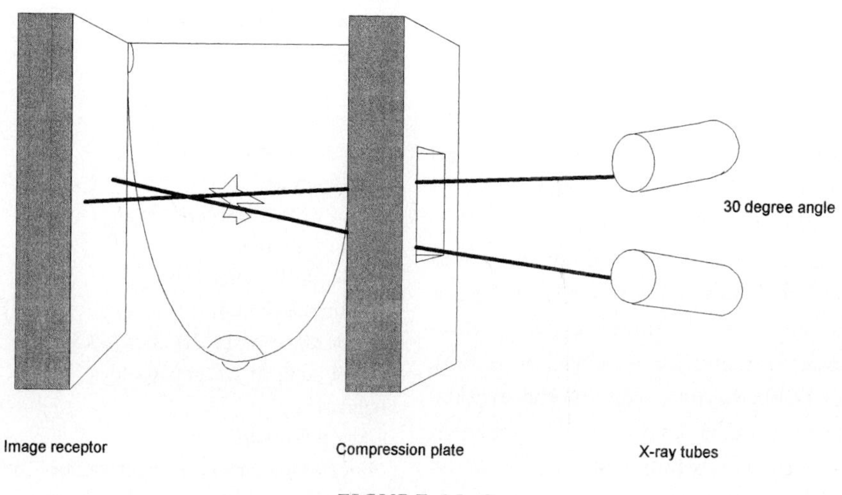

FIGURE 21–3
Method of stereotaxis.

TABLE 21–3.
Comparative evaluation of four commonly used diagnostic procedures after an abnormal mammogram

Parameter	Fine needle	Core needle	Vacuum assisted	Automated excision
Accuracy (%)	80–90	98	98	99
Complications (%)	0	0.1	0.5	1.0
Expenses	$10	$30	$250	$500
Utility	Simple	Intermediate	Intermediate	Complex

Vacuum-Assisted Biopsy

Specially designed needles with a suction and cutting mechanism applied to their sampling chamber are being increasingly used in lieu of spring-loaded needle devices. The advantages are as follows.

1. Usually only one insertion is made into the breast.

2. Tissue samples are large; therefore the pathologist may differentiate in situ from invasive carcinoma, which is advantageous for treatment planning.

The diagnostic accuracy is 98%, with hematoma and infection occurring in fewer than 1% of patients.[18,19] Vacuum-assisted needles can be used with a stereotactic table; their application with ultrasonography may become available in the future.

Automated Cannula Devices

Automated biopsy devices, such as automated breast biopsy instrumentation (ABBI) allow removal of the suspicious breast lesion in one piece, enabling the pathologist to make a full evaluation and diagnosis. These devices are used in conjunction with a stereotactic table and require sterile conditions and a skin incision measuring 5–25 mm.[20] The four diagnostic procedures are compared in Table 21–3.

One must select the technology and tools most suitable for evaluating a mammographic lesion. As a general rule, mammographic mass lesions that are also visualized by ultrasonography may be approached with ultrasound-guided needle biopsy.

Microcalcifications and asymmetric densities are suitable for stereotactic techniques employing a vacuum-assisted or core-needle device. The automated or manual cannula devices employed with the stereotactic table may be used for both masses and calcifications. Wire localization/excisional biopsy still has a place in the management of breast lesions located in the far posterior aspect of the breast, near the axilla, or behind the nipple or when the image-guided sample is inadequate for definitive diagnosis.

Pathology

Cytology

Several earlier reports from Europe and specialized centers in the United States have shown that the accuracy of stereotactic FNA exceeds 90%.[21–23] Some investigators from general community hospitals, however, have reported unacceptably low accuracy and adequacy of sampling.[24] The advantages of FNA are its simplicity, low cost, and availability. FNA is still utilized in conjunction with ultrasonography for the diagnosis of breast masses and cystic lesions.

Histology

Core-needle samples retrieved from a mammographic lesion should be sent for histologic evaluation in 10% formalin solution. Because of artifacts, frozen section is not advisable unless extra samples from a closely targeted area of the breast are obtained. An average of 5 core samples from mass/soft tissue lesions and 8–10 samples from microcalcification targets are deemed adequate. Postbiopsy imaging of the target area in the breast and specimen mammograms of the cores in the case of microcalcifications are essential to document correct sampling. The size and volume of samples from vacuum-assisted probes are twice as large as those retrieved by core-needle biopsy, providing the pathologist more tissue for correct staging (in situ versus invasive) and more precise determination of prognostic factors in case of malignancy. Even larger needles (11 gauge instead of 14 gauge) have now been introduced.[25] Tissue samples obtained by a cannula employing an automated large biopsy device gives the pathologist an even larger piece of tissue in one core instead of multiple cores, allowing easier orientation and more accurate determination of margin involvement. As only 20–25% of mammographic abnormalities are malignant, this technique may not be justified because it is more invasive, expensive, and complex. The following guidelines, as depicted in Table 21–4 may be followed when interpreting the pathology report.

1. Patients with probably benign mammographic abnormalities (BI-RADS 2 and 3) and a definitive histologic diagnosis of fibroadenoma or benign lymph node may be followed at 12-month intervals. In the same patient with an insufficient sample report, the postbiopsy images should be reevaluated for correct needle placement. Repeat biopsy or a shorter follow-up (6 months) is advised.

2. Patients with mammographic BI-RADS 2 and 3 lesions and core samples revealing atypia, lobular carcinoma in situ, or frank malignancy should undergo wire localization/excisional biopsy for full evaluation.

TABLE 21–4.
Image–tissue correlation and management

Mammography (BI-RADS)	Ultrasonography	Core-needle biopsy	Plan
2, 3	Benign	Benign/ insufficient	Mammography in 6–12 months
2, 3	Benign	Atypical, in situ, cancer	Localize and excise
4	Indeterminate	Benign	Mammography in 6 months
4	Indeterminate	Atypical	Localize and excise
5	Malignant	Benign/atypical/ insufficient	Localize and excise
4, 5	Malignant	Cancer	Discuss cancer treatment

3. For patients with indeterminate mammographic and sonographic images and definitely benign histology, diagnostic mammograms should be obtained in 6 months. However, those with indeterminate images and atypical histology should undergo excisional biopsy.

4. Patients with highly suspicious mammographic and ultrasound images and a needle biopsy confirming malignancy have the opportunity to discuss and plan one-step surgery. If the needle biopsy report is benign, atypical, or insufficient in a BI-RADS 5 lesion, wire localization and excision should be undertaken. This is a relatively uncommon situation that may occur in a patient with a radial scar or who underwent irradiation following previous lumpectomy.

Conclusions

Because management of patients with abnormal mammograms is multidisciplinary, it is important that one person collates the data, coordinates the diagnostic steps, communicates the results to physicians and the patient, and supervises the follow-up.

References

1. American Cancer Society Cancer Risk Report: Prevention and Control. 1998:24.
2. Shapiro S. Periodic Screening for Breast Cancer: The Health Insurance Plan Project and Its Sequelae, 1963–1986. Baltimore: Johns Hopkins University Press, 1988.
3. Tabar L, Vitak B, Chen HH, et al. The Swedish Two-County Trial twenty years later. Updated mortality results and new insights from long-term follow-up. Radiol Clin North Am 2000;38(4);625–651.
4. Hall FM, Storella JM, Silverstone DZ, Wyshak G. Nonpalpable breast lesions: recommendations for biopsy based on suspicion of carcinoma at mammography. Radiology 1988;167:353–358.
5. Yankaskas BC, Knelson MH, Abernetty ML, et al. Needle localization biopsy of occult lesions of the breast: experience in 199 cases. Invest Radiol 1988;23:729–733.
6. Fischer U, Kopka L, Grabbe E. Magnetic resonance guided localization and biopsy of suspicious breast lesions. Top Magn Reson Imaging 1998;9(1):44–59.
7. Davis PL, McCarty KS Jr. Sensitivity of enhanced MRI for the detection of breast cancer: new, multi-center, residual and recurrent. Eur Radiol 1997; 7(suppl):289–298.
8. Khalkhali I, Iraniha S, Diggles LE, et al. Scintimammography: the new role of technetium-99m sestamibi imaging for the diagnosis of breast carcinoma. Q J Nucl Med 1997;41:231–238.
9. Sickles EA. Periodic mammographic follow-up of probably benign lesions: results in 3184 consecutive cases. Radiology 1991;179:463–468.
10. Bolmgren J, Jacobson B, Nordenstrom R. Stereotaxic instrument for needle biopsy of the mamma. Am J Radiol 1977;129:121–125.
11. Nordenstrom B, Azjicek J. Stereotaxic needle biopsy and preoperative indication of nonpalpable mammary lesions. Acta Cytol 1977;21:350–351.
12. Svane G. Stereotaxic needle biopsy of nonpalpable breast lesion: a clinical and radiological follow-up. Acta Radiol Diagn 1983;24:385–390.
13. Dowlatshahi K, Jokich PM, Schmidt R, et al. Diagnosis of occult breast lesions using stereotaxic needle cytology. Arch Surg 1987;122:1343–1346.
14. Elvecrog EL, Lechner MC, Nelson MT. Nonpapable breast lesions: correlation of stereotaxic large core needle biopsy and surgical biopsy results. Radiology 1993;188:453–455.
15. Parker SH, Burbank F, Jackman RJ, et al. Percutaneous large core breast biopsy: a multi-institutional study. Radiology 1994;193:359–364.
16. Meyer JE, Smith DN, Lester SC, et al. Large-core needle biopsy of nonpalpable breast lesions. JAMA 1999;281:1638–1641.
17. Jackman RJ, Nowels KW, Shepard JR, et al. Stereotactic large-core needle biopsy of 450 nonpalpable breast lesions with surgical correlation in lesions with cancer or atypical hyperplasia. Radiology 1994;193:91–95.
18. Jackman RJ, Burbank F, Parker SH, et al. Atypical ductal hyperplasia diagnosed at stereotactic breast biopsy: improved reliability with 14-gauge, directional vacuum-assisted biopsy. Radiology 1997;204:485–488.
19. Bernstein JR. Role of stereotactic breast biopsy. Semin Surg Oncol 1996; 12:290–299.
20. Kelley WE Jr, Bailey R, Bertelsen C, et al. Stereotactic automated surgical biopsy using the ABBI biopsy device: a multicenter study. Breast J 1998; 4:302–306.
21. Gent HJ, Sprenger E, Dowlatshahi K. Stereotaxic needle localization and cytological diagnosis of occult breast lesions. Ann Surg 1986;204:580–584.

22. Azavedo E, Svane G, Aver G. Stereotactic fine-needle biopsy in 2594 mammographically detected non-palpable lesions. Lancet 1989;8446: 1033–1036.
23. Mitnick JS, Vazquez MF, Roses DF, et al. Stereotaxic localization for fine needle aspiration breast biopsy: initial experience with 300 patients. Arch Surg 1991;126:1137–1140.
24. Jackson P, Reynolds HE. Stereotaxic needle-core biopsy and fine needle aspiration cytologic evaluation of nonpalpable breast lesions. Radiology 1991;181:633–634.
25. Lieberman L, Smolkin JH, Dershaw DD, et al. Calcification retrieval at stereotactic, 11 gauge, directional, vacuum-assisted breast biopsy. Radiology 1998;208:251–260.

Chapter 22

Carcinoma In Situ

THEODORE N. TSANGARIS

A. Epidemiology and Etiology

No cancer from any site provokes more diverging intellectual and emotional responses or calms and unsettles people like ductal carcinoma in situ (DCIS). Its various names—ductal carcinoma in situ, noninvasive ductal carcinoma, preinvasive ductal carcinoma—provide a glimpse into its controversy. Four factors contribute to its controversial nature. First and foremost is its relatively unknown biologic behavior. Second is the increasing incidence of the disease despite the fact that not all consider this entity to be cancer. Third, the true natural history of the disease is uncertain. Finally, the best management for the disease, given its excellent prognosis regardless of treatment regimen, is not clear. We may find that the disease is truly heterogeneous not because of its own intrinsic properties but because of the human host in whom it presents. We may also find that we are better served treating the patient and not the disease.

The concept of in situ cancer was first proposed by Broders,[1] who attempted to define a transition between benign and malignant epithelium. Abnormal cells confined to their original boundaries is a property associated with in situ cancers at all organ sites. In 1941 Foote and Stewart[2] applied the term "*in situ*" to lobular carcinoma in situ; they considered it in an intermediate state between normal epithelium and invasive malignant disease. Progression to cancer was considered unavoidable, and aggressive treatment seemed an obvious course of action for the surgeon.

Over the years, as the incidence of DCIS has increased, we have been forced to reevaluate our earlier concepts of the biology, malignant potential, and treatment of the disease. This increased incidence clearly parallels the increased utilization of screening mammography, which frequently detects the disease in asymptomatic individuals.[3,4] Swansen et al.[5] reported that the incidence of DCIS increased 213% in Caucasians and 153% in African-Americans between 1983 and 1989. DCIS accounts for 30–40% of mammographically detected breast cancers.[6–8] Ernster et al.[9] analyzed data on DCIS reported to the National Cancer Institute's Surveillance, Epidemiology, and End Results (SEER) program between 1973 and 1992. They noted an increase in DCIS incidence beginning during the early 1980s. The average annual increases in rates between 1973 and 1983 and between 1983 and 1992 changed

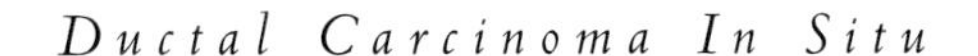

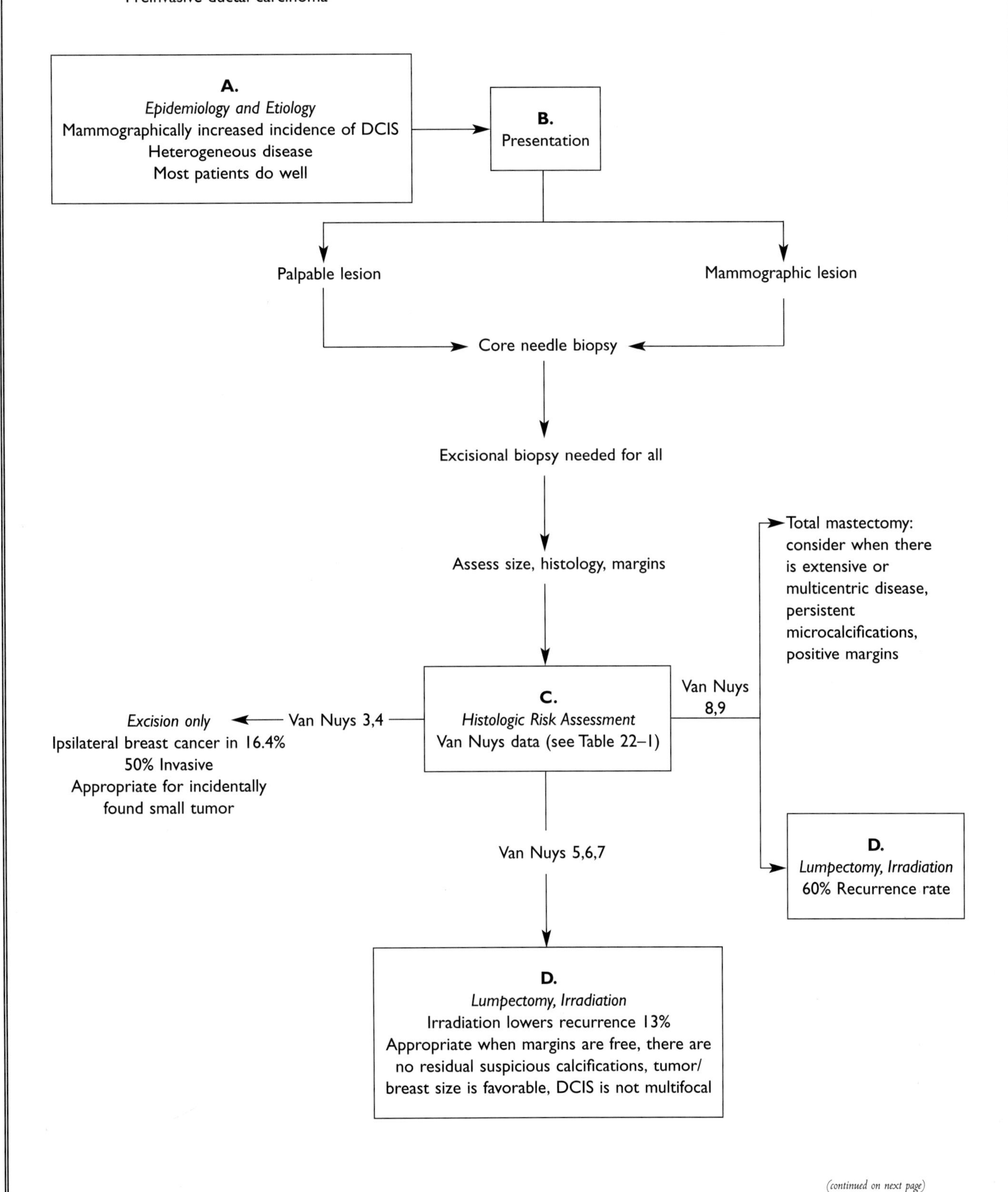

(continued on next page)

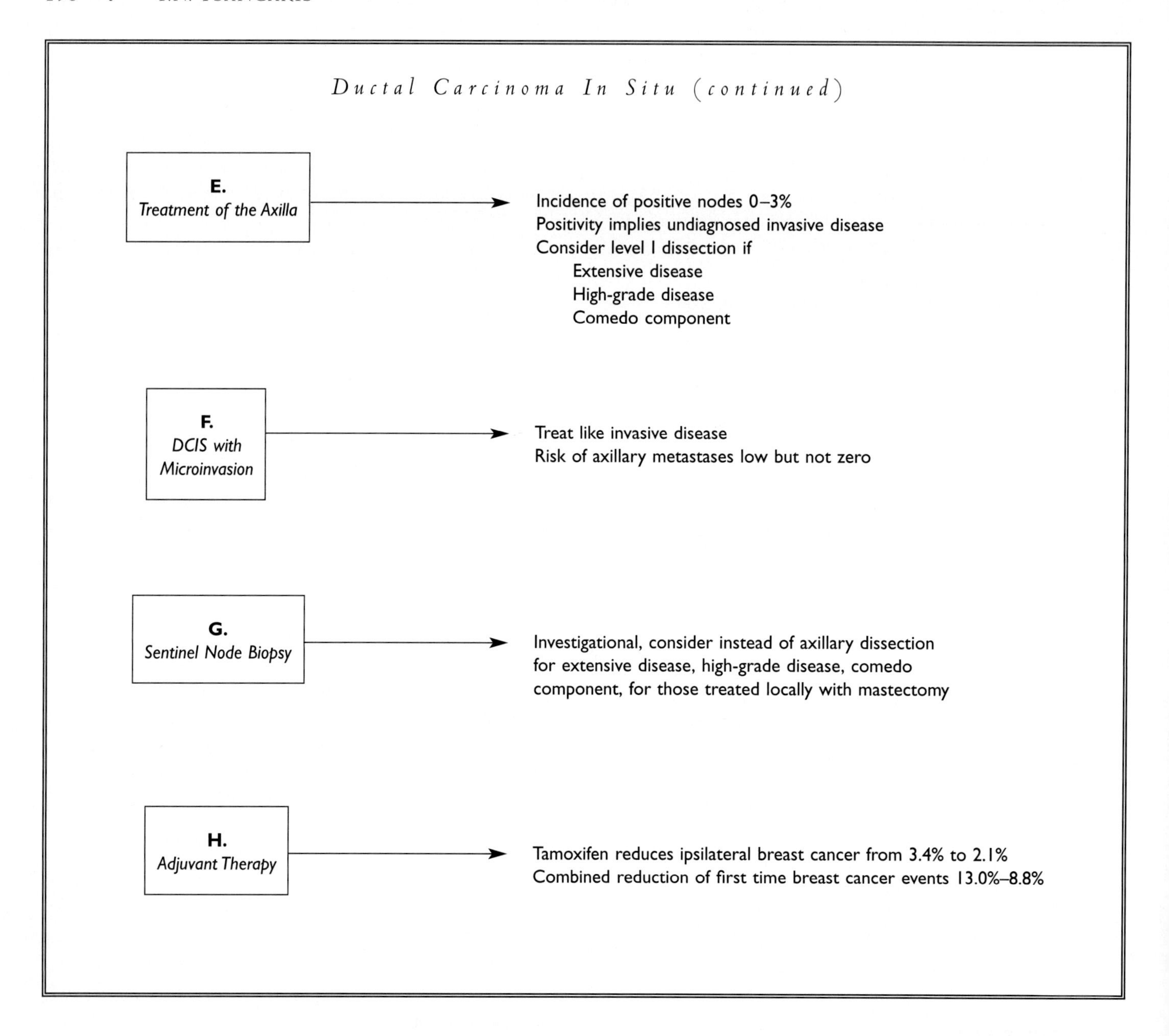

from 0.3% to 12.0% among women aged 30–39 years, from 0.4% to 17.4% among women aged 40–49 years, and from 5.2% to 18.1% among women aged 50 years or older. In 1999 more than 36,000 new cases of DCIS were diagnosed in the United States.[10]

B. Presentation

As the incidence of DCIS increased, its presentation changed. Initially, DCIS was a disease that presented clinically as a palpable lesion.[11–13] After 1985 it was more likely to be asymptomatic and discovered mammographically.[6–8] Treatment is determined by the initial presentation, method of diagnosis, and extent of disease. DCIS within a palpable lesion may be diagnosed by excisional or core biopsy; the same is true for mammographically discovered lesions. Ultimately, complete excision is needed to assess important factors, such as size, histology, margins, and the presence of residual disease.[14]

Previously, mastectomy was the treatment of choice for DCIS,[9] whereas breast conservation is preferred today. This transition has been a slow process, paradoxically lagging behind the change in surgical treatment seen for invasive cancer. This is probably because of two factors: uncertainty of the natural history of the disease and the desire to eradicate the disease completely in the name of a 100% cure. Both of these reasons are poor excuses for promoting mastectomy.

There have been many reports of retrospective and small prospective studies on the utility of breast conservation with or without radiation therapy for DCIS,[15–24] but it was the National Surgical Adjuvant Breast and Bowel Project (NSABP) B-17 study that showed the utility of this approach in a large, prospective fashion.

Gump at Columbia-Presbyterian was one of the first physicians to suggest that the treatment of DCIS might be individualized based on the clinical and histologic presentation[25]: Gross DCIS could be treated with mastectomy or lumpectomy plus irradiation, and microscopic disease found incidentally could be watched or treated in several ways.

C. Histologic Risk Assessment and Treatment

Much has changed since the above treatment was proposed during the mid-1980s. Silverstein et al.[26] and Lagios et al.[27] carefully studied DCIS in patients treated at the Van Nuys Breast Center in California, and in 1995 they introduced their classification (Van Nuys pathologic classification). This system is based on nuclear grade and the presence or absence of comedo-type necrosis.[26] A high nuclear grade is associated with a worse prognosis regardless of whether comedo-type necrosis is present. Low-grade DCIS is subclassified into two groups, depending on the presence or absence of comedo necrosis. In 394 patients treated with breast conservation, the probability of local recurrence was greatest for high-grade lesions followed by low-grade lesions with comedo necrosis and then low-grade lesions without comedo necrosis. This phenomenon has been observed in other series.[27–35]

Combining the Van Nuys pathologic classification with tumor size and margin width produced the Van Nuys prognostic index (VNPI)[36–39] (Table 22–1). Tumor size and margin width are important prognostic factors and provide information on the extent of disease.[39] This is important when discussing treatment options. The VNPI assigns a score ranging from 1 to 3 for tumor size, margin, and pathologic classification; the sum is the prognostic index score. Treatment options may be suggested using the VNPI. A tumor with a score of 3 or 4 suggests that excision alone is appropriate. A score of 5, 6, or 7 implies that the patient would benefit from irradiation. A score of 8 or 9 suggests a definite benefit from irradiation, with mastectomy also strongly considered for this group.

As of 1997, a total of 394 patients had been followed for local recurrence-free survival utilizing the VNPI.[39] Those with low scores (3 or 4) had low local recurrence rates, and irradiation was of little benefit when given after excision. Patients with intermediate scores (5, 6, 7) appeared to benefit from irradiation; a 13% average decrease in local recurrence rate in irradiated patients was seen when compared to the excision-alone group. Patients with high scores (8 or 9) benefited the most from radiation therapy, although local recurrence rates were still high. A 60% recurrence rate was seen in this group, suggesting that mastectomy might be the most appropriate treatment. This prognostic tool is a helpful addition to the management of DCIS. Ultimately, however, both patients and physicians involved in the decision-making process realize that precise categories and risk stratification do not apply to every case or individual. Patients with DCIS may benefit from rescoring or "down"-scoring by reexcision, as suggested by the Van Nuys group. Essentially, reexcision may improve the margin status of selected patients, thereby lowering their final score.

TABLE 22–1.
Three categories of the Van Nuys prognostic index

Score	Size (mm)	Margins (mm)	Pathologic classification
1	≤15	≥10	Non-high-grade (1–2) without necrosis
2	16–40	1–9	Non-high-grade (1–2) with necrosis
3	≥41	<1	High-grade (3) with or without necrosis

Implications of Van Nuys prognostic index scores

3, 4	Favorable score: suggests excision only
5, 6, 7	Intermediate score: suggests lumpectomy plus irradiation
8, 9	Poor score: suggests mastectomy

Down-scoring can be accomplished with reexcision and improving margin status.

D. Lumpectomy and Irradiation

In 1985 the NSABP began a randomized clinical trial to see if lumpectomy with radiation therapy was more effective than local excision alone. Women with localized DCIS were eligible, whereas those with multifocal DCIS were not. Margins had to be histologically tumor-free. Patients with diffuse microcalcifications were eligible if they were histologically benign. A total of 814 patients were enrolled in the study.

The results of the NSABP B-17 study were reported in 1993.[40] Among the women treated with lumpectomy alone, ipsilateral breast cancer developed in 16.4%, and among those treated with lumpectomy and breast irradiation ipsilateral breast cancer developed in 7.0%. Not only did breast irradiation after lumpectomy decrease the incidence of ipsilateral breast cancer, it made it more likely that recurrence would be non-invasive. That is, of the 16.4% who developed breast cancer with lumpectomy alone, 50% of the lesions were noninvasive. The addition of irradiation produced a noninvasive/invasive ratio of approximately 3:1.

Although radiation therapy had a clearly favorable result, this study has been criticized. There was no mastectomy arm, but this seems an appropriate omission because local recurrence rates following this procedure are already understood. To answer the critics, the NSABP analyzed the data based on pathologic subgroups.[41] The presence of moderate/marked comedo necrosis was a significant independent predictor of ipsilateral tumor recurrence. Uncertain or involved margins were also a statistically significant independent predictor. Radiation treatment was beneficial in reducing ipsilateral breast tumor recurrences for all size tumors, from small (1.0 cm) to large. Nuclear grade did not seem to be a significant factor predicting recurrence.

Comedo carcinoma is regarded as an independent prognostic factor, and quantifying the degree of comedo necrosis seems appropriate because of the difference in recurrence rates between tumors with a moderate/marked component and those with slight/absent comedo patterns. The conclusions suggest that radiation therapy is appropriate treatment for both subgroups.

In 1997 the NSABP presented updated results from the B-17 study.[42] After 8 years the cumulative incidences of noninvasive and invasive ipsilateral breast recurrence as first events were reduced by radiation therapy to 8.2% and 3.9%, respectively.

E. *Treatment of the Axilla*

By definition, DCIS is noninvasive, and metastases to ipsilateral lymph nodes should not occur. Most studies, including the NSABP B-17,[40] did not include positive nodes as an inclusion criterion. The assumption is that the presence of metastases in axillary lymph nodes implies the presence of an undiagnosed invasive component. In patients with DCIS who are treated with mastectomy, positive lymph nodes are occasionally found in level I lymph nodes, even though no invasive component was found in the breast. The incidence of axillary node metastases is 0–3% when there is no evidence of invasion on routine hematoxylin and eosin (H&E)-stained preparations.[3,43–49] It therefore appears that treatment of the axilla by surgery or irradiation overtreats 97% of patients[50] and perhaps is not indicated.[51] Others have conceded that extensive disease, high-grade disease, or the presence of comedo carcinoma warrants axillary sampling because these subgroups have an increased likelihood of axillary involvement.

F. *Microinvasive Disease*

The special and increasingly seen clinical presentation of DCIS with microinvasion merits discussion. Moriya and Silverberg[53] looked at pure DCIS and tumors with different proportions of infiltrating carcinoma. In their series the presence of lymph node metastases correlated with the proportion of infiltrating carcinoma in the primary tumor. When the percentage of DCIS in the primary tumor was 100%, lymph node metastases occurred in 3%. If the DCIS component was less than 10%, there was a 78% rate of lymph node involvement. Between these two extremes, various percentages of lymph node metastases were noted. Strikingly impressive was the observation that even with a 90% or greater component of DCIS in the primary tumor, there was a 10% incidence of nodal involvement. Lymph node metastases in this series did not correlate with various histologic subtypes of DCIS.

The Brown University group looked retrospectively at more than 1126 patients with minimally invasive disease.[53] In this series, nodal positivity was seen in 9.8% of patients with T1a lesions. It was suggested by the authors that even patients with small invasive cancers should undergo axillary sampling.

Silverstein et al.[54] presented single-institution data. In their study none of the 189 Tis (DCIS) patients who underwent axillary dissection had positive nodes. Altogether, 96 patients with T1a lesions (<5 mm) were included in this study, 46 of whom had extensive intraductal disease with one or more foci of invasion measuring ≤1 mm. These tumors would be considered by some as intraductal carcinomas with microinvasion rather than T1a lesions. Regardless, only 3% of the patients had positive axillary nodes. Silverstein et al. concluded that DCIS patients clearly should not undergo axillary dissection, and that patients with T1a lesions or DCIS with microinvasion probably did not require axillary sampling.

G. *Sentinel Node Biopsy*

The emergence of sentinel lymph node biopsy as a reliable alternative to axillary dissection[55–58] may solve the problem of axillary sampling in DCIS patients with microinvasion. Preliminary data were presented at the 52nd Cancer Symposium of the Society of Surgical Oncology regarding this approach for patients with DCIS.

The Moffit Cancer Center presented 87 patients with DCIS who underwent lymphatic mapping.[59] The sentinel lymph nodes were examined by cytology, H&E histology, and immunohistochemistry of cytokeratin. Of the 87 patients, 5 (6%) had positive sentinel lymph nodes. One of the five patients had comedo disease and one had extensive low-grade disease. The sentinel lymph node was positive only by cytokeratin histochemistry in three and cytokeratin and H&E in two. Only the sentinel lymph node was positive in these five patients. The authors concluded that for DCIS patients sentinel lymph node biopsy is an accurate, minimally invasive method of detecting micrometastatic disease to the regional nodes.

The Moffit Cancer Center also retrospectively reviewed 70 patients between 1986 and 1993 who had DCIS (n = 53) or

DCIS with microinvasion (n = 17).[60] Immunohistochemical staining of archived tissue for cytokeratin found that 7.5% of DCIS patients and 11.7% of the DCIS patients with microinvasion had micrometastatic nodal disease. It should be noted, however, that there was no significant difference in recurrence or survival between patients with microinvasion and those without. It appears that further studies of the clinical significance of axillary lymph node status in DCIS are warranted. Sentinel lymph node mapping may be the appropriate vehicle because of its minimally invasive approach and its accuracy.

H. Adjuvant Therapy

As the controversies of local and regional treatments for DCIS continue, adjuvant therapy for DCIS has emerged as a new concept to consider. Two studies completed and recently reported have brought this question to the forefront.

The NSABP B-24 study, which followed the B-17 study, approached the question directly.[61] Between 1991 and 1994 more than 1800 patients with DCIS were treated with lumpectomy and radiation therapy. They were then randomized to tamoxifen versus placebo. The results after an average of 62 months of follow-up were as follows. With tamoxifen the incidence of ipsilateral invasive breast cancer was reduced from 3.4% to 2.1%. All first-time breast cancer events, including those from the contralateral breast, were reduced from 13.0% to 8.8%. Subset analysis is not available, as the data were presented in abstract form; however, the study is intriguing if only for its report of reduced contralateral breast cancer.

The question was indirectly approached by the NSABP P-1 trial.[62] In this trial 13,388 women identified as being at high risk for developing breast cancer were randomly assigned to receive tamoxifen 20 mg/day or placebo for 5 years. In addition to reducing the incidence of invasive breast cancer by 49%, the reduction in risk of noninvasive breast cancer was 50% through 69 months of follow-up. This reduction was observed for all age groups and risk categories.

The importance of adjuvant therapy for DCIS patients may be as important for the contralateral breast as it is for the ipsilateral breast. Clinically, the risk of synchronous bilateral cancers or contralateral breast cancer is uncertain. Alpers and Wellings[63] found contralateral DCIS in 48% of their series, but the 20-year risk of contralateral breast cancer may be closer to 12–13%.[64,65]

Tamoxifen is a welcome addition to the treatment arsenal. The risk versus benefit of adjuvant therapy for DCIS probably must be individualized perhaps based on the estrogen receptor/progesterone receptor (ER/PR) status or other tumor markers. Hopefully, subject analysis and further studies will shed light on the most appropriate use of adjuvant therapy in DCIS patients.

Future treatment options for DCIS promise to be as exciting as the current modalities remain controversial. Many of the cooperative study groups are developing new protocols to answer lingering questions. For example, would lumpectomy plus tamoxifen with or without radiation therapy be a better approach? Ultimately, better prognostic markers and subset analyses of DCIS patients, such as the margin status, will hopefully guide clinicians as they address this heterogeneous entity called noninvasive breast cancer.

References

1. Broders AC. Carcinoma in-situ contrasted with benign penetrating epithelium. JAMA 1932;99:1670–1674.
2. Foote FW, Stewart FW. Lobular carcinoma in situ: a rare form of mammary cancer. Am J Pathol 1941;17:491–496.
3. Gump FE, Jicha DL, Ozello L. Ductal carcinoma in situ (DCIS): a revised concept. Surgery 1987;102:790–795.
4. Bassett L. Mammographic analysis of calcifications. Radiol Clin North Am 1992;30:93–105.
5. Swansen GM, Ragheb NE, Lin CS, et al. Breast cancer among black and white women in the 1980's. Cancer 1993;72:788–798.
6. Kerlikowske K, Grady D, Barclay J, Sickles EA, Eaton A, Ernster V. Positive predictive value of screening mammographically by age and family history of breast cancer. JAMA 1993;270:2444–2450.
7. Lynde JF. Low-cost screening mammography: results of 21,141 consecutive examinations in a community program. South Med J 1993;86:338–343.
8. Rebner M. Non-invasive breast cancer. Radiology 1994;190:623–631.
9. Ernster VL, Barclay J, Kerlikowske K, Grady D, Henderson C. Incidence of and treatment for ductal carcinoma in situ of the breast. JAMA 1996;275:913–918.
10. Parker SL, Tong T, Bolden S, et al. Cancer statistics, 1997. CA Cancer J Clin 1997;47:5–27.
11. Morrow M, Schnitt SJ, Harris JR. Ductal carcinoma in situ. In: Harris JR, Lippman ML, Morrow M, et al. (eds) Diseases of the Breast. Philadelphia: Lippincott-Raven, 1995;355–368.
12. Ashikari R, Hadju Si, Robbins GF. Intra-ductal carcinoma of the breast. Cancer 1971;28:1182–1187.
13. Barth A, Brenner J, Giuliano AE. Current management of ductal carcinoma in situ. West J Med 1995;163:360–366.
14. Morrow M, Bland K, Foster R. Breast cancer surgical practice guidelines. Oncology 1997;11:877–886.
15. Fisher ER, Sass R, Fisher B, Wickerham L, Paik SM. Pathologic findings from the National Surgical Adjuvant Breast Project (Protocol 6): intraductal carcinoma (DCIS). Cancer 1986;57:197–208.
16. Page DL, Dupont WD, Rogers LW, Jensen RA, Schuyler PA. Continued local recurrence of carcinoma 15–20 years after a diagnosis of low grade ductal carcinoma in situ of the breast treated only by biopsy. Cancer 1995;26:1197–1200.
17. Lagios MD, Page DL. Radiation therapy for in situ or localized breast cancer [letter]. N Engl J Med 1993;21:1577–1578.
18. Page DL, Lagios MD. Pathologic analysis of the NSABP B-17 trial: unanswered considering current concepts of ductal carcinoma in situ. Cancer 1995;75:1219–1222.

19. Recht A, Danoff BS, Solin LJ, et al. Intraductal carcinoma of the breast: results of treatment with excisional biopsy and irradiation. J Clin Oncol 1995;3:1339–1343.
20. Solin LJ, Fouble BL, Schultz DJ, Yeh I-T, Kowalyshyn MJ, Goodman RL. Definitive irradiation for intraductal carcinoma of the breast. Int J Radiat Oncol Biol Phys 1990;19:843–850.
21. Solin LJ, Recht A, Fourguet A, et al. Ten-year results of breast-conserving surgery and definitive irradiation for intraductal carcinoma (ductal carcinoma in situ) of the breast. Cancer 1991;68:2337–2344.
22. Silverstein MJ, Waisman JR, Gierson ED, Colburn W, Gamigami P, Lewinsky BS. Radiation therapy for intraductal carcinoma: is it an equal alternative? Arch Surg 1991;126:424–428.
23. Bornstein BA, Recht A, Connolly JL, et al. Results of treating ductal carcinoma in situ of the breast with conservative surgery and radiation therapy. Cancer 1991;67:7–13.
24. McCormick B, Rosen PP, Kinne D, Cox L, Yahalom J. Ductal carcinoma in situ of the breast: an analysis of local control after conservation surgery and radiotherapy. Int J Radiat Oncol Biol Phys 1991;21:289–292.
25. Gump FE. In situ cancers. In: Harris JR, Hellman S, Henderson IC, Kinne DW (eds) Breast Diseases. Philadelphia: Lippincott-Raven, 1987;359–368.
26. Silverstein MJ, Poller DN, Waisman JR. Prognostic classification of the breast ductal carcinoma in situ. Lancet 1995;345:1154–1157.
27. Lagios NM, Margolin FR, Westdahl PR, et al. Mammographically detected duct carcinoma in situ: frequency of local recurrences following lumpectomy and prognostic effect of nuclear grade on local recurrence. Cancer 1989;63:619–624.
28. Holland R, Peterse JL, Millis R, et al. Ductal carcinoma in situ: a proposal for a new classification. Semin Diagn Pathol 1994;11:167–180.
29. Barnes DM, Meyer JS, Gonzalez JG, et al. Relationship between c-erb B-2 immunoreactivity and thymidine labeling index in breast carcinoma in situ. Breast Cancer Res Treat 1991;18:11–17.
30. Lagios MD, Westdahl PR, Margolin FR, et al. Duct carcinoma in situ: relationship of extent of non-invasive disease to the frequency of occult invasion, multicentricity lymph node metastases, and short-term treatment failures. Cancer 1982;50:1309–1314.
31. Solin LJ, Yet IT, Kurtz J, et al. Ductal carcinoma in situ (intraductal carcinoma) of the breast treated with breast conserving surgery and definitive irradiation: correlation of pathologic parameters with outcome of treatment. Cancer 1993;71:2532–2542.
32. Poller DN, Silverstein MJ, Galea M, et al. Ductal carcinoma in situ of the breast: a proposal for a new simplified histological classification association between cellular proliferation and c-erb B-2 protein expression. Med Pathol 1994;7:257–262.
33. Bellamy COC, McDonald C, Salter DM, et al. Non-invasive ductal carcinoma of the breast: the relevance of histologic categorization. Hum Pathol 1993;24:16–23.
34. Sloane JP, Ellman R, Anderson TJ, et al. Consistency of histopathological reporting of breast lesions detected by breast screening: findings of the UK national external quality assessment (EQA) scheme. Eur J Cancer 1994;30:1414–1419.
35. Douglas-Jones AG, Gupta SK, Attanoos RL, et al. A critical appraisal of six modern classifications of ductal carcinoma in situ of the breast (DCIS): correlation with grade of associated invasive disease. Histopathology 1996;29:397–409.
36. Silverstein MJ, Poller DN, Craig PH, et al. A prognostic index for breast ductal carcinoma in situ [abstract]. Breast Cancer Res Treat 1996;37:34.
37. Silverstein MJ, Lagios MD, Craig PH, et al. The Van Nuys Prognostic Index for ductal carcinoma in situ. Breast J 1996;2:38–40.
38. Silverstein MJ, Lagios MD, Craig PH, et al. A prognostic index for ductal carcinoma in situ of the breast. Cancer 1996;77:2267–2274.
39. Silverstein MJ, Lagios MD. Use of predictors of recurrence to plan therapy for DCIS of the breast. Oncology 1997;11:393–410.
40. Fisher B, Costantino J, Redmond C, et al. Lumpectomy compared with lumpectomy and radiation therapy for the treatment of intraductal breast cancer. N Engl J Med 1993;328:1581–1586.
41. Fisher E, Costantino J, Fisher B, Palekar AS, Redmond C, Mamounas E. Pathologic findings from the National Surgical Adjuvant Breast Project (NSABP) protocol B-17. Cancer 1995;75:1310–1319.
42. Mamounas E, Fisher B, Dignam J, Wickerman DL, Margolese R, Womark N. Effect of breast irradiation following lumpectomy in intraductal breast cancer (DCIS): updated results from NSABP B-17. Proc Soc Surg Oncol 1997;50:7.
43. Ashikari R, Hadju SI, Robbins GF. Intraductal carcinoma of the breast (1960–1969). Cancer 1971;28:1182–1187.
44. Fentiman IS, Fagg N, Millis RR, et al. In situ ductal carcinoma of the breast: implications of disease pattern and treatment. Eur J Surg Oncol 1986;12:261–266.
45. Kinne DW, Petrek JA, Osborne MP, et al. Breast carcinoma in situ. Arch Surg 1989;124:33–36.
46. Lagios MD, Margolin FR, Westdahl PR, et al. Mammographically detected duct carcinoma in situ: frequency of local recurrence following tylectomy and prognostic effect of nuclear grade on local recurrence. Cancer 1989;63:618–624.
47. Silverstein MJ, Rosser RJ, Gierson ED, et al. Axillary lymph node dissection for intraductal breast carcinoma: is it indicated? Cancer 1987;59:1819–1824.
48. Von Rueden DG, Wilson RE. Intraductal carcinoma of the breast. Surg Obstet Gynecol 1984;158:105–111.
49. Westbrook KC, Gallagher HS. Intraductal carcinoma of the breast: a comparative study. Am J Surg 1975;130:667–670.
50. Fentiman IS. The treatment of in situ breast cancer. Acta Oncol 1989;28:923–926.
51. Gallagher WJ, Koerner FC, Wood WC. Treatment of intraductal carcinoma with limited surgery: long-term follow-up. J Clin Oncol 1989;7:376–380.
52. Moriya T, Silverberg SG. Intraductal carcinoma (ductal carcinoma in situ) of the breast: a comparison of pure noninvasive tumors with those including different proportions of infiltrating carcinoma. Cancer 1994;74:2972–2978.
53. White RE, Vezeridis MP, Konstadoulakis M, Cole BF, Wanebo HJ, Bland KI. Therapeutic options and results for the management of minimally invasive carcinoma of the breast: influence of axillary dissection for treatment for T1a and T1b lesions. J Am Coll Surg 1996;183:575–582.
54. Silverstein MJ, Gierson ED, Waisman JR, Senofsky GM, Colburn WJ, Gamagami P. Axillary lymph node dissection for T1a breast carcinoma. Cancer 1994;73:664–667.
55. Giuliano AE, Kirgan DM, Guenther JM, Morton DL. Lymphatic mapping and sentinel lymphadenectomy for breast cancer. Ann Surg 1994;220:391–401.
56. Giuliano AE, Dale PS, Turner RR, Morton DL, Evans SW, Krasne DL. Improved axillary staging of breast cancer with sentinel lymphadenectomy. Ann Surg 1995;222:394–401.
57. Krag DN, Weaver DL, Alex JC, Fairbank JT. Surgical resection and radiolocalization of the sentinel lymph node in breast cancer using a gamma probe. Surg Oncol 1993;2:335–340.
58. Albertini JJ, Lyman GH, Cox CH, et al. Lymphatic mapping and sentinel node biopsy in the patient with breast cancer. JAMA 1996;276:1818–1822.
59. Pendas S, Dauway E, Giuliano R, Ku NK, Cox CE, Reintgen DS. Sentinel node biopsy in DCIS patients. Proc Soc Surg Oncol 1999;52:28.
60. Dauway EL, Pendas S, Giuliano R, et al. DCIS or Tmic: what is the clinical significance of micrometastases detected by cytokeratin analysis? Proc Soc Surg Oncol 1999;52:40.

61. Fisher B, Dignam J, Wolmark N, et al. Tamoxifen in treatment of intraductal breast cancer: National Surgical Adjuvant Breast and Bowel Project B-24 randomized controlled trial. Lancet 1999;353:1993–2000.
62. Fisher B, Costantino JP, Wickerham DL, et al. Tamoxifen for prevention of breast cancer: report of the National Surgical Adjuvant Breast and Bowel Project P-1 study. J Natl Cancer Inst 1998;90:1371–1388.
63. Alpers CH, Wellings SR. The prevalence of carcinoma in situ in normal and cancer-associated breasts. Hum Pathol 1985;16:796–807.
64. Robbins GF, Berg JW. Bilateral primary breast cancers: a prospective clinicopathological study. Cancer 1964;17:1501–1527.
65. Jotti GS, Petit JY, Contesso G. Minimal breast cancer: a clinically meaningful term? Semin Oncol 1986;13:384–392.

Chapter 23

Early Invasive Breast Cancer

THOMAS R. WITT

The appropriate options for management of a patient with breast cancer change with the invasiveness and clinical stage of the cancer. At one end of the spectrum of breast neoplasia is lobular carcinoma in situ for which the patient may require only careful observation as a "high risk" individual. At the other end of the spectrum is distant metastatic disease, for which local intervention is reserved for diagnostic or palliative purposes. In the large spectrum between these two extremes are the operable, or nonmetastatic, cancers. A small number of them are "locally advanced"; and because of their high risk for systemic disease, the management algorithm may differ significantly from that utilized for the larger proportion of "early invasive cancers."

The purpose of this chapter is to outline the management of early invasive breast cancer. A full understanding of this management requires knowledge of the epidemiology, risk factors, screening techniques, physical and radiographic evaluation of the breast, and staging. Techniques and options of locoregional surgical therapy, radiation therapy, reconstruction, adjuvant systemic therapy, posttreatment follow-up, prognosis, and prevention of cancer in the high risk patient are important concepts to understand as well.[1]

A. *Epidemiology*

Breast cancer is the most common nonskin cancer in women and is the second leading cause of cancer deaths in women (44,000 deaths were expected to occur in the United States in 1999).[2] Approximately 176,000 new U.S. cases were expected to be diagnosed in 1999. This represents a modest decline in incidence over the past several years and may be due to the fact that increased early utilization of mammography over the past 10–15 years has resulted in the mammographic detection of many breast cancers that would otherwise not have been detected until they became clinically apparent during more recent years. The incidence of breast cancer increases with advancing age up to the eighth decade and then levels off. There are both socioeconomic and geographic/ethnic variations in the incidence: It is found more commonly among high socioeconomic groups and in the United States and United Kingdom; it is relatively uncommon in Japan. Approximately 1% of breast cancers occur in men.

Early Breast Cancer

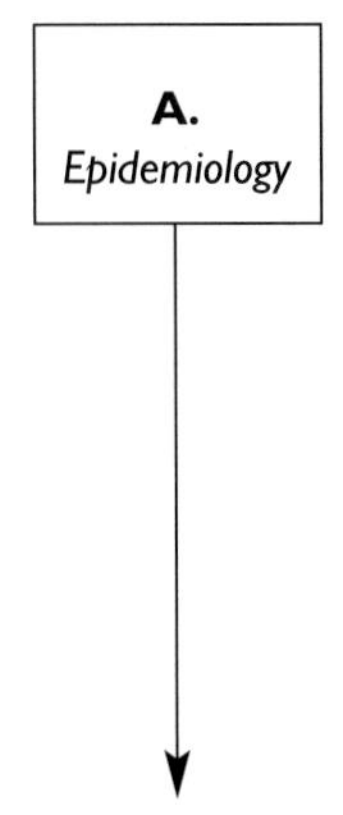

Most common nonskin
  cancer in women
  176,000 cases/year;
  44,000 deaths/year; number 2
  cause of cancer death in women
Female : male = 100 : 1
Incidence $\uparrow$ with age up to 8th
  decade
More common in high
  socioeconomic groups
Geographic/ethnic variation:
  common in U.S. and U.K.,
  uncommon in Japan

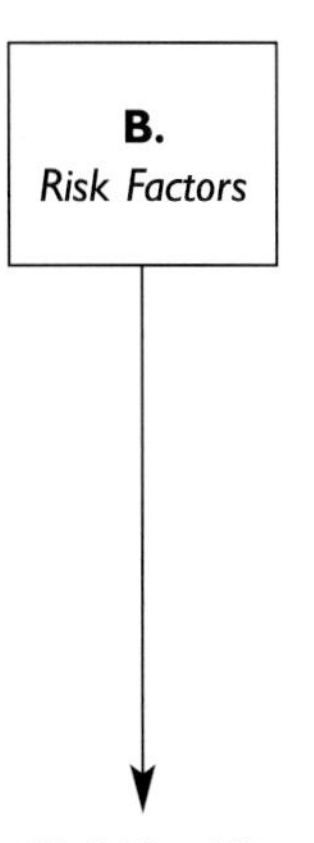

Genetic: BRCA1, BRCA2, p53 mutations
Family history:
  1st degree vs more distant relative
  premenopausal vs post menopausal
  bilateral vs unilateral disease
  (all three) $\uparrow$ risk up 5 fold
Preexisting breast disease:
  severe hyperplasia: 1.5–2 $\times \uparrow$ risk
  atypical hyperplasia: 4–5 $\times \uparrow$ risk
  lobular CA in situ: 8–10 $\times \uparrow$ risk
Endocrine influences:
  early menarche
  nulliparity or late 1st pregnancy
  late menopause
  prolonged oral contraceptive use
  prolonged hormone replacement therapy
Previous breast cancer:
  1%/year risk of new cancer

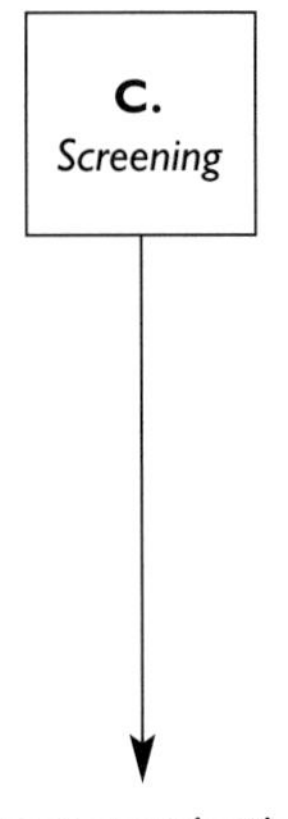

Clinical breast examination
  Age 20–40: every third year
  Age > 40: annually
Mammography
  Age 35–40: first mammography
  Age 40–50: every 1–2 years
  Age > 50: annually
Self-examination
  Age > 20: monthly

(continued on next page)

Early Breast Cancer (continued)

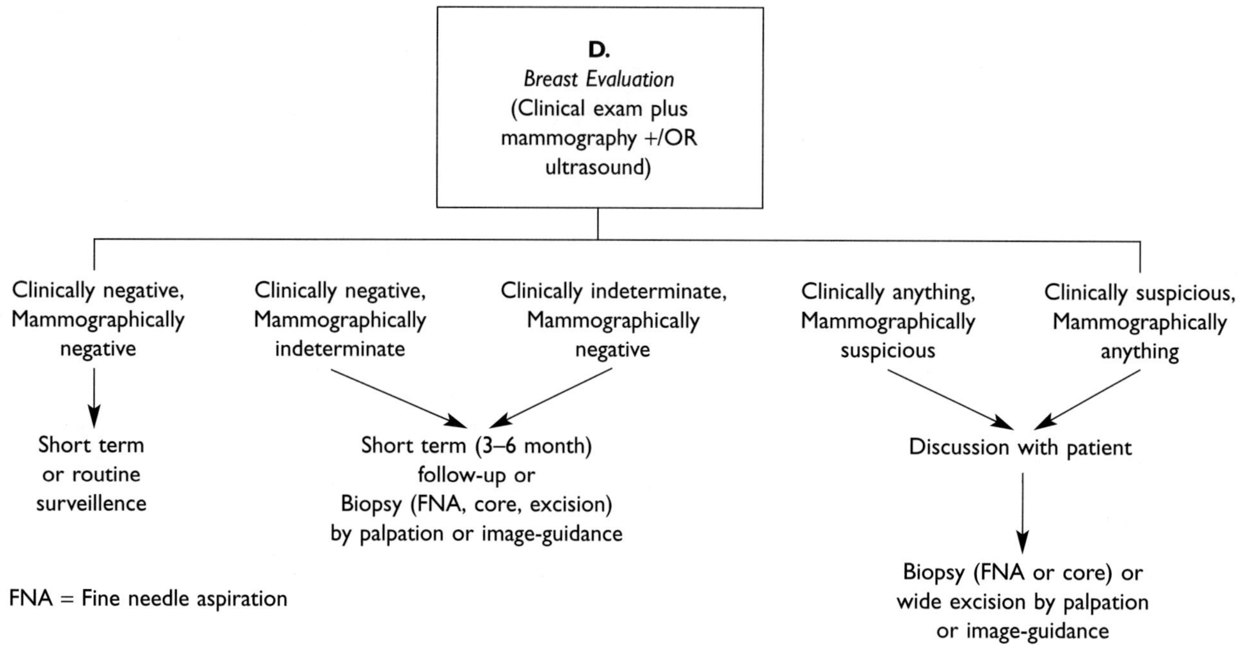

D.
Breast Evaluation
(Clinical exam plus mammography +/OR ultrasound)

- Clinically negative, Mammographically negative → Short term or routine surveillence
- Clinically negative, Mammographically indeterminate / Clinically indeterminate, Mammographically negative → Short term (3–6 month) follow-up or Biopsy (FNA, core, excision) by palpation or image-guidance
- Clinically anything, Mammographically suspicious / Clinically suspicious, Mammographically anything → Discussion with patient → Biopsy (FNA or core) or wide excision by palpation or image-guidance

FNA = Fine needle aspiration

E.
Tissue Diagnosis

- FNA by palpation
- Core biopsy by palpation
- FNA by image guidance
- Core biopsy by image guidance
- Incisional biopsy
- Marginal excisional biopsy
- Wide excision (partial mastectomy)

F.
Staging Work-Up

Routine: History
Clinical examination
Bilaterial diagnostic mammography
Chest X-ray
CBC + platelet count
Blood chemstries (liver function tests)

Selective: Bone scan
CT chest
CT liver
Other scans as clinical indicated

G.[5]
Staging (TNM)
AJCC 1997

Stage	*TNM*
0	Tis N0 M0
I	T1 N0 M0
IIA	T0 N1 M0
	T1 N1 M0
	T2 N0 M0
IIB	T2 N1 M0
	T3 N0 M0
IIIA	T0 N2 M0
	T1 N2 M0
	T2 N2 M0
	T3 N1–2 M0
IIIB	T4 Any N M0
	Any T N3 M0
IV	Any T Any N M1

Primary Tumor (T)

Tx		tumor not assessed
T0		no evidence of primary tumor
Tis		carcinoma in situ
T1		≤ 2 cm
	T1mic	≤ .1 cm
	T1a	> .1 cm; ≤ .5 cm
	T1b	> .5 cm; ≤ 1.0 cm
	T1c	> 1.0 cm; ≤ 2.0 cm
T2		> 2.0 cm; ≤ 5.0 cm
T3		> 5.0 cm
T4		any size with direct extension to chest wall or skin

Regional Lymph Nodes (N)

N0	no lymph node mets
N1	movable, ipsilateral
N2	fixed, ipsilateral
N3	internal mammary

Metastases (M)

M0	no metastases
M1	distant metastases (includes ipsilateral supraclavicular)

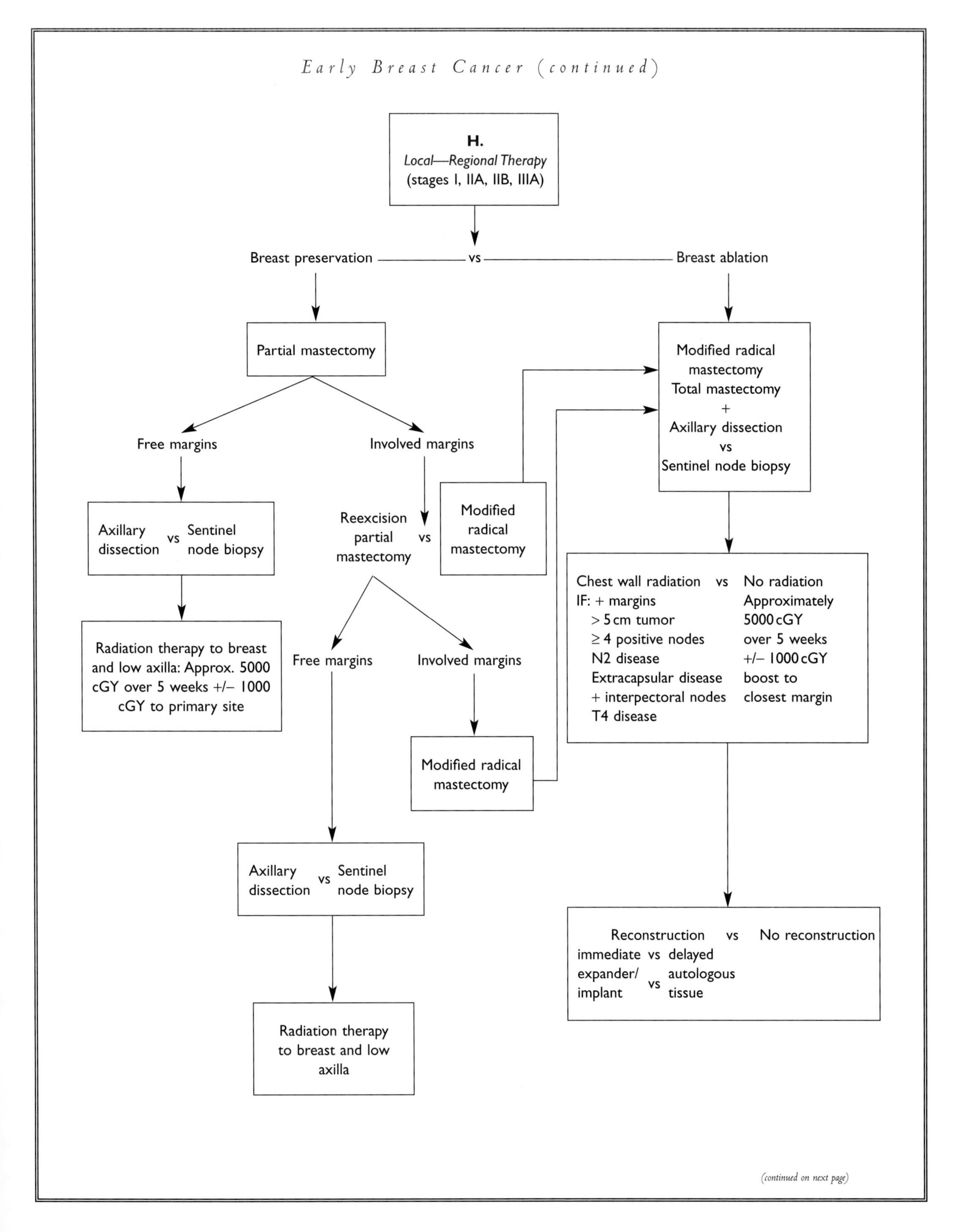

(continued on next page)

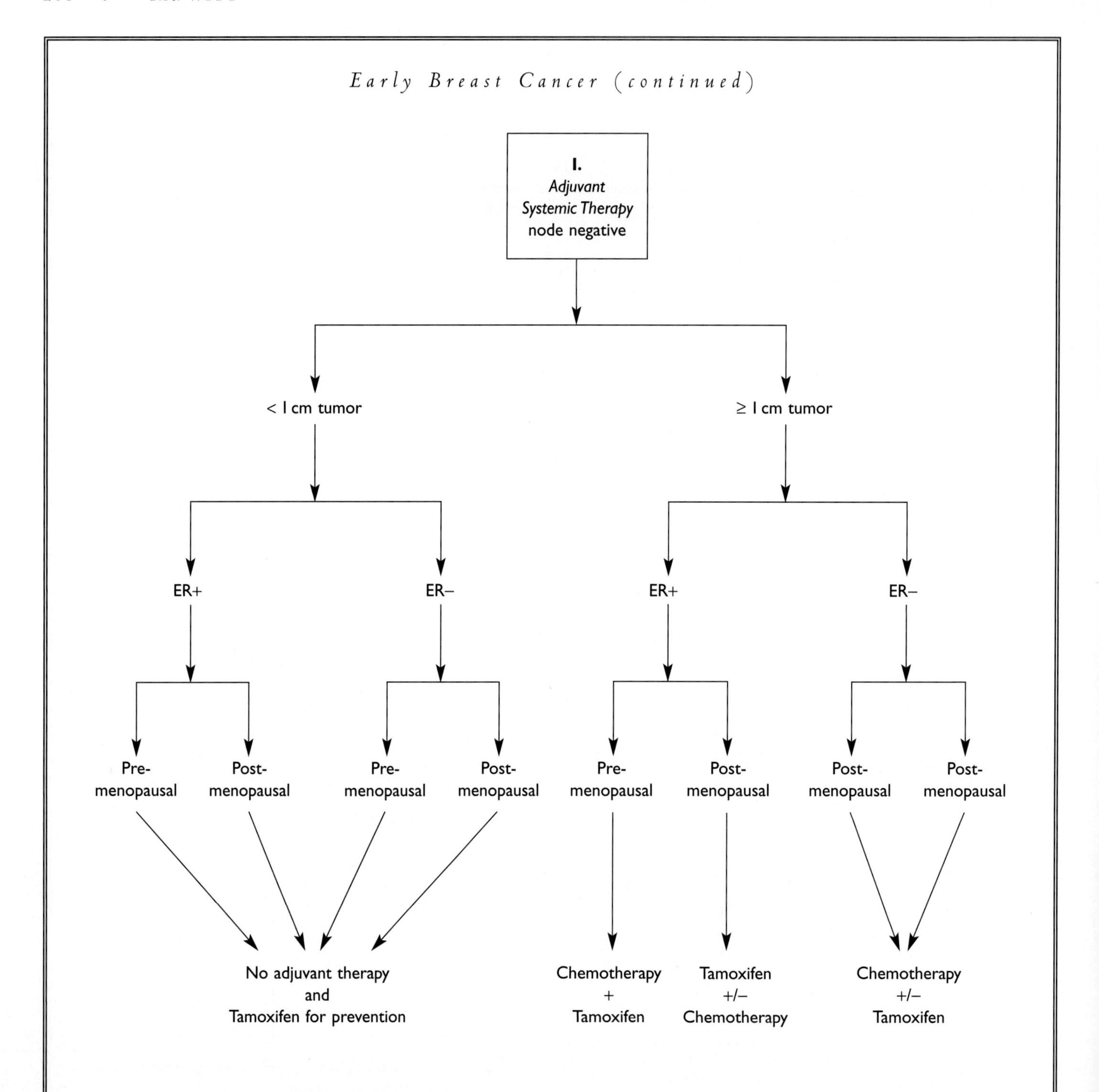

Chemotherapy options: AC (adriamycin + cytoxan) every 3 weeks × 4 cycles
CMF (cytoxan, methotrexate, 5-FU) every 4 weeks × 6 cycles

Tamoxifen: 20 mg/day × 5 years

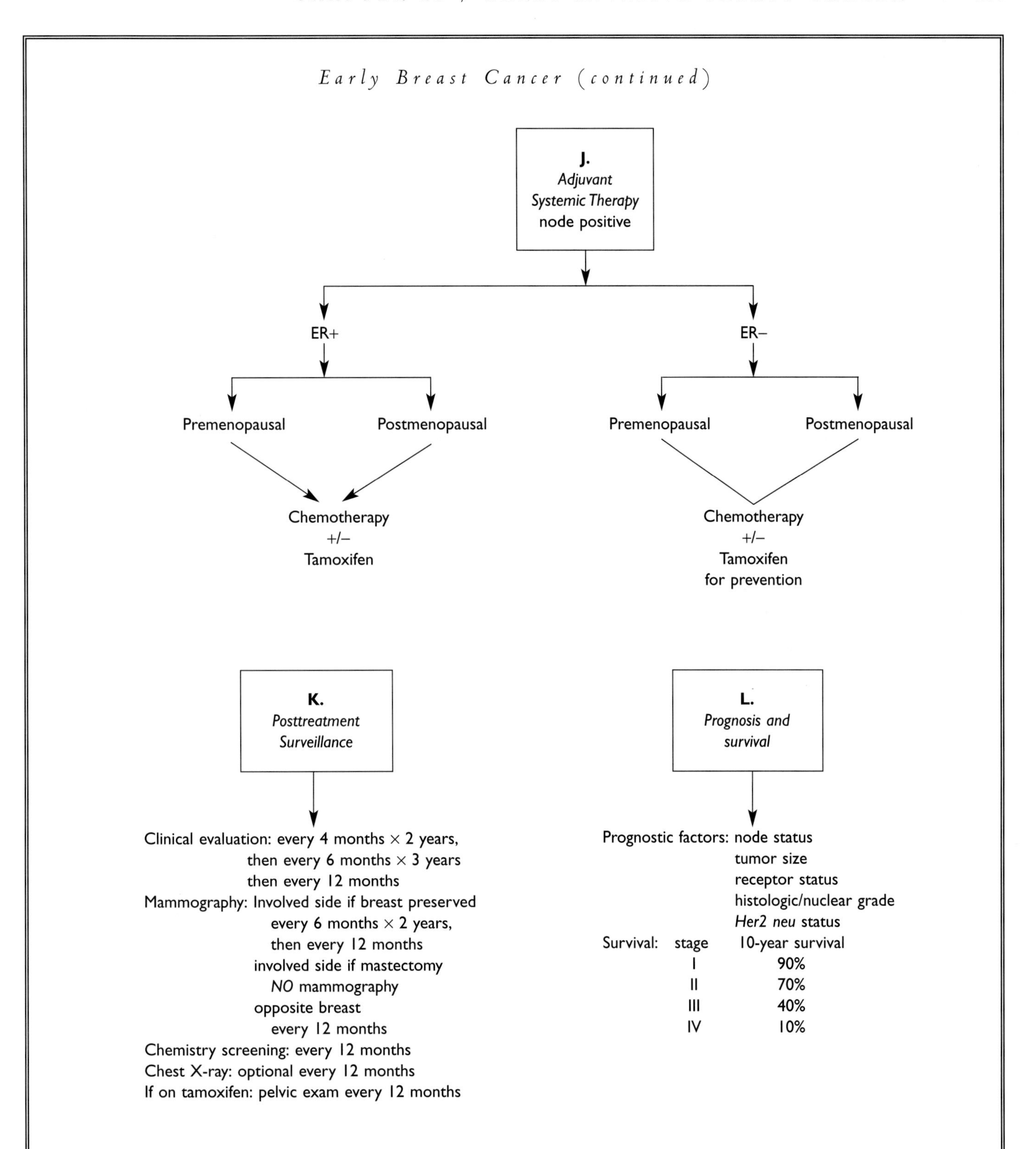
Early Breast Cancer (continued)
J.
Adjuvant
Systemic Therapy
node positive
ER+
ER–
Premenopausal
Postmenopausal
Premenopausal
Postmenopausal
Chemotherapy
+/–
Tamoxifen
Chemotherapy
+/–
Tamoxifen
for prevention
K.
Posttreatment
Surveillance
L.
Prognosis and
survival
Clinical evaluation: every 4 months × 2 years,
then every 6 months × 3 years
then every 12 months
Mammography: Involved side if breast preserved
every 6 months × 2 years,
then every 12 months
involved side if mastectomy
NO mammography
opposite breast
every 12 months
Chemistry screening: every 12 months
Chest X-ray: optional every 12 months
If on tamoxifen: pelvic exam every 12 months
Prognostic factors: node status
tumor size
receptor status
histologic/nuclear grade
Her2 neu status
Survival: stage 10-year survival
I 90%
II 70%
III 40%
IV 10%

B. Risk Factors

A number of risk factors have been shown independently to predict a higher likelihood of developing breast cancer.[3] Identifiable specific genetic mutations represent the most accurately predictable risk factors and yet are found in only approximately 5% of all women with breast cancer. A mutation in the *BRCA1* (*br*east *ca*ncer) gene leads to an approximately 85% lifetime risk of developing breast cancer and a 40% lifetime risk of developing ovarian cancer. These cancers are usually found at a much earlier age than cancers not associated with this mutation. Mutation in the *BRCA2* gene leads to a similar increase in the likelihood of breast cancer and an approximately 20% risk of ovarian cancer. Ten percent of men with *BRCA2* gene mutations develop breast cancer. Mutation in the *p53* gene leads to the Li-Fraumeni syndrome, which includes a constellation of malignancies of the breast, soft tissues, brain, adrenal cortex, and hemopoietic system.

A family history of breast cancer, excluding cases where a genetic mutation has been identified, is also a significant risk factor. The closer the genetic link to the index case, the more likely it is that a patient will develop breast cancer. If the relative is premenopausal or has bilateral breast cancer, the risk is increased further. Thus a first-degree relative with premenopausal, bilateral breast cancer may confer a fivefold increased risk above the average likelihood of developing breast cancer over an at-risk individual's lifetime.

Most forms of fibrocystic change do not confer an increased risk of subsequent breast cancer. However, if there is severe hyperplasia of the ductal or lobular epithelium, there may be a modest increase in risk. Dysplasia or atypical hyperplasia confers a four- to fivefold increased risk. Lobular carcinoma in situ confers an 8- to 10-fold increased risk of subsequently developing invasive breast cancer.

A number of endocrine influences are associated with an increased risk of developing breast cancer, including early menarche, nulliparity or late first pregnancy, and late menopause. Somewhat controversial has been the possible role of oral contraceptive use and hormone replacement therapy as risk factors for breast cancer. Large meta-analyses of data regarding these issues suggest that there indeed is an increased risk of breast cancer associated with prolonged use of these drugs.

Of note also is that a history of breast cancer confers approximately 1% increased risk of developing a second, unrelated breast cancer per year. This makes sense based on the fact that all of that individual's breast parenchyma has presumably been exposed to the same environmental and genetic influences that may have been involved in formation of the initial cancer.

C. Screening and Early Detection

The purpose of "screening" for breast cancer is detection of cancer at an earlier and therefore more curable stage. Finding a primary tumor when it is small also enhances the likelihood that breast-conserving techniques can be utilized for locoregional treatment.

Screening is accomplished by (1) breast self-examination, which is recommended monthly beginning at age 20; (2) clinical breast examination, which is recommended every 3 years between the ages of 20 and 40 and annually after age 40; and (3) mammography. The frequency of mammography is controversial and has been the subject of numerous clinical trials and intense debate.[4] Most organizations recommend an initial screening mammogram between the ages of 35 and 40 and annual mammography after age 50. Between the ages of 40 and 50, mammography every 1–2 years seems appropriate, depending on risk factors. There have been conflicting results, however, as to whether there is a survival benefit from annual screening mammography for women in their forties.

A suspicious mass should always be evaluated by mammography at virtually any age; but *screening* mammography for patients less than 35 years of age is of little benefit owing to the density of the breast and the low likelihood of a cancer being present in the absence of significant physical findings.

D. Breast Evaluation

Proper management of the patient with breast cancer begins with breast evaluation. The ultimate outcome can be adversely affected by poor judgment during the early "evaluation" stage of the process. For example, inappropriate marginal excision of a clearly malignant-appearing mass almost certainly necessitates reexcision, as the margin is likely positive. For the small-breasted woman this may render mastectomy inevitable or at least cause significant breast deformity as a consequence of the second "lumpectomy." In such a case, wide excision would have been the more appropriate choice, even though the diagnosis of cancer had not yet been established.

Clinical breast evaluation usually involves a combination of physical examination and imaging. Mammography with or without ultrasonography is the most useful method for imaging the breast and suffices in most patients. Other imaging techniques [magnetic resonance imaging (MRI), position emission tomography (PET), and radionuclide imaging] are available but have relatively limited applicability for most patients. The key principle for breast evaluation is that management be generally dictated by the more suspicious finding whether detected by physical examination or radiographic tests. A normal mammogram, for example, should not negate the need for biopsy of a clinically suspicious palpable nodule.

If both the clinical and radiographic findings are *not suspicious*, the patient can be observed with follow-up evaluation on a short-term or routine annual basis, depending on other factors, such as the patient's underlying risk profile. If the clinical or radiographic findings are *indeterminate* (not obviously benign or malignant), short-term follow-up may be considered, but it is better to err on the side of biopsy. Sampling the lesion with image-guided needle biopsy may be appropriate, rather than total excision, in such indeterminate cases; but the patient must be followed carefully with short-term reevaluation. For *highly suspicious* lesions based on clinical examination or mammographic findings, biopsy is definitely indicated; the technique chosen may vary with the ultimate treatment plan. For example, a clinically suspicious mass in a patient who wants a mastectomy as her definitive local therapy would be better biopsied by the needle technique than by excision, as it is less invasive, and the breast is going to be removed anyway once cancer is proven. Conversely, a highly suspicious mammographic finding in a patient who wants breast conservation would be better biopsied by wire localization and wide excision than by stereotactic core biopsy, as excision is warranted anyway once cancer is proven. If a stereotactic core biopsy failed to prove the presence of cancer in such instances, the lesion would still have to be excised because of its highly suspicious nature and the concern over a false-negative biopsy or sampling error. Therefore, whenever possible, for a patient with findings that are extremely suspicious for cancer, a discussion regarding her preferences for local therapy may lead to a clearer understanding of the most appropriate biopsy technique.

As suggested above, one must always remember that in the case of highly suspicious findings a negative sampling biopsy must always be followed by either a repeat needle biopsy or an open biopsy because of the risk of sampling error.

E. Tissue Diagnosis

There are several methods for obtaining tissue. Fine-needle aspiration (FNA) utilizes a small needle (20–22 gauge) passed through a wide area of the tumor numerous times. A relatively small volume of tissue is obtained, and the histologic architecture of the lesion cannot be assessed. Needle placement can be guided by palpation or, in cases of nonpalpable lesions, by mammography (including stereotactic techniques) or ultrasonography. It is the simplest, least painful, and least expensive biopsy technique but provides a cytologic rather than histologic diagnosis. Some surgeons are reluctant to perform mastectomy based on FNA cytology alone; but in the presence of classically malignant findings by both clinical and mammographic assessment, a positive FNA interpretation by an experienced cytologist should be considered diagnostic. Modern immunohistochemical techniques allow hormone receptor analysis on FNA samples.

Core biopsies utilize larger needles (usually 11–15 gauge) that remove a solid piece of tissue for a histologic diagnosis. A considerably larger volume of tissue can be removed, with some forms of core biopsy techniques capable of essentially "removing" entire small abnormal areas. Core biopsy can be guided by palpation, ultrasound quidance, or stereotactic imaging.

Incisional biopsy is an open technique usually done under local anesthesia with or without sedation. It is a "sampling" technique utilized to remove small portions of large abnormal areas. It is not commonly used, as core biopsy techniques are almost as accurate while being less invasive and less costly. It has applicability in patients with large cancers requiring mastectomy when the core biopsy was nondiagnostic.

Marginal excisional biopsy is a technique whereby the entire lesion is essentially removed without a margin of normal tissue around it. It is inappropriately used to manage highly suspicious lesions because if mastectomy is planned the less invasive core biopsy is better suited; and if breast preservation is planned, a wide excision would be necessary to provide free margins. It is appropriately utilized to remove lesions that are most likely benign, when preservation of as much breast tissue as possible is desired.

Wide excision (lumpectomy, quadrantectomy, partial mastectomy) is utilized as both a diagnostic and therapeutic biopsy technique in cases of highly suspicious lesions for patients desiring breast preservation. It can usually be performed under local anesthesia with sedation. Some surgeons are reluctant to utilize this technique for lesions that are not proven to be cancer because of the fear of creating a deformity. What is not appreciated by some surgeons, however, is that relatively large volumes of breast tissue can be removed, especially from the central and upper portions of the breast, with little or no resulting contour change provided the deep tissues are not reapproximated and a drain is not used. Reexcising a previously inadequately excised cancer to achieve free margins creates much more of a tissue deficit than if an appropriately wide excision had been performed in the first place.

F. and G. Staging

In all cases, therapy depends on properly staging the cancer. It would be inappropriate, for example, to perform a mastectomy on a patient with known distant metastases unless the mastectomy were required for palliative purposes. The minimal workup required to stage a breast cancer includes a detailed clinical history and physical examination including examination of both breasts and axillary and supraclavicular lymph node basins. Bilateral diagnostic mammography is also required to rule out multicentric disease in the ipsilateral breast and an occult tumor in the contralateral breast. A complete blood count (CBC) with platelet count, a chest radiograph (to rule out pulmonary metastases), and a blood chemistry profile for transaminase and alkaline phosphatase elevations, which may signal liver and bone metastases, respectively, complete the basic workup. Some clinicians routinely order a bone scan and computed tomography (CT) scan of the chest and liver to rule out metastatic disease. These tests are probably better performed on a selective basis. They are certainly indicated in cases where there is clinically positive axillary adenopathy. They should be performed preoperatively because if distant metastatic disease is found an inappropriately performed mastectomy can be avoided. Other indications for these scans include clinical symptoms or signs suggestive of lung, liver, or bone metastases, an abnormal chest radiography, or elevated transaminases or alkaline phosphatase.

Once the staging workup has been completed, the patient is then *clinically staged*. This is done utilizing the most current TNM staging system,[5] which allows consistent assessment of patients and reporting of treatment outcomes. Of note in this system is that the presence of positive supraclavicular nodes constitutes distant metastatic disease (M1) rather than advanced regional disease (N3). Also, actual skin invasion rather than puckering or nipple inversion is required for the T4 designation. The latter two findings can be due to tumors much deeper in the breast, causing foreshortening of Cooper's ligaments. Tethering of the skin in this manner does not substantially alter the staging or prognosis. Similarly, invasion of the pectoralis major muscle does not constitute chest wall involvement, which is defined as involvement of the ribs, intercostal muscles, or serratus anterior muscle.

H. *Local–Regional Therapy*

After patients have been evaluated and staged, those whose lesions fall into the category of "early invasive cancer" (stages I, IIA, IIB, IIIA) should undergo local–regional therapy. Trials evaluating the issue of neoadjuvant systemic therapy (i.e., chemotherapy prior to surgery) for "early-stage disease" have shown equivalent survival curves when compared with the standard therapy of local–regional treatment first followed by adjuvant therapy. This is still considered the standard of care.

With rare exceptions (e.g., elderly patients or those with significant medical co-morbidity or disability) local–regional therapy for early invasive breast cancer consists of breast *preservation* [defined as partial mastectomy (lumpectomy), axillary dissection, and radiation therapy to the breast] or breast *ablation* (modified radical mastectomy).

Numerous clinical trials have shown equivalent survival comparing these two treatments when certain entry criteria are met. Probably the best such trial in this regard is the B-06 trial of the National Surgical Adjuvant Breast Project (NSABP). With data now matured well beyond 12 years of follow-up,[6] the survival of patients undergoing lumpectomy, axillary dissection, and radiation therapy versus mastectomy is statistically equal. To enter this trial there had to be unifocal disease of ≤ 4 cm and not centrally (retroareolarly) located. Free margins of excision were required, but microscopically these margins could be just one high-powered microscopic field. These "rules" have been changed to allow more patients the opportunity for breast preservation. For example, tumors > 4 cm can be successfully treated with breast preservation if the breast is large enough to permit a margin-free excision with a reasonable cosmetic result. Tumors in the retroareolar location can likewise be treated with breast preservation if the patient is willing to have the nipple–areolar complex sacrificed during lumpectomy. Diffuse cancers are still a contraindication to breast preservation, but discreet multicentric cancers can be successfully treated with breast preservation, provided free margins can be achieved around each tumor. The B-06 trial also confirmed the benefit of postoperative radiation therapy in the breast preservation group; local recurrence rates dropped from approximately 40% in patients not irradiated to only 10% in those receiving radiation.

Partial Mastectomy

The first step in breast preservation is the performance of a partial mastectomy. It can be combined with axillary dissection as a single operation, especially when the surgeon believes that the likelihood of obtaining a free margin around the primary tumor is high. For the purpose of this discussion, however, these two procedures are considered as separate operations.

The purpose of the partial mastectomy is to remove the entire tumor with a margin of uninvolved breast tissue around it. An extremely wide margin (e.g., quadrantectomy for a relatively small tumor) does not obviate the need for radiation therapy or lead to better survival. Therefore it does not seem necessary.

There are several important technical considerations pertinent to partial mastectomy. First, the skin incision should be oriented in the most cosmetically appealing manner. Although the classic recommendation has been for the incision to be parallel to the areolar border in the upper hemisphere of the breast and radially oriented in the lower hemisphere, curvilinear primarily transversely oriented incisions yield excellent results in both the upper and lower breast. The skin immediately over the tumor need not be sacrificed unless the tumor is superficial, raising the fear of a positive superficial margin.

How wide to go peripherally around the tumor is a matter of judgment and clinical experience. The depth of excision required is frequently underestimated, resulting in a positive deep margin. This almost never needs to happen, as dissecting down to the pectoralis fascia is a simple maneuver that actually facilitates the rest of the lumpectomy procedure, enhances the likelihood of a negative deep margin, and has negligible impact on the cosmetic outcome. Closure of the deep tissues or placing a drain should be avoided, as it frequently lead's to puckering of the breast. Hematoma and infection rates are each in the 1% range and are not significantly changed by drainage or deep tissue closure. Because large amounts of breast tissue can be removed without cosmetic consequences, one should generally err on the side of removing more rather than less tissue. In cases where the likelihood of achieving a negative margin is in doubt, partial mastectomy should be done separately from the axillary dissection. If a positive margin is found, necessitating mastectomy, the mastectomy is better performed if the axillary dissection has not yet been carried out.

Axillary Dissection Versus Sentinel Lymph Node Biopsy

Some form of axillary assessment is required in most cases of early invasive breast cancer. When clinically suspicious axillary lymph nodes are present, a formal axillary dissection should be performed for therapeutic purposes. When the axilla is clinically negative, axillary dissection is considered by most to be of primarily diagnostic significance (i.e., done to determine stage and prognosis). This is supported by the NSABP B-04 trial that showed no survival advantage whether the axilla was dissected, irradiated, or observed and then dissected if it became clinically positive. Others still hold that there may be some modest therapeutic benefit to elective axillary dissection.

The classic complete axillary dissection removes the axillary fat pad from the latissimus dorsi muscle laterally to Halsted's ligament (the subclavius muscle tendon) medially and from inferior to the axillary vein and superficial to the subscapularis muscle. A variable amount of the tail of the breast is removed as the inferior margin. In the past, the pectoralis minor muscle was removed or divided to facilitate exposure to the axilla, but this is rarely required because suspending the arm across the clavicular area relaxes the pectoralis major muscle, allowing adequate exposure to the high axilla.

The standard of care currently requires that level I tissue (up to the lateral border of the pectoralis minor) and a variable amount of level II tissue (underneath the pectoralis minor) be removed. A level III dissection (tissue medial to the pectoralis minor) is rarely required unless clinically evident disease is detected there. The interpectoral nodes (those lying along the thoracocromial vessels on the undersurface of the pectoralis major) should be assessed, as occasionally they are the only positive lymph nodes present.

Actual dissection of the axillary fat pad is done with identification and preservation of the axillary vein, long thoracic nerve, thoracodorsal nerve and vessels, and medial pectoral neurovascular pedicle. Preservation of the sensory nerves in the axilla, especially the second intercostal brachiocutaneous nerve, is optional but is being done with increasing frequency and is usually easily accomplished if there are no clinically suspicious lymph nodes near the nerve.

Postoperative consequences of axillary dissection include temporary shoulder stiffness, variable degree of sensory loss to the periaxillary skin, and the possibility of developing lymphedema in the ipsilateral arm. This edema is significant from a cosmetic and comfort standpoint in approximately 5% of cases. Because of the morbidity associated with axillary dissection, especially lymphedema, it is not performed in selected cases of invasive cancer (e.g., the elderly, those whose systemic adjuvant therapy recommendations are not affected by the outcome, and those with extremely small primary tumors).

Interest in finding a less morbid way to assess the axilla has led to utilization of the sentinel lymph node biopsy in selected patients with invasive breast cancer. This technique is based on the presumption that a given area of the breast drains lymph first and preferentially to a specific lymph node. If this lymph node can be identified via injection of a radioactive tracer or vital dye, removed, and proven to be cancer-free, the rest of the lymph nodes in the axilla must be cancer-free as well, obviating the need for a formal axillary dissection. If the sentinel lymph node is positive for cancer, it is generally held (though somewhat controversially) that a more formal axillary dissection should be performed to determine how many lymph nodes are involved and if there is extracapsular extension of the axillary disease. In approximately 5% of cases localizing techniques fail to identify a specific sentinel node. In such cases axillary dissection should be performed. Finally, the false-negative rate may be as high as 10%, where the node thought to be the sentinel node fails to reveal the cancer, which is actually present in another axillary node. This is the most significant problem associated with the sentinel lymph node technique, as it leads to understaging and possible undertreatment of the patient from an adjuvant systemic therapy standpoint. Despite these potential drawbacks, sentinel lymph node biopsy is growing in popularity and, upon completion of some clinical trials currently under way, may become the standard of care for axillary assessment, especially with small primary tumors (T1a, T1b).[7]

Postlumpectomy Irradiation

The final component of breast conservation therapy is irradiation of the ipsilateral breast.[8] This is necessitated by the fact that there is often clinically occult multicentric cancer present in the involved breast and that a histologically "free" margin does not guarantee total tumor removal. As stated under Logal–Regional Therapy, above, radiation therapy after lumpectomy significantly reduces the in-breast tumor recurrence rate. A typical course of radiation is approximately 5000 cGy delivered over 5 weeks (one fraction per day, 5 days per week) to the entire breast and low axilla to include the axillary tail. A "boost" of 1000 cGy over 1 week can be optionally delivered to the lumpectomy site if the margins were close. The higher axilla and supraclavicular areas are usually not irradiated, reducing the risk of lymphedema, unless there is significant axillary involvement or extracapsular nodal extension. The internal mammary chain also is not usually included unless the tumor was located medially and had metastasized to axillary lymph nodes. Current treatment planning techniques involve delivery of radiation tangentially to the chest wall to minimize the amount of lung and heart tissue exposed to radiation. The most common side effects of radiation therapy are skin changes, tenderness in the involved area, and fatigue. Hair loss and nausea do not occur with breast irradiation.

Modified Radical Mastectomy

The other approach to local–regional management of early invasive breast cancer is removal of the entire breast and axillary contents (modified radical mastectomy). Prior to the acceptance of breast-conserving techniques, modified radical mastectomy was the standard of care for several decades. It had supplanted the more aggressive muscle-removing Halsted radical mastectomy when it became clear that there was no survival advantage to the more aggressive surgery.

Current indications for modified radical mastectomy include the presence of a tumor too large in relation to breast size to permit an acceptable cosmetic result after lumpectomy, positive margins after attempted lumpectomy, multicentric or diffuse breast involvement, contraindications to radiation therapy, or personal preference by the patient.

The technique involves removing the entire breast and a variable amount of the axillary fat pad usually up to or including level II tissue. The pectoralis major muscle is preserved, which facilitates postmastectomy reconstruction and provides more cosmetically acceptable chest wall appearance, even when reconstruction is not performed. The skin incision is usually a modified elliptical one oriented transversely or obliquely across the chest wall. It is designed to include the nipple–areolar complex, the skin affected by previous needle or open biopsies of the cancer, and any skin thought to be too close to the primary tumor to be spared. Current techniques support sparing as much skin as possible in patients in whom reconstruction is to be performed. Otherwise, sufficient additional skin is removed to allow a tension-free closure but without leaving redundant folds of skin.

The axillary dissection portion of the modified radical mastectomy is performed according to the same considerations outlined above, except the axillary tissue is removed in continuity with the breast. Sentinel lymph node techniques can be utilized during a mastectomy but seem somewhat less applicable, as removal of the entire tail of the breast necessitated by the mastectomy requires significant exposure and dissection of the low axillary area anyway. The complications of modified radical mastectomy include those already mentioned for axillary dissection plus possible flap necrosis, hematoma, infection, and the obvious cosmetic and functional sequelae attendant to loss of the breast.

Postmastectomy Chest Wall Irradiation

Occasionally radiation therapy to the chest wall is recommended following mastectomy (5–10% of cases). Indications include positive mastectomy margins, a primary tumor > 5 cm, four or more positive axillary lymph nodes, matted lymph nodes or extracapsular nodal involvement, positive interpectoral lymph nodes, or skin or chest wall involvement. Some of these indications are flexible, but positive margins after mastectomy would be an absolute indication for chest wall irradiation. The technique is somewhat similar to that described for postlumpectomy irradiation (see above) in which 5000 cGy is delivered over a 5-week period. An additional 1000 cGy may be optionally delivered as a boost to the closest margin of excision. The regional lymph nodes, including the supraclavicular nodes, are usually included in the field. An internal mammary port can be added for a medially oriented primary tumor with positive axillary lymph nodes. The side effects of the radiation therapy are those discussed above.

It had been believed that chest wall irradiation after mastectomy improved the local control rate but had little impact on overall survival. Some recent studies, however, suggest that there may also be a survival advantage to chest wall irradiation in selected groups of patients, especially those who are node-positive.[8–10]

Reconstruction

After mastectomy the patient has the option of undergoing surgical reconstruction of the breast. It can be done immediately (i.e., at the same time as the mastectomy) or in a delayed fashion in which several months pass to allow the inflammation of the mastectomy to subside. The most common technique for breast reconstruction is placement of a subpectoral tissue expander. Postoperatively, this device is slowly expanded by sequential saline injections to create a mound that most closely approximates the size of the opposite breast. The expander is then later removed and replaced with a permanent implant.

The breast mound can also be reconstructed utilizing autologous tissue. One option in this regard is use of the transverse rectus abdominis myocutaneous (TRAM) flap. This procedure involves transposing a portion of the rectus abdominis muscle with its overlying skin and subcutaneous tissue as a free flap necessitating a microvascular anastomosis or as a rotation flap based on the superior epigastric vessels. This operation requires several hours of surgery, and the recovery and rehabilitation time

after it is considerably longer. However, it yields excellent cosmetic results and avoids the need for a prosthetic implant in the chest wall area. Alternatively, a myocutaneous flap utilizing the latissimus dorsi muscle can be rotated around into the anterior chest wall area, but it usually requires placement of a tissue expander or implant. The nipple (utilizing local skin) and the areola (most often tattooed) can be reconstructed later if the patient so chooses.

Possible complications of reconstruction include flap necrosis, implant rupture or migration, or capsule formation around the implant. Patient factors that may adversely affect the outcome of reconstruction include arteriosclerotic vascular disease, diabetes, a history of smoking, and a history of irradiation of the chest wall.

I. and J. Adjuvant Systemic Therapy

The indications for systemic therapy have broadened significantly over the past three decades. Cytotoxic chemotherapy was originally used only to treat documented systemic disease. Later, its value in the adjuvant setting in reducing the recurrence rate among node-positive patients was recognized. More recently similar value has been demonstrated among select groups of node-negative patients. The antiestrogen agent tamoxifen was developed during this evolution. Intensive evaluation of its utility likewise demonstrated effectiveness in the same settings of distant metastatic disease and both node-positive and node-negative adjuvant therapy. It has even shown effectiveness as a chemopreventive agent, reducing the risk of developing breast cancer among high-risk individuals. Cytotoxic chemotherapy and hormone therapy (primarily tamoxifen) are frequently combined in the adjuvant treatment of selected groups of breast cancer patients.

The criteria used to plan adjuvant therapy includes nodal status, size of the primary tumor, hormone receptor status, and menopausal status of the patient (age ≥ 50 when the menopausal status cannot be assessed). Other measures of tumor aggressiveness (e.g., ploidy, S-phase fraction, histologic/nuclear grade, *Her 2 neu*) play only a secondary role in equivocal cases.

A large number of randomized prospective clinical trials have led to our current understanding of the effectiveness of adjuvant systemic therapy and the guidelines used to make adjuvant treatment recommendations.[11,12] As a broad generalization, the benefit of adjuvant therapy is an approximate 30–40% reduction in the risk of systemic recurrence. The absolute benefit depends on the initial likelihood of recurrence after local–regional therapy has been completed. For example, for a favorable stage I cancer, the likelihood of systemic recurrence may be only 10%. Therefore only approximately 3% of these patients who receive adjuvant therapy benefit. In contradistinction, an aggressive stage II cancer may be associated with a 45% likelihood of systemic recurrence, in which case adjuvant systemic therapy would benefit approximately 15% of patients so affected. Thus even though virtually every patient with early invasive breast cancer may benefit from combinations of chemotherapy or tamoxifen (or both), the likelihood of benefit in some cases is so small it is not worth the morbidity associated with the treatment. This morbidity includes neutropenia, hair loss, and nausea with adriamycin and cyclophosphamide; neutropenia, variable hair loss, esophagitis, and weight gain with cyclophosphamide, methotrexate, and 5-fluorouracil; and an increased incidence of endometrial cancer and thromboembolic phenomena with tamoxifen.

Node-Negative Patients (I)

Among node-negative patients, if the tumor is < 1 cm there is insufficient benefit from systemic therapy to warrant its routine use regardless of receptor or menopausal status. The exception is tamoxifen when used as a chemopreventive agent.

Among node-negative patients with tumors ≥ 1 cm, those with estrogen receptor (ER)-negative tumors are advised to undergo chemotherapy, with tamoxifen optionally added for prevention. For similar patients with ER-positive tumors who are premenopausal, a combination of chemotherapy and tamoxifen is recommended; and for those who are postmenopausal tamoxifen with chemotherapy frequently added is recommended if the patient's general medical status permits.

Node-Positive Patients (J)

In general and with the exception of elderly patients (> 70 years old) and those with co-morbid medical conditions, it is recommended that all patients with positive axillary lymph nodes be given chemotherapy. Among these patients, those with ER-positive tumors also benefit from addition of tamoxifen. Those with ER-negative tumors may also benefit from tamoxifen in its role as a chemopreventive agent.

Currently, two chemotherapy regimens are considered standard for adjuvant systemic therapy. One regimen is AC (i.e., adriamycin 60 mg/m^2 IV and cyclophosphamide 600 mg/m^2 IV every 3 weeks for a total of four cycles). Another regimen is CMF (cyclophosphamide 100 mg/m^2 PO each day for 14 days, methotrexate 40 mg/m^2 on days 1 and 8, and 5-fluorouracil 500–600 mg/m^2 IV on days 1 and 8). The CMF regimen is then cycled every 4 weeks for a total of six cycles. There have been no randomized trials to prove the superiority of CMF versus AC. Many patients prefer AC because of its shorter duration (9 weeks versus 6 months), although hair loss is more likely to occur with AC.

K. Posttreatment Surveillance

There is considerable variability in the routine for posttreatment surveillance of patients with early invasive breast cancer. This algorithm represents the broadly accepted plan for surveillance.

It is of note that some clinicians believe that breast cancer patients should be followed clinically every 6 months for life because of their being at high risk for developing a second primary tumor. The value of systemic screening with chemistry profiles and chest radiographs has been questioned by the assertion that survival after detection of systemic disease is not enhanced by finding the disease preclinically, in contrast to detecting it on the basis of clinical signs and symptoms. Routine gynecologic evaluation for those on tamoxifen is important because of its modestly increased incidence of endometrial cancer among postmenopausal patients. The accepted follow-up is an annual clinical pelvic examination and Papanicolaou smear. Pelvic ultrasonography; transvaginal ultrasonography; and endometrial biopsies may be used if indicated based on the pelvic examination or postmenopausal vaginal bleeding, but they are not routinely needed.

L. Prognosis and Survival

A number of variables have been shown to predict outcome and survival independently after treatment of early invasive breast cancer. Of those listed in this algorithm, nodal status is the most important prognostic determinant. Large tumor size, negative ER status, high histologic and nuclear grade, and *Her2 neu* overexpression also predict a worse prognosis.

Because breast cancer frequently recurs after 5 years, survival data are usually based on the 10-year follow-up. The numbers presented in this algorithm are broad generalizations but reflect the general worsening of the prognosis with advanced stages of the disease.

Management of the High Risk Patient

Our knowledge of the risk factors that predict the likelihood of developing breast cancer, especially our ability to identify predisposing genetic mutations (see above), have allowed identification of subsets of individuals who are at extremely high risk of developing breast cancer. Until recently, either careful clinical and mammographic surveillance or prophylactic bilateral total mastectomy were the only options available to these patients.

Tamoxifen has been shown to be a reasonably effective chemopreventive agent, reducing the risk of future development of breast cancer among high risk individuals by nearly 50%.[13] The dose of tamoxifen is 20 mg by mouth each day for 5 years. When making the decision to use tamoxifen in this way, one must weigh the possible morbidity associated with tamoxifen use (an increased incidence of endometrial cancer and thromboembolic phenomena) against the statistical likelihood that the individual patient will develop breast cancer. Entry criteria for the tamoxifen chemoprevention trial (NSABP-1) took into account the presence of lobular carcinoma in situ, the patient's age, age at menarche, age at first live birth, the number of first-degree relatives with breast cancer, the number of previous breast biopsies, and the number of biopsy specimens with atypical hyperplasia. A risk profile was then generated.

Conclusions

Breast cancer is the second leading cause of cancer death in women. Identifiable risk factors include mutations in the *BRCA1* and *BRCA2* genes; a positive family history; a prior biopsy showing atypical hyperplasia, or in situ changes; various endocrine changes; and a history of breast cancer. Screening is performed with self and clinical breast examinations and mammography. For the patient with a suspicious palpable or mammographic finding, biopsy is indicated, the planning of which must be carefully thought out as it relates to the patient's desire for breast preservation. For early breast cancer, survival is similar whether the patient is treated with modified radical mastectomy or lumpectomy and breast irradiation. The clinically positive axilla should be treated with axillary dissection. The clinically negative axilla may be alternately approached using sentinel node biopsy techniques, reserving formal axillary dissection for cases where the sentinel node is positive. Histologically confirmed lymph node metastasis mandates systemic chemotherapy with tamoxifen added therapeutically for ER/PR-positive tumors or as a chemopreventive agent (NSABP P-1 trial). Node-negative patients with primary tumors < 1 cm do not require adjuvant therapy, although tamoxifen can be used for prevention. Premenopausal women with node-negative tumors ≥ 1 cm are treated primarily by chemotherapy with tamoxifen added for prevention. Postmenopausal women with node-negative, ER/PR-positive tumors ≥ 1 cm are treated by tamoxifen primarily with chemotherapy added, depending on the patient's overall condition. Following mastectomy, chest wall irradiation is indicated if the margins are positive, the tumor is > 5 cm, four or more axillary nodes are positive, there are matted lymph nodes or extracapsular nodal extension by tumor, or there is skin or chest wall involvement.

References

1. Carlson RW, Anderson BO, Densinger W, et al. Update: NCCN practice guidelines for the treatment of breast cancer; NCCN proceedings. Oncology 1999;13(5A):41–66.
2. Landis S, Murray T, Bolden S, Wingo P. Cancer statistics, 1999. CA Cancer J Clin 1999;49:8–31.
3. Harris J, Lippman M, Morrow H, Hellman S (eds) Diseases of the Breast. Philadelphia: Lippincott-Raven, 1996.
4. Report of the Organizing Committee and Collaborators, Falun Meeting. Falun, Sweden (March 1996). Breast cancer screening with mammography in women aged 40–49 years. Int J Cancer 1996;68:693–699.

5. Fleming ID, Cooper JS, Henson DE, et al. (eds) AJCC Staging Manual, 5th ed., Philadelphia: Lippincott Williams & Wilkins, 1997.
6. Fisher B, Anderson S, Redmond CK, Wolmark N, Wickerham DL, Cronin WM. Reanalysis and results after 12 years of follow-up in a randomized clinical trial comparing total mastectomy with lumpectomy with or without irradiation in the treatment of breast cancer. N Engl J Med 1995;333(22): 1456–1461.
7. Krag D, Weaver D, Ashikaga T, et al. The sentinel node in breast cancer —a multicenter validation study. N Engl J Med 1998;339(14):941–946.
8. Perez CA, Brady LW (eds). Principles and Practice of Radiation Oncology, 3rd ed. Philadelphia: Lippincott-Raven, 1998.
9. Overgaard M, Hansen PS, Overgaard J, et al. Postoperative radiotherapy in high-risk premenopausal women with breast cancer who receive adjuvant chemotherapy. Danish Breast Cancer Cooperative Group 82b Trial. N Engl J Med 1997;337(14):949–955.
10. Ragaz J, Jackson SM, Le N, et al. Adjuvant radiotherapy and chemotherapy in node-positive premenopausal women with breast cancer. N Engl J Med 1997;337(14):956–962.
11. Early Breast Cancer Trialists' Collaborative Group. Polychemotherapy for early breast cancer: an overview of the randomised trials. Lancet 1998;352:930–941.
12. Early Breast Cancer Trialists' Collaborative Group. Tamoxifen for early breast cancer: an overview of the randomised trials. Lancet 1998;351:1451–1467.
13. Fisher B, Costantino J, Wickerham D, et al. Tamoxifen for prevention of breast cancer: report of the National Surgical Adjuvant Breast and Bowel Project P-1 study. J Nat Cancer Inst 1998;90:1371–1388.

CHAPTER 24

Locally Advanced Breast Cancer

ELIZABETH MARCUS

Approximately 185,000 women were diagnosed with breast cancer in 1999 in the United States. Despite recent advances in public awareness and improvements in compliance with screening programs for early detection, approximately 10–15% of women with breast cancer presented with locally advanced disease.[1] In certain populations, particularly the medically underserved, the percentage of patients presenting with locally advanced breast cancer (LABC) may be higher. For example, at Cook County Hospital, which serves the medically indigent of Chicago and Illinois' Cook County, nearly 25% of the patients are diagnosed with cancer when their disease is already locally advanced. Nearly every surgeon who treats patients with breast cancer encounters locally advanced cases, underscoring the need to understand the options related to the management of this disease.

Historically, patients with LABC did extremely poorly in terms of local control and overall survival. For many years surgery alone was the standard of care for LABC, and 5-year survival rates were far from satisfactory. Surgical treatment typically consisted of a Halstead radical mastectomy; despite this radical approach, patients had high local recurrence rates and developed distant metastatic disease. The 5-year survival rates with surgery alone varied from 5% to 55% depending on the series.[2–4] Many of these series included a mix of patients, and naturally the series with better results tended to include more patients with less advanced disease at presentation. Much like the experience with surgery alone, radiation therapy alone was also found to be ineffective, with 5-year survival rates even lower, ranging from 18% to 28%.[5–7] It was not until the 1970s and the advent of neoadjuvant chemotherapy and other multimodality therapeutic strategies that an improvement in outcome was seen. It is fair to say that multimodality therapeutic strategies (including a combination of chemo/hormonal therapy, surgery, and radiation therapy) are the standard of care for this disease. A number of controversies still exist, however, about optimal management including the best timing and sequencing of treatment modalities, surgical procedure to be utilized, and the chemo/hormonal agents to be prescribed. These points are the decision points in the management algorithm.

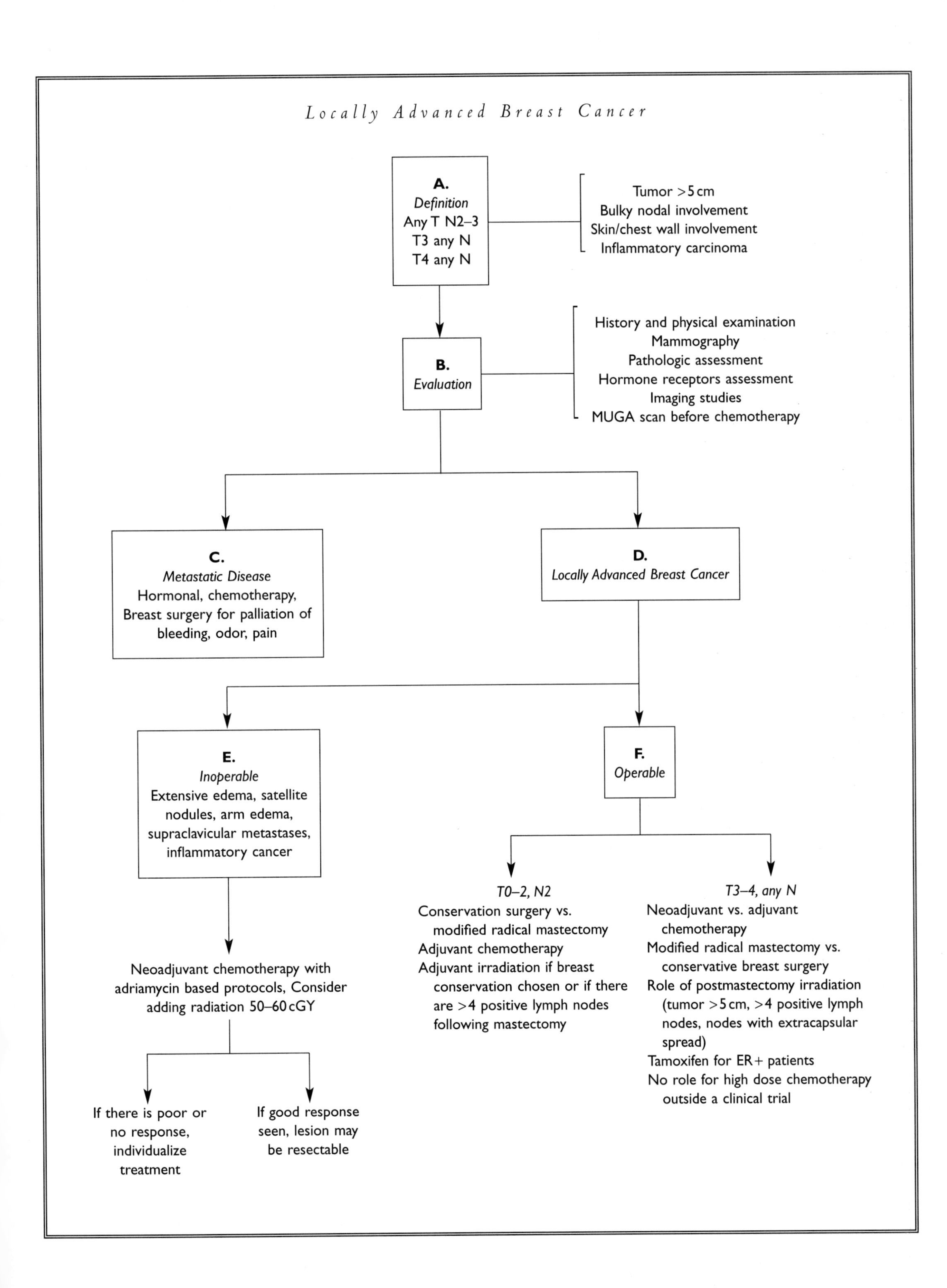

Locally Advanced Breast Cancer
A.
Definition
Any T N2–3
T3 any N
T4 any N
Tumor >5 cm
Bulky nodal involvement
Skin/chest wall involvement
Inflammatory carcinoma
B.
Evaluation
History and physical examination
Mammography
Pathologic assessment
Hormone receptors assessment
Imaging studies
MUGA scan before chemotherapy
C.
Metastatic Disease
Hormonal, chemotherapy, Breast surgery for palliation of bleeding, odor, pain
D.
Locally Advanced Breast Cancer
E.
Inoperable
Extensive edema, satellite nodules, arm edema, supraclavicular metastases, inflammatory cancer
F.
Operable
Neoadjuvant chemotherapy with adriamycin based protocols, Consider adding radiation 50–60 cGY
If there is poor or no response, individualize treatment
If good response seen, lesion may be resectable
T0–2, N2
Conservation surgery vs. modified radical mastectomy
Adjuvant chemotherapy
Adjuvant irradiation if breast conservation chosen or if there are >4 positive lymph nodes following mastectomy
T3–4, any N
Neoadjuvant vs. adjuvant chemotherapy
Modified radical mastectomy vs. conservative breast surgery
Role of postmastectomy irradiation (tumor >5 cm, >4 positive lymph nodes, nodes with extracapsular spread)
Tamoxifen for ER+ patients
No role for high dose chemotherapy outside a clinical trial

A. Definition

The definition of what constitutes LABC has changed over the years with the evolving staging systems, making interpretation of the literature difficult. When evaluating the literature on LABC, it is important to understand how the authors have defined the disease and exactly which patients they have included in their studies. In general, the term LABC is applied to patients who have large tumors (>5 cm), bulky nodal involvement, or skin or chest wall involvement. It also includes patients diagnosed with inflammatory breast cancer. Using the American Joint Commission on Cancer (AJCC) staging system, this includes some IIB patients (T3 N0) and patients with IIIA (anyT N2, T3 N1, T3 N2) or IIIB (T4 anyN, anyT N3) disease. By definition, these patients do not have metastatic disease. Patients with supraclavicular nodal involvement are considered to have metastatic disease, even if this is the sole site of metastasis.

B. Evaluation

When a patient presents with a suspected LABC, the initial decision points are (1) Is this a cancer? (2) Is it metastatic or simply LABC? The first step is always a thorough history and physical examination. In particular, the practitioner should ask about the duration of symptoms, family history of breast or ovarian cancer, ongoing use of hormone replacement therapy (which should be stopped), and if there are systemic symptoms (i.e., bone pain, shortness of breath), which may point to the presence of metastatic disease. Evaluation with bilateral mammography is essential, as disease in the contralateral breast, which may alter management, may be missed on simple physical examination.

A tissue diagnosis must be established. Options for establishing the diagnosis include fine-needle aspiration (FNA) biopsy, core biopsy, and incisional biopsy (excisional biopsy is rarely possible in the face of LABC). Although FNA biopsy has the advantage of minimal discomfort for the patient, it cannot definitively determine the invasiveness of the malignancy. A large ductal carcinoma in situ (DCIS) is unusual in this day and age, but it may still be seen. Furthermore, FNA biopsy may not provide enough tissue for other studies, such as evaluation of the estrogen and progesterone receptor status and assessment of the overamplification (by immunohistochemistry staining) or gene amplification [by fluorescent in situ hybridization (FISH)] of c-*erbB2/Her2neu*. Assessment of the tumor for these factors may have implications for future treatment options. If it is decided to give the patient neoadjuvant chemotherapy, the possibility exists that a complete pathologic response will occur following treatment and there will be no tumor present for assessment after surgery. Core needle biopsy, which has the advantage of allowing these tests to be run on the tumor, can be performed in the clinic or office setting with minimal discomfort to the patient when a local anesthetic is utilized. In addition, it can be performed while preserving all future surgical options. There is rarely need to subject the patient to an incisional biopsy, which is reserved for those rare situations where an invasive cancer cannot be diagnosed by core needle biopsy.

Once a diagnosis has been established, the next step is to rule out metastatic disease. Evaluation should include a full history and physical examination. The presence of bone pain, shortness of breath, or supraclavicular lymphadenopathy suggests metastatic disease. Laboratory evaluation should include a complete blood count (CBC), platelet count, liver function tests, and chest radiography. Although some practitioners still perform extensive imaging [i.e., total body computed tomography (CT) scans], the most recent National Comprehensive Cancer Network (NCCN) guidelines consider this practice to be somewhat controversial.[8]

The NCCN guidelines recommend bone scans in the face of symptoms or elevated alkaline phosphatase and CT scans as indicated by abnormalities of other screening tests (i.e., liver function tests or chest radiography). CT of the chest may be useful for assessing the extent of chest wall involvement when there is extensive local disease. In addition to staging, a multiple gated acquisition (MUGA) scan should be obtained to evaluate cardiac function prior to adriamycin-based therapy owing to the potential cardiac toxicity of the chemotherapeutic regimens.

C. Metastatic Disease

The natural history of breast cancer is varied; but once metastatic disease is discovered, long-term cure becomes unlikely. However, the disease may follow an indolent course that includes long-term remissions, and it is difficult to know what course the patient's disease will take. Patients should be treated initially with systemic therapy; therapeutic strategies include *hormonal* treatment with antiestrogens, aromatase inhibitors, progestational agents (i.e., megestrol acetate), medical oophorectomy with luteinizing hormone-releasing agonists (i.e., goserelin), or surgical oophorectomy. In addition, many *chemotherapeutic agents* and dosing regimens active against breast cancer have been used to treat metastatic disease. The new agents and therapeutic strategies are promising, and many clinical trials are open to patients with metastatic disease. Inclusion in a clinical trial should be one of the options for these patients.

If there is a good response to therapy, it may be reasonable to address the issue of local control. Another reason to perform *surgery* in the patient with metastatic disease is to palliate symptoms such as ulceration, bleeding, odor, or pain due to local disease. Treatment should be individualized based on the extent of disease, the patient's overall physical condition, and the patient's wishes. The emphasis during treatment of metastatic disease is palliation of symptoms and prolongation of apparent disease-free intervals.

D. *Locally Advanced Breast Cancer*

Once the diagnosis of LABC has been made, and metastatic disease has been excluded, the first decision is whether the patient has operable disease. The classic description of inoperability comes from the work of Haagensen and Stout published in 1943.[2] They included as inoperable any patient with: (1) extensive edema of the skin over the breast; (2) satellite nodules in the skin over the breast; (3) intercostal or parasternal nodules; (4) edema of the arm; (5) proven supraclavicular metastases (now considered metastatic disease); or (6) inflammatory-type carcinoma. They thought that the local recurrence rates and the high risk of distant failure in this group of patients predicted the futility of a surgical procedure for controlling the disease. In the age of multimodality therapy the term "inoperable" has become one of surgical judgment: The question is can the patient technically undergo a surgical procedure with negative margins? Many of Haagensen and Stout's original criteria may still be applied when assessing operability, as they indicate a situation in which surgical extirpation is unlikely to yield negative margins.

E. *Inoperable Disease*

If patients have inoperable disease, they are treated with neoadjuvant chemotherapy, usually a doxorubicin-containing regimen if their cardiac status allows it. The response is assessed during chemotherapy. If at the completion of treatment the patient has an operable status, surgical resection can be performed. A course of radiation therapy (50–60 Gy) should be considered followed by surgery if a favorable response to irradiation is seen. The use of irradiation as the only modality for local control results in local recurrence rates of 40–70%. In one study at the M.D. Anderson Cancer Center the addition of surgery to chemotherapy and irradiation improved local control for patients with stage IIIB inflammatory breast cancer who had a complete response (local recurrence 0% vs. 20%) or a partial response (local recurrence 12% vs. 30%) to their chemotherapy regimen.[9] Patients with a poor response to induction chemotherapy and who never become operable have a poor prognosis and do not benefit from the addition of surgical resection. In these instances, treatment should be individualized; alternatives include a different chemotherapy regimen, hormonal therapy for patients with hormonally sensitive disease, or inclusion in clinical trials of new treatment regimens.

F. *Operable Disease*

For patients with technically operable disease, there are many choices with regard to treatment. For patients with small tumors and bulky nodal disease (T0–2, N2 disease) it is reasonable to operate promptly; choices include breast conservation or a modified radical mastectomy. Breast conservation consists of lumpectomy with negative margins, as positive margins are associated with high local recurrence rates even with the addition of radiation therapy. A therapeutic axillary node dissection should be included to remove all gross disease. Once information is available concerning the tumor size and nodal status, decisions can be made concerning appropriate adjuvant chemo/hormonal therapy for the patient. Irradiation should be standard local adjuvant therapy if breast conservation has been elected.

For more extensive disease (T3 and T4 lesions) the use of combined-modality regimens in recent years, including surgery, chemotherapy, and irradiation, have improved survival rates from 5–55% with single-modality regimens to 50–75%.[10–12] The question remains as to the optimal sequencing of these combined-modality regimens. Many controversies still exist and are outlined below.

Neoadjuvant Versus Adjuvant Chemotherapy

The question of sequencing chemotherapy and surgery remains an unanswered one. There are potential advantages to each. The advantage of surgery followed by adjuvant chemotherapy is that it provides more accurate staging in terms of tumor size and nodal status, which may be of prognostic value. The potential advantage of neoadjuvant (or "induction") chemotherapy includes downstaging the tumor, thereby possibly allowing breast conservation and providing an opportunity to assess tumor response in vivo. Although some staging information (i.e., true nodal status at diagnosis) is lost with the use of the neoadjuvant approach, the preoperative response of a tumor to induction therapy is prognostic of outcome.[13,14]

In addition, there had been some hope that there would be a survival advantage to neoadjuvant/induction chemotherapy. The theoretic advantage was that early treatment of presumed micrometastatic disease and prevention of the emergence of drug-resistant cell lines would decrease failure rates and improve survival. Another theoretic advantage came from experiments in animal models suggesting that the presence of the primary tumor inhibited the growth of micrometastatic disease; it follows, then, that treatment of the micrometastases prior to removing the primary tumor should improve survival.

However, as is often the case, what is true in vitro may not be true in vivo. There are few randomized clinical trials that compare neoadjuvant chemotherapy to postoperative adjuvant therapy.[13,15–17] It is important to note that these trials must be interpreted carefully, as they have different definitions of "locally advanced breast cancer." Some include tumors as small as 3 cm, which may be biologically different from larger tumors. Extrapolating these results to patients with large tumors must be done with caution. Despite that admonition, none of these trials has shown a clear survival advantage of one strategy or another. In the absence of a clear survival advantage, either neoadjuvant or adjuvant chemotherapy is reasonable to consider.

One other potential benefit of the neoadjuvant chemotherapy strategy is that it provides a model for studying the effects of new treatments on tumor response and biology. The clinical and pathologic response to new treatment regimens is readily assessable in a shorter period of time than the classic adjuvant chemotherapy model. In addition, with the collection of tumor specimens both before and after treatment, biologic and molecular markers may be studied for their predictive value, which may allow future tailoring of therapy for the individual patient. They may also be studied for their responses to new treatments, thereby suggesting new targets for therapeutic interventions.

Breast Conservation Versus Modified Radical Mastectomy

The original intent of breast conservation therapy in the face of locally advanced breast cancer was to spare patients a surgical procedure that would not affect their survival. Because patients with locally advanced disease had a poor prognosis, why put them through a deforming procedure that did not stand to improve their outcome? In recent years with the more widespread use of breast-conserving therapy for early-stage disease and the increased use of neoadjuvant chemotherapy, the question has become: Could extensive disease be converted to less extensive disease, transforming the patient to a conservation candidate? Several studies have sought to answer this question.

One report on this strategy came from Bonnadonna et al. in 1990.[18] Patients with locally advanced breast cancer underwent neoadjuvant chemotherapy followed by surgery and irradiation. The criterion for eligibility for breast conservation was that the tumor had to be <3 cm following chemotherapy. Of the 157 patients in this study, 127 (81%) were able to have breast-conserving therapy. In a report from Touboul et al. from France,[19] 50 of 82 patients (61%) with LABC became candidates for breast conservation with either lumpectomy + irradiation (n = 18) or irradiation alone (n = 32) (in the absence of palpable tumor). The group treated with lumpectomy plus irradiation had a 16% local failure rate, and 25% of the patients treated with irradiation alone had local failure, either by itself or in combination with regional or distant failure. The group treated with mastectomy had distant failure as some component of their initial site of failure (37%); local failure was part of this recurrence in only 6% of patients treated by mastectomy. The study concluded that although neoadjuvant chemotherapy permitted selecting a group of patients technically eligible for conservation, the impact on long-term outcome remained to be determined.

Other institutions have also reported on the feasibility of breast conservation following administration of neoadjuvant chemotherapy.[20–23] The patient populations varied, with some studies including some stage IIB patients. In addition, different studies have different criteria for characterizing a patient as a conservation candidate. Keeping this in mind, the breast-conservation rates range from 27% to 81%. All of these studies have shown the feasibility of this strategy: that many patients can be down-staged by initial administration of chemotherapy.

The question remains, however, whether a large breast cancer made small with neoadjuvant chemotherapy behaves like one that is small at diagnosis. Are they biologic equivalents, and can the results from breast conservation trials on early-stage disease be extrapolated to LABC that has a good response to neoadjuvant chemotherapy? Many of the reported studies lack extended long-term follow-up. Although they do not seem to show an increase in locoregional failure, many of the studies included patients who presented at lower stages of disease; and evaluating subgroups of large tumors may reveal increased local recurrence rates in those treated with breast conservation therapy. Whereas those treated with conservation have a distant failure rate similar to that of studies where mastectomy was routinely employed, as improvements are made in systemic therapy it is not clear whether improving local control affects survival. All of these issues make it difficult to draw clear conclusions as to the role of breast conservation in LABC. With the lack of conclusive evidence as to its safety or harm, it remains an option for patients who are down-staged by neoadjuvant chemotherapy.

Role of Postmastectomy Irradiation

The role of postmastectomy irradiation is another issue that essentially questions how best to improve local control during treatment of LABC. Until recently the conventional wisdom, extrapolated from trials of breast conservation in early disease, was that improved local control did not affect survival. During the last few years, however, the role of radiation therapy following mastectomy has been reexamined. The primary question is whether improvements in local control affect survival and, if so, in which group of patients the advantage is seen.

Two recent studies, one from British Columbia[24] and the other from the Danish Breast Cancer Group,[25] confirmed the benefit of postmastectomy irradiation in patients with large tumors (>5 cm), more than four positive lymph nodes, and the presence of nodes with extracapsular extension. The patients with these features were at increased risk (30–40%) of local recurrence. The difference in distant recurrence rates between patients undergoing postmastectomy irradiation and those who did not was approximately 10%, favoring the group with irradiation. This corresponded with improved survival in patients with irradiation following mastectomy.

In both of these studies the group of patients with one to three positive nodes failed to show statistically significant improvement in survival, although this may have been due to the fact that the numbers were too small to show a difference. This group did benefit in terms of local control, although it is not clear whether this benefit translates into an improvement in survival. Further research is needed to answer this question.

Although these studies were performed on patients treated with mastectomy initially prior to adjuvant chemotherapy or radiation therapy, it is not clear whether the subgroups identified (tumor >5 cm, more than four positive nodes) apply to patients who undergo neoadjuvant chemotherapy. For example, should the patient's inclusion in a high risk group be based on the tumor size at presentation or tumor size after chemotherapy? Again, there are no randomized trials to guide management. However, extrapolating the data from these studies make the addition of irradiation to mastectomy for locally advanced breast cancer a reasonable option, even following neoadjuvant chemotherapy. Whether there are groups of patients for whom irradiation or surgery may be omitted without sacrificing local or distant control remains a question for future studies.

Adjuvant Hormonal Therapy

Patients whose tumors are estrogen receptor-positive (ER^+) benefit from the addition of tamoxifen, a nonsteroidal antiestrogenic compound, to their regimen. In the meta-analysis performed by the Early Breast Cancer Trialists' Collaborative Group (EBCTCG),[26] who evaluated all of the trials of tamoxifen versus no therapy, the use of tamoxifen reduced the risk of breast cancer recurrence by 26% ± 4% for women with node-negative disease. In women with node-positive disease, addition of tamoxifen reduced the risk of recurrence by 28% ± 2%. The 1995 update of the EBCTCG study, which included data on approximately 30,000 women, demonstrated continued benefit with the use of tamoxifen.[27] Even with the use of adjuvant chemotherapy, there was an additional benefit to the use of tamoxifen. It is recommended as adjuvant therapy for patients with ER^+ tumors.

The optimal duration of therapy is still being examined in clinical trials, but the current recommendation is for 5 years of administration. In both the NSABP B-14[28] and the Scottish Tamoxifen Trial,[29] no advantage was found with administration beyond 5 years. Whether less than 5 years of tamoxifen therapy is as beneficial is the subject of ongoing clinical trials. Although these studies primarily involve early-stage breast cancers, it is reasonable to add tamoxifen therapy to the adjuvant treatment of patients with ER^+ locally advanced breast cancer.

Role of High Dose Chemotherapy

During the past several years a good deal of attention has been given to the role of high dose chemotherapy when treating high risk breast cancer patients. For locally advanced disease, the high risk of distant failure has prompted the search for improved systemic therapies. It is only with an improvement in systemic therapy that improvements in survival will be seen. The argument for high dose chemotherapy was that our current systemic therapies do not expose the tumor to high enough doses to eradicate all of the tumor cells and that the dose–response relation seen in vitro would translate into improved tumor kill in vivo. Initial reports from single-institution phase II studies were encouraging and prompted initiation of five phase III randomized clinical trials of high dose chemotherapy versus "standard therapy." These five randomized trials have now produced results.[30–34] Of the five trials, only one was able to show any benefit with high dose chemotherapy; and it was subsequently found that the results of this study were based on fraudulent data, so the results have been discounted.[32] There may be a subgroup of patients who ultimately benefit from this treatment strategy, but it is fair to say that currently, outside the context of a well designed clinical trial, there is no role for high dose chemotherapy in the treatment of breast cancer.

References

1. Wingo PA, Tong T, Bolden S. Cancer statistics, 1995. CA Cancer J Clin 1995;45:8–30.
2. Haagensen C, Stout A. Carcinoma of the breast. II. Criteria of operability. Ann Surg 1943;118:859–870.
3. Scottenfeld D, Nash AG, Robbins GF, Beattie EJ Jr. Ten-year results of the treatment of primary operable carcinoma: a summary of 304 patients evaluated by the TNM system. Cancer 1976;38:1001–1007.
4. Arnold DJ, Lesnick GJ. Survival following mastectomy for stage III breast cancer. Am J Surg 1979;137:362–366.
5. Harris JR, Sawicka J, Gelman R, Hellman S. Management of locally advanced carcinoma of the breast by primary radiation therapy. Int J Radiat Oncol Biol Phys 1983;9:345–349.
6. Rao DV, Bedwinek J, Perez C, Lee J, Fineberg B. Prognostic indicators in stage III and localized stage IV breast cancer. Cancer 19982;50:2037–2043.
7. Rubens RD, Armitage P, Winter PJ, Tong D, Hayward JL. Prognosis in inoperable stage III carcinoma of the breast. Eur J Cancer 1977;13:805–811.
8. Update of the NCCN guidelines for the treatment of breast cancer: NCCN proceedings. Oncology 1997;11:199–200.
9. Fleming RY, Asmar L, Buzdar AU, et al. Effectiveness of mastectomy by response to induction chemotherapy for control in inflammatory breast carcinoma. Ann Surg Oncol 1997;4:452–461.
10. Hortobagyi GN, Singletary SE, McNeese MD. Treatment of locally advanced and inflammatory breast cancer. In: Harris JR, Lippman ME, Morrow M, Hellman S (eds) Diseases of the Breast. Philadelphia: Lippincott-Raven, 1996:585–599.
11. Colozza M, Gori S, Mosconi AM, et al. Induction chemotherapy with cisplatin, doxorubicin, and cyclophosphamide (CAP) in a combined modality approach for locally advanced and inflammatory breast cancer: long-term results. Am J Clin Oncol 1996;19:10–17.
12. Buzdar AU, Singletary SE, Booser DJ, Frye DK, Wasaff B, Hortobagyi GN. Combined modality treatment of stage III and inflammatory breast cancer: M.D. Anderson Cancer Center experience. Surg Oncol Clin N Am 1995;4:715–734.
13. Fisher B, Bryant J, Wolmark N, et al. Effect of preoperative chemotherapy on the outcome of women with operable breast cancer. J Clin Oncol 1998;16:2672–2685.
14. Kuerer JM, Newman LA, Smith TL, et al. Clinical course of breast cancer patients with complete pathologic primary tumor and axillary lymph node response to doxorubicin-based neoadjuvant chemotherapy. J Clin Oncol 1999;17:460–469.
15. Mauriac L, Durand M, Avril A, Dilhuydy JM. Effects of primary chemotherapy in conservative treatment of breast cancer patients with operable tumors larger than 3 cm: results of a randomized trial in a single centre. Ann Oncol 1991;2:347–354.
16. Scholl SM, Forquest A, Asselain B, et al. Neoadjuvant versus adjuvant chemotherapy in premenopausal patients with tumors considered too large for breast conserving surgery: preliminary results of a randomized trial: S6. Eur J Cancer 1994;30A:645–652.
17. Powles TJ, Hickish TF, Makris A, et al. Randomized trial of chemoendocrine therapy started before or after surgery for treatment of primary breast cancer. J Clin Oncol 1995;13:547–552.
18. Bonnadonna G, Veronesi U, Brambilla C, et al. Primary chemotherapy to avoid mastectomy in tumors with diameters of three centimeters or more. J Natl Cancer Inst 1990;82:1539–1545.
19. Touboul E, Lefranc JP, Blondon J, et al. Multidisciplinary treatment approach to locally advanced non-inflammatory breast cancer using chemotherapy and radiotherapy with or without surgery. Radiother Oncol 1992;25:167–175.
20. Singletary S, McNeese M, Hortobagyi G. Feasibility of breast-conservation surgery after induction chemotherapy for locally advanced breast carcinoma. Cancer 1992;69:2849.
21. Merajver SD, Weber BL, Cody R, et al. Breast conservation and prolonged chemotherapy for locally advanced breast cancer: the University of Michigan experience. J Clin Oncol 1997;15:2873–2881.
22. Schwartz GF, Birchansky CA, Komarnicky LT, et al. Induction chemotherapy followed by breast conservation for locally advanced carcinoma of the breast. Cancer 1994;73:362–390.
23. Calais G, Descamps P, Chapet S, et al. Primary chemotherapy and radiosurgical breast-conserving treatment for patients with locally advanced operable breast cancers. Int J Radiat Oncol Biol Phys 1993;26:37.
24. Ragaz J, Jackson SM, Le N, et al. Adjuvant radiotherapy and chemotherapy in node-positive premenopausal women with breast cancer. N Engl J Med 1997;337:956–962.
25. Overgaard M, Hansen PS, Overgaard J, et al. Postoperative radiotherapy in high-risk premenopausal women with breast cancer who receive adjuvant chemotherapy: Danish Breast Cancer Cooperative Group. N Engl J Med 1997;337:949–955.
26. Early Breast Cancer Trialists' Collaborative Group. Systemic treatment of early breast cancer by hormonal, cytotoxic, or immune therapy: 133 randomised trials involving 31,000 recurrences and 24,000 deaths among 75,000 women. Lancet 1992;339:1–15.
27. Early Breast Cancer Trialists' Collaborative Group. Tamoxifen for early breast cancer: an overview of the randomised trials. Lancet 1998;351: 1451–1467.
28. Fisher B, Dignam J, Bryant J, et al. Five versus more than five years of tamoxifen therapy for breast cancer patients with negative lymph nodes and estrogen receptor-positive tumors. J Natl Cancer Inst 1996;88:1529–1542.
29. Stewart HJ, Forrest AP, Everington D, et al. Randomised comparison of 5 years of adjuvant tamoxifen with continuous therapy for operable breast cancer: the Scottish Cancer Trials Breast Group. Br J Cancer 1996; 74:297–299.
30. Rodenhuis S, Richel DJ, van der Wall E, et al. Randomised trial of high-dose chemotherapy and haemopoietic progenitor-cell support in operable breast cancer with extensive axillary lymph-node involvement. Lancet 1998;352:515–521.
31. Hortobagyi GN, Budzar AU, Bodey GP, et al. High-dose induction chemotherapy of metastatic breast cancer in protected environment: a prospective randomized study. J Clin Oncol 1987;5:178–184.
32. Bezwoda W. Randomised, controlled trial of high dose chemotherapy (HD-CVVp) versus standard dose (CAF) chemotherapy for high risk, surgically treated, primary breast cancer [abstract 4]. Proc Am Soc Clin Oncol 1999;18:2a.

33. Scandinavian Breast Cancer Study Group. Results from a randomized adjuvant breast cancer study with high dose chemotherapy with CTCb supported by autologous bone marrow stem cells versus dose escalated and tailored FEC therapy [abstract 3]. Proc Am Soc Clin Oncol 1999; 118:2a.

34. Peters W, Rosner G, Vredenburgh J, et al. A prospective, randomized comparison of two doses of combination alkylating agents (AA) as consolidation after CAF in high-risk primary breast cancer involving ten or more axillary lymph nodes (LN): preliminary results of CALGB 9082/SWOG 9114/NCIC MA-13 [abstract 2]. Proc Am Soc Clin Oncol 1999;18:1a.

Section 5

Cutaneous Malignancies

Chapter 25

Melanoma

JAMES S. ECONOMOU

The incidence of cutaneous melanoma is increasing. The typical melanoma patient has a fair complexion and a tendency to sunburn. Individuals who have had a prior melanoma or who have multiple dysplastic nevi are at greater risk. Familial melanoma is uncommon but has been well documented and underscores the genetic component to this disease.

Melanomas can occur anywhere in the body but tend to be found more commonly on the lower extremities in women and on the trunk in men. Signs and symptoms of melanoma include a change in the size of a preexisting lesion or appearance of a new lesion, irregular shape, and irregular color with a variety or shades of brown and black. Minor features include a diameter >7 mm, inflammation, oozing, crusting or bleeding, or a change in sensation.

A. Growth Patterns

There are four major growth patterns of melanoma. Seventy percent of melanomas are the *superficial spreading* type. These lesions generally arise in a preexisting nevus, and there is frequently a history of a slow change in the precursor lesion over several years. Superficial spreading melanomas evolve from having a flat to an irregular surface with both vertical and lateral asymmetry.

Nodular melanoma is the second most common growth pattern, found in 15–30% of patients. These melanomas tend to be more biologically aggressive and develop more rapidly. They tend to occur during middle age, appear on the trunk or head/neck, and are more common in men. Nodular melanomas may have a diameter of 1–2 cm and tend to arise de novo in uninvolved skin. They tend to be darker than superficial spreading melanomas and are more raised, as the name implies. They may be blue-black or have shades of red, gray, or purple; 5% are amelanotic. These tumors tend to have discrete borders without the irregular perimeter characteristic of superficial spreading melanomas.

Lentigo maligna melanomas (4–10%), located on the face of older patients, are generally large, flat lesions and tend to be present for many years. These skin cancers may display prominent irregularity of margins with areas of regression.

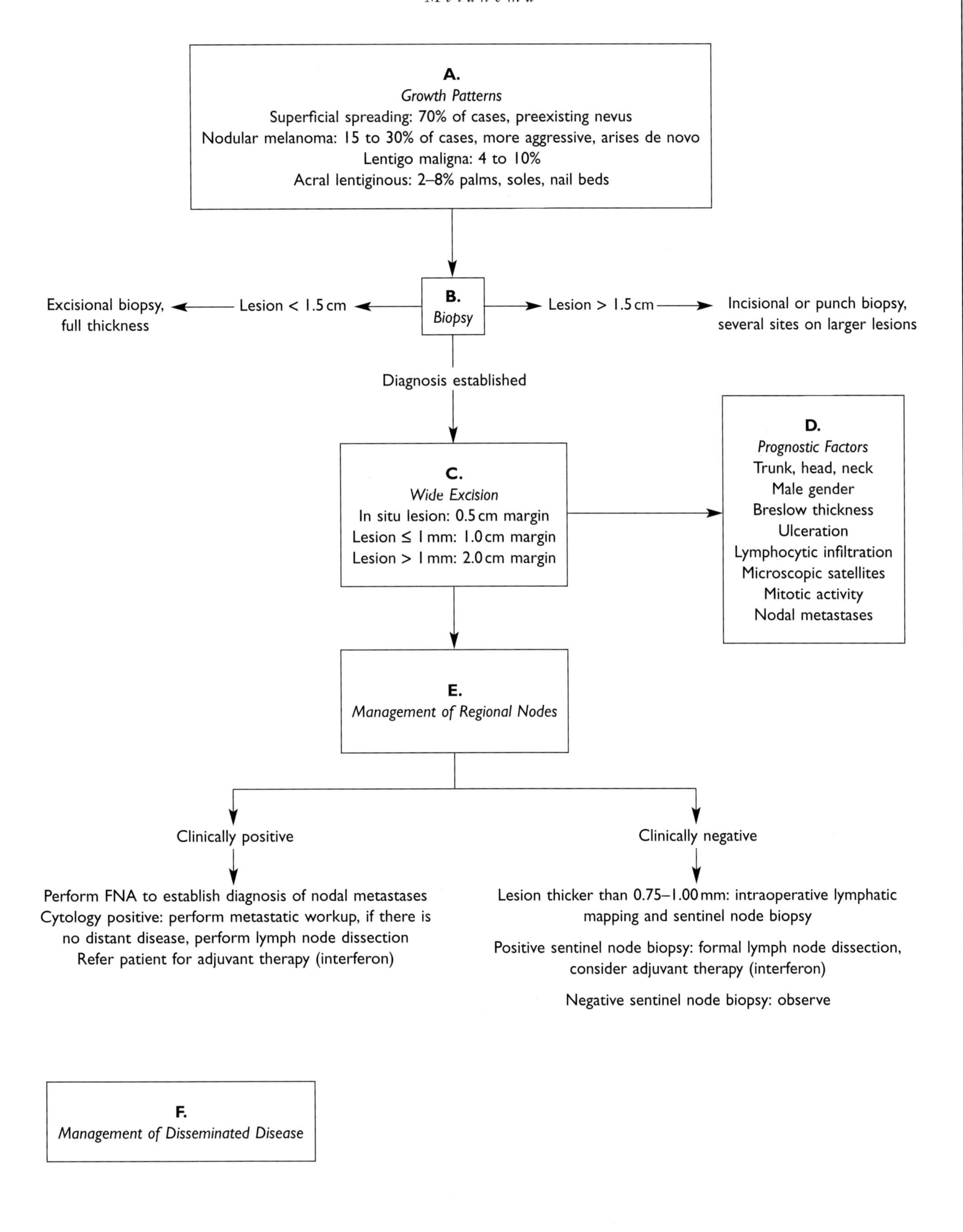

Melanoma
A.
Growth Patterns
Superficial spreading: 70% of cases, preexisting nevus
Nodular melanoma: 15 to 30% of cases, more aggressive, arises de novo
Lentigo maligna: 4 to 10%
Acral lentiginous: 2–8% palms, soles, nail beds
B.
Biopsy
Lesion < 1.5 cm
Excisional biopsy, full thickness
Lesion > 1.5 cm
Incisional or punch biopsy, several sites on larger lesions
Diagnosis established
C.
Wide Excision
In situ lesion: 0.5 cm margin
Lesion ≤ 1 mm: 1.0 cm margin
Lesion > 1 mm: 2.0 cm margin
D.
Prognostic Factors
Trunk, head, neck
Male gender
Breslow thickness
Ulceration
Lymphocytic infiltration
Microscopic satellites
Mitotic activity
Nodal metastases
E.
Management of Regional Nodes
Clinically positive
Perform FNA to establish diagnosis of nodal metastases
Cytology positive: perform metastatic workup, if there is no distant disease, perform lymph node dissection
Refer patient for adjuvant therapy (interferon)
Clinically negative
Lesion thicker than 0.75–1.00 mm: intraoperative lymphatic mapping and sentinel node biopsy
Positive sentinel node biopsy: formal lymph node dissection, consider adjuvant therapy (interferon)
Negative sentinel node biopsy: observe
F.
Management of Disseminated Disease

Finally, *acral lentiginous melanomas* occur on the palms or soles or underneath nail beds. They occur in only 2–8% of Caucasian patients, with a higher incidence in patients with darker skin coloration. Most are located on the sole of the foot and are generally large. They have a relatively short evolution.

B. Biopsy

Full-thickness biopsy of a suspicious pigmented lesion must be performed for accurate microstaging. Excisional biopsies for small lesions (<1.5 cm) are appropriate, and the orientation of the biopsy incision should be made in anticipation of the possible need for a subsequent wider excision. Incisional or punch biopsies are appropriate for large lesions, particularly those on the face and hands. It may be prudent to obtain more than one biopsy sample from large lesions.

Microstaging the primary lesion is a critical component of managing this disease (see below). The Breslow microstaging method measures the thickness using an ocular micrometer. The total vertical height of the melanoma is measured and expressed in millimeters. The Clark microstaging method categorizes the level of invasion in terms of penetration into the dermal layers of the skin.

The revised staging system recently approved by the American Joint Committee on Cancer (to be implemented in January 2003) is shown in Tables 25–1 and 25–2.

TABLE 25–1.
AJCC definition of TNM for cutaneous melanoma

T classification	Thickness	Ulceration status
T1	≤1.0 mm	a: without ulceration and level II/III b: with ulceration or level IV/V
T2	1.01–2.0 mm	a: without ulceration b: with ulceration
T3	2.01–4.0 mm	a: without ulceration b: with ulceration
T4	>4.0 mm	a: without ulceration b: with ulceration

N classification	No. of metastatic nodes	Nodal metastatic mass
N1	1 node	a: micrometastasis* b: macrometastasis†
N2	2–3 nodes	a: micrometastasis* b: macrometastasis† c: in transit met(s)/ satellite(s) without metastatic nodes
N3	4 or more metastatic nodes, or matted nodes, or in transit met(s)/satellite(s) with metastatic node(s)	

M classification	Site	Serum lactate dehydrogenase
M1a	Distant skin, subcutaneous, or nodal mets	Normal
M1b	Lung metastases	Normal
M1c	All other visceral metastases	Normal
	Any distant metastasis	Elevated

* Micrometastases are diagnosed after sentinel or elective lymphadenectomy.
† Marcrometastases are defined as clinically detectable nodal metastases confirmed by therapeutic lymphadenectomy or when nodal metastasis exhibits gross extracapsular extension.
SOURCE: Balch CM, Buzaid AC, Soong S-S, et al. Final version of the American Joint Committee on Cancer staging system for cutaneous melanoma. J. Clin. Oncol. 2001;19:3635–3648. Note: The above TNM classification system will be implemented in January 2003 and will appear in the AJCC® Cancer Staging Manual, 6th edition (2002) published by Springer-Verlag New York, Inc.

C. Wide Excision

Local control of primary melanoma requires wide excision with a margin of normal-appearing skin. The risk of local recurrence is a function of tumor thickness. A melanoma in situ may be reexcised with a margin of 0.5 cm. Thin melanomas, measuring ≤ a millimeter in thickness, may be excised with a 1 cm margin. Intermediate and thick melanomas measuring >1 mm in depth should be excised with a margin of 2 cm. Several randomized clinical trials have shown that these more conservative margins may be safely employed with a low incidence of local recurrence. Melanomas arising on the fingers and toes may require amputation. Not uncommonly, excision of facial lesions requires surgical judgment, as excisions with a >1 cm margin may compromise cosmesis and function. Local recurrences tend to be a harbinger of the subsequent development of metastatic disease. In most cases, however, this likely is a reflection of the biology of the disease rather than the inadequacy of the initial excision margins.

D. Prognostic Factors

A number of factors are known to predict the risk for metastatic disease and melanoma. Patients with melanomas on the extremities have a better survival rate than those with melanoma of the trunk or head/neck. Women have a better survival rate than men, primarily because their melanomas occur more commonly on the extremities. The vertical height (Breslow thickness) is the single most important prognostic factor. Ulcerated melanomas are more aggressive biologically.

TABLE 25-2.
AJCC stage grouping for cutaneous melanoma

	Clinical staging			Pathologic staging†		
	T	N	M	T	N	M
0	Tis	N0	M0	Tis	N0	M0
IA	T1a	N0	M0	T1a	N0	M0
IB	T1b	N0	M0	T1b	N0	M0
	T2a	N0	M0	T2a	N0	M0
IIA	T2b	N0	M0	T2b	N0	M0
	T3a	N0	M0	T3a	N0	M0
IIB	T3b	N0	M0	T3b	N0	M0
	T4a	N0	M0	T4a	N0	M0
IIC	T4b	N0	M0	T4b	N0	M0
III‡	Any T	N1	M0			
		N2				
		N3				
IIIA				T1–4a	N1a	M0
				T1–4a	N2a	M0
IIIB				T1–4b	N1a	M0
				T1–4b	N2a	M0
				T1–4a	N1b	M0
				T1–4a	N2b	M0
				T1–4a/b	N2c	M0
IIIC				T1–4b	N1b	M0
				T1–4b	N2b	M0
				Any T	N3	M0
IV	Any T	Any N	Any M1	Any T	Any N	Any M1

* Clinical staging includes microstaging of the primary melanoma and clinical/radiologic evaluation for metastases. By convention, it should be used after complete excision of the primary melanoma with clinical assessment for regional and distant metastases.
† Pathologic staging includes microstaging of the primary melanoma and pathologic information about the regional lymph nodes after partial or complete lymphadenectomy. Pathologic stage 0 or stage 1A patients are the exception; they do not require pathologic evaluation of their lymph nodes.
‡ There are no stage III subgroups for clinical staging.
SOURCE: Balch CM, Buzaid AC, Soong S-S, et al. Final version of the American Joint Committee on Cancer staging system for cutaneous melanoma. J. Clin. Oncol. 2001;19:3635–3648. Note: The above TNM classification system will be implemented in January 2003 and will appear in the AJCC® Cancer Staging Manual, 6th edition (2002) published by Springer-Verlag New York, Inc.

Nodular melanomas have a reputation for carrying the worst prognosis among the four histologic subtypes, which appears to be due to a preponderance of thick lesions at presentation. When nodular melanomas are matched with superficial spreading melanomas interms of lesion thickness, there is no survival difference between these two melanomas. Other pathologic features such as lymphocytic infiltration, microscopic satellites, and mitotic activity also have an influence on survival. The most significant prognostic factor for survival is the presence or absence of lymph node metastasis.

E. Management of Regional Lymph Nodes

Until 1990 the only way to determine if a clinically negative regional lymph node basin harbored micrometastatic disease was to perform a staging or elective lymph node dissection. Much effort was spent identifying patients at high risk and determining if an elective lymph node dissection conferred a survival advantage. This strategy was based on the premise that malignant melanoma metastasized in an orderly fashion from the primary site to its regional lymph node basin and then systemically. It was hypothesized that by performing a formal lymph node dissection in patients with clinically negative but microscopically positive lymph node basins, a larger percentage of these patients would enjoy a survival advantage than if a dissection was performed when metastatic disease became clinically evident. Although this biological view is intuitively attractive, it has been difficult to prove in randomized trials and even more difficult to justify the unnecessary performance of lymphadenectomy in almost 80% of patients.

This controversy was entirely supplanted in 1990 by the introduction of intraoperative lymphatic mapping and sentinel lymph node biopsy. The sentinel lymph node is the first draining lymph node on a direct lymphatic drainage pathway from the primary tumor site. It is the lymph node most likely to receive metastasis from the primary tumor. Lymphatic mapping was initially performed using a blue vital dye, isosulfan blue, which when injected intradermally rapidly enters the lymphatics and stains one or a few lymph nodes in the relevant lymph node basin. Many properly conducted clinical trials have now shown that this technique has high accuracy and sensitivity for identifying patients with lymphatic disease. The false-negative rate of this technique (patients whose sentinel nodes were negative but who had microscopically positive nonsentinel nodes) is low. The sensitivity of identifying small numbers of microscopic melanoma cells in these lymph nodes has been significantly improved with the use of immunohistochemical stains for S-100 and HMB-45. Use of the reverse polymerase chain reaction to detect messenger RNA for various melanoma antigens such as tyrosinase is still viewed as investigational.

The identification of lymphatic dye-stained sentinel nodes has been made technically easier with the introduction of radiolymphoscintigraphy. Just prior to surgery, technetium-labeled sulfur colloid is injected around the primary site of the cutaneous melanoma. Radioactive lymph nodes in the appropriate lymph node basin can be visualized using scintigraphic images obtained with a large-field, low-energy, general-purpose collimated digital camera system. These radioactive nodes can usually be defined within a half-hour after radioactive probe injection. Use of an intraoperative gamma detecting probe allows precise placement of a biopsy incision and a greater than 98% success rate in retrieval of radioactive nodes. In most series there is a high concordance in the simultaneous tracking of radioactive probe and lymphatic dye to the same lymph node. There are reports in a small percentage of patients of apparently divergent pathways with incomplete or no overlap of these two mapping agents. In these patients it appeared that the blue lymphatic dye was more accurately predictive. The current standard of practice is to use both agents with the radiocolloid to allow precise placement of a small biopsy incision and to direct dissection, with the blue dye used as a visual aid. The radioactive nodes retrieved should be examined for blue dye and the radioactivity counted. Any residual radioactivity above background in the lymph node basin or any retrieval of nonblue radioactive nodes should prompt a further search for radioactive or blue-stained nodes.

Radiolymphoscintigraphy also identifies the appropriate lymph node basin for lesions on the trunk and head and neck. It is frequently difficult to predict whether midline trunk or head lesions will drain to more than one lymph node basin. If drainage is to more than one basin, sentinel node biopsy can be performed in each of these areas. Moreover, in the head/neck region, where the use of small incisions is desirable, the technical advantages of this mapping agent are clear.

The current standard of practice is to perform a formal lymph node dissection in patients in whom the sentinel node is microscopically positive. The presence of metastatic disease in secondary and tertiary echelon nodes within the same lymph node basin is approximately 25%.

The introduction of intraoperative lymphatic mapping and sentinel lymph node biopsy has satisfied both the critics and opponents of elective lymph node dissection. The morbidity associated with sentinel lymph node biopsy is minor, but it yields the most important prognostic information for this disease. Only patients with histologically proven metastatic disease are subjected to formal regional lymph node dissection, and these patients are identified as being at high risk for harboring systemic metastatic disease and may be eligible for adjuvant therapy. This approach is also appropriate for patients with thick lesions even though their chances of harboring systemic disease is considerable. Nevertheless, whether the early identification and aggressive surgical treatment of patients with microscopic regional disease in fact confers a survival advantage must await properly conducted clinical trials.

A small percentage of patients with malignant melanoma on initial presentation have clinically positive regional disease or systemic metastatic disease (or both). Pathologic confirmation of clinically suspicious nodes can be readily achieved with fine-needle aspiration cytology. These patients should undergo a careful metastatic workup prior to the performance of putative therapeutic lymph node dissection. In a small percentage of these patients the primary lesion cannot be identified and may have undergone spontaneous regression.

Patients with regional disease are viewed as being at high risk for having systemic microscopic disease and should be considered for adjuvant therapy. Interferon-α is the only adjuvant therapy shown to reduce disease-free recurrences in high risk patients, but not all cooperative studies have shown a clear benefit. Other therapies must be considered investigational, the most promising of which are immune-based.

Isolated limb perfusion allows regional delivery of high concentrations of chemotherapy or biologic therapy in patients with advanced extremity disease. Currently, the most effective regimen is hyperthermic melphalan. Complete clinical responses can be achieved in two-thirds of patients, but a lower percentage are cured as they generally have systemic disease.

F. *Management of Disseminated Disease*

Metastases from melanoma can occur in almost any area of the body. The mean survival for patients with systemic metastatic melanoma is about 6 months. Systemic biological and/or chemotherapy can produce significant responses in a minority of patients.

Surgical excision of metastatic disease in the appropriate patient can provide for excellent palliation.

Conclusions

The algorithm for management of primary cutaneous melanoma is straightforward. A full-thickness, excisional or incisional biopsy is required for diagnosis and microstaging. The margin of excision of the wide excision is governed by the thickness and anatomic site. Intraoperative lymphatic mapping with sentinel lymph node biopsy can be justified for patients with invasive melanomas. Patients with thin melanomas have a low incidence of metastatic disease, but the precise depth at which lymphatic mapping should not be offered to patients has not been firmly established. The current convention is to recommend this staging technique to patients with lesions thicker than 0.75 to 1.0 mm. Formal lymph node dissection is reserved for patients who have microscopically or clinically positive lymph node basins. These patients are at high risk for harboring systemic metastatic disease and should be considered for some form of adjuvant therapy.

Suggested Readings

Albertini JJ, Cruse CW, Rapaport D, et al. Intraoperative radiolymphoscintigraphy improves sentinel lymph node identification for patients with melanoma. Ann Surg 1996;223:217–224.

Balch CM. Surgical management of melanoma: results of prospective randomized trials. Ann Surg Oncol 1998;5:301–309.

Balch CM, Soong S-J, Bartolucci AA, et al. Efficacy of an elective regional lymph node dissection of 1 to 4 mm thick melanomas for patients 60 year of age and younger. Ann Surg 1996;224:255–266.

Balch CM, Soong S-J, Gershenwald JE, et al. Prognostic factors analysis of 17,600 melanoma patients: validation of the American Jaint Committee on Cancer Melanoma Staging System. J. Clin Oncol 2001;19:3622–3634.

Kirkwood JM, Strawderman MH, Ernstoff MS, Smith TJ, Borden EC, Blum RH. Interferon alfa-2b adjuvant therapy of high-risk resected cutaneous melanoma: the Eastern Cooperative Oncology Group trial EST 1684. J Clin Oncol 1996;14:7–17.

Leong SP, Steinmetz I, Habib FA, et al. Optimal selective sentinel lymph node dissection in primary malignant melanoma. Arch Surg 1997;132: 666–673.

Morton DL, Wen D-R, Wong JH, et al. Technical details of intraoperative lymphatic mapping for early stage melanoma. Arch Surg 1992;127:392–399.

Mudun A, Murray DR, Herda SC, et al. Early stage melanoma: lymphoscintigraphy, reproducibility of sentinel node detection, and effectiveness of the intraoperative gamma probe. Radiology 1996;199:171–175.

Strom EA, Ross MI. Adjuvant radiation therapy after axillary lymphadenectomy for metastatic melanoma: toxicity and local control. Ann Surg Oncol 1995;2:445–449.

Vrouenraets BC, Klaase JM, Kroon BBR, van Geel BN, Eggermont AMM, Franklin HR. Long-term morbidity after regional isolated perfusion with melphalan for melanoma of the limbs. Arch Surg 1995;130:43–47.

Chapter 26

Nonmelanotic Skin Cancer

STEVEN D. BINES

Squamous Cell Cancer

A. Epidemiology

Squamous cell carcinoma is the second most common skin cancer, ranking behind basal cell carcinoma. Its incidence is approximately 20–25% of that of basal cell carcinoma, and it constitutes 20% of cutaneous malignancies. More than 100,000 new cases are diagnosed each year. The tumor generally occurs in mid to late life (usually after age 40), most commonly affecting areas of sun exposure. Men are affected more often than women, with an incidence of approximately 900 versus 300 per 100,000, respectively.

The typical squamous cell carcinoma presents as a hyperkeratotic, skin-colored or darkly pigmented papule, nodule, or plaque. Occasionally it is erythematous. These lesions most frequently develop on the face, arm, back, neck, and dorsum of the hand. Squamous cell cancers may be associated with significant subcutaneous extension, and the clinical impression of subcutaneous fullness or invasion must be considered when planning treatment. Pain at the time of presentation implies the presence of perineural extension from the primary tumor site.

B. Histology

A number of variables must be considered when evaluating a squamous cell carcinoma. They relate to the lesion's ability to recur locally and to metastasize.

Location is an important variable. The central zone of the face is considered a high risk area for subclinical extension because of its anatomy; lesions located in this area are therefore at high risk for local recurrence. Subcutaneous tumor growth along resistance planes, such as the perichondrium of the auricular and nasal cartilages and the tarsal plates of the eyelids, allow the tumor to spread in directions that are difficult to predict based solely on the clinical appearance of the primary lesion and the surface anatomy of the region involved. Lesions of the temple, dorsum of the hand, lips, scalp, and penis are associated with a high risk of metastatic disease. Patients with lesions in these areas must be carefully examined for evidence of regional lymphadenopathy.

Squamous Cell Carcinoma

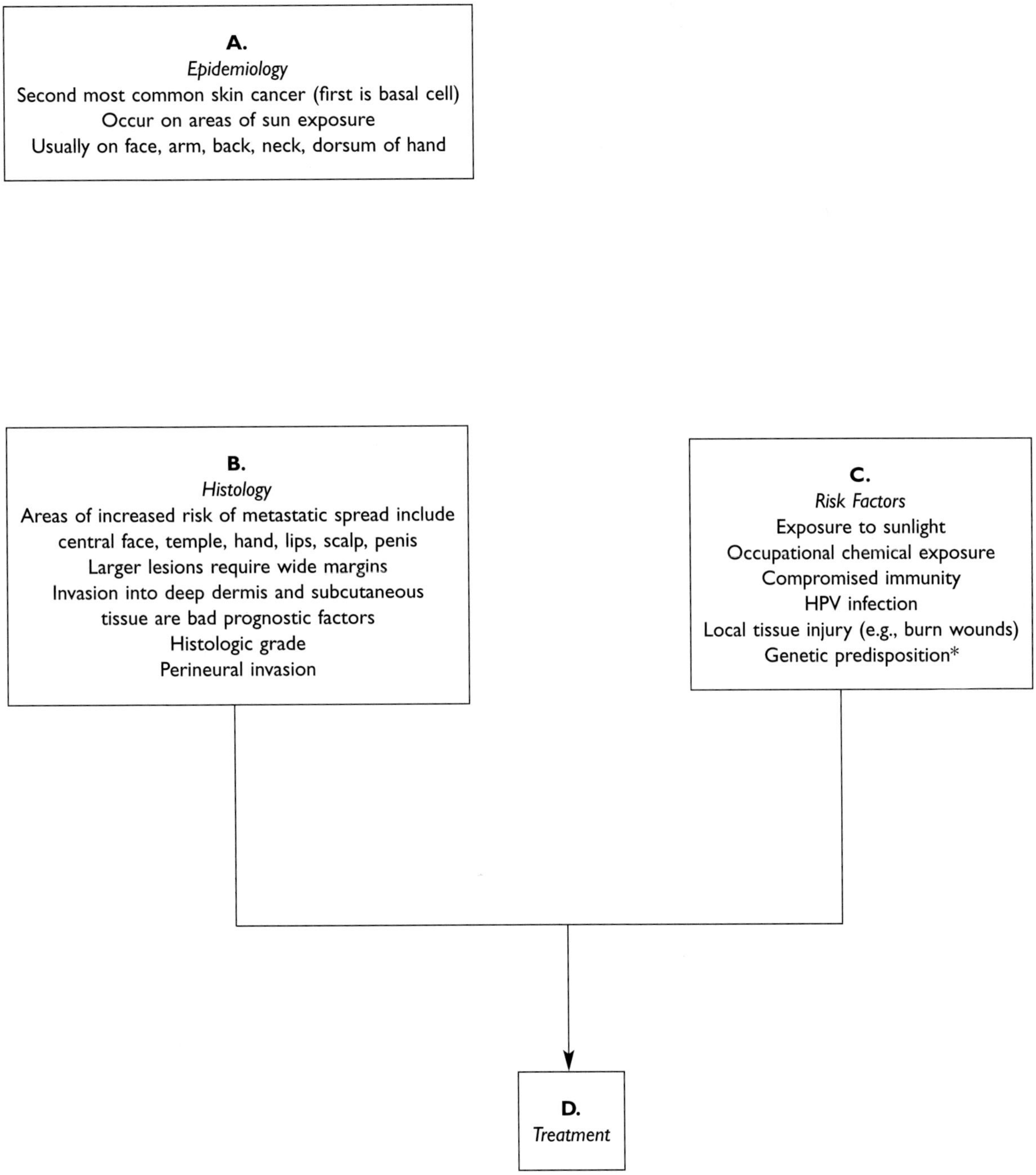

A.
Epidemiology
Second most common skin cancer (first is basal cell)
Occur on areas of sun exposure
Usually on face, arm, back, neck, dorsum of hand

B.
Histology
Areas of increased risk of metastatic spread include central face, temple, hand, lips, scalp, penis
Larger lesions require wide margins
Invasion into deep dermis and subcutaneous tissue are bad prognostic factors
Histologic grade
Perineural invasion

C.
Risk Factors
Exposure to sunlight
Occupational chemical exposure
Compromised immunity
HPV infection
Local tissue injury (e.g., burn wounds)
Genetic predisposition*

D.
Treatment

*Xeroderma pigmentosum
Epidermal dysplasia
Recessive dystrophic epidermolysis bullosa
Occulocutaneous albinism

(continued on next page)

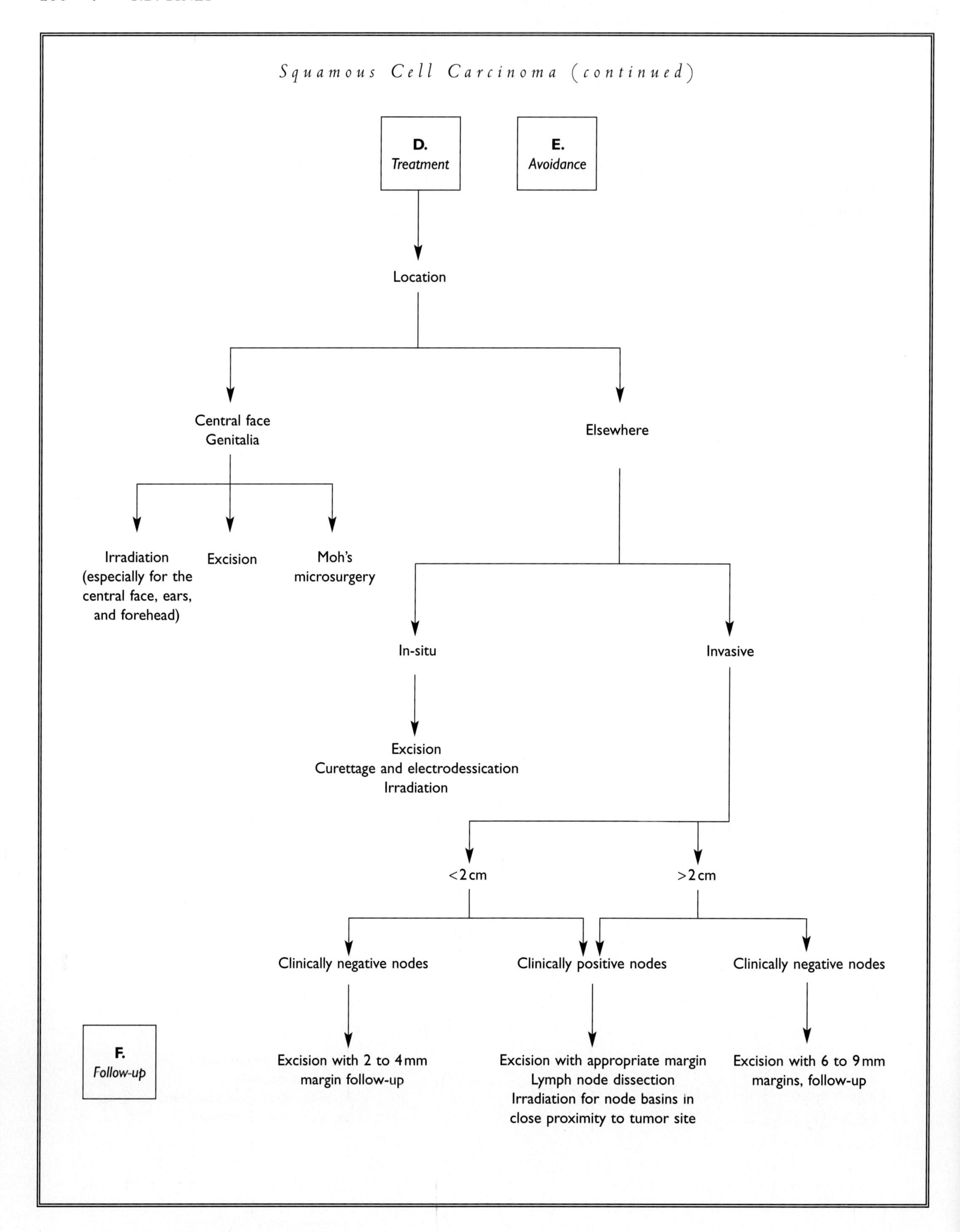
Squamous Cell Carcinoma (continued)
D. Treatment
E. Avoidance
Location
Central face
Genitalia
Elsewhere
Irradiation (especially for the central face, ears, and forehead)
Excision
Moh's microsurgery
In-situ
Invasive
Excision
Curettage and electrodessication
Irradiation
<2 cm
>2 cm
Clinically negative nodes
Clinically positive nodes
Clinically negative nodes
Excision with 2 to 4 mm margin follow-up
Excision with appropriate margin
Lymph node dissection
Irradiation for node basins in close proximity to tumor site
Excision with 6 to 9 mm margins, follow-up
F. Follow-up

Size is an important variable when assessing the biologic behavior of a squamous cell carcinoma: the larger the lesion, the greater the chance for local recurrence. As a consequence, excision margins are selected according to tumor size. Although guidelines vary, a 4- to 5-mm margin for lesions <2 cm in diameter and a 6- to 9-mm margin for lesions >2 cm in diameter have been recommended.

Depth of invasion and *histologic grade* are associated with recurrence and metastases. Invasion into the deep dermis or subcutaneous tissue and a Broder's grade 2 or higher are associated with higher recurrence rates. Squamous cell cancers demonstrate a propensity to invade along perineural planes. Tumors that have *perineural invasion* are therefore at much higher risk for local recurrence. The nerves act as a venue for subclinical extension, necessitating a wider margin of excision when this finding is present.

The *immunosuppressed* or *immunocompromised patient* has an increased risk for local recurrence or metastasis. Metastasis is typically to regional lymph nodes. Hematogenous spread is rare but can occur.

The verrucous squamous cell cancer is a clinicopathologic subtype that is low grade and indolent and carries a low risk for metastasis. It presents with an exophytic wart-like appearance and often arises on the foot or glans penis and anal canal (giant condyloma of Buschke-Lowenstein). Histologically, there is no invasion of the dermis associated with the verrucous-type lesions.

Pathologic evaluation may reveal different histologic subtypes. These subtypes bear little relation to their biologic behavior, in contrast to basal cell cancers where subtypes may behave differently. Squamous cell carcinomas, which are typically a proliferation of atypical squamous cells arising from the epidermis, are generally divided into spindle cell and acantholytic types. Spindle cell tumors may appear similar to malignant melanoma or superficial malignant fibrocytomas; immunohistologic staining can help make this differentiation. Squamous cell cancers are positive for cytokeratin and negative for S-100; melanomas are S-100-positive and cytokeratin-negative. Acantholytic-type squamous cell cancers usually arise from acantholytic solar keratoses.

C. Risk Factors

The pathogenesis of squamous cell cancer is interesting. The single most significant event associated with the development of squamous cell cancer is cumulative lifetime exposure to sunlight. Ultraviolet B radiation (290–320 mm) is known to cause squamous cell cancers in rodent models. Observations that support the significance of sun exposure in humans include the facts that Whites are far more likely than Blacks to develop squamous cell carcinoma, the incidence of squamous cell carcinoma is inversely correlated with latitude, fair-skinned individuals who burn easily (skin type I and II) are at greatest risk for developing squamous cell carcinoma, and squamous cell carcinomas most commonly arise on sun-exposed skin.

Occupational *chemical exposure* is also a causative factor for squamous cancer. The first such causative relation was described by Percival Potts, who studied scrotal tumors in chimney sweeps. He concluded that soot was the causative agent. Other hydrocarbons, including paraffin, tar, shell oil, and creosote oil, have been associated with squamous cell carcinoma. Chronic arsenic exposure and exposure to radiation are also associated with an increased incidence.

Compromised immunity is associated with an increased incidence of squamous cell cancer. This is seen in transplant patients receiving immunosuppression medication, patients whose immunity is suppressed by lymphoreticular malignancy, and patients who are human immunodeficiency virus (HIV)-positive. The ratio of the incidence of basal cell cancer to squamous cell cancer is reversed in these patients. *Human papilloma virus* (HPV) exposure has been associated with squamous cell carcinoma. HPV types 16 and 18 have been implicated in the pathogenesis of squamous cell carcinoma of the cervix and the anus. Other factors play a role in the development of these cancers as well; HPV infection alone does not seem to be the sole factor responsible.

Local tissue changes associated with thermal injury, chronic ulceration, sinus tracts, hidradenitis suppurativa, and chronic cutaneous lupus erythematosus are all associated with an increased risk for squamous cell cancer. Squamous cell cancer arising in these injured areas have a high propensity for metastases and local recurrence. There is also a *genetic predisposition* to developing squamous cell carcinoma. It is noted in patients with xeroderma pigmentosum, epidermal dysplasia, and recessive dystrophic epidermolysis bullosa and oculocutaneous albinism. Finally, there is a well known association with squamous cell carcinoma of the mucocutaneous surface of the mouth and oral pharynx in patients with a history of heavy *alcohol and tobacco use*.

D. Treatment

Treatment options for squamous cell carcinoma are generally divided into excisional therapies and superficial ablative therapies. In general, squamous cell carcinoma requires a more aggressive approach to treatment than basal cell carcinoma. All patients with squamous cell cancer require close follow-up to monitor for local recurrence and metastases.

Tumor location, size, depth of invasion, and histologic differentiation affect treatment choices. A number of interventions are at the disposal of the treating physician, including surgical excision, curettage and electrodesiccation, cryotherapy, topical laser therapy, Moh's micrographic surgery, and radiation therapy. When considering wide excision, the appropriate margins have been already suggested: 4–5 mm for lesions <2 cm in diameter and 6–9 mm for larger lesions.

Tumors at high risk for local recurrence and metastases are those >1–2 cm in diameter that have invaded the mid-dermis or deeper. Those involving cartilage and bone are extremely high risk. Squamous cell carcinoma of the lip, ear, temple, and genitalia and lesions associated with the preexisting conditions previously discussed are also high risk. For these high risk lesions, excision with a frozen section margin check should be used to assess the adequacy of excision. Nonexcisional superficial ablative techniques should be used only on squamous cell carcinoma in situ (Bowen's disease) or on lesions that invade no deeper than the superficial dermis.

Proper surgical staging requires full-thickness excisional biopsy. Frequently, the diagnosis is made by shave biopsy, which provides insufficient information for complete staging. In such cases, clinical examination becomes extremely important. Tumors that are indurated and have undermined the skin laterally and those with associated local pain may be deeply invasive and should be treated by excision.

Curettage and electrodesiccation may be used for superficial squamous cell cancers; this technique should not be used for lesions with aggressive histology, large size, or high risk anatomic location (central face). First, curettage is performed by paring down the lesion to normal tissue, after which electrodesiccation is used to destroy potential tumor nests at the base. *Cryotherapy* freezes tissue to −195.5°C with liquid nitrogen and can be used for small lesions (<2 cm) on the eyelid, ear, chest, back, or tip of the nose. It is also used for recurrent tumors with definable margins. Cryotherapy should not be used for eyelid free margins, the vermilion border of the lip, ala nasi, scalp, and tumors >3 cm. *Surgical excision* is an effective treatment for all lesions in nearly every location and allows histologic assessment of all margins.

Radiation therapy has been valuable for treating squamous cell carcinoma. Cure rates approach 92%. It is of particular value in the central face, ear, and forehead, where excisional therapy is potentially deforming. It has the advantage of treating a wide region around the tumor with excellent local control and good cosmetic outcome.

Prior to initiating therapy, a biopsy should be obtained for both histologic confirmation and evaluation of tumor thickness. A lead shield is fashioned with a portal large enough to encompass the entire clinical margin plus 0.5 cm. Most tumors are treated with a dose of 4000–6000 cGy to the superficial skin. The dose is usually divided over 3–4 weeks to prevent complications. Short term, the most troublesome sequelae after irradiation is "burn" to the area. Long-term sequelae include destruction of hair follicles and sweat glands, radiation dermatitis leading to changes in skin pigmentation (hyper- or hypopigmentation), and the development of radiation-induced precancerous lesions.

High risk tumors have the capability of spreading to regional lymph nodes. Generally, regional lymph node dissection is not offered to patients unless there is clinically evident disease. Radiation therapy, however, can be used to include regional lymph nodes when they are in close proximity to the primary tumor being irradiated.

E. Avoidance

With society's continued exposure to ultraviolet (UV) radiation from sunlight and tanning booths and with the ongoing depletion of the ozone layer, the incidence of nonmelanotic skin cancer is likely to increase over the next several years. It is thought that a reduction in solar exposure starting during early childhood is likely to reduce the incidence of squamous cell carcinoma in high risk individuals. Sunscreen (15 SPF minimum), lip screen, broad-brimmed hats, and proper clothing can provide this protection. Limiting tobacco and alcohol use reduces the incidence of oral squamous cell carcinoma. Use of condoms may reduce HPV infection rates and therefore reduce the rates of genital squamous cell carcinoma.

F. Follow-up

The chance of developing a second skin cancer within 5 years after treatment of the original basal cell or squamous cell cancer is as high as 50%. Careful periodic skin examination is indicated for a minimum of 5 years after diagnosis; and a program of skin examination every 4–6 months with aggressive biopsy of any suspicious skin lesions should be offered to all patients who have undergone excision of a basal cell or squamous cell cancer.

Basal Cell Cancer

G. Epidemiology

Basal cell cancer is a malignancy of basaloid epithelial cells and is the most common cancer, outnumbering cutaneous squamous cell cancer 4 : 1. Approximately 500,000 new cases are diagnosed each year. It most often affects light-skinned people, and rarely affects those with dark skin. As such, more than 90% of these lesions occur in Caucasians. The development of this tumor is clearly related to chronic exposure to UV radiation. It develops mainly on sun-exposed areas, the incidence varying directly with increasing accumulated sun exposure and inversely with increasing skin pigmentation. More than 80% develop on the head and neck. It tends to occur more frequently in men, usually after age 40. Those with type I skin (burn, never tan) are most susceptible.

Prior injury (trauma, burns, vaccination sites), radiation therapy, and exposure to inorganic arsenic can predispose to the development of basal cell cancer. Several genetic syndromes are

Basal Cell Carcinoma

G.
Epidemiology
Most common tumor
Areas of sun exposure such as head, neck
Caucasians >> dark skinned individuals

H.
Histology
Nodular:
most common,
ulcerated ("rodent ulcer")
Morpheaform:
flat, scar-like,
undermined edges,
high recurrence rate
Superficial:
trunk and extremities,
erythematous patches
Pigmented:
differentiate from melanoma

I.
Risk Factors
Size >2 cm
Location: central face
Perineural invasion
Histologic subtype

J.
Treatment

Curettage and electrodesiccation
Small, favorable lesions (less aggressive basal cell cancers, superficial lesions)
Multiple superficial lesions
No margin control
Suitable for the forehead, cheeks, and trunks
Not suitable for hands, digits, shoulders

Cryotherapy
Margin control not possible

Excision
Standard therapy for larger lesions
Able to histologically check margins

Moh's
High cure rates with better cosmesis
Ideal for high risk lesions (e.g., morpheoform type, micronodular type, poorly differentiated, perineural invasion, indistinct margins, basal cell >2 cm, squamous cell >1 cm)
Especially good for recurrent or incompletely removed tumors

Irradiation
Good cosmesis
Central facial lesion and lesions of eyelids, nose, lips, forehead

K.
Metastasis
Extremely rare

associated with an increased risk for basal cell cancer, including xeroderma pigmentosum, nevoid basal cell syndrome, albinism, and Bazex syndrome. Certain developmental skin lesions are associated with an increased risk of basal cell cancer development including nevus sebaceous and linear unilateral basal cell nevus.

H. Histology

Unlike squamous cell cancer, there are several distinctive clinical subtypes that correlate with histology and biologic potential. In addition, these subtypes affect treatment choices. Histologic subtypes include nodular basal cell cancer (most common), morpheaform, superficial, fibroepitheliomatous, and infundibulocystic.

Nodular basal cell cancer is the most frequent form of basal cell cancer. It often appears as an elevated papule with overlying telangiectasia. It can become ulcerated as it enlarges, giving the appearance of having been nibbled at, leading to its name "rodent ulcer." Pigmented basal cell cancer is a variant of nodular basal cell cancer that, because of its dark pigment, must be differentiated from melanoma. This type often occurs in dark-skinned individuals.

Morpheaform or sclerosing basal cell cancers (also known as fibrosing or desmoplastic) have a flat, scar-like appearance. Some demonstrate endophytic growth leading to a true tumor margin that is larger than the visible margin. These lesions should be palpated carefully to assess the true extent of tissue induration. This biologic feature leads to a higher recurrence rate and makes morpheaform basal cell cancer one that is considered aggressive.

Superficial basal cell cancers tend to appear on the trunk and extremities. They appear as erythematous patches, although some have an overlying patchy scale-like or pigmented appearance. They are the most common type of basal cell cancer, seen with chronic arsenism and in radiation fields. In these two instances the cancer can affect broad areas and be present in discontinuous patches.

I. Risk Factors

The risk a given basal cell carcinoma presents to the individual is based on a number of parameters.

Location: the central zone of the face is an area at high risk for subclinical extension. This is due to the presence of resistance planes and fusion zones that allow subclinical spread by these indolently growing tumors.

Size: Tumors >2 cm have lower cure rates.

Histology: Basal cell cancer is not histologically homogeneous like squamous cell cancer. The more dangerous subtypes include the micronodular, infiltrative, and morpheaform basal cells. These subtypes have a higher recurrence rate than those with nodular or superficial histology.

Perineural involvement: Tumors found to have perineural involvement are associated with a high recurrence rate.

J. Treatment

Treatment options include excision, curettage and electrodesiccation, cryotherapy, radiation therapy, and Mohs' microsurgical therapy. Tumors with an aggressive infiltrative growth pattern, such as morpheaform, micronodular, and infiltrative variants, require excision with a margin check; they should not undergo superficial treatments such as curettage or cryotherapy. With less aggressive, more circumscribed growth patterns, including small nodular basal cell cancers and superficial basal cell cancers, adequate treatment can be achieved with curettage and electrodesiccation or cryotherapy. It is apparent, then, that size, location, and histologic subtype (determined by a pretreatment biopsy) combined with the experience of the treating physician determine the treatment a patient receives.

Curettage and electrodesiccation can be used for less aggressive growth pattern basal cell carcinomas and superficial squamous cell cancers. It is best used on flat areas such as the forehead, cheek, or trunk. The technique combines the use of curettage with electrodesiccation of the wound margin. The wounds heal by secondary intention, which sometimes provides better cosmetic results for large lesions of the trunk than can be achieved with excision. The same is true for some small lesions on flat surfaces of the face.

This technique does not allow margin control and should not be used on squamous cell cancers except those shown by biopsy to be extremely superficial. Hypertrophic scarring can occur when using this technique on the dorsum of the hands, digits, and shoulders. Excision is usually preferred in these areas. The technique is of special value when treating small multiple superficial basal cell carcinomas arising in areas of chronic radiation dermatitis.

Cryotherapy uses liquid nitrogen administered by spray, cotton-tipped applicator, or probe. Like curettage and electrodesiccation, margin control is not possible, so a pretreatment biopsy is necessary to determine if suitable and favorable histology is present. With both curettage/electrodesiccation and cryotherapy, scars are often hypopigmented. Any sign of recurrence after use of these treatment modalities must be treated by surgical excision.

Surgical excision has been the standard therapy. It is against this procedure that results of the other techniques have been compared. Margin checks at the time of excision are mandatory for optimizing results, especially when dealing with aggressive basal cell and deeply invasive squamous cell cancers. Full-thickness excision followed by careful, layered, tension-free closure usually provides excellent cosmetic results. Large lesions of the eyelid or commissure of the mouth are best treated with excision. Deeply invasive tumors involving cartilage and bone are, in the opinion of some, best treated by excision. Carcinomas arising in sinus tracts, ulcers, and scars are best treated by excision. The margin of excision for basal cell cancers <1 cm in diameter should be 4–5 mm wide. The margin should be increased up to 9 mm for aggressive growth pattern basal cell cancer and those >1 cm in diameter.

Some advocate using curettage prior to excision to better define the true extent of tumor and minimize the loss of normal tissue. This requires experience on the part of both surgeon and pathologist. Clearly, selective use of excisional therapy can be applied without curettage.

Irradiation for the treatment of basal cell cancer can provide excellent results. It is associated with cure rates of 96% and a favorable cosmetic outcome for small lesions of the central face including the eyelids, nose, and lips. It is capable of controlling large lesions and has been used successfully for extensive tumors of the scalp and forehead. With proper fractionization and shielding, damage to underlying cartilage and bone and adjacent normal tissue can be minimized and complications avoided.

Consideration should be given to including the regional lymph nodes in the radiation field when treating large basal cancers and invasive squamous cell cancers, particularly when it can be done in continuity. This is more convenient in some areas of the body than others, such as the cervical and preauricular areas, and for lesions of the genitalia. To be effective, the radiation must penetrate at least 2–5 mm. The radiation dose varies between 100 and 300 kV per day and is given according to several fractionation schedules. Typically, 15–17 fractions are given for tumors ≤2 cm in diameter, increased to 20–22 fractions for tumors >2 cm in diameter, and increased to 30–33 fractions for larger lesions involving cartilage.

Mohs' micrographic surgery (MMS) was described in 1941 by Frederick Mohs. The technique originally used 20% zinc chloride paste to fix tumor-bearing tissue in situ followed by excision and evaluation of the excisional margins. This combination of zinc and surgery led to the technique known as Mohs' chemosurgery. In 1970 Theodore Tromovitch developed the fresh tissue technique that eliminated the zinc oxide paste. It is an exacting technique that requires extensive training to master. Selecting cases best treated by MMS requires sophisticated clinical judgment.

The MMS technique is used most commonly to treat basal cell and squamous cell cancers. Its main advantages are high cure rates and minimal tissue loss. What sets it apart from the other surgical excision techniques is the mapping of the lesion and horizontal sectioning of the specimen, which allows examination of 100% of the surgical margin. This ability to optimize tissue preservation is important in areas where maintaining function and cosmetic appearance is difficult, such as the nose, eyelids, lips, ears, digits, and genitalia.

The ability to check 100% of the margin makes it a useful procedure for treating lesions with a high risk of recurrence. Such lesions include morpheaform, infiltrative, and micronodular basal cell cancer; poorly differentiated invasive squamous cell cancers; tumors with perineural invasion; tumors with indistinct clinical margins; basal cell cancers >2 cm in diameter; and squamous cell cancers >1 cm in diameter. MMS is the treatment of choice for recurrent or incompletely removed tumors. In practice, most basal cell cancers and squamous cell cancers can be treated successfully with less extensive, less expensive treatment, but MMS should be seriously considered for basal cell and squamous cell cancers in difficult locations with a high risk for recurrence or when recurrence has already developed.

K. Metastasis

Metastasis from basal cell cancers is rare but is occasionally seen with the basalosquamous basal cell cancer that is a variant of nodular basal cell cancer. The duration and size of the lesion affect its propensity to metastasize. Recurrent lesions should also heighten awareness of possible metastatic disease. The lung, followed by bone, lymph nodes, and liver, are the most frequent sites of metastatic disease.

Selected Reading

Squamous Cell Carcinoma

Arndt FA, LeBoit PE, Robinson JF, Wintron BU (eds) Cutaneous Medicine and Surgery: An Integrated Program in Dermatology. Philadelphia: Saunders, 1996;1383–1431.

Freedberg IM, Eisen AZ, Wolff K, et al (eds). Fitzpatrick's Dermatology in General Medicine, 5th ed, vol 1. New York: McGraw-Hill, 1999;840–856.

Friedman RJ, Rigel DS, Kopf AL, Harrison MN, Barber D (eds) Cancer of the Skin. Philadelphia: Saunders, 1991;35–73.

Henriksen T, et al. Ultraviolet-radiation and skin cancer: effect of an ozone layer depletion. Photochem Photobiol 1990;51:579.

Basal Cell Carcinoma

Arndt FA, LeBoit PE, Robinson JF, Wintron BU (eds) Cutaneous Medicine and Surgery: An Integrated Program in Dermatology. Philadelphia: Saunders, 1996;1383–1431.

Cottell WI, Proper S. Mohs' surgery, fresh tissue technique: our technique with a review. J Dermatol Surg Oncol 1982;8:576–587.

Drake LA, Ceilley RI, Cornelison RL, et al. Guidelines of care for basal cell carcinoma. J Am Acad Dermatol 1992;26:117.

Freedberg IM, Eisen AZ, Wolff K, et al (eds) Fitzpatrick's Dermatology in General Medicine, 5th ed, vol 1. New York: McGraw-Hill, 1999;840–856.

Friedman RJ, Rigel DS, Kopf AL, Harrison MN, Barber D (eds) Cancer of the Skin. Philadelphia: Saunders, 1991;35–73.

Henriksen T, et al. Ultraviolet-radiation and skin cancer: effect of an ozone layer depletion. Photochem Photobiol 1990;51:579.

Johnson TM, Tromovitch TA, Swanson NA. Combined curettage and excision: a treatment method for primary basal cell carcinoma. J Am Acad Dermatol 1991;24:613.

McGrouther DAM. Treatment of basal cell carcinoma: a plastic surgeon's view. Br J Dermatol 1987;117:399.

Section 6

Gastrointestinal Malignancies

Chapter 27

Cancer of the Esophagus

KEITH W. MILLIKAN
LAUREL A. LITTRELL
JONATHAN A. MYERS

A. Epidemiology and Etiology

Incidence

The worldwide geographic variation in incidence for esophageal cancer is greater than for any other cancer. In the United States and Canada, Whites have an incidence of fewer than 5 cases per 100,000 people. In Linxian County, China, the age-adjusted incidence reaches 500 per 100,000, making esophageal cancer the leading cause of death in that county. There is great variation within individual countries as well. In the United States rates in urban areas are consistently higher than in rural areas, with men affected more commonly than women.[1,2] Comparatively, esophageal cancer occurs over three times more frequently in the Black population than in the White population.[3]

Causes

In westernized countries, alcohol and tobacco intake are thought to be the major causes of esophageal cancer. Alcohol, especially hard liquor such as whiskey, vodka, and moonshine contain carcinogenic *N*-nitroso compounds.[4] Heavy alcohol consumption increases the risk of developing esophageal cancer up to 50-fold. Tobacco also contains *N*-nitroso derivatives as well as carcinogenic lactones, epoxides, and polycyclic aromatic polyhydrocarbons.[5] The death rates due to esophageal cancer in smokers are five- to tenfold times greater than in nonsmokers. Cigar and pipe smokers have fourfold increases in death rates compared to nonsmokers. The combination of alcohol and tobacco use has an additive effect, with increases in incidence reaching 100-fold.

Other conditions predisposing to the development of esophageal cancer include achalasia (risk increased 14–16%), Barrett's esophagus, esophageal diverticula, esophageal webs, tylosis, and infectious agents such as human papilloma virus.[6] Caustic injury from lye ingestion may cause esophageal

Esophageal Cancer

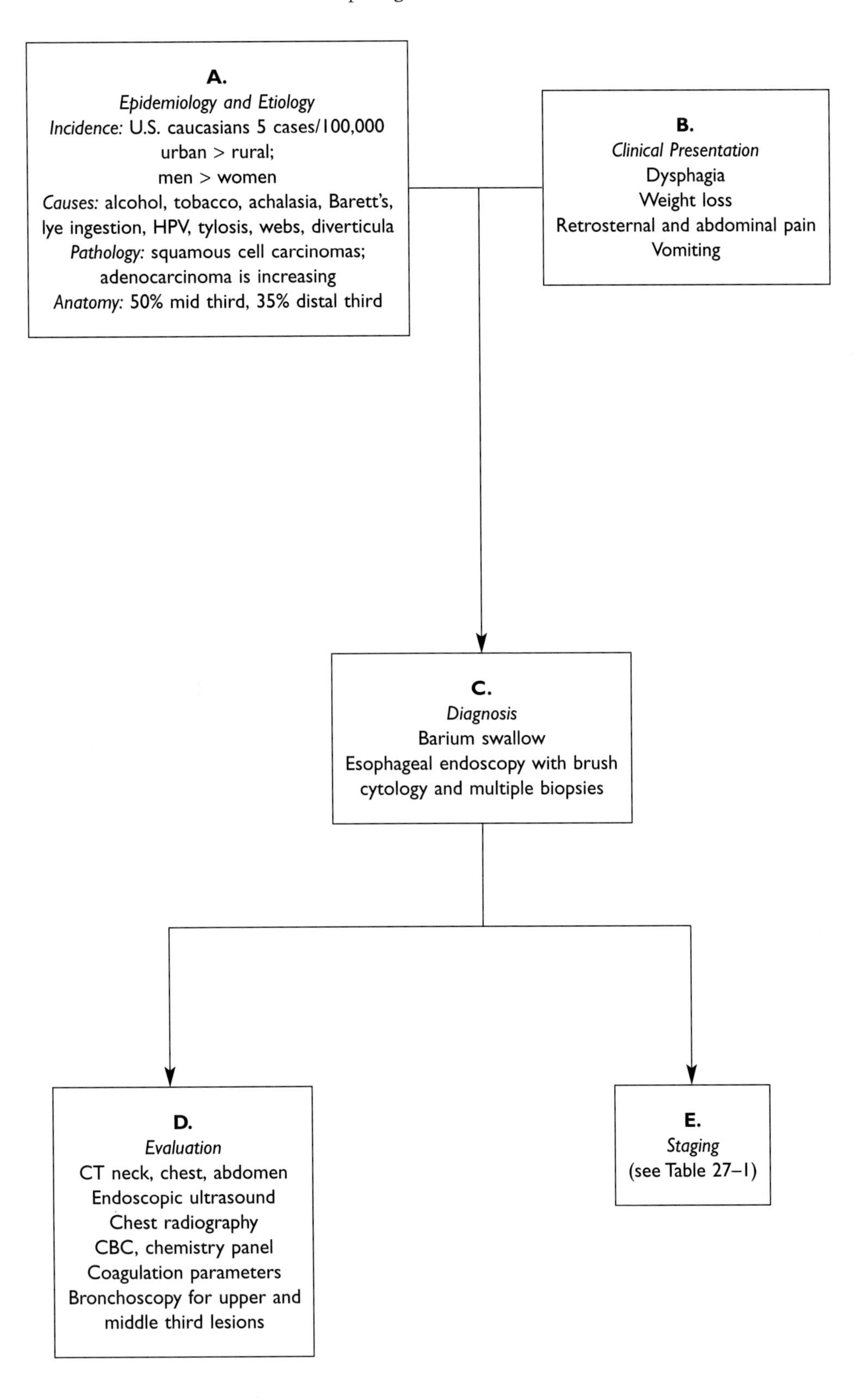

(continued on next page)

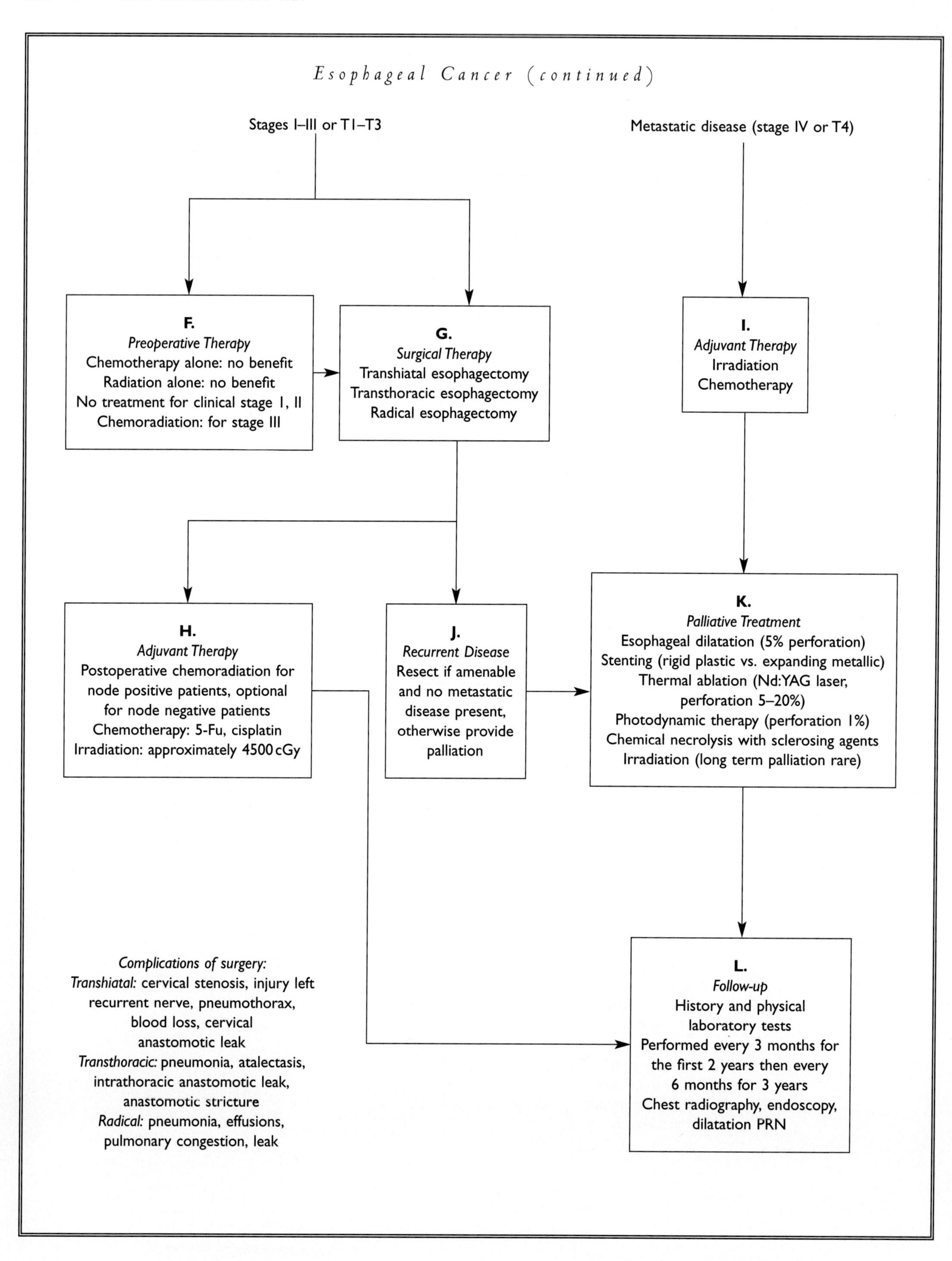
Esophageal Cancer (continued)
Stages I–III or T1–T3
Metastatic disease (stage IV or T4)
F.
Preoperative Therapy
Chemotherapy alone: no benefit
Radiation alone: no benefit
No treatment for clinical stage I, II
Chemoradiation: for stage III
G.
Surgical Therapy
Transhiatal esophagectomy
Transthoracic esophagectomy
Radical esophagectomy
I.
Adjuvant Therapy
Irradiation
Chemotherapy
H.
Adjuvant Therapy
Postoperative chemoradiation for node positive patients, optional for node negative patients
Chemotherapy: 5-Fu, cisplatin
Irradiation: approximately 4500 cGy
J.
Recurrent Disease
Resect if amenable and no metastatic disease present, otherwise provide palliation
K.
Palliative Treatment
Esophageal dilatation (5% perforation)
Stenting (rigid plastic vs. expanding metallic)
Thermal ablation (Nd:YAG laser, perforation 5–20%)
Photodynamic therapy (perforation 1%)
Chemical necrolysis with sclerosing agents
Irradiation (long term palliation rare)
Complications of surgery:
Transhiatal: cervical stenosis, injury left recurrent nerve, pneumothorax, blood loss, cervical anastomotic leak
Transthoracic: pneumonia, atalectasis, intrathoracic anastomotic leak, anastomotic stricture
Radical: pneumonia, effusions, pulmonary congestion, leak
L.
Follow-up
History and physical laboratory tests
Performed every 3 months for the first 2 years then every 6 months for 3 years
Chest radiography, endoscopy, dilatation PRN

carcinoma many years later, and such individuals should be screened regularly, especially more than 20 years after the injury.[7]

Pathology

In the past, squamous cell carcinoma was by far the most common cell type of esophageal cancer. However, in the United States there has been a rapid rise in the incidence of adenocarcinoma of the esophagus, whereas rates for squamous cell carcinoma have remained relatively stable.[8] The incidence of squamous cell carcinoma is decreasing in white men, but adenocarcinoma is increasing steadily in both Blacks and Whites at a rate of 5–10% per year.[9] Reports have shown that adenocarcinoma makes up 28% to more than one-half of the cases of esophageal cancer in North America.[10,11] Advanced squamous cell carcinoma and adenocarcinoma comprise approximately 95% of all primary esophageal malignancies, with undifferentiated carcinoma contributing about 3–4%. Among squamous cell carcinomas, polypoid lesions are most common (60%) and then ulcerative lesions (25%); the remaining infiltrative, stenosing lesions.[12] Variants of squamous cell carcinoma include basaloid squamous cell and squamous cell with sarcomatoid features. Verrucous squamous cell cancer is rare in the esophagus. Mucoepidermoid and adenosquamous lesions are other variants that are histologically similar to the salivary gland or squamous cell varieties with some glandular component, respectively. Exceedingly rare cancers of the esophagus include small cell carcinomas, carcinoid tumors, malignant melanomas, sarcomas, choriocarcinomas, extramedullary plasmacytomas, and collision tumors. Most of these lesions have been reported only in case reports.[9]

Anatomy

Esophageal malignancies arise most frequently in the middle third of the esophagus (approximately 50%) and occur least frequently in the proximal, or cervical, esophagus (15%). Approximately 35% of esophageal cancer arises in the distal third.[2] Because the incidence of adenocarcinoma is on the rise, cases involving the distal one-third of the esophagus are increasing as well.[2,10] The rich lymphatic system and lack of serosa surrounding the esophagus results in metastatic spread of esophageal malignancies to any area of the thorax or its draining nodal beds. Cancers from the upper third tend to drain into the internal jugular, cervical, and supraclavicular areas. The middle third drains into peritracheal, hilar, subcarinal, paraesophageal, periaortic, and pericardial regions. The distal third drains into the perigastric nodes along the lesser curvature of the stomach, left gastric artery, and celiac plexus. However, celiac nodes may be involved in 10% of upper-third cancers and in nearly half of patients with middle-third lesions.[7]

B. *Clinical Presentation*

Because esophageal cancer is relatively asymptomatic in its early stages and once symptoms begin their onset is insidious, patients often present with late disease, precluding a chance for surgical cure. At presentation 50–75% of patients have unresectable disease and require palliative measures.[7,13] Regardless of where the lesion is located, patients commonly report difficulty swallowing (96%), weight loss, and retrosternal pain. For patients with a lesion in the upper one-third of the esophagus, additional symptoms include having the sensation of a lump or pain in the throat and cough or hoarseness. For lesions in the middle and lower thirds, the most common additional symptoms are upper abdominal pain and vomiting.[13] A history of anorexia and weight loss is extremely important, as weight loss of less than 10% of total body weight is considered a favorable prognostic factor, associated with increased long-term survival. Because of the association with alcohol and tobacco use, these patients often have concomitant hepatic, renal, and cerebral dysfunction, which are associated with significantly increased operative risk. In fact, cirrhotic patients undergoing resection have an operative mortality of 20%, which is even higher in the presence of ascites, a contraindication to esophagogastrectomy. Cardiovascular and pulmonary disease are frequently present and contribute greatly to postoperative morbidity.

C. *Diagnosis*

When esophageal cancer is suspected, contrast esophagraphy, or barium swallow, is useful for initial visualization of esophageal anatomy, especially before instrumentation with an endoscope. Double-contrast esophagrams provide maximum distension and good visualization of morphology of both obvious and small lesions and can provide insight as to whether the mass is mucosal or extramucosal.[12] In a retrospective study of 50 cases of esophageal cancer, 98% of the lesions were demonstrated with barium studies, and esophageal carcinoma was diagnosed or suspected in 96% of the patients.[14]

After a lesion has been seen and the anatomy visualized with barium studies, endoscopy with biopsy should be performed. Barium studies alert the endoscopist regarding the site and extent of the lesion and any areas of high-grade obstruction. Flexible endoscopy permits magnified visualization, as well as histologic sampling. During endoscopy malignant areas are seen as either polypoid exophytic lesions or infiltrating fibrotic areas of friable mucosa.[11] Both brush cytology and multiple biopsies should be performed. Increasing the number of biopsies from one to six increases the diagnostic yield from 93% to 98–100%.[15] The accuracy of brush cytology alone ranges from 80% to 95%, and that of biopsy alone is approximately 89%.[11,16]

D. Evaluation

Once a diagnosis of esophageal cancer has been established with barium studies, endoscopy, and biopsy, patients should undergo computed tomography (CT) of the neck, chest, and abdomen to stage the primary tumor, regional nodes, and distant metastases. The CT scan is particularly good for determining direct extension into adjacent structures and the presence of distant metastases, especially in lung and liver. Extension into adjacent structures is seen as a loss of fat planes, and the CT scan has 70–100% specificity for determining when adjacent structures have been invaded.[11] Its value for evaluating nodal involvement is controversial. According to Chandawarkar et al., the CT scan is best for nodal groups in the left paratracheal, lower paraesophageal, cervical paraesophageal, and supraclavicular regions.[17] Although accuracy and sensitivities are fairly high for all nodal groups, the sensitivity of the CT scan for detecting nodal metastases in the periaortic, mid-paraesophageal, lower posterior mediastinal, paracardiac, lesser curvature, and left gastric areas is less.[17]

Magnetic resonance imaging (MRI) has been evaluated in the workup of esophageal cancer and thus far has not proven to be superior to CT scans.[17] Endoscopic ultrasonography (EUS) has distinct advantages compared to CT in terms of its ability to assess the size, shape, margins, and internal echogenicity of the nodes. Overall accuracy for assessing nodes was 89%, and sensitivity was consistently higher than with CT.[17] Further studies have demonstrated that EUS is more accurate than CT for assessing depth and tumor infiltration into the esophageal wall and adjacent structures. The overall accuracy of EUS was 82% compared to 50% with CT. Additionally, EUS was found to be superior for diagnosing regional lymph node metastasis and staging.[18] In 20% of cases, however, the EUS probe cannot pass through a malignant stricture; in these patients the CT scan is preferable to EUS for assessing locoregional disease.[18] Ninety percent of patients with an obstructing lesion have stage III or IV disease.[19] CT scanning should always be done to rule out distant metastases, as they are a contraindication to resection. EUS should be performed if nodal status would determine whether chemoradiation therapy or surgery is the next treatment option.

Conventional chest radiographs provide an assessment of lung parenchyma. They also allow visualization of the azygoesophageal recess, which may be abnormal in patients with esophageal cancer. Widening of the mediastinum or posterior indentation of the trachea may also be seen. However, the plain chest radiograph is frequently normal in patients with esophageal cancer.[12]

Bronchoscopy is recommended for upper- and middle-third tumors to rule out invasion of the airway.[20] A complete blood count (CBC), coagulation studies, and chemistry panels should also be assessed during evaluation of patients with esophageal carcinoma.

E. Staging

A standardized system for staging esophageal cancer is essential. Improved imaging techniques, such as those described above, permit preclinical staging of esophageal cancer, but surgical pathology remains the most accurate method. The current staging system in use is the tumor-node-metastasis (TNM) system developed by the American Joint Committee on Cancer in 1983 and updated in 1988 (Table 27–1).[21] "T" refers to the depth of invasion of the primary tumor; "N" refers to the presence or absence of regional lymph node involvement; and "M" describes whether distant metastases are present. The "T" status is the critical prognostic factor for patients without nodal involvement (N0) or distant metastases (M0). Patients with intraepithelial carcinoma (Tis) or intramucosal T1 carcinomas have 5-year survival rates of 80–85% after surgery.[22] Once the tumor extends beyond the muscularis propria (T3), survival rates fall to less than 25% at 5 years.[19] After regional nodal involvement or distant metastasis has occurred, survival rates drop dramatically.

Operable Cancer (Stages I–III or T1–T3)

F. Preoperative Treatment

After diagnosis and staging, the treating physician must decide whether patients with operable cancer (stages I–III or T1–T3) should be treated with surgery or undergo an initial course of preoperative radiation, chemotherapy, or both followed by surgery at a later date.

Preoperative Radiation Therapy Radiation therapy is used in an attempt to improve locoregional control of esophageal tumors. It has been used alone, in combination with surgery, and in combination with both chemotherapy and surgery. When used with surgery, radiation therapy may be applied preoperatively, postoperatively, and intraoperatively. In a review by Thomas, six randomized trials comparing preoperative (neoadjuvant) radiation therapy to surgery alone failed to demonstrate a survival benefit.[4] Doses of radiation typically ranged between 20 and 40 Gy at 1.75–3.3 Gy/fraction.[4] In a study of 106 patients by Huang et al., 5-year survival rates with surgery alone were 25% compared with 46% for patients receiving doses of 40 Gy at 2 Gy/fraction.[23] Although some studies have demonstrated a 60–70% response rate and even 15–25% pathologic complete response rates, in general this has not translated into a clinically significant survival advantage. Hence currently there are no conclusive data recommending the

TABLE 27–1.
AJCC definition of TNM and stage grouping for esophageal cancer

Primary Tumor (T)

TX	Primary tumor cannot be assessed
T0	No evidence of primary tumor
Tis	Carcinoma *in situ*
T1	Tumor invades lamina propria or submucosa
T2	Tumor invades muscularis propria
T3	Tumor invades adventitia
T4	Tumor invades adjacent structures

Regional Lymph Nodes (N)

NX	Regional lymph nodes cannot be assessed
N0	No regional lymph node metastasis
N1	Regional lymph node metastasis

Distant Metastasis (M)

MX	Distant metastasis cannot be assessed
M0	No distant metastasis
M1	Distant metastasis

Tumors of the lower thoracic esophagus:
- M1a Metastasis in celiac lymph nodes
- M1b Other distant metastasis

Tumors of the midthoracic esophagus:
- M1a Not applicable
- M1b Nonregional lymph nodes and/or other distant metastasis

Tumors of the upper thoracic esophagus:
- M1a Metastasis in cervical nodes
- M1b Other distant metastasis

For tumors of midthoracic esophagus use only M1b, since these tumors with metastasis in nonregional lymph nodes have an equally poor prognosis as those with metastasis in other distant sites.

Stage Grouping

Stage	*T*	*N*	*M*
0	Tis	N0	M0
I	T1	N0	M0
IIA	T2	N0	M0
	T3	N0	M0
IIB	T1	N1	M0
	T2	N1	M0
III	T3	N1	M0
	T4	Any N	M0
IV	Any T	Any N	M1
IVA	Any T	Any N	M1a
IVB	Any T	Any N	M1b

SOURCE: Used with the permission of the American Joint Committee on Cancer (AJCC®), Chicago, IL. The original source for this material is the AJCC® Cancer Staging Manual, 5th edition (1997) published by Lippincott Williams & Wilkins Publishers, Philadelphia, PA.

use of preoperative radiation therapy for potentially curable esophageal cancer.[24]

PREOPERATIVE CHEMOTHERAPY Four prospective randomized trials have compared survival rates in patients receiving preoperative (neoadjuvant) chemotherapy to those undergoing surgery alone. The National Cancer Institute study randomized patients to a surgical resection arm and to an arm treated both preoperatively and postoperatively with chemotherapy. No survival benefit was shown by the study when *all* randomized patients were compared, although there was a threefold median survival increase from 6.2 months to 20.0 months in patients who responded to chemotherapy.[25] Another trial from the University of Heidelberg also demonstrated a survival benefit only in chemotherapy responders (13 months compared to 5 months).[26] The Second Scandinavian Trial in Esophageal Cancer involved 187 patients randomized to one of the following four treatment arms: surgery alone, preoperative chemotherapy, preoperative radiation therapy, and preoperative chemoradiation. Three-year survival rates for the group receiving preoperative chemotherapy showed a survival disadvantage.[27] The North American GI Intergroup trial compared surgical treatment alone to three cycles of preoperative cisplatin and 5-fluorouracil (5-FU) followed by surgery and postoperative cisplatin and 5-FU. Results did not show an improvement in overall survival in patients with epidermoid cancer or adenocarcinoma of the esophagus.[28] In addition to no survival benefit noted from the above studies, operative mortality was increased in two of the trials after giving preoperative chemotherapy. Preoperative chemotherapy alone has not been documented to increase long-term survival and should be considered only in clinical trials.

Preoperative Chemoradiation Chemotherapy and radiation therapy are often used together in combination with surgery in an attempt to obtain better regional and distant control of esophageal cancer. Several nonrandomized clinical phase II cooperative multiinstitution trials have compared the results of preoperative chemoradiation to surgery alone. The Radiation Therapy Oncology Group (RTOG) and the Southwest Oncology Group (SWOG) independently tested the combination of preoperative cisplatin, 5-FU, and 30 Gy of radiation. Resection rates were similar (66% and 63%, respectively). The median survival was 13 months in the RTOG study and 14 months in the SWOG trial. Three-year survival rates were slightly better in the SWOG study (16%) than in the RTOG study (8%), but neither was any better than historical rates for surgery alone. In both groups approximately one-fourth of patients undergoing surgery after chemoradiation had a complete response, and these patients showed improved survival rates. Treatment toxicity was primarily hematologic and resulted in mortality rates of 5–15%.[29,30] Although most patients had squamous cell carcinoma, the Eastern Cooperative Oncology Group (ECOG) studied 46 patients with adenocarcinoma of the esophagus who received preoperative chemoradiation at doses of 60 Gy at 2 Gy/fraction, mitomycin C (10 mg/m^2 on day 1), and 5-FU (1000 mg/m^2/day on days 2–5 and 28–31). Resection rates were 72%. One-fourth of patients undergoing resection had a complete pathologic response. Median survival was 16.8 months, which was slightly better than in the RTOG/SWOG studies.[31]

Several single-institution nonrandomized trials have been performed, and the results have usually been more favorable than the multiinstitutional results; the phase II multiinstitution trials generally reported more favorable results than phase III trials. Naunheim et al., from St. Louis University, reported on 29 patients with squamous cell carcinoma and 18 with adenocarcinoma ($n = 47$) who received preoperative chemoradiation consisting of simultaneous cisplatin, 5-FU, and 3000–3600 cGy of radiation. The results were promising when compared to a group of historical controls. Total resectability was 72% after preoperative chemoradiation. The overall median survival was improved by 1 year (10.5 months in historical controls and 23 months with preoperative chemoradiation). The 3-year actuarial survival was 40% with preoperative chemoradiation compared to 0% in historical controls.[32]

Another promising study came from the University of Michigan where Forastiere et al. treated 43 patients (22 with squamous cell carcinoma, 21 with adenocarcinoma) with preoperative chemoradiation. Patients received a 5-FU continuous infusion for 21 days and cisplatin and vinblastine on days 1–5 and 17–21. Radiation therapy at doses of 3750–4500 cGy was also given during this intensive 21-day inpatient chemotherapy treatment. Patients underwent surgical resection 3–4 weeks later. In all, 84% underwent potentially curative resections, with no residual tumor found in 24%. The median survival for these patients was 29 months compared to 12 months for historical controls. The 5-year survival was 34%. Sixty percent of patients with complete response were alive at 5 years and had a median survival of 70 months.[33]

Five randomized trials have evaluated preoperative chemoradiation, two utilizing sequential chemotherapy and radiation followed by surgery and three utilizing concomitant preoperative chemoradiation. Nygaard et al., from Norway, performed a four-arm randomized clinical trial in which patients with squamous cell carcinoma were randomized to one of the following four arms: surgery alone, preoperative cisplatin and bleomycin, preoperative radiation of 3500 cGy, or preoperative sequential chemoradiation. The number of patients in each arm was relatively small, but the results showed no significant difference in the 3- and 5-year survival rates for any of the three modalities compared to surgery alone.[27] The 3-year survival rates were significantly higher for any modality that utilized radiation therapy; however, as previously mentioned, the number of patients in each arm was small. Moreover, three times the number of patients in the radiotherapy groups were lost to follow-up, which may have been a confounding factor.[34]

In another randomized trial from Rennes, France, 86 patients with squamous cell carcinoma underwent surgery alone or were given preoperative cisplatin and 5-FU followed by 2000 cGy of radiation followed by another cycle of cisplatin and 5-FU before surgery. The study stopped early after 104 patients were enrolled, and there was no improvement in survival after 3 years of evaluation. The lack of a difference between the two groups may have been due to the relatively mild nature of the chemoradiation given (low radiation dose).[35]

The University of Michigan studied 100 patients, 75 with adenocarcinoma and 25 with squamous cell carcinoma. The patients were randomized to transhiatal resection alone or preoperative concomitant chemoradiation consisting of cisplatin (20 mg/m^2 on days 1–5 and 17–21), vinblastine (1 mg/m^2 on days 1–4 and 17–20), 5-FU (300 mg/m^2/day continuous infusion for 21 days), and radiation doses of 45 Gy (1.5 Gy bid for 3 weeks). The mortality rate attributed to chemoradiation was 0%; however, nearly 80% of patients had grade 3 or 4 neutropenia, thrombocytopenia, or both. Ninety percent of patients in each arm underwent total resection. Twenty-eight percent of patients receiving chemoradiation had complete pathologic responses, although at the 2-year follow-up there was no difference in median survival.[36] An updated review of the data demonstrates a twofold increase in 3-year survival: 32% for those receiving chemoradiation versus 15% for those undergoing surgery alone.[37] Final conclusions have yet to be drawn.

In a study of 113 patients with adenocarcinoma from Dublin, Walsh et al. compared surgery alone to preoperative concomitant chemoradiation. Patients in the chemoradiation arm received cisplatin (75 mg/m^2 on day 7) and 5-FU (15 mg/kg/day on days 1–5) during weeks 1 and 6 while receiving radiation therapy to a dose of 40 Gy at 2.67 Gy/fraction. The median survival rates were significantly higher for the multimodality group (16 months versus 11 months for the surgery-alone group). The 3-year survival rates were 32% for the patients receiving chemoradiation and only 6% for those in the surgery-alone group. The complete pathologic response rate for patients receiving chemoradiation was 25%.[38]

In a study from Germany, 25 patients with locally advanced squamous cell carcinoma or adenocarcinoma received preoperative sequential chemotherapy and chemoradiotherapy followed by surgery. Two courses of six weekly doses of 5-FU (2 g/m^2 over 24 hours) and folinic acid (500 mg/m^2 over 2 hours) combined with cisplatin (50 mg/m^2 over 1 hour) given twice weekly. Then 30 Gy of irradiation was given concurrently with one course of cisplatin and etoposide. Partial remission with subjective improvement was seen in 60% (6/10) of patients with squamous cell carcinoma and 66% (10/15) of those with adenocarcinoma. Of 19 patients undergoing surgery, 16 had a complete resection. Ten of these sixteen (62%) had a complete pathologic response; 43% were alive at a median follow-up of 20 months. Side effects were mild to moderate and were usually related to mucositis. Unfortunately, the operative mortality rate was 16%.[39]

There is still no consensus regarding preoperative chemoradiation. The toxicities are high, and no convincing long-term survival has been shown. The principal benefit of preoperative chemoradiation is for the node-positive patient. At present, EUS should be performed to determine nodal status. A clinical trial should then randomize node-positive patients into preoperative chemoradiation or surgery alone. Until more clinical trials are completed, preoperative chemoradiation should be considered in this context.

G. Surgical Therapy

Whether preoperative chemoradiation is utilized, the next step for patients without metastatic disease is surgery. The goal of treatment is eradication of disease, including the entire tumor with regional lymph nodes, and relief of dysphagia. Surgical treatment is considered the gold standard of therapy and generally provides a 20% five-year survival in most studies.[11]

The choice of surgical procedure depends mainly on the preference of the surgeon and location of the tumor, although body habitus, prior irradiation, previous operations, and the condition of the patient also influence this decision.[40] Cervical esophageal cancers frequently do not undergo operation; instead only chemoradiation is utilized, as 5-year survival rates are low and surgical morbidity is significant. When treated surgically, pharyngolaryngectomy, extrathoracic esophagectomy, and gastric interposition are usually the procedures of choice.[11] Thoracic inlet tumors are generally resected via extrathoracic esophagogastrectomy without laryngectomy if possible. For middle- or lower-third tumors, combined thoracic and abdominal approaches are usually used, especially the Ivor Lewis procedure or transhiatal esophagectomy.[11]

Ivor Lewis Esophagogastrectomy The Ivor Lewis procedure (combined laparotomy and right thoracotomy) is the most commonly used procedure for resecting a middle- or lower-third esophageal tumor. The stomach is fully mobilized through a midline epigastric incision after the abdomen is explored for liver metastases or unresectable retroperitoneal nodes. If either is present, palliation of symptoms becomes the primary concern and total tumor resection is abandoned. If resection is undertaken, the right gastric and gastroepiploic arteries are spared. The greater omentum is divided along the greater curvature, leaving a small piece of omentum on the curvature for later use to wrap around the anastomosis. The stomach is elevated, and the short gastric vessels are clamped and tied. After the stomach is mobilized, the hiatus is enlarged and the lower esophagus is dissected. The stomach and omentum should be advanced into the posterior mediastinum before the abdomen is closed.[40]

With the patient in the left lateral decubitus position, a standard right posterolateral thoracotomy is performed through the fourth or fifth interspace. The right lung is deflated and retracted anteriorly to allow exposure for the esophageal dissection and anastomosis.[40] The amount of esophagus resected depends on the extent and location of the tumor. Proximal and distal margins 5 cm beyond the tumor are obtained. During dissection of the esophagus, paraesophageal tissues and all nodal groups around the esophagus should be included with the specimen, especially the periesophageal, subcarinal, perigastric, and celiac nodes.[11] The stomach is then pulled into the chest, and the lesser curvature is resected, forming a tubular structure. The anastomosis is performed with an end-to-side esophagogastrostomy.[11] In-hospital mortality rates are reported to be 2–4%, resulting mainly from pneumonia or anastomotic leaks.[11,41,42] In a review by Muller et al., however, mortality rates ranged from 4% to as high as 18%.[43]

Because the anastomosis is intrathoracic, it is the most critical part of the procedure in regard to the success of the operation and morbidity. Intrathoracic anastomotic leaks can be catastrophic. Mathisen et al. had no leaks in their series,[41] and Lee and Miller[11] reported leak rates of 1–2%. Lozac'h et al. reported rates of almost 7%.[42] One-third to one-half of the anastomotic leaks resulted in death. Because of the gravity of a leak, patients should be kept *nil per os* (NPO) after surgery until a barium swallow 1 week after surgery demonstrates no evidence of a leak. A nasogastric tube in place distal to the anastomosis site is also wise. If a leak is present but is small and well drained by the chest tube, the patient should be kept NPO. Antibiotic therapy and nutritional support should be continued, followed by repeat barium swallow in 1 week.[40] Fluid collections identified by CT should be drained percutaneously. Massive leaks require surgical intervention, usually resection of devitalized tissue with cervical esophagostomy. Reanastomosis should be done later. According to Mathisen et al., leaks can be minimized by using the two-layer technique for the experienced surgeon or the stapled anastomosis for those less experienced in the former technique.[41]

Additional complications after the Ivor Lewis operation include anastomotic strictures, which occur in 5–16% of patients. They are usually effectively treated by endoscopic dilatation. Late benign narrowing, however, has been reported in up to 35% of patients, and strictures from cancer recurrence at the anstomosis have occurred in 5–7% of patients.[41,42,44]

Pulmonary complications, usually pneumonia, are the most common cause of postoperative morbidity, with rates typically 12–15%.[40,41,42] Atelectasis and respiratory insufficiency are also common pulmonary complications.[40] Gastric dysfunction and outlet obstruction occurs in approximately 3–9% of patients. One-third of these patients require surgery.[41,42]

In a 1990 review Muller et al. found that survival rates depended solely on the cancer stage at the time of diagnosis, rather than the surgical procedure chosen.[43] In the study by Mathisen et al., 5-year survival rates for patients who underwent resection via the Ivor Lewis procedure were 8.0% for the 73 patients with adenocarcinoma and 33.2% for the 31 patients with squamous cell carcinoma (patients with squamous cell cancer were given preoperative chemotherapy).[41] Lozac'h et al. found that the actuarial survival at 24 months was 68% for patients who underwent Ivor Lewis procedures with stage I or II disease and only 23% for patients with stage III disease.[42]

Transhiatal Esophagectomy Transhiatal esophagectomy (THE) has been championed by many as an appropriate alternative to transthoracic approaches. By avoiding thoracotomy and utilizing a cervical anastomosis, the combined physiologic insult and morbidity associated with both thoracic and abdominal incisions are alleviated, and the risk of an intrathoracic esophagogastric anastomotic leak is eliminated.[45] Because of the nature of the procedure, wide resection of the esophagus along with its contiguous soft tissues and lymph nodes is not possible, although sampling of accessible subcarinal, paraesophageal, and celiac lymph nodes is done routinely by many proponents THE.[45]

The procedure has three phases: abdominal, cervical, and mediastinal. The abdominal phase is through a supraumbilical incision. The stomach is mobilized as in the Ivor Lewis procedure, celiac lymph nodes are biopsied, and a pyloromyotomy is performed to a avoid delayed gastric emptying after vagotomy. The distal esophagus is mobilized from the posterior mediastinum. At this time it is necessary to ascertain that the esophagus is not fixed to any mediastinal structures such as the aorta. The cervical phase is then begun, making an incision on the left side of the neck from the suprasternal notch up to the level of the cricoid cartilage parallel to the left sternocleidomastoid muscle. The esophagus is dissected posteriorly to the prevertebral fascia and by blunt finger dissection into the superior mediastinum. Care should be taken not to injure the left recurrent laryngeal nerve as the esophagus is dissected away from the trachea. The esophagus is retracted superiorly, and blunt dissection continues to the level of the carina through the neck incision if possible. The mediastinal phase consists of continued blunt dissection of the mediastinum through both the neck incision and the abdominal incision until mobilization of the entire thoracic esophagus is complete. The upper esphagus is divided through the cervical incision. The stomach and thoracic esophagus are delivered into the abdominal wound, the proximal stomach is divided with a linear stapler, and the esophagus and proximal stomach are removed completely from the field. The remaining gastric portion is then pushed up through the hiatus and pulled through the posterior mediastinum. After the abdominal incision is closed, the cervical esophagogastric anastomosis is performed, suturing the remaining esophagus to a small button-hole stoma made on the anterior surface of the stomach.[46]

In a retrospective study of 583 patients undergoing THE (417 for malignant disease) by Orringer et al., intraoperative complications included pneumothoraces treated with chest tubes in 74% of patients, tracheal lacerations in four patients, and splenectomy due to injury in 4% of patients.[47] Another criticism of this procedure is difficulty with hemostasis due to poor exposure. Orringer et al. reported average intraoperative blood losses of 875 ml (excluding four patients who had blood losses ranging from 6600 to 18,000 ml) compared to 500 ml measured by Mathisen et al. using the Ivor Lewis procedure.[41,47] Millikan et al. demonstrated less blood loss for THE than for transthoracic procedures, although the results were not statistically significant.[48]

Cervical anastomotic leaks occur more frequently with THE than do thoracic anastomotic leaks with the Ivor Lewis procedure. Orringer et al. reported a 9% leak rate in cervical anastomoses for carcinoma.[47] Millikan et al. reported a 7% leak rate.[48] Transthoracic procedures have reported leak rates of 0–7%, but cervical leaks are less serious.[11,41,42] More than 90%

of cervical leaks are managed at the bedside by opening and packing the wound until the leak heals.

Left recurrent nerve injury is much more common with THE as well, with 9% of the patients suffering hoarseness; one-third of them have true vocal cord paralysis.[47] Cervical dysphagia requiring occasional dilatation occurs in 52% of patients. Severe dysphagia requiring regular dilatation occurs in 5%, and true fibrotic anastomotic strictures occur in fewer than 2% of patients.[47]

In-hospital mortality rates are 4–5%, which is similar to the rates reported for transthoracic procedures in many studies.[47,48] In contrast to transthoracic procedures, a significantly smaller percentage of deaths are due to respiratory complications. This is probably due to avoidance of a thoracotomy as well as great attention to pulmonary status preoperatively.[47,48]

Orringer et al. reported that 41% of patients were alive at 2 years, and the overall 5-year survival rate was 27%.[47] These results are not much different than those obtained with transthoracic procedures. Shahian et al. found there was no statistical difference in median survival for patients undergoing transthoracic resection (14.1 months) or extrathoracic resection (12.6 months) (p = 0.48).[49] Orringer et al. found that overall survival depended more on the cancer stage than on the choice of operation. Survival rates are slightly better for distal-third tumors. Millikan et al. indicated that transhiatal esophagectomy offers the least morbidity and has stage-specific survival equal to that seen with transthoracic approaches.[48]

RADICAL EN BLOC ESOPHAGOGASTRECTOMY Although THE may be curative for patients with early disease, Skinner and others argue that patients treated with radical esophagogastrectomy have the greatest chance at long-term survival and therefore should undergo as extensive a procedure as possible. The procedure is performed transthoracically and includes resection of all the affected esophagus, right and left parietal pleura, pericardium, thoracic duct, azygos vein, segments of the right intercostal arteries, and bilateral segments of the intercostal veins. Because the resection is so extensive, patients chosen for en bloc resection by Skinner et al. are first assessed as to whether they are medically able to undergo such a procedure. Patients chosen also had esophageal cancer staged both clinically and operatively as stage IIB or less.[50]

A left thoracotomy incision in the sixth intercostal space is performed for tumors of the gastric cardia or lower esophagus. The entire procedure is performed through this incision. Retracting the diaphragm allows visualization and dissection of the soft tissues and lymph nodes of the upper abdomen, including the hepatic and splenic artery nodes and all retroperitoneal tissues cephalad to the pancreas up to the level of the hiatus. For tumors of the upper, middle, or lower esophagus that are within 10 cm of the aortic arch, a right posterolateral thoracotomy is performed at the fifth interspace. If no evidence of metastatic disease is found during inspection of the liver, lungs, and mediastinum, the en bloc resection is begun. The full length of the mediastinal intrathoracic pleura is incised. The azygos vein and thoracic duct are ligated as they enter the mediastinum through the diaphragm. Pericardium is incised until the entire esophageal specimen is freed anteriorly. All tissues contiguous with the esophagus that lie anteriorly over the aorta are carefully dissected. The left pleural cavity is then entered, and the esophagus is divided 10 cm proximally if possible and at the esophageal hiatus. The esophagus, almost completely covered by soft tissues, can then be removed. The thoracotomy is closed, and cervical lymph node and scalene fat pad dissection is performed through bilateral U-shaped incisions over the lower one-third of the sternomastoid muscles. When utilizing a right thoracotomy, a laparotomy must be performed if cure is still thought possible. After full lymph node dissection, the stomach is mobilized if it is to be used for the anastomosis. Skinner often uses a segment of left and transverse colon for the reconstruction. The stomach or segment of colon to be used is pushed through the posterior mediastinum, and a cervical anastomosis is performed.[51]

Postoperatively, right and left chest tubes and respiratory support are managed in the intensive care unit. Aggressive fluid management is needed because of pulmonary sequestration and congestion secondary to removal of lymphatics. The patient should be kept NPO for 4–5 days, at which time a barium swallow is performed to determine if the patient is ready for clear fluids.[51] Postoperative complications occur in 43% of patients; they are mainly pulmonary in nature, including pneumonia, persistent pleural effusion, and atelectasis. There is a high rate of arrhythmias as well.[50] The in-hospital postoperative mortality reported by Skinner et al. was 9.7%.[50]

Skinner's studies have demonstrated comparatively high survival rates. The overall 1-year survival rates were almost twice that of standard esophagectomy (65% vs. 33%), although en bloc resections were done only on patients with early, minimal disease. Skinner found that survival rates changed drastically when factors such as the degree of wall invasion and the quantity of lymph nodes involved were taken into account.

Overall, stage for stage, THE has the same long-term survival rate as is seen with transthoracic approaches to esophagectomy. THE has lower morbidity (especially pulmonary) and similar operative mortality, and it should be considered the procedure of choice for esophageal cancer. Transthoracic approaches should be considered only when the cancer may be dangerously close to structures that are difficult to separate during a transhiatal approach (i.e., the aortic arch or carina in upper middle-third lesions).

H. Adjuvant Therapy: Chemotherapy and Irradiation

Irradiation, chemotherapy, and chemoradiation are often used postoperatively in an attempt to improve the prognosis of patients with esophageal cancer.

Postoperative Radiation Therapy Two prospective randomized trials of postoperative radiation completed to date have not shown any improvement in survival when compared to surgery alone. In a randomized study by Teniere et al. patients received either postoperative radiation doses of 45–55 Gy or surgery alone. Postsurgical relapse was decreased from 30% to 15% with the addition of radiation; unfortunately, the 5-year survival rates were only 19% for both groups.[52] The study by Fok et al. actually noted decreased median survival rates after postoperative irradiation as a result of irradiation-related death.[53]

Postoperative Chemotherapy Combination therapy with cisplatin and 5-FU is the accepted regimen when utilizing chemotherapy to treat esophageal cancer. With squamous cell carcinoma of the esophagus, this combination has an overall response rate of 50% for local disease and 35% for distant disease.[54] Trials comparing postoperative chemotherapy to surgery alone have been discouraging so far. A multicenter two-arm randomized trial of 120 patients, with the chemotherapy group receiving eight cycles of postoperative cisplatin and 5-FU, was compared to a group undergoing resection alone. The results demonstrated similar survival rates and an 8% mortality rate due to the chemotherapy.[55] Currently, postoperative chemotherapy is being studied in most trials when given in conjunction with irradiation.

Postoperative Chemoradiation The combination of chemotherapy and irradiation in multimodality therapy after surgery seems to show promise over individual therapies used alone. In a nonrandomized study by Ebie et al., 25 patients with biopsy-proven esophageal carcinoma (10 squamous cell carcinoma, 15 adenocarcinoma) underwent transhiatal esophagogastrostomy after no distant metastases were found on CT. After surgery, patients received concomitant chemoradiation therapy consisting of induction therapy with cisplatin (100 mg/m^2/day on day 1) and 5-FU (1.0 g/m^2/24 hr on days 1–5). Approximately 2 weeks after the initial therapy, patients began concurrent chemotherapy and radiation therapy on an every other week schedule: cisplatin (60 mg/m^2/day on day 1), 5-FU (800 mg/m^2/24 hr on days 1–5), and radiation at a total dose of 45 Gy in doses of 150–200 cGy bid. About 43–50% of patients suffered grade 3 leukopenia, resulting in decreased doses or unscheduled breaks of chemotherapy in 9 of the 25 patients. The median survival was 19 months, which was better than that of historical controls at the same institution. Twenty percent of patients showed no evidence of disease at follow-up of 33–70 months. Local control was excellent (84% with local control, 0% of patients had recurrences in the esophageal bed).[56]

The University of Pennsylvania has also had success with postoperative chemoradiation. After surgical resection, radiation therapy was given at doses of 54 Gy if all the tumor had been resected or 59–63 Gy if residual disease was present. Postoperative modulated 5-FU was given during the first and last weeks of radiation therapy. The 3-year survival was 39%, and teatment-related mortality was 7%.[57]

Metastatic Disease

I. Adjuvant Therapy

For patients with tumors invading adjacent structures (T4) or metastatic to distant sites (stage IV), surgery is not recommended. In a review of 10 studies, Thomas found that patients who had undergone radiation therapy had 2-year survival rates of only 3–27% and 5-year survival rates of 0–20%.[4] Some patients have palliation of dysphagia with radiation therapy; half are palliated for at least 2 months, but fewer than 15% remain improved after a year.[58] In addition to receiving 50–60 Gy of radiotherapy, patients with unresectable carcinoma may be treated concurrently with 5-FU plus cisplatin or 5-FU plus mitomycin.[20] If chemotherapy is selected for patients with metastatic disease, they should also be encouraged to enroll in available clinical trials.

J. Recurrent Disease

If a patient develops locoregional relapse after surgery, chemoradiation, or both for esophageal cancer, it must be determined if the relapse is technically resectable. If the disease is resectable and the patient is medically fit, surgery remains an option. If the above criteria are not met or the patient has a second relapse, palliative treatment should be instituted.[20]

K. Palliative Treatment

Most cases of esophageal cancer are diagnosed at incurable stages or patients are too debilitated to undergo surgery or intensive courses of radiation, chemotherapy, or both. Therefore other palliative measures to relieve dysphagia and improve quality of life are necessary.

Endoscopic *dilatation* of malignant strictures has been used successfully for years. It is easy to perform and is fast and inexpensive. Most patients are able to resume eating a soft or regular diet. Repeated dilatations are usually necessary, and perforation rates have been reported to be as high as 5%.[59]

Rigid plastic *stents* and expandable metal stents are available; they are easy to place and can provide long-term relief of dysphagia. Rigid stents, which are typically placed after endoscopic dilatation, are used less frequently because they are more difficult to place and have a higher perforation rate than expanding stents. Complications associated with rigid stents include the following: migration (15%), perforation (7%), obstruction (6%), pressure necrosis (3%), and bleeding (1%).[60] Self-expanding stents are easier to place because they do not require as much dilatation as the rigid stents. Because they are made of wire mesh, tumor ingrowth and reocclusion may occur. Migration is less likely, however.

Thermal ablation (destruction) with the neodynium:yttrium-aluminum-garnet (Nd:YAG) laser can be directed at the tumor under endoscopic visualization to vaporize tissue for temporary palliation. However, it is expensive and requires frequent treatments.[61] Dysphagia is relieved in 70–80% of patients in most studies; but bleeding, perforation, or fistula formation occurs in 5–20% of patients.[59] Intraluminal, short strictures and proximal lesions are better suited for laser ablation.

Photodynamic therapy is accomplished using a photosensitizing agent that accumulates in malignant tissue. It results in oxygen free radical formation when activated by light. This in turn causes selective destruction and necrosis without heat, which results in a lower incidence of perforation (1% with photodynamic therapy compared to up to 7% with laser). Fewer sessions were needed with photodynamic therapy, but there were more side effects, including sunburn (19%), fever (16%), pleural effusion (10%), and nausea (8%).[62]

Chemical necrolysis may be of benefit. Sclerosing agents, such as alcohol, can be injected directly into the tumor endoscopically. This therapy is inexpensive and widely available. Complications include stricture formation in normal tissue, bleeding, and perforation. Most patients in small, uncontrolled studies have been able to eat solid food again after the procedure.[59]

External beam radiation can be used for palliation. Most squamous cell carcinomas respond to irradiation, but recurrences and side effects are common (esophagitis, skin burns, pulmonary fibrosis, myelitis). Up to 20% of patients receiving high doses of radiation are not able to complete the course. *Brachytherapy* delivers localized radiation through the endoscopic placement of radioactive seeds. Only 1 cm of tumor necrosis can be achieved, but it is accomplished with less systemic toxicity than external radiation. In small studies fewer than half of the patients were able to advance their diet to solid food.[59]

L. Follow-up

Patients should undergo follow-up on a regular basis after treatment for esophageal carcinoma. In addition to the history and physical examination, a CBC and chemistry panels should be assessed every 3 months for 2 years, then every 6 months for the following 3 years. Chest radiographs should be obtained every 6–12 months after treatment. Additional investigations including endoscopy, upper gastrointestinal radiologic studies, CT scans, and dilatation of strictures should be scheduled as clinically necessary.[20]

References

1. Blot WJ. Epidemiology and genesis of esopphageal cancer. In: Roth JA, Ruckdeschel JC, Weisinburger TH (eds) Thoracic Oncology, 2nd ed. Philadelphia: Saunders, 1995;278–287.
2. Mayer RJ. Overview: the changing nature of esophageal cancer. Chest 1993;103:404S–405S.
3. Blot WJ, Devesa SS, Kneller RW, et al. Rising incidence of adenocarcinoma of the esophagus and gastric cardia. JAMA 1991;265:1287–1289.
4. Thomas CR Jr. Biology of esophageal cancer and the role of combined modality therapy. Surg Clin North Am 1997;77:1139–1167.
5. Launoy G, Milan CH, Faivre J, et al. Alcohol, tobacco and oesophageal cancer: effects of the duration of consumption, mean intake and current and former consumption. Br J Cancer 1997;75:1389–1396.
6. Bremner CG, Bramner RM. Barrett's esophagus. Surg Clin North Am 1997;77:1115–1137.
7. Roth JA, Putnam JB Jr, Rich TA, et al. Cancer of the esophagus. In: Devita VT, Hellman S, Rosenberg SA (eds) Cancer, Principles and Practice of Oncology, 5th ed. Philadelphia: Lippincott-Raven, 1997:980–1021.
8. Chow WH, Blot WJ, Vaughan TL, et al. Body mass index and risk of adenocarcinomas of the esophagus and gastric cardia. J Natl Cancer Inst 1998;90:150.
9. Begin LR. The pathobiology of esophageal cancer. In: Roth JA, Ruckdeschel JC, Weisinburger TH (eds) Thoracic Oncology, 2nd ed. Philadelphia: Saunders, 1995;288–385.
10. Moyana TN, Janoski M. Recent trends in the epidemiology of esophageal cancer: comparison of epidermoid and adenocarcinomas. Ann Clin Lab Sci 1996;26:480–486.
11. Lee RB, Miller JI. Esophagectomy for cancer. Surg Clin North Am 1997;77:1169–1196.
12. Dodd GD, Chasen MH. Diagnostic imaging of esophageal cancer. In: Roth JA, Ruckdeschel JC, Weisinburger TH (eds) Thoracic Oncology, 2nd ed. Philadelphia: Saunders, 1995:368–384.
13. Ojala K, Sorri M, Jokinen K, et al. Symptoms of carcinoma of the esophagus. Med J Aust 1982;1:384–385.
14. Levine MS, Chu P, Furth EE, et al. Carcinoma of the esophagus and esophagogastric junction: sensitivity of radiographic diagnosis. AJR Am J Roentgenol 1997;168:1423–1426.
15. Rice TW. Diagnosis and staging of esophageal carcinoma. In: Roth JA, Ruckdeschel JC, Weisinburger TH (eds) Thoracic Oncology, 2nd ed. Philadelphia: Saunders, 1995:385.
16. Frantz MA, Prolla JC. Correlation of endoscopic cytology and histology in oesophageal cancer: results in Porto Alegre, RS—Brazil. Cytopathology 1996;7:38–53.

17. Chandawarkar RY, Kakegawa T, Fujita H. Comparative analysis of imaging modalities in the preoperative assessment of nodal metastasis in esophageal cancer. J Surg Oncol 1996;61:214–217.
18. Kalantzis N, Kallimanis G, Laoudi F, et al. Endoscopic ultrasonography and computed tomography in preoperative (TNM) classification of oesophageal carcinoma. Endoscopy 1992;24:653.
19. Rice TW, Adelstein DJ. Precise clinical staging allows treatment modification of patients with esophageal carcinoma. Oncology 1997;11(suppl 9):58–62.
20. Ajani JA, Eisenberg B, Emanuel P, et al. NCCN practice guidelines for upper gastrointestinal carcinomas. Oncology 1998;12:179–201.
21. American Joint Committee on Cancer. In: Beahrs OH, Henson DE, Hutter RVP, et al. (eds) Manual for Staging Cancer, 4th ed. Philadelphia: Lippincott, 1992.
22. Sabik JF, Rice TW, Goldblum JR, et al. Superficial esophageal carcinoma. Ann Thorac Surg 1995;60:896–901.
23. Huang GJ, Gu XZ, Wang LJ, et al. Combined preoperative irradiation and surgery for esophageal carcinoma. In: Delarue NC (ed) International Trends in General Thoracic Surgery. St. Louis: Mosby, 1988:315–318.
24. Ajani JA. Current status of new drugs and multidisciplinary approaches in patients with carcinoma of the esophagus. Chest 1998;113(suppl 1):112S–119S.
25. Roth JA, Pass HI, Flanagan MM, et al. Randomized clinical trial of preoperative and postoperative adjuvant chemotherapy with cisplatin, vindesine, and bleomycin for carcinoma of the esophagus. J Thorac Cardiovasc Surg 1988;96:242–248.
26. Schlag PM. Randomized trial of preoperative chemotherapy for squamous cell cancer of the esophagus. Arch Surg 1992;127:1446–1450.
27. Nygaard K, Hagen S, Hansen HS, et al. Preoperative radiotherapy prolongs survival in operable esophageal carcinoma: a randomized, multicenter study of preoperative radiotherapy and chemotherapy: the second Scandinavian trial in esophageal cancer. World J Surg 1992;16:1104–1109.
28. Kelsen DP, Ginsberg R, Pajak TF, et al. Chemotherapy followed by surgery compared with surgery alone for localized esophageal cancer. N Engl J Med 1998;339:1979–1984.
29. Poplin E, Fleming T, Leichman L, et al. Combined therapies for squamous cell carcinoma of the esophagus: a Southwest Oncology Group study (SWOG-8037). J Clin Oncol 1987;5:622–628.
30. Seydel HG, Leichman L, Byhardt R, et al. Preoperative radiation and chemotherapy for localized squamous cell carcinoma of the esophagus: a RTOG study. Int J Radiat Oncol Biol Phys 1988;14:33–35.
31. Keller SM, Coia LR, Ryan L, et al. Chemo-radiation followed by esophagectomy for adenocarcinoma of the esophagus and gastroesophageal junction: results of a phase II study of the Eastern Cooperative Oncology Group. Proc Am Soc Clin Oncol 1995;14:196.
32. Naunheim KS, Petruska P, Roy TS, et al. Preoperative chemotherapy and radiotherapy for esophageal carcinoma. J Thorac Cardiovasc Surg 1992;103:887–893.
33. Forastiere AA, Orringer MB, Perez-Tomayo C, et al. Concurrent chemotherapy and radiation therapy followed by transhiatal esophagectomy for local-regional cancer of the esophagus. J Clin Oncol 1990;8:119–127.
34. Urba S. Combined-modality treatment of esophageal cancer. Oncology 1997;11(suppl 9):63–67.
35. LePrise E, Etienne PL, Meunier B, et al. A randomized study of chemotherapy, radiation therapy, and surgery versus surgery for localized squamous cell carcinoma of the esophagus. Cancer 1994;73:1779–1784.
36. Urba S, Orringer M, Turrisi A, et al. A randomized trial comparing transhiatal esophagectomy to preoperative concurrent chemoradiation followed by esophagectomy in loco-regional esophageal carcinoma. Proc Am Soc Clin Oncol 1995;14:199.
37. Urba S, Orringer M, Turris A, et al. A randomized trial comparing surgery to preoperative concomitant chemoradiation plus surgery in patients with resectable esophageal cancer: updated analysis. Proc Am Soc Clin Oncol 1997;16:277a.
38. Walsh TN, Noonan N, Hollywood D, et al. A comparison of multimodal therapy and surgery for esophageal adenocarcinoma. N Engl J Med 1996;335:462–467.
39. Stahl M, Vanhoefer U, Stuschke M, et al. Preoperative sequential chemo and radiochemotherapy in locally advanced carcinomas of the lower oesophagus and gastrooesophageal junction. Eur J Cancer 1998;34:668–673.
40. Mathisen DJ. Ivor Lewis procedure. In: Pearson FG, Deslauriers J, Ginsberg RJ, et al. (eds) Esophageal Surgery. New York: Churchill Livingstone, 1995:669–676.
41. Mathisen DJ, Grillo HC, Wilkins EW Jr, et al. Transthoracic esophagectomy: a safe approach to carcinoma of the esophagus. Ann Thorac Surg 1988;45:137–143.
42. Lozac'h P, Topart P, Etienne J, et al. Ivor Lewis operation for epidermoid carcinoma of the esophagus. Ann Thorac Surg 1991;52:1154–1157.
43. Muller JM, Erasmi H, Stelzner M, et al. Surgical therapy of oesophageal carcinoma. Br J Surg 1990;77:845–857.
44. King RM, Pairolero PC, Trastek VF, et al. Ivor Lewis esophagogastrectomy for carcinoma of the esophagus: early and late functional results. Ann Thorac Surg 1987;44:119–122.
45. Orringer MB. Transhiatal esophagectomy without thoracotomy for carcinoma of the thoracic esophagus. Ann Surg 1984;200:282–288.
46. Orringer MB. Transhiatal esophagectomy without thoracotomy. In: Pearson FG, Deslauriers J, Ginsberg RJ, et al. (eds) Esophageal Surgery. New York: Churchill Livingstone, 1995:683–708.
47. Orringer MB, Marshall B, Stirling MC. Transhiatal esophagectomy for benign and malignant disease. J Thorac Cardiovasc Surg 1993;105:265–276.
48. Millikan KW, Silverstein J, Hart V, et al. A 15-year review of esophagectomy for carcinoma of the esophagus and cardia. Arch Surg 1995;130:617–624.
49. Shahian DM, Neptune WB, Ellis FH Jr, et al. Transthoracic versus extrathoracic esophagectomy: mortality, morbidity, and long-term survival. Ann Thorac Surg 1986;41:237–246.
50. Skinner DB, Little AG, Ferguson MK, et al. Selection of operation for esophageal cancer based on staging. Ann Surg 1986;204:391–401.
51. Skinner DB. En bloc resection for esophageal carcinoma. In: Pearson FG, Deslauriers J, Ginsberg RJ, et al. (eds) Esophageal Surgery. New York: Churchill Livingstone, 1995:709–718.
52. Teniere P, Hay JM, Fingerhut A, et al. Postoperative radiation therapy does not increase survival after curative resecton for squamous cell carcinoma of the middle and lower esophagus as shown by a multicenter controlled trial. Surg Gynecol Obstet 1991;173:123–130.
53. Fok M, Sham JS, Choy D, et al. Postoperative radiotherapy for carcinoma of the esophagus: a prospective randomized controlled study. Surgery 1993;113:138–147.
54. Ajani JA. Contributions of chemotherapy in the treatment of carcinoma of the esophagus: results and commentary. Semin Oncol 1994;21:474–482.
55. Pouliquen X, Levard H, Hay JM, et al. 5-Fluorouracil and cisplatin therapy after palliative surgical resection of squamous cell carcinoma of the esophagus: a multicenter randomized trial. Ann Surg 1996;223:127–133.
56. Ebie N, Kang HJ, Millikan K, et al. Integration of surgery in multimodality therapy for esophageal cancer. Am J Clin Oncol 1997;20:11–15.
57. Kurtzman SM, Whittington R, Vaughn D, et al. Post-operative chemosensitized radiation with modulated 5-FU following resection of adeno-

carcinoma of the esophagus and esophagogastric junction. Int J Radiat Oncol Biol Phys 1995;32(suppl 1):266.
58. Pearson JG. The value of radiotherapy in the management of esophageal cancer. AJR Am J Roentgenol 1969;105:500–513.
59. Ponec RJ, Kimmey MB. Endoscopic therapy of esophageal cancer. Surg Clin North Am 1997;77:1197–1217.
60. van den Bradt-Gradel V, den Hartog Jager FC, Tytgat GN. Palliative intubation of malignant esophagogastric obstruction. J Clin Gastroenterol 1987;9:290–297.
61. Khandelwal M. Palliative therapy for carcinoma of the esophagus. Compr Ther 1995;21:177–183.
62. Lightdale CJ, Heier SK, Marcon NE, et al. Photodynamic therapy with porfimer sodium versus thermal ablation therapy with Nd:YAG laser for palliation of esophageal cancer: a multicenter randomized trial. Gastrointest Endosc 1995;42:507–512.

CHAPTER 28

Long-Segment and Short-Segment Barrett's Esophagus

PHILIP E. DONAHUE

A. *Epidemiology*

Norman Barrett described an esophageal condition characterized by the presence of columnar epithelium in areas normally lined by squamous epithelium, accounting for its present eponymous designation. The columnar-lined esophagus (CLE) is always an abnormal finding, although there is some disagreement about which varieties of CLE should be called Barrett's esophagus, as described subsequently. There is general agreement, however, that CLE is related to "pathologic" gastroesophageal reflux disease (GER/GERD), the retrograde movement ("reflow") of gastric or intestinal content into the esophagus.[1,2] Abnormal GER is common (5–10% of the population) and is usually associated with a dysfunctional lower esophageal segment that either relaxes inappropriately or fails to adequately contract, allowing gastric contents to make contact with the lower esophageal mucosa. Barrett's esophagus is a result of chronic GER and is the final result of many episodes of injury that culminate in a healing–epithelial metaplasia sequence with the final result a columnar epithelial lining in part of the esophagus. In the past all CLE was termed Barrett's esophagus; at present there is still some uncertainty about terminology, with a few authorities believing that the term Barrett's esophagus should be limited to CLE with the presence of intestinal metaplasia. This is an important point: CLE is itself a condition of metaplasia, but when goblet cells are present within the CLE (CLE-gob), "intestinal metaplasia" has occurred. CLE-gob is significant because of its propensity for the development of epithelial dysplasia and for the possible later development of adenocarcinoma of the esophagus. Whereas some experts reserve the term Barrett's esophagus for CLE-gob, others believe that "Barrett's esophagus" should be used for CLE alone because the presence of a CLE mandates some type of periodic surveillance.[3,4]

Barrett's Esophagus

A.
Epidemiology
Columnar-lined esophagus is always an abnormal finding
Barrett's esophagus is the result of chronic esophageal reflux
Of patients with reflux, 20% have Barrett's
Barrett's reflects advanced reflux disease: surgery indicated;
long-term medical therapy does not retard evolution of Barrett's
Fundoplication may stop progression of metaplasia to dysplasia sequence

↓

B.
Pathogenesis

Long-standing reflux → Mucosal injury, inflammation, ulceration → Metaplasia ± goblet cells → Dysplasia → Neoplasia

C.
Diagnosis

↓

History and physical examination (see Table 28–2)

↓

Heartburn
Regurgitation
Dysplasia
Choking

Endoscopy → Biopsy the esophagus above and below squamocolumnar junction
Biopsy at 1- to 2-cm intervals from the upper gastric rugal folds to the squamous epithelium
Biopsy distal stomach to exclude *H. pylori* infection

pH and motility testing*
Upper GI radiology*
Manometry*
*Useful when atypical symptoms predominate

NOTE: Barrett's esophagus without dysplasia may be followed with surveillance endoscopy every 1–2 years with repeat biopsy.

(continued on next page)

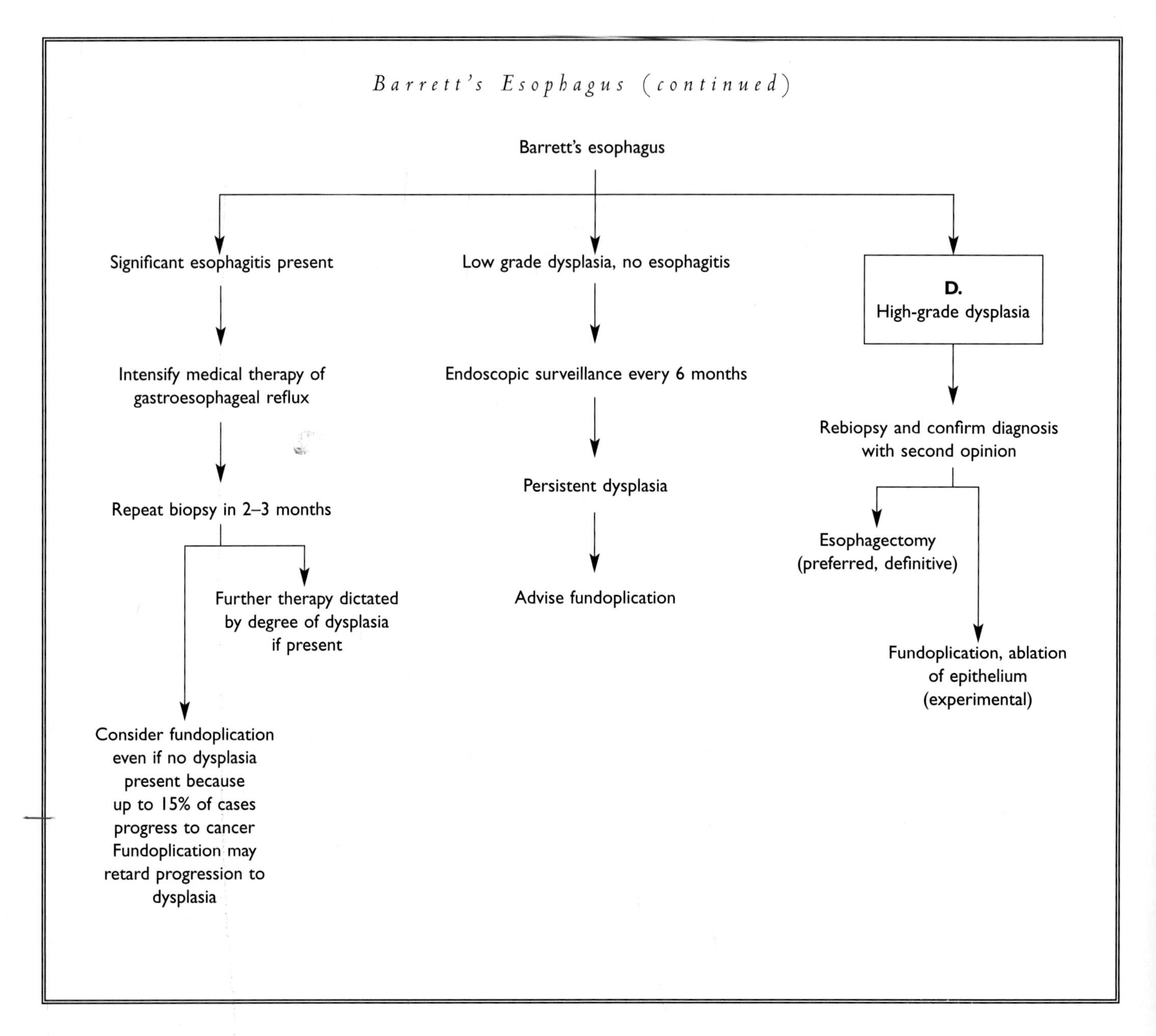

B. *Pathogenesis*

Barrett's Esophagus (CLE) and GER

Long-standing GER leads to mucosal injury, including inflammation (carditis) and ulceration, and eventually esophageal shortening. Among patients who develop a CLE, a subset have an admixture of goblet cells, which are the histologic signature of "intestinal metaplasia." At this time it is known that metaplastic epithelium is sometimes transformed (by a series of genetic changes) into a dysplastic epithelium that has the potential for progression through a spectrum of histopathologic changes including severe dysplasia, carcinoma in situ, and invasive cancer of the esophagus.[3,5] For that reason, the diagnosis of CLE is of great concern to physicians and their patients.

The number of persons with CLE may be substantially higher than previously recognized, as several reports have documented the present of goblet cells in the distal esophagus in 20% of patients with GER; however, there is some uncertainty about these findings, as the status of *Helicobacter* infection in other parts of the stomach has not been completely described.[6–8] Because infections of the gastric antrum and corpus might lead to intestinal metaplasia at this site, it is impossible to draw final conclusions at this time.

Population at Risk for Adenocarcinoma of Esophagus

There is general agreement that the incidence of adenocarcinoma of the esophagus has increased dramatically since the mid-1970s.[9] We do not understand precisely why, although laboratory studies suggest that severe GER and the refluxate composition may be partly responsible. The relation between CLE and esophageal dysplasia is known, as are some of the genetic changes that accompany the transition from CLE to dysplasia of the CLE. The goal of all surveillance strategies is to identify the patient with dysplasia before progression to esophageal adenocarcinoma has occurred.

At present, CLE is not discovered unless endoscopy and esophageal biopsy are performed; alarming recent reports of a 20% incidence of CLE among patients with GER symptoms suggest that millions may be at risk for the subsequent development of adenocarcinoma. On the other hand, it is also possible that a huge at-risk population has existed for years, and the current reports represent late awareness of the medical community about the true incidence of this problem. This is an issue of great importance to patients and of great concern to physicians; each group would like to make decisions based on fact and avoid the worry and uncertainty that accompany the diagnosis of a precancerous condition.[10,11]

Although these individuals require surveillance, the presence of Barrett's epithelium is diagnostic of advanced reflux disease and is itself a sufficient indication for surgical treatment; unfortunately, many physicians believe that control of symptoms is the appropriate target for treatment in patients with CLE.[12] Because fundoplication appears to retard the transition toward severe dysplasia, an increasing number of patients have become candidates for surgical treatment in the recent past.[13] Because laparoscopic procedures are as effective as open operations, and many referring physicians and patients believe that laparoscopic surgery is not associated with major risks, more patients are electing surgical treatment at an earlier stage of disease.

TABLE 28–1.
Causes of gastroesophageal reflux

Underlying problem	Examples
Neonatal period (chalasia)	Frequent vomiting in premature infants
Infants	Pyloric stenosis
Absent LES	Postoperative (after esophageal myectomy or resection of the normal antireflux mechanism)
	Traumatic avulsion of muscles of gastroesophageal segment
Abnormal LES	LES weakened by inflammation, caustic injury, infection, diseased muscle (myopathy, scleroderma)
Displaced sphincter	Weak LES residing in the chest (paraesophageal hernia)
Delayed gastric emptying	Secondary GER: diabetes, gastric atony, gastric outlet obstruction
Abnormal reflex relaxation	Increased "transient relaxations of LES"
Brain/brainstem injury	Dysmotility of pharynx, esophagus, and stomach
Abnormal hormonal milieu	Increased levels of progesterone (pregnancy, BCPs)
Medications that affect LES	Anticholinergic medications, Ca channel-blocking agents

LES, lower esophageal sphincter; GER, gastroesophageal reflux; BCPs, birth control pills.

C. Diagnosis

CLE in Patients with GER

The diagnosis of gastroesophageal reflux has reached a high level of specificity; the routine use of 24-hour pH testing and a heightened awareness that GER is associated with a constellation of typical and atypical symptoms (Table 28–1) has contributed to an increased frequency of diagnosis. Whether other factors such as *Helicobacter* species play a role in the increased diagnosis of GER is less well defined at present.

As discussed above, the importance of biopsy for patients with GER is widely appreciated. Recently there has been renewed interest in the histology and distribution of CLE now that specific dyes (indigocarmine) simplify the recognition or confirm the presence of CLE, resulting in the discovery that CLE is more prevalent than previously thought. The exact incidence of CLE, interestingly, is not precisely known because there are still some problems with definitions regarding the anatomy of the esophageal hiatus and with the nomenclature and histology of the normal gastroesophageal junction.[14,15] Terms such as "hiatus hernia," for example, have a broad definition, and its incidence may be overestimated; moreover, benign diseases such as GER, which do not have "hard" endpoints (e.g., death, amputation, perforation) are often "self-reported," precluding any rigorous analysis of population-based statistics.

Interestingly, the definition of the "gastric cardia" has important implications in any discussion of CLE because the existence of any inflammation of the junctional mucosa between the stomach and the esophagus is highly unusual.[14,15] GER, according to current thinking, may be responsible for inflammation in the cardia and for changes in the lining of the distal esophagus.[16,17] Furthermore, in the esophagus the progression of CLE through phases of early dysplasia, late dysplasia, and carcinoma is associated with a stepwise process of genetic alterations that lead to hyperproliferation, genomic instability, and clonal expansion. Dysplastic epithelial alterations are the histomorphologic feature of this process and the current focus of surveillance activities.[18,19]

Physicians and patients with GER should be informed that CLE occurs as a consequence of years of GER, and that long-term medical therapy does not retard the evolution of CLE.[20] Any patient with CLE should participate in a rational surveillance program and be aware that surgical treatment with effective fundoplication might stop the metaplasia-to-dysplasia sequence.[13] Once metaplasia has progressed to mild or severe dysplasia, other alternatives must be considered, including conventional treatments such as high-dose medical therapy and experimental ones including photodynamic treatment and laser ablation of the abnormal tissues. Surgical procedures to prevent pathologic reflux are appropriate in any patient with CLE and might prevent the progression of CLE to dysplasia. Esophageal resection is the recommended treatment for patients with severe dsyplasia because there is a 50% risk of invasive cancer in such patients.

Diagnosis of Gastroesophageal Reflux

The diagnosis of GER, a condition easily confused with other problems, can be achieved with real specificity in most cases. The diagnostician must consider symptoms of GER as consistent with a variety of foregut conditions as well as cardiac and pulmonary problems (Tables 28–1, 28–2). Diagnosis of GER requires the judicious use of diagnostic tests, including endoscopic observation, pH and motility testing, and upper gastrointestinal (GI) series, among others; the goals of testing are to verify the diagnosis and exclude the possibility that other conditions that might cause similar symptoms are not present.

TABLE 28–2.
Symptoms of gastroesophageal reflux

Symptoms
Typical symptoms
Heartburn (pyrosis)
Regurgitation
Dysphagia/odynophagia
Choking
Atypical symptoms
Severe chest pain
Pulmonary aspiration, asthma (adult onset)
Sinusitis, pharyngitis
Water brash (excess salivation)
Laryngitis, hoarseness, easy fatigability of voice

Causes of LES Failure

Chalasia Chalasia causes vomiting in young children, usually during the neonatal period, and is associated with immaturity of the lower esophageal sphincter (LES); it is quite common in newborn or premature infants. Another condition that may place children at high risk for esophageal inflammation due to reflux is pyloric stenosis. As many as 75% of children with this condition have frank inflammatory changes in the esophagus, occasionally severe enough to cause hematemesis as the presenting complaint.

Surgical, Iatrogenic, or Other Trauma to the LES Surgical excision of the LES is associated with free reflux and severe morbidity; for this reason, all such procedures should include an antireflux mechanism of the inkwell or fundoplication type. Also, when myotomy for achalasia includes myotomy of proximal stomach, an antireflux procedure is necessary to prevent postoperative GER. The GER produced by pneumatic dilation of the esophagus, a procedure loosely analogous to myotomy, eventually occurs in about 50% of the patients so treated. Surgical injury to the diaphragm, including disruption of the phrenoesophageal ligament, the LES, or the esophageal hiatus is another cause of severe GER.

Weakened LES A weakened LES is the most common cause of GER; however, patients with normal pressure in the LES also have GER caused by "inappropriate relaxation" of the sphincter mechanism. Some muscular disorders, including scleroderma and mixed collagen vascular disease, often develop refractory esophagitis and stricture.[17] Modern diagnostic modalities, including endoluminal ultrasonography, may be of use in this setting. Other conditions such as diabetes mellitus, hypothyroidism, or amyloidosis are also associated with abnormalities in the LES, related to the metabolic effects of the primary condition on the muscles that comprise the antireflux barrier.

Gastric Atony Any condition that causes delayed gastric emptying can lead to chronic or episodic gastric distension, thereby setting the stage for (secondary) reflux. Diabetes mellitus is the most common metabolic disorder that affects gastric motility, but other neuropathic conditions may be implicated as well. Acute pancreatitis is a well known cause of gastric ileus, although any inflammatory process in the vicinity of the gastric outlet may be associated with the problem. Gastric and duodenal obstruction by cancer, smooth muscle tumors, or congenital problems can also be associated with severe secondary reflux symptoms. In addition, occasional patients with superior mesenteric artery syndrome, duodenal carcinoma, or other abnormalities may be encountered with severe symptoms of reflux. In all of these instances complete evaluation of the foregut, including barium studies, usually reveals the underlying obstructive lesion as the cause of the reflux condition.

ESOPHAGEAL MANOMETRY Most patients with reflux problems have straightforward disease and do not have exotic or unexpected findings. In the absence of atypical symptoms and with an upper GI series showing a patulous esophageal hiatus with or without hiatus hernia, manometry has low yield and little impact on determining which procedure is done. If the upper GI barium examinations are "normal" and there is no obvious component of esophageal inflammation, comprehensive diagnostic testing is essential for making appropriate decisions.[21,22] Several of our patients with achalasia have had 6- to 18-month periods when their symptoms were interpreted as GER, with the diagnosis becoming obvious after esophageal manometry had been performed.

ENDOSCOPIC EXAMINATION: NEED FOR ROUTINE BIOPSY

Gastroesophageal reflux is a disease in which histology has added little to the diagnosis, excluding those in whom a long-segment Barrett esophagus was suspected because of the typical "shiny and pink" appearance of Barrett's epithelium. The "typical" histologic findings of esophageal inflammation have been considered somewhat superfluous because the cellular evidence of inflammation and basal cell hyperplasia are both nonspecific and subject to interobserver variation. Objective evidence of reflux, however, is useful when it is seen in the typical location just above the gastroesophageal junction. Some patients, however, have marked subjective complaints without visual evidence of inflammation; in these individuals motility and pH testing are extremely important. Recently, however, new information has led to a different approach with respect to endoscopic biopsy of the esophagus. Up to 25% of patients with GER have been found to have columnar lining in the transitional zone (cardia) of the distal esophagus. Because some of these cells are shown to be goblet cells by alcian blue staining methods, the term short-segment Barrett's esophagus has been coined (SS-BE). The emergence of SS-BE merits the full attention of the medical community, as it appears that such segments are at risk for adenocarcinoma, just as long-segment CLE is at risk for this development.

HISTOLOGIC FINDINGS IN THE DISTAL ESOPHAGUS AND PROXIMAL STOMACH

There are specific areas in the distal esophagus and stomach that have been difficult to define precisely because of their inherent mobility, lack of fixation, and dynamic properties: gastric cardia, lower esophageal sphincter, proximal stomach. Some earlier observations about the anatomy of the cardia have been reevaluated by DeMeester and his colleagues in Los Angeles.[13] They proposed that there are some misconceptions about the anatomy and normal histology of the proximal stomach and distal esophagus; the area of the stomach termed "gastric cardia," which has been considered a junctional zone between the esophagus and stomach, may itself have developed as a result of GER because it is covered with acid-resistant columnar epithelium.

The cardia is lined with a "junctional" epithelium that is more resistant to acid reflux than stratified squamous epithelium; although it is logical to suppose that this zone is a buffer area, there are few data to support this thesis. Autopsy series show that many individuals have no transitional zone and, instead, exhibit direct transformation from columnar to stratified squamous epithelium at the esophageal outlet. If this is the case, the very presence of a transitional epithelium with or without inflammation implies that GER is already established. The prevalence of GER therefore, as well as CLE, appears to be much greater than previously appreciated (Table 28–3).

Current Concepts: Barrett's Esophagus

Between 1960 and 1990 Barrett's esophagus was defined as the presence of columnar epithelium at any point 3cm above the gastroesophageal junction; this definition was chosen to avoid confusion about a group of patients with small "tongues" or "flame-like" strands of columnar epithelium extending above the LES.[1,2,8,10,11] The medical community had no consensus about the significance or the relevance of columnar cells so close to

TABLE 28–3.
Epithelial cell types in the esophagus and stomach

Histologic type	Special characteristics
Squamous epithelium	Stratified squamous epithelium
CLE III: intestinal ("specialized") epithelium (Barrett III)	Glands consist of mucus cells and goblet cells (which stain with Alcian blue dyes and are predisposed to adenocarcinoma)
CLE I: cardiac mucosa (Barrett I) "junctional epithelium"	Mucosa has gastric surface and foveolar cells; glands are mucous only
CLE I: acid-cardiac ("fundic") mucosa (Barrett II)	Mucosa has gastric surface and foveolar cells; glands have mucus, acid-producing, and chief cells
Gastric mucosa	Mucosa has gastric surface and foveolar cells, but glands are only acid-producing or chief cells

CLE, columnar lined esophagus.

the upper edge of the sphincter and so close to the "normal" transitional cells; therefore clinicians were left with a "gray" area near the LES. However, all could agree that if columnar cells were seen far above the LES (i.e., 3 cm), an abnormal situation was indeed present; thus the convention regarding the diagnosis of "Barrett's esophagus" came to be recognized. In conjunction with the view of the cardia suggested previously, it is apparent that the prevalence of CLE is much greater than previously recognized; up to 25% of patients with GER are found to have "mutational" GER (as CLE has been termed) if short-segment CLE is considered.

Recommendations for Biopsy during Endoscopic Examinations

The goblet cell, a specialized type of epithelial cell that stains with Alcian blue, is at risk for mutational change and progression to dysplasia and cancer. These cells might be present in the absence of inflammatory changes; therefore it is important that every endoscopic examination include biopsy of the following locations: the esophagus above and below the squamocolumnar junction (when no endoscopic abnormality is seen), at 1- to 2-cm intervals from the upper limit of the gastric rugal folds to the squamous epithelium (when a CLE is seen), and from the distal stomach to assess the presence of *Helicobacter* infection (in all cases).

Discovery of Dysplasia in CLE

When dysplasia has been identified in a biopsy specimen of the CLE, the question for the pathologist is if dysplasia is truly present and, if so, whether the dysplasia is low grade or high grade. If the patient has marked esophagitis, the medical regimen should be intensified (high-dose proton pump inhibitors, such as Prilosec 40–60 mg/day and cisapride in usual dosage); the patient should undergo repeat biopsy at a subsequent time (within 2–3 months), as esophageal inflammation may resolve during the interim, and the previously seen "dysplasia" may simply be a manifestation of an interpretive "overread." If the dysplasia is persistent despite optimal medical management, the patient should be given the option of fundoplication because available evidence suggests that fundoplication may stabilize the dysplastic process. Any patient with dysplasia should undergo repeat endoscopic biopsies at 3-month intervals until the process has stabilized or regressed (Table 28–4).

Recent work associates the inactivation of tumor suppressor genes as a factor in the development and progression of car-

TABLE 28–4.
Endoscopy and biopsy in patients with foregut symptoms

Parameter	Site(s) of biopsy	Expected histologic findings
Endoscopy findings		
No obvious pathology: (±) hiatus hernia; well demarcated esophagogastric junction; no esophagitis	Pre-1998: biopsy optional Present recommendations Gastric corpus/antrum Cardia above/below LES	Occult "carditis" occasionally *Helicobacter* test positive in 20–50% CLE III (25% of those with GER)
Hiatus hernia	Same as above	Same as above
Esophagitis, erosions, ulcerations, or "indistinct" squamocolumnar junction	Same as above	Same as above
Tongues of gastric mucosa extending above LES into esophagus (N.B.: any CLE above LES is potentially dangerous)	Same as above Biopsy tongues of shiny mucosa	CLE III (25% of those with GER) Dysplasia occasionally
Surveillance endoscopy		
Any CLE: endoscopy every 1–2 years (hotly debated issue)	Four quadrants, 2.0-cm intervals	When esophagitis and dysplasia are present, treat GER aggressively and rebiopsy in 2 months. If severe esophagitis is observed, intensive treatment of GER is indicated, as inflammation masquerades as dysplasia/atypia
Known CLE III: endoscopy every 1–2 years (hotly debated issue)	Four quadrants, 2.0-cm intervals	
Mild dysplasia in CLE III: endoscopic surveillance at 6-month intervals	Four quadrants, 2.0-cm intervals	
Severe dysplasia in CLE III: rebiopsy and confirm diagnosis with second opinion	Four quadrants, 2.0-cm intervals	Occult cancer present in approximately 50%

cinomas. Two genes encoding inhibitors of CDK4 and CDK6, *p16* and *p15*, have been identified by positional cloning around gene locus 9p21. Disturbances in some of the genes in this area are associated with deregulation of cell proliferation and the occurrence of genomic instability; interestingly, inactivation of *p16* is almost as common as inactivation of *p53* in human malignancy. Genetic lesions lead to hyperproliferation, genetic instability, and clonal expansion; this process has a histomorphologic counterpart, namely, dysplastic epithelial changes. Inactivation of specific genomic sites can be achieved by several mechanisms, including hypermethylation.[18]

D. Alternatives for Treating a Patient with High-Grade Dysplasia

When high-grade dysplasia has been discovered, the finding should be confirmed by a second biopsy and a second opinion. There are several ways to proceed with the treatment of confirmed high-grade dysplasia, but these approaches are intended to treat the underlying problem as if a cancer is present. There is no effective means, including endoscopic ultrasonography, that can accurately and reliably distinguish between severe dysplasia and dysplastic epithelium containing an occult cancer.

Fundoplication followed by endoscopic ablation of Barrett epithelium is an experimental approach that is made less attractive by the need for repeated endoscopic monitoring of results and by the inability to stage the disease properly. If cancer is present, endoscopic treatment is ineffective and the opportunity for definitive treatment is lost. It is considered an investigational approach at present.[23]

Esophagectomy with esophageal replacement is the standard approach that allows definitive treatment of the underlying problem as well as optimal treatment of the cancer (if present). The choice of the type of resection is at the discretion of the operator.

References

1. Barrett NR. Hiatus hernia: a review of some controversial points. Br J Surg 1954;42:231.
2. Barrett NR. The lower esophagus lined by columnar epithelium. Surgery 1957;41:881–894.
3. Chandrasoma P. Norman Barrett: so close, yet 50 years away from the truth. J Gastrointest Surg 1999;3:7–14.
4. Spechler SJ, Wang HH, Chen YY, et al. Inflammation of the gastric cardia and H. pylori infections are not risk factors for intestinal metaplasia at the esophagogastric junction. Gastroenterology 1997;112:A297.
5. Hirota WK, Loughney TM, Lazas DJ, Maydonovitch CL, Rholl V, Wong RKH. Specialized intestinal metaplasia, dysplasia, and cancer of the esophagus and esophagogastric junction: prevalence and clinical data. Gastroenterol 1999;116:277–285.
6. Pereira AD, Suspiro A, Chaves P, et al. Short segments of Barrett's epithelium and intestinal metaplasia in normal appearing oesophagogastric junctions: the same or two different entities? Gut 1998;42:604–605.
7. Morales TG, Bhattacharyya A, Johnson C, Sampliner RE. Is Barrett's esophagus associated with intestinal metaplasia of the gastric cardia? Am J Gastroenterol 1997;92:1818–1822.
8. Schnell TG, Sontag SJ, Chejfec G. Adenocarcinoma arising in tongues or short segments of Barrett's esophagus. Dig Dis Sci 1992;37:137–143.
9. Cameron AJ. Epidemiology of columnar-lined esophagus and adenocarcinoma. Gastroenterol Clin North Am 1997;26:487–494.
10. Clark GW, Ireland AP, Peters JH, Chandrasoma P, DeMeester TR, Bremner CG. Short-segment Barrett's esophagus: a prevalent complication of gastroesophageal reflux disease with malignant potential. J Gastrointest Surg 1997;1:113–122.
11. Byrne JP, Bhatnagar S, Hamid B, Armstrong GR, Attwood SE. Comparative study of intestinal metaplasia and mucin staining at the cardia and esophagogastric junction in 225 symptomatic patients presenting for diagnostic open-access gastroscopy. Am J Gastroenterol 1999;94:98–103.
12. Sampliner RE. Practice guidelines on the diagnosis, surveillance, and therapy of Barrett's esophagus: the Practice Parameters Committee of the American College of Gastroenterology. Am J Gastroenterol 1998;93:1028–1032.
13. DeMeester SR, Campos GM, DeMeester TR, et al. The impact of an antireflux procedure on intestinal metaplasia of the cardia. Ann Surg 1998;228:547–556.
14. Hayward J. The lower end of the esophagus. Thorax 1961;16:36–41.
15. Csendes A, Maluenda F, Braghetto I, Csendes P, Henriquez A, Quesada MS. Location of the lower esophageal sphincter and the squamous columnar mucosal junction in 109 healthy controls and 778 patients with different degrees of endoscopic oesophagitis. Gut 1993;34:21–27.
16. Paull A, Trier JS, Dalton MD, et al. The histologic spectrum of Barrett's esophagus. N Engl J Med 1976;295:476–480.
17. Falk GW. Reflux disease and Barrett's esophagus. Endoscopy 1999;31:9–16.
18. Klump B, Hsieh C-J, Holzmann K, Gregor M, Proschen R. Hypermethylation of the CDKN2/p16 promoter during neoplastic progression in Barrett's esophagus. Gastroenterology 1999;116:1381–1386.
19. Oberg S, Rfitter MP, Crookes PF, et al. Gastroesophageal reflux disease and mucosal injury with emphasis on short-segment Barrett's esophagus and duodenogastroesophageal reflux. J Gastrointest Surg 1998;2:547–554.
20. Spechler SJ, Goyal RK. The columnar lined esophagus, intestinal metaplasia and Norman Barrett. Gastroenterology 1996;110:614–621.
21. El-Serag HB, Sonnenberg A. Comorbid occurrence of laryngeal or pulmonary disease with esophagitis in United States military veterans. Gastroenterology 1997;113:755–760.
22. Gaynor EB. Otolaryngologic manifestations of gastroesophageal reflux. Am J Gastroenterol 1991;86:801–808.
23. DeMeester SR, DeMeester TR. Columnar mucosa, intestinal metaplasia, and carcinoma of the esophagus and cardia: 50 years of controversy. Ann Surg (1999, in press).

CHAPTER 29

Gastric Cancer

CONSTANTINE V. GODELLAS

A. Epidemiology and Etiology

Cancer of the stomach is a major cause of cancer deaths worldwide. Fortunately, its incidence has decreased in most areas over the last 50 years. Surgery is the mainstay of treatment, but approximately 50% of U.S. patients are not candidates for a curative resection at presentation.

Regions with the highest incidence include the Far East, South America, and eastern Europe. Some public health experts consider the incidence of gastric cancer almost epidemic in Japan, Costa Rica, Chile, and some of the countries of the former Soviet Republic. In the United States 20,000–25,000 new cases are diagnosed annually with 13,000–15,000 deaths. The incidence and mortality have remained fairly stable in the United States over the last 10–15 years. Prior to this, the incidence of gastric cancer in the United States had slowly decreased from being the leading cause of cancer deaths at the beginning of the last century to the number 14 cause today. Nevertheless, the overall prognosis for a patient with stomach cancer diagnosed in the United States is poor, with a 5-year survival rate of less than 20%.

Most authors attribute the high incidence of gastric cancer in the countries listed and the lower rates in Western countries to environmental factors. This is borne out when looking at second- and third-generation immigrants who have moved from countries with a high incidence to countries with a lower incidence. The most significant factor appears to be *diets high in nitrates and nitrites*. Smoked and salted foods were common in early twentieth century America and continue to be common in other countries. It is known that these compounds are broken down into nitrosamines, which are highly carcinogenic. *Socioeconomic status* has also been implicated because of the high incidence found in people with poor refrigeration, unsanitary food preparation, and low quality drinking water. In fact, high concentrations of nitrates and *Helicobacter pylori* have been found in well water. There is a three- to sixfold higher risk of gastric cancer in persons infected with *H. pylori*, and it appears to be independent of the association between *H. pylori* infection and gastric ulcer disease. The mechanism by which these agents appear to lead to gastric cancer is as follows. Infection with *H. pylori* has been shown to result in acute and chronic inflammatory changes, which subsequently lead to mucosal atrophy, metaplasia, and

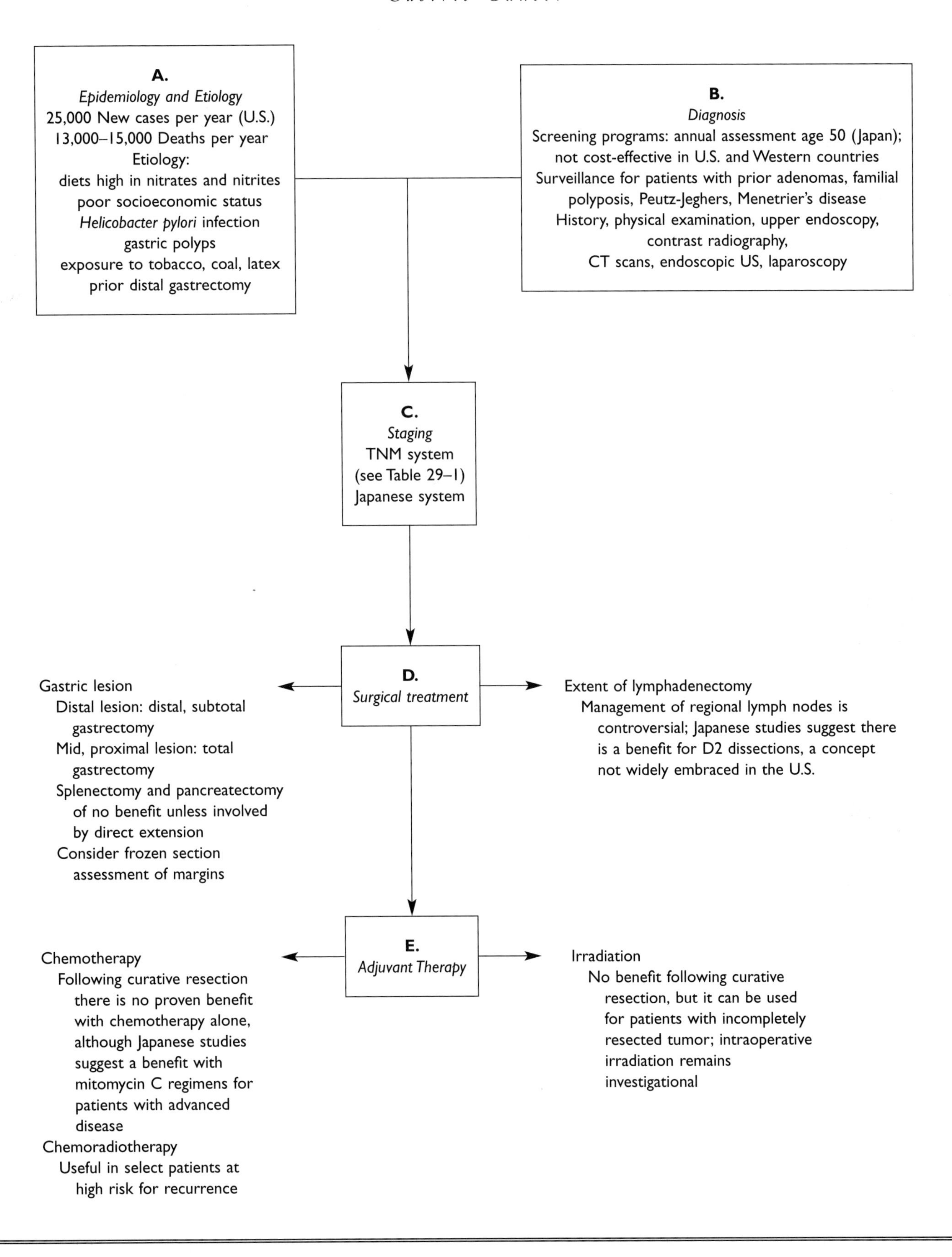
Gastric Cancer
A.
Epidemiology and Etiology
25,000 New cases per year (U.S.)
13,000–15,000 Deaths per year
Etiology:
diets high in nitrates and nitrites
poor socioeconomic status
Helicobacter pylori infection
gastric polyps
exposure to tobacco, coal, latex
prior distal gastrectomy
B.
Diagnosis
Screening programs: annual assessment age 50 (Japan);
not cost-effective in U.S. and Western countries
Surveillance for patients with prior adenomas, familial
polyposis, Peutz-Jeghers, Menetrier's disease
History, physical examination, upper endoscopy,
contrast radiography,
CT scans, endoscopic US, laparoscopy
C.
Staging
TNM system
(see Table 29–1)
Japanese system
D.
Surgical treatment
Gastric lesion
Distal lesion: distal, subtotal gastrectomy
Mid, proximal lesion: total gastrectomy
Splenectomy and pancreatectomy of no benefit unless involved by direct extension
Consider frozen section assessment of margins
Extent of lymphadenectomy
Management of regional lymph nodes is controversial; Japanese studies suggest there is a benefit for D2 dissections, a concept not widely embraced in the U.S.
E.
Adjuvant Therapy
Chemotherapy
Following curative resection there is no proven benefit with chemotherapy alone, although Japanese studies suggest a benefit with mitomycin C regimens for patients with advanced disease
Chemoradiotherapy
Useful in select patients at high risk for recurrence
Irradiation
No benefit following curative resection, but it can be used for patients with incompletely resected tumor; intraoperative irradiation remains investigational

alterations in gastric pH. This allows overgrowth of bacteria in the stomach, which can directly injure the mucosa or cause breakdown of food products into nitrites and nitrosamines, which are highly reactive compounds and can lead to mutagenesis and carcinogenesis.

Gastric polyps are a precursor condition that may confer increased risk for cancer. If found endoscopically, they should be biopsied to determine if they are hyperplastic or adenomatous; only the latter undergo malignant transformation. Risk of cancer increases with larger polyp size and higher number. Polyps >2 cm are associated with a 40% incidence of cancer. Gastrectomy is indicated if histologic review of an endoscopically resected polyp reveals cancer at the margin or if the number of polyps precludes safe endoscopic removal. If endoscopic removal is accomplished, surveillance endoscopy should be performed, as 25–33% of patients develop new polyps.

Proximal gastric and distal esophageal adenocarcinoma has become more prevalent in the United States and other Western countries, constituting approximately 30% of all gastric lesions, in contrast to 10% during the first quarter of the twentieth century. Because of this location, it is frequently difficult to ascertain the true origin of the cancer, and there are some who refer to these as gastroesophageal (GE) junction cancers. Whether this increased incidence is due to the increased use of *gastric acid-lowering drugs* is unclear.

Smoking, work exposure especially in the coal, latex and timber industries, and *prior distal gastrectomy with vagotomy* are other factors associated with an increased risk of developing gastric cancer. With regard to the effect of prior surgery, there is a 15- to 20-year latent period, after which the risk increases three- to sixfold. Therefore endoscopic surveillance should be performed for patients who have undergone prior distal gastrectomy.

B. Diagnosis

The patient with gastric cancer in the United States and most other Western countries usually presents late in the course of their disease. At this point, patients are usually symptomatic. Symptoms, which can be nonspecific and may even mimic ulcer disease, include abdominal pain, weight loss, nausea and anorexia, and early satiety. Patients with advanced disease may have evidence of gastric outlet obstruction, dysphagia (especially with GE junction tumors), constant abdominal pain, and jaundice. In contrast, in countries with a high incidence of gastric cancer and effective screening programs, such as Japan, the tumors are discovered at an early stage and are usually asymptomatic. Because of these screening programs, 50% of gastric cancers are diagnosed at an early stage in Japan, whereas only 10–15% of gastric cancers in the United States and other Western countries are in an early stage at presentation.

In Japan, annual screening with double-contrast air barium radiographs or endoscopy has been advised for patients 50 years of age or older. As stated above, approximately 50% of the gastric cancers diagnosed in Japan are limited to the mucosa and submucosa, and only 10% of these tumors have lymph node metastases. The 5- and 10-year survival rates in Japan exceed 90% and 80%, respectively. The incidence of gastric cancer in the United States is only one-fifth that found in Japan, so mass screening in the United States is not justified. However, high risk groups have been identified who should undergo periodic surveillance: patients with a history of gastric adenoma, familial adenomatous polyposis, Peutz-Jeghers syndrome, or Menetrier's disease.

The physical examination is frequently nondiagnostic in the patient with early gastric cancer. It is possible, however, for a patient to have guaiac-positive stools as an early manifestation of the disease. Late findings include evidence of severe weight loss and muscle wasting. Hematogenous spread of cancer to the liver can cause hepatomegaly and a palpable liver edge. Lymphatic spread through the thoracic duct can lead to adenopathy in the left supraclavicular area (Virchow's node). Local invasiveness of the tumor and fixation to surrounding viscera can produce a large mass that is palpable on physical examination. Gastric cancer can also spread by shedding cells into the peritoneal cavity, leading to a palpable mass at the umbilicus (Sister Mary Joseph's nodule), the pelvic cul-de-sac (Blumer's shelf nodules), and the ovary (Krukenburg tumor). An umbilical mass, if present, should be detected on routine physical examination and should be biopsied by fine-needle aspiration or open biopsy to confirm the presence of malignancy. Blumer's shelf nodules or a Krukenburg tumor can be found on rectal or pelvic examination. Evidence of any of these findings should lead one to suspect a gastrointestinal malignancy in the undiagnosed patient or metastatic disease in the patient previously diagnosed with gastric cancer.

Routine laboratory studies should include a complete blood count (CBC) to determine the presence of anemia. A chemistry panel should be checked for electrolyte disturbances, which can accompany malnutrition or gastric outlet obstruction and emesis. Liver enzymes should be evaluated; if elevated, they suggest metastatic disease in the liver. An albumin level should also be checked, especially in the severely malnourished patient.

Upper endoscopy (esophagogastroduodenoscopy, or EGD) and upper gastrointestinal tract (UGI) barium studies are the two most commonly used methods to diagnose cancer of the stomach. Whereas UGI studies are sensitive and cost-effective, EGD is more specific and can lead to a definitive diagnosis via biopsy at the time of the procedure. This is especially true in the patient with an ulcer that appears malignant on the UGI study but proves to be benign after biopsy. Benign histology, however, does not release the treating physician from the responsibility of adequate follow-up and ensuring that a "benign" ulcer heals. One scenario where EGD is not as accurate as the UGI study or even computed tomography (CT) scanning is when there is diffuse involvement of the gastric wall (linitis plastica), which occurs in approximately 10–15% of cases. In these instances intramural cancer may escape detection with endoscopic biopsy.

In the patient with gastric cancer the CT scan demonstrates thickening of the gastric wall. It can also be utilized to look for regional lymphadenopathy, liver metastases, carcinomatosis, or ascites. Helical CT can distinguish enlarged lymph nodes from vessels during early scanning and detects 72% of nodes >9mm, 45% of nodes 5–9mm, and 1% of nodes <5mm. Large lymph nodes are more likely to harbor metastatic disease; only 5% of nodes <5mm, 21% of nodes 5–9mm, 23% of nodes 10–14mm, and 83% of nodes >14mm are metastatic. Some surgeons believe that it is usually not necessary to obtain a CT scan of the patient with a symptomatic gastric cancer (obstruction, severe bleeding, perforation) because that patient is likely to undergo surgery even if there is evidence of metastatic disease. CT scans can be helpful in the patient with newly diagnosed gastric cancer who is asymptomatic because if there is evidence of metastatic disease curative resection is not possible. This patient would be more likely to undergo chemotherapy than noncurative gastric resection. Clearly, this is a somewhat controversial issue, as some surgeons would operate on the patient with metastatic disease on the basis that eventually the primary cancer would become symptomatic.

Endoscopic ultrasonography is being increasingly utilized to evaluate the depth of wall penetration in patients prior to resection. This is extremely useful for patients enrolled in preoperative chemotherapy protocols. It is not yet perfect for evaluating regional lymphatics outside the immediate perigastric area, however, which makes its widespread use limited at this time.

Laparoscopy has been utilized for the asymptomatic or marginally symptomatic patient to detect unsuspected peritoneal metastatic disease. In recent reports the incidence of peritoneal spread of gastric cancer missed by CT was 24–30%. These asymptomatic patients may be spared unnecessary laparotomy if disseminated disease is discovered laparoscopically. Of course, if the patient is extremely symptomatic and requires gastrectomy for palliation, laparoscopy is probably not warranted.

C. Staging

Gastric cancer is staged in the United States according to the American Joint Committee on Cancer (AJCC) staging classification, most recently updated in 1997. As with most other cancers utilizing this staging system, the primary tumor characteristics (T), whether there are nodal metastases (N), and the presence of distant metastatic disease (M) are all utilized (Table 29–1). The Japanese use a different staging system, with the main difference being the grouping and location of lymph nodes.

TABLE 29–1.
AJCC definition of TNM and stage grouping for gastric cancer

Primary Tumor (T)

TX	Primary tumor cannot be assessed
T0	No evidence of primary tumor
Tis	Carcinoma *in situ*: intraepithelial tumor without invasion of the lamina propria
T1	Tumor invades lamina propria or submucosa
T2	Tumor invades muscularis propria or subserosa*
T3	Tumor penetrates serosa (visceral peritoneum) without invasion of adjacent structures**,***
T4	Tumor invades adjacent structures**,***

**Note*: A tumor may penetrate the muscularis propria with extension into the gastrocolic or gastrohepatic ligaments, or into the greater or lesser omentum without perforation of the visceral peritoneum covering these structures. In this case, the tumor is classified T2. If there is perforation of the visceral peritoneum covering the gastric ligaments or the omentum, the tumor should be classified T3.

***Note*: The adjacent structures of the stomach include the spleen, transverse colon, liver, diaphragm, pancreas, abdominal wall, adrenal gland, kidney, small intestine, and retroperitoneum.

****Note*: Intramural extension to the duodenum or esophagus is classified by the depth of greatest invasion in any of these sites, including stomach.

Regional Lymph Nodes (N)

NX	Regional lymph node(s) canot be assessed
N0	No regional lymph node metastasis
N1	Metastasis in 1 to 6 regional lymph nodes
N2	Metastasis in 7 to 15 regional lymph nodes
N3	Metastasis in more than 15 regional lymph nodes

Distant Metastasis (M)

MX	Distant metastasis cannot be assessed
M0	No distant metastasis
M1	Distant metastasis

Stage Grouping

Stage	*T*	*N*	*M*
0	Tis	N0	M0
IA	T1	N0	M0
IB	T1	N1	M0
	T2	N0	M0
II	T1	N2	M0
	T2	N1	M0
	T3	N0	M0
IIIA	T2	N2	M0
	T3	N1	M0
	T4	N0	M0
IIIB	T3	N2	M0
IV	T4	N1	M0
	T1	N3	M0
	T2	N3	M0
	T3	N3	M0
	T4	N2	M0
	T4	N3	M0
	any T	any N	M1

SOURCE: Used with the permission of the American Joint Committee on Cancer (AJCC®), Chicago, IL. The original source for this material is the AJCC® Cancer Staging Manual, 5th edition (1997) published by Lippincott Williams & Wilkins Publishers, Philadelphia, PA.

This has made comparisons of statistics between groups difficult.

The Japanese system classifies nodes into four major groups.

N1 nodes closest to the primary tumor and along the greater and lesser curvature
N2 nodes along the major vessels from the celiac axis
N3 nodes at the celiac axis, at the base of the superior mesenteric artery, in the hepatoduodenal ligament, peripancreatic
N4 paraaortic and paracaval lymph nodes

Operations that resect N1, N1 and N2, and N1–N3 nodes were formerly called R1, R2, and R3 dissections, respectively. Currently they are termed D1, D2, and D3 resections. N1 nodes are thought to represent the first order of draining nodes along the gastric and perigastric nodal chains; N2 nodes represent the next echelon, depending on the location of the primary tumor. There is no clear advantage to adopting the Japanese staging system; and in the United States the AJCC system continues to be more commonly used.

Gastric cancer is also grouped according to histopathologic type, with adenocarcinoma arising from the mucus-producing glands of the stomach by far the most common. Other types include carcinoid, leiomyosarcoma, primary gastric lymphoma, squamous cell and small cell carcinoma, and undifferentiated carcinoma.

Adenocarcinoma is further subdivided into subtypes based on the Lauren classification, which includes intestinal, diffuse, and mixed types. The intestinal type is usually more well differentiated and is found in areas where the incidence of gastric cancer is high. The diffuse type is more often poorly differentiated and is frequently associated with signet ring type cells.

The most controversial aspect of surgery for gastric cancer is management of the regional lymph nodes. For the patient undergoing purely palliative gastrectomy, this is usually a moot point. For the patient undergoing a potentially curative procedure, however, an extended lymphadenectomy may provide the difference between long-term cure and recurrent disease.

Debate continues as to whether there is any benefit to a D2 resection compared to the lesser lymphadenectomy. Japanese studies support performance of an extended resection, noting improved 5-year survival rates. Western surgeons have been slow to embrace the role of a D2 resection, and no randomized Western studies have demonstrated a clear survival advantage, although data are still being collected. Retrospective and nonrandomized studies at various centers in the United States suggest that D2 resections are associated with no more morbidity than D1 operations and may improve the cure rate. Most surgeons at tertiary centers have adopted this approach.

Thus there is currently ongoing controversy in the United States as to whether a D2 dissection is superior to a D1 dissection. To eliminate variability in the extent of lymphadenectomy among surgeons, there have been attempts to standardize these procedures, but to date no one outside Japan has been able to reproduce the phenomenal results of the Japanese surgeons. Some of this may be due to the diligence of the pathologists looking for all of the lymph nodes or that of the surgeon in marking the various lymph node stations within the resected specimen. The conclusion is that there is probably a benefit of performing a more radical lymph node dissection in selected patients. Removing the spleen or pancreas to accomplish this dissection does not necessarily add to curability and may add markedly to the morbidity.

D. *Surgical Treatment*

The best treatment for gastric cancer is gastrectomy, and the primary goal is a margin-free resection. Intraoperative frozen section analysis of the resection margins should be considered. Unfortunately, many patients are not candidates for curative gastrectomy because of advanced disease at presentation. In the past it was thought that because of the potentially diffuse nature of the disease it was necessary to perform total gastrectomy for all patients. It is now clear that most patients with distal gastric cancer are better served functionally by a distal subtotal gastrectomy so long as the margins of resection are free of tumor. There does not appear to be any difference in survival or recurrence rates for subtotal and total gastrectomy for distal lesions. A subtotal resection involves removing 75–85% of the stomach, the lesser curvature, and a 1- to 2-cm portion of the proximal duodenum. For patients with body and GE junction lesions, it is still frequently necessary to perform a total gastrectomy to obtain free margins.

E. *Adjuvant Therapy*

Despite undergoing apparently curative resections, most U.S. patients die from recurrent disease. As a result, the use of postoperative chemotherapy has been studied extensively. It is beyond the scope of this text to review the literature pertaining to this topic, but the conclusions can be summarized. Postoperative 5-fluorouracil (5-FU) administered alone or in combination with other agents does not confer a survival advantage. Adriamycin-based protocols (concurrent 5-FU and mitomycin C) are also ineffective. Japanese studies have noted a benefit with mitomycin-C in patients with stage II or III disease, but it has not been confirmed in U.S. studies. At the present time, therefore, postoperative chemotherapy alone should not be considered the standard of care following a curative resection.

Postoperative irradiation may play a role in the patient with residual disease following surgery, but it has no proven benefit for the patient who has undergone a curative resection. Intraoperative radiation therapy remains investigational. There is a role for high-fractionation, short-course radiation therapy for the patient with an unresectable tumor that is bleeding or causing near-obstruction. This therapy is purely palliative but may make emergency surgery in this debilitated patient unnecessary.

Recently, postoperative chemoradiotherapy has been shown to significantly improve survival in patients at high risk for recurrence of adenocarcinoma of the stomach. The study utilized fluorouracil and leucouovin chemotherapy before, during, and after the administration of 4500 cGy of radiation. This is one of the first randomized studies to show a survival benefit to postoperative chemoradiotherapy, however, there was a marked toxic effect of the treatment. At the present time this treatment should be used cautiously.

Preoperative neoadjuvant chemotherapy may reduce the size of large lesions and render some lesions operable. Although major responses can be seen in up to 60% of patients, no complete pathologic responses have been found. Significant downstaging can be seen using endoluminal ultrasonography, and peritoneal recurrence may be reduced. A clear survival benefit has not been demonstrated, however, and this form of treatment should be considered investigational.

Follow-up

The prognosis for the patient with gastric cancer is extremely poor, and the overall 5-year survival rate is approximately 20%. Survival is stage-dependent, a fact that is worrisome for patients in the United States and Western countries where most of these patients present with advanced disease. In Japan, where many more patients present with early-stage gastric cancer, the survival is almost 50% at 5 years. Surgical removal remains the treatment of choice with same form of lymph node dissection. Postoperative chemoradiotherapy may prolong survival in select patients.

Selected Reading

Alexander HR, Kelsen DP, Tepper JE. Cancer of the Stomach, in DeVita JP VT, Hellman S, Rosenberg SA. Cancer, Principles and Practice of Oncology 4th ed., JB. Lippincott Philadelphia c. 1993 p 818–848.

Bonnenkamp JJ, Hermans J, Sasako M, van de Velde CJ. Extended lymph-node dissection for gastric cancer: Dutch Gastric Cancer Group. N Engl J Med 1999;340:908–914.

Burke EC, Karpeh MS, Conlon KC, Brennan MF. Laparoscopy in the management of gastric adenocarcinoma. Ann Surg 1997;225:262–267.

Cuschieri A, Fayers P, Fielding J, et al. Postoperative morbidity and mortality after D1 and D2 resections for gastric cancer: preliminary results of the MRC randomised controlled surgical trial. Lancet 1996;347:995–999.

Fink U, Stein HJ, Schuhmacher C, Wilke HJ. Neoadjuvant chemotherapy for gastric cancer: update. World J Surg 1995;19:509–516.

Forman D, Newell DG, Fullerton F, et al. Association between infection with Helicobacter pylori and risk of gastric cancer: evidence from a prospective investigation. BMJ 1991;302:1302–1305.

Ginsberg GG, Al-Kawas FH, Fleischer DE, et al. Gastric polyps: relationship of size and histology to cancer risk. Am J Gastroenterol 1996;91:714–717.

Karpeh MS Jr, Brennan MF. Gastric carcinoma. Ann Surg Oncol 1998; 57:650–656.

Kelsen DP. Adjuvant and neoadjuvant therapy for gastric cancer. Semin Oncol 1996;23:379–389.

Lowy AM, Mansfield PF, Leach SD, Ajani J. Laparoscopic staging for gastric cancer, Surgery 1995;119:611–614.

Parsonnet J, Friedman GD, Vandersteen DP, et al. Helicobacter pylori infection and the risk of gastric carcinoma. N Engl J Med 1991;325:1127–1131.

Sendler A, Dittler HJ, Feussner H, et al. Preoperative staging of gastric cancer as precondition for multimodal treatment. World J Surg 1995;19:501–508.

Siewert JR, Botcher K, Roder JD, et al. Prognostic relevance of systematic lymph node dissection in gastric carcinoma. Br J Surg 1993;80:1015–1018.

Smith JW, Shiu MH, Kelsey L, Brennan MF. Morbidity of radical lymphadenectomy in the curative resection of gastric carcinoma. Arch Surg 1991;126:1469–1473.

Talley NJ, Zinsmeister AR, Weaver A, et al. Gastric adenocarcinoma and Helicobacter pylori infection. J Natl Cancer Inst 1991;83:1734–1739.

Tatsuta M, Iishi H, Okuda S, Taniguchi H, Yokota Y. The association of Helicobacter pylori with differentiated-type early gastric cancer. Cancer 1993;72:1841–1845.

Volpe CM, Koo J, Miloro SM, Driscoll DL, Nava HR, Douglass HO Jr. The effect of extended lymphadenectomy on survival in patients with gastric adenocarcinoma. J Am Coll Surg 1995;181:56–64.

Wanebo HJ, Kennedy BJ, Chmiel J, Steele GD Jr, Winchester DP, Osteen R. Cancer of the stomach: a patient care study by the American College of Surgeons. Ann Surg 1993;218:583–592.

CHAPTER 30

Cancer of the Small Intestine

ROBERT SCHREIBER
DOMENICO COPPOLA
RICHARD KARL

The small intestine constitutes more than 75% of the overall length and 90% of the mucosal surface area of the gastrointestinal tract. It is remarkable that despite the large area at risk the small intestine accounts for less than 2% of all malignant gastrointestinal neoplasms.[1] Approximately 4500 new cases of small intestinal cancer are diagnosed in the United States each year, with a slight male preponderance; and approximately 1200 patients die from disease.[2]

The apparent resistance of the small intestine to malignant neoplasia is an interesting biologic puzzle. Many theories have been posited to explain the low incidence, including: the rapid turnover and death of small intestinal mucosal cells; the lack of bacteria in normal small bowel; rapid stool transit time; immunoglobulin A-mediated immune protection; increased rate of apoptosis; high luminal pH; and detoxifying microsomal enzymes (benzopyrene hydroxylase). None of these theories has been proven, and further molecular research is required to solve this interesting riddle.[3,4]

The molecular mechanisms of colorectal carcinogenesis are the best understood of any solid tumor. Clinical benefits include the discovery of hereditary genetic defects, which provide the opportunity for identifying affected family members, new prognostic factors, and opportunities for novel-directed pharmacologic intervention.[5,6] In comparison, little investigation of small bowel cancer has been done despite the fact that there are many similarities in the characteristics of large and small bowel tumors, most notably the adenoma–carcinoma progression.[7] These similarities should encourage research into the molecular mechanisms involved in small bowel tumorigenesis and may yield an explanation for the markedly lower incidence of cancer development in such an extensive area of apparent risk.[4]

A. Clinical Presentation

The diagnosis of small bowel tumors is often delayed more than 6 months from the time of initial symptoms owing to the insidious nature of their presentation. Malignant tumors are more often symptomatic than their benign counterparts, but patient complaints are often vague or nonspecific. The most frequent symptom is abdominal pain, followed by obstructive symptoms and symptoms of anemia due to occult blood loss. Palpable abdominal masses are rare with benign lesions but are present with about 40% of

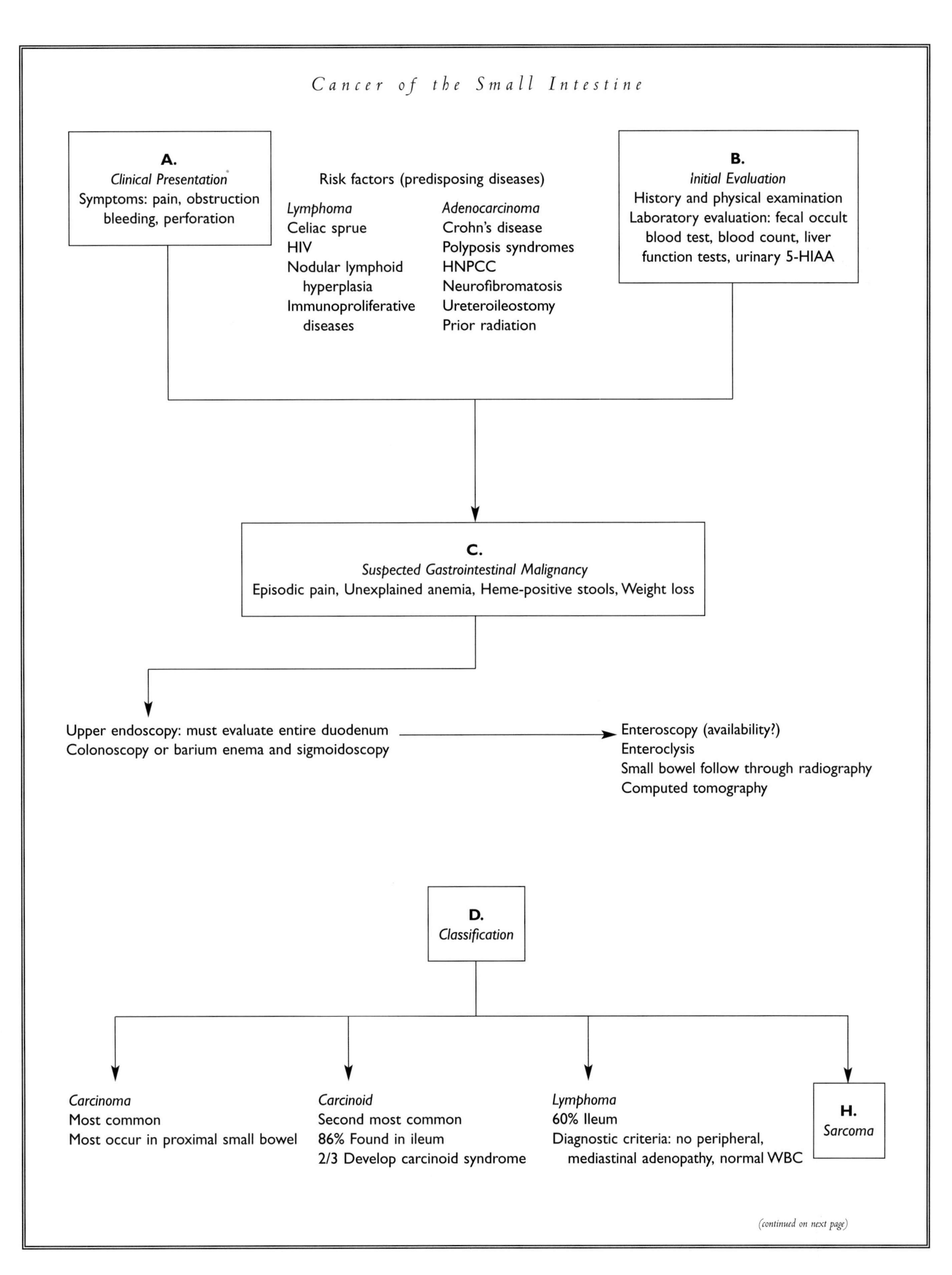

(continued on next page)

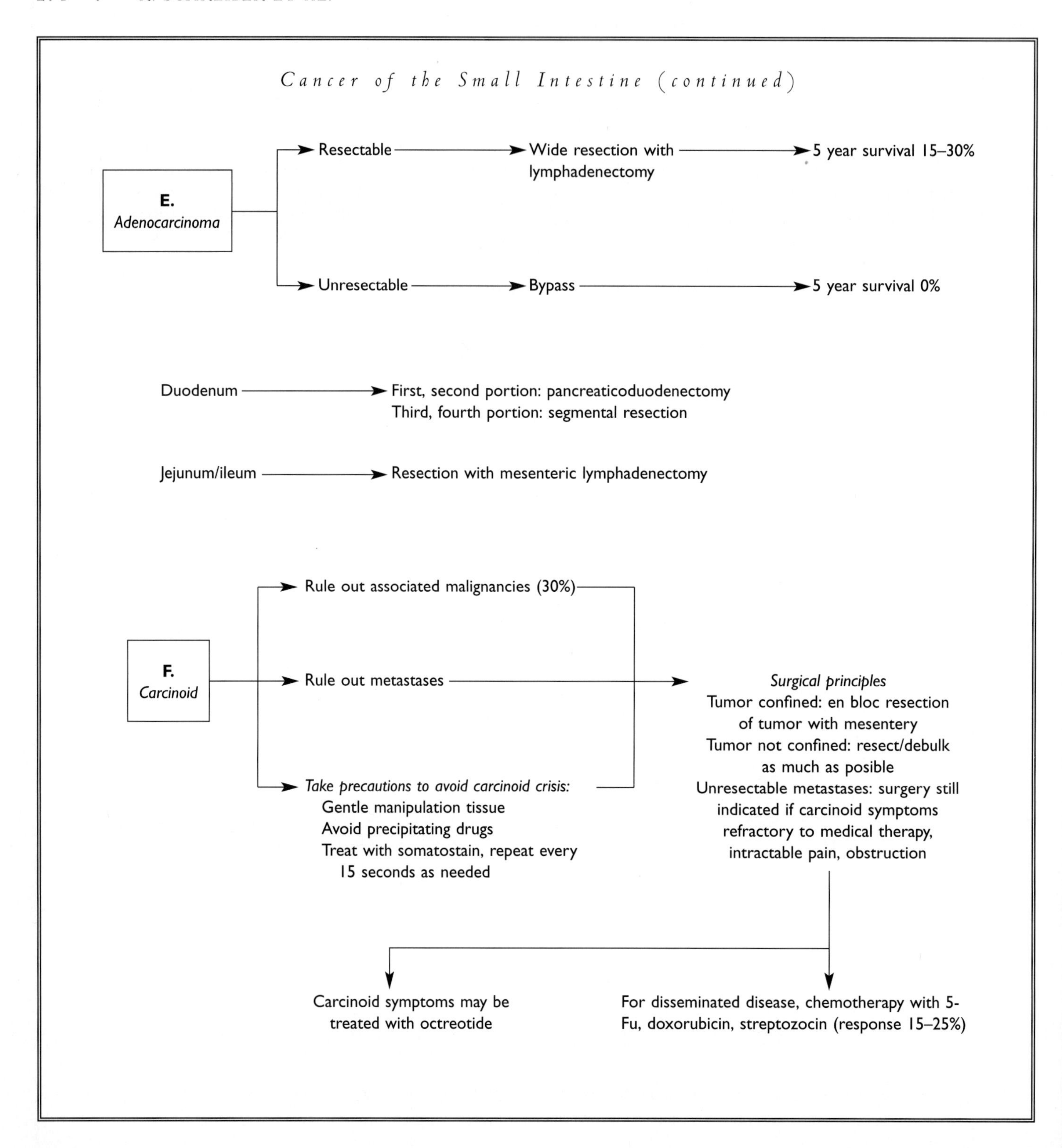

malignant tumors. Perforation is almost exclusively related to lymphomas and leiomyosarcomas. Jaundice occurs in approximately 80% of periampullary tumors due to biliary obstruction. Weight loss and anorexia occur but are rare. The carcinoid syndrome is seen in a small number of cases of metastatic carcinoid from the small intestine[8] (Table 30–1).

The two most common malignant lesions of the small intestine are adenocarcinoma and lymphoma. Immunoproliferative small intestinal disease (Mediterranean lymphoma), celiac sprue, immunodeficiency syndromes (human immunodeficiency virus, or HIV), and nodular lymphoid hyperplasia have been associated with the development of intestinal lymphoma. Patients with

Cancer of the Small Intestine (continued)

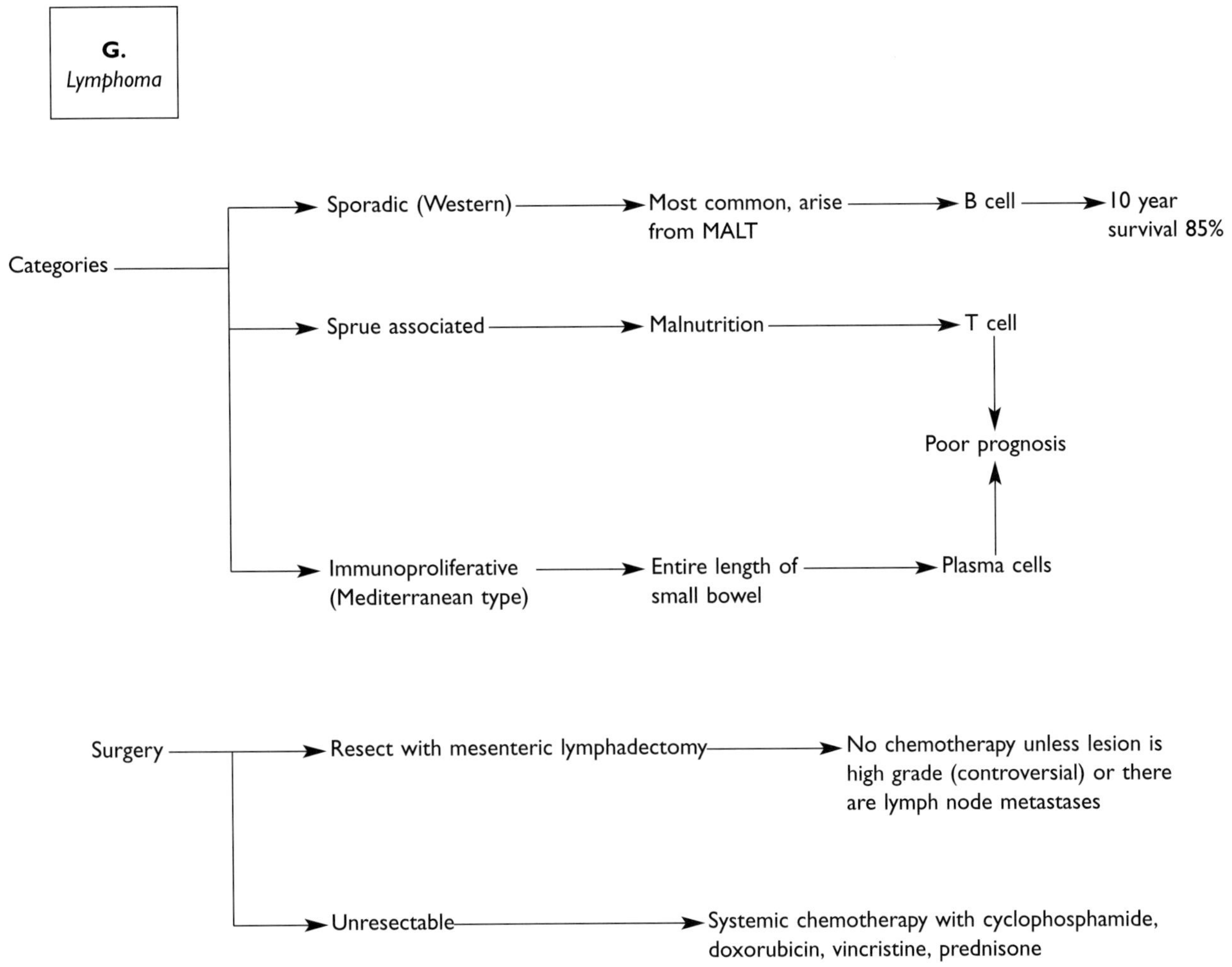

G.
Lymphoma

Categories
- Sporadic (Western) → Most common, arise from MALT → B cell → 10 year survival 85%
- Sprue associated → Malnutrition → T cell → Poor prognosis
- Immunoproliferative (Mediterranean type) → Entire length of small bowel → Plasma cells → Poor prognosis

Surgery
- Resect with mesenteric lymphadectomy → No chemotherapy unless lesion is high grade (controversial) or there are lymph node metastases
- Unresectable → Systemic chemotherapy with cyclophosphamide, doxorubicin, vincristine, prednisone

Crohn's disease, gastrointestinal polyposis syndromes (familial adenomatous polyposis, Gardner syndrome, Peutz-Jeghers syndrome, familial juvenile polyposis), hereditary nonpolyposis colon cancer, neurofibromatosis, or a ureteroileostomy have been shown to be at increased risk for adenocarcinoma.[9] Adenocarcinoma may also develop in an area of small intestinal duplication, a Meckel's diverticulum with heterotopic gastric mucosa, or in an area of previous abdominopelvic irradiation.[10]

B. Initial Evaluation

A high index of suspicion is necessary to establish an early diagnosis of small bowel tumors. The diagnosis is made preoperatively in fewer than 50% of cases. A thorough history may uncover predisposing risk factors, diseases, or family history. Fecal occult blood testing is an essential part of the physical examination despite limited sensitivity and specificity; when positive, it helps direct further interventions.

Laboratory testing may yield clues to the underlying diagnosis. Occult microcytic or iron deficiency anemia suggests chronic gastrointestinal bleeding. Liver function studies may be suggestive of metastatic disease to the liver. Bilirubin determination can detect early obstructive jaundice due to periampullary duodenal lesions. The role of carcinoembryonic antigen (CEA) is not clear, but occasionally an elevation is noted, especially in the presence of hepatic metastases.

TABLE 30–1.
Symptoms of small intestinal tumors[8]

Symptom	Frequency
Abdominal pain	Most common symptom, both benign and malignant
Obstruction	Chronic obstructive symptoms common Adult intussusception: benign lipoma
Abdominal mass	Seen in 40% of malignant cases; rare in benign tumors
Perforation	Seen in 10% of malignant cases, almost exclusively lymphoma or leiomyosarcoma
Jaundice	Seen in 80% of malignant periampullary tumors
Weight loss, anorexia	Rare
Carcinoid syndrome	Seen with a small number of metastatic carcinoid tumors

SOURCE: Reproduced with permission from Lance.[8]

C. Suspected Gastrointestinal Malignancy

Once gastrointestinal (GI) malignancy is suspected, a directed diagnostic workup must be undertaken without delay. Maglinte and Reyes, in a review of 77 patients, found that the delay due to patients failing to seek medical attention was less than 2 months from the onset of symptoms. The delay attributable to the physician failing to order appropriate diagnostic testing was 8.2 months, and failure of the radiologist to establish the diagnosis led to a 12 month delay from the time the patient initially sought medical attention.[11]

When patient symptoms (episodic severe abdominal pain, unexplained anemia, heme-positive stools, unexplained weight loss, nausea, vomiting, bleeding) remain unexplained, further diagnostic workup must be pursued. Upper GI endoscopy is used to exclude lesions proximal to the ligament of Treitz and has replaced upper GI radiography, although careful attention must be paid to the entire duodenum. If the third and fourth portions of the duodenum are not visualized with standard endoscopy, pediatric colonoscopy or a complementary barium study should be undertaken. The colon must be evaluated fully with a combination of flexible sigmoidoscopy and air contrast barium enema or colonoscopy. If the upper and lower tracts are normal, the small bowel must be thoroughly investigated.

Options for small bowel investigation include small bowel enteroscopy, upper GI small bowel follow-through (SBFT), or enteroclysis. Small bowel enteroscopy remains technically challenging and is unavailable in most institutions. Numerous studies have found enteroclysis to be superior to SBFT. In a direct comparison of the two techniques, Bessette et al. found a sensitivity of 61% for SBFT and 95% for enteroclysis. Demonstration of the tumor was achieved in 33% of SBFT studies and 90% of enteroclysis.[12]

Computed tomography (CT) can accurately detect small bowel tumors. Laurent et al.'s study of 35 patients with small bowel tumors showed CT abnormalities in 97% and predicted tumor in 80% of cases. It was also helpful for staging 18 malignant tumors by predicting extramural invasion and liver metastases correctly in 75%.[13] CT may eventually replace enteroclysis and is also indicated for detecting metastatic or recurrent disease.

In the case of GI bleeding of unknown origin, a technetium-99-tagged red blood cell scan may help identify a source within the small bowel. This may be followed by selective visceral arteriography to localize the source. In these difficult cases, superselective injection of methylene blue by the radiologist during arteriography may localize a small bleeding lesion and facilitate its identification by the surgeon intraoperatively.[14]

D. Classification

Based on the Surveillance, Epidemiology, and End Results (SEER) program of the National Cancer Institute's review of nine population-based cancer registries over a 10-year period, malignant tumors of the small intestine are categorized into four histologic types: carcinoma, carcinoid, lymphoma, sarcoma. Combined, 1832 tumors were analyzed in 1828 patients. The overall incidence was 9.6 tumors per million (3.9 per million for carcinomas, 2.9 for carcinoids, 1.6 for lymphomas, 1.2 for sarcomas). The incidence was low in people under 30 years of age but rose dramatically in older individuals. There was a slight male predominance overall, and the incidence of lymphoma among males was almost double that of females. During the decade of observation the only significant change was an increase in the number of carcinoid tumors reported, which was thought to be due to increased detection during the period for some of the more indolent malignant carcinoid tumors.

The distribution of tumors within the length of the small intestine was clearly related to histologic type. In Table 30–2, adapted from the National Cancer Institute's Surveillance Epidemiology and End Results (SEER) study, carcinoid tumors and lymphomas are shown to be concentrated in the distal ileum, whereas carcinomas are much more common in the duodenum, and sarcomas are more evenly distributed.[15]

The fifth edition of the American Joint Commission on Cancer's *AJCC Cancer Staging Manual*, published in 1997, provides staging information on small intestinal cancer (Table 30–3).[16] The classification provided applies only to carcinomas; lymphomas, carcinoids, and visceral sarcomas are not included. Primary lymphomas are staged as extranodal lymphomas. Carcinoid tumors have no staging system, but their size, depth of invasion, regional nodal status, and distant metastases are

TABLE 30–2.
Distribution of small intestinal tumors

Location	Carcinoid	Carcinoma	Sarcoma	Lymphoma
Duodenum	19 (4.6%)	310 (48.4%)	26 (17.7%)	11 (5.3%)
Jejunum	36 (8.7%)	208 (32.5%)	70 (47.6%)	72 (34.4%)
Ileum	361 (86.8%)	123 (19.2%)	51 (34.7%)	126 (60.3%)
Total	416 (~100%)	641 (~100%)	147 (100%)	209 (100%)

TABLE 30–3.
AJCC definition of TNM, stage grouping and histologic grade for small intestinal carcinoma

Primary Tumor (T)

TX	Primary tumor cannot be assessed
T0	No evidence of primary tumor
Tis	Carcinoma *in situ*
T1	Tumor invades lamina propria or submucosa
T2	Tumor invades muscularis propria
T3	Tumor invades through the muscularis propria into the subserosa or into the nonperitonealized perimuscular tissue (mesentery or retroperitoneum) with extension 2 cm or less
T4	Tumor perforates the visceral peritoneum, or directly invades other organs or structures (includes other loops of small intestine, mesentery, or retroperitoneum >2 cm, and abdominal wall by way of serosa; for duodenum only, invasion of pancreas)

Regional Lymph Nodes (N)

NX	Regional lymph nodes cannot be assessed
N0	No regional lymph node metastasis
N1	Regional lymph node metastasis

Distant Metastasis (M)

MX	Distant metastasis cannot be assessed
M0	No distant metastasis
M1	Distant metastasis

Stage Grouping

Stage	T	N	M
0	Tis	N0	M0
I	T1	N0	M0
	T2	N0	M0
II	T3	N0	M0
	T4	N0	M0
III	Any T	N1	M0
IV	Any T	Any N	M1

Histologic grade (G)

GX	Grade cannot be assessed
G1	Well differentiated
G2	Moderately differentiated
G3	Poorly differentiated
G4	Undifferentiated

SOURCE: Used with permission of the American Joint Committee on Cancer (AJCC®), Chicago, IL. The original source for this material is the AJCC® Cancer Staging Manual, 5th edition (1997) published by Lippincott Williams & Wilkins Publishers, Philadelphia, PA.

significant prognostic factors. Sarcomas are grouped under the category of gastrointestinal stromal tumors (GIST) and are discussed below.

E. *Adenocarcinoma*

Adenocarcinoma is the most common malignant tumor of the small intestine. The incidence approaches four cases per million U.S. population annually and accounts for more than 40% of malignant neoplasms of the small bowel. The male/female ratio is 1.4:1.0; altogether, 48% occur in the duodenum, 33% in the jejunum, and 19% in the ileum.[15]

The most common presenting symptom is pain, but in the case of periampullary tumors jaundice due to biliary obstruction is more common. Chronic anemia may be present, but frank hemorrhage is rare. Diagnostic tests include upper gastrointestinal endoscopy with full duodenal inspection, upper GI series with hypotonic duodenography, and enteroclysis. Histologic confirmation of cancer is accomplished with preoperative endoscopy and biopsy.

The difficulty of diagnosis, due to vague symptoms and inexact testing, accounts for an accurate preoperative diagnosis in only 35–72% of cases.[17] If a biopsy is performed it may reveal a tumor with variable degrees of glandular differentiation (establishes epithelial origin) and tumor necrosis. Among the poorly differentiated tumors, where gland formation may be lacking, one may exclude lymphoma or sarcoma with a mucin or cytokeratin stain, which discloses the epithelial nature of the cancer. Occasionally, the exact histologic diagnosis is made only after the tumor has been resected.

Surgery is the most effective form of treatment, but curative resection is possible in only 40–65% of cases. Proximal duodenal lesions require pancreaticoduodenectomy, whereas distal duodenal, jejunal, and ileal lesions may be amenable to wide negative-margin resections with regional lymphadenectomy. Patients with incurable tumors should undergo palliative resection or bypass.[17]

Small bowel adenocarcinomas are radioresistant. Furthermore, it is difficult to irradiate the tumor accurately owing to the mobility of the small bowel and the sensitivity of the remaining normal intestine to radiation toxicity. Intraoperative irradiation may be useful owing to the ability to direct the radiation at the tumor bed and exclude the remaining normal small bowel; however, the benefit of radiation therapy remains to be proven by a multiinstitutional prospective study.

Neugut et al. extensively reviewed the use of chemotherapy and found only 57 reported cases from 1984 to 1997. Chemotherapy was typically reserved for patients with metastatic disease. Most regimens consisted of 5-fluorouracil (5-FU) in combination with a variety of agents such as doxorubicin, mitomycin, lomustine, carmustine, thiopental, cisplatin, or cyclophosphamide. Results of these nonrandomized reports are difficult to interpret. Survival ranges from 3 weeks to 86 months, and 5-year survival rates are 15–30%, increasing to 40–60% in patients whose tumors were resected. Unresectability is uniformly fatal. Additional negative prognostic factors include distant metastases and positive nodal status. Prospective study of this disease is necessary but extremely difficult because of its rarity. Concentration on earlier diagnosis and treatment would make the largest impact on survival.[17]

TABLE 30–5.
Symptoms of carcinoid syndrome

Symptom	Percent of patients, comments
Flushing of head, neck, and chest	Initially 25%; ultimately 90%
Diarrhea, profuse and watery	Initially 25%; ultimately 90%; occurs with flushing
Right-side valvular heart disease	Fibrotic reaction in 10% involving the endocardium, subendocardium
Wheezing, asthma	Bronchospasm 10%
Carcinoid crisis (cardiovascular collapse, intense flush, tachycardia, severe diarrhea, central nervous system manifestations/coma)	Precipitated by general anesthesia, chemotherapy

SOURCE: Reproduced with permission from Grant.[19]

F. *Carcinoid*

Carcinoid tumors are the second most common tumors of the small bowel; they have an annual incidence of 2.9 cases per million population and comprise 30% of all malignancies of the small intestine. The male/female ratio is 1.2:1.0; and 5% are found in the duodenum, 9% in the jejunum, and 86% in the ileum. The SEER study found that the incidence of carcinoid tumors rose 50% over 10 years, which was thought to be a result of improved detection. Table 30–4 illustrates the distribution of carcinoid tumors.

The signs and symptoms of carcinoid tumors (Table 30–5) are often misinterpreted. Many tumors are clinically silent and are discovered incidentally. Symptomatic patients usually present with pain caused by the typical intense desmoplastic reaction surrounding the tumor, leading to foreshortening of the small bowel mesentery and obstructive symptoms. Most cases are correctly diagnosed at exploration for bowel obstruction or liver metastases. Only 10% of **all** carcinoid tumors ever manifest the carcinoid syndrome. Of these, 95% are of midgut origin, including the small bowel, right colon, and appendix, sites that may metastasize to the liver.[19] **Small bowel carcinoids**, in particular, present with the carcinoid syndrome in 15% of cases; ultimately, two-thirds of patients develop the syndrome during the course of their disease.[3]

TABLE 30–4.
Distribution of carcinoid tumors

Tumor site	Cases (%)
Appendix	36.2
Small bowel	28.4
Rectum	16.4
Bronchus	9.9
Colon	6.0
Stomach	2.8
Other	~3.0

SOURCE: Reproduced with permission from Cusack and Tyler.[18]

Carcinoid tumors, being of neuroendocrine origin, secrete a variety of hormones including serotonin, 5-hydroxytryptophan, kallikrein, adrenocorticotropic hormone, histamine, substance P, prostaglandin, catecholamines, gastrin, and insulin. A patient with a history of abdominal pain, intermittent obstructive symptoms, weight loss, diarrhea, or flushing should have their urinary 5-hydroxyindoleacetic acid (5-HIAA) level checked. Serotonin is the principal hormone responsible for the carcinoid syndrome, and 5-HIAA is its urinary metabolite. A normal level is <6 mg/24 hr. Patients with the carcinoid syndrome have levels well over 100 mg/24 hr.[20] Serotonin is effectively degraded in the liver, so it is not until intact hormone escapes into the systemic circulation that the syndrome becomes manifest. The tumor cells are actively synthesizing these products, which account for their reactivity to chromogranin, synaptophysin, argyrophilic, and argentaffinic stains, which are utilized by the pathologist as diagnostic tools. These tumors are characterized by proliferation of monomorphic round to polygonal cells with scant, pink, granular cytoplasm and round, stippled nuclei. They typically exhibit a trabecular or insular growth pattern, which is usually diagnostic.

Carcinoid tumors of the small bowel (compared to those in other locations) have a tendency to metastasize early, despite their small size. In a review by Stinner et al., small bowel carcinoids <1.0 cm had a 44% risk of lymph node metastases, the risk for tumors 1–2 cm rose to 77%, and for those >2 cm it was 85%. In contrast, appendiceal carcinoids rarely metastasize (0.7%) when <2.0 cm.[21] Small bowel carcinoids are often multicentric at the time of operation (30–40%), and hepatic metastases are present in 43% of patients with tumors >2 cm.[20]

The multicentric nature and metastatic potential of small intestinal carcinoids warrants aggressive surgical therapy. A thorough exploration for associated malignancies (present in 30% of patients) followed by en bloc resection with draining lymphatics is the standard of care. Often the metastatic deposits are much larger than the primary lesion, but due to the slow natural progression of the disease (mean survival 8.1 years from onset of symptoms) resection of the primary tumor and metastases is advocated when technically possible. A palliative resection can dramatically increase length of survival and quality of life. The indications for surgery in the presence of disseminated disease include carcinoid symptoms refractory to medical management, intractable pain due to tumor bulk, or obstruction. In patients with unresectable liver metastases, hepatic arterial devascularization or embolization should be considered.[20]

General anesthesia or operative manipulation may precipitate a carcinoid crisis because of the release of vasomotor substances, which manifests as an intense generalized cutaneous flush followed by cardiovascular collapse. This crisis is often unresponsive to typical resuscitative measures, but 50 μg of intravenous somatostatin analogue given immediately and then repeated in 15 seconds should provide dramatic improvement. To avoid this phenomenon, operative management should include gentle manipulation of the tissue, avoidance of all drugs associated with inducing a carcinoid crisis (thiopental, histamine-releasing muscle relaxants such as atracurium and *d*-tubocurarine, adrenergic agents, succinylcholine) and consideration of prophylactic somatostatin analogue administration.[20,21]

The medical management of carcinoid tumors is directed at controlling the symptoms of neuropeptide hypersecretion. This is accomplished with the somatostatin analogue octreotide given subcutaneously. It effectively reduces the symptoms of flushing and diarrhea and in some cases may induce tumor regression; however, surgery remains the mainstay of therapy. Multiple chemotherapeutic agents have been given, but success has been limited. Treatment with 5-Fu, doxorubicin, streptozocin, or combination therapy has yielded response rates on the order of 15–25% with a duration of only 3 months. Recombinant leukocyte A interferon has more promise but is limited by its severe toxicity.[22] Due to the indolent nature of malignant carcinoid tumors, the prognosis of small bowel carcinoid is better than that of adenocarcinoma of the small intestine; the 5-year survival for localized disease is 75%, for regional metastases 59%, and for distant metastases 19%. Overall there is a 54% five-year survival.[23]

In summary, aggressive curative surgical resection should be attempted for carcinoid tumors of the small bowel, even in the face of limited hepatic metastases. When presented with disseminated disease, palliative radical resection should be undertaken to minimize symptoms and prolong life. The somatostatin analogue octreotide should be used perioperatively and postoperatively to avoid carcinoid crisis and ameliorate symptoms. The indolent nature of this disease requires a persistent, aggressive approach to treatment.

G. *Lymphoma*

Lymphoma is the third most common malignant tumor of the small intestine. The incidence is 1.6 cases per million population annually, and it accounts for 17% of all small bowel malignancies. Males are affected twice as often as females (1.9 : 1.0). The distribution of lymphoma in the small intestine parallels the distribution of lymphoid aggregates or Peyer's patches; 5.3% occur in the duodenum, 34.4% in the jejunum, and 60.3% in the ileum.[15] The GI tract is the most common site of extranodal primary lymphoma; 30% of them occur in the small bowel. The criteria for establishing the diagnosis of *primary* small bowel lymphoma are (1) the absence of peripheral or mediastinal adenopathy, (2) a normal white blood cell and differential count, and (3) disease grossly confined to the intestinal segment.[24]

Conditions predisposing to the development of primary small bowel lymphoma are nontropical sprue and Crohn's disease.[25] The most common presenting symptoms are abdominal pain, nausea, vomiting, and partial small bowel obstruction. Lymphoma of the small intestine may grow to a large size, presenting as an abdominal mass. The preoperative diagnosis is established in fewer than one-third of patients, and perforation occurs in up to 25%.

There are three major subtypes of primary small intestinal lymphoma: the sporadic or Western type, sprue-associated lymphoma, and the immunoproliferative or Mediterranean type. The Western type is most common and is found in the distal small bowel. These lesions are B cell lymphomas arising from the mucosa-associated lymphoid tissue (MALT).[26] This type of GI lymphoma affects adults and has no gender predilection; 60% occur in the stomach, 30% in the small intestine, 15% in the proximal colon, and 10% in the distal colon. In their early stage, these tumors are locally confined and are treated by surgical resection. When they relapse, they are usually still confined to the GI tract. This behavior is a reflection of genetic changes peculiar to this type of lymphoma. For example MALTomas do not exhibit translocation of the t[14;18] and t[11;14] loci, commonly seen in other lymphomas. It is speculated that MALT lymphomas arise in the context of chronic mucosal lymphoid stimulation, such as is seen in *Helicobacter*-associated chronic gastritis. The 10-year survival for this type of lymphoma is approximately 85%.[26]

The sprue-associated lymphoma develops in patients with malabsorption syndrome, including gluten-sensitive enteropathy (sprue), usually after 10–20 years of symptomatic disease. This is usually a proximal small bowel T cell lymphoma with poor prognosis.[27]

The Mediterranean lymphoma is characterized by plasma cells that synthesize abnormal α heavy chains. It occurs in children or young adults of Mediterranean ancestry, involves the entire length of small bowel, has involved lymph nodes in 85% of patients, is treated primarily with chemotherapy, and has a poor prognosis. Surgery has a limited role in the management of this variant.

Grossly, small intestinal lymphomas appear as plaque-like thickening of the mucosa and submucosa. They infiltrate the full thickness of the bowel wall and may be ulcerated or polypoid. Histologically, atypical lymphoid cells massively infiltrate the mucosa replacing the glandular epithelium. The monotonous population of cells may consist of follicular center cells, both cleaved and noncleaved, or immunoblasts (or both). B cell lymphomas constitute 95% of the small bowel lymphomas.[28]

Intestinal lymphoma is infrequently diagnosed before surgery. Disease confined to a focal segment of bowel should be resected en bloc with a regional lymphadenectomy, and the remainder of the abdomen is thoroughly explored for additional disease. Adjuvant systemic chemotherapy is indicated when the disease is incompletely resected. When the tumor is completely resected, the role of adjuvant chemotherapy is controversial, but many authors advocate treating intermediate- and high-grade tumors. The standard regimen consists of cyclophosphamide, doxorubicin, vincristine, and prednisone (CHOP). The benefit of irradiation is unproven, as its toxicity appears to outweigh its benefits.

Prognostic factors include tumor grade, stage, resectability, response to therapy, and histologic subtype. Patients with a B cell lymphoma fare better than those with a T cell lymphoma. Coit's review of the literature showed that 5-year survival has improved with the use of multimodality therapy, and many series report 5-year survival rates over 50%.[3]

H. *Sarcoma-Gastrointestinal Stromal Tumors*

Sarcomas are the least common of the four major types of small intestinal cancers, with an annual incidence of 1.2 cases per million population. They account for approximately 13% of small intestinal malignancies, with a nearly equal male/female ratio (1.2 : 1.0). The distribution in the small intestine indicates that 17.7% are in the duodenum, 47.6% in the jejunum, and 34.7% in the ileum.[15] These tumors have now been reclassified as gastrointestinal stromal tumors (GIST) to reflect their cells of origin more accurately.

TABLE 30–6.
Criteria of malignancy in GIST

Condition	Criteria
Benign	No high risk factors
Uncertain malignant potential	One high risk factor
Malignant	One unequivocal or two high risk factors

SOURCE: Modified from Lewin et al.[31]
Unequivocal factors: 1. Metastases
2. Invasion of adjacent organs
High risk factors: 1. Size >5.5 cm. in the stomach and >4 cm. in the small and large bowel
2. Mitoses >5/50 high power field in the stomach and any mitosis in the small or large bowel
3. Any of the following: tumor necrosis, nuclear pleomor phism, dense cellularity, vascular or lamina propria invasion, pattern of growth (epithelioid or alveolar).

GISTs arise from the stroma of the bowel wall, and most (80%) originate within the stomach and small bowel.[29] They are subclassified according to their phenotype as tumors with smooth muscle differentiation (leiomyosarcomas) (43%), tumors with neural differentiation (gastroautonomic nerve tumors, or GANT) (37.5%), tumors with bidirectional neural and smooth muscle differentiation (GIST mixed) (9%), and tumors with no specific differentiation (GIST undifferentiated) (11%).[30,31] All GANT tumors are malignant. GIST tumors may be divided into **benign** and **malignant** according to the criteria of Lewin et al. (Table 30–6).[31] Smooth muscle differentiation can be detected by immunoreactivity for smooth muscle actin and desmin. Neural differentiation is suggested by positivity for neural and neuroendocrine markers (S100, neuron-specific enolase, chromogranin, synaptophysin) but is proven only by electron microscopy in which the tumor cells display cell processes containing intermediate filaments, microtubules, dense-core neurosecretory granules, and synapse-like structures.[32] It has been reported that gastrointestnal pacemaker cell tumors (GIPACT), a subtype of GIST tumors originate from the interstitial cells of Cajal and overexpress the *kit* oncogene receptor.[33]

The criteria to determine the malignant potential of GISTs are listed in Table 30–6.

Sarcomas of the small intestine are generally slow-growing, are locally invasive, and spread to the liver, lungs, and bones via the bloodstream, bypassing the local lymph nodes. They typically present with an abdominal mass, pain, bleeding, or obstructive symptoms and are rarely diagnosed preoperatively.

At the time of exploration, wide resection should be undertaken including neighboring viscera involved by direct extension. A wide mesenteric lymphadenectomy is unnecessary. There is no proven benefit to chemotherapy or irradiation, but it has been used in an adjuvant setting under a protocol for palliation and in an attempt to down-stage tumors to make them resectable.

Lauwers et al. reported the 5-year survival for patients with GISTs to be about 55% and the 10-year survival about 40%.[32] The 5-year survival of those with sarcomas as a whole, prior to any reclassification, is reported to be approximately 20%.[3]

I. Metastases

Metastases to the small bowel are not uncommon. Many tumors have the potential to metastasize to the small bowel, traveling transperitoneally (colorectal, ovarian, gastric, and pancreatic cancer) or hematogenously (lung, breast, cervix, kidney; and most notably melanoma). Bleeding, obstruction, and abdominal pain are the most common presenting symptoms, and treatment is almost certainly palliative. Melanoma is the best studied metastatic tumor. In a review of the Roswell Park experience Ricaniadis et al. reported a 27.6 month survival if patients were "disease-free" after resection, 5.1 months if other metastases were present, and 1.9 months if the patient underwent a bypass procedure. The 5-year survival rate was 28.3% in the complete resection group. There were no survivors in the other two groups.[34] Aggressive treatment has a significant impact on quality of life and may affect long-term survival in those patients who can be rendered free of disease.

References

1. Herbsman H, Wetstein L, Rosen Y, et al. Tumors of the small intestine. Curr Probl Surg 1980;17:121–182.
2. Landis SH, Murray T, Bolden S, Wingo PA. Cancer statistics, 1998. CA Cancer J Clin 1998;48:6–30.
3. Coit DG. Cancer of the small intestine. In: Devita VT, Hellman S, Rosenberg SA (eds) Cancer: Principles and Practice of Oncology, 5th ed. Philadelphia: Lippincott-Raven, 1977:1128–1143.
4. Arber N, Neugut AI, Weinstein B, Holt P. Molecular genetics of small bowel cancer. Cancer Epidemiol Biomarkers Prev 1997;6:745–748.
5. Cho KR, Vogelstein B. Genetic alterations in the adenoma–carcinoma sequence. Cancer 1992;70(suppl):1727–1731.
6. Wargovich MJ. Precancer markers and prediction of tumorigenesis. In: Young GP, Rozen P, Levin B (eds) Prevention and Early Detection of Colorectal Cancer. London: Saunders, 1996:89–101.
7. Levine BA, Kaplan BJ. Polyps and polypoid lesions of the jejunum and ileum. Surg Oncol Clin N Am 1996;5:609–619.
8. Lance P. Tumors and other neoplastic diseases of the small bowel. In: Yamada T (ed) Textbook of Gastroenterology, 2nd ed. Philadelphia: Lippincott, 1995:1696–1713.
9. Ryan JC. Premalignant conditions of the small intestine. Semin Gastrointest Dis 1996;7(2):88–93.
10. Gore RM. Small bowel cancer, clinical and pathologic features. Radiol Clin North Am 1997;35:351–360.
11. Maglinte DDT, Reyes BL. Small bowel cancer radiologic ciagnosis. Radiol Clin North Am 1997;35:361–380.
12. Bessette JR, Maglinte DDT, Kelvin FM, et al. Primary malignant tumors of the small bowel: a comparison of the small bowel enema and conventional follow through. AJR Am J Roentgenol 1989;153:741–744.
13. Laurent F, Raynaud M, Biset JM, et al. Diagnosis and categorization of small bowel neoplasms: role of computer tomography. Gastrointest Radiol 1991; 16:115.
14. Lau WY, Yuen WK, Chu KW, et al. Obscure bleeding in the gastrointestinal tract originating in the small intestine. Surg Gynecol Obstet 1992; 174:119–124.
15. Weiss NS, Yang CP. Incidence of histologic types of cancer of the small intestine. J Natl Cancer Inst 1987;78:653–656.
16. American Joint Committee on Cancer. AJCC Cancer Staging Manual, 5th ed. Philadelphia: Lippincott-Raven, 1997:77–81.
17. Neugut AI, Marvin MR, Rella VA, Chabot JA. An overview of adenocarcinoma of the small intestine. Oncology 1997;11:529–536.
18. Cusack JC, Tyler DS. Small bowel malignancies and carcinoid tumors. In: Berger DH, Feig BW, Fuhrman GM (eds) The M.D. Anderson Surgical Oncology Handbook. Boston: Little Brown, 1995:142–159.
19. Grant C. Carcinoid tumors. Probl Gen Surg 1994;11:58–68.
20. Loftus JP, van Heerden JA. Surgical management of gastrointestinal carcinoid tumors. Adv Surg 1995;28:317–336.
21. Stinner B, Kisker O, Zeilke A, Rothmund M. Surgical management of carcinoid tumors of small bowel, appendix, colon, and rectum. World J Surg 1996;20:183–188.
22. Moertel CG, Rubin J, Kvols LK. Therapy of metastatic carcinoid tumor and the malignant carcinoid syndrome with the recombinant leukocyte A intereferon. J Clin Oncol 1989;7:865–868.
23. Godwin JD, Carcinoid tumors: an analysis of 2837 cases. Cancer 1975; 36:560.
24. Gray GM, Rosenberg SA, Cooper AD, et al. Lymphomas involving the gastrointestinal tract. Gastroenterology 1982;82:143–152.
25. O'Rourke MGE, Lancashire RP, Vattoune JR. Lymphoma of the small intestine. Aust NZ J Surg 1986;56:351.
26. Isaacson PG, Spencer J. Malignant lymphoma of mucosa-associated lymphoid tissue. Histopathology 1987;11:445.
27. Spencer J, Cerf-Bensussan N, Jouvry A, et al. Enteropathy-associated T cell lymphoma (malignant histiocytosis of the intestine) is recognized by a monoclonal antibody (HML-1) that defines a membrane molecule on human mucosal lymphocytes. Am J Pathol 1988;132:1.
28. Isaacson PG, et al. Immunoproliferative small-intestinal disease: an immunohistochemical study. Am J Surg Pathol 1989;13:1023.
29. Antonioli DA. Gastrointestinal autonomic nerve tumors: expanding the spectrum of gastrointestinal stromal tumors. Arch Pathol Lab Med 1989;113:831–833.
30. Erlandson RA, Klimstra DS, Woodruff JM. Subclassification of gastrointestinal stromal tumors based on evaluation by electron microscopy and immunohistochemistry. Ultrastruct Pathol 1996;20:373–393.
31. Lewin KJ, Riddell RH, Weinstein WM. Mesenchymal tumors. In: Gastrointestinal Pathology and Its Clinical Implications. New York: Igaku-Shoin, 1992:284–241.
32. Lauwers GY, Erlandson RA, Casper ES, Brennan MF, Woodruff JM. Gastrointestinal autonomic nerve tumors: a clinicopathological, immunohistochemical and ultrastructural study of 12 cases. Am J Surg Pathol 1993;17:887–897.
33. Kindblom LG, Remotti HE, Aldenborg F, Meis-Kindblom JM. Gastrointestinal pacemaker cell tumor (GIPACT): gastrointestinal stromal tumors show phenotypic characteristics of the interstitial cell of Cajal. Am J Pathol 1998;152:1259–1269.
34. Ricaniadis N, Konstadoulakis MM, Walsh D, Karakousis CP. Gastrointestinal metastases from malignant melanoma. Surg Oncol 1995;4:105–110.

Chapter 31

Periampullary Malignancies

Constantine V. Godellas

Primary cancers of the periampullary region include cancer of the pancreatic head (including the uncinate process), ampullary cancer, distal bile duct cancer, and duodenal cancer. Patients with periampullary cancer most commonly present with jaundice. Whereas these cancers have similar treatment, their prognoses are vastly dissimilar.

A. Epidemiology

Most periampullary cancers originate in the pancreatic head (75%), with the remainder arising from the distal bile duct (10%), ampulla (10%), and duodenum (5%). Because of the proximity of these tumors to one another, the exact origin of the cancer is sometimes unclear. This makes data on incidence and survival difficult to obtain. The major histologic type of all of these cancers is adenocarcinoma. Endocrine malignancies (i.e., gastrinoma), lymphoma, sarcoma, and metastases from other sources may also be found but make up a much smaller percentage and are not discussed here. The reader is encouraged to consult elsewhere in this textbook concerning gastrinoma (see Chapter 13) and insulinoma (see Chapter 14).

Cancer of the exocrine pancreas is a leading cause of death in the United States and western Europe; in fact, it is the fifth leading cause of cancer deaths in the United States. Because its mortality rate is extremely high, the incidence and mortality rates are nearly identical. The incidence of pancreatic cancer worldwide has increased slightly, whereas it has remained essentially stable in the United States. There is a slightly higher incidence in men than in women, and most occur after age 65 years. The highest incidence rates in the world appear to be among African-American men. Because the number of patients who develop the other periampullary malignancies is small, it is difficult to obtain clear incidence rates. However, there do not appear to have been any major changes in incidence or mortality rates over the last several years.

Periampullary Cancer

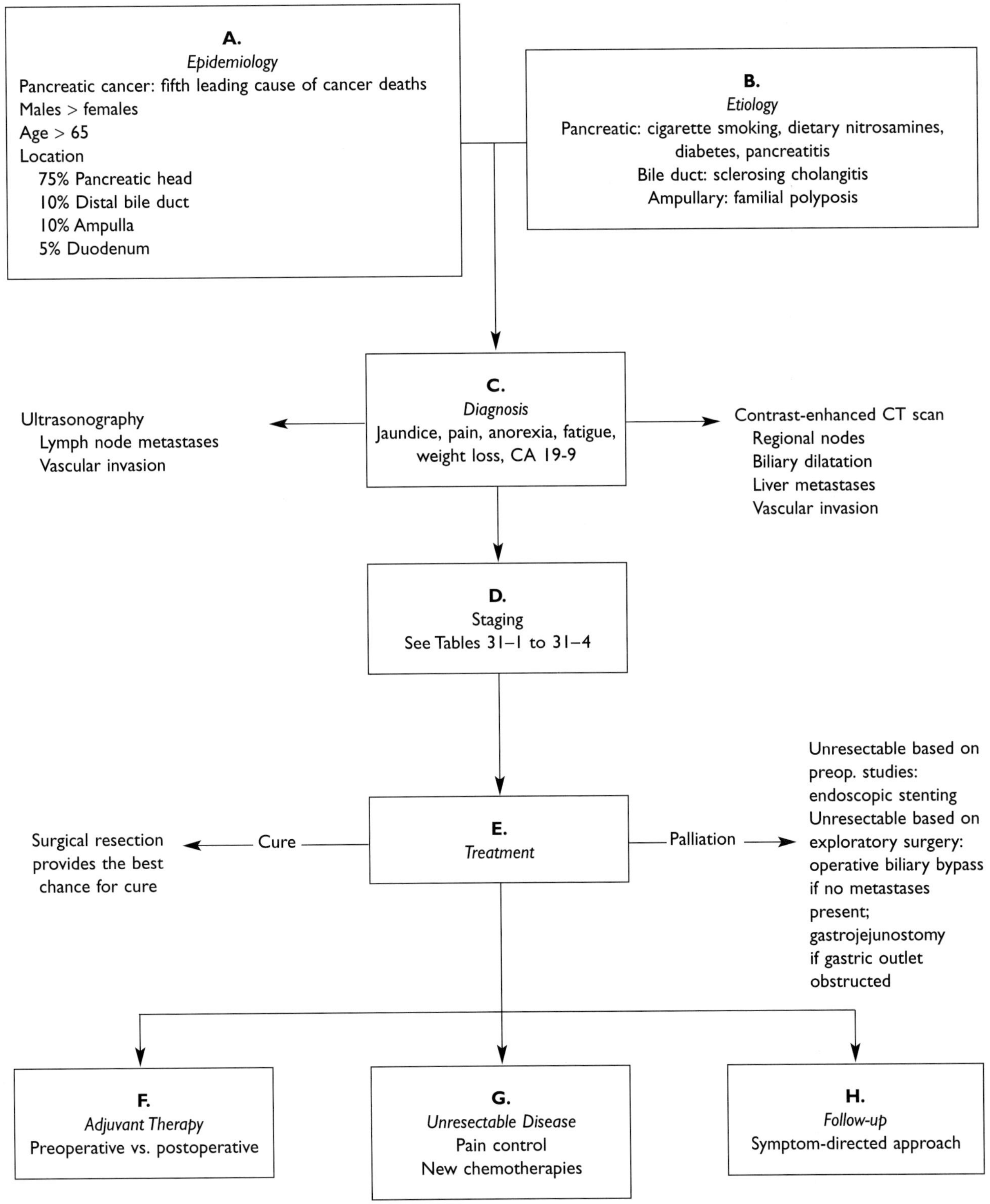

A.
Epidemiology
Pancreatic cancer: fifth leading cause of cancer deaths
Males > females
Age > 65
Location
- 75% Pancreatic head
- 10% Distal bile duct
- 10% Ampulla
- 5% Duodenum

B.
Etiology
Pancreatic: cigarette smoking, dietary nitrosamines, diabetes, pancreatitis
Bile duct: sclerosing cholangitis
Ampullary: familial polyposis

C.
Diagnosis
Jaundice, pain, anorexia, fatigue, weight loss, CA 19-9

Ultrasonography
- Lymph node metastases
- Vascular invasion

Contrast-enhanced CT scan
- Regional nodes
- Biliary dilatation
- Liver metastases
- Vascular invasion

D.
Staging
See Tables 31–1 to 31–4

E.
Treatment

Cure → Surgical resection provides the best chance for cure

Palliation → Unresectable based on preop. studies: endoscopic stenting
Unresectable based on exploratory surgery: operative biliary bypass if no metastases present; gastrojejunostomy if gastric outlet obstructed

F.
Adjuvant Therapy
Preoperative vs. postoperative

G.
Unresectable Disease
Pain control
New chemotherapies

H.
Follow-up
Symptom-directed approach

B. Etiology

Epidemiologists have identified cigarette smoking as the risk factor most strongly associated with adenocarcinoma of the pancreas. The mechanism is presumed secondary to N-nitroso compounds from cigarette smoke causing activation of oncogenes such as K-*ras*. Cigarette smoke has not been clearly linked as a risk factor to any of the other periampullary malignancies.

Diets high in the consumption of red meat, fat, and smoked or cured foods have been implicated in causing cancer of the pancreas, bile duct, ampulla, and small intestine. The main causative agent here again appears to be nitrosamines. The mechanism may be different from that for cigarette smoking, as it is known that K-*ras* mutation levels in patients with cholangiocarcinoma and ampullary cancer are much lower than are seen in patients with pancreatic cancer.

There appears to be an association between *diabetes mellitus* and pancreatic cancer and between *chronic pancreatitis* and pancreatic cancer, but no cause and effect has been documented for either of these factors. There is a known association between *sclerosing cholangitis* and cholangiocarcinoma. It is thought that a chronic inflammatory condition causes changes in cell repair and structure that may eventually lead to malignancy.

As with other malignancies, a number of patients have an inherited susceptibility to developing periampullary malignancies. The most well established and understood genetic trait is found in patients with familial adenomatous polyposis (FAP), who are prone to develop ampullary adenomas. These adenomas may undergo malignant transformation in a manner similar to the adenoma–carcinoma sequence known to exist for colon cancer. Other hereditary syndromes that may predispose patients to pancreatic cancer include *hereditary nonpolyposis colorectal cancer*, *hereditary pancreatitis*, and *ataxia telangiectasia*. There is even evidence to suggest that there may be a familial predisposition to pancreatic cancer that has not been designated a specific syndrome, but preliminary reports refer to it as the *familial pancreatic cancer syndrome*.

C. Diagnosis

Jaundice is one of the most common presenting signs in patients with periampullary malignancy. Obstruction of the bile duct occurs early in ampullary and distal bile duct cancers owing to their location. Even small cancers of the pancreatic can present early with jaundice if their location is close to the intrapancreatic bile duct. Duodenal and pancreatic cancers farther away from the bile duct that cause obstruction and jaundice late in their course usually have a less favorable prognosis if jaundice is the presenting feature. Because bile duct obstruction associated with malignancy is gradual in onset, the jaundice may be painless and not associated with cholangitis.

Pain is frequently associated with periampullary cancer and may be described as a dull, difficult to characterize vague epigastric discomfort. When the disease is advanced, the pain progresses to a constant, severe low thoracic or upper lumbar pain (mid-back). This pain pattern usually implies a locally advanced tumor or lymphatic metastases invading the celiac nerve plexus. Other symptoms include *anorexia* and *fatigue*. Severe *nausea/emesis* are more commonly seen in patients with duodenal/gastric outlet obstruction from a locally advanced mass. *Weight loss* can be seen early, related to the anorexia, but is more pronounced later in the course in patients with advanced disease.

Clinical signs other than jaundice can be a palpable gallbladder and hepatomegaly. Painless jaundice and a palpable mass (gallbladder) in the right upper quadrant is known as Courvoisier's sign and implies a periampullary malignancy. A palpable nodule at the umbilicus (Sister Mary Joseph's sign) or a mass felt in the pelvic cul-de-sac (Blumer's shelf nodule) on rectal or bimanual pelvic examination implies peritoneal metastases from a gastrointestinal (GI) malignancy. A positive left supraclavicular node (Virchow's node) implies distant spread of disease. Guaiac-positive stool may be found, especially in patients with duodenal tumors, large ampullary cancers, or pancreatic cancers that have invaded the duodenum. Migratory superficial thrombophlebitis, or Trousseau's sign, is also a feature of advanced disease, as is evidence of ascites.

Laboratory studies may demonstrate several abnormalities. Patients may exhibit anemia and low albumin levels, reflecting both the chronic nature of the disease and the nutritional sequelae. Frequently, patients have increased alkaline phosphatase, α-glutamyl transferase, and bilirubin levels secondary to biliary obstruction. Marked elevation of the hepatic transaminases implies severe liver injury secondary to long-standing biliary obstruction or metastatic disease. The prothrombin time is frequently elevated in patients with long-standing biliary obstruction. Tumor markers such as carcinoembryonic antigen (CEA) and CA 19-9 are helpful in some patients. CEA is a marker frequently used for GI malignancies and is commonly elevated in patients with periampullary malignancies. However, it has low specificity, being increased also in conditions such as biliary obstruction and pancreatitis. CA 19-9, another GI tumor marker, is much more specific and sensitive for pancreatic cancer than CEA but less so for ampullary and duodenal cancers. A host of other tumor markers have been studied in serum, endoscopic retrograde cholangiopancreatography (ERCP) brushings, and feces looking for shed tumor cells. No one has clearly proven itself as yet.

The radiologic test of choice for a patient with a periampullary cancer is the contrast-enhanced computed tomogra-

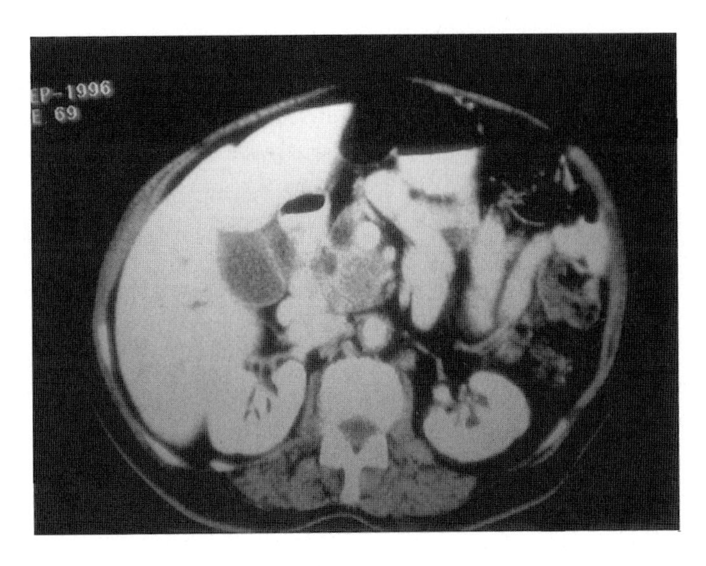

FIGURE 31–1.
Computed tomography scan.

phy (CT) scan with fine cuts through the periampullary region (Fig. 31–1). This scan allows accurate measurement of the size and location of the primary tumor. It is also extremely valuable in the evaluation of: (1) the surrounding lymph nodes; (2) the extra- and intrahepatic biliary system for ductal dilatation; (3) the liver for metastases; and (4) the portal vein and superior mesenteric artery for evidence of invasion. New advances in magnetic resonance imaging (MRI) technology may supplant CT as the preferred test. Super-fast, contrast-enhanced MRI allows better evaluation of the liver and peritoneum for metastatic disease. The location of the primary tumor and its relation to associated vascular structures is also better visualized. The main advance, however, is the ability to assess the biliary ductal system. Magnetic resonance cholangiopancreatography (MRCP) allows noninvasive visualization of the ductal system and is being used increasingly in centers that have the technology.

For the patient with a resectable periampullary mass, no metastatic disease, and no encasement of the major blood vessels, ERCP is not necessary. ERCP may facilitate biliary stenting for the patient with unresectable disease and is also useful for obtaining brushings of the duct from a patient with a stricture but no clear mass. ERCP can diagnose and even treat an impacted stone in the distal common bile duct, a situation that mimics a periampullary malignancy.

Endoscopic ultrasonography (EUS) has gained popularity for preoperative evaluation of these patients. EUS provides more accurate information regarding tumor size, lymph node involvement, and vascular invasion than CT. Fine-needle aspiration (FNA) or biopsy can also be performed for a lesion deemed unresectable, or in patients who require tissue diagnosis prior to enrollment in preoperative protocols.

Diagnostic laparoscopy is another test used by some for preoperative evaluation of patients with periampullary malignancies. Some surgeons prefer to perform laparoscopy preoperatively, and others use it as the first step of a planned resection on the same day. Although high quality CT scans have led to improved resectability rates, approximately 20–40% of lesions are found to be unresectable on open exploration. Laparoscopic evaluation could potentially spare these patients a major abdominal incision. The experienced laparoscopic surgeon can even perform biliary-enteric or gastroenteric bypass in the patient with unresectable disease.

D. Staging

The American Joint Committee on Cancer (AJCC) TNM classification is utilized for periampullary malignancies. Unfortunately, it is difficult to apply this system to these patients, especially for those who do not undergo resection. Each of the four tumor types has its own staging system, which means that the exact tumor location must be known. This knowledge is sometimes not available even after examining of the resected specimen. This difficulty is further compounded in patients who have unresectable tumors because of the criteria mentioned previously. The four staging classifications are presented in Tables 31–1 through 31–4.

E. Treatment

Complete surgical extirpation of these tumors provides the only chance for cure and the best option for long-term survival. The operation for resecting these tumors has not changed appreciably during the last 25 years, although the advent of minimally invasive surgery has expanded our surgical options, especially for palliative surgery. The surgical procedure used is pancreaticoduodenectomy or the Whipple procedure, with a modification being that of pyloric preservation. The main goal of these operations is to remove the head of the pancreas, the attached duodenum, the distal bile duct, and surrounding/adjacent lymph nodes and connective tissue. This is done to obtain complete tumor clearance; complete resection is not always possible, however, because of locally advanced disease or metastatic disease. The possibility that a tumor is resectable depends on the primary tumor type. Patients with distal bile duct and ampullary cancers have higher resectability rates because of earlier diagnosis, whereas patients with duodenal and pancreatic cancer present later and therefore have lesions that are more likely to be unresectable. For patients with small tumors, the pylorus may be preserved, which has been shown by some to lead to better long-term function.

TABLE 31–1.
AJCC definition of TNM and stage grouping for extrahepatic bile duct cancer

Primary Tumor (T)

TX	Primary tumor cannot be assessed
T0	No evidence of primary tumor
Tis	Carcinoma *in situ*
T1	Tumor invades subepithelial connective tissue or fibromuscular layer
T1a	Tumor invades subepithelial connective tissue
T1b	Tumor invades fibromuscular layer
T2	Tumor invades perifibromuscular connective tissue
T3	Tumor invades adjacent structure(s), liver, pancreas, duodenum, gallbladder, colon, stomach

Regional Lymph Nodes (N)

NX	Regional lymph nodes cannot be assessed
N0	No regional lymph node metastasis
N1	Metastasis in cystic duct, pericholedochal and/or hilar lymph nodes (i.e., in the hepatoduodenal ligament)
N2	Metastasis in peripancreatic (head only), periduodenal, periportal, celiac, and/or superior mesenteric and/or posterior pancreaticoduodenal lymph nodes

Distant Metastasis (M)

MX	Distant metastasis cannot be assessed
M0	No distant metastasis
M1	Distant metastasis

Stage Grouping

Stage	*T*	*N*	*M*
0	Tis	N0	M0
I	T1	N0	M0
II	T2	N0	M0
III	T1	N1	M0
	T1	N2	M0
	T2	N1	M0
	T2	N2	M0
IVA	T3	Any N	M0
IVB	Any T	Any N	M1

SOURCE: Used with the permission of the American Joint Committee on Cancer (AJCC®), Chicago, IL. The original source for this material is the AJCC® Cancer Staging Manual, 5th edition (1997) published by Lippincott Williams & Wilkins Publishers, Philadelphia, PA.

TABLE 31–2.
AJCC definition of TNM and stage grouping for pancreatic cancer

Primary Tumor (T)

TX	Primary tumor cannot be assessed
T0	No evidence of primary tumor
Tis	Carcinoma *in situ*
T1	Tumor limited to the pancreas 2 cm or less in greatest dimension
T2	Tumor limited to the pancreas more than 2 cm in greatest dimension
T3	Tumor extends directly into any of the following: duodenum, bile duct, peripancreatic tissues
T4	Tumor extends directly into any of the following: stomach, spleen, colon, adjacent large vessels

Regional Lymph Nodes (N)

NX	Regional lymph nodes cannot be assessed
N0	No regional lymph node metastasis
N1	Regional lymph node metastasis
pN1a	Metastasis in a single regional lymph node
pN1b	Metastasis in multiple regional lymph nodes

Distant Metastasis (M)

MX	Distant metastasis cannot be assessed
M0	No distant metastasis
M1	Distant metastasis

Stage Grouping

Stage	*T*	*N*	*M*
0	Tis	N0	M0
I	T1	N0	M0
	T2	N0	M0
II	T3	N0	M0
III	T1	N1	M0
	T2	N1	M0
	T3	N1	M0
IVA	T4	Any N	M0
IVB	Any T	Any N	M1

SOURCE: Used with the permission of the American Joint Committee on Cancer (AJCC®), Chicago, IL. The original source for this material is the AJCC® Cancer Staging Manual, 5th edition (1997) published by Lippincott Williams & Wilkins Publishers, Philadelphia, PA.

TABLE 31–3.
AJCC definition of TNM and stage grouping for duodenal cancer

Primary Tumor (T)

TX	Primary tumor cannot be assessed
T0	No evidence of primary tumor
Tis	Carcinoma *in situ*
T1	Tumor invades lamina propria or submucosa
T2	Tumor invades muscularis propria
T3	Tumor invades through the muscularis propria into the subserosa or into the nonperitonealized perimuscular tissue (mesentery or retroperitoneum) with extension 2 cm or less*
T4	Tumor perforates the visceral peritoneum, or directly invades other organs and structures (includes other loops of small intestine, mesentery, or retroperitoneum more than 2 cm, and the abdominal wall by way of the serosa; for the duodenum only includes invasion of the pancreas)

**Note*: The nonperitonealized perimuscular tissue is, for jejunum and ileum, part of the mesentery and, for duodenum in areas where serosa is lacking, part of the retroperitoneum.

Regional Lymph Nodes (N)

NX	Regional lymph nodes cannot be assessed
N0	No regional lymph node metastasis
N1	Regional lymph node metastasis

Distant Metastasis (M)

MX	Distant metastasis cannot be assessed
M0	No distant metastasis
M1	Distant metastasis

Stage Grouping

Stage	T	N	M
0	Tis	N0	M0
I	T1	N0	M0
	T2	N0	M0
II	T3	N0	M0
	T4	N0	M0
III	Any T	N1	M0
IV	Any T	Any N	M1

SOURCE: Used with the permission of the American Joint Committee on Cancer (AJCC®), Chicago, IL. The original source for this material is the AJCC® Cancer Staging Manual, 5th edition (1997) published by Lippincott Williams & Wilkins Publishers, Philadelphia, PA.

TABLE 31–4.
AJCC definition of TNM and stage grouping for ampullary cancer

Primary Tumor (T)

TX	Primary tumor cannot be assessed
T0	No evidence of primary tumor
Tis	Carcinoma *in situ*
T1	Tumor limited to the ampulla of Vater or sphincter of Oddi
T2	Tumor invades duodenal wall
T3	Tumor invades 2 cm or less into pancreas
T4	Tumor invades more than 2 cm into pancreas and/or into other adjacent organs

Regional Lymph Nodes (N)

NX	Regional lymph nodes cannot be assessed
N0	No regional lymph node metastasis
N1	Regional lymph node metastasis

Distant Metastasis (M)

MX	Distant metastasis cannot be assessed
M0	No distant metastasis
M1	Distant metastasis

Stage Grouping

Stage	T	N	M
0	Tis	N0	M0
I	T1	N0	M0
II	T2	N0	M0
	T3	N0	M0
III	T1	N1	M0
	T2	N1	M0
	T3	N1	M0
IV	T4	Any N	M0
	Any T	Any N	M1

SOURCE: Used with the permission of the American Joint Committee on Cancer (AJCC®), Chicago, IL. The original source for this material is the AJCC® Cancer Staging Manual, 5th edition (1997) published by Lippincott Williams & Wilkins Publishers, Philadelphia, PA.

These operations are technically difficult and previously carried high mortality rates. Current mortality rates in centers commonly performing this operation are less than 5%. Morbidity rates are still high, however, with problems occurring in up to 25% of patients. Common postoperative complications include delayed gastric emptying and anastomotic leaks, especially at the pancreatic anastomosis. For a more detailed description of these operations, the reader is encouraged to review a surgical atlas.

Planned palliative resection is not recommended for periampullary tumors. Palliative surgery of any sort in this patient population actually has a higher mortality rate than resective surgery. For this reason, endoscopic stenting is preferred over operative biliary bypass for the patient with metastatic disease whose mean survival is only 6 months. For locally advanced tumors without metastases, operative biliary bypass may still have a role, as the mean survival for these patients approaches 12 months. Sometimes this decision is made at the time of laparotomy when the patient is found to have unresectable disease but has already been subjected to an open procedure, whereas the patient found to have locally advanced unresectable disease during the preoperative workup may just undergo endoscopic stenting.

The last major issue in palliative surgery is whether to perform a prophylactic gastrojejunostomy. Most pancreatic surgeons perform gastrojejunostomy only in the patient with advanced disease presenting with gastric outlet obstruction.

F. Adjuvant Therapy

Any therapy given in addition to surgery for patients with periampullary cancer is considered adjuvant. Chemotherapy is usually given in combination with radiation therapy. There has been increasing use of preoperative (neoadjuvant) therapy with chemoradiation. The potential benefits are to reduce the incidence of local recurrence after resection, increase the likelihood of complete surgical excision, and decrease the likelihood that manipulation of the tumor will cause tumor cell implantation at distant sites.

Another potential use for neoadjuvant therapy is to render an initially unresectable tumor an operable one. To date there are no good data to suggest that preoperative therapy is better than postoperative chemoradiation in patients with completely resected lesions. Furthermore, its usefulness for converting nonresectable tumors into resectable ones has not yet been clearly delineated. Intraoperative adjuvant radiation therapy can also be given to the periampullary region. Although there appears to be many potential benefits to this therapy, the increased operative time and cost appear to outweigh the fact that there is no clear benefit over external beam postoperative radiation therapy.

The most convincing data supporting the use of adjuvant therapy comes from studies of postoperative chemoradiation using 5-fluorouracil (5-FU) and 40 Gy of external beam radiation therapy, as in the gastrointestinal tumor study group (GITSG) trial. Although the numbers are small, patients with pancreatic cancer treated with postoperative adjuvant therapy survived longer (median survival 11 months versus 20 months). Subsequent studies appear to validate this initial experience, although the median survival for all patients with pancreatic cancer is still less than 2 years. The 5-year survival rate for patients with pancreatic cancers that are completely resected is less than 25%. Clearly, better chemotherapeutic agents are needed.

The survival rates for completely resected distal bile duct and ampullary cancers are better (30% and 50% at 5 years, respectively); and those for duodenal cancer are somewhat worse (20% at 5 years). The main reason for this is that the former patients tend to present earlier than those with pancreatic and duodenal cancers. The 5-year survival rate for all of the periampullary malignancies deemed unresectable is essentially 0%, with the median survival ranging from 6 months for patients with metastatic disease to approximately 12 months for those with locally advanced, nonmetastatic disease.

G. Unresectable Disease

Much of the subject of unresectable disease has already been covered in the preceding paragraphs. Patients with unresectable disease must be categorized into two categories: (1) those with locally advanced, nonmetastatic disease; and (2) those with peritoneal or liver metastases (or both). As mentioned, the survival is markedly different. The main surgical options for these patients are palliative, as mentioned. An important consideration is control of their pain. This can be done in one of several ways. Oral medication is one of the first steps when addressing the pain of these patients; additional methods include administration of pain medication by transdermal patch and sublingual routes. In the patient with severe pain who does not obtain relief by one of these routes, percutaneous chemical ablation of the celiac plexus can usually provide substantial pain relief.

One of the biggest advances made in the last 10 years in the treatment of pancreatic cancer has been utilization of a new chemotherapeutic agent, gemcitabine. In multiple studies, this drug has appeared to prolong survival of patients with unresectable disease. It also acts as a radiosensitizer and is sometimes used in conjunction with radiation therapy for locally advanced tumors. Gemcitabine has also been used for other periampullary cancers, but most of the published data refer to its use in pancreatic cancer. More recently, gemcitabine is being used as postoperative therapy in patients who have undergone complete resection and in those who develop metastatic disease after resection.

Over the last few years there was initial excitement in the use of matrix metalloproteinase inhibitors for the treatment of pancreatic cancer. This has not yet proven beneficial. The use of immunologic and biologic agents is still new in the treatment of periampullary malignancies. Again, most of this work has been done to treat patients with pancreatic malignancies.

H. Follow-up

Patients with tumors that have been resected should be followed by history and physical examination on a regular basis postoperatively. Routine use of CT scanning to evaluate for recurrent disease or metastatic disease is not cost-effective and not necessary. Serum tumor markers are sometimes used, but because resection of metastatic disease is usually not an option and chemotherapy is not yet effective this is more of an intellectual exercise. Follow-up is therefore directed by the patient's symptoms; new or progressive pain or weight loss should be investigated with CT scans of the abdomen. Patients rarely live long enough for stenosis at the bile duct anastomosis to become an issue, but in the long-term survivor this may be seen and may require dilatation or revision. Pancreatic anastomotic stenosis can sometimes lead to pancreatic insufficiency, and these patients may require pancreatic enzyme supplementation. It is also not uncommon for these patients to have pancreatic insufficiency secondary to long-standing pancreatic duct obstruction, and they therefore require enzyme supplementation after resection.

Conclusions

Periampullary malignancies are mostly of pancreatic origin. Tumors that obstruct the bile duct early, leading to jaundice, tend to have a more favorable prognosis because they are more likely to be diagnosed at an early stage and therefore are resected. Resection offers the best chance for cure. Adjuvant therapy is not yet optimal. Even with resection, the prognosis with most of these cancers is extremely poor.

Selected Reading

Brennan MF, Kinsella TJ, Casper ES. Cancer of the Pancreas, in DeVita JP VT, Hellman S, Rosenberg SA. Cancer, Principles and Practice of Oncology 4th ed., JP Lippincott, Philadelphia c. 1993 p 849–882.

Lotze, MT, Flickinger JC, Carr BI, Hepatobiliary Neoplasms, in DeVita, JP VT, Hellman S, Rosenberg SA. Cancer, Principles and Practice of Oncology 4th ed., JP Lippincott, Philadelphia, c. 1993, p 883–914.

Howard J, Idezuki Y, Ihse I, Prinz R (eds) Surgical Diseases of the Pancreas, 3rd ed. Baltimore: Williams & Wilkins, 1998, Sections 9, 10, and 12.

CHAPTER 32

Carcinoma of the Body and Tail of the Pancreas

CARLOS FERNÁNDEZ-DEL CASTILLO

A. General Considerations

Cancer of the head of the pancreas has a reputation as a tumor with a poor prognosis, but carcinoma of the body and tail of the pancreas is even worse, with long-term survival being so rare that when it occurs it has been the subject of case reports.[1] Approximately 28,000 new cases of pancreatic adenocarcinoma are diagnosed each year in the United States,[2] and of these only 15–20% occur in the distal gland. Not only is this entity less common, but the diagnosis is established late in the course of the disease when the tumor is usually no longer resectable.

Unlike carcinoma of the head of the pancreas, which commonly presents with jaundice, the symptoms of cancer of the pancreatic body and tail are insidious, consisting of vague abdominal discomfort evolving into pain over the course of several months, accompanied by unexplained weight loss. In the Johns Hopkins series, 90% of 113 patients had abdominal pain at the time of presentation, 54% had weight loss, and 16% had nausea or vomiting.[3] Only 4% had jaundice, likely related to extension of the tumor into the head of the gland or more commonly to extensive liver metastases. Recent-onset diabetes mellitus is not unusual, and a palpable mass is identified in as many as 20% of patients.[3,4] Back pain, another frequent symptom, usually portends invasion into the celiac plexus.[5]

A mass in the distal pancreas is not necessarily ductal adenocarcinoma; and because any other diagnosis is a welcome finding, other possibilities should always be considered. They include neuroendocrine tumors, mucinous cystic neoplasms, serous cystadenomas, solid and papillary tumors, lymphoma, sarcoma, and even metastatic tumors. In our experience, resection is performed three times more frequently for any of these indications than for ductal adenocarcinoma.[6] Chronic pancreatitis can be limited to the tail of the pancreas, present clinically as a mass, and be radiographically indistinguishable from carcinoma. Conversely, what is believed to be chronic pancreatitis can harbor cancer. Over a 6-year period we performed 16 distal pancreatic resections for presumed chronic pancreatitis, and 20% of the specimens contained ductal adenocarcinoma.[7]

Occasionally, patients are diagnosed when a tumor is found by computed tomography (CT) or ultrasonography performed for unrelated reasons or at the time of laparotomy. Theoretically, these

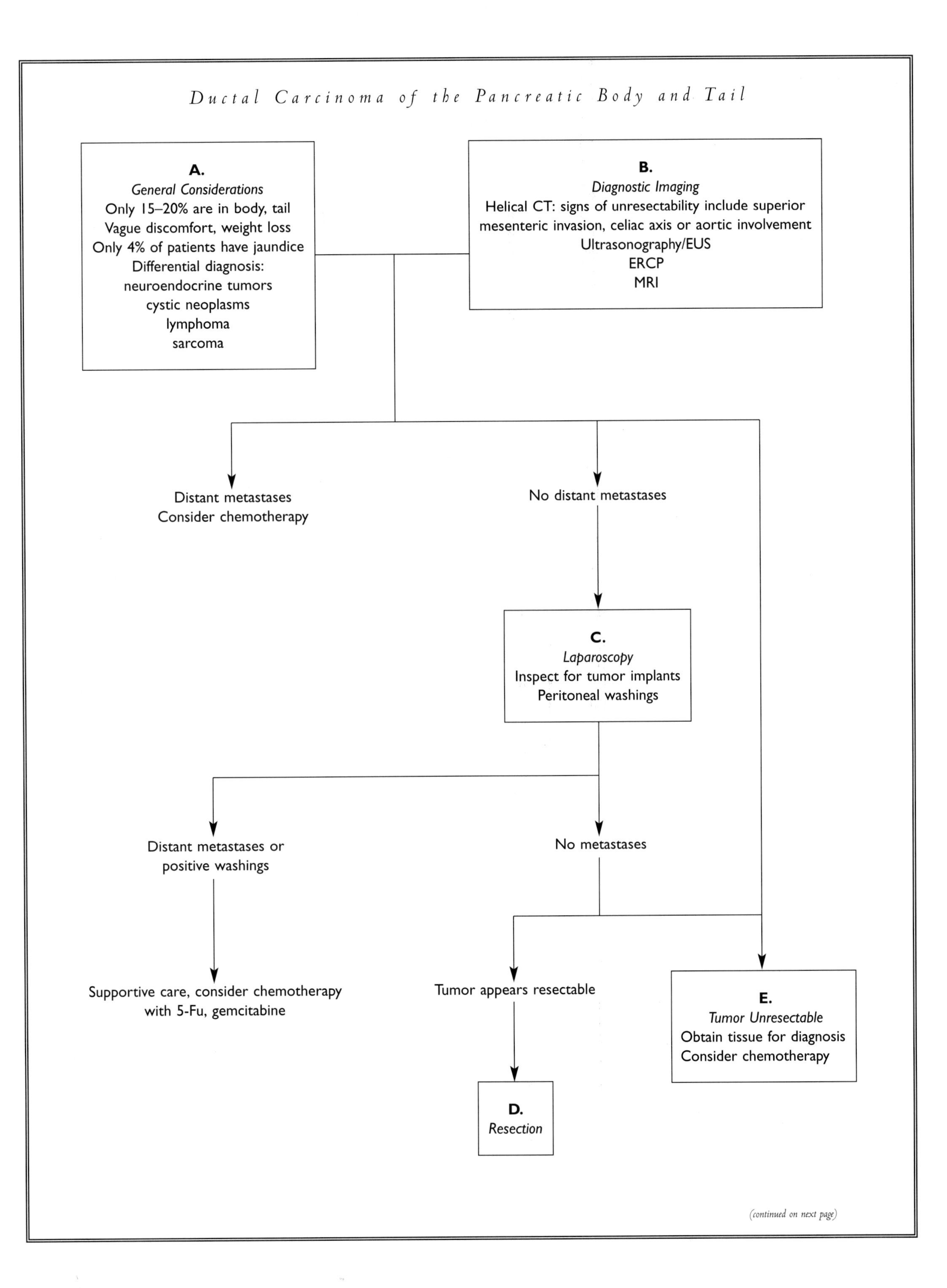

(continued on next page)

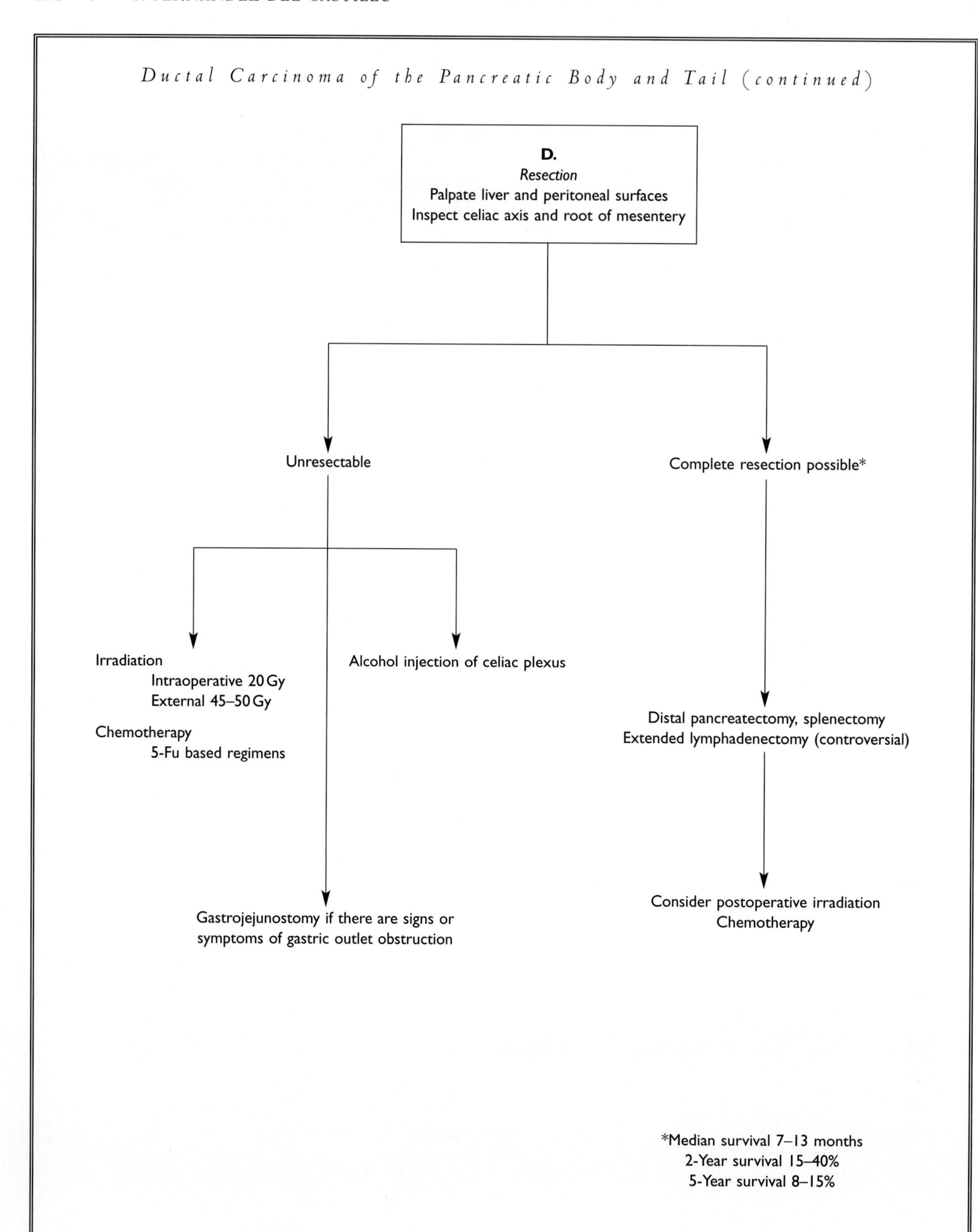
Ductal Carcinoma of the Pancreatic Body and Tail (continued)
D.
Resection
Palpate liver and peritoneal surfaces
Inspect celiac axis and root of mesentery
Unresectable
Complete resection possible*
Irradiation
Intraoperative 20 Gy
External 45–50 Gy
Chemotherapy
5-Fu based regimens
Alcohol injection of celiac plexus
Distal pancreatectomy, splenectomy
Extended lymphadenectomy (controversial)
Gastrojejunostomy if there are signs or
symptoms of gastric outlet obstruction
Consider postoperative irradiation
Chemotherapy
*Median survival 7–13 months
2-Year survival 15–40%
5-Year survival 8–15%

asymptomatic patients have a better prognosis, and one should proceed with staging as described below. In these circumstances, the larger the tumor, the lower is the likelihood of the mass being ductal adenocarcinoma; therefore biopsy should be part of the workup. However, if the mass is small and helical CT shows no signs of unresectability, laparoscopy and resection should follow.

B. Diagnostic Imaging

Computed tomography is the single most important test for diagnosis of pancreatic cancer and is almost indispensable when staging it. It provides an assessment of tumor size and local extension, contiguous organ involvement, peripancreatic nodal metastases, vascular encasement, hepatic metastases, and consequently resectability.[8] In most patients with advanced pancreatic cancer, it provides all the information needed for staging if it shows extensive local disease or metastases (Fig. 32–1). However, it is limited in its ability to identify small liver and peritoneal metastases and is also unable to detect microinvasion and to differentiate inflammatory lymph node enlargement from metastatic nodes. Several studies have shown that although it is highly accurate for predicting *unresectability* (average 94%), it is not as accurate for predicting *resectability* (average 60%).[9] Advances in CT technology, including thin-section and spiral CT scans, may improve accuracy by providing more detailed images during the bolus phase of contrast enhancement. Spiral CT has the added advantage of acquiring a volume of data (rather than individual slices) that can be subsequently manipulated to depict vascular anatomy and to assess better the vascular involvement.

Specific to tumors of the body and tail of the pancreas, CT signs of unresectability include invasion of the superior mesenteric vessels or celiac axis and aortic involvement. Because both the splenic artery and vein are removed with the specimen, their involvement per se does not preclude resection. However, complete encasement of any of these two vessels is usually associated with extensive retroperitoneal invasion.

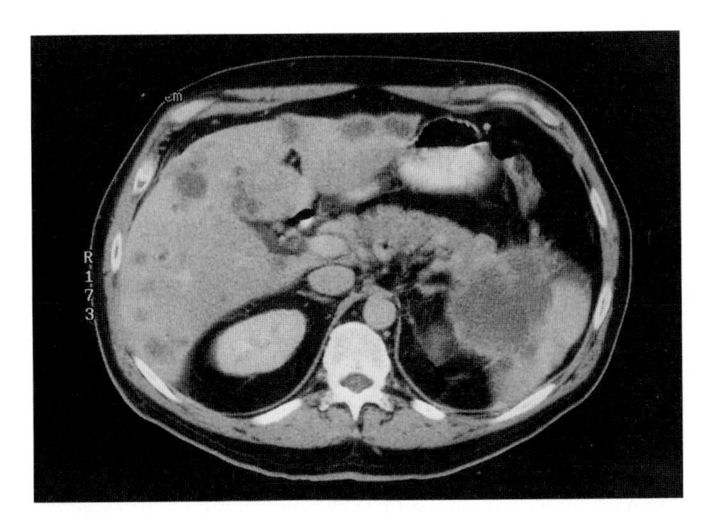

FIGURE 32–1
Computed tomography (CT) demonstrating a large mass in the tail of the pancreas with multiple liver metastases.

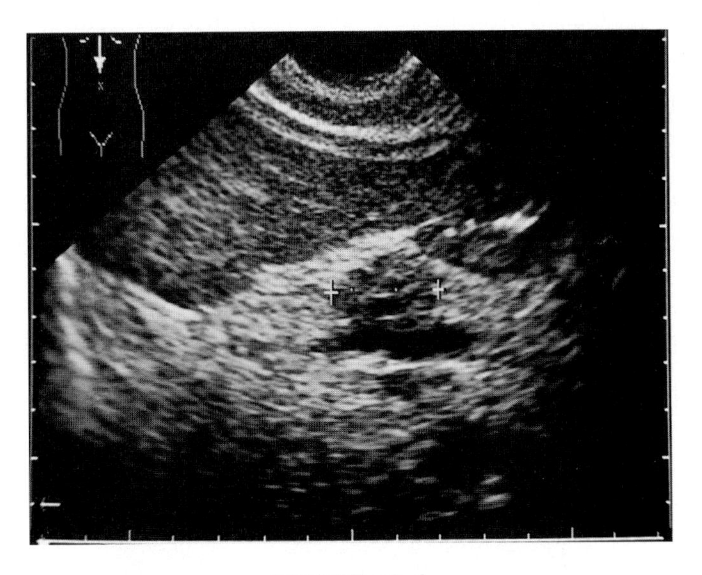

FIGURE 32–2
Ultrasonography demonstrating a tumor in the body of the pancreas, adjacent to the splenic vein.

As with pancreatic head tumors, the sensitivity of CT for carcinoma of the distal pancreas is not 100%, which means that a normal CT cannot entirely exclude this diagnosis. By relying on changes in echogenicity rather than in the contour of the gland, ultrasonography sometimes detects small lesions not seen by CT (Fig. 32–2). Endoscopic ultrasonography (EUS) has overcome the limitations that bowel gas and morbid obesity pose for transabdominal ultrasonography. The most sensitive test for the diagnosis of this malignancy, however, is endoscopic retrograde pancreatography, which demonstrates an abnormal pancreatic duct in practically all cases of ductal adenocarcinoma. Magnetic resonance imaging (MRI) is emerging as a useful tool for evaluating the pancreas and the biliary and pancreatic ducts; and in the future it may become the procedure of choice for diagnosing and staging this disease.[10]

C. Laparoscopy

If precise preoperative staging for pancreatic cancer is required, laparoscopic examination is indispensable. Many studies have shown that 22–48% of patients who have apparently localized disease by CT have evidence of metastatic spread by laparoscopy.[11–16] Typically, the lesions identified by laparoscopy are 1–2 mm in diameter and are located on the parietal peritoneum and the liver surface; occasionally there are large deposits in the omentum or mesentery (Fig. 32–3).

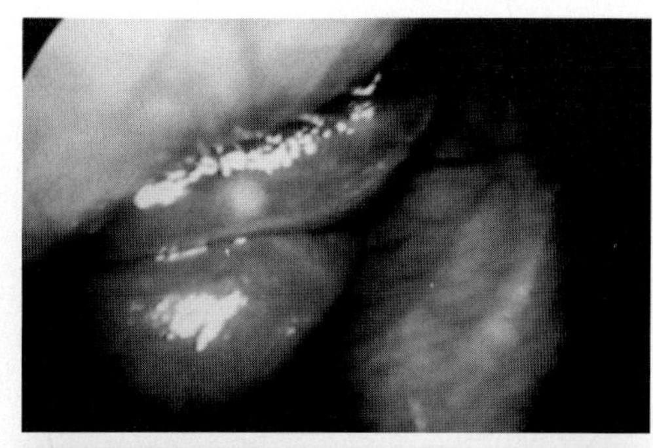

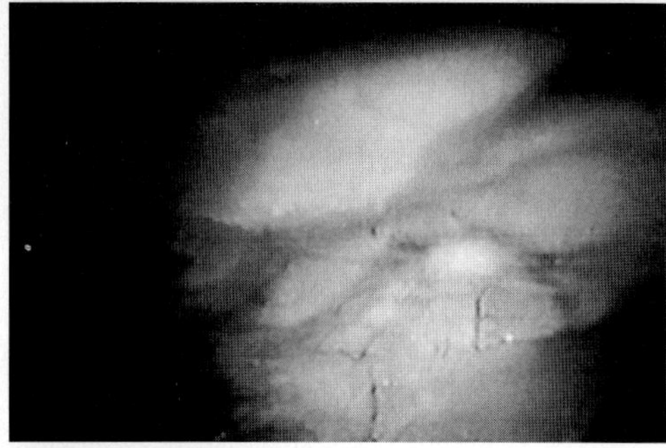

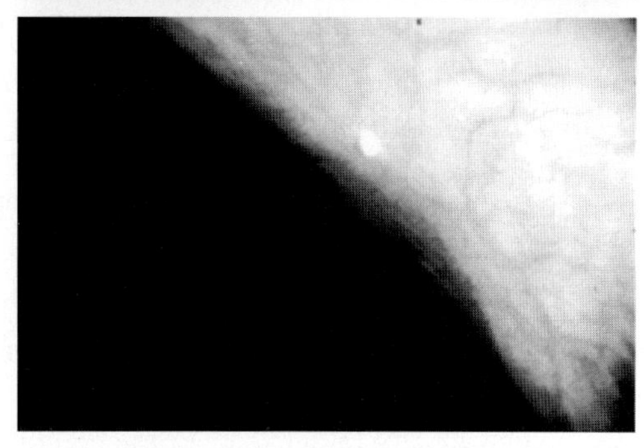

FIGURE 32–3
Laparoscopic detection of liver (top), omental (middle), and peritoneal (bottom) metastases from pancreatic cancer.

In our experience with 200 patients over a 12-year period, laparoscopy detected metastases in 31%.[16] The yield is much higher for tumors of the body and tail of the pancreas (29/54, 53%) than for tumors of the pancreatic head (33/146, 22%), perhaps reflecting the delay in diagnosis of distal pancreatic tumors. Even though the prevalence of intraabdominal spread detected by laparoscopy has been decreasing significantly over time, our most recent experience still shows that 44% of patients with cancers of the body and tail who have no CT evidence of metastatic spread are found by laparoscopy to have such spread. This fully justifies the addition of laparoscopy to the staging of these patients, as the cost, discomfort, and potential risks of unnecessary laparotomy can be avoided.

In addition to giving an assessment of the presence or absence of visible tumor implants, laparoscopy provides the opportunity to perform peritoneal washings. This procedure discloses the presence of an additional 8% of patients with micrometastases.[17] In a recent study, we found that the survival of patients with malignant cells found in peritoneal washings and absence of visible metastases is as poor as that of patients with macroscopic implants, and that they derive no benefit from treatment aimed at local control (i.e., surgical resection or irradiation).[18]

Others have expanded the use of laparoscopy in pancreatic cancer staging to investigate vessel and lymph node invasion.[15,19] This is accomplished by extended laparoscopic dissection or the concomitant use of laparoscopic ultrasonography. The benefits of this type of assessment have yet to be compared to the information obtained with helical CT.

D. *Resection*

Resection offers the only possibility of cure and perhaps the best palliation for patients with cancer of the body and tail of the pancreas. Resection should be considered if there is no sign of metastatic disease and complete tumor removal can be accomplished. At the time of exploration, after searching for liver and peritoneal metastases attention should be directed to the presence of enlarged lymph nodes in the celiac axis and root of the mesentery. Although lymphatic clearance of these areas is possible, bulky lymphadenopathy is a sign of advanced disease, and negative margins cannot usually be achieved. The same can be said of contiguous invasion of the posterior gastric wall or the mesocolon; and unless the involvement is focal, an extensive resection in rarely justified. If resection is pursued, the operation includes removal of the spleen and the splenic vessels, as well as the appropriate portion of the pancreas, usually with division at the level of the neck of the gland.

Pancreatic cancer is characterized by tumor spread via neural structures and lymph nodes. A study from Japan that included 20 patients who underwent distal pancreatectomy with extensive lymphatic dissection demonstrated lymph node invasion and neural plexus invasion in 80% and 70% of cases, respectively.[5] The lymph nodes most frequently affected were those along the splenic artery (50%), common hepatic artery (25%), and paraaortic region (25%).[5] This is an important observation because lymphatic clearance of the latter two sites is not routinely done in the United States for distal pancreatic tumors. As with cancers of the pancreatic head, the impact of extensive lymphatic dissection on survival has yet to be proven.

Even though there are no data to support the use of adjuvant treatment for resected carcinoma of the distal pancreas, our policy at Massachusetts General Hospital is to recommend postoperative radiation and 5-fluorouracil (5-FU) to all patients, extrapolating from the Gastrointestinal Tumor Study Group (GITSG) studies supporting the use of this treatment for cancer of the pancreatic head.[20,21]

TABLE 32–1.
Ductal adenocarcinoma of the pancreatic body and tail

Study	Institution	No. of patients	No. of resections	Median survival (months)	Survival (%)	
					2 years	5 years
Nordback[3]	Johns Hopkins	113	9 (8%)	7	22	11
Dalton[4]	Mayo Clinic	N.S.	26	10	15	8
Johnson[22]	Mannheim	105	13 (12%)	13	38	—
Brennan[23]	MSKCC	331	34 (10%)	12	15	14

There were no operative deaths.
N.S., not stated.

The results of four recent series of resected adenocarcinoma of the pancreatic body and tail are shown in Table 32–1.[3,4,22,23] They demonstrate that resectability rates are lower than for pancreatic head tumors, that the operation can be done safely, and that 5-year survival, although less than that for proximal pancreatic tumors, is not dismal and certainly possible for some patients. Because of the small number of patients in single series, the only significant predictor of survival that has been identified is tumor differentiation.[23] As expected, survival has been better in patients with small tumors and no lymph node metastases, but it does not reach statistical significance.[22,23]

Patients whose tumors are found to be unresectable at laparotomy should undergo alcohol ablation of the celiac plexus. This technique significantly facilitates pain control or delays the onset of pain if it is not already present. It has also been associated with better survival for reasons that are poorly understood but may be related to improved functional status.[24] Depending on the location of the tumor, consideration should be given to a gastrojejunostomy, as obstruction of the fourth portion of the duodenum at the level of the ligament of Treitz occurs in up to 20% of patients as the disease progresses. Performing gastrojejunostomy is controversial, but few would argue its utility if there are signs of gastric or duodenal obstruction at laparotomy for planned, but aborted, pancreaticoduodenectomy. Prophylactic gastrojejunostomy for the asymptomatic patient with localized unresectable disease is not indicated.

If a mass in the body and tail of the pancreas appears unresectable, tissue confirmation of adenocarcinoma should be obtained using the least invasive means possible. This is a prerequisite before proceeding with irradiation and chemotherapy, and it helps rule out other diagnoses that may have a better prognosis and different treatment. Other entities that can present as a mass in the distal pancreas include islet cell tumors, lymphoma, cystadenocarcinoma, solid and papillary tumors, and metastatic lesions. Fine-needle and core biopsies can be obtained under CT guidance and via endoscopic ultrasonography. If the mass appears resectable, however, obtaining a preoperative histologic diagnosis is not necessary.

E. *Unresectable Disease*

Localized Disease

External-beam radiation therapy in combination with 5-FU therapy can significantly extend survival for patients with unresectable but localized pancreatic ductal adenocarcinoma.[25] This is true for tumors of the head of the pancreas and those of the distal part of the gland. In the GITSG study[25] patients were randomized to receive 40 Gy plus 5-FU, 60 Gy plus 5-FU, or 60 Gy without chemotherapy. The radiation was administered as a split course with 20 Gy over 2 weeks followed by a 2 week rest. The 5-FU was given intravenously as a bolus dose of 500 mg/m^2/day for the first 3 days of each 20 Gy cycle and then weekly following completion of irradiation. Randomization was performed after surgical exloration confirmed unresectability but the disease was confined to the peripancreatic tissue and regional nodes. For each of the chemoradiation groups the median survival was 10 months; for the radiation-only group the median survival was 6 months. Approximately 80% of patients completed chemoradiation. The patients most likely to benefit from treatment were those with a high performance status and minimal symptoms.

Intraoperative radiation therapy (IORT) offers the possibility of delivering a high dose to the cancer without injuring neighboring tissues. Either before or after fractionated external radiotherapy, a 20 Gy boost is delivered directly to the surgically exposed tumor by an electron beam through a field-limiting cone.[26,27] Higher doses can cause duodenal ulceration, perforation, or upper gastrointestinal hemorrhage due to radiation duodenitis. Usually IORT is followed or preceded by external beam irradiation; and the median survival ranges from 12 to 15 months. If 5-FU is given in conjunction with external beam radiation, survival may be extended even further. At the Massachusetts General Hospital, this is currently done in a dedicated operating room suite. We have treated more than 200 pancreatic cancer patients with IORT. In our first report the median survival was 16.5 months;[26] subsequently the survival has been about 13 months with excellent local control. Twenty percent have lived beyond 2 years, and six patients are alive 5 years or more after diagnosis (all histologically confirmed). One additional benefit of IORT is relief of pain in 50–93% of patients.[27,28] Analysis of our experience shows that tumor location (head versus body or tail) is irrelevant, although tumor size is one of the most important predictors of survival, and the average tumors from the distal pancreas are larger than those in the head of the gland.

Metastatic Disease

The prognosis is especially dismal for patients who have distant metastases at the time of diagnosis. Unfortunately, it occurs in 50% of patients with cancer of the pancreatic body and tail. 5-FU is the most widely used chemotherapeutic agent; response rates vary and may approach 30%. Gemcitabine is a deoxycytidine with lipophilic properties that give the drug enhanced membrane permeability. It may be superior to 5-FU for patients with metastatic pancreatic cancer; however, median survival is less than 6 months, and only 18% of patients survive longer than a year after diagnosis.[29] We have seen a few patients treated with gemcitabine whose disease has remained stable for more than 12 months with few or no side effects from the chemotherapy.

Conclusions

In contrast to cancers of the head of the pancreas (jaundice), cancers of the pancreatic body and tail do not have heralding signs. The principal clinical features are pain and weight loss. Although the diagnosis of pancreatic cancer carries a grave prognosis, it is not a uniformly fatal disease, even when located in the body and tail. Resection offers the best chance for cure; resectability can be determined preoperatively using CT and laparoscopy. Metastatic disease to the liver, peritoneal surfaces, and omentum and peritoneal washings are contraindications to pancreatectomy. For localized unresectable disease, symptoms can be palliated and survival prolonged with combined irradiation (external beam or intraoperative) and chemotherapy.

References

1. Saltzman A, Horvitz A, Dyckman J. Survival for 25 years following partial pancreatectomy for carcinoma of the body of the pancreas. Mt Sinai J Med 1987;54:427–428.
2. National Cancer Institute. Annual Cancer Statistics Review 1973–1989. National Institutes of Health Publication 92-2789. Bethesda: US Department of Health and Human Services, 1992.
3. Nordback IH, Hruban RH, Boitnott JK, Pitt HA, Cameron JL. Carcinoma of the body and tail of pancreas. Am J Surg 1992;164:26–31.
4. Dalton RR, Sarr MG, van Heerden JA, Colby TV. Carcinoma of the body and tail of the pancreas: is curative resection justified? Surgery 1992;111: 489–494.
5. Kayahara M, Nagakawa T, Futagami F, Kitagawa H, Ohta T, Miyazaki I. Lymphatic flow and neural plexus invasion associated with carcinoma of the body and tail of the pancreas. Cancer 1996;78:2485–2491.
6. Fernández-del Castillo C, Rattner DW, Warshaw AL. Standards for pancreatic resection in the 1990's. Arch Surg 1995;130:295–300.
7. Rattner DW, Fernández-del Castillo C, Warshaw AL. Pitfalls of distal pancreatectomy for relief of pain in chronic pancreatitis. Am J Surg 1996;171: 142–146.
8. Freeny PC, Traverso W, Ryan JA. Diagnosis and staging of pancreatic adenocarcinoma with dynamic computed tomography. Am J Surg 1993;165: 600–606.
9. Andersen HB, Effersoe H, Tjalve E. CT for assessment of pancreatic and periampullary cancer. Acta Radiol 1993;34:569–572.
10. Trede M, Rumstadt B, Wendl K, et al. Ultrafast magnetic resonance imaging improves the staging of pancreatic tumors. Ann Surg 1997;226: 393–407.
11. Cuschieri A, Hall AW, Clark J. Value of laparoscopy in the diagnosis and management of pancreatic carcinoma. Gut 1978;19:672–677.
12. Ishida H. Peritoneoscopy and pancreas biopsy in the diagnosis of pancreatic diseases. Gastrointest Endosc 1983;29:211–218.
13. Warshaw AL, Tepper JE, Shipley WU. Laparoscopy in the staging and planning of therapy for pancreatic cancer. Am J Surg 1986;151:76–80.
14. Warshaw AL, Gu Z-Y, Wittenberg J, Waltman AC. Preoperative staging and assessment of resectability of pancreatic cancer. Arch Surg 1990;125: 230–233.
15. Bemelman WA, de Wit LT, van Delden OM, et al. Diagnostic laparoscopy combined with laparoscopic ultrasonography in staging of cancer of the pancreatic head region. Br J Surg 1995;82:820–824.
16. Fernández-del Castillo C, Rattner DW, Warshaw AL. Further experience with laparoscopy and peritoneal cytology in staging for pancreatic cancer. Br J Surg 1995;82:1127–1129.
17. Fernández-del Castillo C, Warshaw AL. Laparoscopic staging and peritoneal cytology (in pancreatic cancer). Surg Oncol Clin N Am 1998;7: 135–142.
18. Makary MA, Warshaw AL, Centeno BA, Willett CG, Rattner DW, Fernández-del Castillo C. Implications of peritoneal cytology for pancreatic cancer management. Arch Surg 1998;133(4):361–365.
19. Conlon KC, Dougherty E, Klimstra DS, Coit DG, Turnbull ADM, Brennan MF. The value of minimal access surgery in the staging of patients with potentially resectable peripancreatic malignancy. Ann Surg 1996;223: 134–140.
20. Kalser MH, Ellenberg SS. Pancreatic cancer: adjuvant combined radiation and chemotherapy following curative resection. Arch Surg 1985;120: 899–903.
21. Gastrointestinal Tumor Study Group. Further evidence of effective adjuvant combined radiation and chemotherapy following curative resection of pancreatic cancer. Cancer 1987;59:2006–2010.
22. Johnson CD, Schwall G, Flechtenmacher J, Trede M. Resection for adenocarcinoma of the body and tail of the pancreas. Br J Surg 1993;80: 1177–1179.
23. Brennan MF, Moccia RD, Klimstra D. Management of adenocarcinoma of the body and tail of the pancreas. Ann Surg 1996;223:506–512.
24. Lillemoe KD, Cameron JL, Kaufman HS, Yeo CJ, Pitt HA, Sauter PK. Chemical splanchnicectomy in patients with unresectable pancreatic cancer. Ann Surg 1993;217:447–457.
25. Gastrointestinal Tumor Study Group. Therapy of locally unresectable pancreatic carcinoma: a randomized comparison of high dose (6000 rads) radiation alone, moderate dose radiation (4000 rads + 5-fluorouracil), and high dose radiation + 5 fluorouracil. Cancer 1981;48:1705–1710.

26. Dobelbower RR, Konski AA, Merrick HW, Bronn DG, Schifeling D, Kamen C. Intraoperative electron beam radiation therapy (IOEBRT) for carcinoma of the exocrine pancreas. Int J Radiat Oncol Biol Phys 1991;20:113–119.
27. Shipley WU, Wood WC, Tepper JE, et al. Intraoperative electron beam irradiation for patients with unresectable pancreatic carcinoma. Ann Surg 1984;200:289–294.
28. Heijmans HJ, Hoekstra HJ, Mehta DM. Is adjuvant intra-operative radiotherapy (IORT) for resectable and unresectable pancreatic carcinoma worthwhile? Hepatogastroenterology 1986;36:474–477.
29. Rothenberg ML, Moore MJ, Cripps MC, et al. A phase II trial of gemcitabine in patients with 5-FU refractory pancreas cancer. Ann Oncol 1996;7:347–353.

Chapter 33

Proximal Bile Duct Cancer

J. LAWRENCE MUNSON

The management of carcinoma originating in the proximal biliary tree is controversial and its cure elusive. Even though imaging techniques have improved and are increasingly available, the diagnosis of this entity is often late. Despite improved preoperative management, technologically advanced surgical tools, complex resectional techniques, and specialized monitoring and postoperative care units, the overall prognosis of patients with proximal biliary carcinoma remains discouragingly poor. Nonetheless, surgical extirpation of the disease offers the patient the only hope of lasting survival or perhaps even cure.[1–3]

An algorithmic approach to proximal bile duct cancer is not meant to be the final word in the management of these neoplasms. Instead, it provides a logical template for patient assessment, staging, and treatment. Understanding that each patient is unique allows the surgeon to modify his or her approach as the patient is guided through the frightening process of facing this slow-growing but relentless cancer.

A. *Epidemiology and Etiology*

The incidence of bile duct cancer in the United States is approximately 1/100,000, with 3000 to 4500 new cases diagnosed per year.[4] On the basis of autopsy series, the incidence of biliary carcinoma is 0.01–0.46%, which attests to the fact that this slow-growing entity may or may not be the cause of death.[5–8]

Historically, carcinoma of the extrahepatic biliary tree has been noted in the literature[7,9] for more than a century, with the first reported study of bile duct cancer credited to Durand-Fardel in 1840. Musser reported 18 cases in 1889.[7] Although Altmeier et al.[10] reported three cases of perihilar malignancy in 1957, most physicians attribute the description of tumors of the hepatic duct bifurcation to Klatskin,[11] who reported 13 such cases in 1965. In fact, primary bile duct cancer arising at the hepatic bifurcation is often called a "Klatskin" tumor.

The cause of proximal bile duct cancer is unknown, but definite common links exist in specific high risk groups (Table 33–1). The common denominators are bile stasis, chronic inflammation, and biliary calculi.

Proximal Bile Duct Cancer

A.
Epidemiology
3000–4500 New cases per year

B.
Histology
95% Adenocarcinoma (solid vs. cystadenocarcinoma)
Solid patterns:
papillary—intraluminal growth
nodular—mid or upper third of duct, diffuse

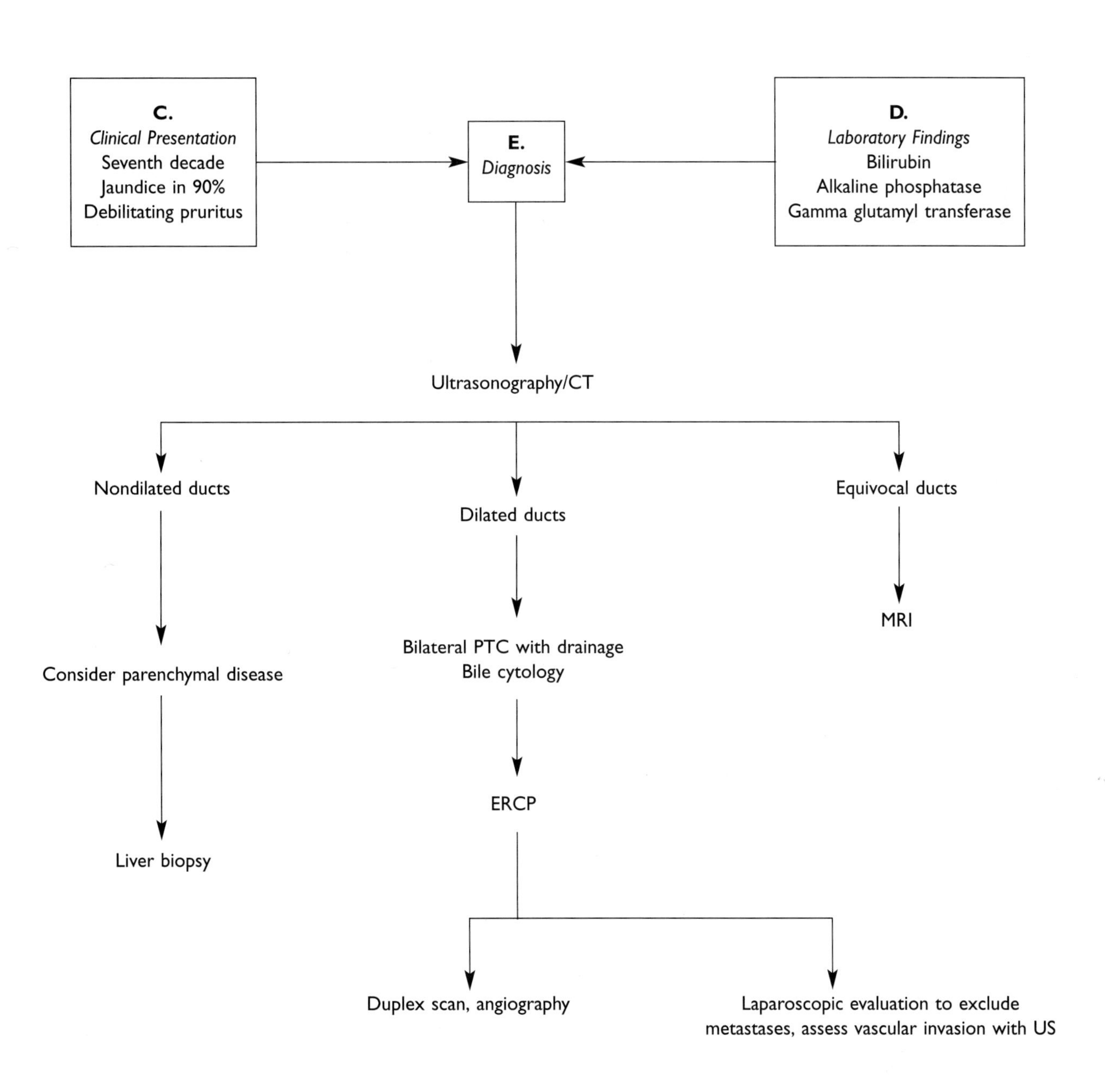

(continued on next page)

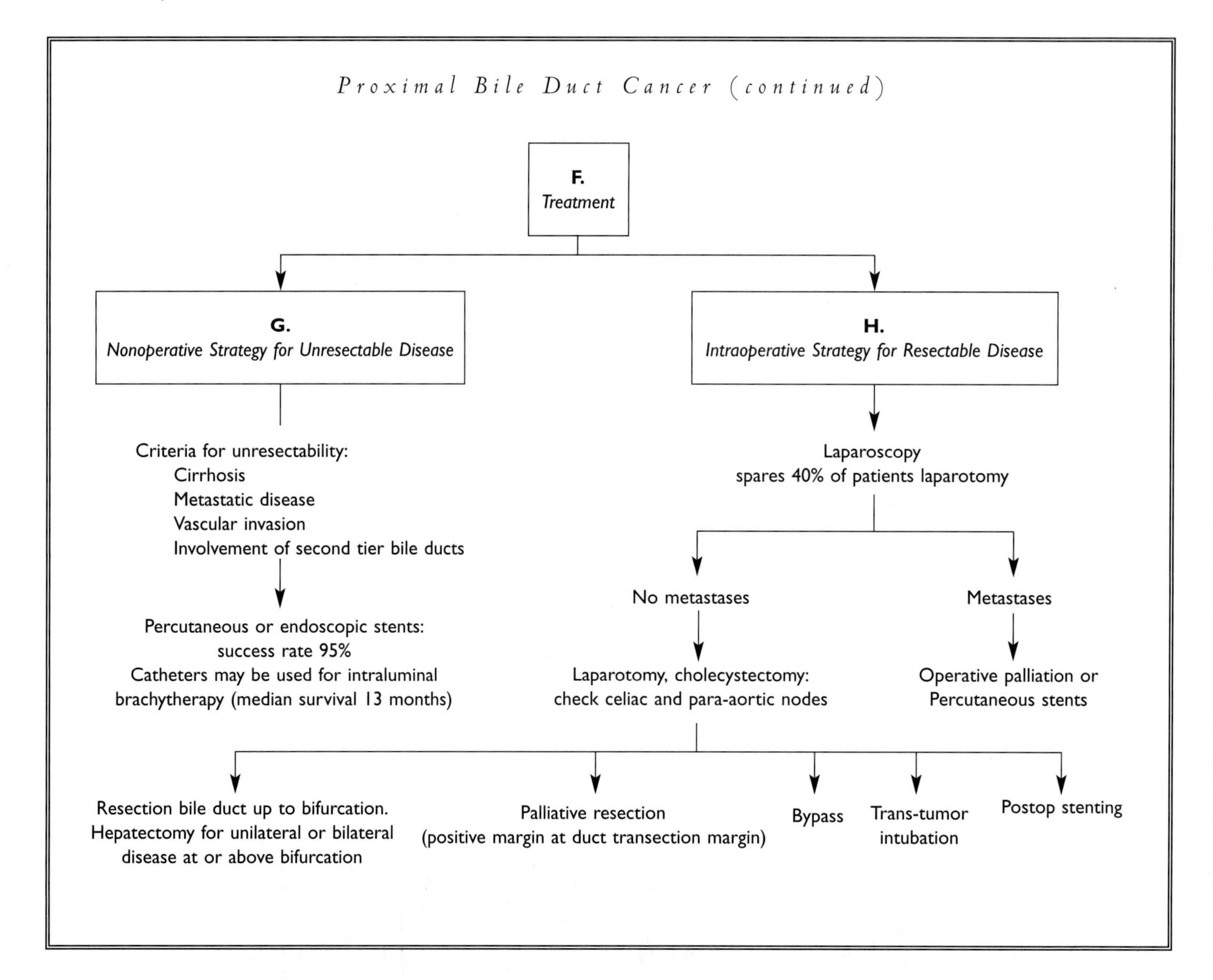

B. Histology

Histologically, most (95%) bile duct cancers are adenocarcinomas (cholangiocarcinomas). Other cell types include squamous cell carcinoma, mucoepidermoid carcinoma, leiomyosarcoma, rhabdomyosarcoma, granular cell carcinoma, and carcinoid. The adenocarcinomas may be further subdivided into solid and cystadenocarcinoma subtypes. The former are the most common, constituting approximately 90% of all biliary cancers. The solid forms are characterized into papillary, nodular, and diffuse forms. The papillary type grows intraluminally, sometimes showing multicentricity, and is most often found in the distal bile duct. The *nodular* type tends to be located in the middle or upper third of the extrahepatic biliary tree and presents as a small, hard, well localized mass. The *diffuse* infiltrative type exhibits thickened duct walls with an extensive desmoplastic or sclerosing response that may encase all of the portal structures.[5–7]

Lesions proximal to the cystic duct comprise 30–76% of bile duct cancers.[6,12] These proximal tumors tend to be slow-growing and may develop neural, perineural, lymphatic, and subepithelial spread. Although distant metastases are distinctly uncommon, lymph node spread is seen in 30% of patients.[8] Blood-borne metastases may become more common as local control improves. The slow-growing, locally invasive nature of these tumors continually frustrates the surgeon, who believes these factors should make this disease more easily controllable, if not curable.

C. Clinical Presentation

The typical patient presenting with proximal bile duct cancer is in his or her seventh decade. Patients in the high risk groups tend to be seen two decades earlier. Jaundice, the most common clinical sign, is present in more than 90% of patients.[8,13,14] Because these tumors are slow-growing, jaundice may not occur until quite late in the course of the disease. Tumors obstructing only one side of the bifurcation may never cause jaundice, but

TABLE 33–1.
High risk factors

Cystic dilation of the bile duct (choledochal cyst and Caroli's disease)
Clonorchiasis
Hepatolithiasis
Sclerosing cholangitis
Ulcerative colitis
Thorium dioxide exposure (Thorotrast)
Suspected risk factors
Asbestosis
Dioxin exposure
Nitrosamines
Polychlorinated biphenyls
Oral[18]

they may cause atrophy of the affected side by obstructing the portal vein and the hepatic duct. This may result in compensatory hypertrophy of the contralateral lobe, as seen on computed tomography (CT).[8]

Along with jaundice, most patients have debilitating pruritus and on presentation may have diffuse excoriations from uncontrollable scratching. Other symptoms, such as malaise, mild weight loss, upper abdominal discomfort (due to mild liver distension), anorexia, and fatigue, tend to be vague.[15] Physical examination tends to reveal only jaundice and evidence of excoriations, although mild hepatomegaly may be detected. A distended (Courvoisier) gallbladder is not present with proximal tumors. Late findings with proximal cancers may be ascites or splenomegaly, suggesting portal vein occlusion with portal hypertension. Fevers, chills, or rigors associated with cholangitis are uncommon unless some form of biliary instrumentation has been performed.

D. *Laboratory Findings*

Laboratory findings with proximal bile duct cancer are few; elevated levels of direct bilirubin, alkaline phosphatase, and γ-glutamyl transferase suggest biliary epithelial injury. With unilateral duct obstruction, only the latter two levels may be elevated. Tumor markers such as carcinoembryonic antigen (CEA), CA 19-9, and α-fetoprotein, are usually normal. Mild anemia may be present. At this time no early screening test exists for proximal bile duct cancer.

E. *Diagnosis*

Jaundice may be due to a variety of diagnoses, enumerated in Table 33–2. A number of these conditions are also associated with the development of bile duct cancer; that is, they are part of the high risk conditions.

Radiography

Radiographic tests are the diagnostic mainstay of proximal bile duct cancer. Any patient presenting with jaundice should first undergo ultrasonography of the liver and biliary tree to exclude stone disease. Ultrasonography can identify the level of biliary obstruction and accurately determine the presence of calculi. A Doppler study of the porta hepatis is performed during the ultrasound study if the radiologist sees evidence of obstruction and dilation. The Doppler study may show involvement of the portal vessels by direct tumor extension.

Computed tomography is usually the next test after calculi have been ruled out.[16] This study often shows a mass at the porta hepatis, but it also shows the hepatic parenchyma and the caudate lobe, which is frequently invaded early in the course of this disease. The presence of lobar atrophy is important when determining the operative strategy and planning preoperative drainage. CT findings of bilateral parenchymal involvement or extrahepatic metastases exclude any but palliative procedures.

The newest noninvasive modality is magnetic resonance cholangiography and pancreatography (MRCP). Our experience with this technique is limited at this time, although it may

TABLE 33–2.
Differential diagnosis of jaundice

Cystic disease of the bile duct
Choledochal cyst[a]
Caroli's disease[a]
Inflammatory strictures
Sclerosing cholangitis[a]
Chronic pancreatitis
Ischemic strictures
Postradiation strictures
Chemotherapy-induced strictures
Calculus disease
Mirizzi syndrome
Postoperative/traumatic strictures
Acquired immunodificiency syndrome (AIDS)-related strictures
Neoplastic strictures
Benign tumors of the bile duct
Biliary cystadenomas
Malignant tumors involving the bile ducts
Periampullary tumors
Pancreatic ductal cancer
Islet cell tumors
Metastatic tumors to the porta hepatis
Lymphoma
Metastatic adenocarcinoma
Infections/infestations
Clonorchis sinensis[a]
Ascariasis

High risk factor.

well replace percutaneous transhepatic cholangiography (PTC) and endoscopic retrograde cholangiopancreatography (ERCP) when preoperative drainage is not needed. Preimaging ingestion of an iron-containing solution effectively eliminates the bowel signal and demonstrates the entire biliary tree, regardless of whether obstruction is present.

If proximal biliary carcinoma is strongly suspected at this point, the standard study is PTC. If the lesion involves the bifurcation of the hepatic ducts, it may be necessary to perform bilateral PTC so all intrahepatic branches may be studied. The presence of bilateral disease that has extended into the secondary bile ducts indicates that the cancer is likely unresectable. The most controversial issue with PTC is whether to establish bilateral biliary drainage at the time of the study.[2,6,17–29] Several studies of preoperative drainage have failed to show substantial benefit with the procedure. Furthermore, instrumentation of this type may precipitate cholangitis with virulent, resistant organisms. Advocates of preoperative drainage note that the cholestatic liver tolerates warm ischemia less well than a healthy, functioning one.[4] Beazley et al.[17] cited studies demonstrating a 13–28% mortality with major surgery on patients with serum bilirubin levels higher than 10 mg/dl. In addition, there are several benefits of a more subjective nature. First, on presentation, these patients tend to have debilitating pruritus, which can be treated only with prompt biliary drainage. Second, nutritionally depleted patients can be helped by relieving the obstruction, providing vitamin K, and improving liver function to permit restoration of synthetic function. Third, the infrequent but dangerous development of bile peritonitis can be prevented or treated by establishing free biliary drainage. Fourth, preoperative placement of bilateral catheters through the hepatic bifurcation to the distal bile duct or duodenum permits easy identification of the hepatic ducts at the porta hepatis. Easy though the identification of the bile ducts may be during hepatic resection for *liver* tumors, the desmoplastic reaction associated with *cholangiocarcinoma*, sclerosing cholangitis, or postoperative biliary strictures can prove daunting. Lastly, these stents can be used safely to draw large Silastic drainage catheters through the liver for postoperative anastomotic protection or palliative prolonged drainage. Biliary tract surgeons in Japan[18] use preoperative biliary drainage as a prerequisite to resection. If the bilirubin level does not drop to 3 mg/dl after 6 weeks of bilateral drainage, the patient is referred for palliative treatment only.

Preoperative selective hepatic angiography and portography may be used to determine vascular invasion, although in the thin patient duplex scanning may be as accurate and is less invasive. Arteriography is perhaps most useful when other preoperative studies suggest that major hepatic resection is required.

Laparoscopic evaluation of the porta hepatis and liver with intraoperative ultrasonography may be performed as an outpatient procedure to rule out metastatic disease. This may spare the patient a major laparotomy.[20] Laparoscopic ultrasonography can help assess vascular invasion and guide biopsy studies.

Preoperative Tissue Diagnosis

The need to establish a tissue diagnosis of cholangiocarcinoma before surgery is controversial. Certainly, the goal of therapy is to relieve jaundice, preferably by complete surgical excision of the strictured area. It may help the patient cope with the process preoperatively by knowing whether malignancy is present. If establishing a histologic diagnosis can help the patient decide on a course of action, pursuit of a tissue diagnosis is justifiable.

Cytologic examination of bile obtained through percutaneous catheters may reveal tumor cells. The addition of brush cytology may improve the diagnostic yield; fine-needle aspiration of the strictured area may be rewarding as well. Intraoperatively, it is not necessary to establish a tumor diagnosis to proceed with curative resection of the biliary tree. However, if surgical bypass or palliative stenting only is performed, it is best to have biopsy proof of cancer. Any subsequent decisions regarding palliative treatment with chemotherapy or irradiation usually require proof of the presence of malignancy.

Classification of Proximal Bile Duct Cancer

In 1988 Bismuth et al.[21] described a system of classifying proximal bile duct tumors by the extent of ductal involvement (Fig. 33–1). This system has fairly wide acceptance and is useful when comparing data from different institutions.[22] This classification gives us an anatomic description of the tumors, but more formal staging of the lesion is preferably done with the TNM system (Table 33–3).

The natural history of proximal bile duct cancer is that of progressive liver failure and death an average of 3 months after diagnosis. Percutaneous biliary bypass can extend the mean survival for another 2–3 months. Surgical resection for palliation (positive margins macroscopically or microscopically) may result in a 5-year survival rate of 0–15%, whereas curative resection (defined by negative macroscopic and microscopic margins) may yield 5-year survival rates of 17–44%.[2,4,12,23]

F. Treatment

G. Nonoperative Strategy for Unresectable Disease

Some patients are clearly not candidates for an extensive resection because of coexisting medical problems that place them at risk for surgical complications. The presence of cirrhosis is a relative contraindication to hepatic resection unless the procedure can be limited to segmentectomy. Metastatic disease, bilateral or extensive vascular invasion (portal veins, hepatic arteries, or contralateral combination of both), and tumor involving the second-order biliary ducts bilaterally or contralateral to a point of vascular invasion are contraindications to resection.

These patients are best served with percutaneous or endoscopically placed stents, with a functional success rate of approximately 95%.[24] If resectability is in doubt, exploration is the most reliable method for assessing the extent of disease.

H. Intraoperative Strategy for Resectable Disease

Our initial operative procedure usually begins with laparoscopy to rule out carcinomatosis or extensive local tumor spread. Laparoscopy can spare at least 40% of patients an immediate laparotomy.[20] If extrahepatic disease is discovered, the decision is then whether to proceed with operative palliation or percutaneous decompression. If percutaneous stents had been placed preoperatively, the latter is chosen and expandable metal stents can be placed without formal laparotomy.

After laparoscopy, a laparotomy is performed if this option is chosen. After abdominal exploration, cholecystectomy is done, permitting better access to the porta hepatis. The hilar plate is dropped for full exposure of the bifurcation of the hepatic ducts. Resection usually begins at the distal duct, dissecting circumferentially to free it from the portal vein and the hepatic artery. After the Kocher maneuver has been performed, the foramen of Winslow is opened to assess retroperitoneal tumor growth. Lymph nodes in the extrahepatic tissues, including those outside the planned resection site, such as the celiac and paraaortic nodes, are sampled.

With the completion of intraoperative staging the therapeutic options to be considered are resection with curative intent by skeletonization of the hepatoduodenal ligament, possibly with partial hepatectomy; palliative resection with hepati-

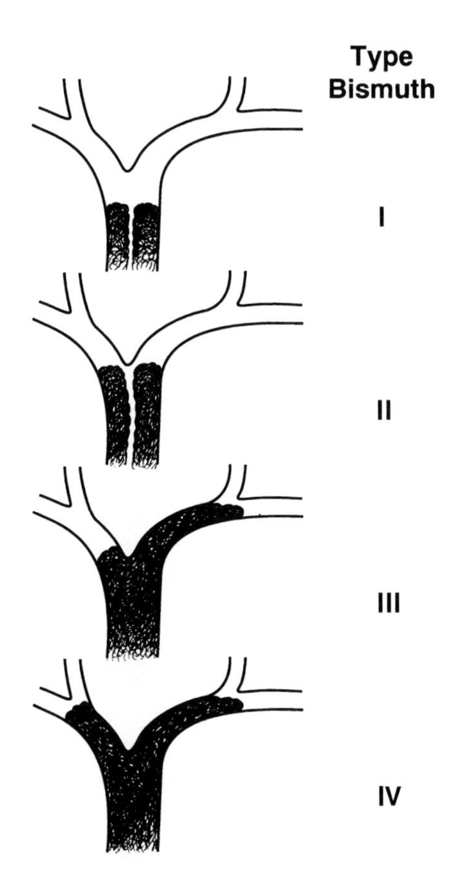

FIGURE 33–1
Classification of proximal bile duct cancer. (Reprinted with permission of the Lahey Clinic, Burlington, MA.)

TABLE 33–3.
AJCC definition of TNM and stage grouping for extrahepatic bile duct cancer

Primary Tumor (T)	
TX	Primary tumor cannot be assessed
T0	No evidence of primary tumor
Tis	Carcinoma *in situ*
T1	Tumor invades subepithelial connective tissue or fibromuscular layer
T1a	Tumor invades subepithelial connective tissue
T1b	Tumor invades fibromuscular layer
T2	Tumor invades perifibromuscular connective tissue
T3	Tumor invades adjacent structure(s): liver, pancreas, duodenum, gallbladder, colon, stomach
Regional Lymph Nodes (N)	
NX	Regional lymph nodes cannot be assessed
N0	No regional lymph node metastasis
N1	Metastasis in cystic duct, pericholedochal and/or hilar lymph nodes (i.e., in the hepatoduodenal ligament)
N2	Metastasis in peripancreatic (head only), periduodenal, periportal, celiac, and/or superior mesenteric and/or posterior pancreaticoduodenal lymph nodes
Distant Metastasis (M)	
MX	Distant metastasis cannot be assessed
M0	No distant metastasis
M1	Distant metastasis

Stage Grouping

Stage	*T*	*N*	*M*
0	Tis	N0	M0
I	T1	N0	M0
II	T2	N0	M0
III	T1	N1	M0
	T1	N2	M0
	T2	N1	M0
	T2	N2	M0
IVA	T3	Any N	M0
IVB	Any T	Any N	M1

[a] Sarcomas and carcinoid tumos are not included.
SOURCE: Used with permission of the American Joint Committee on Cancer (AJCC®), Chicago, IL. The original source for this material is the AJCC® Cancer Staging Manual, 5th edition (1997) published by Lippincott Williams & Wilkins Publishers, Philadelphia, PA.

cojejunostomy; palliative bypass with hepaticojejunostomy to segment III or V ducts; transtumoral intubation; and biopsy of the tumor with planned postoperative intubation. Total hepatectomy with transplantation has fallen out of favor because of limited donor resources. However, Pichlmayr et al.[25] found no significant survival differences in patients undergoing resection and those undergoing transplantation.

Bismuth I and II tumors may be managed with resection by skeletonization of the bile duct up to uninvolved proximal ducts above the bifurcation followed by bilateral hepaticojejunostomy. Resection of the caudate lobe (segment I) may prove beneficial because the caudate ducts drain at about the level of the bifurcation.[4,18,25,26] Tumor that invades anteriorly to segment IV may be resected with the bifurcation. Our technique divides the bile duct at the level of the superior border of the pancreas. The duct and the investing soft tissue and lymphatics about the hepatic artery and the portal vein are elevated cephalad. Proximal to the bifurcation, the ducts are divided and the margins assessed microscopically. If the hepatic duct is affected unilaterally or there is direct unilateral extension of tumor in the liver or vascular structures, hepatic resection in addition to the skeletonization resection is possible. If tumor has involved the bifurcation, as in a Bismuth III type tumor, extended hepatic resection with the extrahepatic biliary tree is performed. A Bismuth type IV tumor may be excised with palliative intent with bilateral hepaticojejunostomy, bypassed proximally to the segment III duct or segment V duct, intubated transhepatically, or biopsied only. The operative resection performed at the Lahey Clinic is shown in Fig. 33–2.

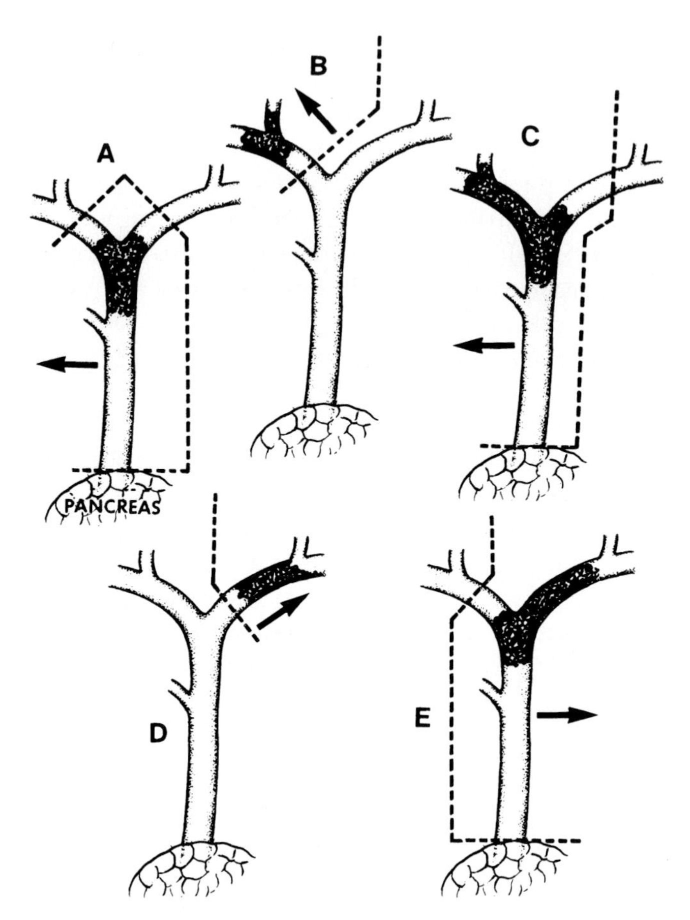

FIGURE 33–2
Various extents and locations of tumor involvement that determine therapeutic options are shown. (A) Skeletonian resection. (B, C) Extended right hepatectomy. (D, E) Left hepatectomy. (Reprinted with permission of the Lahey Clinic, Burlington, MA.)

Patients whose tumors are considered unresectable based on preoperative scans or intraoperative findings should undergo bilateral ductal stenting. The catheters may be used as access for intraluminal brachytherapy with iridium seeds or wire sources.[27–29] Hayes et al.[30] treated patients with nonresectable bile duct cancer with iridium-192 (^{192}Ir), achieving a median survival time of about 13 months. We recommend placing metal expandable intraluminal stents to achieve internal drainage regardless of whether irradiation is considered.

The use of adjuvant radiotherapy remains controversial, although many studies have shown its benefit and value as a possible adjunct. Hayes et al.[30] treated patients with unresectable bile duct cancer with ^{192}Ir, achieving a median survival of 13 months. The most significant surgical series is that of Pitt et al.[31] from Johns Hopkins, which studied the use of external beam radiation for both resected and palliated tumors. In this study survival was longest for the patients undergoing complete resection, with no significant improvement in either the length or quality of survival in patients receiving radiation.

Eschelman et al.[32] placed metal stents in 22 patients with unresectable cholangiocarcinomas or extrahepatic bile duct cancers and then added intraluminal ^{192}Ir brachytherapy (mean dose 25 Gy); external beam radiation was given in addition to ^{192}Ir in 11 patients. Patients with cholangiocarcinoma had an extended mean stent patency of 19.5 months and a mean survival of 22.6 months. In contrast, patients with extrahepatic bile duct cancers had a mean stent patency of 4.8 months and a mean survival of 5.3 months.

Milella et al.[33] treated 111 inoperable patients with cholangiocarcinoma with transhepatic stenting and external irradiation (10 patients), external and brachytherapy irradiation (12 patients), or no further treatment (89 patients). Patients treated with combined external and intraluminal irradiation had the longest survival and best quality of life. In contrast, Roayaie et al.[34] found no benefit when adjuvant chemotherapy and radiation were administered, but this therapy was given only to patients with positive margins, nodal metastases, or unresectable disease.

Currently, we do not advise adjuvant irradiation following complete resection with negative margins and nodes. If the tumor is unresectable, there may be a survival advantage with stenting with or without irradiation compared to no treatment at all. We have adopted a strategy of palliation with intraluminal expandable metal stents and high dose intraluminal brachytherapy of 15 Gy delivered at 1.0 cm in conjunction with 4500 cGy external beam radiation.

Chemotherapy has produced disappointing results for patients with biliary carcinoma. The most commonly used agents are 5-fluorouracil (5-FU), mitomycin C, adriamycin, and intraarterial floxuridine (FUDR) infusion, which offers a partial response of up to 30% without improvement in survival.[6,15,28]

Carcinoma of the proximal biliary tree is slow-growing but relentless and allows few patients a chance of cure. Resective procedures, whether for cure or palliation, offer the longest, least complicated survival.[2,18,35] As elusive as cure remains, surgery in combination with stenting and irradiation may afford patients with cholangiocarcinoma relief from jaundice, pruritus, and cholangitis and gives them the best quality of life possible.

References

1. Emond JC, Mayes JT, Rouch DA, Thistlethwaite JR, Broelsch CE. Experience with radial resection in the management of proximal bile duct cancer. HPB Surg 1989;1:297–307.
2. Pinson CW, Rossi RL. Extended right hepatic lobectomy, left hepatic lobectomy, and skeletonization resection for proximal bile duct cancer. World J Surg 1988;12:52–59.
3. Rossi RL, Gagner M, Heiss FW, Shea JA. Resective operations for biliary carcinoma. Jpn J Surg 1990;20:613–619.
4. Pichlmayer R, Weimann A, Kempnauer J, et al. Surgical treatment in proximal bile duct cancer: a single-center experience. Ann Surg 1996;224:628–638.
5. Yeo CJ. Bile duct cancer. In Cameron JL (ed) Current Surgical Therapy, 5th ed. St. Louis: Mosby-Year Book, 1995:380–385.
6. Gallinger S, Gluckman D, Langer B. Proximal bile duct cancer. Adv Surg 1990;23:89–118.
7. Yeo CJ, Pitt HA, Cameron JL. Cholangiocarcinoma. Surg Clin North Am 1990;70:1429–1447.
8. Kuvshinoff BW, Fong Y, Blumgart LH. Proximal bile duct tumors. Surg Oncol Clin N Am 1996;5:317–336.
9. Gardner B. Resection of proximal bile duct cancer involving hepatic artery with five-year survival. N J Med 1989;86:797–799.
10. Altemeier WA, Gall EA, Zinninger MM, Hoxworth PI. Sclerosing carcinoma of the major intrahepatic bile ducts. Arch Surg 1957;75:450–461.
11. Klatskin G. Adenocarcinoma of the hepatic duct at its bifurcation within the porta hepatis: an unusual tumor with destructive clinical and pathological features. Am J Med 1965;38:241–256.
12. Boerma EJ. Research into the results of resection of hilar bile duct cancer. Surgery 1990;108:572–580.
13. Lai EC, Tompkins RK, Roslyn JJ, Mann LL. Proximal bile duct cancer: quality of survival. Ann Surg 1987;205:111–118.
14. Callery MP, Meyers WC. Bile duct cancer. In: Cameron JL (ed) Current Surgical Therapy, 6th ed. St. Louis: Mosby-Year Book, 1998:455–461.
15. Broe PJ, Cameron JL. The management of proximal biliary tract tumors. Adv Surg 1981;15:47–91.
16. Engels JT, Balfe DM, Lee JK. Biliary carcinoma: CT evaluation of extrahepatic spread. Radiology 1989;172:35–40.
17. Beazley RM, Hadjis N, Benjamin IS, Blumgart LH. Clinicopathological aspects of high bile duct cancer: experience with resection and bypass surgical treatments. Ann Surg 1984;199:623–636.
18. Nimura Y. Hepatectomy for proximal bile duct cancer. In: Braasch JW, Tompkins RK (eds) Surgical Disease of the Biliary Tract and Pancreas: Multidisciplinary Management. St. Louis: Mosby-Year Book, 1994:251–264.
19. Su CH, Tsay SH, Wu CC, et al. Factors influencing postoperative morbidity, mortality, and survival after resection for hilar cholangiocarcinoma. Ann Surg 1996;223:384–394.
20. Nieveen van Dijkum EJ, de Wit LT, van Delden OM, et al. The efficacy of laparoscopic staging in patients with upper gastrointestinal tumors. Cancer 1997;79:1315–1319.
21. Bismuth H, Castaing D, Traynor O. Resection or palliation: priority of surgery in the treatment of hilar cancer. World J Surg 1988;12:39–47.
22. Wilker DK, Izbicki JR, Rohloff R, Knoefel WT, Mandelkow H, Schweiberer L. Is aggressive surgical palliation of proximal bile duct cancer with involvement of both main hepatic ducts worthwhile? HPB Surg 1992;5:235–249.
23. Grove MK, Hermann RE, Vogt DP, Broughan TA. Role of radiation after operative palliation in cancer of the proximal bile ducts. Am J Surg 1991;161:454–458.
24. Wagner HJ, Knyrim K. Relief of malignant obstructive jaundice by endoscopic or percutaneous insertion of metal stents. Bildgebung 1993;60:76–82.
25. Pichlmayer R, Ringe B, Lauchart W, Bechstein WO, Gubernatis G, Wagner E. Radical resection and liver grafting as the two main components of surgical strategy in the treatment of proximal bile duct cancer. World J Surg 1988;12:68–77.
26. Taat CW, van Lanschot JJ, Gouma DJ, Obertop H. Role of extended lymph node dissection in the treatment of gastrointestinal tumours: a review of the literature. Scand J Gastroenterol 1995;30(suppl 212):109–116.
27. Alden ME, Waterman FM, Topham AK, Barbot DJ, Shapiro MJ, Mohiuddin M. Cholangiocarcinoma: clinical significance of tumor location along the extrahepatic bile duct. Radiology 1995;197:511–516.
28. Fortner JG, Vitelli CE, Maclean BJ. Proximal extrahepatic bile duct tumors: analysis of a series of 52 consecutive patients treated over a period of 13 years. Arch Surg 1989;143:1275–1279.
29. Minsky B, Botet J, Gerdes H, Lightdale C. Ultrasound directed extrahepatic bile duct intraluminal brachytherapy. Int J Radiat Oncol Biol Phys 1992;23P:165–167.
30. Hayes JK Jr, Sapozink MD, Miller FJ. Definitive radiation therapy in bile duct carcinoma. Int J Radiat Oncol Biol Phys 1988;15:735–744.
31. Pitt HA, Nakeeb A, Abrams RA, et al. Perihilar cholangiocarcinoma: postoperative radiotherapy does not improve survival. Ann Surg 1995;221:788–798.
32. Eschelman DJ, Shapiro MJ, Bonn J, et al. Malignant biliary duct obstruction: long-term experience with Gianturco stents and combined-modality radiation therapy. Radiology 1996;200:717–724.
33. Milella M, Salvetti M, Cerrotta A, et al. Interventional radiology and radiotherapy for inoperable cholangiocarcinoma of the extrahepatic bile ducts. Tumori 1998;84:467–471.
34. Roayaie S, Guarrera JV, Ye MQ, et al. Aggressive surgical treatment of intrahepatic cholangiocarcinoma: predictors of outcomes. J Am Coll Surg 1998;187:365–372.
35. Rossi RL, Heiss FW, Beckmann CF, Braasch JW. Management of cancer of the bile duct. Surg Clin North Am 1995;65:59–78.

Chapter 34

Cancer of the Gallbladder

Daniel J. Deziel

Gallbladder cancer occurs in 6000–7000 new patients each year in the United States.[1] Approximately 90% of these tumors are adenocarcinomas. Occasional histologic variants include anaplastic, adenosquamous, squamous, neuroendocrine, or undifferentiated carcinomas. Other malignancies such as melanoma, sarcoma, and lymphoma may rarely occur. Gallbladder cancer spreads by local growth into the liver and adjacent viscera; through lymphatic drainage to the hepatoduodenal, pancreatic, celiac, mesenteric, and periaortic nodes; through venous drainage to the liver and hepatoduodenal/portal circulation; and by direct peritoneal dissemination. Extraabdominal disease is generally a late occurrence. About 75% of gallbladder cancers are considered beyond the confines of curative resection when diagnosed; about 10% are limited to the gallbladder, and about 15% have locoregional spread that is resectable.[2] In a large French survey, 85% of gallbladder cancers were T3 or T4 tumors, and the overall median survival was 3 months.[3]

Epidemiologically, gallbladder cancer is three to four times more frequent in women than in men (bile duct cancer has a slight male predominance). The mean age of patients is 65 years. The incidence is high in certain populations, particularly southwest Native Americans, Mexican and Alaskan natives, northern Japanese, northeastern Europeans, Israelis, Bolivians, and Chileans. Chronic inflammation is a likely etiologic factor as evidenced by the typical association with gallstones (70–90%) and by the increased risk in individuals with large gallstones (>3 cm), a calcified gallbladder wall ("porcelain gallbladder"), cholecystoenteric fistula, xanthogranulomatous cholecystitis, and chronic typhoid bacillus infection. Gallbladder adenomas are considered premalignant, as are adenomatous polyps elsewhere in the gastrointestinal tract; the likelihood of a malignant polyp increases with size >1 cm and with the age of the patient. Gallbladder cancer is also seen in association with bile duct cysts, abnormal anatomic junctions of the pancreatic duct with the common bile duct, and ulcerative colitis. A statistical association with obesity and estrogens exists just as it does for gallstones. Finally, environmental carcinogens may play a role; workers in rubber plants may have a higher risk, and experimental studies have demonstrated that nitrosamines and azotoluene are carcinogenic.

Although gallbladder cancer can be suspected preoperatively in some patients, the diagnosis is often made during or after cholecystectomy. The prognosis depends critically on two factors: (1) the extent

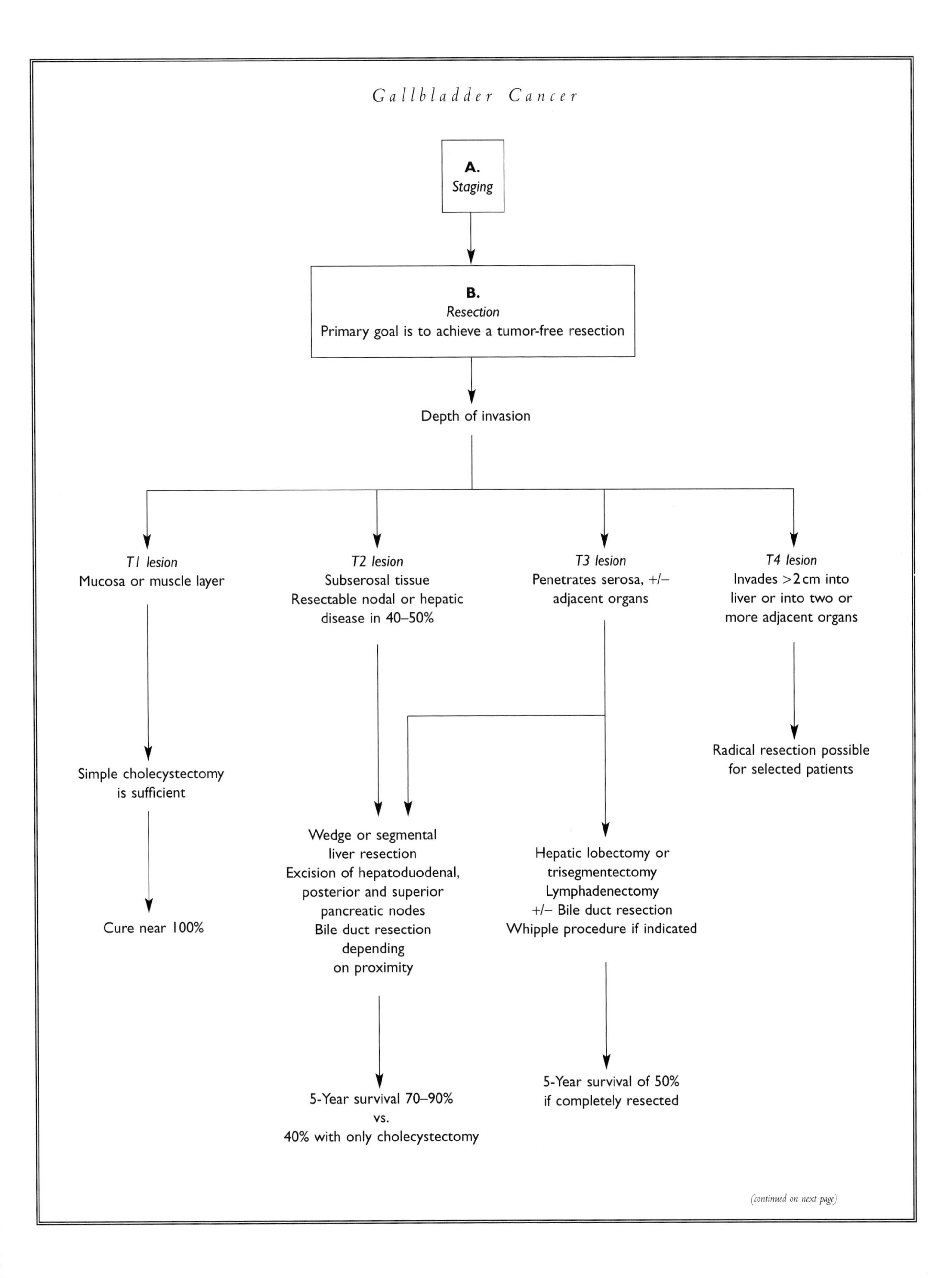

(continued on next page)

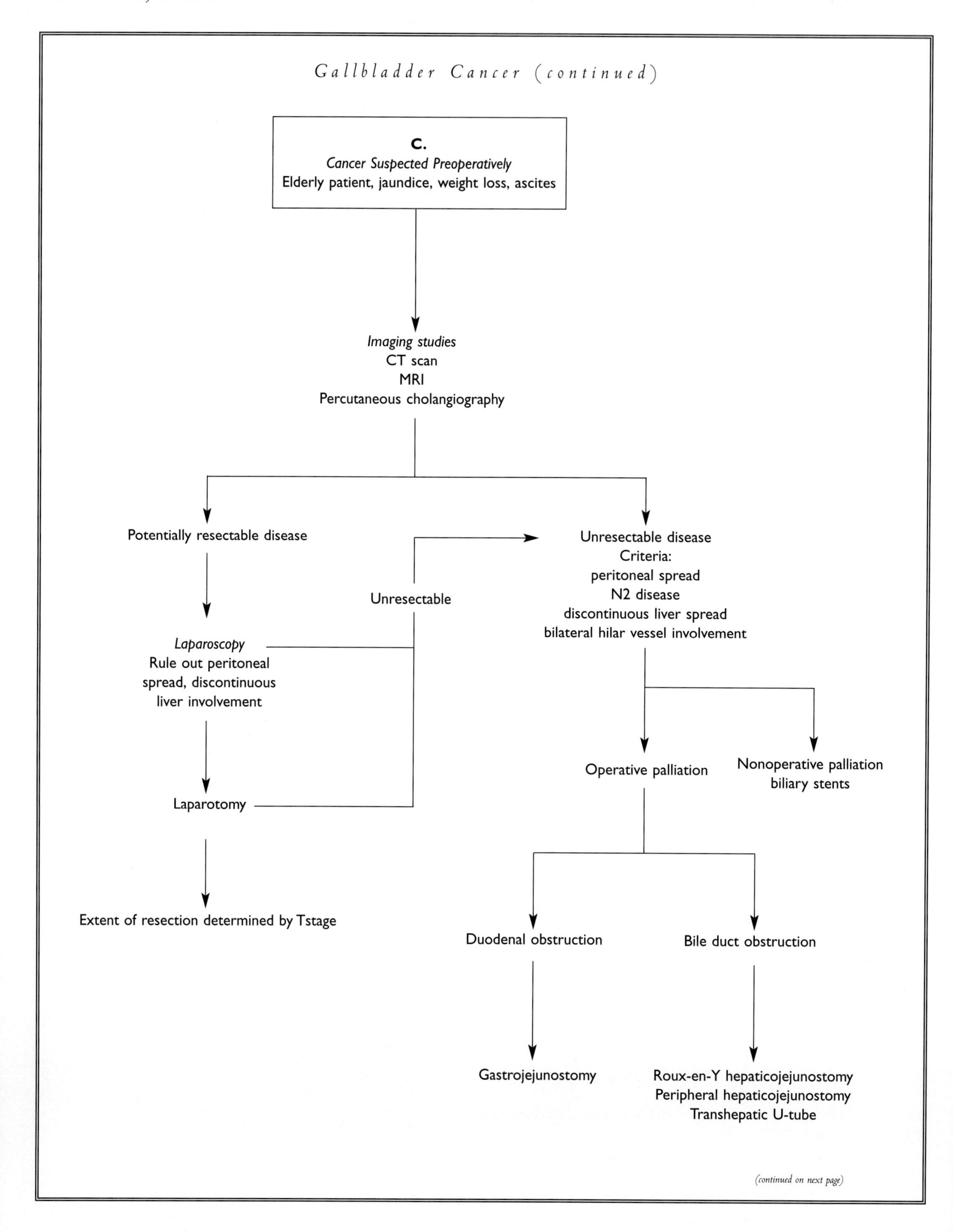

(continued on next page)

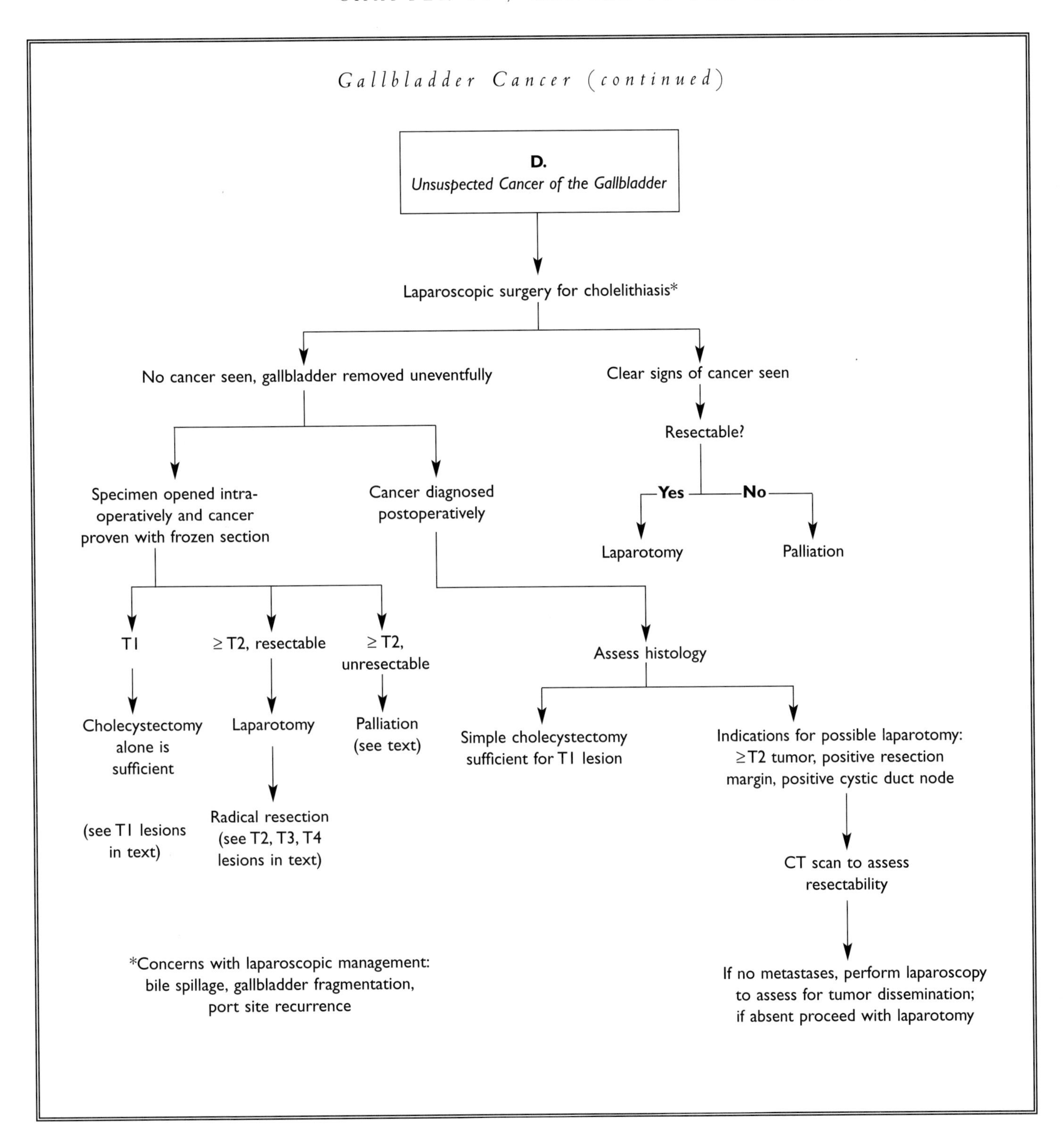

of disease at the time of diagnosis and (2) the extent of the surgical resection. Limited cancers are usually cured by cholecystectomy alone. For patients with locally advanced cancer, the appropriate extent of resection is a key determinant of outcome. Tumors that are regionally advanced or that have distant metastases are not cured by any single or combined modalities. Treatment for patients in this last group is purely palliative. For the most part, chemotherapy and radiation therapy have not been effective in the treatment of gallbladder cancer.

Most cholecystectomies are now accomplished laparoscopically. While the benefit of laparoscopic cholecystectomy has been apparent for patients with benign calculous gallbladder disease, its application to patients with possible neoplastic

TABLE 34–1.
AJCC definition of TNM and stage grouping for gallbladder cancer

Primary Tumor (T)

TX	Primary tumor cannot be assessed
T0	No evidence of primary tumor
Tis	Carcinoma *in situ*
T1	Tumor invades lamina propria or muscle layer
T1a	Tumor invades lamina propria
T1b	Tumor invades muscle layer
T2	Tumor invades perimuscular connective tissue; no extension beyond serosa or into liver
T3	Tumor perforates the serosa (visceral peritoneum) or directly invades one adjacent organ, or both (extension 2 cm or less into liver)
T4	Tumor extends more than 2 cm into liver, and/or into two or more adjacent organs (stomach, duodenum, colon, pancreas, omentum, extrahepatic bile ducts, any involvement of liver)

Regional Lymph Nodes (N)

NX	Regional lymph nodes cannot be assessed
N0	No regional lymph node metastasis
N1	Metastasis in cystic duct, pericholedochal, and/or hilar lymph nodes (i.e., in the hepatoduodenal ligament)
N2	Metastasis in peripancreatic (head only), periduodenal, periportal, celiac, and/or superior mesenteric lymph nodes

Distant Metastasis (M)

MX	Distant metastasis cannot be assessed
M0	No distant metastasis
M1	Distant metastasis

Stage Grouping

Stage	T	N	M
0	Tis	N0	M0
I	T1	N0	M0
II	T2	N0	M0
III	T1	N1	M0
	T2	N1	M0
	T3	N0	M0
	T3	N1	M0
IVA	T4	N0	M0
	T4	N1	M0
IVB	Any T	N2	M0
	Any T	Any N	M1

SOURCE: Used with permission of the American Joint Committee on Cancer (AJCC®), Chicago, IL. The original source for this material is the AJCC® Cancer Staging Manual, 5th edition (1997) published by Lippincott Williams & Wilkins Publishers, Philadelphia, PA.

lesions is much debated. The management of patients who have had gallbladder cancer diagnosed incidentally following laparoscopic cholecystectomy also poses some unresolved dilemmas.

A. *Staging*

The American Joint Commission on Cancer (AJCC) staging of gallbladder cancer is shown in Table 34–1. An understanding of the pathologic criteria for staging the primary tumor is important because the depth of tumor invasion is an essential consideration when determining which patients should undergo resection and which resection is appropriate. The normal gallbladder wall consists of epithelium, lamina propria (underlying connective tissue), lamina muscularis (a thin layer of smooth muscle), subserosal connective tissue (adventitia), and serosa. The epithelial layer and lamina propria constitute the mucosa. The wall of the gallbladder differs from that of the intestine in that it lacks muscularis mucosa and submucosa.

An earlier staging system proposed by Nevin et al.[4] and a modified version[5] are described in Table 34–2. The modified Nevin system with five stages may correlate better with survival than the AJCC system but does not differentiate between T2 and T3 lesions. It has been suggested that the AJCC system be modified to include T4N0 tumors as stage III based on the longer-term survival observed in some patients following resection of T4 tumors with negative nodes.[6] Other staging systems have been used in Japan and elsewhere.[7]

B. *Resection*

The indications for and extent of surgical resection are determined primarily by the T stage of the tumor. The goal is to achieve a tumor-free resection.

T1 Lesions

The T1 tumors are nearly always cured by cholecystectomy alone.[6,8,9] This certainly holds true for T1a lesions, which are limited to the mucosa. Although this is also probably true for most T1b tumors, which involve the muscular layer, most reports of inapparent gallbladder cancers include only a small number of T1b lesions. A small proportion of these patients may have additional disease, and there have been occasional reports of

TABLE 34–2.
Staging gallbladder cancer

Stage	Nevin system[4]	Modified Nevin system[5]
I	Intramucosal	In situ carcinoma
II	Mucosa and muscularis	Mucosal or muscularis invasion
III	All layers	Transmural invasion, direct liver invasion
IV	All layers and cystic lymph node	Lymph node metastases
V	Direct liver invasion or metastases	Distant metastases

recurrence and death following cholecystectomy alone.[10] Until more data are available, the decision to perform simple cholecystectomy or a more radical operation for a T1b gallbladder cancer should be made on an individual basis.

T2 Lesions

There is consensus that the prognosis for patients with T2 tumors (subserosal connective tissue) can be improved by more radical resection.[6,9,11–13] Optimal treatment includes en bloc resection of the adjacent liver and lymphadenectomy of the hepatoduodenal and posterosuperior pancreatic nodes with or without resection of the common bile duct. Traditionally, a nonanatomic wedge resection of 2–3 cm of liver adjacent to the gallbladder fossa has been described. A segment-oriented liver resection of anatomic segments IVb and V may be oncologically preferable and is simple and safe when performed by experienced surgeons.[6] Bile duct resection should be considered when the tumor is located in proximity to the common hepatic duct or common bile duct. Bile duct resection may also be necessary in reoperative cases where inflammation and fibrosis along the hepatoduodenal ligament render identification of uninvolved margins difficult; however, bile duct resection has more operative morbidity.[6] About 40–50% of patients undergoing radical resection of T2 tumors have resectable nodal or hepatic disease.[6,9,14,15] The 15-year survival rate for T2 gallbladder cancer treated by radical resection is 70–90% compared to 40% when treated by cholecystectomy alone.[6,9]

T3 Lesions

Most patients with T3 tumors have residual disease after cholecystectomy, and essentially none is cured by removing the gallbladder alone. The surgical approach is similar to that for T2 lesions. The need to perform an extended liver resection (lobectomy or trisegmentectomy) depends on the status of the vessels at the hepatic hilum in terms of tumor involvement or difficulty of dissection. At more advanced T stages, a larger proportion of tumors are unresectable due to metastatic or nodal disease; nonetheless, 5-year survival rates of 50% or more have been obtained for patients with T3 tumors that are completely resected.[6,11,12]

T4 Lesions

Extended resections for T4 tumors are controversial. Formal hepatic lobectomy or trisegmentectomy is typically required, and pancreaticoduodenectomy may be necessary for duodenal invasion; however, few patients with T4 disease are suitable for such resections. Many of these tumors are unresectable due to metastatic disease, or co-morbid conditions may render the patient physiologically unfit for a major resection. Although there is no predictable 5-year survival following resection of T4 tumors, some longevity has been obtained.[6,9,11] The prognosis may be particularly favorable for patients with bulky disease but negative lymph nodes.[6]

Whether patients with gallbladder cancer benefit from radical resection if they have nodal disease is incompletely settled. Shirai et al. reported 5-year survival rates of 85% for patients with negative nodes and 45% for positive nodes.[16] Among the node-positive patients, survival was 69% when complete resection was accomplished but 0% when there was microscopic or macroscopic residual disease. Thus resection appears beneficial for node-positive patients provided complete resection is possible. Others have demonstrated improved survival for patients with N1 disease but have failed to demonstrate survival benefit when N2 disease was present.[6,12]

C. *Cancer Suspected Preoperatively*

The clinical presentation of gallbladder cancer largely determines the initial management. Malignant disease may be suspected preoperatively in patients with jaundice, abnormal imaging studies (mass, thickened gallbladder wall), or manifestations of advanced malignancy including systemic symptoms of malaise and weight loss and abdominal findings such as ascites, a palpable mass, or gastrointestinal obstruction or bleeding.[17] Malignancy should particularly be considered when elderly patients exhibit these features.

Imaging Studies

If a biliary tract malignancy is suspected, a high quality, contrast-enhanced CT scan is usually obtained. Magnetic resonance imaging can also be useful for assessing the extent of ductal or vascular involvement.[18] Percutaneous transhepatic cholangiography may be necessary to define the proximal extent of duct involvement. Angiography is not typically necessary.

Laparoscopy

If imaging studies demonstrate potentially resectable disease and the patient is physiologically fit for the resection required, an operation is performed. Laparoscopic cholecystectomy is not indicated if gallbladder cancer is suspected, but laparoscopy can be performed prior to laparotomy to identify peritoneal or hepatic spread not detectable by preoperative scans.[19] Gallbladder cancers have a greater propensity for peritoneal spread than do bile duct cancers. Laparoscopy is logical only if it can minimize the rate of *nontherapeutic* laparotomies. If laparotomy is needed (even if for *palliation* of unresectable disease), laparoscopy is unnecessary.

Laparotomy

The tumor is assessed at laparotomy to determine if it is completely resectable. Criteria of unresectability include peritoneal spread, N2 disease, discontinuous liver metastases, and bilateral involvement of the hilar vessels. Intraoperative ultrasonography has proved valuable for evaluating the extent of hepatic involvement.[20]

Palliation

When operative evaluation demonstrates unresectable disease, whether a palliative procedure is required and the optimum method of palliation should be determined. Patients with unresectable gallbladder cancer have limited life expectancy, so the least morbid means of palliation is preferred. When unresectable gallbladder cancer results in bile duct obstruction, the site of obstruction is usually high and surgical access to the hilum of the liver may be difficult if not impossible. A Roux-en-Y hepaticojejunostomy to the left hepatic duct in segment III of the liver or peripheral hepaticojejunostomy can be an effective solution to this problem.[21,22] Operatively placed transhepatic U-tubes can also provide durable, safe decompression.[23] Cholecystojejunostomy is not appropriate for gallbladder cancers, although it is useful for many patients with unresectable malignant obstruction of the distal common bile duct.

Patients with established or impending duodenal obstruction from a tumor are treated by gastrojejunostomy. Limited experience has been reported with endoscopic deployment of metal stents for palliation of malignant duodenal obstruction.

The surgeon may choose to rely on biliary stents placed nonoperatively by endoscopic or percutaneous approaches for definitive biliary decompression in a patient with unresectable biliary tract cancer. This is particularly applicable when functioning stents have been placed preoperatively or when surgical anastomosis or intubation of the bile duct is not feasible.

Patients who are physiologically unfit to undergo a major operation or who have advanced unresectable disease (determined by preoperative imaging studies) receive palliative treatment. Bile duct obstruction is treated by endoscopic or percutaneous stent placement. *Endoscopic stents* are associated with a lower rate of early complications but are less often successful in traversing proximal sites of obstruction compared to *transhepatic stents*. All nonoperative biliary stents are associated with more frequent problems of occlusion, cholangitis, and recurrent jaundice; and they produce a greater need for subsequent interventions and hospitalizations than do surgically created biliary enteric anastomoses. However, nonoperative stents are preferable to the morbidity of operative intervention in patients with known unresectable proximal malignant obstruction and limited anticipated survival. Pain is managed by narcotic analgesics, percutaneous celiac nerve block, and occasionally irradiation.

Radiation treatment and chemotherapy can be considered on an individual basis for patients with unresectable disease but have had little demonstrable efficacy in the treatment of gallbladder cancer. These modalities cannot substitute for effective mechanical decompression of biliary obstruction.

D. Unsuspected Cancer of the Gallbladder

Gallbladder cancer is most frequently discovered unexpectedly at the time of cholecystectomy for benign disease or during postoperative histologic examination of the gallbladder specimen. When a gallbladder has been removed, the surgeon should always open the specimen in the operating room to inspect it visually and palpably. Frozen sections should be obtained from any unusual mass or mucosal lesions. If cancer is identified, the decision to perform additional resection at the time is determined by the apparent T stage of the tumor, the condition of the patient, and the capability of the surgeon. Ideally, definitive resection at that time would be preferred for technical reasons and would spare the patient a second operation, but there are issues regarding informed consent. Reoperative procedures are more difficult owing to postoperative inflammatory changes and are more likely to necessitate a major liver or bile duct resection. If the tumor appears to be a T1 lesion, the procedure is terminated to await permanent sections. The liver and peritoneal surfaces should be inspected and the hepatoduodenal ligament and hilum palpated if the cholecystectomy was performed via an open approach. If the operative findings suggest malignancy prior to cholecystectomy and the surgeon is not capable of performing a definitive resection (if indicated), the procedure should be concluded without biopsy.[24] Biopsy risks tumor dissemination and may prohibit definitive resection for which the patient should be referred.

When a cancer of the gallbladder is diagnosed by postoperative histology, the pertinent issue is whether reoperation for a more radical resection should be performed. If the patient is not physiologically fit for such resection, the issue is null. For operable patients, a second operation should be considered for histologic findings of: (1) a T2 or deeper lesion; (2) positive cystic duct node; (3) positive cystic duct margin. Depth of invasion is the best indicator for reoperation. Shirai et al. identified a cystic duct node in 36 of 98 gallbladder specimens with inapparent cancer.[9] Reoperation was proposed for patients with cystic node metastases based on the observation that no patient with a positive node survived 5 years following cholecystectomy, whereas the 5-year survival was 84% for patients without metastases to the cystic duct node. Thus involvement of the cystic duct node can be considered a marker for residual disease potentially amenable to curative resection. A positive surgical margin is an indicator for reoperation regardless of tumor depth. Resection of the extrahepatic bile duct should be anticipated for patients with a positive cystic duct margin.

Prior to a second operation for radical resection, a high quality computed tomography (CT) scan is advisable to rule out liver metastases. Postoperative inflammatory changes complicate dissection of the hepatic hilum and hepatoduodenal ligament. Benign fibrosis may not be grossly distinguishable from malignancy; second operations for definitive resection are therefore more likely to require bile duct resection or extended hepatic resection to ensure tumor clearance.

The management of inapparent cancer diagnosed in gallbladders removed laparoscopically is problematic. Bile or stone spillage occurs during a substantial proportion of laparoscopic cholecystectomies and may not be documented. Spillage may result in early peritoneal dissemination and death of patients with otherwise curable tumors.[24–26] There is no effective therapy for peritoneal metastases from gallbladder cancer. Tumor recurrence at laparoscopic port sites is another concern, as it has typically indicated a fatal outcome.[15,24,25,27,28] Such recurrence has not been limited to the port site from which the specimen was extracted, implicating potential tumor contamination of other sites from laparoscopic instruments or uncharacterized oncologic effects of the pneumoperitoneum. Excision of port sites has been recommended during reoperation. There is little indication that it has been widely practiced, however, and there are no available data regarding its efficacy. There is a tendency to leave longer cystic duct stumps during laparoscopic cholecystectomy than during traditional open cholecystectomy. This practice has fostered concern that the cystic duct margin should be removed laparoscopically.[27] Because of the possibility of peritoneal spread, laparoscopy may be particularly useful prior to laparotomy for patients being considered for resection after laparoscopic cholecystectomy.

Currently, the possibility of gallbladder cancer is considered a contraindication to laparoscopic cholecystectomy. This contraindication includes polypoid lesions of the gallbladder >1 cm in size, which have a higher risk of harboring malignancy. Certainly, laparoscopic cholecystectomy can be curative for benign polyps and early T1a cancers.[15,28,29] However, spillage of gallbladder contents during laparoscopic cholecystectomy is predictably common and is not necessarily preventable. The oncologic consequences of laparoscopic events can be deadly. Furthermore, the long-term results of reoperation for radical resection of gallbladder cancer removed laparoscopically are not yet known.

References

1. Landis SH, Murray T, Bolden S, et al. Cancer statistics, 1998. CA Cancer J Clin 1998;48:6–29.
2. Adson M. Carcinoma of the gallbladder. In: Moody FG (ed) Advances in Diagnosis and Surgical Treatment of Biliary Tract Disease. Chicago: Year Book, 1983.
3. Cubertafond P, Gainant A, Cucchiaro G. Surgical treatment of 724 carcinomas of the gallbladder: results of the French Surgical Association survey. Ann Surg 1994;219:275–280.
4. Nevin J, Moran T, Kay S, et al. Carcinoma of the gallbladder: staging, treatment, and prognosis. Cancer 1976;31:141–148.
5. Donahue J, Nagorney D, Grant C, et al. Carcinoma of the gallbladder: does radical resection improve outcome? Arch Surg 1990;125:237–241.
6. Bartlett D, Fong Y, Fortner J, et al. Long-term results after resection for gallbladder cancer: implications for staging and management. Ann Surg 1996;224:639–646.
7. Yamaguchi K, Enjoji M. Carcinoma of the gallbladder: a clinicopathology of 103 patients and a newly proposed staging. Cancer 1988;62:1425–1432.
8. Yamaguchi K, Tsuneyoshi M. Subclinical gallbladder carcinoma. Am J Surg 1992;163:382–386.
9. Shirai Y, Yoshida K, Tsukada K, et al. Inapparent carcinoma of the gallbladder: an appraisal of a radical second operation after simple cholecystectomy. Ann Surg 1992;215:326–331.
10. Kimura W, Shimada H. A case of gallbladder carcinoma with infiltration into the muscular layer that resulted in relapse and death from metastasis to the liver and lymph nodes. Hepatogastroenterology 1990;37:86–89.
11. Matsumoto Y, Fujii H, Aoyama H, et al. Surgical treatment of primary carcinoma of the gallbladder based on the histologic analysis of 48 surgical specimens. Am J Surg 1992;163:239–245.
12. Chijiwa K, Tanaka M. Carcinoma of the gallbladder: an appraisal of surgical resection. Surgery 1994;115:751–756.
13. Ouchi K, Suzuki M, Saijo S, et al. Do recent advances in diagnosis and operative management improve the outcome of gallbladder carcinoma? Surgery 1993;113:324–329.
14. De Aretxabala X, Roa I, Araya JC, et al. Operative findings in patients with early forms of gallbladder cancer. Br J Surg 1990;77:291–293.
15. Suzuki K, Kimura T, Ogawa H. Is laparoscopic cholecystectomy hazardous for gallbladder cancer? Surgery 1998;123:311–314.
16. Shirai Y, Yoshida K, Tsukada K, et al. Radical surgery for gallbladder carcinoma: long-term results. Ann Surg 1992;216:565–568.
17. Piehler J, Crichlow R. Primary carcinoma of the gallbladder. Arch Surg 1977:112:26–30.
18. Sagoh T, Itoh K, Togashi K, et al. Gallbladder carcinoma: evaluation with MR imaging. Radiology 1990;174:131–136.
19. Callery MP, Strasberg SM, Doherty GM, et al. Staging laparoscopy with laparoscopic ultrasonography: optimizing resectability in hepatobiliary and pancreatic malignancy. J Am Coll Surg 1997;185:33–39.
20. Clarke MP, Kane RA, Steele G. Prospective comparison of preoperative imaging and intraoperative ultrasonography in the detection of liver tumors. Surgery 1989;106:849–855.
21. Dudley S, Edis AJ, Adson MA. Biliary decompression in hilar obstruction: round ligament approach. Arch Surg 1979;114:519–522.
22. Schlitt H, Weimann A, Klempnauer J, et al. Peripheral hepatojejunostomy as palliative treatment for irresectable malignant tumors of the liver hilum. Ann Surg 1999;229:181–186.
23. Millikan KW, Gleason TG, Deziel DJ, et al. The current role of U-tubes for benign and malignant biliary obstruction. Ann Surg 1993;218:621–629.
24. Fong Y, Brennan M, Turnball A, et al. Gallbladder cancer discovered during laparoscopic surgery: potential for iatrogenic tumor dissemination. Arch Surg 1993;128:1054–1056.
25. Wibbenmeyer L, Wade T, Chen R, et al. Laparoscopic cholecystectomy can disseminate in situ carcinoma of the gallbladder. J Am Coll Surg 1995;181:504–510.
26. Ohtani T, Tankano Y, Shirai Y, et al. Early intraperitoneal dissemination after radical resection of unsuspected gallbladder carcinoma following laparoscopic cholecystectomy. Surg Laparosc Endosc 1998;8:58–62.
27. Shirai Y, Ohtani T, Hatakeyama K. Is laparoscopic cholecystectomy indicated for early gallbladder cancer? Surgery 1997;122:120–121.
28. Yamaguchi K, Chijiiwa K, Ichimiya H, et al. Gallbladder carcinoma in the era of laparoscopic cholecystectomy. Arch Surg 1996;131:981–984.
29. Kubota K, Yasutsugu B, Noie T, et al. How should polypoid lesions of the gallbladder be treated in the era of laparoscopic cholecystectomy? Surgery 1995;117:481–487.

CHAPTER 35

Hepatocellular Cancer

PIERRE F. SALDINGER
YUMAN FONG

Hepatocellular cancer (HCC) is the most prevalent cancer worldwide, killing an estimated 1.25 million people annually. The incidence has nearly doubled in the United States since the 1980s, although it remains more common in such areas as Japan, Southeast Asia and Sub-Saharan Africa. There does not appear to be a genetic basis for the increased susceptibility in certain geographic areas; rather, risk is related to environmental exposure. Chronic liver disease of any type increases the risk of HCC, with infection with hepatitis B and C virus being the best known and documented in the United States. These two viruses are independent risk factors but may act synergistically. Other risk factors include alcoholic cirrhosis, repeated ingestion of aflatoxin (wheat, soybeans, corn, rice, oats, bread, milk, cheese, peanuts), androgenic steroids, parasites, α_1-antitrypsin deficiency, and possible oral contraceptives.

Once a high risk patient has been identified, a screening program consisting of periodic ultrasonographic scans and serum α-fetoprotein (AFP) determinations has been advised by the National Institutes of Health. Whereas ultrasonography is useful as a screening tool, computed tomography (CT) scanning is the procedure of choice for further study of mass lesions. Magnetic resonance imaging (MRI) is preferred by many, and arteriography is reserved for situations where vascular encasement is suspected or arterial anatomy is to be studied prior to resection.

The care of patients with HCC is a challenging task for gastroenterologists, oncologists, interventional radiologists, and surgeons. Surgical excision remains the therapy of choice, but it can be offered only to certain patients who suffer from this disease. Ablative therapy and transplantation are available options for those who are not surgical candidates because of limited hepatic reserve. Patients with HCC often have some degree of liver insufficiency and cirrhosis and are therefore best managed by a multidisciplinary team. The range of treatment options that can be offered to the patient directly depend on the patient's liver function and extent of tumor.

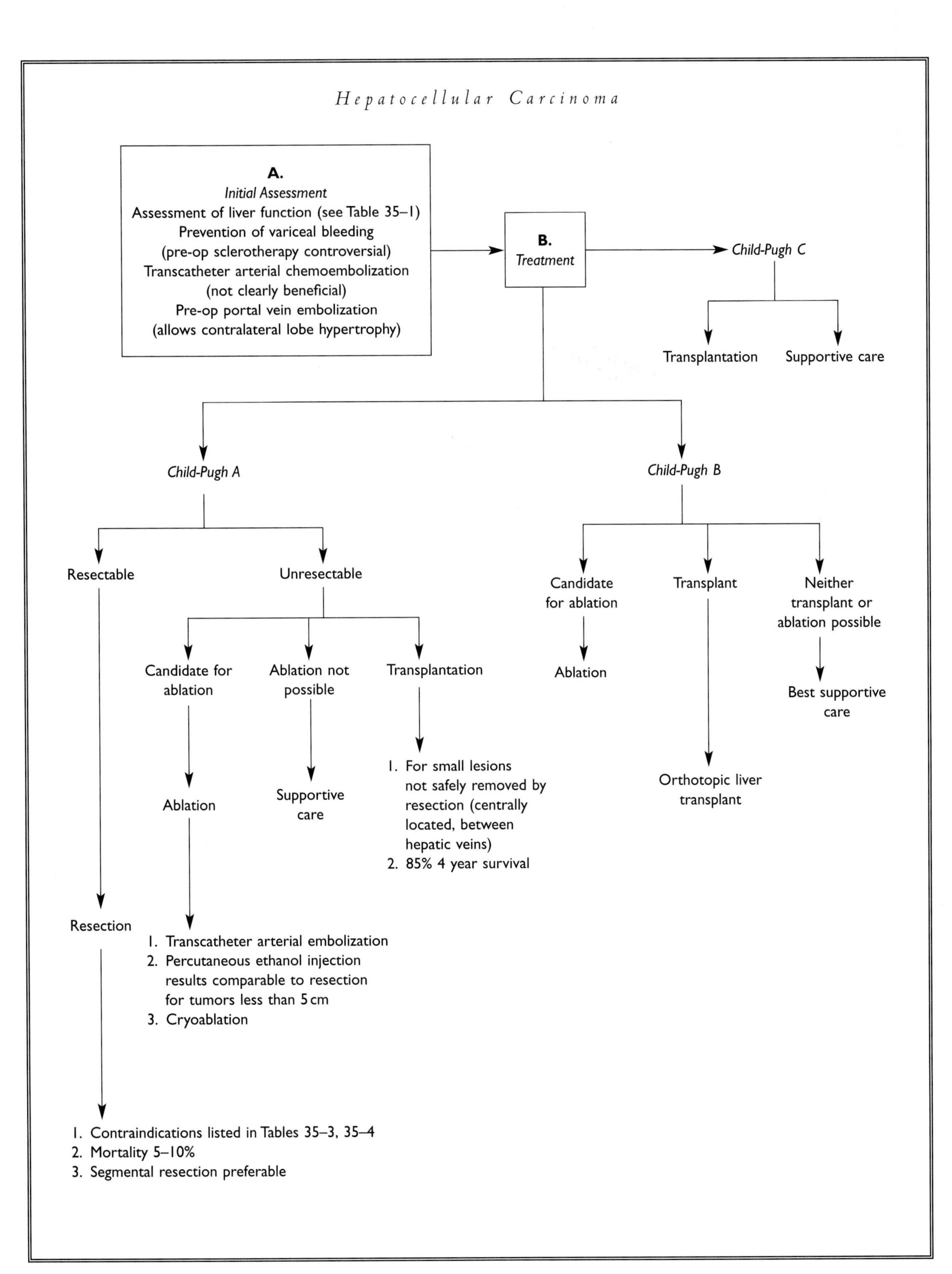
Hepatocellular Carcinoma
A.
Initial Assessment
Assessment of liver function (see Table 35–1)
Prevention of variceal bleeding
(pre-op sclerotherapy controversial)
Transcatheter arterial chemoembolization
(not clearly beneficial)
Pre-op portal vein embolization
(allows contralateral lobe hypertrophy)
B.
Treatment
Child-Pugh C
Transplantation
Supportive care
Child-Pugh A
Child-Pugh B
Resectable
Unresectable
Candidate for ablation
Ablation not possible
Transplantation
Ablation
Supportive care
1. For small lesions not safely removed by resection (centrally located, between hepatic veins)
2. 85% 4 year survival
Resection
1. Transcatheter arterial embolization
2. Percutaneous ethanol injection results comparable to resection for tumors less than 5 cm
3. Cryoablation
1. Contraindications listed in Tables 35–3, 35–4
2. Mortality 5–10%
3. Segmental resection preferable
Candidate for ablation
Transplant
Neither transplant or ablation possible
Ablation
Best supportive care
Orthotopic liver transplant

TABLE 35–1.
Preoperative tests for evaluation of liver reserve

Preoperative assessment of liver function	References
Child-Pugh grading	3, 5–9
Serum alanine transferase	8
Indocyanine green clearance test	1, 5, 7, 10
Amino acid clearance test	1
Aminopyrine breath test	1, 5
Urea nitrogen synthesis	4
Portal pressure	11

A. *Initial Assessment*

Assessment of Liver Function

Patients with HCC can present with different stages of liver function, ranging from normal liver function and intact parenchyma to liver insufficiency and advanced cirrhosis. Mortality and long-term morbidity after resection or ablation are usually related to underlying cirrhosis and progressive liver failure.[1–5] Careful assessment of liver function prior to any therapeutic intervention is essential to identify patients for whom surgical intervention carries prohibitive risk. Therefore a variety of tests are used to evaluate liver function reserve (Table 35–1). Most investigators use the Child-Pugh score (Table 35–2) or modifications thereof to evaluate the functional reserve of patients with HCC. Child-Pugh grading generally overestimates the functional reserve, as most of the parameters are not directly linked to liver function or are difficult to assess objectively. Serum albumin can be influenced by many factors other than just the synthetic capacity of the liver, whereas encephalopathy and ascites are difficult to quantify objectively, especially in borderline cases. Serum bilirubin is the only variable in the Child-Pugh grading that reflects liver function in a constant fashion. A Child-Pugh score of more than 8 is generally accepted as a contraindication for major hepatic resection.[6] The Child-Pugh classification fails to identify patients who, despite a favorable score, may experience significant alteration in liver function postoperatively. As many as 50% of Child's A patients can develop liver failure after resection, some of whom never recover.[11] Despite its lack of accuracy, the Child-Pugh classification remains the most commonly used and useful means for assessing liver function.

Several authors have used other tests to improve the ability to predict whether patients can sustain a major hepatic resection. Indocyanine green (ICG) clearance can be added to the preoperative assessment[13,14] to further classify Child's A patients. The ICG clearance of Child's A patients varies widely, and increased retention has correlated with hospital mortality in some studies.[5,7,15] The aminopyrine breath test and the amino acid clearance test do not have the same discriminative power in Child's A patients.[1] One study showed that twofold elevation of serum alanine transferase (ALT) is associated with a marked increase in morbidity and mortality in Child's A patients.[8] Urea nitrogen synthesis rate can also be used to assess Child's A and B patients.[4] A promising but more invasive method is measurement of the hepatic portal venous pressure gradient. Bruix et al. found that all patients who had a pressure gradient of more than 10 mm Hg preoperatively developed decompensated liver failure after resection.[11] This was the only significant predictor of hepatic failure in a multivariate analysis. Serum bilirubin, blood urea nitrogen, platelet count, and IGG clearance were significant predictors in a univariate analysis only. Interestingly, the preoperative mean bilirubin concentration of both groups, though different, were within normal limits. This clearly indicates that a normal bilirubin does not necessarily place a patient in a low risk category.

Active inflammation of the liver secondary to infection with hepatitis C virus (HCV) or hepatitis B virus (HBV) can increase morbidity and mortality after liver resection as shown in two reports.[2,16] Whether active hepatitis should be treated preoperatively to diminish inflammation and improve liver function has not been addressed.

The Child-Pugh classification and its modifications are still used by most investigators.[3,5–9] The alternative methods described above discriminate between Child's A patients who can tolerate a major hepatectomy and those who will not (Table 35–3). There have been no prospective studies of any of these methods showing their superiority to the Child-Pugh classification. At this point it is difficult to justify the additional cost and, in some cases, associated risk these tests entail.

TABLE 35–2.
Pugh's modification of the Child score

	Criteria, by no. of points		
Parameter	1	2	3
Bilirubin (mg/dl)	<2	2–3	>3
Albumin (g/dl)	>3.5	2.8–3.5	<2.8
Prothrombin time (seconds over normal)	1–3	4–6	>6
Ascites	None	Mild	Moderate
Encephalopathy	None	I–II	III–IV

Grade A: 5–6 points
Grade B: 7–9 points
Grade C: 10–15 points

SOURCE: Pugh et al.[12]

TABLE 35–3.
Limits for major hepatic resection

Test	Ref.	Contraindication for major resection
Child-Pugh	Franco[6]	Score > 8
Serum alanine transferase	Noun[8]	ALT > twofold upper limit of normal value
Indocyanine green clearance	Lau[1]	Retention rate at 15 minutes > 15%
	Makuuchi[14]	Retention rate at 15 minutes > 10%
	Fan[5]	Retention rate at 15 minutes > 14%
	Wu[7]	Retention rate at 15 minutes > 10%
	Hasegawa[13]	Retention rate at 15 minutes > 10%
	Hemming[15]	Clearance < 5 mL/min/kg
Urea nitrogen synthesis	Paquet[4]	< 6 g/day
Hepatic venous pressure gradient	Bruix[11]	> 10 mm Hg

Prevention of Variceal Bleeding

An increase in portal pressure after liver resection places cirrhotic patients at risk for variceal bleeding. Upper endoscopy and possible sclerotherapy is routinely performed as part of the preoperative workup by some,[4,7] whereas others treat only patients with large varices.[13] No prospective data are available on this subject, and there are reports of postoperative variceal bleeding that requires intervention despite preoperative sclerotherapy.[4] We do not routinely perform endoscopy on patients preoperatively unless there is a history of bleeding.

Preoperative Transcatheter Arterial Chemoembolization

Several studies have shown no benefit for preoperative transcatheter arterial chemoembolization (TAE) of HCC.[17,18] In fact, postembolization complications were observed in as many as 50% of the patients, and no survival benefit was reported. It is our opinion that TAE can be helpful as a temporizing measure for patients awaiting liver transplantation. Its neoadjuvant use in conjunction with resection has not proved useful.

Preoperative Portal Vein Embolization

The portal vein branch supplying the tumor may be percutaneously embolized prior to surgery. Hypertrophy of the contralateral lobe is measured 4–6 weeks later by computed tomography (CT scan). Preoperative hypertrophy of the spared liver may thus permit resection deemed too extensive prior to embolization.[19–23] There have been a few reports of applying this technique to patients with cirrhotic livers or impaired liver function with apparent success.[24–26] It is indeed an intriguing technique that allows testing of the regenerative potential of part of the liver before surgery. The indications for this procedure must be defined more precisely to establish its usefulness and safety.

B. Treatment

Liver Resection

Once it is established that a patient can tolerate a liver resection with acceptable risk, the resectability of the lesion must be determined. Contraindications for liver resection in patients with preserved liver function are listed in Table 35–4. Management of unresectable lesions is discussed later in the chapter.

Surgical Considerations Most patients undergoing liver resection for HCC have some degree of cirrhosis. The challenge lies in removing as little functional parenchyma as possible to avoid postoperative liver failure while removing all of the cancer with clear margins. Most groups accept a tumor-free margin of at least 10 mm.[27] Major resections of large tumors are well tolerated, as little functional parenchyma is removed. Small tumors are by far more difficult to manage. A deep, centrally located small lesion might necessitate an extended resection for anatomic reasons, depriving the patient of much needed functional liver. Whenever feasible, a limited anatomic resection such as segmentectomy is preferable for small lesions,

TABLE 35–4.
Contraindications for liver resection in patients with preserved liver function

Systemic spread
Lung metastasis
Extrahepatic abdominal metastases
Tumor too extensive for resection
Local factors
Prospective remnant too small (i.e., segment)
Tumor in contact with all three hepatic veins
Tumor in contact with right and left branches of the portal vein
Tumor growth into main portal vein

TABLE 35–5.
Operative mortality for liver resection in patients with hepatocellular cancer

Study	Year	No.	Operative mortality (%)	
			Overall	Cirrhosis
Hasegawa[13]	1987	204	[a]	8
Chen[28]	1989	120	4	7
Choi[29]	1990	174		13
Franco[6]	1990	72	7	7
Takenaka[2]	1990	126	*	19
Tsuzuki[30]	1990	119	9	21
Paquet[4]	1991	23	*	13
Hemming[15]	1992	22	*	18
Nagasue[31]	1993	229	7	12
Capussotti[9]	1994	33	*	3
Fan[5]	1995	54	*	13
Vauthey[32]	1995	106	6	14
Fuster[33]	1996	48	*	4
Wu[7]	1996	70	*	2
Noun[8]	1997	108	*	8

[a] All patients have cirrhosis.

sparing as much functional parenchyma as possible. If this is not possible, ablative therapies or orthotopic liver transplantation (OLT) must be considered.

Cirrhosis, if present, renders the liver resection technically difficult. The liver parenchyma in this case is hard and makes retraction of the liver difficult. Moreover, anatomic landmarks become distorted and difficult to find owing to fibrosis and atrophy/hypertrophy. In addition, portal hypertension and tissue friability contribute to increased blood loss during mobilization and parenchymal transection. All these factors increase the level of complexity compared to resection in a normal liver.

Major resections of at least one lobe of the liver can be performed in patients with HCC with an overall mortality of 5–10%. Patients with cirrhosis have higher mortality (Table 35–5). Major resections are indicated for patients whose large tumors replace most of one lobe, who have acceptable liver function, and who have no atrophy of the uninvolved lobe, resulting in minimal removal of functional parenchyma.

Segmental resection is chosen whenever feasible to spare as much functional parenchyma as possible. In theory, resection of each segment is possible, individually[34–36] or in various combinations, to avoid a full lobectomy.[37,38] We prefer cryo-assisted resection to wedge resections if an anatomic resection is not possible. Vessels are difficult to control during nonanatomic resection, and hemorrhage from deep vessels is not infrequent. Clear margins are difficult to obtain under such circumstances. To facilitate these resections we use a cryo-assisted technique.[39] The cryoprobe is thereby not used for its tumoricidal action but as a handle during dissection to improve visualization of vessels (Fig. 35–1). The specimen once removed is cut open to ensure adequate margins. Freezing the specimen at least 1 cm beyond the tumor margins prior to parenchymal transection also helps ensure a negative resection margin. We have used this method successfully in 37 patients.

We favor a right subcostal incision with midline extension to the xiphoid ("hockeystick") for all types of liver resection. Bifurcated incisions and thoracotomies are to be avoided because of their propensity to leak ascites. Inflow control is obtained by the intermittent Pringle maneuver. The portal triad can be clamped for long times in cirrhotic patients without increasing morbidity or mortality.[40–45] It is essential to keep a low central venous pressure and a Trendelenburg position during parenchymal dissection to prevent bleeding from the hepatic veins.[46] The hepatic veins are controlled and transected extrahepatically whenever possible. We and most authors use the Kelly fracture technique for the parenchymal transection.[47] Although the ultrasonic dissector might facilitate skeletonization of pedicles, it is cumbersome to use and does not offer any significant advantages over the crushing technique. The harmonic scalpel is proving useful as an alternative for transection in the fibrotic or cirrhotic patient. Abdominal drains can be a source of major postoperative fluid losses and a source of infection. Drainage after liver resection is not necessary,[48] particularly in a cirrhotic patient.[49,50] It is our practice not to use drains unless biliary reconstruction or thoracotomy has been performed.

POSTOPERATIVE CARE It is not uncommon for patients with HCC to develop transient liver decompensation postoperatively, especially those with cirrhosis. There is no need

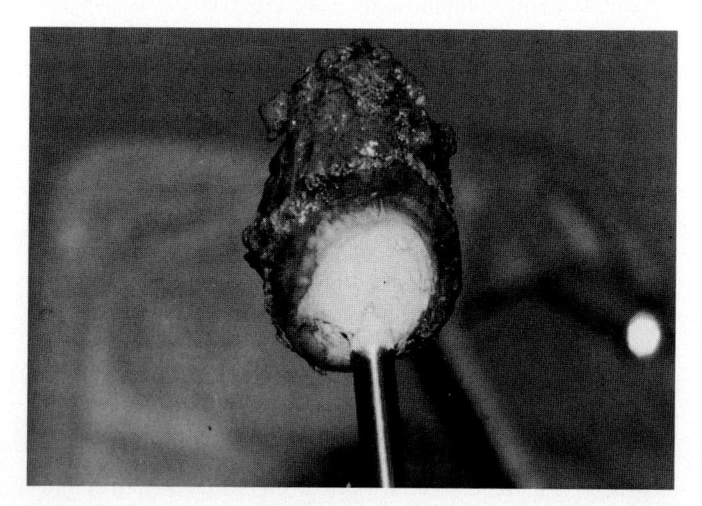

FIGURE 35–1
Specimen after cryo-assisted resection. The specimen is still frozen to the cryoprobe. It will be removed and cut in two to assess for tumor-free clearance.

for fluid or sodium restriction during the first 24 hours after surgery. Crystalloid administration must be sufficient to maintain a normal urine output.[51] Patients are subjected to water and sodium restriction after the first postoperative day. In patients with cirrhosis, spironolactone is used as soon as peroral administration is tolerated. Furosemide can be added for further control of ascites. The prothrombin time can be elevated, and correction with fresh frozen plasma might be required to avoid bleeding complications during the early postoperative phase.

Orthotopic Liver Transplantation

Liver transplantation may be considered for two categories of patient: Child's A patients with lesions ≤5 cm that cannot be safely removed by liver resection and patients with small lesions whose liver function does not permit resection. Total hepatectomy and liver transplantation has the potential to cure the cancer and the underlying liver disease. Mazzaferro et al. reported 85% four-year survival after transplantation without any adjuvant treatment.[52] Some argue that patients with Child's A cirrhosis, even if resection is possible, should undergo liver transplantation.[53] We prefer partial hepatectomy for patients with small lesions and Child's A cirrhosis unless the lesion is centrally located, in which care OLT or other ablative therapies would be more suitable.

Ablative Therapies

Ablative therapies, such as percutaneous alcohol injection (PEI) or transcatheter arterial embolization (TAE) can be considered in patients with preserved or moderately impaired liver function.

Transcatheter Arterial Embolization Transcatheter arterial embolization is performed by selectively catheterizing the hepatic arterial branch feeding the tumor and embolizing it with Gelfoam or other means. The portal blood flow to that portion of the liver should be preserved to avoid massive liver necrosis. Consequently, patients with ipsilateral portal vein occlusion must be considered for PEI or are offered no therapy. We do not embolize patients with Child's C cirrhosis because of the unacceptable mortality rate.[54]

Percutaneous Ethanol Injection Necrosis is induced by percutaneous injection of absolute alcohol into the tumor. It is a safe ablative modality for patients with cirrhosis and has minimal morbidity and mortality.[55] PEI can be highly effective and produces results comparable to resection in tumors <5 cm (Table 35–6).[56] Adding PEI to TAE seems to be beneficial in causing tumor necrosis of large lesions,[57] and it might increase survival compared to use of TAE alone.[58,59]

Cryoablation Cryosurgery can be performed with acceptable morbidity and mortality for patients with hepatocellular carcinoma, including patients with cirrhosis.[60] Cryoablation may offer an alternative to resection for patients whose liver function do not permit resection. Our current practice is to perform cryoablation for patients with HCCs considered unresectable based on *intraoperative* findings, as these patients already have incurred the risks of anesthesia and laparotomy. For all other patients we favor PEI, which does not require an anesthetic or an operation. Cryoablation may be considered if the tumor grows despite PEI or embolization.

TABLE 35–6.
Comparison of surgery, PEIT, and no therapy for HCC <5 cm in patients with Child's A and B cirrhosis

	3-year survival (%)		
Child classification	Surgery	ETOH injection	No therapy
A	79	71	26
B	40	41	13

PEIT, percutaneous alcohol injection therapy
SOURCE: Livraghi et al.[56]

Radiofrequency Ablation Radiofrequency ablation can also be performed with low morbidity and mortality either laparoscopically or during laparotomy. The indications and use parallel those for cryotherapy; there may be advantages with radiofrequency ablation with respect to ease of application, size of probe used, and time required to complete the treatment.

Chemotherapy

Systemic chemotherapy for HCC has produced poor results and considerable side effects. In fact, none of the regimens has had a response rate of more than 10%. We do not use chemotherapy for HCC unless within the confines of a study of patients who are not candidates for other treatment modalities.

Conclusions

Determining the correct therapy for patients with HCC is a challenge. Surgery, if feasible, remains the gold standard for suitable patients. Patients with inoperable, large lesions and Child's A or B status can benefit from ablative therapies to halt tumor progression.

There is ongoing debate regarding the correct treatment for patients with small lesions and intact or mildly altered liver function. OLT achieves the best results, but organ shortage limits its use. In uncontrolled studies, PEI yields results comparable to those seen with resection without the need for anesthesia and operation. Its controlled comparison to resection and OLT would be important.

We apply an algorithm for managing patients with HCC. Management of Child C patients poses no major dilemma because their course is characterized by deteriorating liver function and OLT is the only possible therapy. Child's A patients can qualify for any of the modalities. Improved preoperative assessment of liver function may allow classification of this group with more refinement to allow selection of the appropriate therapy. Child's B patients can qualify for ablative therapies (PEI, TAE) or OLT. In this patient group, any intervention can precipitate deterioration of liver function, and the potential to control the tumor must be weighed against the risks of progressive liver failure.

References

1. Lau H, Man K, Fan ST, Yu W-C, Lo CM, Wong J. Evaluation of preoperative hepatic function in patients with hepatocellular carcinoma undergoing hepatectomy. Br J Surg 1997;84:1255–1259.
2. Takenaka K, Kanematsu T, Fukuzawa K, Sugimachi K. Can hepatic failure after surgery for hepatocellular carcinoma in cirrhotic patients be prevented? World J Surg 1990;14:123–127.
3. Nagasue N, Yukaya H, Kohno H, Chang YC, Nakamura T. Morbidity and mortality after major hepatic resection in cirrhotic patients with hepatocellular carcinoma. HPB Surg 1988;1:45–56.
4. Paquet KJ, Koussouris P, Mercado MA, Kalk JF, Muting D, Rambach W. Limited hepatic resection for selected cirrhotic patients with hepatocellular or cholangiocellular carcinoma: a prospective study. Br J Surg 1991; 78:459–462.
5. Fan ST, Lai EC, Lo CM, Ng IO, Wong J. Hospital mortality of major hepatectomy for hepatocellular carcinoma associated with cirrhosis. Arch Surg 1995;130:198–203.
6. Franco D, Capussotti L, Smadja C, et al. Resection of hepatocellular carcinomas: results in 72 European patients with cirrhosis. Gastroenterology 1990;98:733–738.
7. Wu CC, Ho WL, Yeh DC, Huang CR, Liu TJ, P'eng FK. Hepatic resection of hepatocellular carcinoma in cirrhotic livers: is it unjustified in impaired liver function? Surgery 1996;120:34–39.
8. Noun R, Jagot P, Farges O, Sauvanet A, Belghiti J. High preoperative serum alanine transferase levels: effect on the risk of liver resection in child grade A cirrhotic patients. World J Surg 1997;21:390–394.
9. Capussotti L, Borgonovo G, Bouzari H, Smadja C, Grange D, Franco D. Results of major hepatectomy for large primary liver cancer in patients with cirrhosis. Br J Surg 1994;81:427–431.
10. Noguchi T, Imai T, Mizumoto R. Preoperative estimation of surgical risk of hepatectomy in cirrhotic patients. Hepatogastroenterology 1990;37: 165–171.
11. Bruix J, Castells A, Bosch J, et al. Surgical resection of hepatocellular carcinoma in cirrhotic patients: prognostic value of preoperative portal pressure. Gastroenterology 1996;111:1018–1022.
12. Pugh RNH, Murray-Lyon IM, Dawson JL, Pietroni MC, Williams R. Transection of the oesophagus for bleeding oesophageal varices. Br J Surg 1973; 60:646–649.
13. Hasegawa H, Yamazaki S, Makuuchi M, Elias D. Hepatectomy for hepatocarcinoma on a cirrhotic liver: decision plans and principles of perioperative resuscitation: experience with 204 cases (in French). J Chir (Paris) 1987;124:425–431.
14. Makuuchi M, Kosuge T, Takayama T, et al. Surgery for small liver cancers. Semin Surg Oncol 1993;9:298–304.
15. Hemming AW, Scudamore CH, Shackleton CR, Pudek M, Erb SR. Indocyanine green clearance as a predictor of successful hepatic resection in cirrhotic patients. Am J Surg 1992;163:515–518.
16. Higashi H, Matsumata T, Adachi E, et al. Influence of viral hepatitis status on operative morbidity and mortality in patients with primary hepatocellular carcinoma. Br J Surg 1994;81:1342–1345.
17. Wu CC, Ho YZ, Ho WL, Wu TC, Liu TJ, P'eng FK. Preoperative transcatheter arterial chemoembolization for resectable large hepatocellular carcinoma: a reappraisal. Br J Surg 1995;82:122–126.
18. Harada T, Matsuo K, Inoue T, Tamesue S, Nakamura H. Is preoperative hepatic arterial chemoembolization safe and effective for hepatocellular carcinoma? Ann Surg 1996;224:4–9.
19. De Baere T, Roche A, Elias D, Lasser P, Lagrange C, Bousson V. Preoperative portal vein embolization for extension of hepatectomy indications. Hepatology 1996;24:1386–1391.
20. De Baere T, Roche A, Vavasseur D, et al. Portal vein embolization: utility for inducing left hepatic lobe hypertrophy before surgery. Radiology 1993; 188:73–77.
21. Kawasaki S, Makuuchi M, Miyagawa S, Kakazu T. Radical operation after portal embolization for tumor of hilar bile duct. J Am Coll Surg 1994; 178:480–486.
22. Kawasaki S, Makuuchi M, Kakazu T, et al. Resection for multiple metastatic liver tumors after portal embolization. Surgery 1994;115:674–677.
23. Nagino M, Nimura Y, Kamiya J, et al. Changes in hepatic lobe volume in biliary tract cancer patients after right portal vein embolization. Hepatology 1995;21:434–439.
24. Shimamura T, Nakajima Y, Une Y, et al. Efficacy and safety of preoperative percutaneous transhepatic portal embolization with absolute ethanol: a clinical study. Surgery 1997;121:135–141.
25. Lee KC, Kinoshita H, Hirohashi K, Kubo S, Iwasa R. Extension of surgical indications for hepatocellular carcinoma by portal vein embolization. World J Surg 1993;17:109–115.
26. Wakabayashi H, Okada S, Maeba T, Maeta H. Effect of preoperative portal vein embolization on major hepatectomy for advanced-stage hepatocellular carcinomas in injured livers: a preliminary report. Surg Today 1997;27: 403–410.
27. Yoshida Y, Kanematsu T, Matsumata T, Takenaka K, Sugimachi K. Surgical margin and recurrence after resection of hepatocellular carcinoma in patients with cirrhosis: further evaluation of limited hepatic resection. Ann Surg 1989;209:297–301.
28. Chen MF, Hwang TL, Jeng LB, Jan YY, Wang CS, Chou FF. Hepatic resection in 120 patients with hepatocellular carcinoma. Arch Surg 1989; 124:1025–1028.
29. Choi TK, Edward CS, Fan ST, Francis PT, Wong J. Results of surgical resection for hepatocellular carcinoma. Hepatogastroenterology 1990;37:172–175.
30. Tsuzuki T, Sugioka A, Ueda M, et al. Hepatic resection for hepatocellular carcinoma. Surgery 1990;107:511–520.
31. Nagasue N, Kohno H, Chang YC, et al. Liver resection for hepatocellular carcinoma: results of 229 consecutive patients during 11 years. Ann Surg 1993;217:375–384.
32. Vauthey JN, Klimstra D, Franceschi D, et al. Factors affecting long-term outcome after hepatic resection for hepatocellular carcinoma. Am J Surg 1995;169:28–34.
33. Fuster J, Garcia-Valdecasas JC, Grande L, et al. Hepatocellular carcinoma and cirrhosis: results of surgical treatment in a European series. Ann Surg 1996;223:297–302.

34. Franco D, Smadja C, Kahwaji F, Grange D, Kemeny F, Traynor O. Segmentectomies in the management of liver tumors. Arch Surg 1988;123: 519–522.
35. Franco D, Bonnet P, Smadja C, Grange D. Surgical resection of segment VIII (anterosuperior subsegment of the right lobe) in patients with liver cirrhosis and hepatocellular carcinoma. Surgery 1985;98:949–954.
36. Nagasue N, Yukaya H, Ogawa Y, Hirose S, Okita M. Segmental and subsegmental resections of the cirrhotic liver under hepatic inflow and outflow occlusion. Br J Surg 1985;72:565–568.
37. Makuuchi M, Hasegawa H, Yamazaki S, Takayasu K. Four new hepatectomy procedures for resection of the right hepatic vein and preservation of the inferior right hepatic vein. Surg Gynecol Obstet 1987;164:68–72.
38. Makuuchi M, Mori T, Gunven P, Yamazaki S, Hasegawa H. Safety of hemihepatic vascular occlusion during resection of the liver. Surg Gynecol Obstet 1987;164:155–158.
39. Polk W, Fong Y, Karpeh M, Blumgart LH. A technique for the use of cryosurgery to assist hepatic resection. J Am Coll Surg 1995;180:171–176.
40. Nagasue N, Uchida M, Kubota H, Hayashi T, Kohno H, Nakamura T. Cirrhotic livers can tolerate 30 minutes ischaemia at normal environmental temperature. Eur J Surg 1995;161:181–186.
41. Wu CC, Hwang CR, Liu TJ, P'eng FK. Effects and limitations of prolonged intermittent ischaemia for hepatic resection of the cirrhotic liver. Br J Surg 1996;83:121–124.
42. Kim YI, Kobayashi M, Aramaki M, Nakashima K, Mitarai Y, Yoshida T. "Early-stage" cirrhotic liver can withstand 75 minutes of inflow occlusion during resection. Hepatogastroenterology 1994;41:355–358.
43. Kim YI, Nakashima K, Tada I, Kawano K, Kobayashi M. Prolonged normothermic ischaemia of human cirrhotic liver during hepatectomy: a preliminary report. Br J Surg 1993;80:1566–1570.
44. Smadja C, Kahwaji F, Berthoux L, Grange D, Franco D. Value of total pedicle clamping in hepatic excision for hepatocellular carcinoma in cirrhotic patients. Ann Chir 1987;41:639–642.
45. Elias D, Desruennes E, Lasser P. Prolonged intermittent clamping of the portal triad during hepatectomy. Br J Surg 1991;78:42–44.
46. Cunningham JD, Fong Y, Shriver C, Melendez J, Marx WL, Blumgart LH. One hundred consecutive hepatic resections: blood loss, transfusion, and operative technique. Arch Surg 1994;129:1050–1056.
47. Lin TY. A simplified technique for hepatic resection: the crush method. Ann Surg 1974;180:285–290.
48. Fong Y, Brennan MF, Brown K, Heffernan N, Blumgart LH. Drainage is unnecessary after elective liver resection. Am J Surg 1996;171:158–162.
49. Smadja C, Berthoux L, Meakins JL, Franco D. Patterns of improvement in resection of hepatocellular carcinoma in cirrhotic patients: results of a non drainage policy. HPB Surg 1989;1:141–147.
50. Franco D, Smadja C, Meakins JL, Wu A, Berthoux L, Grange D. Improved early results of elective hepatic resection for liver tumors: one hundred consecutive hepatectomies in cirrhotic and noncirrhotic patients. Arch Surg 1989;124:1033–1037.
51. Tsuge H, Mimura H, Orita K, Sugawara M, Hashimoto K, Ochiai Y. Evaluation of preoperative and postoperative sodium and water loading in patients undergoing hepatectomy for liver cirrhosis complicated by hepatocellular carcinoma. Hepatogastroenterology 1991;38(suppl 1):56–62.
52. Mazzaferro V, Regalia E, Doci R, et al. Liver transplantation for the treatment of small hepatocellular carcinomas in patients with cirrhosis. N Engl J Med 1996;334:693–699.
53. Schwartz ME, Sung M, Mor E, et al. A multidisciplinary approach to hepatocellular carcinoma in patients with cirrhosis. J Am Coll Surg 1995;180: 596–603.
54. Bismuth H, Morino M, Sherlock D, et al. Primary treatment of hepatocellular carcinoma by arterial chemoembolization. Am J Surg 1992;163: 387–394.
55. Livraghi T, Giorgio A, Marin G, et al. Hepatocellular carcinoma and cirrhosis in 746 patients: long-term results of percutaneous ethanol injection. Radiology 1995;197:101–108.
56. Livraghi T, Bolondi L, Buscarini L, et al. No treatment, resection and ethanol injection in hepatocellular carcinoma: a retrospective analysis of survival in 391 patients with cirrhosis: Italian Cooperative HCC Study Group. J Hepatol 1995;22:522–526.
57. Tanaka K, Okazaki H, Nakamura S, et al. Hepatocellular carcinoma: treatment with a combination therapy of transcatheter arterial embolization and percutaneous ethanol injection. Radiology 1991;179:713–717.
58. Tanaka K, Nakamura S, Numata K, et al. Hepatocellular carcinoma: treatment with percutaneous ethanol injection and transcatheter arterial embolization. Radiology 1992;185:457–460.
59. Yamamoto K, Masuzawa M, Kato M, et al. Evaluation of combined therapy with chemoembolization and ethanol injection for advanced hepatocellular carcinoma. Semin Oncol 1997;24:S6-50–S6-55.
60. Adam R, Akpinar E, Johann M, Kunstlinger F, Majno P, Bismuth H. Place of cryosurgery in the treatment of malignant liver tumors. Ann Surg 1997;225:39–50.

CHAPTER 36

Colorectal Hepatic Metastasis

JOSÉ M. VELASCO
TINA J. HIEKEN
NADER YAMIN
ALEXANDER DOOLAS

A. Epidemiology

Colorectal cancer is the fourth most common malignant disease in the Western world, and its incidence is increasing. Approximately 50% of patients die from recurrent disease following curative resection of the primary tumor, and the liver is the most frequent site of recurrence. Liver metastases can be found in up to 35% of patients at the time of resection during their initial presentation, and up to 40% of all patients thought to be rendered disease-free eventually develop hepatic metastases. Only 25% of these patients have recurrence confined to the liver and are therefore potential surgical candidates. Untreated patients with liver metastases have variable survival rates but invariably die from disease, the median survival being less than 12 months. Initial uncontrolled data strongly suggest that carefully selected patients benefit from liver resection, with 5-year survival rates of 25–35%.[1]

There is a lack of consensus concerning the most appropriate postoperative follow-up for patients at risk of hepatic metastases and how to select patients who can benefit from liver resection. Given the current state of knowledge, it is generally accepted that a single, accessible, metachronous metastasis in a good risk patient whose primary lesion is controlled and has no evidence of extrahepatic disease should be resected. On the other hand, multiple, inaccessible, asymptomatic lesions in the presence of extrahepatic disease should not be resected. Moreover, a poor prognosis after resection of liver metastases is likely when there are more than three metastatic lesions, positive surgical margins, extrahepatic disease, nodal involvement at the primary tumor site, and poor differentiation. Liver resection should be undertaken at centers with documented favorable mortality and morbidity for these procedures. By today's standards mortality should be less than 5%. Alternative forms of therapy are not substitutes for resection but should be considered as adjuncts to an operation.[2]

Colorectal cancers are a heterogeneous group of tumors consisting of multiple subpopulations of cells with different properties. To produce metastases, tumor cells must succeed with invasion, embolization, survival in the circulation, arrest in a distant capillary bed, and extravasation into and multiplication within an organ. The outcome depends on the interaction of metastatic cells with multiple host factors. The predilection for colorectal cancer to metastasize to the liver is due partly to portal venous

Colorectal Hepatic Metastasis

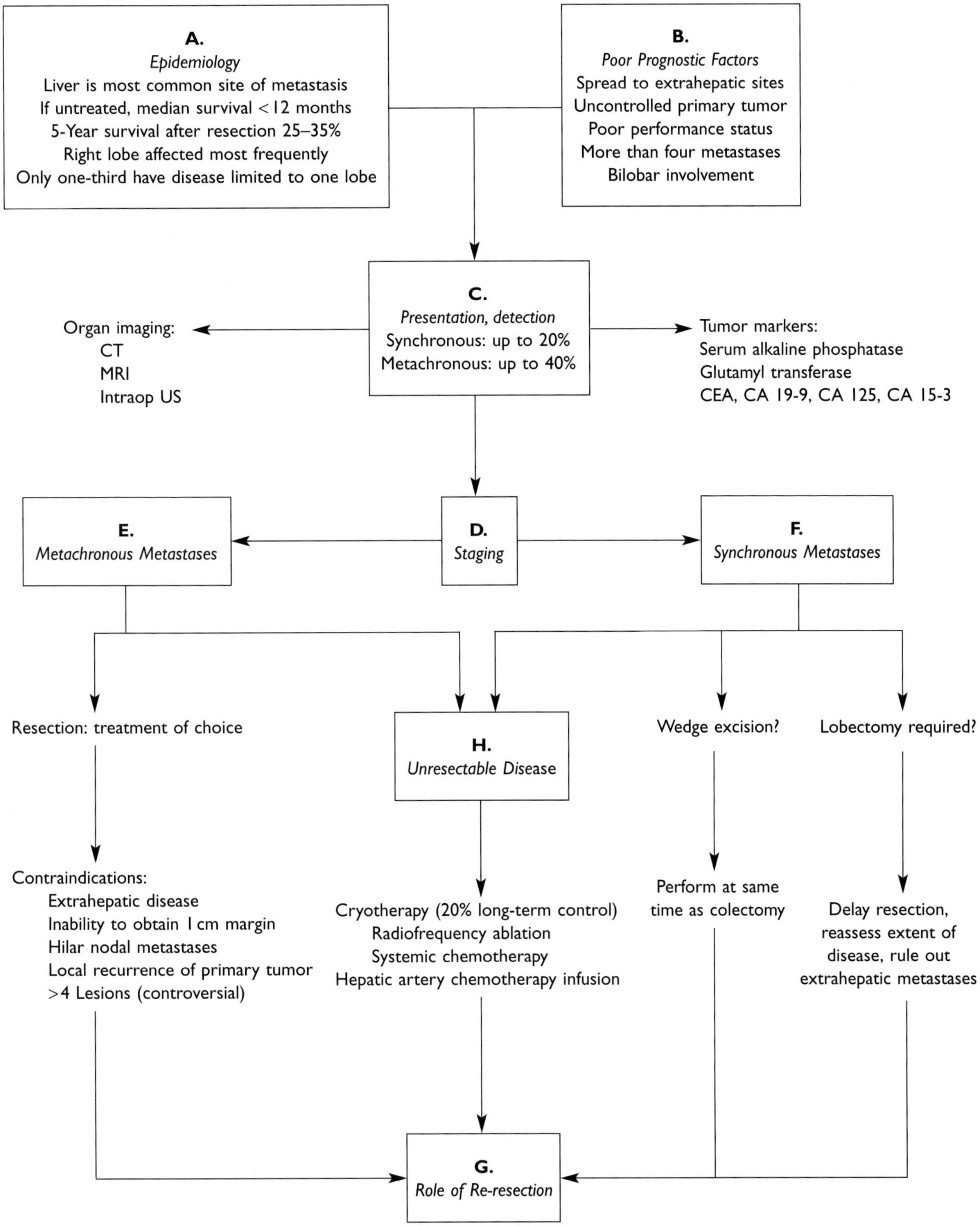

A.
Epidemiology
Liver is most common site of metastasis
If untreated, median survival <12 months
5-Year survival after resection 25–35%
Right lobe affected most frequently
Only one-third have disease limited to one lobe

B.
Poor Prognostic Factors
Spread to extrahepatic sites
Uncontrolled primary tumor
Poor performance status
More than four metastases
Bilobar involvement

C.
Presentation, detection
Synchronous: up to 20%
Metachronous: up to 40%

Organ imaging:
- CT
- MRI
- Intraop US

Tumor markers:
- Serum alkaline phosphatase
- Glutamyl transferase
- CEA, CA 19-9, CA 125, CA 15-3

D.
Staging

E.
Metachronous Metastases

Resection: treatment of choice

Contraindications:
- Extrahepatic disease
- Inability to obtain 1 cm margin
- Hilar nodal metastases
- Local recurrence of primary tumor
- >4 Lesions (controversial)

F.
Synchronous Metastases

Wedge excision?

Perform at same time as colectomy

Lobectomy required?

Delay resection, reassess extent of disease, rule out extrahepatic metastases

H.
Unresectable Disease

Cryotherapy (20% long-term control)
Radiofrequency ablation
Systemic chemotherapy
Hepatic artery chemotherapy infusion

G.
Role of Re-resection

drainage. The virtual absence of metastasis to cirrhotic livers may be explained by diminished portal flow.[3] The right lobe of the liver is involved with metastasis most frequently, for unclear reasons. It may be due to regional blood flow distribution, portal vein streaming, or a proportionally larger segmental volume. One-third of patients have disease limited to one lobe. Intrahepatic invasion of the portal vein is thought to be responsible for intrahepatic spread of tumor (satellite lesions). Approximately 10% of patients with liver metastasis, who are potential candidates for liver resection, have metastases spread to extrahepatic lymph nodes, which excludes the possibility of cure. Isolated lung metastasis may result from tumor emboli into the thoracic duct or from cancer cells traversing the liver.[4–6]

Compared to the hematogenous route, the lymphatic pathway plays a limited role in the development of liver metastases. Tumor cells may invade sequential nodes, spread through venolymphatic communications, or pass directly to the vena cava via the thoracic duct. It is uncommon to find involvement of the lymph nodes along the hepatic artery in the absence of lymph node involvement at the primary site. Although some metastatic blood supply is derived from the portal vein, their chief supply is derived from the hepatic artery. Angiographic studies of liver metastases have shown great variability in their blood supply, which bears important implications for local therapies such as chemoperfusion, hepatic artery ligation, and chemoembolization.[7]

The growth rate and age of liver metastases have not been fully elucidated. Scheele et al.[8] assessed tumor doubling times with serial computed tomography (CT) scans, finding a mean of 155 days for clinically overt metastases and a mean of 86 days for "occult" metastases. Assuming Gompertzian growth, the mean (±SD) age of overt metastases was 3.7 ± 3.1 years and that of occult metastases 2.3 ± 2.0 years. These calculations show that there is a large variation in the growth pattern of liver metastasis. A more precise definition of the growth rate is needed.[9]

B. Natural Course and Prognostic Factors

The median survival of patients with untreated liver disease is 12 months or less. Survival from the time of diagnosis is longer for patients with solitary lesions (10–21 months). Abnormally elevated serum alkaline phosphatase and carcinoembryonic antigen (CEA) levels have been identified as prognostic factors in most studies; other accepted poor prognostic factors include spread to extrahepatic sites and primary tumors that have not been resected. Rougier et al.[10] proposed a classification system based on *performance status* and the *number of involved segments*. A normal performance status and three or fewer involved segments was associated with a 1-year survival of 58% compared with 18% for symptomatic patients and those with more than three segments involved. Survival beyond 5 years is rare.[1,7]

Improved operative technique and perioperative care have introduced a selection bias that makes analysis of the natural course of the disease extremely difficult. It is distinctly uncommon for patients not to receive therapy of some sort, whether operative or nonoperative. The prognostic impact of tumor biology on untreated hepatic metastasis has not been investigated extensively, although *ploidy* has been proposed as a possible factor. Quality of life assessment may be of value for predicting survival and even for selecting patients suitable for resection. *Disease-free interval* has been used as a selection criterion; hepatic resection is technically feasible in only 10% of patients with synchronous metastasis and in 25% of patients with metachronous metastasis.

Considering that 75% of patients surviving liver resection die during the next 5 years, physicians have avoided operating on patients with short disease-free intervals. With the advent of more accurate imaging tests [e.g., positron emission tomography (PET) scanning] to detect extrahepatic and intrahepatic disease and improved surgical technique that allows re-resection of metastases, most physicians have fortunately abandoned this expectant attitude.[11]

C. Presentation/Detection

Liver metastases are described as *synchronous* if detected at the time of diagnosis of colorectal cancer or at the time of resection of the primary tumor. *Metachronous* metastases appear any time after primary tumor presentation. The incidence of synchronous liver metastasis is difficult to determine because of variable institutional practices and means of pursuing the possibility of metastatic disease. Three population-based studies showed an incidence ranging from 16.3% to 19.4%. After a curative operation, metachronous liver metastases appear as the *initial* site of failure in 15% of patients, but up to 40% of patients eventually develop liver metastases. The incidence of true metachronous lesions depends on the ability to detect occult synchronous metastasis. Measuring CEA in bile and determining the Doppler perfusion index at the time of primary tumor resection may facilitate more accurate identification of patients at risk.[1,7,11]

Most liver metastases are initially silent; it has been estimated that the subclinical phase of a liver metastasis may be 2.5–5.0 years. Alternatively, patients may present with fever, thromboembolism, pain, weight loss, or malaise. Hepatomegaly often indicates advanced disease, as do manifestations of hepatic failure. The median survival once ascites or jaundice appears is measured in weeks.[1,7]

During their asymptomatic phase, detection of liver metastases may be problematic. Blood tests may be normal if patients with metastatic disease have adequate functional liver reserve. Levels of serum alkaline phosphatase and serum γ-glutamyl transferase provide the greatest sensitivity (90%) and specificity (93%). Serum CEA levels are used during the follow-up of patients and are frequently elevated in the presence of liver metastases. Other tumor markers, such as CA 19-9, CA 15-3, and CA-125, may be elevated but are not specific.[7,11,12]

Organ imaging remains the most sensitive method for detecting liver metastases. The resolution of conventional imaging techniques such as ultrasonography, CT, and magnetic resonance imaging (MRI) continues to improve, but the ability of these techniques to detect small metastases (<1 cm) is limited. In general, the CT scan is accepted as the most useful tool for evaluating liver lesions and extrahepatic disease. Technical enhancements (bolus dynamic, helical scans, and the use of portography) have increased the sensitivity of CT up to 90%. CT arterial portography (CTAP) is highly sensitive, but it has low specificity because of the false positives created by perfusion defects. The limited availability and expense of MRI have rendered ultrasonography and CT the most widely used examinations, although in certain circumstances MRI can provide better definition of segmental and vascular involvement by liver lesions.[7,11]

The best method for imaging patients at high risk for liver metastases remains to be determined. Hepatic flow scanning and duplex color ultrasonography allow calculation of the hepatic perfusion index, which has high sensitivity but undefined specificity for detecting liver metastases. Doppler color scanning is being investigated as an alternative to intraoperative ultrasonography (IOUS) when screening for liver metastases, but it is operator-dependent and its results are not easily reproduced. PET scans and immunoscintigraphy show great promise but are not readily available and remain investigational.[7]

Intraoperative ultrasonography performed during laparotomy or laparoscopy has high sensitivity and specificity. Laparoscopy with ultrasonography (LUS) permits accurate evaluation of the liver, peritoneal surfaces, and lymph nodes; if extrahepatic disease is found, patients may be spared unnecessary laparotomy. Although percutaneous liver biopsy should not be used routinely because of the risk of tumor spill, it may be indicated when a diagnosis must be established without the risk of a laparotomy (e.g., for the elderly patient or the patient with several co-morbid conditions).[13]

D. *Staging*

If liver resection is being contemplated, the preoperative workup must assess the primary tumor site for possible recurrent cancer, the extent of liver involvement, and whether extrahepatic disease is present. From a practical point of view, chest radiography, ultrasonography, and enhanced CT should provide enough information. MRI may be useful in equivocal cases and to further delineate the location of the lesions relative to major vessels. Preoperative CEA and CA 19-9 levels provide a baseline and may be used as prognostic indicators. CT volumetry may facilitate operative decisions, particularly for patients with heavy tumor burden and undefined liver reserve.[7,12]

Several staging systems for colorectal liver metastasis have been proposed, but no single system has been universally accepted. Gayowski et al. proposed a system incorporating tumor size, tumor distribution, number of metastatic lesions, and the extent of extrahepatic disease. This study confirmed that patients with nodal or extrahepatic involvement have a poor prognosis following liver resection.[14] In a report of 416 patients with resectable colorectal metastases, Jarnagin et al.[13] proposed a preoperative scoring system to identify patients likely to have unresectable disease. Resectability ranged from 95% for patients with a score of 0 (unilobar, solitary lesions) to 62% for those with a score of 3 (multiple, bilobar). Of the factors analyzed, only the estimated number of lesions was an independent predictor of unresectable disease. This held true for patients with extrahepatic metastases and those with extensive intrahepatic disease.[11,13,14]

E. *Metachronous Metastases*

Surgical resection is the treatment of choice for colorectal liver metastases, with reported 5-year survival rates ranging from 22% to 48% and the operative mortality less than 5%. Eligible patients should be free of serious co-morbid conditions that preclude a life expectancy of at least 18–24 months; ideally, the operative mortality remains less than 3%, particularly in the elderly. Therefore assessment of factors influencing survival after liver resection is crucial. Improved results in recent years have led to liberalization of indications for liver resection.[1,7,11,12,15,16]

In 1986 Ekberg et al. proposed three contraindications to liver resection: the presence of four or more metastases, synchronous extrahepatic disease, and the inability to obtain a resection margin of at least 1 cm.[17] Foster and Berman determined that the stage of the primary disease had little bearing on survival, as did the extent of resection and the interval between primary tumor and liver resection.[18] They claimed that multiple nodules in one lobe of the liver did not affect the outcome adversely, but bilobar involvement worsened the prognosis. Nordlinger et al. proposed a prognostic scoring system based on a retrospective multicenter review of 1568 patients with resected liver metastases from colorectal cancer. They were attempting to study expected survival, estimated operative risk, and ultimate outcome. The 5-year survival and operative mortality were 28.0% and 2.3%, respectively; outcome was affected by age (≥60 years), stage of the primary tumor, time from diagnosis of primary tumor to metastasis (≥2 years), size of the largest metastasis (≥5 cm), number of metastases (four or more), and disease-free margin (≥1 cm).[19] Others argue that a smaller margin may be all that is needed.[1,13,20,21] Cady et al. proposed a scoring system based on the number of metastases, disease-free interval, CEA level, margin of resection, and specimen weight.[22] Other, more controversial prognostic factors include blood loss, site of the primary tumor, gender, extent of liver resection (wedge versus lobe versus trisegmentectomy), and synchronous versus metachronous metastases.[11,12,15]

At the present time there is a strong consensus that hepatic resection should be considered whenever technically possible, provided patients are fit enough to tolerate such a procedure, do not have major morbidity, and ideally have normal liver function. Absolute contraindications include inability to obtain clear margins (≥1 cm), lymph node metastases at the hilum of the liver, distant extrahepatic disease, lung metastases, and unresectable local recurrence. Direct tumor extension into surrounding structures other than the diaphragm is usually associated with other negative factors such as large tumor mass or poor tumor differentiation. It is reasonable to consider resection for more than three metastases if the procedure can be undertaken with low mortality and morbidity and the lesions are concentrated in an adequate segment amenable to resection. The lobar distribution and size of metastases probably do not affect survival.[12,15]

With respect to the operative approach, anatomic resections guided by IOUS are advisable and are most likely to achieve clear margins. IOUS facilitates identification of satellite lesions and tumor infiltration into surrounding vascular structures.[11] Because patients with three or more metastases and bilobar involvement have occult unresectable disease in up to 40% of cases, laparoscopy and LUS are being utilized increasingly to avoid unnecessary celiotomy.[13] If more radical procedures (trisegmentectomy) are required to achieve free margins, the mortality is higher and the prognosis is worse, although 5-year survival is still possible.[23,24]

Liver resection is performed under general anesthesia. Packed red blood cells, fresh frozen plasma, and platelets should be ready if needed. The patient is positioned on the operating room table tilted toward the left to permit easy access to the flank in case the incision must be extended. Typically, a bilateral subcostal incision with a vertical midline extension is used, which provides excellent exposure. Once the abdomen is entered, any adhesions in the right upper quadrant are taken down, the liver palpated bimanually, and the hilum and retroperitoneum inspected for adenopathy (metastases are a contraindication for resection). Adhesions from prior surgery may make exploration of the remainder of the abdomen difficult, and this step can be avoided provided preoperative imaging studies did not reveal abnormal or suspicious areas. Once the liver is fully exposed and one has access to the dome and posterior surfaces, IOUS is performed to determine the number and location of the lesions and their relation to major branches of the portal and hepatic veins. If ablative therapy is being performed, ultrasonography may help direct the surgeon to the safest "window" of passage through the parenchyma.

If the decision is made to proceed with hepatic lobectomy, dissection is undertaken in the hilum to isolate the right and left branches of the hepatic artery, portal vein, and bile ducts. The corresponding hepatic vein must also be isolated and at the appropriate time oversewn with a running suture of permanent monofilament suture. Once the hilar vessels and hepatic veins have been controlled, the liver parenchyma is transected, which can be accomplished with an ultrasonic dissector or the finger fracture technique. The operation must proceed in a deliberate team-oriented fashion among the surgeon, first assistant, and scrub person. Liberal use of suture material, hemostatic clips, and topical hemostatic agents is important. Attempts should be made to preserve the middle hepatic vein, and a margin of at least 1 cm is considered essential. Once the specimen has been removed, the cut edge of the liver is inspected for bleeding or loss of bile from small biliary tributaries.

If operative and ultrasonographic findings indicate that a wedge resection(s) would be sufficient, extensive dissection in the hilum can be avoided; however, the major vessels must be accessible for the Pringle maneuver. One must not underestimate the magnitude of a wedge resection or the potential for blood loss, especially when dealing with lesions in the dome and posterior surface where exposure is somewhat limited. The goal of the operation is a surgical margin of at least 1 cm. Multiple wedge excisions can be performed if indicated. Again, liberal use of suture-ligature and topical hemostatic agents facilitates the operation and minimizes blood loss.

F. Synchronous Metastases

Patients who present with synchronous liver metastases may require palliative resection of an advanced primary tumor to relieve obstruction or bleeding. In the presence of extensive bilobar tumor producing hepatomegaly or ascites or low serum albumin, an operation may not be warranted provided the lesion is not bleeding or causing obstruction. Alternatively, patients may be found to have potentially resectable liver metastases on a preoperative CT scan or on inspection and palpation during the primary operation. Prospective comparison of palpation and inspection, CT scans, and IOUS confirm the benefit of IOUS for detecting additional metastases. Occult tumor may be found using a gamma probe to detect radiolabeled monoclonal antibodies.[11,15]

The decision to resect hepatic metastases at the time of primary tumor surgery is influenced by the experience of the institution and the operating surgeon, the extent and location of the metastases, and the extent of the operation required to remove the primary tumor. As a general rule, wedge or segmental resections can be done concomitantly with colectomy. Lobar resections should be done 2–6 weeks later after thorough investigation to rule out metastases elsewhere, such as in the contralateral lobe of the liver or the chest. If tumor distribution mandates resection of more than 50% of the liver parenchyma, this observation is especially prudent. On the other hand, a lesion that is solitary and >4 cm probably could be resected.[11,12,15,25] Because there is no conclusive evidence to support a waiting period or early resection in these patients, accepted guidelines include a combination of liver resection and right colon procedures and a combination of any colorectal procedure with removal of two or less Couinaud segments.[12]

G. *Role of Re-resection*

Tumor relapse after liver resection occurs in 75% of patients, mainly within the first 2 years. Approximately 20% of these patients have liver-only recurrence and may be candidates for re-resection. During the interim from the first liver resection some patients may have developed lung metastases that are detectable with CT imaging. Repeat liver resection is safe with an operative mortality of less than 10% and a median survival of 30–40 months, in contrast to 4 months without resection.

Recently, 5-year survival rates for more than 45% of patients have been reported for those who underwent a curative resection following an initial liver resection with clear margins.[26,27] The presence of synchronous lung metastases lowers the survival rate to 32% after resection of liver and lung metastases.[12] Serum CEA levels provide a valuable marker for detecting recurrent tumors; liver function tests have debatable usefulness. Because of mortality and morbidity rates similar to those for the initial liver resection, it seems reasonable to continue aggressive surveillance with regular serum CEA levels, chest radiography, and CT scans of the liver and lungs after hepatic resection.[12,15]

H. *Unresectable Disease*

Ablative Therapy

Unfortunately, most patients with metastatic liver disease are not candidates for resection. Furthermore, many patients experience liver recurrences following resection and few of those are candidates for re-resection. For these reasons, increasing interest has been focused on ablative techniques: cryotherapy, radiofrequency thermal ablation (RAF), laser and microwave ablation.

Cryotherapy

Cryosurgical ablation involves in situ freezing (without resection) of neoplastic lesions. Modern liquid nitrogen delivery systems and recirculating probes have been developed that allow treatment of tumors in virtually any hepatic segment. Real-time ultrasonography permits identification of liver lesions, including their relation to surrounding vascular and biliary structures, accurate placement of cryosurgery probes, and monitoring of the iceball or cryolesion. Cryosurgery acts by destroying cells directly as a result of physicochemical effects and indirectly by affecting surrounding vessels. Liquid nitrogen circulates at −196°C through a probe in direct contact with the tissue to be treated; rapid freezing and slow thawing enhances cell damage. In the liver a temperature of −15°C is lethal; nevertheless, studies have suggested that exposure of all areas of the tumor to at least −40°C is necessary to minimize the potential for local recurrence and to account for errors in judgment concerning tumor margins. The cycle is repeated more than once so any remaining viable tumors cells are destroyed.

The goal of cryotherapy is eradication of all liver lesions with a 1 cm margin. The lesions shrink after 3–6 months, and in most cases an area of fibrosis persists. Conventionally, cryotherapy requires laparotomy to assess intrahepatic and extrahepatic disease and for direct application of the probes under ultrasound guidance, although laparoscopy can be used in certain circumstances.[28]

Initially, hepatic cryotherapy was used in patients with unresectable metastases, but some authors suggest that it may have a potentially curative role in the treatment of liver metastases.[29] Indications have not been clearly defined, but patients with unresectable metastases because of bilobar or anatomic location and patients with small lesions in the contralateral lobe during resection of a large metastasis might be considered for cryotherapy. Extrahepatic disease is considered a contraindication, and cryotherapy is usually not helpful for patients with multiple liver metastasis (more than five lesions).

The abdominal incision and exposure of the liver generally proceed in a fashion similar to hepatectomy; in fact, resection and cryotherapy can be combined in the same patient. Once extrahepatic disease has been ruled out, ultrasonography is performed to determine the number and location of the lesions and their relation to major vessels. Under ultrasound guidance, a needle is placed in the lesion and a guidewire passed through the needle. A dilator and peel-away catheter are then advanced over the guidewire. When satisfactory placement has been obtained, the cryotherapy probe is inserted. Ultrasound is used to guide each of these steps and to monitor iceball formation, ensuring that the tumor edges are encompassed by the ice zone. Large lesions are treated with a large probe; alternatively, multiple small probes may be inserted into a single large tumor. When the last freeze-thaw cycle has been completed, the probe is gently withdrawn and the track packed with topical hemostatic agents.

Follow-up of patients is carried out using CT scans and tumor markers. Based on worldwide experience concerning colorectal metastases to the liver, it appears that long-term control is possible in 20% of cases. Among the patients who fail subsequent to cryotherapy, approximately 70% have extrahepatic disease; one-third have recurrence in the untreated liver and only 10% at the cryosurgery-treated site. The mortality and morbidity rates are less than 1% and 5%, respectively. Adjuvant therapy with hepatic arterial infusion of chemotherapy may reduce the failure rate in the liver.[28,30]

The complications in patients with colorectal hepatic metastasis treated with cryotherapy are comparable to the complications following liver resection. Coagulopathy, with an elevated prothrombin time and variable thrombocytopenia, often develops. Platelet transfusion is indicated for platelet counts less than 7500/mm^3; and fresh frozen plasma and vitamin K are indicated in the presence of clinically evident bleeding. Significant hypothermia and myoglobinuria commonly occur. Both conditions can be prevented and their effects minimized by actively warming the patient and by vigorous alkaline diuresis. Virtually all patients develop pleuropulmonary complications (i.e., atelectasis, pleural effusion). Finally, hepatic abscesses and bile duct injuries may occur, albeit infrequently.

Radiofrequency Thermal Ablation

Radiofrequency ablation is becoming the most commonly utilized ablative modality because it allows greater preservation of healthy liver parenchyma, it may be applied to multiple, bilobar lesions, to those centrally located, or in areas not technically respectable, and it may be applicable in some patients with isolated hepatic recurrence. RFA appears to result in comparable if not better outcomes than cryotherapy at a lower cost and associated morbidity.[31–33]

Thermal ablation uses high-frequency electrical, alternating current (200–1200KHz) delivered by inserting a needle electrode into the tumor under ultrasound or CT guidance. Components common to all devices include a single or, best, multiprong, monopolar electrode, a dispersive electrode, and a generator controlled manually or linked to a computer. The tip of the needle optimally contains a thermistor for temperature monitoring since tissue must be heated at least to greater than 45°C before necrosis occurs as cellular protein denatures and cell structure is lost. The temperature generated by the radiofrequency pulse and by the probe dimensions determines ablation size. The heat generated is the difference between that generated by the current within the tissue and the heat loss through conduction and convection. The latter is the main mechanism of heat loss from the lesion and acts as a protective measure to prevent damage to vessel walls. Initially, single needles caused a cylindrical lesion in the range of 1.0–1.5 cm in maximal diameter; complete ablation often required multiple or simultaneous insertions at 0.5–1.5 cm intervals. In an effort to increase the size, change the shape of the thermal lesions, and decrease the number of needles used, multiprong electrodes have been developed, resulting in a spherical area of coagulation necrosis. Moreover, the principal limitation of ablation size has been obviated by the usage of 5.0 cm electrodes. Evolving technology facilitates the use of modified electrodes, including cooled-tip needles so that greater local current densities can be applied to tissues in a shorter time. The exposure time ranges from 6 to 12 minutes per needle. With multiple prong needles, the output of the generator is adjusted to keep temperatures between 95°C and 105°C. In larger tumors, the "pull-back" technique allows repeated applications by reactivating the generator at each location without having to reintroduce the needle, hence, minimizing sticks and tumor seeding. Dedicated software and IOUS records the temperature curves obtained and the location and size of the thermal injury respectively.[31,34]

Thermal ablation can be administered through percutaneously inserted electrodes under local anesthesia with conscious sedation or, best, under general anesthesia via celiotomy or laparoscopy depending on the lesion size, number, location, and planned track. Laparotomy or laparoscopy are preferred because they allow use of IOUS to detect additional lesions, further define those identified and to monitor the ablation; this is paramount in cases of close proximity to other organs, including the bile ducts. In addition, these approaches permit simultaneous modalities of therapy such as resection, cryotherapy and hepatic arterial inflow control.[33]

Ultrasonography demonstrates a homogeneous, hyperechoic area at the needle tip(s) when the temperature reaches 90°C. Because of the lower vascularity and the less well-defined edges of metastatic disease when compared to hepatomas, US with color-doppler capabilities is not entirely reliable. Even spiral CT and dynamic MRI may not be as accurate as in other types of tumors. Therefore, it is imperative to depict an area of necrosis exceeding the original lesion; at least a 0.5 cm margin of coagulative necrosis should be seen all around the lesion. Spiral CT and MRI may show the presence of a "halo" which enhances in the arterial phase, caused by the peritumoral inflammatory reaction. Postoperatively, regular imaging surveillance at 1 week and 3 month intervals, should demonstrate a progressive decrease in the size of the lesion.[32,35]

Patients eligible for RFA should have disease limited to the liver. Ideally, the tumor should be nodular, single, or if multiple, limited to three or four nodules, and with a maximal diameter of 3–4 cm, even though larger lesions have been successfully treated.[31,33]

Complications seem to be few. They include pain, skin burns, transient elevation of transaminases and low mortality. Short-term results are encouraging with local control rates of 80% and 43% of patients are disease free at a median of 9 months.[32] Predictors of failure include lack of lesion enlargement at 1 week, progressive lesion shrinkage, large size, adenocarcinoma or sarcoma histology, and vascular invasion on US.[32]

RFA is particularly suited for inoperable metachronous lesions, preferably solitary or less than 4 in number, smaller than 3–5 cm, alone or in combination with other modalities: resection, intraarterial chemotherapy.[36,37]

Systemic Chemotherapy

Systemic chemotherapy alone is associated with a 10–20% clinical, objective response rate (≤50%), but no clear benefit exists with regard to survival or quality of life.[38] The most widely used agent is 5-fluorouracil (5-FU). Its benefit as an adjuvant after liver resection is unclear, although some retrospectives studies have suggested that adjuvant systemic therapy may improve survival.[39] Following intravenous chemotherapy, Bismuth et al. resected liver metastases initially considered unresectable in 53 patients. They reported a 3-year survival of 53%.[40] New chemotherapeutic agents administered systemically or via hepatic artery infusion, immunotherapy, and preoperative chemoembolization must be evaluated in clinical trials. At the present time, neoadjuvant treatment should be investigated as a means to improve the outcome of liver resection for hepatic metastases or to down-stage patients to make them suitable operative candidates.[40]

Regional Chemotherapy

Because hepatic metastases derive their blood supply mainly from the hepatic artery, hepatic artery infusion (HAI) of chemotherapy using an implantable pump to deliver fluorodeoxyuridine (FUDR) directly into the liver has been studied since the late 1970s. Currently, HAI is an option for treatment of unresectable liver metastases and can be considered adjuvant therapy following liver resection or ablative treatment such as cryotherapy. Patients with low-volume tumor burden (<20%) and those with relatively normal liver function have benefited the most.[41]

Hepatic response rates with HAI for patients with unresectable disease are higher than for those receiving systemic chemotherapy, but a clear benefit in survival has not been demonstrated consistently. A meta-analysis of six trials of HAI used in 654 patients showed a tumor response rate for HAI and systemic therapies of 41% and 14%, respectively. The first site of failure was the liver in 39% of patients who received HAI versus 74% of those treated with intravenous chemotherapy; the survival advantage was modest.[42] Kemeny et al. conducted a randomized trial of a small group of patients treated with adjuvant HAI following resection. Their results suggested that lower recurrence rates in the liver and a longer median survival could be achieved with HAI.[43] Selective injection of cytotoxic drugs together with an occluding agent into the hepatic artery (chemoembolization) is based on the hypothesis that embolization may promote arterial perfusion of underperfused metastases while concurrently blocking the arterial blood supply to healthy liver, producing increased cytotoxicity.[44] No survival advantage has been demonstrated using this treatment in patients with unresected lesions.[15,44]

The main complications seen after HAI include chemical hepatitis, gastritis, duodenitis, and cholecystitis (33% incidence).[45] Preoperative angiography is required to define the numerous variations of the hepatic arterial blood supply. Cholecystectomy should be done routinely, and the vessels around the pylorus and lesser curvature of the stomach should be ligated to reduce the likelihood of misperfusion.

Investigational Cytoreductive Therapy

Other techniques used to palliate patients with unresectable hepatic metastasis include ethanol injection, thermotherapy, and interstitial radiotherapy. A disadvantage, common to all of them, is the lack of monitoring tissue destruction and the size of lesions that can be treated. For instance, laser-induced thermotherapy produces incomplete necrosis of lesions >20 mm. High-dose interstitial irradiation, selective internal irradiation, and high-dose intraoperative brachytherapy have been investigated as adjuvants to resection or as alternatives for patients with unresectable metastasis.[15,46]

Conclusions

The treatment of choice for patients with colorectal hepatic metastases is resection; the other therapies mentioned herein are not substitutes. Resection is undertaken provided certain selected criteria have been met: The patient must be a suitable operative candidate free of serious medical co-morbidities; the patient should be free of local tumor recurrence and extrahepatic disease; and there must be sufficient liver reserve to sustain life after resection. At the time of surgery IOUS is essential and may change the operative approach in a significant number of cases. Five-year survival rates of approximately 30% can be expected following resection. Re-resection can be offered to patients who have failure confined to the liver. Local ablative techniques such as cryotherapy or RFA can be offered to patients whose metastases are not resectable. Intraarterial chemotherapy, as the sole treatment or as an adjunct to resection or cryotherapy, continues to play a role.

References

1. Norstein J, Silen W. Natural history of liver metastasis from colorectal carcinoma. J Gastrointest Surg 1997;1:398–407.
2. SSAT, AGA, ASLD, ASGE, AHPBA Consensus Panel. Treatment of hepatic metastasis from colorectal metastasis. J Gastrointest Surg 1997;1: 396–397.
3. Lieber MM. The rare occurrence of metastatic carcinoma in the cirrhotic liver. Am J Med Sci 1957;233:145–152.
4. Sugarbaker PH, Hughes K. Surgery for colorectal metastasis in the liver. In: Wanebo HJ (ed) *Colorectal Cancer*. St. Louis: Mosby, 1993:405–414.
5. Weiss L. Metastatic inefficiency. Adv Cancer Res 1990;54:159–211.
6. Gutman M, Fidler IJ. Biology of human colon cancer metastasis. World J Surg 1995;19:226–234.
7. Hugh TJ, Kinsella AR, Poston GJ. Management strategies for colorectal liver metastasis. Part I. Surg Oncol 1997;6:19–30.
8. Scheele J, Stangl R, Altendorf-Hofmann A. Hepatic metastasis from colorectal carcinoma: impact of surgical resection on the natural history. Br J Surg 1990;77:1241–1246.
9. Finlay IG, Meek D, Brunton F, et al. Growth rate of hepatic metastasis in colorectal carcinoma. Br J Surg 1988;75:641–644.
10. Rougier P, Milan C, Lazorthes F, et al. Prospective study of prognostic factors in patients with unresected hepatic metastases from colorectal cancer. Br J Surg 1995;82:1397–1400.
11. Millikan KW, Staren ED, Doolas A. Invasive therapy of metastatic colorectal cancer to the liver. Surg Clin North Am 1997;77:27–48.
12. Scheele J, Stangl R, Altendorf-Hofmann A. Resection of liver metastasis revisited. J Gastrointest Surg 1997;1:408–422.
13. Jarnagin WR, Fong Y, Ky A, et al. Liver resection for metastatic colorectal cancer: assessing the risk of occult irresectable disease. J Am Coll Surg 1999;188:33–42.
14. Gayowski TJ, Iwatsuki S, Madariaga JR, et al. Experience in hepatic resection for metastatic colorectal cancer: analysis of clinical and pathologic risk factors. Surgery 1994;116:703–711.
15. Hugh TJ, Kinsella AR, Poston GJ. Management strategies for colorectal liver metastasis. Part II. Surg Oncol 1997;6:31–48.
16. Foster JH, Berman MM. Literature survey. In: Solid Liver Tumors. Philadelphia: Saunders, 1977:214.
17. Ekberg H, Tranberg KG, Andersson R, et al. Determinants of survival in liver resection for colorectal secondaries. Br J Surg 1986;73:727–731.
18. Foster JH, Berman MM. Long-term survival; colon and rectal metastasis. In: Solid Liver Tumors. Philadelphia: Saunders, 1977:221–225.
19. Nordlinger B, Jaeck D, Guiget M, et al. Surgical resection of liver metastasis: multicentric retrospective study by the French Association of Surgery. In: Nordlinger B, Jaeck D (eds) *Treatment of Hepatic Metastasis of Colorectal Cancer*. Paris: Springer, 1992:129–161.
20. Yamamoto J, Sugihara K, Kosuge T, et al. Pathologic support for limited hepatectomy in the treatment of liver metastasis from colorectal metastasis. Ann Surg 1995;221:74–78.
21. Elias D, Lasser P, Rougier P, et al. Nouvel echec dans la tentative de definition des indications d'exerese des metastasis hepatiques d'origine colorectale. J Chir (Paris) 1992;129:59–65.
22. Cady B, Stone MD, McDermott WV, et al. Technical and biological factors in disease-free survival after hepatic resection for colorectal metastasis. Arch Surg 1992;127:561–569.
23. Wanebo HJ, Chu LD, Vezerides MP, et al. Patient selection for hepatic resection of colorectal metastasis. Arch Surg 1996;131:322–329.
24. Iwatsuki S, Esquivel CO, Gordon RD, et al. Liver resection for metastatic colorectal cancer. Surgery 1986;100:804–810.
25. Vogt P, Raab R, Ringe B, et al. Resection of synchronous liver metastasis from colorectal cancer. World J Surg 1991;15:62–67.
26. Wanebo HJ, Chu QD, Avradopoulos KA, et al. Current perspectives on repeat hepatic resection for colorectal carcinoma: a review. Surgery 1996; 119:361–371.
27. Nordlinger B, Vaillant JC, Guiguet M, et al. Survival benefit of repeat liver resections for recurrent colorectal metastases: 143 cases. J Clin Oncol 1994; 12:1491–1496.
28. Ravikumar TS, Sotomayor R, Goel R. Cryosurgery in the treatment of liver metastasis from colorectal cancer. J Gastrointest Surg 1997;1:426–432.
29. Morris DL, Horton MDA, Dilley AV, et al. Treatment of hepatic metastases by cryosurgery and regional cytotoxic perfusion. Gut 1993;34:1156–1157.
30. Preketes AP, Caplehorn JR, King J, et al. Effect of hepatic artery chemotherapy on survival of patients with metastases from colorectal carcinoma treated with cryotherapy. World J Surg 1995;19:768–771.
31. Lencioni R, Cioni D, Goletti O, et al. Radiofrequency thermal ablation of liver tumors: state-of-the-art. Cancer J 2000;60:S304–S315.
32. Siperstein A, Garland A, Engle K, et al. Local recurrence after laparoscopic radiofrequency thermal ablation of hepatic tumors. Ann Surg Oncol 2000; 7:106–113.
33. Wood TF, Rose DM, Chung M, et al. Radiofrequency ablation of 231 unresectable hepatic tumors: indications, limitations, and complications. Ann Surg Oncol 2000;7:593–600.
34. Scudamore C. Volumetric radiofrequency ablation: technical considerations. Cancer J 2000;6:S316–S318.
35. Jiao LR, Hansen PD, Havlik R, et al. Clinical short-term results of radiofrequency ablation in primary and secondary liver tumors. Am J Surg 1999; 177:303–306.
36. Scudamore CH, Shung IL, Patterson EJ, et al. Radiofrequency ablation followed by resection of malignant liver tumors. Am J Surg 1999;177:411–417.
37. Kainuma O, Asano T, Aoyama H. Combined therapy with radiofrequency thermal ablation and intra-arterial infusion chemotherapy for hepatic metastases from colorectal cancer. Hepatograstroenterology 1999;46:1071–1077.
38. Rougier P, Lasser P, Elias D. Chemotherapy of hepatic metastasis of colorectal origin. In: Nordlinger B, Jaeck D (eds) *Treatment of Hepatic Metastasis of Colorectal Cancer*. Paris: Springer, 1992:109–128.
39. Hughes KS, Foster J. The role of adjuvant chemotherapy following curative hepatic resection of colorectal metastases. Proc Am Soc Clin Oncol 1991; 10:145–150.
40. Bismuth H, Adam R, Farabos CH, et al. Resection of unresectable hepatic metastases from colorectal metastases with neoadjuvant chemotherapy. Eur J Cancer 1995;31A:S209.
41. Kemeny MM. Hepatic artery infusion as treatment of hepatic metastases from colorectal cancer. J Gastrointest Surg 1997;1:423–425.
42. Meta-Analysis Group in Cancer. Reappraisal of hepatic arterial infusion in the tratment of nonresectable liver metastases from colorectal cancer. J Natl Cancer Inst 1996;88:252–258.

43. Kemeny M, Goldberg DA, Beatty JD, et al. Results of a prospective randomized trial of continuous regional chemotherapy and hepatic resection as treatment of hepatic metastases from colorectal primaries. Cancer 1986;57: 492–498.
44. Lang EK, Brown CL. Colorectal metastases to the liver: selective chemoembolization. Radiology 1993;189:417–422.
45. Kemeny MM, Battifora H, Blaney D, et al. Sclerosing cholangitis after hepatic artery infusion of FUDR. Ann Surg 1985;202:176–181.
46. Nag S, Martinez-Monge R, Mills J, et al. Intraoperative high dose rate brachytherapy in recurrent or metastatic colorectal carcinoma. Ann Surg Oncol 1998;5:16–22.

CHAPTER 37

Colon Cancer

MARC I. BRAND

We have learned a great deal about the biology, prevention, and treatment of colon cancer, the second most deadly cancer in the United States. For example, there is both clinical and genetic evidence supporting the adenoma–carcinoma sequence, which states that nearly all colorectal cancers arise from a preexisting adenoma. Colonoscopy may interrupt this sequence by identifying and removing polyps, thereby reducing the incidence of colorectal cancer. Various levels of risk for colorectal cancer have been identified, and several methods for screening the population have been developed. There is evidence that these screening programs reduce colorectal cancer incidence and mortality. Unfortunately, implementation of screening strategies is reaching less than half of the population. Genetic testing for hereditary colorectal cancer syndromes is currently available commercially. Chemotherapeutic treatment of advanced disease is receiving a great deal of attention, and many new strategies for its use are being developed, including oral fluoropyrimidines, metalloproteinase inhibitors, topoisomerase inhibitors, and various antiangiogenesis agents. Unfortunately, assessment of colorectal cancer risk is often overlooked until advanced disease produces obvious symptoms.

A. Screening Strategies for Colorectal Cancer

Colorectal cancer screening implies the use of a particular strategy to identify individuals likely to have colon cancer or adenomatous polyps at a presymptomatic stage. The initial step in establishing a screening program is to assess the patient's risk for developing the disease.

Patients at *high risk* for colorectal cancer (5–10% of total colorectal cancer burden) include those with a family history of familial adenomatous polyposis, hereditary nonpolyposis colorectal cancer, or inflammatory bowel disease. Screening for these patients is described in Chapter 38. Patients at *moderate risk* for colorectal cancer (15–20% of total colorectal cancer burden) include those with a family history of colorectal cancer or a personal history of colorectal cancer or polyps. Screening for those with a positive family history is described in Chapter 38. Surveillance for patients with a personal history is described here. Patients at *average risk* for colorectal cancer are those who have reached the age of 50 years, have no symptoms referable to the bowel, have no personal or family history of colorectal cancer,

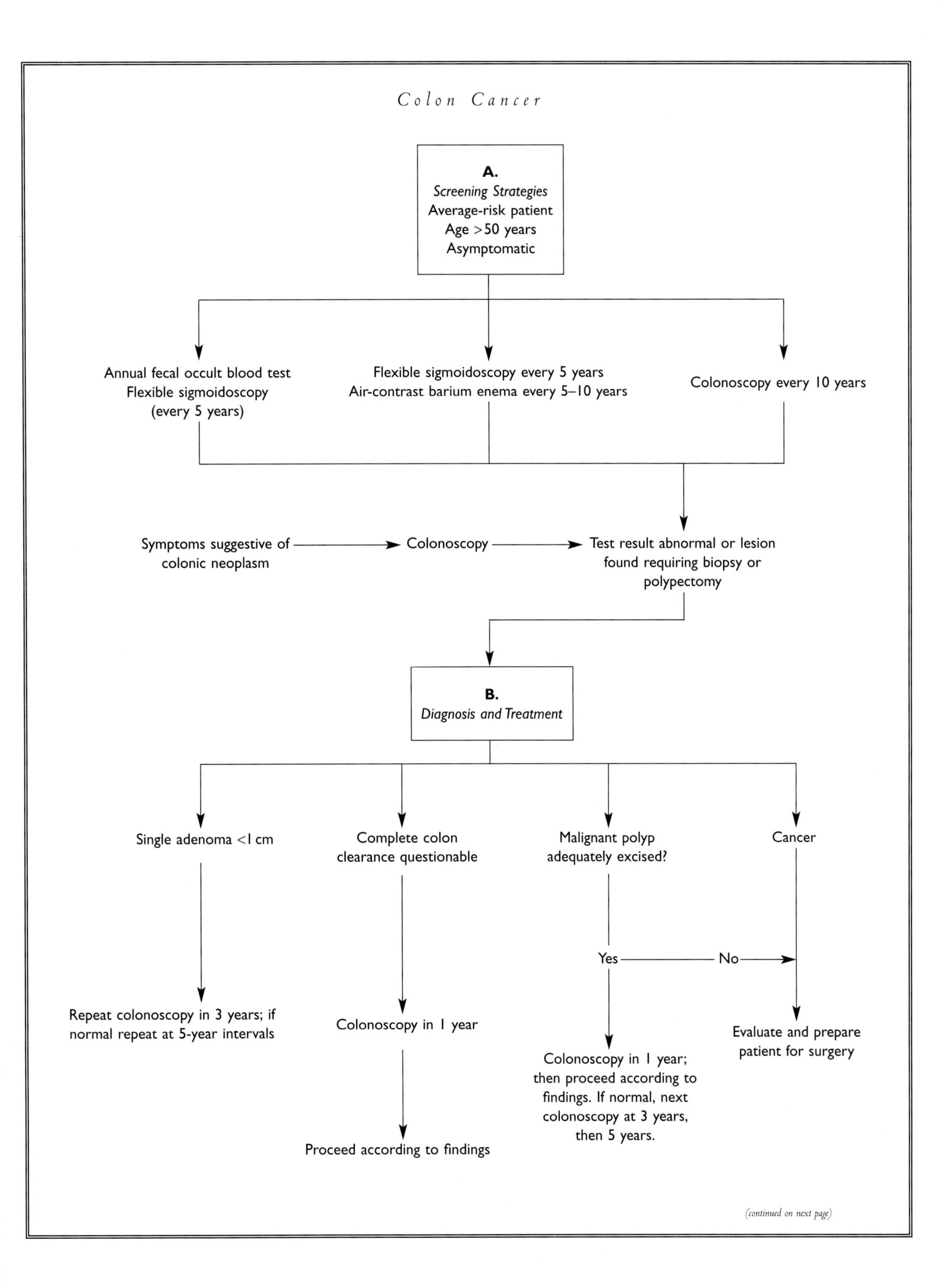

(continued on next page)

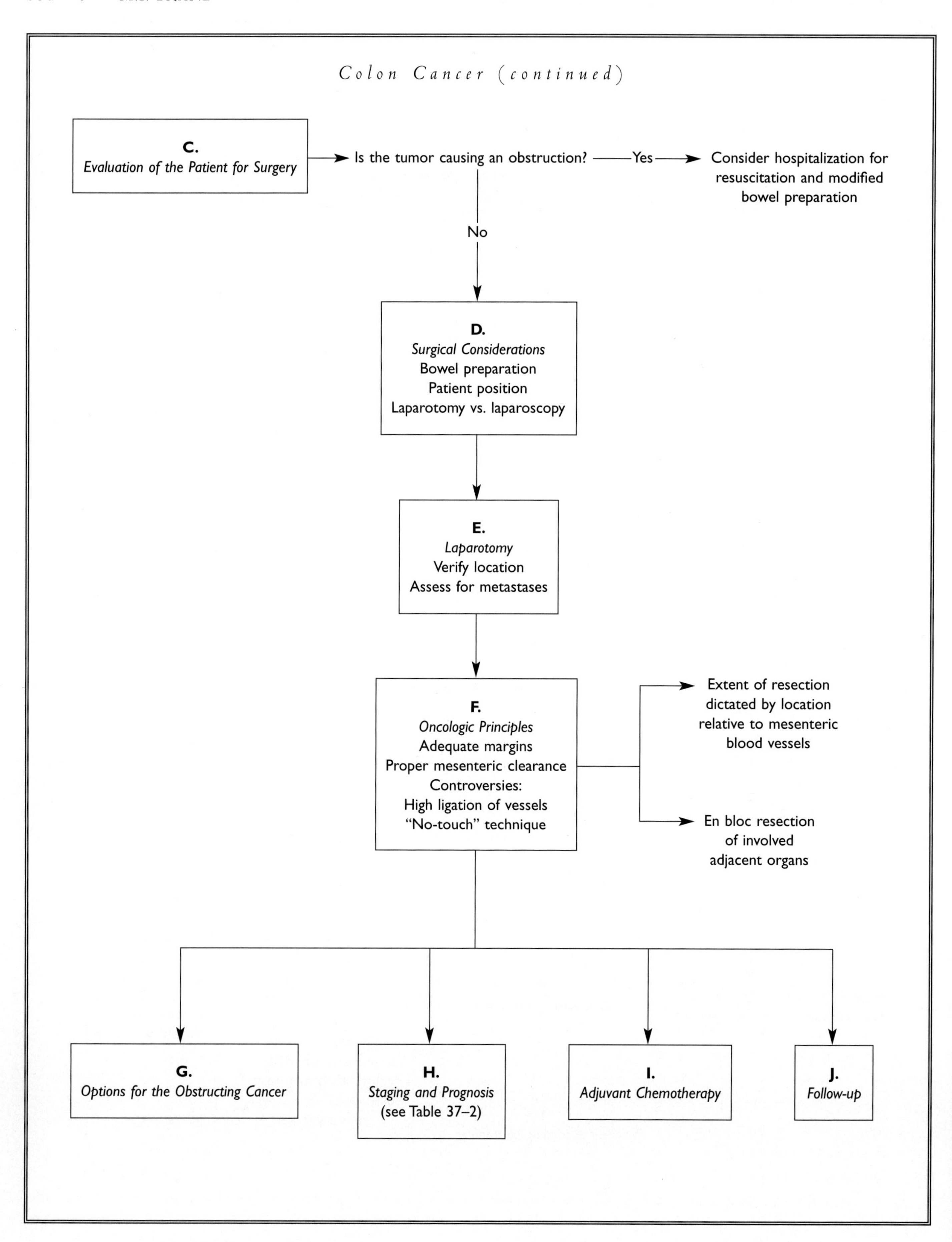
Colon Cancer (continued)
C.
Evaluation of the Patient for Surgery
Is the tumor causing an obstruction?
Yes
Consider hospitalization for resuscitation and modified bowel preparation
No
D.
Surgical Considerations
Bowel preparation
Patient position
Laparotomy vs. laparoscopy
E.
Laparotomy
Verify location
Assess for metastases
F.
Oncologic Principles
Adequate margins
Proper mesenteric clearance
Controversies:
High ligation of vessels
"No-touch" technique
Extent of resection dictated by location relative to mesenteric blood vessels
En bloc resection of involved adjacent organs
G.
Options for the Obstructing Cancer
H.
Staging and Prognosis
(see Table 37–2)
I.
Adjuvant Chemotherapy
J.
Follow-up

and do not have inflammatory bowel disease. Colorectal cancer in patients at average risk for the disease accounts for the remaining 70–80% of the total colorectal cancer burden. It is this group of individuals, everyone over age 50, to which the following discussion of colorectal cancer screening is directed. The recommendations that follow are based on colorectal cancer screening guidelines reported in 1997 by the American Cancer Society[1] and the American Gastroenterological Association.[2]

Fecal Occult Blood Test/Flexible Fiberoptic Sigmoidoscopy

One acceptable option for average risk screening is the combination of fecal occult blood testing (FOBT) annually and flexible fiberoptic sigmoidoscopy (FFS) every 5 years. FOBT has been shown to reduce the colorectal cancer mortality rate by 33% among individuals given the test annually compared to controls.[3] Additional benefits seen in this study include a 17% increase in 5-year survival (from 59% in controls to 69% in annually screened patients) and a trend toward fewer cases of metastatic disease at the time of cancer diagnosis (9.3% in annually screened patients and 16.5% in control patients).

It is important to note that the performance of this test depends on following a specified protocol. Dietary restrictions (abstinence from red meat, turnips, horseradish) and medication restrictions (abstinence from salicylates and vitamin C) should be imposed for at least 2 days before and during the study. Two samples from different areas of each of three consecutive stools should be obtained, as bleeding tends to be intermittent and blood is unevenly distributed in the stool. Cards should be stored at room temperature until testing, which should be performed within 4 days of obtaining the sample. Before testing, the slides are rehydrated by adding a drop of water to each test window; this step increases the sensitivity (and decreases specificity) of the test. The sensitivity of rehydrated FOBT for detection of colorectal cancer is estimated to be 88–92% with a specificity of 90–92%. A test is considered positive if any one of the six windows displays a blue color.

Using the 60 cm sigmoidoscope, FFS should be performed every 5 years. This instrument retains the benefits of the other instruments available for sigmoidoscopy (25 cm rigid scope and 35 cm flexible scope) but allows the greatest depth of insertion.[4] Its benefits include simple bowel preparation (saline laxative enema 1–2 hours before the examination), no need for sedation, and the ability to biopsy a polyp. The 60 cm scope can visualize all of the sigmoid colon in more than 90% of cases.[4] It is estimated that FFS identifies 40–60% of all the adenomas that can be found at colonoscopy and that approximately 66% of patients with adenomas are identified. FFS is considered positive if a cancer or any polyp >1 cm in diameter is found. A single adenoma <1 cm in diameter is not thought to increase the risk of finding more proximal, or future, neoplastic lesions. Although FOBT has a high sensitivity for detecting colorectal cancer, it is relatively insensitive for identifying adenomas. In 210 average-risk patients with negative FOBT, colonoscopy identified adenomas in 25%.[5] Therefore the addition of FFS to FOBT provides useful, complementary information for colorectal cancer risk assessment. An interval of every 5 years is recommended based on data demonstrating that the protective effect of FFS lasts 6 years.[6] This screening program is currently reimbursed by Medicare for average risk patients over age 50.[7]

FFS/Air Contrast Barium Enema

The second option for colorectal cancer screening is the combination of FFS every 5 years and air-contrast barium enema (ACBE) every 5–10 years. The ACBE examination is more involved and demanding on the patient and radiologist than the single-column barium enema, but it improves the visualization of mucosal detail. It allows complete evaluation of the colon in 90–95% of procedures. The sensitivity and specificity of ACBE are somewhat lower than for colonoscopy (Table 37–1). FFS is recommended in addition to ACBE because it has been shown to be more sensitive than ACBE in the rectosigmoid region.[7] An abnormal result (polyp >1 cm, mass, stricture) should be further evaluated by colonoscopy. This screening program is currently reimbursed by Medicare for average risk patients over age 50.[7]

Colonoscopy

The third option for colon cancer screening in the average risk population is colonoscopy every 10 years. This test is obviously more involved for the patient (complete bowel preparation, intravenous sedation/analgesia, discomfort during the procedure, and the need to be driven home after the test) but has several benefits. The entire colon (to the cecum) may be directly visualized in up to 95% of cases performed by experienced endoscopists. Polyps may be biopsied, which allows distinction between adenomatous and nonadenomatous polyps. Furthermore, complete colonoscopic polypectomy is curative for that polyp, and clearance of the colon on a regular (every 3 years) basis has been shown to reduce the incidence of colorectal cancer.[8] Finally, colonoscopy is the most sensitive test for identifying small (<1 cm) polyps, although the clinical impact of this is not known for the average risk population. The 10-year interval between normal colonoscopic examinations is based on polyp dwell time (the time during which adenoma is present but has not yet become a cancer).

Symptoms

Although screening strategies for colorectal cancer are recommended for all persons of average risk over age 50, colorectal cancer for this population is expected to present outside of

TABLE 37–1.
Sensitivity and effectiveness of various screening tests for colorectal polyps and cancer

		Sensitivity (%)			Effectiveness[a]		
Screening test	Frequency (years)	Polyps <1 cm	Polyps >1 cm	Cancer	Expected cancers	Cancers prevented	Decrease in cancer deaths
FOBT	1			60.0	2610	2378	1330
FFS[b]	5	73.3	96.7	96.7	3013	1976	967
FOBT/FFS	1/5				1901	3087	1609
ACBE	5	67.0	82.0	84.0	1604	3384	1663
FFS/ACBE	5/5	99.0	99.0	98.0			
C'scopy	10	78.5	85.0	96.7	1418	3570	1763

FOBT, fecal occult blood testing; FFS, fiberoptic flexible sigmoidoscopy; ACBE, air-contrast barium enema; C'scopy, colonoscopy.
[a] Expected incidence of 4988 cases of colorectal cancer per 100,00 population, based on a simulation model of patients at average risk for colon cancer and the reported performance of the various investigations.
[b] Sensitivity for lesions in the rectum and sigmoid colon, not the entire colon.

screening programs as well. Colorectal cancers diagnosed outside a colorectal screening program may be due to failure of the screening strategy and tests (Table 37–1), lack of participation in the screening program, development of interval cancers since the last screening examination, or early age of onset of the colorectal cancer, before screening is initiated.

The U.S. Centers for Disease Control and Prevention (CDC) recently interviewed more than 50,000 members of the U.S. population over age 50 to estimate the utilization of colorectal cancer screening strategies. Only 19.8% of persons questioned had undergone FOBT during the last year, and only 30.4% had undergone FFS during the last 5 years. A strikingly low 9.5% of persons reported having had both tests at the recommended time intervals.[9] The use of barium enema and colonoscopy was not investigated, nor was the indication for the test (screening or diagnosis) examined.

Patients may be diagnosed with (1) colorectal cancer outside a screening program, (2) interval cancer within a screening program, or (3) at an early age of onset due to evaluation of symptoms or findings on examination. Symptoms may be gradual in onset (bleeding, change in bowel habits, abdominal pain) or acute (obstruction, localized abscess, free perforation).

Bleeding is the most common symptom and may be occult or visible. *Occult bleeding* should be evaluated by colonoscopy, as a colonic etiology is found in as many as 50% of patients[10] with neoplasia being found in 33% of cases. Visible bleeding may be classified as hemorrhagic, suspicious, or outlet types.[10] *Hemorrhagic bleeding* (large-volume rectal bleeding requiring hospitalization) is due to colorectal neoplasia in approximately 10% of cases. *Suspicious rectal bleeding* may be seen as dark blood, blood streaked on (or mixed in) the stool, any bleeding associated with a change in bowel habits, or any bleeding in a patient with a personal or family history of colorectal neoplasia. Colorectal neoplasia has been found in 40% of patients with suspicious rectal bleeding: 15% was proximal to the splenic flexure and 25% proximal to the sigmoid colon. Thus colonoscopy is thought to be a better diagnostic test than FFS for suspicious rectal bleeding. *Outlet-type rectal bleeding* is seen as bright blood (related to a bowel movement) on the toilet paper or in the toilet water. Patients with this bleeding pattern who also have a change in bowel habits or a positive personal or family history for colorectal neoplasia are considered to have suspicious-type rectal bleeding. Colorectal neoplasia was found in 21% of patients with outlet-type rectal bleeding, with only one lesion (2%) found proximal to the splenic flexure. Therefore FFS is adequate for the evaluation of outlet-type rectal bleeding as defined above.

Various changes in bowel habits may be seen in patients with colorectal neoplasia. Examples are new-onset constipation or diarrhea (as a deviation from the patient's normal pattern), progressive narrowing of stool caliber, or mucus found on (or in) the stool.

Colonoscopy may identify one of several degrees of neoplasia, including polyps or a mass. Normal mucosa may also be found. A normal colonoscopy (complete to the cecum) should return the patient to the average risk category and continued use of the average risk screening guidelines.

B. Diagnosis and Treatment

Varying degrees of polyp formation have different implications for future risk of colorectal neoplasia. Although there are many histologic types, only adenomatous polyps are thought to carry a risk of future malignant transformation. Therefore a diagnosis of colorectal polyps without histologic evidence of adenomatous tissue does not alter a person's level of risk.

A single, small (1 cm) tubular or tubulovillous adenoma has not been shown to increase the risk for subsequent neoplasia.

However, the potential for neoplastic change has been demonstrated, and the possibility of a missed lesion exists. Therefore, repeat colonoscopy is recommended in 3 years.[1] Colonoscopy every 5 years is suitable follow-up if the 3-year colonoscopy is normal.

Several circumstances may be encountered that raise greater concern for the possibility of residual adenomatous tissue following colonoscopy with or without polypectomy. Consequently, the certainty that the colon and rectum have been completely cleared of neoplasia is not ensured. Repeat colonoscopy may be performed at 1 year rather than at 3 years. These circumstances include suboptimal mucosal visibility due to poor bowel preparation, removal of multiple adenomas, removal of a large sessile adenoma, and concern about the completeness of polypectomy.[11] Patients with multiple adenomas demonstrate a greater tendency to develop colorectal neoplasia; and the likelihood of small, missed adenomas is increased. Removal of large sessile adenomas or the need for advanced polypectomy techniques (piecemeal polypectomy, submucosal elevation) raise the probability of incomplete polypectomy and residual adenomatous tissue at the polypectomy site.

Early repeat colonoscopy (within 1 year) should be continued until the colon and rectum are confidently cleared of adenomatous tissue. Once this is achieved, colonoscopy should be repeated in 3 years. If the colonoscopy performed at 3-years does not reveal adenomatous tissue, repeat colonoscopies every 5 years are adequate.

The management decisions regarding malignant polyps removed endoscopically may be difficult. Colon resection should be recommended when the risk of residual cancer at the polypectomy site or the risk of lymph node metastasis is greater than the operative risk. It is important to distinguish between a truly invasive carcinoma and other lesions that erroneously suggest an invasive component (carcinoma in situ, intramucosal carcinoma, severe dysplasia). The latter lesions do not carry a significant risk of lymph node metastases. The malignant polyp is defined as an adenomatous polyp that contains an invasive (submucosal) component.[12] Direct discussion between the pathologist and surgeon or review of the slides by a pathologist with whom the surgeon is familiar is often helpful.

Surgical resection is indicated for all sessile malignant polyps and for pedunculated polyps with unfavorable histology. Unfavorable histology may be classified in one of two ways. The "Haggitt classification," proposed in 1985,[13] describes the level of cancer invasion into the stalk or base. Cancer invasion in pedunculated polyps is divided into four levels. Level 1 invasion is characterized by cancer found in the submucosa confined to the head of the polyp. Level 2 invasion penetrates the submucosa to the junction between the head and neck of the polyp. Level 3 invasion extends into the stalk of the polyp itself. Cancer found in the submucosa of the bowel wall below the stalk is described as level 4 invasion. Invasive carcinoma arising in a sessile polyp is, by definition, classified as level 4 invasion, as the only submucosa present is in the bowel wall underneath the polyp. Using this classification, an adverse outcome (lymph nodes positive for cancer in a colectomy specimen and the development of colorectal cancer) occurred in 8 of 64 patients. Seven of these adverse outcomes were in patients with level 4 invasion. Level 4 invasion was associated with a 25% chance of an adverse outcome, whereas a lesser degree of invasion was associated with a 1% chance of an adverse outcome. Based on these data, formal hemicolectomy is indicated for malignant polyps with level 4 invasion.

An alternative definition of unfavorable histology was suggested by Cranley et al.[14] These authors reviewed the course of 38 patients with 40 malignant polyps removed endoscopically. Unfavorable histology was defined as tumor at or near the cautery line, poorly differentiated carcinoma, or lymphatic invasion by the cancer. Of the 24 patients with unfavorable histology, 10 (42%) had residual cancer at the polypectomy site, locally recurrent cancer, or metastatic cancer during follow-up; 14 patients with favorable histology in a malignant polyp had no adverse cancer events. Invasive cancer at or near the cautery line was most predictive of an adverse cancer event. These authors recommend a formal colectomy for malignant polyps that demonstrate this type of unfavorable histology. The advantage of this classification is that it does not require inclusion of submucosa from the underlying bowel wall to assess level 4 invasion, which is often difficult or dangerous to obtain.

Surgery is indicated for patients found to have a mass suspicious for cancer, regardless of whether it has been proven histologically. Surgery is also indicated for patients found to have an adenomatous polyp too large for endoscopic removal or one that appears to be a polypoid cancer. Polyps generally too large for colonoscopic removal occupy more than one-third the circumference of the bowel lumen or cross two haustral folds.[15] Colotomy and polypectomy is an option for removing these lesions when they appear benign, but it is rarely used because the reduction in morbidity is minimal and the potential for an inadequate cancer operation is much higher. Polyps likely to be a polypoid cancer are recognized endoscopically by their harder appearance (assessed by probing the lesion with the tip of the scope or biopsy instrument) relative to that of benign adenomas, their irregular appearance, and their friability.[4]

C. *Evaluation of Patient for Surgery*

Planning for surgery follows identification of a lesion that requires colectomy for safe, effective cancer control. Preoperative evaluation is directed at assessing the level of symptomatology produced by the lesion, staging the lesion as much as is feasible, and a general medical evaluation in regard to fitness for major surgery.

The need for accurate preoperative staging is less important for colon cancer than it is for rectal cancer. There are more treatment options for local control of rectal cancer (tumor ablation, local resection, formal proctectomy), and the morbidity associated with each approach is quite different. In contrast, the options for local control of colon cancer are limited, as is the morbidity. Therefore complete knowledge of the tumor stage is not as crucial to the decision-making process for colon cancer as it is for rectal cancer. The necessary preoperative information for patients with colon cancer includes complete evaluation of the colon (barium enema and colonoscopy), chest radiography, and preoperative blood tests, which are used as a baseline for postoperative follow-up. Whenever feasible, the colon should be completely evaluated prior to operation. Altogether, 3–8% of patients with colon cancer have a synchronous colon cancer,[16] and it is an obvious disservice to the patient to perform colectomy and leave a cancer remaining in the colon. Preoperative chest radiography provides information regarding lung metastases that would not otherwise be learned at the time of the operation. Diffuse lung metastases may alter the decision to operate or alter (minimize) the planned operation.

Preoperative computed tomography (CT) of the abdomen to determine the presence of liver metastases is controversial. Without preoperative knowledge of the local stage of the disease, it is difficult to estimate the likelihood of liver metastases being present. Consequently, CT scans of the abdomen are necessary in nearly all patients with colon cancer (even those at low risk for metastases) to find the patients with liver metastases. Second, the liver may be assessed intraoperatively (unlike the lungs) with inspection, bimanual palpation, and intraoperative ultrasonography (IOUS) if deemed necessary. The intraoperative assessment of the liver by both of these measures is as accurate as the CT scan.[17] Third, the wisdom of synchronous liver resection for metastases at the time of formal colectomy has been debated. Thus routine preoperative CT scans of the abdomen could be described as an expensive, not always needed study that offers little information over that obtained at the time of laparotomy (or laparoscopy); and it does little to change the planned approach to a colon cancer. The major benefit of preoperative CT scans of the abdomen is for patients expected to have a locally advanced tumor involving adjacent structures, knowledge of which may change the operative approach to the tumor. The tumor may be seen invading the musculature of the abdominal wall or flank, the duodenum and pancreas, or the urinary tract. The use of a medial-to-lateral approach to mobilize the colon (preliminary lymphovascular ligation, "no-touch" isolation technique) often makes resection of such lesions technically easier (see below). Similarly, preoperative knowledge of an extensive metastatic burden in the liver may mitigate against any operation at all;[18] however, such extensive involvement would be suggested by hepatomegaly, weight loss, or markedly abnormal serum liver function tests.

It is important to identify patients who have significant symptoms due to a colon cancer, as the symptoms may have an impact on preoperative preparation or operative approach. Chronic bleeding may produce chronic, compensated anemia that requires preoperative blood transfusion. Patients with abdominal, flank, or back pain may have local invasion of the tumor into surrounding structures (muscles, ureter) or perforation of the tumor. The perforation may be contained and associated with an abscess, or it may be freely perforated. Imaging studies (acute abdominal series, CT scans of the abdomen and pelvis, abdominal ultrasonography, intravenous pyelography) that may not be routinely obtained for patients with colon cancer may be useful in these patients. Finally, symptoms suggestive of colonic obstruction (nausea and vomiting, crampy abdominal pain, obstipation, abdominal distension) may require altering the technique of preoperative bowel preparation, planned operative procedure (including a possible stoma), or preoperative hospitalization and resuscitation.

D. Surgical Considerations

Final considerations prior to proceeding with colectomy involve bowel preparation, patient position, and the surgical approach (laparotomy versus laparoscopy). Bowel preparation, intended to reduce the incidence of postoperative wound infection, involves both mechanical and antibiotic preparation. A multitude of regimens have been employed over the years to cleanse the colon of stool and bacteria mechanically. Current regimens use either large-volume (4 liters) colonic lavage with an orally administered polyethylene glycol (PEG)-based solution or a hypertonic sodium phosphate laxative (Fleets PhosphoSoda) administered the day before surgery along with restricting oral intake to clear liquids only. The PEG solution has the advantage of not causing any fluid or electrolyte imbalances at the expense of a large volume of unpleasant liquid. The PhosphoSoda preparation has the advantage of a much smaller volume to be taken (4 ounces twice) and better patient tolerance,[19] but it may cause dehydration and other fluid problems in patients with congestive heart failure or hyperphosphatemia in those with renal insufficiency. The goal of this mechanical preparation is to reduce the fecal load in the colon and reduce the quantity of bacteria in it. The concentration of bacteria in the stool is not affected by the mechanical preparation.[20–22] Antibiotic preparation may be given orally or intravenously. Oral antibiotics are chosen that are effective against the colonic flora, gram-negative rods, and anaerobes and that maintain a high level in the colonic lumen. A common regimen is to administer neomycin 1 g and erythromycin base 1 g at 1 p.m., 2 p.m., and 11 p.m. the day before surgery. The bowel preparation should be taken between the second and third doses. Intravenous antibiotics are administered against the same spectrum of organisms during the 30 minutes preceding the incision.

Patient positioning for surgery on colon cancer is an important consideration. The main advantage when altering the patient's position is to provide access to the anus, rectum, and left colon by placing the patient in the modified lithotomy position. This allows the use of transanal circular stapling techniques if a distal anastomosis is to be performed. A second advantage to the modified lithotomy position is the ease of performing intraoperative colonoscopy. This may be necessary to document the location of the area in question or examine the proximal colon in instances when it could not be examined preoperatively. Finally, if intraoperative findings suggest that the ureters are in jeopardy, the lithotomy position facilitates placement of stents.

Laparoscopic colorectal surgery is becoming increasingly more feasible and popular. Many concerns remain as to whether laparoscopic techniques offer significant advantages over the open, conventional techniques with respect to cost, speed of recovery, and resumption of gut function. When considering laparoscopic colectomy for malignancy, additional questions about the oncologic efficacy of laparoscopic techniques and port-site recurrences have been raised. Prospective clinical trials are currently under way to answer these questions; and until they are answered, laparoscopic colectomy for colon cancer should continue to be performed by highly skilled laparoscopic colorectal surgeons within the context of these trials.

E. *Laparotomy*

The surgical management of colon cancer begins with exploration of the abdomen. The primary tumor is assessed for its location and extent of local organ invasion. It is not uncommon for colonoscopic localization of a tumor to be inaccurate. Landmarks in the colon are not constant; varying degrees of colonoscopic insertion place the tip at the same location in the colon based on the degree of bowing and looping of the colonoscope, but the colonic length is variable among patients. Therefore it is of utmost importance to ensure that the proposed segment of the colon harboring the cancer is indeed the site involved. The extent of local organ invasion is another important factor to assess prior to dividing the colonic lumen or the blood supply to the colon. It is an unfortunate circumstance to be in a situation where these structures have been divided, only to find out that the degree of local organ invasion prevents resection.

In addition to assessing the primary tumor, the remainder of the abdomen is explored for distant disease. The liver is examined by inspection and bimanual palpation. The peritoneal surfaces are examined for implantation suggestive of carcinomatosis. The pelvis should also be examined with specific attention paid to the ovaries and pouch of Douglas. Suspicious lesions should be biopsied by wedge excision or core needle biopsy to provide a tissue diagnosis of disseminated disease.

F. *Oncologic Principles*

Prior to initiating resection, certain oncologic principles should be considered. The proximal and distal margins of resection and the level of vascular ligation must be determined. Other factors to consider are the utility of the "no-touch" isolation technique of resection and methods to reduce intraluminal tumor cells at the lines of resection to be used for anastomosis.

The *distal margin* is based on concern about distal, intramural spread of the tumor. This spread may occur through submucosal lymphatics but has rarely been seen to exceed 4 cm.[23] Consequently, when it is easy to obtain this distal margin, as it is in the colon, a 5 cm distal margin is recommended. The *proximal margin* of resection is generally based on the level of vascular ligation performed. The concern is that well vascularized bowel be used for the anastomosis. The level of vascular ligation depends on the location of the primary lesion, such that the draining lymph node basins are removed en bloc with the specimen. Therefore lesions involving the cecum and ascending colon require ligation of the ileocolic and right colic arteries. A right hemicolectomy with anastomosis between the terminal ileum and proximal transverse colon is performed. Lesions involving the transverse colon, from the hepatic to the splenic flexure, require extended right hemicolectomy. This involves ligation of the ileocolic, right colic, middle colic, and ascending branch of the left colic arteries. Anastomosis is performed between the terminal ileum and well vascularized descending colon. Lesions involving the splenic flexure and descending colon are managed by left hemicolectomy. The inferior mesenteric artery and left branch of the middle colic artery are ligated. Anastomosis is performed between the midportion of the transverse colon and the rectum. Lesions involving the sigmoid colon require ligation of the inferior mesenteric artery and the ascending branch of the left colic artery at its origin. The colon is divided at this level, which roughly corresponds to the junction of the descending and sigmoid colons, and the proximal rectum. The vascular supply to the proximal colon may be tenuous, as it is based only on the marginal artery originating from the left branch of the middle colic artery, and should be carefully assessed prior to using it for an anastomosis. The anastomosis is performed between the descending colon and proximal rectum.

The extent of lymphatic dissection and the level of vascular ligation must also be considered. Controversy exists as to whether more extensive dissection provides the patient with any survival benefit or reduced rate of local recurrence, and if there is more morbidity associated with more extensive dissection. Bacon et al.[24] performed a detailed study of lymph node involvement in specimens removed with an extensive lymphatic dissection. A total of 80 patients with left colon cancer were studied, 11 (14%) of whom had lymphatic metastases between the left colic artery and the origin of the inferior mesenteric artery. Of these 11 patients, 3 achieved 5-year survival, which would not be anticipated if the tumor-bearing lymph nodes were not resected. In another study Malassagne et al.[25] prospectively evaluated the outcome of patients undergoing radical excision of colon cancer with vascular ligation at the origin of the vessels. A significant impact on prognosis was noted for patients who had apical lymph node involvement. Specifically, the presence of apical lymph node involvement decreased the 5-year survival rate from 45% to 17%. Although it is unclear whether vascular ligation at the origin of the major colonic vessels actually improves survival, evidence suggests that assessment of apical lymph node involvement may at least improve prognostic abilities.

Other areas of investigation regarding the need for lymphatic dissection and evaluation have been directed at the minimum number of lymph nodes required to enable accurate assessment of lymph node involvement. This is an important question, as adjuvant therapy would not be recommended for patients who are inaccurately diagnosed as having node-negative disease. Hernanz et al.[26] estimated the minimum number of lymph nodes to be evaluated so the pathologic staging of the specimen reflects its true lymph node stage. A mathematic model was used to calculate the probability of finding at least one positive lymph node in a particular sample size of lymph nodes with a defined proportion of positive lymph nodes. Using this model, the authors determined that a minimum of six lymph nodes should be examined to provide a 95% probability that the lymph node status is accurately assessed. Increasing the minimum number of lymph nodes assessed to ten would increase the probability of an accurate lymph node staging to 99%. In another study, Caplin et al.[27] hypothesized that patient survival is improved if seven or more lymph nodes are examined. The study contained 211 patients with node-negative disease (82 patients with six or fewer lymph nodes examined) and 145 patients with node-positive disease. The 5-year survival for patients with node-negative disease and six or fewer lymph nodes examined was 49%, similar to that of node-positive patients in this series. The 5-year survival rate for patients with node-negative disease who had seven or more lymph nodes examined was 68%, and this difference was found to be statistically significant. The implication is that survival is improved by the degree of accuracy of defining these patients as node-negative. The worse prognosis (in patients with node-negative disease having six or fewer lymph nodes examined) is thought to be due to understaging the pathologic stage.

In summary, these studies suggest that wide excision of the mesocolon along with the primary tumor to include the greatest number of lymph nodes and the apical lymph nodes, at the very least, allows better pathologic staging and determination of prognosis. Consequently, high ligation at the origin of the vascular supply to the tumor-bearing segment is considered to be an important component of hemicolectomy for cancer.

The "no-touch" isolation technique of colonic resection, first described by Barnes in 1952[28] and popularized by Turnbull et al.,[29] was developed because of concern that manipulation of the tumor-bearing segment may result in dissemination of tumor emboli into the portal circulation and ultimately metastases. Fisher and Turnbull[30] demonstrated tumor cells in the portal venous blood in 8 of 25 patients undergoing colectomy for cancer.

The technique begins with lymphovascular ligation, proximal and distal division of the bowel, and then mobilization of the colon and tumor-bearing segment from its attachments. The first two maneuvers isolate the tumor from its access to the vascular system and colonic lumen *before* the tumor is manipulated during mobilization. This differs from a conventional approach to colectomy, which is initiated by mobilizing the colon and then dividing the bowel and blood supply. The details of the technique are beautifully described by Jagelman and Turnbull.[31] Whether the "no-touch" isolation technique results in a decreased incidence of metastases and improved outcome remains controversial.

Turnbull et al.[29] presented their results in 896 patients operated on for colon cancer between 1950 and 1964. They compared the outcome of 664 patients treated by Turnbull using the "no-touch" technique with 232 patients undergoing conventional resection performed by other surgeons at the Cleveland Clinic. A major benefit in patient survival was found for patients with node-positive disease. The 5-year survival rate was 58% for patients undergoing the "no-touch" technique, whereas the patients undergoing conventional resection had a 5-year survival rate of 28%. Although these results are impressive, the technique has received a great deal of criticism. This study contains a degree of bias in that the "no-touch" technique was performed by only one surgeon (not by random allocation) whose clinical skill, rather than the technique, may be responsible for the difference noted in 5-year survival rates.

Turnbull also compared his results of the "no-touch" technique with a group of historical controls undergoing conventional resection during the 3 years preceding his adoption of the "no-touch" technique.[32] The corrected 5-year survival rate for node-positive patients undergoing the "no-touch" technique ($n = 104$) was 78%, compared with 51% for 52 patients undergoing conventional resection. Although this difference is found in a series of patients operated on by the same surgeon using different techniques, the comparison is marred by the use of historical controls. Others have attempted to reproduce the dramatic results of Turnbull without success.[33,34] Although the efficacy of the technique remains controversial, the potential benefits are significant at a minimal expense, and the technique warrants further consideration.[35]

The primary tumor may be locally advanced and invading neighboring structures. Several series have demonstrated that 40–60% of adherent tumors have histologically proven malignant adhesions. Despite the locally advanced nature, 5-year survival rates of 40–60% have been achieved when a wide, en bloc dissection has been performed. Invasion into fixed structures (abdominal wall, duodenum, kidney, ureter) adds a significant level of difficulty to performing an oncologic colectomy. The problem is that the colon is fixed in two locations: the site of local organ invasion and the mesentery. When this is the case, the tumor should be approached from a relatively normal, easily mobilized segment of the colon. This may involve mobilizing the colon from both its proximal and distal ends, although the colon remains adherent to the involved structure and the mesentery. It is often difficult to free the tumor circumferentially without either entering the tumor or injuring the neighboring structure (which is problematic in the duodenum, kidney, and ureter). Even if entering the tumor or injuring neighboring structures is avoided, the wrong plane of dissection is often entered, making the dissection bloodier and more difficult than it might otherwise be.

An alternative approach is to mobilize the colon from a medial to lateral direction. The first maneuver is to divide all the major vessels to that segment of the colon at their origin. The mesentery is then bluntly dissected lateral to the tumor and proximal and distal to the planned lines of resection. Once this is achieved, the only remaining attachments are those of the tumor to the structure it has invaded. The specimen may then be elevated on this attachment, and the area can be seen much more clearly, allowing a safe, wide en bloc dissection. This technique is essentially the "no-touch" technique, and the increased visibility and preservation of tumor attachments are some of the undeniable advantages of this technique.

G. *Options for the Obstructing Cancer*

Colorectal cancer is the most common cause of colonic obstruction in the United States, with obstruction present in 8–30% of patients with colorectal cancer.[36] The presence of colonic obstruction may necessitate changes in the preoperative bowel preparation and operative procedure, and it potentially requires a diverting stoma.

Bowel preparation, as discussed above, is an integral part of the preoperative preparation for colon surgery. The type of bowel preparation used in the presence of colonic obstruction may have to be tailored to the patient's degree of obstruction and symptoms. Patients who are found to have an obstructing lesion on the basis of endoscopic or radiologic inability to pass a scope or contrast material through the lesion are described as having "retrograde obstruction." These patients most likely have been given, and tolerated, a bowel preparation for the examination, and it is reasonable to use the same preparation for surgery. In contrast, patients who are found to have an obstructing colorectal cancer and who manifest signs and symptoms of colonic obstruction (nausea, vomiting, colicky pain, abdominal distension, dilated proximal colon on abdominal radiographs) are described as having "antegrade obstruction." In this setting, the use of an aggressive bowel preparation (large volume PEG colonic lavage or a hypertonic sodium phosphate laxative solution) may be hazardous and result in bowel perforation. In this setting a slower, gentler preparation should be considered. Options include 3 days of clear liquids with repeated use of mild laxatives for mildly symptomatic patients or no bowel preparation for severely symptomatic patients. The patient should also be counseled to proceed cautiously with any of these options and to stop the use of any laxatives if symptoms worsen significantly.

The surgical options available for the management of obstructing colon cancer are the same as those for colonic obstruction in general. They include proximal diversion and delayed resection, segmental resection without anastomosis, segmental resection with intraoperative colonic lavage and primary anastomosis, subtotal colectomy with ileorectal anastomosis, or bypass of the obstructed segment. The site of the obstruction (right versus left), the stage of the cancer, and the degree of acute and chronic illness are important deciding factors. Patients who are acutely ill due to the colonic obstruction and those who are debilitated from chronic illness, may be best served by relieving the obstruction with proximal diversion and delaying resection of the obstructing lesion until the patient's medical condition is optimized. Alternatively, bypassing the obstructed segment may be the best option in patients with unresectable disease. Right hemicolectomy and primary anastomosis or end-ileostomy for obstructing right-sided colon cancer has been shown to be equally safe, with comparable anastomotic leak rates (10% and 6%, respectively).[37] The same is not true for left-sided obstructing colon cancer. An anastomotic leak rate as high as 18% has been reported in patients undergoing left hemicolectomy and primary anastomosis in the setting of left-sided colonic obstruction.[38] Segmental resection and proximal diversion is a safe alternative, but it has the disadvantages of a significant complication rate associated with subsequent surgery for reanastomosis, and as many as 30% of patients do not achieve colostomy reversal.[36] In an attempt to avoid these disadvantages, attempts have been made to restore continuity with a primary anastomosis at the time of resection. Two equally safe options have emerged: (1) segmental colectomy, intraoperative colonic lavage, and primary anastomosis; or (2) subtotal colectomy and ileorectal anastomosis. These two techniques have been found to have acceptable anastomotic leak rates of approximately 5% and 9%, respectively.[39] Subtotal colectomy has the advantage of being able to address synchronous disease in the proximal colon that requires resection (synchronous colon cancer, ischemia of the cecum secondary to obstruction) but has the disadvantage of tending to have a higher anastomotic leak rate. It also results in more frequent bowel movements.

In medically suitable patients with left-sided colonic obstruction, segmental resection, intraoperative colonic lavage,

TABLE 37–2.
Staging systems for colorectal cancer

Degree of involvement	Duke's 1935[a]	Astler-Coller 1954[b]	ACPS 1983	AJCC TNM 1997	
				TNM	Stage
Depth of primary tumor					
Lamina propria or muscularis mucosa	—	A	O	T0 = Tis	0
Submucosa	A	B1	A	T1,	I
Muscularis propria				T2	
Subserosa or pericolic fat			B	T3,	II
Adjacent organ or free tumor perforation	B	B2		T4	
Nodal metastases					
None	—	—	—	N0	—
1–3 Positive nodes	C1, C2	C1, C2	C	N1,	III
>3 Positive nodes	C1, C2	C1, C2		N2	
Distant metastases					
None	—	—	—	M0	—
Present	—	—	D	M1	IV

ACPS, Australian Clinicopathological Staging System.
[a] C1, epicolic nodes only; C2, involved nodes adjacent to level of vessel ligation.
[b] C1, primary lesion confined to bowel wall (i.e., B1) with any positive nodes; C2, primary lesion through bowel wall (i.e., B2) with any positive nodes.

and primary anastomosis is becoming the procedure of choice. Subtotal colectomy and ileorectal anastomosis is a reasonable option that should be reserved for patients who require synchronous proximal colectomy and do not have fecal peritonitis. Segmental resection without anastomosis is best reserved for patients with additional risk factors, such as poor nutritional status, immunosuppression, and perforation with fecal peritonitis.[36]

H. Staging and Prognosis

Several staging systems have been devised to help predict the outcome of patients with colon cancer. The importance of staging tumors is that it allows determination of patient prognosis and selection of additional therapies. Moreover, it affords the opportunity to compare the outcome of various treatments for patients with a similar expected outcome.

The first staging system was devised by Dukes in 1930.[40] He recognized the importance of three major factors that determine outcome: depth of tumor invasion, the presence of lymph node metastases, and the presence of distant metastases. These factors were combined into different stages described by the letters A, B, and C. Since his initial description, there have been many modifications of the original staging system; each uses the same letters (with the letter D added) as well as numbers to divide these stages into subgroups. The end result is a confusing collection of staging systems that have similar names and descriptors with different implications (Table 37–2). Alternatively, the AJCC has devised the TNM classification scheme based on the same factors.[41]

Additional factors have been identified as having prognostic significance, although they are not as strong determinants of survival as tumor invasion, nodal status, and presence of distant metastases.[42] Some of the more commonly known factors that adversely affect survival include a poorly differentiated tumor, lymphovascular invasion, symptomatic presentation (perforation or obstruction), and an inexperienced surgeon.

I. Adjuvant Chemotherapy

Adjuvant chemotherapy is provided to patients without evidence of disease as a "prophylactic" measure following potentially curative resection of the primary cancer. The impetus for this step is based on the significant variability in patient outcome following apparently curative resection.[43] Despite apparently complete surgical removal of the primary tumor and no evidence of metastatic disease, patients may ultimately die of recurrent, distant disease, suggesting that systemic metastases existed at the time of surgery but were not identifiable at that time, so-called micrometastases. These systemic metastases are amenable to systemic therapy. It is hypothesized that chemotherapy after cura-

TABLE 37–3.
Adjuvant chemotherapy for colon cancer: standards of care in 1999

TNM stage	Regimen	Drug	Dose	Schedule
II	No consensus on benefit of adjuvant therapy; individualize use to patients with other unfavorable features.			
III	6 Months: low-dose leucovorin	5-FU	425 mg/m^2/day IV bolus × 5 days	Every 4–5 weeks; repeat 6 cycles
		Leucovorin	20 mg/m^2/day IV bolus × 5 days	
	12 Months: high-dose leucovorin	Leucovorin	500 mg/m^2/day IV over 2 hours, then 5-FU	Every week × 6, 3 weeks rest, repeat 4–6 cycles
		5-FU	500 mg/m^2/day IV bolus × 5 days	

SOURCE: Macdonald.[53]

tive resection has the greatest chance of being effective when the metastatic burden is thought to be low. The problem is how to identify patients with the greatest likelihood of having micrometastases. Chemotherapy can be given to patients who may benefit from it the most, and those with a low probability of micrometastases would not be subjected to the morbidity of chemotherapy without potential benefit. There are no tests available to identify these patients. Therefore patients are encouraged to accept adjuvant chemotherapy based on the pathologic stage of the primary tumor. Tumors that have penetrated the entire bowel wall [T3 and T4 (stage II) lesions] and node-positive [N1 or N2 (stage III)] tumors are associated with a higher risk of recurrence.

Current chemotherapeutic regimens for colon cancer are based on the thymidylate synthase inhibitor 5-fluorouracil (5-FU). Although this drug has been used to treat colon cancer patients since its discovery in 1957,[44] its efficacy has only recently been elucidated. Several studies during the 1990s demonstrated the survival advantage of 5-FU-based regimens for patients with node-positive colon cancer. The first major study to alter the futile view of adjuvant chemotherapy for colon cancer was reported by Laurie et al.[45] in 1990 and updated in 1995.[46] This report detailed the results of the intergroup trial INT-0035, which compared surgery alone, surgery plus levamisole, and surgery plus 5-FU and levamisole in the treatment of stage III colon cancer. Levamisole is an anthelmintinic agent with a presumed immunomodulatory effect. The combination of surgery plus 5-FU and levamisole was superior to the other two treatment arms, with a 41% reduction in relapse rate and a 33% decrease in the death rate. After 7 years of follow-up the survival advantage persisted, with 60% of patients receiving adjuvant therapy surviving compared to 46% undergoing surgery alone. Thus adjuvant 5-FU plus levamisole became the standard of care for patients with stage III colon cancer. Subsequent studies have used this regimen as the gold standard against which new treatment strategies are tested.

The next major area of study evaluated the gold standard of adjuvant 5-FU plus levamisole against 5-FU with high- or low-dose leucovorin with or without levamisole.[47–52] Leucovorin was used as a biochemical modulator of 5-FU activity by stabilizing the 5-FU–thymidylate synthase complex and the resultant enzyme inhibition. Studies have shown that adjuvant chemotherapy using a 5-FU-based regimen results in higher 5-year disease-free and overall survival rates than surgery alone for patients with stage III colon cancer, and that several regimens have equal efficacy. Recent recommendations for adjuvant chemotherapy for stage III colon cancer are listed in Table 37–3.[53]

In addition to the progress made with the use of 5-FU in the treatment of stage III colon cancer, several other agents are being actively investigated. The agents being evaluated include topoisomerase inhibitors (irinotecan, topotecan, 9-aminocamptothecin), thymidylate synthase inhibitors (raltitrexed), oxaliplatin (a third-generation platinum complex), and 5-FU "prodrugs" (capecitabine, tegafur).[54] It is too early to incorporate these agents into standard practice, but it is likely they will be used in the near future.

J. Follow-up

The post operative follow-up of patients after curative resection for colon cancer is both crucial and controversial. The purpose of follow-up is to identify recurrent disease (local or distant) at its earliest stage such that the likelihood of potential curative resection is increased. As many as 40% of patients develop a recurrence following curative resection of a primary colon cancer, and most of these recurrences are diagnosed within the

TABLE 37–4.
Potential impact of follow-up after curative treatment of colon cancer

Study Follow-up regimen	No. of patients	Curative re-resection rate		Cumulative 5-year survival (%)	
Rosen[56a]					
Intensive	795	76/295 (25.8%)	$p = 0.0001$	61.6	$p = 0.003$
Conventional	725	25/284 (8.5%)		47.9	
Pietra[57b]					
Intensive	104	17/26 (65%)	$p < 0.01$	73.1	$p < 0.02$
Conventional	103	2/20 (10%)		58.3	

[a] Meta-analysis of two randomized and three comparative cohort studies.
[b] Prospective randomized study.

first 2 years after surgery.[55] Proponents of intensive follow-up cite improved resectability rates and better survival rates; opponents of intensive follow-up describe it as a program of unproven benefit at a great expense.[56] A recent meta-analysis evaluating the benefit of intensive follow-up after curative resection of colorectal cancer was reported by Rosen et al. in 1998.[56] These authors combined the results of two randomized, controlled clinical trials and three comparative-cohort studies. Each of these studies compared intensive follow-up programs that included a frequent history, physical examination, and CEA monitoring with traditional follow-up based on symptoms only and provided a minimum of 2 years of quantitative follow-up of patients with recurrent cancer. A statistically significant benefit was seen in the group of patients undergoing intensive follow-up with respect to curative re-resection rates, 5-year survival after recurrence, and cumulative 5-year survival rates (Table 37–4). Another study reported in 1998 described the results of a prospective, randomized controlled clinical trial of conventional and intensive follow-up of patients with colorectal cancer at a single institution.[57] This study also demonstrated a statistically significant advantage for patients in the intensive follow-up program with respect to curative re-resection rates and 5-year survival rates (Table 37–4).

Although these studies show promise for the benefit of intensive follow-up programs, many issues must still be resolved. The potential benefit has been demonstrated, but two major issues require further investigation. The first issue is who should undergo intensive follow-up after potentially curative resection (based on disease stage, site of primary lesion, and other factors). The second issue relates to the structure of the follow-up program (the tests to use and the frequency of testing) that are most beneficial and cost-effective. Once these issues are settled, the controversial nature of follow-up after curative resection for colorectal cancer will likely be eliminated.

References

1. Byers T, Levin B, Rothenberger D, Dodd GD, Smith RA. American Cancer Society guidelines for screening and surveillance for early detection of colorectal polyps and cancer: update 1997. CA Cancer J Clin 1997; 47:154–160.
2. Winawer SJ, Fletcher RH, Miller L, et al. Colorectal cancer screening: clinical guidelines and rationale. Gastroenterology 1997;112:594–642.
3. Mandel JS, Bond JH, Church TR, et al. Reducing mortality from colorectal cancer by screening for fecal occult blood. N Engl J Med 1993; 328:1365–1371.
4. Church JM. Flexible endoscopy insertion technique. In: Endoscopy of the Colon, Rectum, and Anus. New York: Igaku-Shoin, 1995:287.
5. Rex DK, Lehman GA, Hawes RH, Ulbright TM, Smith JJ. Screening colonoscopy in asymptomatic average-risk persons with negative fecal occult blood tests. Gastroenterology 1991;100:64–67.
6. Muller AD, Sonenberg A. Protection by endoscopy against death from colorectal cancer. Arch Intern Med 1995;155:1741–1748.
7. Coverage of Colorectal Cancer Screening. In: Illinois/Michigan Medicare B Bulletin, December 1987:22.
8. Winawer SJ, Zauber AG, Ho MN, et al. Prevention of colorectal cancer by colonoscopic polypectomy. N Engl J Med 1993;329:1977–1981.
9. Screening for colorectal cancer—United States, 1997. MMWR Morb Mortal Wkly Rep 1999;48:116–121.
10. Church JM. Colonoscopy for the diagnosis and treatment of colorectal bleeding. Semin Colon Rectal Surg 1992;3:42–48.
11. Markowitz AJ, Winawer SJ. Management of colorectal polyps. CA Cancer J Clin 1997;47:93–112.
12. Nivatvongs S. Benign neoplasms of the colon and rectum. In: Gordon PH, Nivatvongs S (eds) Principles and Practice of Surgery for the Colon, Rectum, and Anus. St. Louis: Quality Medical, 1999:548.
13. Haggitt RC, Glotzbach RE, Soffer EE, Wruble LD. Prognostic factors in colorectal carcinomas arising in adenomas: implications for lesions removed by endoscopic polypectomy. Gastroenterology 1985;89:328–336.
14. Cranley JP, Petras RE, Carey WD, Paradis K, Sivak MV. When is endoscopic polypectomy adequate therapy for colonic polyps containing invasive carcinoma? Gastroenterology 1986;91:419–427.
15. Waye JD. Polypectomy from A to Z. In: Syllabus Book, ASGE 15th Interim Postgraduate Course, New York, 1999:34.

16. Gordon PH. Malignant neoplasms of the colon. In: Gordon PH, Nivatvongs S (eds) Principles and Practice of Surgery for the Colon, Rectum, and Anus. St. Louis: Quality Medical, 1999:613.
17. Jerby BL, Milsom JW. Role of laparoscopy in the staging of gastrointestinal cancer. Oncology (Huntingt) 1998;12:1353–1360.
18. Liu SK, Church JM, Lavery IC, Fazio VW. Operation in patients with incurable colon cancer—is it worthwhile? Dis Colon Rectum 1997;40:11–14.
19. Vanner SS, MacDonald PH, Paterson WG, Prentice RSA, DeCosta LR, Beck IT. A randomized prospective trial comparing oral sodium phosphate with standard polyethylene glycol-based lavage solution (GoLYTELY) in the preparation of patients for colonoscopy. Am J Gastroenterol 1990; 85:422–427.
20. Raahave D, Hansen OH, Carstensen HE, et al. Septic wound complications after whole bowel irrigation before colorectal operations. Acta Chir Scand 1982;147:215–218.
21. Arabi Y, Dimock F, Burdon DW, et al. Influence of bowel preparation and antimicrobials on colonic microflora. Br J Surg 1978;65:555–559.
22. Weidema WF, van den Bogaard ARJM. Whole gut irrigation and antimicrobial prophylaxis in elective colorectal surgery [thesis]. Utrecht: Bohn, Scheltema & Holkema, 1984.
23. Fengler SA, Pearl PK. Technical considerations in the surgical treatment of colon and rectal cancer. Semin Surg Oncol 1994;10:200–207.
24. Bacon HE, Dirbas F, Myers TB, Ponce de Leon F. Extensive lymphadenectomy and high ligation of the inferior mesenteric artery for carcinoma of the left colon and rectum. Dis Colon Rectum 1985;1:457–465.
25. Malassagne B, Valleur P, Serra J, et al. Relationship of apical lymph node involvement to survival in resected colon carcinoma. Dis Colon Rectum 1993;36:645–653.
26. Hernanz F, Revuelta S, Redondo C, Madrazo C, Castillo J, Gomez-Fleitas M. Colorectal adenocarcinoma: quality of the assessment of lymph node metastases. Dis Colon Rectum 1994;37:373–377.
27. Caplin S, Cerottini JP, Bosman FT, Constanda MT, Givel JC. For patients with Dukes' B (TNM stage II) colorectal carcinoma, examination of six or fewer lymph nodes is related to poor prognosis. Cancer 1998;83:666–672.
28. Barnes JP. Physiologic resection of the right colon. Surg Gynecol Obstet 1952;94:723.
29. Turnbull RB Jr, Kyle K, Watson FR, Spratt J. Cancer of the colon: the influence of the no-touch isolation technic on survival rates. Ann Surg 1967; 166:420–427.
30. Fisher ER, Turnbull RB Jr. The cytologic demonstration and significance of tumor cells in the mesenteric venous blood in patients with colorectal carcinoma. Surg Gynecol Obstet 1955:100:102.
31. Jagelman DG, Turnbull RB Jr. Colectomy for malignant disease of the colon: the "no-touch" isolation technique. In: Todd, Fielding (eds) Rob & Smith's Operative Surgery. London: Butterworth, 1983:270–282.
32. Turnbull RB Jr. The no-touch isolation technique of resection. JAMA 1975;231:1181–1182.
33. Wiggers T, Jeekel J, Arends JW, et al. No-touch isolation technique in colon cancer: a controlled prospective trial. Br J Surg 1988;75:409–415.
34. Slanetz CA Jr. Effect of no-touch isolation on survival and recurrence in curative resections for colorectal cancer. Ann Surg Oncol 1998;5:390–398.
35. Beart RW Jr. To touch or not to touch [editorial]. Ann Surg Oncol 1998;5:389.
36. Lopez-Kostner F, Hool GR, Lavery IC. Management and causes of acute large-bowel obstruction. Surg Clin North Am 1997;77:1265–1290.
37. Phillips RK, Hittinger R, Fry JS, Fielding LP. Malignant large bowel obstruction. Br J Surg 1985;72:296–302.
38. Corman ML (ed). Carcinoma of the colon. In: Colon and Rectal Surgery, 4th ed. Philadelphia: Lippincott-Raven, 1998:668.
39. SCOTIA Study Group. Single-stage treatment for malignant left-sided colonic obstruction: a prospective randomized clinical trial comparing subtotal colectomy with segmental resection following intraoperative irrigation. Br J Surg 1995;82:1622–1627.
40. Dukes CE. The spread of cancer of the rectum. Br J Surg 1930;17:643.
41. Rösch T. Endoscopic guidelines: the new TNM classification in gastroenterology (1997). Endoscopy 1998;30:643–649.
42. Nathanson SD. Is there a role for clinical prognostic factors in staging patients with colorectal cancer? Semin Surg Oncol 1994;10:176–182.
43. Fuchs CS, Mayer RJ. Adjuvant chemotherapy for colon and rectal cancer. Semin Oncol 1995;22:472–487.
44. Heidelberger C, Chanakari NK, Danenberg PV, et al. Fluorinated pyrimidines: a new class of tumor inhibitory compounds. Nature 1957;179: 663–666.
45. Laurie JA, Moertel CG, Fleming TR, et al. Surgical adjuvant therapy of large-bowel carcinoma: an evaluation of levamisole and the combination of levamisole and fluorouracil. J Clin Oncol 1989;7:1447–1456.
46. Moertel CG, Fleming TR, Macdonald JS, et al. Fluorouracil plus levamisole as effective adjuvant therapy after resection of stage III colon carcinoma: a final report. Ann Intern Med 1995;122:321–326.
47. O'Connell MJ, Mailliard JA, Kahn MJ, et al. Controlled trial of fluorouracil and low-dose leucovorin given for 6 months as postoperative adjuvant therapy for colon cancer. J Clin Oncol 1997;15:246–250.
48. International Multicentre Pooled Analysis of Colon Cancer Trials (IMPACT) Investigators. Efficacy of adjuvant fluorouracil and folinic acid in colon cancer. Lancet 1995;345:939–944.
49. Francini G, Petrioli R, Lorenzini L, et al. Folinic acid and 5-fluorouracil as adjuvant chemotherapy in colon cancer. Gastroenterology 1994;106:899–906.
50. Haller DG, Catalano PJ, Macdonald JS, Mayer RJ. Fluorouracil (FU), leucovorin (LV) and levamisole (LEV) adjuvant therapy for colon cancer: preliminary results of INT-0089 [abstract]. Proc Am Soc Clin Oncol 1996;15:496.
51. Wolmark N, Rockette H, Mamounas EP, et al. The relative efficacy of 5-FU + leucovorin (FU-LV), 5-FU + levamisole (FU-LEV), and 5-FU + leucovorin + levamisole (FU-LV-LEV) in patients with Dukes' B and C carcinoma of the colon: first report of NSABP C-04 [abstract]. Proc Am Soc Clin Oncol 1996;15:460.
52. O'Connell JM, Laurie JA, Shepherd L, et al. A prospective evaluation of chemotherapy duration and regimen as surgical adjuvant treatment for high-risk colon cancer: a collaborative trial of the North Central Cancer Treatment Group and The National Cancer Institute of Canada Clinical Trials Group [abstract]. Proc Am Soc Clin Oncol 1996;15:478.
53. Macdonald JS. Adjuvant therapy of colon cancer. CA Cancer J Clin 1999;49:202–219.
54. Punt CJA. New drugs in the treatment of colorectal carcinoma. Cancer 1998;83:679–689.
55. Galandiuk S, Wieand HS, Moertel CG, et al. Patterns of recurrence after curative resection of carcinoma of the colon and rectum. Surg Gynecol Obstet 1992;174:27–32.
56. Rosen M, Chan L, Beart RW Jr, Vukasin P, Anthone G. Follow-up of colorectal cancer: a meta-analysis. Dis Colon Rectum 1998;41:1116–1126.
57. Pietra N, Sarli L, Costi R, Ouchemi C, Grattarola M, Peracchia A. Role of follow-up in management of local recurrences of colorectal cancer: a prospective, randomized study. Dis Colon Rectum 1998;41:1127–1133.

Chapter 38

High Risk Premalignant Colorectal Conditions

Marc I. Brand
James M. Church

Colorectal cancer (CRC) remains a major health threat as we enter the twenty-first century. It is responsible for the third highest rate of cancer deaths in both men and women in the United States. Two major events during the last few decades of the twentieth century greatly enabled us to better understand the genesis of CRC and to identify individuals at higher than average risk for its development: the advent of flexible colonoscopy with polypectomy and the identification of genetic mutations in both sporadic and hereditary forms of CRC. Colonoscopy with polypectomy has enabled us to identify and remove colorectal adenomas before the development of CRC. This practice has been shown to reduce the incidence of CRC in the National Polyp Study[1] and may be partly responsible for the overall decreased incidence of CRC in the United States.[2] Advances in molecular genetics have identified some of the mutations that underlie the transformation of normal colorectal mucosa to adenomas and finally cancer (the adenoma–carcinoma sequence)[3] as well as transmissible germline mutations in the syndromes of familial adenomatous polyposis and hereditary nonpolyposis colorectal cancer. The recommendations in this chapter are based on current information and may well be refined as knowledge increases. The emphasis of this chapter is on patients with a risk for CRC higher than that of the general population: those with familial colorectal cancer, mucosal ulcerative colitis, and the hereditary CRC syndromes of hereditary nonpolyposis colorectal cancer and familial adenomatous polyposis.

Familial Colorectal Cancer

The term familial colorectal cancer (FCC) refers to clustering of CRC in a single family. The pattern of clustering suggests the presence of some common causative factor but does not fit the criteria for a dominantly inherited syndrome. The causative factors that underlie this clustering are unknown but are thought to be a combination of environmental and hereditary factors. It is estimated that 10% of adults in the Western world have a first-degree relative (FDR) with CRC.[4,5]

Several studies have demonstrated an increased risk of CRC if an individual has an FDR with CRC. The risks have been summarized by Allen[6] and are as follows.

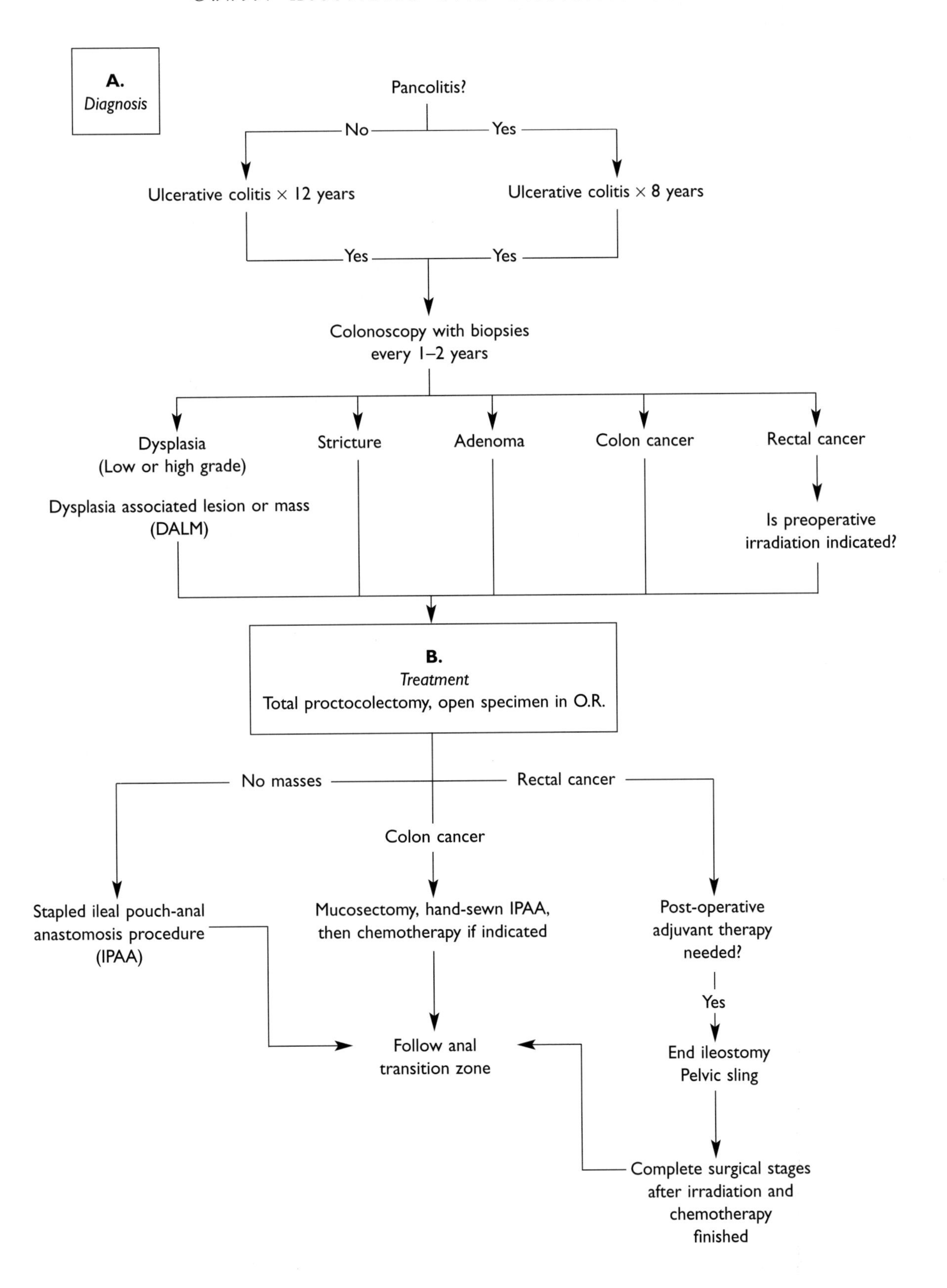

Cancer Associated with Ulcerative Colitis
A.
Diagnosis
Pancolitis?
No
Yes
Ulcerative colitis × 12 years
Ulcerative colitis × 8 years
Yes
Yes
Colonoscopy with biopsies every 1–2 years
Dysplasia (Low or high grade)
Dysplasia associated lesion or mass (DALM)
Stricture
Adenoma
Colon cancer
Rectal cancer
Is preoperative irradiation indicated?
B.
Treatment
Total proctocolectomy, open specimen in O.R.
No masses
Rectal cancer
Colon cancer
Stapled ileal pouch-anal anastomosis procedure (IPAA)
Mucosectomy, hand-sewn IPAA, then chemotherapy if indicated
Post-operative adjuvant therapy needed?
Yes
End ileostomy
Pelvic sling
Follow anal transition zone
Complete surgical stages after irradiation and chemotherapy finished

1. Average risk adult: 1 in 50
2. CRC in one FDR at any age: 1 in 17
3. Neoplastic polyp in one FDR at age <60 years: 1 in 14
4. CRC in one FDR at age <50: 1 in 10
5. CRC in two FDRs at any age: 1 in 6

Little is known about the genetic defects responsible for FCC. However, a recent publication has demonstrated a relation between a novel mutation and FCC in Jewish people of Ashkenazic (eastern European) descent.[7] The inherited mutation is located at codon 1307 of the *APC* (adenomatous polyposis coli) gene and consists of a single nucleotide transversion (T to A). This results in a single amino acid substitution (lysine for isoleucine) and transcription of a full-length protein product (not a stop codon and truncated protein product as commonly happens in familial adenomatous polyposis. Interestingly, a somatic mutation (not inherited in the germline but acquired after conception) was found close to the inherited codon 1307 mutation in 48% of tumor specimens in which the codon 1307 mutation was present. This second, somatic mutation resulted in a truncated protein product. The codon 1307 mutation is thought to create an unstable sequence (hypermutable tract), which predisposes this segment of the *APC* gene to somatic, protein truncating mutations, which are then pathogenetic. This study also found that the codon 1307 mutation was found only in Ashkenazi Jews and not in non-Jewish controls. In fact, the greater the family CRC history, the higher was the percentage of individuals with the mutation. The mutation was found in 6.1% of Ashkenazim without CRC (mean age 34.2 years), 10.4% of all Ashkenazim with CRC, 16% of Ashkenazim age less than 66 years of age with CRC, and 28% of Ashkenazim with CRC and a positive family history. These results are intriguing for an association between this mutation and FCC in Ashkenazim, but more study is necessary to show the reproducibility of the association and to strengthen it. Furthermore, the positive predictive value of this mutation within a family for the ultimate development of colorectal neoplasia in gene carriers must be determined.

Current recommendations for unaffected, at-risk patients with a positive family history for CRC are fairly straightforward.[6] It is anticipated that they will be refined as our understanding of the *APCI* 1307 K and other mutations increases. Patients with a single FDR with CRC (age >60 years) undergo the average risk screening regimen reported by the American Cancer Society but beginning at age 40 years.[8] Patients with a single FDR with CRC (age <60 years) or an additional relative with CRC should undergo colonoscopic screening 10 years earlier than the youngest affected relatives with CRC. It is currently unknown whether these patients from a FCC family develop CRC from normal mucosa more rapidly than in patients with sporadic CRC (10 years).[9] Therefore the currently recommended interval between screening examinations is 5 years.[6]

Cancer Associated with Ulcerative Colitis

A. Diagnosis

Pancolitis The association between mucosal ulcerative colitis (MUC) and CRC has been recognized for more than half a century. Debate remains as to the magnitude of the risk as well as the utility of a surveillance program for early detection of precancerous changes or even cancer itself. Epidemiologic evidence suggests that the greatest cancer risk is associated with pancolitis (disease proximal to the splenic flexure), and that the risk increases exponentially with duration of disease. A community-based study found the cumulative risk of cancer for patients with pancolitis to be 7.2% after 20 years of disease and 16.5% after 30 years of disease, a relative risk 19 times that of the general population.[10] The risk of cancer in those with proctosigmoiditis was significantly less (1.8% vs. 11.9% at 20 years of symptoms) than that of pancolitis in a study of 1248 patients.[11] Current evidence suggests that coexisting primary sclerosing cholangitis (PSC) is an independent risk factor for cancer in MUC. A study from the Cleveland Clinic found that 12.9% (17/132) of MUC patients with PSC developed CRC, whereas only 2.6% (5/196) of a randomly selected group of MUC patients (of similar disease duration and extent) without PSC developed CRC.[12] The development of cancer complicating MUC differs from sporadic cancer in its earlier age of onset (mean age 43 years) and its multicentricity (13.5%).[11]

Prevention of cancer or cancer mortality requires prophylactic removal of all mucosa at risk. There is currently no effective chemopreventive agent. The timing of surgery may be based on entry into a higher risk category (e.g., development of PSC, defined duration of disease). Such a policy would result in frequent removal of colons without cancer or precancerous change, many of which would be from relatively asymptomatic patients. Alternatively, surgery may be recommended once a precancerous state is found. This is the basis of current surveillance programs, but there is currently no strong evidence to support the effectiveness of these programs in reducing the cancer mortality rate. A decision analysis showed that proctocolectomy only for low-grade dysplasia was nearly as effective at reducing cancer-related mortality as prophylactic colectomy in the absence of dysplasia.[13] Most authors recognize the importance of a surveillance program with regularly scheduled colonoscopy and random biopsy. The factors assessed should include dysplasia (low grade, high grade), a dysplasia-associated lesion or mass (DALM), stricture, adenoma, or cancer.

One recommended surveillance program involves colonoscopy beginning 8 years after the onset of pancolitis or 12 years after the onset of left-sided colitis. Colonoscopy is performed every 1–2 years with four-quadrant random biopsies every 10 cm. Additionally, areas endoscopically suspicious for flat dysplasia (discolored mucosa, velvety villous appearance, fine nodular thickening), DALM, (firm polypoid structures, irregular nodularity, discolored mucosa), or strictures should also be biopsied.[14] It is important to recognize that dysplasia, and even cancer, can develop in relatively bland-appearing mucosa and may not have any distinguishing endoscopic features.

DYSPLASIA The association between dysplasia and cancer in MUC was first noted by Morson and Pang in 1967.[15] A great deal of discussion has since been directed at the histologic definition of dysplasia and its relation to cancer. It is now recognized that dysplasia can be patchy, multifocal, remote from the site of malignancy, and hidden in relatively normal-appearing mucosa. It has been estimated that a minimum of 33 random biopsies from the entire colon must be obtained to have a 95% chance of sampling from dysplastic mucosa when it is present.[16] Hence the recommendations for conducting surveillance colonoscopy have been offered as described above. Studies have shown that 40% of patients found to have high grade dysplasia were also found to have a cancer on subsequent total proctocolectomy (TPC).[17] Similarly, 50% of patients found to have low grade dysplasia are expected to develop high grade dysplasia or a cancer within the next 5 years.[18] The presence of a DALM was associated with a cancer in 43% of cases.[17] A word of caution about dysplasia is advisable: The histologic diagnosis of dysplasia in ulcerative colitis can be confusing, and variability among pathologists reviewing the same specimen can be significant.[19]

STRICTURE A stricture is worrisome and may herald the presence of cancer. Provided Crohn's disease and spasm had been excluded, a stricture was associated with cancer in 6 of 15 (40%) cases; only two of these six cancers were diagnosed preoperatively. Neoplasia (low-grade dysplasia, high-grade dysplasia, cancer) was found in 13 of 15 (86%) of cases.[20] Consequently, finding a stricture in MUC warrants prophylactic surgery.

ADENOMA One of the more difficult situations to manage is an adenoma arising in colitic epithelium. The confusion is whether it represents a sporadic adenoma (for which the entire population is theoretically at risk) or a DALM in MUC. There are no good studies to help solve this problem. The current recommendation is that if the patient is less than 50 years of age the likelihood of a sporadic adenoma is low and the adenoma should be considered MUC-related. Additionally, if the adenoma has developed in a background of acute, chronic, or quiescent colitis it should be considered MUC-related.[21] This then represents an indication for prophylactic surgery.

The presence of a colonic or rectal cancer may jeopardize sphincter preservation. For the latter, especially if located in the distal rectum, one must not compromise oncologic principles in the hope of completing an ileoanal anastomosis; and if sphincter excision is indicated, it should be performed without hesitation.

B. TREATMENT

The operation of choice for CRC prophylaxis in MUC is proctocolectomy to remove the colonic and rectal mucosa completely. The basis for this recommendation is the multicentric nature of MUC-related cancer. Alternatively, total abdominal colectomy and ileorectal anastomosis (TAC/IRA) has been used for surgical management of MUC; long-term follow-up of these patients has revealed a cancer risk of 6% at 20 years, 15% at 30 years, and 32% at 43 years.[22] Only complete mucosal excision eliminates this risk.

An important component of prophylactic surgery is intraoperative assessment of the colorectal mucosa. The specimen should be opened and rinsed for adequate visual and tactile examination of the mucosa, inspecting for any masses or ulceration suspicious for cancer. Any areas that are equivocal should be evaluated by frozen section.

If no malignancy is found on pre- or intraoperative inspection of the mucosa, we recommend an ileal pouch/anal anastomosis (IPAA) via a double-stapled anastomosis with preservation of the anal transition zone (ATZ) (Fig. 38–1). Preservation of the ATZ is associated with better functional results, a lower leak rate, and a shorter operation than mucosectomy with a handsewn anastomosis. The theoretic disadvantage of ATZ preservation is whether the remaining diseased

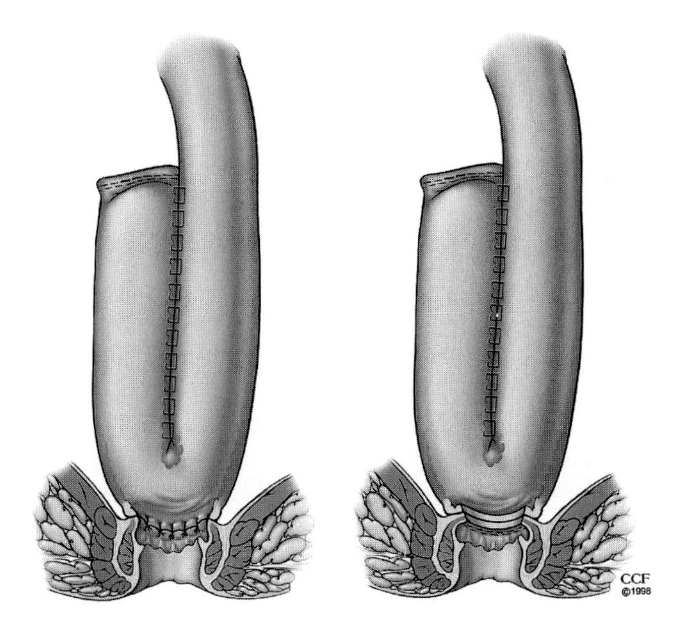

FIGURE 38–1
Ileal pouch-anal anastomosis: mucosectomy followed by handsewn anastomosis (left), double-stapled technique (right) without mucosectomy. (Reprinted with permission from the Clevel and Clinic Foundation.)

mucosa is at risk for carcinoma. Although the length of follow-up is relatively short, no case of cancer in the ATZ following a double-stapled anastomosis has been described. The Cleveland Clinic has reviewed their experience with slightly more than 200 patients having a stapled anastomosis between 1987 and 1992 with 5–10 years of follow-up and biopsy of the ATZ.[23] Only eight patients were found to have dysplasia in the ATZ, seven of whom had low-grade dysplasia. No cancers were identified.

If a colon cancer is present, we recommend mucosectomy and handsewn ileoanal anastomosis (Fig. 38–1). This is based on the above-mentioned study from the Cleveland Clinic,[23] which indicated a trend for the development of ATZ dysplasia in patients with colon or rectal cancer. If chemotherapy is indicated, it is wise to delay closure of the loop ileostomy until chemotherapy is completed. If disseminated intraabdominal cancer is found, survival is compromised; and it is probably best to construct an end-ileostomy alone and not construct a pouch at this time.

If a mid or distal rectal cancer is present in the proctocolectomy specimen that was not diagnosed preoperatively and it appears advanced enough that it may require postoperative adjuvant therapy (stage II or III), it is wise to delay construction of the ileoanal pouch. As one might expect, a radiated pouch has significantly worse long-term function.[24] Instead, we recommend performing a proctocolectomy with end-ileostomy and to quarantine the small bowel from the pelvis (and radiation field) with the use of a pelvic sling, utilizing omentum or an absorbable mesh. Once radiotherapy is completed, the ileoanal pouch can be constructed and a mucosectomy with handsewn anastomosis performed. As stated previously, the presence of a distal rectal cancer (especially if advanced) argues against sphincter preservation.

The long-term effects of using small bowel to create the ileoanal pouch are not known. Pouches are subject to fecal stasis and with time frequently show chronic inflammation and colonic metaplasia of the mucosa. In fact, dysplasia in the pouch has been described. Therefore we recommend continued annual surveillance of the ATZ (if retained) and the pouch with endoscopy and biopsy of both areas. Low-grade dysplasia of the ATZ found on surveillance biopsy may represent true dysplasia or MUC-related inflammatory/reparative changes. Treatment consists of topical antiinflammatory agents and repeating the biopsies at 3 months. Persistent dysplasia is treated with mucosectomy, pouch advancement, and handsewn neo-IPAA, which may be accomplished through a transanal approach. If high-grade dysplasia is found, prompt mucosectomy is indicated without repeating the biopsy.

Hereditary Nonpolyposis Colorectal Cancer

Hereditary nonpolyposis colorectal cancer (HNPCC) is inherited in an autosomal dominant fashion. This syndrome, like other forms of hereditary CRC, produces CRC at a significantly earlier stage in life than sporadic CRC. HNPCC is associated with a high lifetime risk of CRC (approximately 80%) despite the formation of relatively few polyps.[25] Affected individuals lack physical features (multiple colonic polyps, pigmentation changes) to provide an early clue to the diagnosis of HNPCC and susceptibility to cancer. Although this syndrome is thought to represent only 5–10% of all CRCs, its recognition is crucial for appropriate screening, timely surgery, and counseling of family members. The critical tools necessary to diagnose HNPCC are a thorough family cancer history and a high index of suspicion when confronted with certain cardinal features.[26]

1. Early age of onset (mean age 44 years, earliest age 20 years)
2. Proximal location of CRC (70% of cancers are proximal to the splenic flexure)
3. High rate of synchronous or metachronous CRC (45% if initial treatment was less than subtotal colectomy)
4. Certain histologic features (poor differentiation, abundant extracellular mucin, signet-ring cells, peritumoral lymphoid response)
5. Multiple primary epithelial (endometrial, ovarian, small bowel, renal, gastric) cancers

C. Diagnosis

The clinical diagnosis of HNPCC is based on the application of criteria proposed by the International Collaborative Group on Hereditary Non-Polyposis Colorectal Cancer (ICG-HNPCC) at a 1990 meeting in Amsterdam.[27] These criteria, known as the Amsterdam criteria, were established to describe a familial pattern of CRC that exhibits an autosomal dominant inheritance pattern and is extremely unlikely to occur by chance alone.[28] These criteria are easily remembered by the "3-2-1-0" rule and are summarized as follows.

1. At least *three* relatives with histologically confirmed CRC, with at least one individual being an FDR of the other two
2. CRC involving at least *two* generations
3. At least *one* case of CRC diagnosed before age 50
4. Syndrome is *not* familial adenomatous polyposis (FAP)

Although the last criterion seems obvious, there may be some confusion between an "aggressive" case of HNPCC and an attenuated form of familial adenomatous polyposis (FAP). A patient belonging to an "Amsterdam family" should be evaluated as being at risk for HNPCC.

A patient may also present for evaluation of CRC risk because of a relative with an HNPCC-related cancer and a

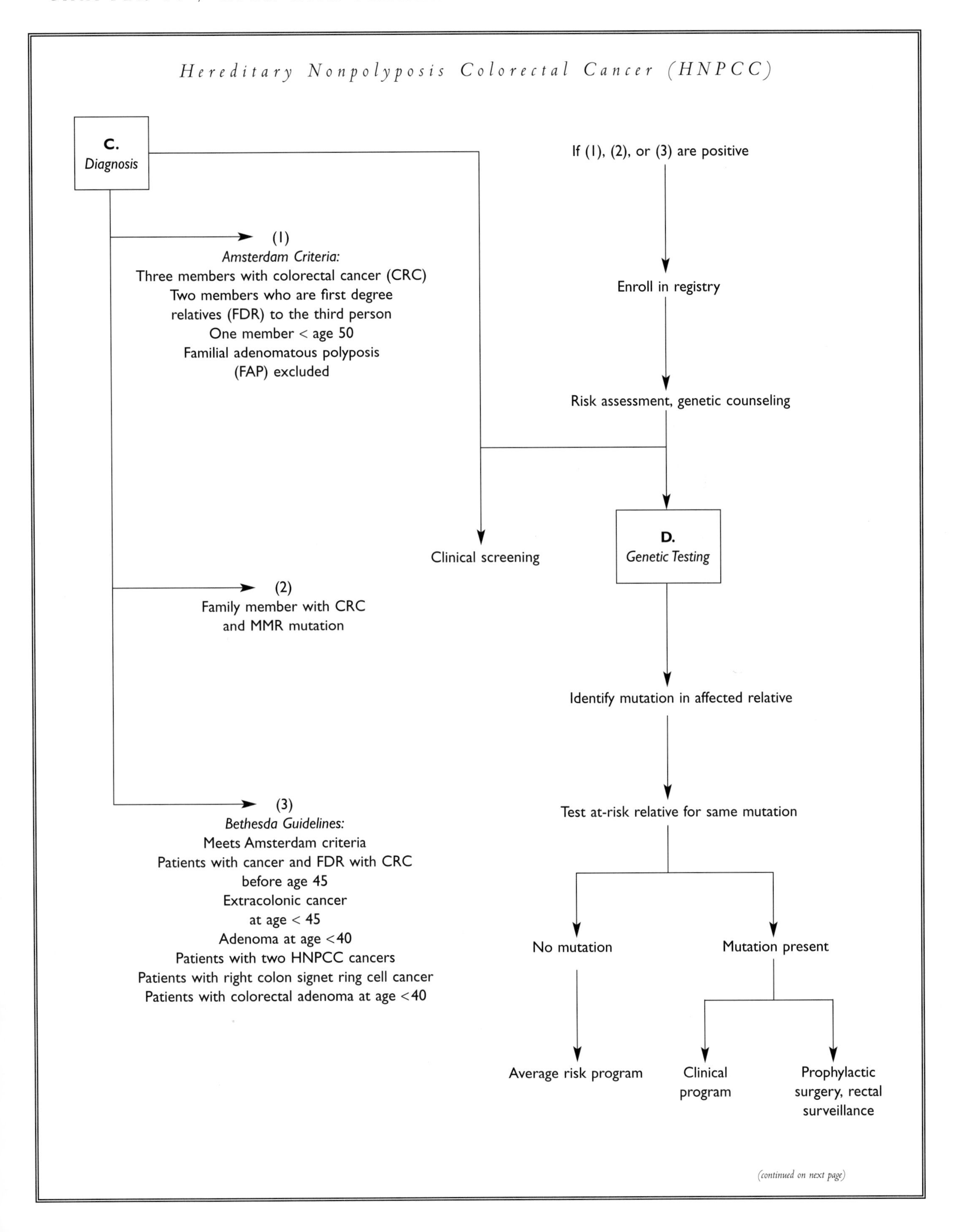

(continued on next page)

Hereditary Nonpolyposis Colorectal Cancer (HNPCC) (continued)

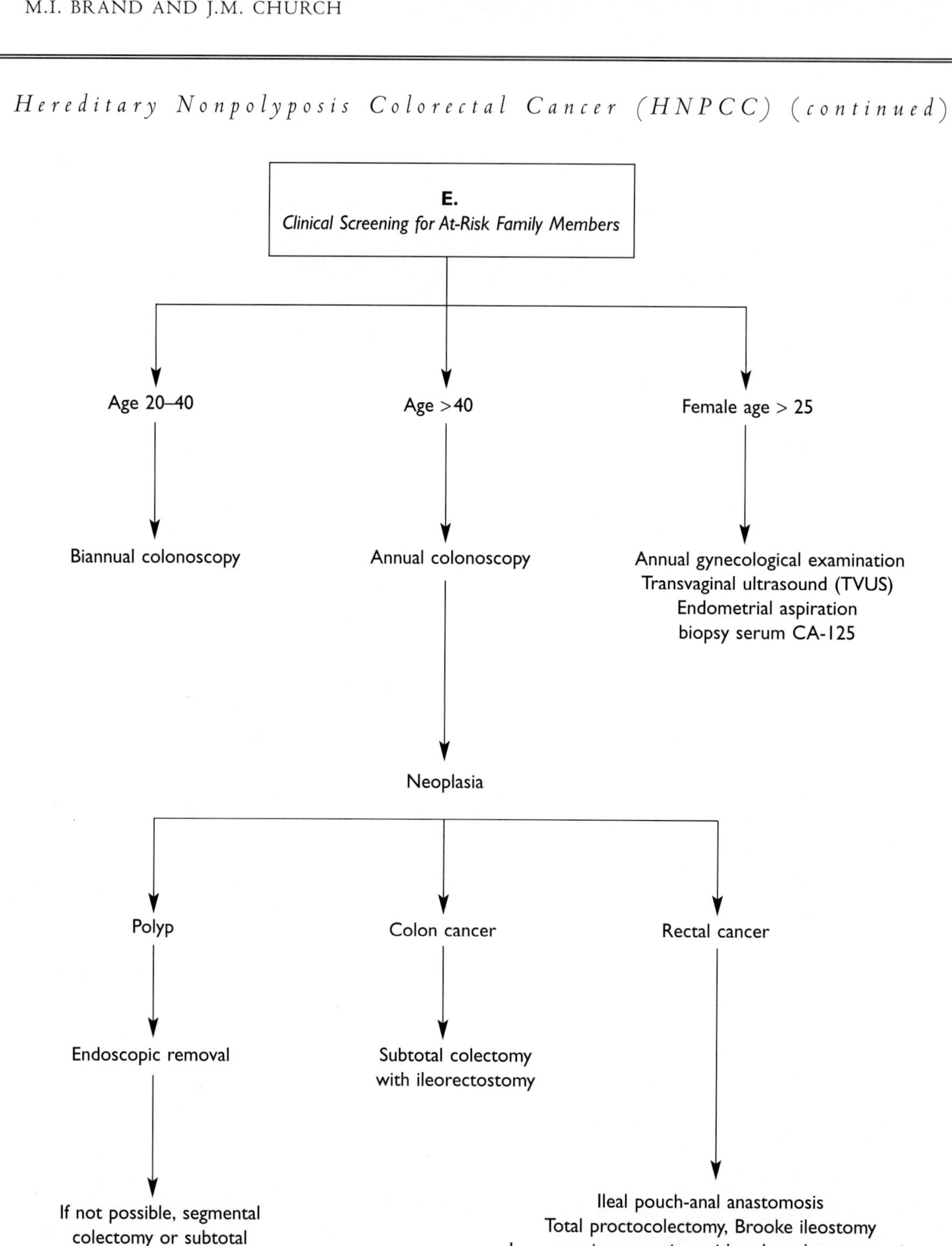

mutation implicated in HNPCC (see below). That patient likely belongs to an HNPCC family. Such patients and family members at risk for HNPCC should be evaluated with that concern in mind.

Criticism has been directed at the *Amsterdam criteria* on several grounds, all of which reflect the difficulty of making an early diagnosis of HNPCC.

1. A small kindred may not have an adequate number of relatives at risk to fulfill the Amsterdam criteria at the time of presentation.[29]

2. Families may be unable to provide complete information due to:[6]
   a. Early death of relatives from noncancer causes, prior to the onset of cancer which may have ultimately developed.
   b. Lack of knowledge of all existing relatives at risk.
   c. Lack of knowledge of the health issues of other relatives at risk.

3. Extracolonic cancers are not addressed by the Amsterdam criteria.[30]

About 50% of Amsterdam-positive families have a mutation.

A central question is how to identify HNPCC families that do not (yet) meet the Amsterdam criteria. In response to this concern, guidelines were established to identify patients who should undergo testing of the tumor for microsatellite instability (see below), the molecular phenotype of HNPCC tumors. Identification of microsatellite instability would then warrant germline *MMR* gene mutation analysis. These guidelines originate from a workshop of the Early Detection Branch of the National Cancer Institute held in Bethesda in 1996.[31] These guidelines have become known as the "Bethesda Guidelines" and are summarized as follows.

1. Patients whose family meets the Amsterdam criteria

2. Patients with CRC and an FDR with
   a. CRC diagnosed before age 45, *or*
   b. An estracolonic, HNPCC-related, cancer diagnosed before age 45, *or*
   c. A colorectal adenoma diagnosed before age 40

3. Patients with two HNPCC-related cancers (two synchronous or metachronous CRCs or CRC and HNPCC-related cancer)

4. Patients with signet-ring cells or right-sided, undifferentiated CRC diagnosed before age 45

5. Patients with endometrial cancer diagnosed before age 45

6. Patients with a colorectal adenoma diagnosed before age 40

The presence of any one of these six items is sufficient to warrant testing for MSI.

Patients who have been found to belong to an HNPCC family or are suspected of it on the basis of meeting the Bethesda Guidelines should be referred to a hereditary colorectal cancer registry. *Registries* have made a significant impact on the understanding and management of familial adenomatous polyposis and will undoubtedly prove to be a great resource for HNPCC families and their treating physicians.

Patients identified as belonging to an HNPCC family (on the basis of having met the Amsterdam criteria or the Bethesda Guidelines or because of a relative with an HNPCC-related cancer and an appropriate mutation) should undergo extensive counseling. The counseling must discuss cancer risk and genetic testing for both the patient and all at-risk relatives. Discussions with family members require the understanding, permission, and assistance of the patient; without this level of patient involvement, a breach of confidentiality and lack of understanding of family dynamics may result in suboptimal care.

A major breakthrough in the application of molecular genetics to the study of HNPCC occurred in 1993[32,33] when genetic linkage to a locus on chromosome 2p was demonstrated in two large HNPCC families from North America and New Zealand. The molecular defect resulting from this mutation caused a lack of recognition of errors in DNA replication, the so-called DNA mismatch repair (MMR) system. Five MMR genes have currently been identified: *hMLH1*, *hMSH2*, *hPMS1*, *hPMS2*, and *hMSH6*. These five genes account for 60–70% of HNPCC mutations, and it is anticipated that other mutations will be found in other areas of the MMR system. Among these genes, 90% of mutations in HNPCC have been identified in *hMLH1* and *hMSH2*. Although numerous and unique mutations have been identified, the end result of the mutation is a truncated protein product in approximately 70% of mutations.[34,35]

The molecular phenotype of cells that harbor defective MMR is known as a replication error (RER) or microsatellite instability (MSI). Microsatellites are segments of DNA with repetitive base sequences, which may be as little as two bases long. These microsatellites are prone to slippage of the DNA strands during replication, producing an abnormal number of basepairs. MSI itself is not the cause of cancer but is reflective of the cells' overall inability to correct errors in DNA replication. It is these "other errors" that can affect oncogenes and tumor suppressor genes, resulting in carcinogenesis. Studies have demonstrated that 77–95% of HNPCC tumors demonstrate MSI, in contrast to only 13–20% of sporadic tumors.[36]

D. Genetic Testing

Once genetic testing has been chosen as the means for initial evaluation of an Amsterdam or Bethesda family, testing should begin with one of the patient's affected relatives. Three approaches can be taken: (1) identify the genetic defect (direct gene sequencing of all the MMR genes); (2) identify the structurally abnormal gene product [protein truncation testing (PTT) or immunohistochemistry (IHC)] using any tumor tissue; or (3) identify the functional loss of the mutated gene product (MSI) using a sample of tumor and normal tissue. A practical approach to the initial evaluation is to study an affected relative first. In Bethesda families, if both normal and tumor tissue is available from this person, MSI testing should be performed to document the defective MMR system. This is a relatively simple, inexpensive technique that can be performed on any parafin-embedded tissue block or normal cell including white blood cells. PTT or IHC of the MMR gene protein products is another simple and inexpensive technique that can define the presence of a mutation and localizes the affected gene in approximately 70% of identifiable mutations.[35] Genetic sequencing to identify the exact mutation can then be applied to the gene responsible for the truncated protein. Having identified the exact mutation, subsequent family members can easily be tested for the same mutation. Genetic sequencing for HNPCC is commercially available (Myriad Genetic Laboratories, Salt Lake City, UT) and cost about $2000 for the initial analysis. Testing at-risk relatives once the mutation in a family is known costs about $350. MSI testing is now commercially available (Johns Hopkins Medical Laboratories, Baltimore) and costs about $300.

Mutations involving a change in a single base may not produce a truncated protein (negative PTT) and may or may not be associated with HNPCC. Therefore if the PTT is negative but the tumor is MSI-positive, direct gene sequencing of MMR genes is warranted. Given that 90% of mutations are in the *hMLH1* and *hMSH2* genes,[35] it is prudent to begin with sequencing these two genes first. If the mutation is identified, subsequent family members can be tested for the same mutation. However, it is possible for initial genetic testing of a family to identify a MSI^+ tumor but not a genetic mutation. This result should be interpreted as a false negative (i.e., HNPCC is present but the involved gene has not yet been identified). That family should pursue a clinical screening program (see below).

If a mutation has been identified in the family, all at-risk relatives should be tested for that mutation. Having already identified the mutation, it is a relatively simple task to study any cell in an at-risk relative for that mutation by direct genetic sequencing of that gene. The sample used is from peripheral blood.

The relatives who test negative for a known mutation have not inherited the syndrome and do not carry the high risk of cancer associated with HNPCC. These individuals are spared the rigorous lifetime screening program and constant health concern (for themselves and their offspring) they would have otherwise had to endure. This is one of the major benefits of genetic testing. They do, however, carry the same risk as the general population and should be enrolled in an average risk CRC screening program.

Individuals who test positive for the mutation have inherited the syndrome and carry an 80% chance of developing CRC. Management of these patients may be expectant and conservative by enrolling them in a clinical screening program tailored to the natural history of HNPCC (see below).

Conversely, management may be aggressive and prophylactic, consisting of a subtotal colectomy and ileorectal anastomosis (STC/IRA).[37] There are no studies available that demonstrate the utility (survival benefit, cancer prevention, cost-effectiveness) of prophylactic STC/IRA, but it is justifiable on the basis of an 80% chance of developing colorectal neoplasia over the patient's lifetime. Factors to be considered when contemplating prophylactic colectomy include the patient's age, fear of cancer, medical co-morbidity, anal sphincter function, and compliance with a clinical screening program. Total proctocolectomy and ileal pouch-anal anastomosis (TPC/IPAA) cannot be justified as a prophylactic procedure for HNPCC because proctectomy significantly increases the operative morbidity.

It is important to remember that a prophylactic STC/IRA does not entirely eliminate the possibility of cancer. This risk of rectal cancer after STC/IRA is estimated to be 12% at 12 years.[38] It is imperative that both the physician and patient recognize this and that continued rectal cancer surveillance with annual proctoscopy be maintained in addition to the rest of the clinical screening program (see below).

E. Clinical Screening for At-Risk Family Members

Clinical screening programs for HNPCC effectively reduce the incidence of CRC and help diagnose CRC at an earlier stage. Furthermore, screening has been shown to reduce CRC-related mortality and improve the 5-year survival rate.[39,40] Three questions must be answered: Which organ systems (if more than one) are at sufficient risk and require screening? What is the appropriate test to screen each system? What is the appropriate age to begin and the best time interval between screening examinations?

As previously indicated, patients with HNPCC are at increased risk for cancers in many of the epithelial-lined organs, including the colon, uterus, ovaries, small bowel, urinary tract, biliary tree, and pancreas. The colon is by far the most frequently involved organ; 32% of HNPCC mutation-positive patients develop CRC by age 40, and nearly 90% develop CRC by age 75.[6] The earliest CRC has been diagnosed at about age 16 years.[40] Second in frequency is endometrial cancer, with approximately one-third of women developing this cancer by age 70. Ovarian cancer is the third most frequent HNPCC-related malignancy; 10% develop ovarian cancer by age 70. These three cancers occur at a sufficient rate to warrant regular screening.[6] The remainder of the extracolonic cancers occur with a lifetime risk of less than 5%; and for these cancers a history, physical examination, and basic laboratory studies are all that is needed.

For example, the biliary tree can be assessed by seeking evidence of cholestasis, and the urinary tract can be assessed by seeking evidence of gross or microscopic hematuria at the regularly scheduled screening tests.

Colonoscopy is the study of choice for CRC screening in HNPCC patients. The entire colon must be evaluated, as 70% of CRCs are proximal to the splenic flexure. It is estimated that each polyp has a 50% chance of progressing to cancer and can do so while still <1 cm in size.[28] The greater sensitivity of colonoscopy (compared to barium enema) for small polyps and the ability to destroy the polyp through the colonoscope makes colonoscopy a more effective screening tool.

The recommended age to begin CRC screening is 20–25 years of age or 10 years before the age of diagnosis of the youngest affected relative. This timing is based on the observation that it is rare for CRC to develop before age 20. The frequency of examinations has not been standardized, and most authorities recommend an interval of 1–3 years. Interval cancers have been reported within 2 years of the previous total colonic screening examination,[40] and it is thought that HNPCC adenomas may have a more rapid growth rate. Additionally, the potential of adenomas <10 mm to be missed and to harbor malignant potential exists.[41] Therefore a reasonable schedule of colonoscopic screening allows a longer interval earlier in the schedule (when the risk of CRC developing is lower) and a shorter interval when the risk of developing CRC is higher. One such schedule employs colonoscopy every 2 years for HNPCC patients age 20–39 years and then annual colonoscopy after age 40. The age at which to discontinue the high risk screening program and return to an average risk program is not well defined. As many as 8% of CRCs present after the age of 60,[42] and most authorities recommend continuing high risk screening until co-morbidity is such that an aggressive approach is unwarranted.

Screening guidelines for endometrial and ovarian cancer are even less well studied, and there is no reliable means (family history, specific mutation) to determine which women with HNPCC will develop either of these cancers. Endometrial cancer screening is performed with endometrial aspiration and transvaginal ultrasonography (TVUS) (82–98% sensitivity).[43] Ovarian cancer screening includes TVUS and serum CA-125 measurement. The recommended age to begin screening is at 25–35 years based on a mean age of 40 years at diagnosis. The frequency with which these tests should be performed is not well established, but current recommendations are for annual evaluation.

After completion of the appropriate screening examinations, patients who have not been found to have neoplasia should be encouraged to return for the next screening examination(s) and to report any new and persistent symptoms that may develop in the interim. This may generate some unnecessary phone calls, but it keeps the patient cognizant of the risk of cancer and the need for continued screening. Patients who have been found to have neoplasia on screening examination require further management to eliminate the neoplastic growth, and the options must be individualized based on the neoplasm and the patient.

If the identified neoplasm is a colonic *polyp*, it should be biopsied or removed endoscopically, if possible. Endoscopic polypectomy alone is adequate therapy for the completely removed adenoma and even for polyps harboring cancer, provided the margin is not involved, the cancer is well differentiated, and it lacks lymphovascular invasion. If the patient has large or multiple polyps or if a malignant polyp lacks the above favorable features, options include a segmental resection or STC/IRA. The latter effectively reduces the risk of cancer and makes subsequent surveillance of the large bowel much easier without increasing the operating time or morbidity. Therefore if surgery is indicated for a colonic polyp in the setting of HNPCC, STC/IRA should be performed in most cases.

If a *cancer* is found, operative choices are segmental colectomy, STC/IRA, and TPC/IPAA. Studies have shown a 40% rate of metachronous colon cancer at 10 years in HNPCC patients treated by segmental resection,[44] making this option undesirable in young patients. The added complexity and morbidity of proctectomy and IPAA make this procedure a second choice after STC/IRA. It is most appropriate for individuals with a high degree of anxiety regarding the potential of a metachronous rectal cancer and those in whom compliance with subsequent rectal surveillance is expected to be low.

Patients found to have a *rectal cancer* pose similar concerns about the extent of resection. In this case, the choice is among proctectomy/coloanal anastomosis (CAA), TPC/IPAA, and TPC/ileostomy. The morbidity associated with proctectomy is equally present for all three options, with progressively more altered bowel function for the three options as listed. If the patient is young and suitable for sphincter preservation, TPC/IPAA is the best alternative because it eliminates the risk of metachronous cancer and preserves bowel continuity. Construction of the ileal pouch should be delayed if postoperative radiotherapy is anticipated.

Female patients undergoing operative management of colonic neoplasia should be counseled regarding the risk of endometrial and ovarian cancer and be given the opportunity to decide on a concomitant total abdominal hysterectomy and bilateral salpingoophorectomy (TAH/BSO). Strong consideration for TAHBSO should especially be given for patients who are postmenopausal or those who have completed childbearing.

Familial Adenomatous Polyposis

Familial adenomatous polyposis (FAP), like HNPCC, is a hereditary form of CRC that is inherited in an autosomal dominant fashion. FAP is estimated to occur in 1:8000 live births and is thought to be responsible for 1% of the CRC burden in the United States.[45] The natural history of the disease is punctuated by the certain development of CRC at a young age (usually before age 40 years) and the variable development of extracolonic manifestations. Gardener syndrome (colonic polyposis, osteomas, epidermoid cysts, desmoid tumors) and Turcot syndrome (colonic polyposis, brain tumors) are now known to represent variations of FAP and its extracolonic manifestations. The latter are beyond the scope of this chapter and are not discussed in any detail.

F. Diagnosis

The clinical diagnosis of FAP rests on identifying multiple (>100) adenomatous colorectal polyps. This definition is based on the phenotypic expression of the disease and does not require a family history of FAP (20% of patients lack a family history).[46] This is in sharp contrast to the clinical diagnosis of HNPCC (Amsterdam criteria). Attenuated FAP has been recognized as a variant of FAP, where the patient develops fewer than the minimum 100 polyps (usually 20–100 polyps) used to diagnose FAP.[47]

In at-risk relatives of known FAP patients (parents, siblings, children), FAP may be diagnosed with less stringent criteria. Specifically, the presence of one or more adenomatous polyps at an early age (<50 years) in an at-risk relative is sufficient for the diagnosis. Similarly, the presence of an extracolonic manifestation in an at-risk relative can be used to diagnose FAP prior to the onset of colonic polyps.

The diagnosis of FAP has significant implications for both the patient initially diagnosed and all family members at risk for FAP. The patient and his or her family face significant health concerns, insurance and employment limitations, and family planning issues. Enrollment in a registry devoted to the care of families with hereditary CRC is a vital component in the complete care of the patient and family. The registry is composed of, or has access to, health professionals with dedicated interest in FAP from multiple specialties including surgery, gastroenterology, genetics, and social work. This team approach provides the FAP family with guidance about proper screening and surveillance programs, tracing extended family members at risk for FAP, and psychosocial support. The United Kingdom experience during the initiation of two registries during the late 1980s demonstrates the importance of a registry in identifying at-risk relatives in need of screening. The West Midlands Polyposis Register found that only 52% of at-risk relatives were in a screening program,[48] and the Northern Region Polyposis Registry found only 6.5% of at-risk relatives were being screened for FAP.[49] The registry also complements the resources and medical care provided by the patients' treating physician(s) so all the needs of the FAP family are fulfilled. Finally, the registry provides the necessary link between clinical management, research, and education. Therefore every family with a diagnosis of FAP should be referred to, and encouraged to enroll in, a polyposis registry.

G. Risk Assessment

The initial role of the treating physician (or registry) is to ensure that the initial presenting member of a FAP family (proband) is properly educated about FAP. This includes discussion about the natural history of FAP, the patient's risk for CRC, duodenal polyps, and desmoid tumors, current knowledge of molecular genetics and testing for FAP, and the recommended surveillance and treatment programs. The proband should be educated about the 50% risk of FAP in his or her FDRs; and consent to contact at-risk relatives should be obtained from the patient. Similar education is provided to these at-risk relatives.

Once a FAP family with at-risk relatives is identified, the proband and his or her relatives can be approached regarding genetic testing. Genetic testing is available through several commercial laboratories (www.genetests.org) and is based on recent advances in our understanding of the molecular defects responsible for FAP. The gene responsible for FAP was localized to the long arm of chromosome 5 by Herrera and colleagues in 1986[50] and is now known as the adenomatous polyposis coli (*APC*) gene. The *APC* gene is large (8500 kb pairs), and its protein product provides a tumor suppressor function that when lost by inactivating gene mutations sets the stage for epithelial neoplasia. The ultimate pathway to CRC in FAP is thought to be the same pathway that leads to sporadic CRC and involves mutations in several other genes.[51] Most *APC* mutations result in a premature stop codon and consequently a truncated protein product that can be detected by the protein truncation test (PTT) in 80% of FAP patients.[52] The PTT is performed on a peripheral blood sample and is considered positive when two protein products of differing size (normal and truncated) are detected. The size of the truncated protein can be used as a guide to the point in the large *APC* gene where the mutation is located for subsequent genetic sequencing and direct mutational analysis. This initial analysis costs about $500 and takes about 2 weeks to complete at the Allogen Laboratories. Once the specific mutation is identified, at-risk relatives can easily be tested for that same mutation at a cost of about $250.

Before embarking on genetic testing, the requesting physician must be able to identify the proper indications for genetic testing for FAP and the proper sequence and interpretation of the genetic tests; and the physician must also be prepared to provide the necessary psychosocial support for the family undergoing genetic testing. A study evaluating the clinical use of genetic testing for FAP demonstrated that 83% of the 177 individuals tested had appropriate indications for testing, but 32% of the test results were misinterpreted by the ordering physician.[53]

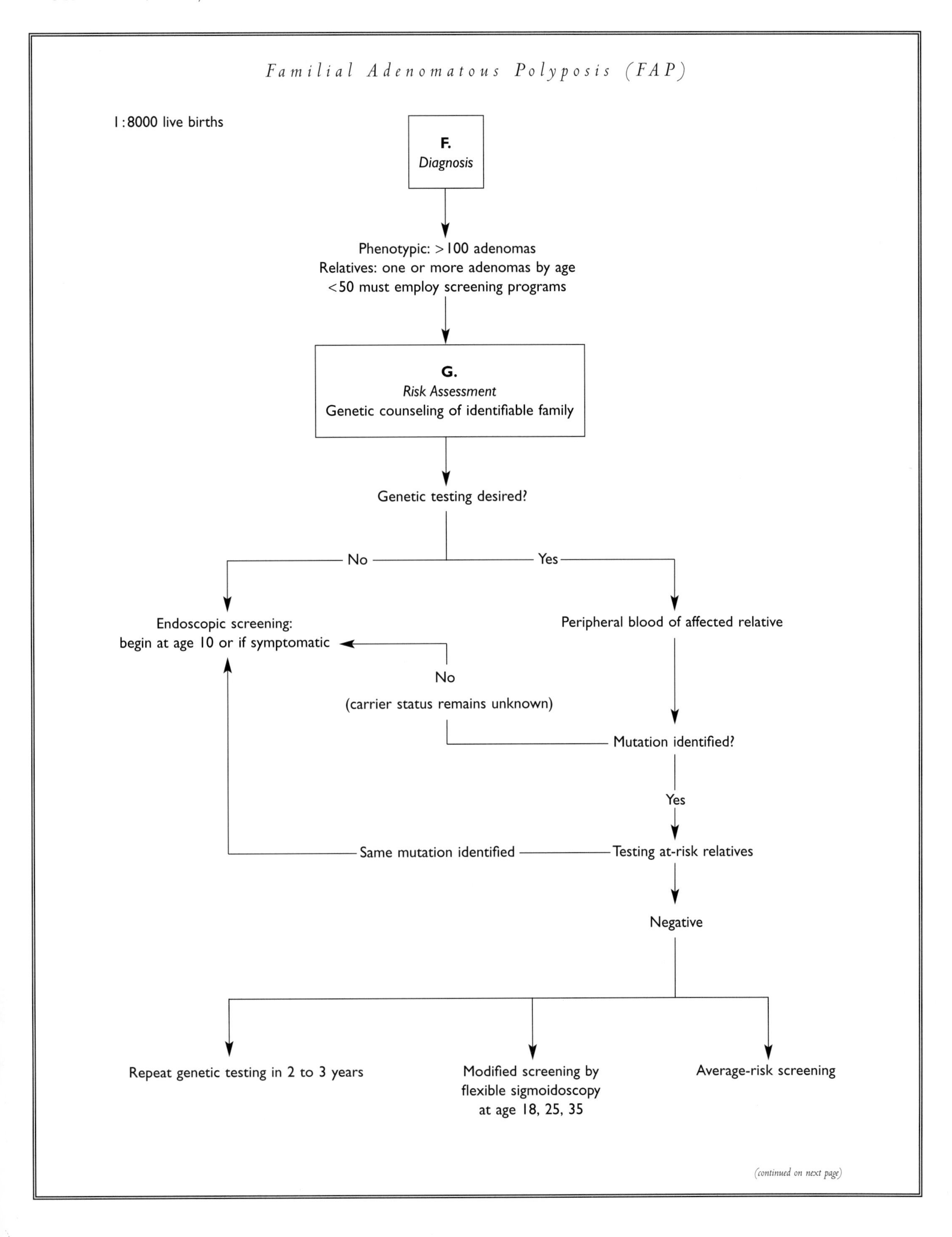

(continued on next page)

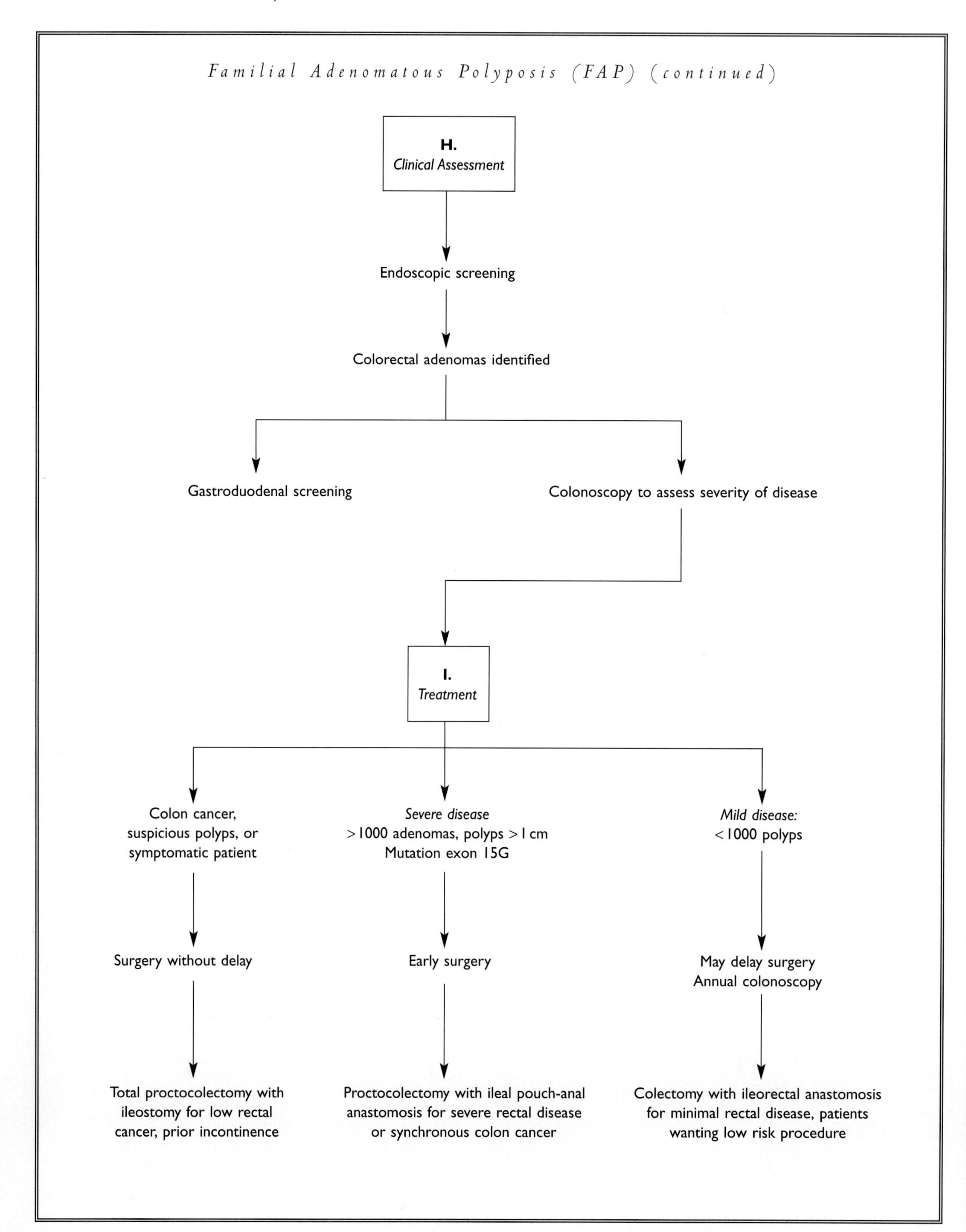
Familial Adenomatous Polyposis (FAP) (continued)
H.
Clinical Assessment
Endoscopic screening
Colorectal adenomas identified
Gastroduodenal screening
Colonoscopy to assess severity of disease
I.
Treatment
Colon cancer, suspicious polyps, or symptomatic patient
Severe disease
>1000 adenomas, polyps >1 cm
Mutation exon 15G
Mild disease:
<1000 polyps
Surgery without delay
Early surgery
May delay surgery
Annual colonoscopy
Total proctocolectomy with ileostomy for low rectal cancer, prior incontinence
Proctocolectomy with ileal pouch-anal anastomosis for severe rectal disease or synchronous colon cancer
Colectomy with ileorectal anastomosis for minimal rectal disease, patients wanting low risk procedure

Genetic testing for FAP is indicated when knowledge of presymptomatic carrier status can alter the approach to FAP on the part of the patient or ordering physician. At-risk relatives may be more compliant with surveillance programs if a positive carrier status is identified, or they may make family planning decisions based on this information. The ordering physician may be able to reduce the frequency of examinations significantly in the endoscopic screening program of at-risk relatives who do not carry the mutation. Occasionally, the diagnosis of FAP may be in doubt (attenuated FAP), and identification of a germline *APC* mutation can secure the diagnosis of FAP. The proper sequence and interpretation of testing is addressed below. The results of genetic testing may have profound psychosocial implications (confidentiality, guilt, alterations in family relationships, and limitations in employment and insurance opportunities). These issues require pre- and posttest counseling as well as written informed consent. The previously mentioned study of clinical FAP gene testing found these issues neglected in more than 80% of patients tested.[53]

After providing appropriate counseling, obtaining written informed consent, and completion of the family pedigree, testing the FAP family (or a portion of the family) that desires genetic testing may commence. Testing begins with a peripheral blood sample from an affected relative before studying at-risk relatives. This strategy is used to increase the yield of positive results on the first person tested. Testing an affected individual first has an 80% chance of identifying the mutation.[52] Conversely, initial testing of a presymptomatic at-risk relative is anticipated to have half that chance (40%), as this individual has only a 50% chance of having FAP. When protein truncation is not present, the presence of various phenotypes can be used to screen associated "hot spots" in the gene, as several genotype-phenotype correlations have been identified.[54] Specifically, severe polyposis (>1000 polyps) is associated with mutations on exon 15E. Conversely, attenuated FAP is localized to exons 3, 4, and the 3′ end of exon 15. Families with congenital hypertrophy of the retinal pigment epithelium (CHRPE) have mutations localized between exons 9 and 15G.

If initial genetic testing identified the *APC* mutation, predictive testing of presymptomatic at-risk relatives can be performed. Results can then be given as positive or negative for inheritance of FAP. However, if genetic testing does not identify a mutation in the *APC* gene and the in vitro synthesized protein (IVSP) assay does not demonstrate a truncated protein product, testing is uninformative. Other tests to identify the mutation may be performed (linkage analysis, direct gene sequencing) if desired. However, no prediction of FAP inheritance can be made by testing subsequent presymptomatic family members until a mutation has been found, and further testing should not be done until then. Instead, these FAP families must be evaluated by an endoscopic screening program.

Once the mutation is identified in the family, subsequent testing of all at-risk relatives in whom testing is desired can be undertaken at a significantly lower cost and with a more meaningful interpretation. Testing of children should begin just before the time for the first screening endoscopy examination, usually at age 10–12 years. If testing detects the same mutation in an at-risk relative, endoscopic surveillance should start immediately (see below) because the penetrance is near 100%. If testing does not detect the same mutation, the individual has not inherited FAP and has a CRC risk similar to that of the general population. Opinions vary as to the appropriate CRC screening of these patients, as there is a theoretic risk of a false-negative result. Therefore options for screening include repeating the genetic test in 2–3 years, undertaking a modified screening program (flexible sigmoidoscopy at ages 18, 25, and 35 years), or simply instituting an average risk screening program.

H. Clinical Screening

A clinical screening program is necessary for every relative at risk for developing polyposis. Individuals who have declined the option of genetic testing require screening because their carrier status is unknown and they carry a 50% risk of inheriting FAP. Similarly, in families where genetic testing has been uninformative (no mutation found), the carrier status remains unknown and the risk of FAP remains at 50%. Finally, an individual identified as carrying the *APC* mutation on genetic testing has inherited the syndrome and must be evaluated in a screening program.

The purpose of a clinical screening program is to identify the onset of polyposis in a presymptomatic phase. The screening program should be predicated on the natural history of the disease, such as age at which polyps first appear, where they appear, and when cancers may start. Polyp formation is rarely noted before the age of 7 years, but nearly 20% of FAP patients have polyps by age 10.[55] The distribution of polyps is relatively homogeneous throughout the colon and rectum and can be reliably identified by rigid proctoscopy or flexible sigmoidoscopy. The earliest age of cancer diagnosis in the literature is 12 years,[56] with 7% of untreated patients developing cancer by age 21.[5] Consequently, colorectal polyps can be reliably detected before malignant degeneration in most patients by performing proctosigmoidoscopy (rigid or flexible) annually beginning at age 10. The importance of presymptomatic screening of at-risk relatives has been shown in several studies. Comparison of CRC rates between probands and call-up cases (screening done because of at-risk status) underscore this importance. Bussey demonstrated a 66.2% CRC rate in FAP probands that was significantly reduced to 9.4% in the call-up group.[57] Results of the Finnish registry reveal similar efficacy, with CRC present in 65.5% of probands but in only 6.6% of the call-up group.[58]

The presence of a single adenomatous polyp in a young patient with FAP indicates the onset of phenotypic expression of FAP for that patient. Before focusing on management of the colon and rectum, it is important to recognize the potential for duodenal neoplasia and institute an appropriate screening protocol. An excellent review of duodenal polyposis has been reported from the St. Mark's Prospective Foregut Surveillance Programme.[59] Duodenal polyps are common in FAP, affecting 90% of patients, and are almost always adenomatous. Only a small number of patients ultimately develop a malignancy, but it still represents the second most common cause of cancer death associated with FAP after CRC.[60] The periampullary region is involved in almost all cases, although the neoplasia may be microscopic. A side-viewing endoscope is used to improve visualization of the periampullary region, and multiple biopsies of grossly visible polyps are obtained. A staging system (based on polyp number, size, histologic pattern, presence of dysplasia) can then be applied to the endoscopic and histologic results to classify the severity of the duodenal polyposis.[61]

Duodenal screening should begin by age 25 years. Patients with early-stage duodenal polyposis (Spigelman stage I or II based on number, size, and histology of the adenomas)[61] should be reexamined every 3 years. If there is no progression in the stage of duodenal polyposis, it is reasonable to reexamine the patient in 5 years. Patients with advanced duodenal polyposis should be examined biannually (stage III) or annually (stage IV). If the stage has progressed since the last examinations, a shorter interval between examinations (1 year) is recommended. Finally, interval development of symptoms or signs relating to upper intestinal pathology (epigastric pain, occult gastrointestinal bleeding, pancreatitis, jaundice) indicate early reexamination, as they may reflect an underlying malignancy. Management of duodenal polyposis remains under study and in evolution. Patients with large villous adenomas, severely dysplastic adenomas, or duodenal cancer should be considered for a pancreaticoduodenectomy.

Once a single colorectal adenomatous polyp is identified histologically, the entire colon and rectum should be evaluated by colonoscopy. Although the diagnosis of FAP is now confirmed and the need for surgery determined, more information is needed to refine the surgical recommendation. Evidence suggesting severe polyposis (>1000 polyps), advanced stage of polyp formation (>1 cm), or the presence of cancer mandate prompt surgical intervention. If surgery is to be delayed longer than 1 year after diagnosis, colonoscopy should be performed annually to prevent delay in surgery if these features have developed in the interim.

I. Treatment

Surgery without delay is indicated for patients who have a colon cancer. Furthermore, it is prudent to recommend surgery without delay in patients who have a polyp suspicious for cancer (but not proven histologically), as sampling error may give a false sense of security. Similarly, several studies have shown a 65% rate of cancer at the initial evaluation of patients presenting with symptoms[57,58]; therefore symptomatic patients should also undergo prompt surgical intervention.

Patients who manifest evidence of severe or advanced FAP should be advised to have surgery during the next few months. Severe disease may be phenotypic (>1000 adenomas) or genotypic (mutations in exon 15G) and has been associated with twice the cancer rate of patients with mild disease.[54,62] Additionally, the presence of large polyps (>1 cm) suggests and advanced stage of polyposis and need for surgery in the near future.

Surgery may be offered at a convenient time for patients with mild polyposis (<1000 polyps). This may mean delaying surgery a few years for young children until the patient's psychosocial and physical development is more conducive to surgery. Annual colonoscopy should be performed until the time of surgery, so progression of disease to severe polyposis or cancer is not allowed to persist for an extended period of time.

Colonic surgery for FAP is performed with both curative and prophylactic intent. Every colectomy should be conducted according to oncologic principles, and the surgeon should assume that an occult cancer is present and a curative operation must be performed. Surgery is also prophylactic, being meant to provide a significant, durable reduction in cancer incidence without excess operative or functional morbidity. The three major options for realizing these goals are total proctocolectomy with either an end-ileostomy or ileal pouch-anal anastomosis (TPC/IPAA) and total abdominal colectomy with ileorectal anastomosis (TAC/IRA).

TPC with end-ileostomy has the advantage of entirely eliminating the risk of CRC with low operative morbidity, but this is achieved with significant functional morbidity because of the permanent ileostomy and the potential genitourinary dysfunction associated with a proctectomy. Both of these functional morbidities can be devastating to the young patient undergoing prophylactic surgery for FAP. Therefore it has generally been relegated to cases of absolute necessity when the anal sphincter cannot be salvaged as a result of low rectal cancer or poor preoperative sphincter function.

TPC/IPAA is an excellent operation for FAP. It virtually eliminates the risk of CRC, especially when a rectal mucosectomy is performed. The functional morbidity of a permanent stoma is eliminated, but patients with previously normal bowel function are still faced with several stools per day and potential problems with continence. The operative morbidity is increased owing to multiple anastomotic lines in the pouch and the potential for an anastomotic leak. Therefore this operation is often reserved for those high risk situations when it is not wise to retain the rectum: severe polyposis (>1000 polyps),[63] significant rectal polyposis (>20 polyps),[64] a large rectal polyp, and a synchronous colon cancer. The presence of a cancer, even in the colon, should prompt proctectomy, as the mucosa in at least one area has sustained enough genetic insult to have caused a cancer.

TAC/IRA is another option for FAP in selected cases. It is associated with lower operative and functional morbidity than TPC/IPAA, but there is a delayed increased risk of rectal cancer and need for proctectomy. The reported incidence of rectal cancer following TAC/IRA varies widely, ranging between 3.6% and 59.0%; most series report an incidence of 10–20%.[65] These reports are difficult to compare because many factors affect the incidence of cancer, including the length of the remaining rectosigmoid stump, status of the rectum at colectomy, and follow-up intensity/compliance.

Patients with an IRA or IPAA require continued follow-up for CRC surveillance. The potential for rectal polyps and cancer following IRA is obvious. In fact, rectal cancer has even been noted after apparent regression of rectal polyps.[66] Several cases of anal transitional zone (ATZ) polyps following ATZ-preserving IPAA have been reported.[67,68] Ileal pouch adenomas[68,69] and even ileal pouch carcinoma[70] have been reported as well. Thus there is a definite need for continued surveillance of either the retained rectum following IRA or the ileal pouch and ATZ following IPAA if subsequent advanced cancer is to be prevented. Regular examination of this area with a rigid or flexible scope and biopsy or fulguration of any polyps is recommended. The initial intervals should be relatively short (3 months) until the area at risk is free of polyps for two examinations. At that time the interval can be extended to every 6 months and then ultimately annually.

One of the most intriguing prospects for FAP is chemoprevention of polyp formation. Sulindac is the most promising of the currently evaluated agents. A study from Germany[71] demonstrated encouraging results in polyp regression, with 78% of patients having complete polyp regression and the remaining 22% showing partial regression. Moreover, molecular markers of the antiproliferative effect of sulindac were seen as well. This therapy is in its infancy and, although exciting, is not recommended in place of a close endoscopic surveillance program.

References

1. Winawer SJ, Zauber AG, Ho MN, et al. Prevention of colorectal cancer by colonoscopic polypectomy: the National Polyp Study Workgroup. N Engl J Med 1993;329:1977–1981.
2. Landis SH, Murray T, Bolden S, Wingo PA. Cancer statistics, 1998. CA Cancer J Clin 1998;48:6–29.
3. Vogelstein B, Fearon ER, Hamilton SR, et al. Genetic alterations during colorectal-tumor development. N Engl J Med 1988;319:525–532.
4. Burt RW, Petersen GM. Familial colorectal cancer: diagnosis and management. In: Young GP, Rozen P, Levin B (eds) Prevention and Early Detection of Colorectal Cancer. London: Saunders, 1996;171–194.
5. Burt RW. Familial risk and colorectal cancer. Gastroenterol Clin North Am 1996;25:793–803.
6. Allen JI. Practical applications of the molecular revolution for colorectal cancer prevention. Semin Colon Rectal Surg 1998;9:73–82.
7. Laken SJ, Petersen GM, Gruber SB, et al. Familial colorectal cancer in Ashkenazim due to a hypermutable tract in APC. Nat Genet 1997; 17:79–83.
8. Byers T, Levin B, Rothenberger D, Dodd GD, Smith RA. American Cancer Society guidelines for screening and surveillance for early detection of colorectal polyps and cancer: update 1997: American Cancer Society detection and treatment advisory group on colorectal cancer. CA Cancer J Clin 1997;47:154–160.
9. Bond JH. Interference with the adenoma–carcinoma sequence. Eur J Cancer 1995;31A:1115–1117.
10. Gyde SN, Prior P, Allan RN, et al. Colorectal cancer in ulcerative colitis: a cohort study of primary referral from three areas. Gut 1988;29:206–217.
11. Mir-Madjlessi SH, Farmer RG, Easley KA, Beck GJ. Colorectal and extracolonic malignancy in ulcerative colitis. Cancer 1986;58:1596–1574.
12. Shetty K, Rybicki L, Brzezinski A, Carey W, Lashner BA. Primary sclerosing cholangitis increases the risk of colorectal cancer in ulcerative colitis patients [abstract]. Am J Gastroenterol 1997;92:1688.
13. Provenzale D, Kowdley KV, Arora S, Wong JB. Prophylactic colectomy or surveillance for chronic ulcerative analysis? A decision analysis. Gastroenterology 1995;109:1188–1196.
14. Tytgat GN, Dhir V, Gopinath N. Endoscopic appearance of dysplasia and cancer in inflammatory bowel disease. Eur J Cancer 1995;31A:1174–1177.
15. Morson BC, Pang LS. Rectal biopsy as an aid to cancer control in ulcerative colitis. Gut 1967;8:423–434.
16. Rubin CE, Haggitt RC, Burmer GC, et al. DNA aneuploidy in colonic biopsies predicts future development of dysplasia in ulcerative colitis. Gastroenterology 1992;103:1611–1620.
17. Bernstein CN, Shanahan F, Weinstein WM. Are we telling patients the truth about surveillance colonoscopy in ulcerative colitis? Lancet 1994; 343:71–74.
18. Connell WR, Lennard-Jones JE, Williams CB, Talbot IC, Price AB, Wilkinson KH. Factors affecting the outcome of endoscopic surveillance for cancer in ulcerative colitis. Gastroenterology 1994;107:934–944.
19. Melville DM, Jass JR, Morson BC, et al. Observer study of the grading of dysplasia in ulcerative colitis: comparison with clinical outcome. Hum Pathol 1989;20:1008–1014.
20. Lashner BA, Turner BC, Bostwick DG, Frank PH, Hanauer SB. Dysplasia and cancer complicating strictures in ulcerative colitis. Dig Dis Sci 1990; 35:349–352.
21. Torres C, Antonioli D, Odze RD. Polypoid dysplasia and adenomas in inflammatory bowel disease: a clinical, pathologic, and follow-up study of 89 polyps from 59 patients. Am J Surg Pathol 1998;22:275–284.
22. Baker WN, Glass RE, Ritchie JK, Aylett SO. Cancer of the rectum following colectomy and ileorectal anastomosis for ulcerative colitis. Br J Surg 1978;65:862–868.
23. O'Riordain MG, Fazio VW, Lavery IC, et al. Incidence and natural history of dysplasia of the anal transitional zone (ATZ) after ileal pouch-anal anastomosis (IPAA): results of a 5–10 year follow-up. Dis Colon Rectum 2000;43(12):1660–1665.
24. Radice E, Nelson H, Devine RM, et al. Ileal pouch-anal anastomosis in patients with colorectal cancer: long-term functional and oncologic outcomes. Dis Colon Rectum 1998;41:11–17.
25. Vasen HF, Wijnen JT, Menko FH, et al. Cancer risk in families with hereditary nonpolyposis colorectal cancer diagnosed by mutation analysis. Gastroenterology 1996;110:1020–1027. Erratum: Gastroenterology 1996;111:1402.
26. Lynch HT, Smyrk T, Lynch J, Fitzgibbons RJ, Lanspa S, McGinn T. Update on the differential diagnosis, surveillance and management of hereditary non-polyposis colorectal cancer. Eur J Cancer 1995;31A:1039–1046.

27. Vasen HF, Mecklin JP, Khan PM, Lynch HT. The International Collaborative Group on Hereditary Non-Polyposis Colorectal Cancer (ICG-HNPCC). Dis Colon Rectum 1991;34:424–425.
28. Lynch HT, Smyrk TC, Watson P, et al. Genetics, natural history, tumor spectrum, and pathology of hereditary nonpolyposis colorectal cancer: an updated review. Gastroenterology 1993;104:1535–1549.
29. Percesepe A, Anti M, Roncucci L, et al. The effect of family size on estimates of the frequency of hereditary non-polyposis colorectal cancer. Br J Cancer 1995;72:1320–1323.
30. Beck NE, Tomlinson IP, Homfray T, et al. Genetic testing is important in families with a history suggestive of hereditary nonpolyposis colorectal cancer even if the Amsterdam criteria are not fulfilled. Br J Surg 1997;84:233–237.
31. Rodriguez-Bigas MA, Boland CR, Hamilton SR, et al. A National Cancer Institute workshop on hereditary nonpolyposis colorectal cancer syndrome: meeting highlights and Bethesda guidelines. J Natl Cancer Inst 1997; 89:1758–1762.
32. Peltomaki P, Aaltonen LA, Sistonen P, et al. Genetic mapping of a locus predisposing to human colorectal cancer. Science 1993;260:810–812.
33. Aaltonen LA, Peltomaki P, Leach FS, et al. Clues to the pathogenesis of familial colorectal cancer. Science 1993;260:812–816.
34. Hirsch B. DNA repair and its malfunctions. Semin Colon Rectal Surg 1998;9:21–29.
35. Liu B, Parsons R, Papadopoulos N, et al. Analysis of mismatch repair genes in hereditary non-polyposis colorectal cancer patients. Nat Med 1996; 2:169–174.
36. Green SE, Bradburn DM, Varma JS, Burn J. Hereditary non-polyposis colorectal cancer. Int J Colorectal Dis 1998;13:3–12.
37. Church JM, Prophylactic colectomy in patients with hereditary nonpolyposis colorectal cancer. Ann Med 1996;28:479–482.
38. Rodriguez-Bigas MA, Vasen HF, Pekka-Mecklin J, et al. Rectal cancer risk in hereditary nonpolyposis colorectal cancer after abdominal colectomy: international collaborative group on HNPCC. Ann Surg 1997;225: 202–207.
39. Jarvinen HJ, Mecklin JP, Sistonen P. Screening reduces colorectal cancer rate in families with hereditary nonpolyposis colorectal cancer. Gastroenterology 1995;108:1405–1411.
40. Vasen HF, Taal BG, Nagengast FM, et al. Hereditary nonpolyposis colorectal cancer: results of long-term surveillance in 50 families. Eur J Cancer 1995;31A:1145–1148.
41. Rex DK, Cutler CS, Lemmel GT, et al. Colonoscopic miss rates of adenomas determined by back-to-back colonoscopies. Gastroenterology 1997; 112:24–28.
42. Vasen HF, Taal BG, Griffioen G, et al. Clinical heterogeneity of familial colorectal cancer and its influence on screening protocols. Gut 1994;35:1262–1266.
43. van den Bosch, Vandendael A, van Schoubroeck D., Wranz PA, Lombard, CJ. Combining vaginal ultrasonography and office endometrial sampling in the diagnosis of endometrial disease in postmenopausal women. Obstet Gynecol 1995;85:349–352.
44. Fante R, Roncucci L, Di GC, et al. Frequency and clinical features of multiple tumors of the large bowel in the general population and in patients with hereditary colorectal carcinoma. Cancer 1996;77:2013–2021.
45. Stern HS, Smith A. Recognition, screening, and medical management of familial adenomatous polyposis. Semin Colon Rectal Surg 1995;6:19–24.
46. Rustin RB, Jagelman DG, McGannon E, Fazio VW, Lavery IC, Weakley FL. Spontaneous mutation in familial adenomatous polyposis. Dis Colon Rectum 1990;33:52–55.
47. Lynch HT, Smyrk T, McGinn T, et al. Attenuated familial adenomatous polyposis (AFAP): a phenotypically and genotypically distinctive variant of FAP. Cancer 1995;76:2427–2433.
48. Morton DG, Macdonald F, Haydon J, et al. Screening practice for familial adenomatous polyposis: the potential for regional registers. Br J Surg 1993;80:255–258.
49. Rhodes M, Chapman PD, Burn J, Gunn A. Role of a regional register for familial adenomatous polyposis: experience in the northern region. Br J Surg 1991;78:451–452.
50. Herrera L, Kakati S, Gibas L, Pietrzak E, Sandberg AA. Gardner syndrome in a man with an interstitial deletion of 5q. Am J Med Genet 1986;25: 473–476.
51. Madoff RD, Wong KS. The multistep model of colorectal carcinogenesis. Semin Colon Rectal Surg 1998;9:30–37.
52. Powell SM, Petersen GM, Krush AJ, et al. Molecular diagnosis of familial adenomatous polyposis. N Engl J Med 1993;329:1982–1987.
53. Giardiello FM, Brensinger JD, Petersen GM, et al. The use and interpretation of commercial APC gene testing for familial adenomatous polyposis. N Engl J Med 1997;336:823–827.
54. Church JM. Anatomy of a gene: functional correlations of APC mutation. Semin Colon Rectal Surg 1998;9:49–52.
55. Murday V, Slack J. Inherited disorders associated with colorectal cancer. Cancer Surv 1989;8:139–157.
56. Abramson DJ. Multiple polyposis in children: a review and a report of a case in a 6-year-old child who had associated nephrosis and asthma. Surgery 1967;61:288–301.
57. Bussey HJR. Familial Polyposis Coli: Family Studies, Histopathology, Differential Diagnosis, and Results of Treatment. Baltimore: Johns Hopkins University Press, 1975.
58. Jarvinen HJ. Epidemiology of familial adenomatous polyposis in Finland: impact of family screening on the colorectal cancer rate and survival. Gut 1992;33:357–360.
59. Spigelman AD, Phillips RKS. The upper gastrointestinal tract. In: Phillips RKS, Spigelman AD, and Thomson JPS (ed) Familial Adenomatous Polyposis and Other Polyposis Syndromes. London: Edward Arnold, 1994;106–127.
60. Jagelman DG, DeCosse JJ, Bussey HJ. Upper gastrointestinal cancer in familial adenomatous polyposis. Lancet 1988;1:1149–1151.
61. Spigelman AD. Familial adenomatous polyposis and the upper gastrointestinal tract. Semin Colon Rectal Surg 1995;6:26–28.
62. Debinski HS, Love S, Spigelman AD, Phillips RK, Iwama T, Mishima Y. Colorectal polyp counts and cancer risk in familial adenomatous polyposis: factors affecting the risk of rectal cancer following rectum-preserving surgery in patients with familial adenomatous polyposis. Gastroenterology 1996; 110:1028–1030.
63. Iwama T, Mishima Y. Factors affecting the risk of rectal cancer following rectum-preserving surgery in patients with familial adenomatous polyposis. Dis Colon Rectum 1994;37:1024–1026.
64. Sarre RG, Jagelman DG, Beck GJ, et al. Colectomy with ileorectal anastomosis for familial adenomatous polyposis: the risk of rectal cancer. Surgery 1987;101:20–26.
65. Jagelman DG. Choice of operation in familial adenomatous polyposis. World J Surg 1991;15:47–49.
66. Feinberg SM, Jagelman DG, Sarre RG, et al. Spontaneous resolution of rectal polyps in patients with familial polyposis following abdominal colectomy and ileorectal anastomosis. Dis Colon Rectum 1988;31:169–175.
67. Malassagne B, Penna C, Parc R. Adenomatous polyps in the anal transitional zone after ileal pouch-anal anastomosis for familial adenomatous polyposis: treatment by transanal mucosectomy and ileal pouch advancement. Br J Surg 1995;82:1634.
68. Ziv Y, Church JM, Oakley JR, McGannon E, Schroeder TK, Fazio VF. Results after restorative proctocolectomy and ileal pouch-anal anastomosis in patients with familial adenomatous polyposis and coexisting colorectal cancer. Br J Surg 1996;83:1578–1580.

69. Nugent KP, Spigelman AD, Nicholls RJ, et al. Pouch adenomas in patients with familial adenomatous polyposis. Br J Surg 1993;80:1620.
70. Palkar VM, deSouza LJ, Jagannath P, Naresh KN. Adenocarcinoma arising in "J" pouch after total proctocolectomy for familial polyposis coli. Indian J Cancer 1997;34:16–19.
71. Winde G, Schmid KW, Brandt B, Muller O, Osswald H. Clinical and genomic influence of sulindac on rectal mucosa in familial adenomatous polyposis. Dis Colon Rectum 1997;40:1156–1168.

CHAPTER 39

Rectal Cancer

THEODORE J. SACLARIDES

This chapter focuses on the management of rectal cancer. High risk acquired and inherited conditions that place patients at high risk for colorectal cancer are covered in Chapter 38, and the reader is encouraged to review that material for the necessary information. It cannot be overemphasized that all average risk asymptomatic patients over the age of 50 should be enrolled in a screening program and that surveillance of higher risk patients should be performed at an earlier age.

A. Epidemiology

Rectal cancer is distinctly different from colon cancer in terms of its biologic behavior and treatment. Higher recurrence rates have been noted with rectal cancer than with similar-stage colon cancer. Because these lesions are accessible transanally and the sequelae of surgically penetrating the extraperitoneal tissue are not as catastrophic as penetrating the abdominal cavity, there are more options for both curative and palliative treatment. Patient-related concerns unique to rectal cancer include the fear of incontinence, permanent stomas, and genitourinary dysfunction; and the patient's attitude toward these issues frequently determines treatment despite advice rendered by the surgeon. Surgeon-related issues include technical skill deep in the pelvis, the ability to spare the anal sphincter and the nerves governing genitourinary function, and the ability to perform the proper mesorectal excision to keep recurrence rates as low as possible. Outcome is directly related to surgical expertise, and rectal cancer in most instances should be treated only by physicians whose practice has a high volume of these patients.

Rectal cancers found in asymptomatic patients during screening usually present at an earlier stage, and so the prognosis is better and transanal therapy may be an option. More advanced lesions may cause symptoms such as the passage of bloody stools, tenesmus, or the urge to defecate constantly, a feeling of obstructed defecation, or pain when the sphincter is involved by tumor. Patients who present with any of these symptoms should undergo a digital rectal examination and proctosigmoidoscopy regardless of age.

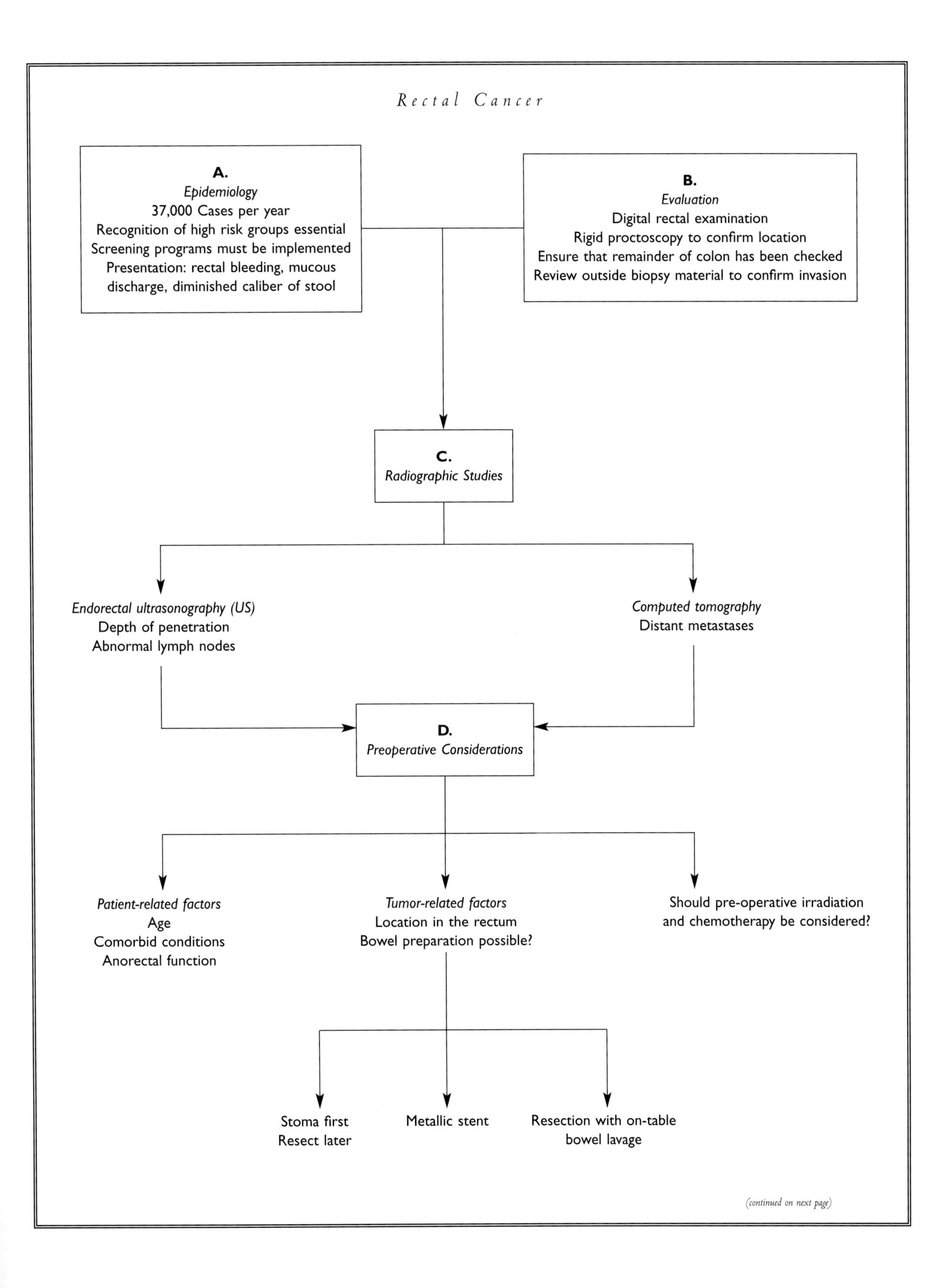
Rectal Cancer
A.
Epidemiology
37,000 Cases per year
Recognition of high risk groups essential
Screening programs must be implemented
Presentation: rectal bleeding, mucous discharge, diminished caliber of stool
B.
Evaluation
Digital rectal examination
Rigid proctoscopy to confirm location
Ensure that remainder of colon has been checked
Review outside biopsy material to confirm invasion
C.
Radiographic Studies
Endorectal ultrasonography (US)
Depth of penetration
Abnormal lymph nodes
Computed tomography
Distant metastases
D.
Preoperative Considerations
Patient-related factors
Age
Comorbid conditions
Anorectal function
Tumor-related factors
Location in the rectum
Bowel preparation possible?
Should pre-operative irradiation and chemotherapy be considered?
Stoma first
Resect later
Metallic stent
Resection with on-table bowel lavage
(continued on next page)

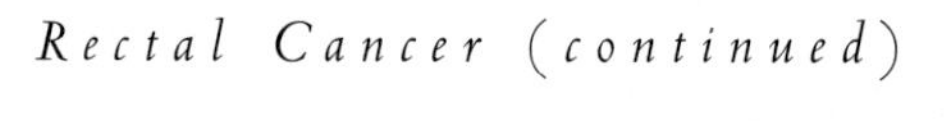

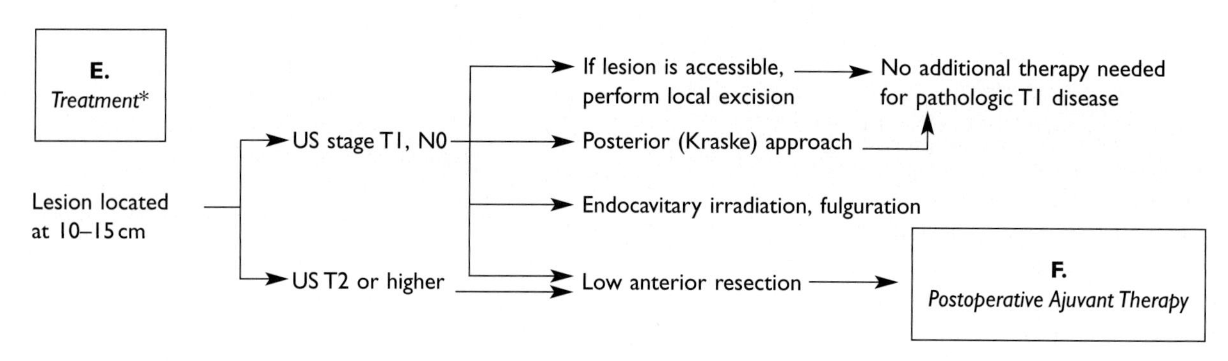

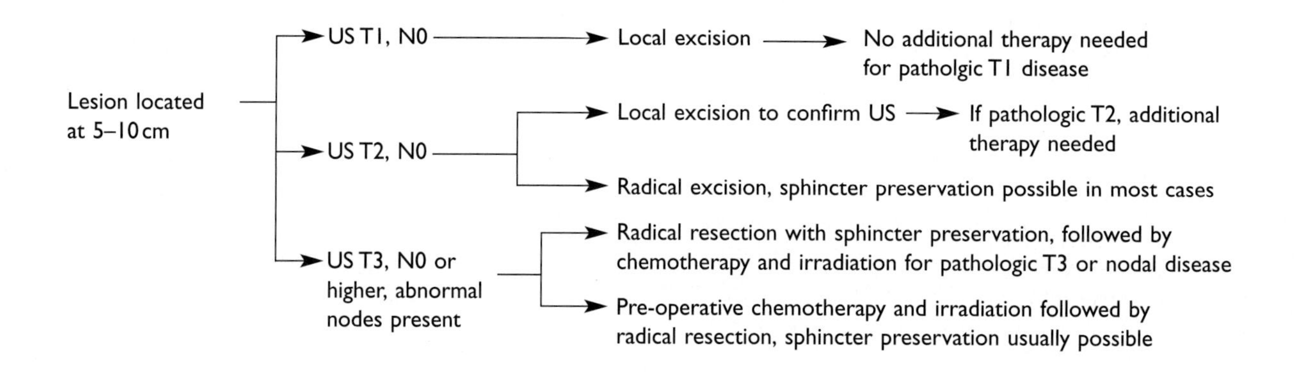

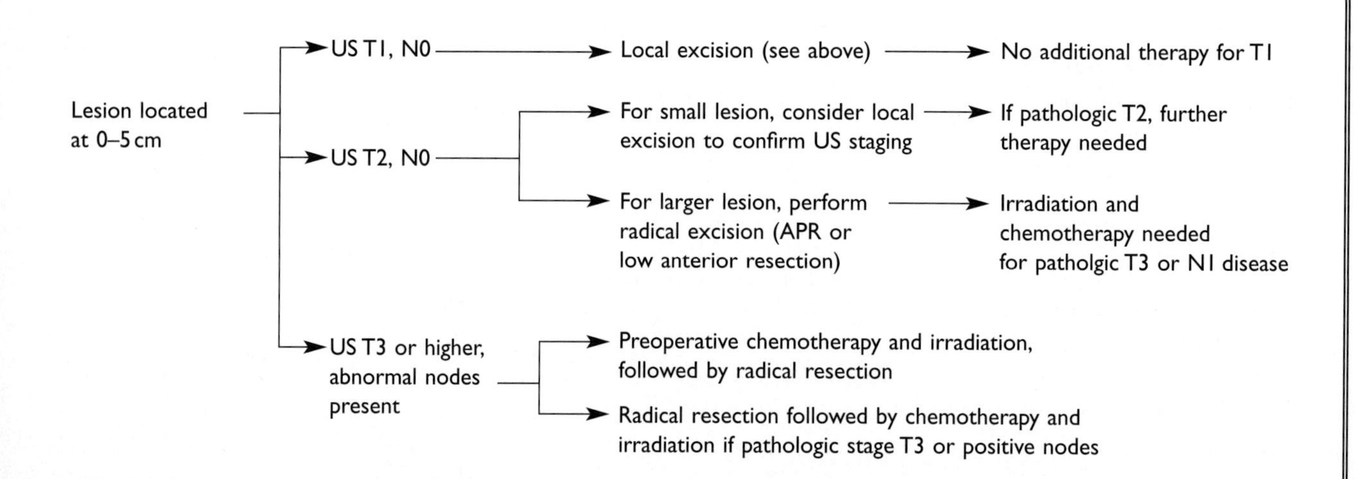

*Predicated on availability of ultrasonography

An algorithmic approach to patient management provides a template that can be adjusted, added to, or even subtracted from, depending on various regional and institutional practices. It does not provide the only acceptable pathway and certainly should not be considered the standard of care. This is certainly the case with rectal cancer, where the availability of diagnostic tests such as endoluminal ultrasonography and computed tomography (CT) scans may affect decision making. Furthermore, a patient's concerns and desire to avoid a permanent stoma and other factors such as body habitus and preoperative sphincter dysfunction influence the choice of treatment yet cannot be accounted for in an algorithm. This chapter assumes that rectal ultrasonography is available, and it is used to stratify the patient into various treatment groups.

B. Evaluation

The digital rectal examination may show that the tumor has become fixed to neighboring structures and, when performed by an experienced examiner, can be used to estimate the degree of rectal wall involvement. The physician should sweep his or her finger across the broad surface of the sacrum and in doing so may feel nodal metastases in the mesorectum. Perhaps the single most important test the surgeon responsible for the patient's care should perform is *rigid proctoscopy*. The distance from the anal verge determines the choice of operation, and this is best assessed with a rigid instrument rather than with a flexible, fiberoptic scope, which may loop or bend in the rectum thereby skewing the measurement. In addition, the anteroposterior orientation of the tumor and its possible relation to the peritoneal reflection is determined. Many surgeons believe local (transanal) excision of a penetrating anterior lesion in the mid or upper rectum of a woman is not appropriate. The degree of circumferential involvement may influence treatment in that a nearly complete obstruction lends a different sense of urgency than a smaller lesion. The remainder of the colon should be assessed with either *colonoscopy* or *barium studies* to exclude synchronous polyps or cancer. If the diagnosis was established at an outside institution, the biopsy material may have to be *reviewed by another pathologist*, especially in cases where the degree of invasion or differentiation may affect treatment decisions. Examples include those instances where a lesion was completely removed endoscopically, there is no residual tumor endoscopically, and there is doubt as to whether the lesion is an invasive or an in situ cancer. In the latter instance, close observation may be appropriate. Also, transanal excision is less preferable to a radical operation if the tumor is poorly differentiated or has invaded lymphatic channels or blood vessels in the rectal wall.[1] In such cases the probability of mesorectal metastases is higher and, if present, would go untreated by transanal excision. An experienced gastrointestinal pathologist should be sensitive to these issues and may provide invaluable assistance to the surgeon. Lastly, the *overall medical condition* of the patient should be assessed. The presence of several co-morbid conditions may adversely affect the patient's ability to undergo a major resection.

C. Radiographic Studies

Endorectal ultrasonography has had a significant impact on the treatment of patients with rectal cancer in that the depth of penetration and the presence of lymph node metastases can be determined with reasonable accuracy. This examination is well tolerated by patients, minimal preparation is required, and no sedation is needed. The test is usually performed with a rigid ultrasound probe that provides a 360 degree image of the rectum. If the lesion is located in the mid or distal rectum, the probe may be passed blindly above the lesion and scanning performed as the instrument is withdrawn. If the lesion is small and likely to be passed over too quickly or if it is located in the upper rectum, the probe may be passed under direct vision through a specially designed 2 cm diameter proctoscope to verify accurate placement. Alternatively, scanning can be performed with the flexible fiberoptic probe popular with gastroenterologists who study upper gastrointestinal diseases. More important than which probe is used is the appreciation by the ultrasonographer that the information obtained directly affects treatment.

As stated above, the important information provided by ultrasonography is depth of penetration and the presence of lymph node metastases. For the former, ultrasonography has an accuracy of 90–95% in most hands and in this regard is more sensitive and accurate than CT or magnetic resonance imaging (MRI).[2–5] Normal lymph nodes are generally not detected by ultrasonography because of their similar echotexture with the mesorectal fat. Metastatic nodes are hypoechoic and spherical, in contrast to inflammatory nodes, which are usually hyperechoic and oval. The positive predictive value is influenced by node size, with hypoechoic nodes ≥ 1 cm being metastatic in most instances. Smaller nodes have less predictive value, but most physicians view a hypoechoic structure of any size with suspicion.

Deciding which patient with rectal cancer undergoes ultrasonography is controversial, although one could argue that nearly all patients newly diagnosed with this malignancy should have it. Need is determined by regional and personal practices with respect to preoperative neoadjuvant therapy and the capability of performing transanal excision. The current trend suggests that lesions that have penetrated the perirectal fat or adjacent viscera or have metastasized into neighboring lymph nodes should be treated with preoperative irradiation and chemotherapy followed by surgery. Reduced local recurrence rates and improved chances of sphincter preservation can be expected with this plan. Ultrasonography is certainly capable of making this determination as well as selecting patients with T2 N0 lesions, who may undergo prompt surgery without preoperative therapy. In addition, local (transanal) excision may be chosen for patients with superficial accessible lesions and avoided in those instances where deeper penetration implies that mesorectal disease would go untreated with this approach. Ultrasonography therefore can play a role in the management of most patients. The exception is the elderly or infirm patient whose only surgical option for a small lesion is transanal excision or fulguration regardless of what the ultrasound scan shows.

Computed tomography scans of the chest and abdomen also influence decision making and should probably be obtained in most if not all surgical patients. In contrast to lesions located above the peritoneal reflection, rectal cancers may be aggressively treated with a variety of transanal methods, such as excision, electrodesiccation, or laser ablation without fear of penetrating the peritoneal cavity. Although their use as curative therapy is debatable, these options are suitable for the patient with widely unresectable metastatic disease in the liver or lungs found by CT scanning. If a solitary metastasis is found in either of these locations, a staged approach may be considered whereby the rectal cancer is resected first at which time the extent of intraabdominal disease is determined. The metastatic tumor is then addressed at a later surgery provided the liver or lung component has remained stable and there is adequate reserve remaining in the involved organ to sustain life.

D. Preoperative Considerations

Tumor-related factors influence treatment decisions, and many of these factors have been addressed. They pertain to the distance of the tumor from the anal verge, potential for sphincter preservation, need for preoperative neoadjuvant therapy, presence of metastatic disease, and whether the bowel can be adequately cleansed for resection. With regard to the latter, treatment of a nearly complete obstruction may require an initial colostomy followed by resection soon thereafter once co-morbid conditions such as electrolyte abnormalities and nutritional deficiencies have been addressed. Alternatively, the tumor could be resected and intraoperative bowel lavage performed before reestablishing bowel continuity.[6,7] For the patient with unresectable metastatic disease, metallic expandable stents can be placed under endoscopic control to reestablish and maintain luminal patency and thereby avoid a colostomy.[8] Patency can also be maintained by transanal fulguration of the tumor whereby the surface of the lesion is shaved with electrocautery. This may require repetitive sessions depending on the bulk of the tumor, the patient's longevity, and the response of the primary and metastatic disease to systemic therapy or radiation if given.

If surgery is undertaken to resect the primary tumor the patient should undergo mechanical bowel cleansing with oral cathartics or lavage with a nonabsorbable electrolyte solution. Nonabsorbable oral antibiotics are given as well as intravenous antibiotics in most instances. These patients are at risk for deep venous thrombosis because of their cancer and the fact that pelvic surgery is being performed and the operation may be lengthy. Additional risk factors may include obesity and a history of thrombotic episodes. Consequently, proper prophylaxis should be considered and may consist of low-dose subcutaneous injections of heparin or its low-molecular-weight counterpart; alternatively, sequential compression devices may be used on the lower extremities. With respect to the latter, there is no conclusive evidence that these devices lower the incidence of pulmonary embolism, but they are frequently used in conjunction with heparin for the patient at high risk for deep venous thrombosis. Ureteral stents are not routinely used by most experienced surgeons, but they should be considered in instances where there has been a history of prior pelvic surgery or the tumor is large and possibly fixed to adjacent structures.

Patient-related Factors

The patient's age and co-morbid conditions must be considered before embarking on a major resection. A thorough history may reveal a history of prior myocardial infarction, exercise intolerance, or unstable angina, all of which should be evaluated by a cardiologist. If necessary, rectal surgery should be delayed until cardiac stress testing and even cardiac catheterization are performed.

The adequacy of sphincter function should be determined prior to surgery. If there is a history of fecal incontinence, there is no reason to believe that it will improve after surgery unless one thinks that the tumor itself is responsible for the deranged bowel function. However, incontinence temporally related to a specific event such as an obstetric injury or hemorrhoid or fistula surgery or that is due to aging or a systemic illness such as diabetes will likely persist and may sway the surgeon to consider a permanent colostomy.

Preoperative Chemotherapy and Irradiation

The treatment of rectal cancer has evolved substantially over the last two decades and is usually multidisciplinary in nature. The debate centers around the sequence of administering adjuvant therapy in relation to surgery (i.e., whether it should be given preoperatively or postoperatively). All would agree that the main risk factors for recurrence of cancer following surgery are transmural penetration by the cancer and metastatic disease in the mesorectal lymph nodes. To reduce recurrence rates, the U.S. National Institutes of Health (NIH) issued a consensus statement stating that the presence of these risk factors mandates *postoperative* chemotherapy and irradiation;[9] it established the standard of care in the United States and is still widely practiced to this day.

The trend is shifting toward *preoperative* therapy, facilitated by the use of endorectal ultrasonography to identify patients with adverse tumor-related factors. Preoperative adjuvant therapy with irradiation alone has been studied, and lower recurrence rates compared to patients undergoing surgery alone have been noted.[10] No improvement in survival was seen until the 1997 Swedish Rectal Cancer Trial demonstrated both reduced recurrence rates *and* enhanced survival. Again, the control arm consisted of patients treated with surgery alone; no patient received chemotherapy.[11] Currently, most centers using preoperative therapy combine irradiation with chemotherapy, citing the latter's ability to potentiate the effects of irradiation and its ability to treat systemic disease promptly. Proponents of combined preoperative therapy cite lower recurrence rates, the ability to down-stage tumors, the ability to render large bulky lesions more easily resectable, enhanced likelihood of sphincter preservation, and better functional results because the irradiated segment is to be removed. No clear improvement in survival was demonstrated until a recent Swedish study that compared pre- and postoperative therapy; this study has been criticized, however, because of different radiation doses in the treatment arms. The preoperative group received 2500 cGy in five fractions, whereas the postoperative group received 4500 cGy.

The NSABP R-03 protocol was designed to compare treatment groups receiving equivalent radiation doses. The preliminary results have been reported, but patient accrual has been a problem. Of the 116 patients randomized, treatment toxicity has been similar in the treatment groups, and a 60% increase in sphincter preservation was noted in the group receiving preoperative therapy. A complete pathologic response was seen in 8% of the patients. All patients received seven cycles of 5-fluorouracil (5-FU)/leucovorin bolus infusion. Radiation consisted of 4500 cGy over 25 fractions (180 cGy/fraction) in both treatment groups.[12] other studies have also noted a complete pathologic response in a significant portion of patients.[13–16]

Regardless of the degree of response, radical surgery should be performed because no reliable factors have been identified to predict whether nodal metastases are present in patients without palpatory, endoscopic, or sonographic[16] evidence of residual disease. Perhaps future studies can determine which patients with a complete response can undergo local excision or observation alone.

E. Treatment

As stated above, the algorithm presented herein is predicated on the availability of ultrasonography, which is used to identify patients with lesions amenable to transanal excision and to identify those who should be treated with preoperative irradiation and chemotherapy. This approach also assumes that the concept of preoperative therapy has been embraced by the treating physician, an assumption that may not be valid. Most surgeons agree that preoperative irradiation should be applied if the rectal cancer is fixed to surrounding structures; however, debate continues as to whether it should be given for the locally advanced lesion that has not become fixed or adherent. Although it is not considered state of the art to administer preoperative therapy, the trend in clinical practice is certainly leaning in this direction in the United States and abroad. If preoperative therapy is given, most advise continuing with chemotherapy postoperatively because the original pathologic stage of the tumor was not known. If preoperative therapy is not given, one should follow the NIH recommendations that radiation and chemotherapy should be given postoperatively for the tumor that has either penetrated the perirectal fat or metastasized to regional lymph nodes.

Lesions in the Upper Rectum

Lesions 10–15 cm from the anus are treated similarly to sigmoid cancers in that preoperative radiation and chemotherapy are generally not given. The reason is that fixation to surrounding pelvic structures such as bone or prostate is not as likely to happen with upper rectal cancers, and one must be concerned about exposing small bowel to radiation. Biologically, upper rectal cancers have recurrence rates comparable to those of sigmoid lesions, which are generally lower than recurrence rates seen with mid and distal rectal cancers. Also, their location in the upper rectum render them less amenable to transanal excision unless the surgeon is adept at performing this operation. Furthermore, because these tumors are close to the peritoneal reflection, operative choices are limited and are determined primarily by the stage of the lesion.

If the lesion is confined to the mucosa and submucosa, as seen by ultrasonography, transanal excision may be considered, although accessibility is an issue that must be overcome. Conventional instrumentation provides easy access to lesions in the mid and distal rectum; such instrumentation has limited use for upper rectal lesions because of poor exposure and limited reach. Transanal endoscopic microsurgery (TEM) overcomes some of these limitations. TEM procedures use a 40 mm diameter rectoscope, available in lengths of 12 and 20 cm, and long shafted instruments that are operated and inserted in parallel through the facepiece of the scope. Carbon dioxide is continuously insufflated, and a combined endosurgical unit regulates gas insufflation, suction, and saline irrigation so the intrarectal pressure is maintained at approximately 15 cm H_2O; the rectal lumen then remains constantly distended, providing improved visibility compared to that using conventional instrumentation.[17]

With transanal excision, full-thickness excision of the rectal wall is performed so the pathologist can comment on the depth of penetration. An alternative to transanal excision is local excision through a posterior or transsacral approach. Described by Kraske in 1885, this approach is performed through an incision made between the anus and the coccyx. Dissection continues until the posterior wall of the rectum is exposed; the rectum is then opened, the lesion removed with a full-thickness excision, the rectal wall sutured, and the wound closed. The most feared complication of this approach is a fecal fistula through the wound, which generally mandates performing a temporary colostomy until the fistula heals. Although this approach is still utilized selectively by surgeons, its use is generally not necessary if TEM is available.

If histologic review after transanal excision confirms that the lesion is confined to the mucosa and submucosa, no further treatment is required. If the lesion has penetrated the muscularis propria or beyond, further treatment is required because of the high likelihood that nodal metastases are present. The preferred treatment in these instances is low anterior resection; for the patient who is not a candidate for radical surgery, irradiation and chemotherapy may be considered. Studies of small numbers of patients with pathologic T2 lesions have shown that irradiation and chemotherapy following transanal excision provide acceptable cure rates, but such treatment should not be considered standard therapy at this time.[18–20] If no further treatment is given following transanal excision of a pathologic T2 lesion, recurrence rates of approximately 30% can be expected—thus the recommendation that further therapy must be given.

Other forms of transanal therapy include endocavitary irradiation and fulguration; proper patient selection is essential if these modalities are to be used with curative intent. Tumors must be small (no larger than 3 cm), accessible, and superficial. Endocavitary radiation is administered directly down the shaft of a specially designed proctoscope that is placed in contact with the cancer. High-dose radiation is given in multiple sessions until the total dose reached is approximately 12,000 cGy; treatment sessions are well tolerated and administered on an outpatient basis. The depth of penetration by the radiation is 6 mm, so this form of treatment is suitable only for superficial cancers.[21] Endocavitary irradiation may be combined with external beam irradiation.[22] Fulguration is performed in the operating room and consists of repetitively debulking the tumor with an electrical current until normal tissue at the tumor base is reached. Because the lesion is not excised with either of these techniques, the exact depth of penetration is not known with certainty; therefore decisions regarding the need for further treatment cannot be based on precise clinical information. Close patient follow-up with digital rectal examination and proctoscopy is mandatory.

Low anterior resection is advised for lesions in the upper rectum that penetrate the muscularis propria (T2), as seen by ultrasonography. This approach is also undertaken for lesions that have penetrated the wall or have metastatic nodes. Preoperatively, patients undergo a bowel cleansing regimen with oral cathartics, enemas, or oral lavage with a nonabsorbable solution. Antibiotics are given orally, intravenously, or by both routes.

A lower midline incision is made and the abdomen is inspected for evidence of metastatic disease in the liver and on the peritoneal surfaces. The sigmoid colon is mobilized from its lateral attachments; the left ureter and gonadal vessels are identified; and the presacral space is entered in its avascular plane. The lateral extent of the dissection follows the pelvic side walls along the ureters and iliac vessels. The superior rectal vascular pedicle is ligated at its base, just distal to the origin of the left colic artery from the inferior mesenteric artery. The mesentery of the upper sigmoid colon is sequentially ligated, and the distal descending colon is then transected. Spillage of colonic contents should be avoided, which can be accomplished with occlusive clamps or stapling devices that simultaneously transect and close the colon. In the pelvis, dissection continues outside the fascia propria of the rectum until several centimeters below the inferior edge of the tumor. One should strive to attain a distal margin of at least 2 cm; there is no survival or recurrence benefit in obtaining a larger margin. At the chosen point of rectal transection, the mesentery is dissected and the rectum divided. There is no need to perform a complete mesorectal excision for lesions in the upper rectum; in fact, doing so may unnecessarily increase the risk of anastomotic leak by jeopardizing the blood supply to the remaining rectal segment, and it may worsen postoperative bowel function. Some surgeons advocate total mesorectal excision for all rectal cancers, but most have not adopted this aggressive approach, instead limiting the use of total mesorectal excision to tumors in the mid and distal rectum. Intestinal continuity is reestablished by a handsewing or stapling technique. Postoperative adjuvant therapy may be needed depending on tumor stage; this subject is covered in detail below.

Lesions in the Mid Rectum

For lesions in the mid rectum (i.e., 5–10 cm from the anus), the choice of operation should again be individualized and is based on the clinical examination and ultrasound findings. The indications for transanal excision are the same as mentioned above; that is, the tumor should be small, superficial, accessible, and well differentiated, and it should lack lymphatic or vascular invasion. Adhering to these selection criteria minimizes the risk of untreated lymph node metastases in the mesorectum. As stated above, local excision is considered curative for pathologic T1 lesions, but additional treatment is required for pathologic T2 or T3 lesions. Such treatment may consist of low anterior resection or irradiation and chemotherapy depending on the overall health of the patient.

If ultrasonography reveals that a mid-rectal cancer has penetrated the perirectal fat, has nodal metastases, or has become adherent to surrounding pelvic side walls or adjacent viscera, radiation and chemotherapy are administered preoperatively. The benefits are enumerated above. Surgical technique and the experience of the surgeon have been identified as extremely important factors as they relate to outcome and recurrence rates. The efforts of Heald et al. (Basingstoke, U.K.) have focused attention on how proctectomy for cancer should be conducted: that dissection in the pelvis should follow avascular tissue planes outside the mesorectum, and that the surgeon should not slant his or her dissection *through* the mesentery until the distal point of transection is reached.[23,24] Rather, a total mesorectal excision (TME) is performed for mid and distal lesions to reduce the likelihood of leaving residual cancer. This is accomplished by dissecting within the avascular tissue planes and by completely removing the posterior extension of the mesenteric fat down to the levator plate.[25–27] Surgeons in the United States argue that this technique has been the standard of care for years, but the low recurrence rates achieved by Heald and colleagues have certainly helped underscore the importance of proper surgical technique. Concerns surrounding TME include a potentially higher anastomotic leak rate from devascularization, worse function because of the low nature of the resection and anastomosis, and the ineffectiveness of this operation to deal with positive lateral margins (a problem shared with non-TME approaches).

Preoperative irradiation and chemotherapy lead to tumor shrinkage in most instances. As such, the distal extent of the lesion is not easily palpable intraoperatively, and the surgeon may resort to division of the rectum at the level of the pelvic floor. A coloanal anastomosis is created in these instances by a stapling or handsewing technique, but temporary fecal diversion may be required especially if a colonic reservoir is made. Bowel function and continence can be improved by constructing a J-shaped colonic reservoir to reduce stool frequency, urgency, and incontinence.[28,29] The procedure is analogous to the J-shaped ileal reservoir created during total proctocolectomy for chronic ulcerative colitis. The diverting stoma is subsequently closed in approximately 3 months, provided the reservoir has healed satisfactorily. Following surgery, chemotherapy is given regardless of the histologic stage of the tumor. No further radiation is prescribed.

For the patient whose tumor partially penetrates the muscularis propria and has not metastasized to regional lymph nodes, as shown by ultrasonography, prompt surgery without preoperative therapy may be prescribed. Postoperative irradiation and chemotherapy are applied if adverse histologic features are subsequently identified (i.e., transmural penetration or nodal metastases; see below). The same holds true for the patient who did not receive preoperative therapy because of local practice patterns or ideology.

Lesions in the Lower Rectum

For lesions located up to 5 cm from the anus, the principles outlined above with respect to indications for and treatment following transanal excision and indications for preoperative irradiation and chemotherapy still apply. If preoperative treatment was not given, the indications for postoperative therapy also apply. The chief concern with tumors in this location is if sphincter preservation is possible; usually it is not if the tumor presented at an advanced stage regardless of the response to preoperative treatment. If a distal margin of at least 2 cm can be obtained and the sphincter muscle itself is unharmed by the dissection, one may consider a low anterior resection with coloanal anastomosis with or without a colonic reservoir. If sphincter preservation is not possible, an abdominoperineal resection (APR) should be performed. Originally described in 1908 by Miles, the APR as we know it today consists of a combined abdominal and perineal approach whereby the sigmoid colon and its mesentery, the rectum and mesorectum, a portion of the pelvic floor, and the anal canal are resected. A permanent colostomy is created. Although a synchronous approach is possible, generally the abdomen is explored first to determine the extent of local and distant disease. A TME is performed, with care taken to protect the ureters and gonadal vessels; an end-sigmoid colostomy is then created through the patient's left lower quadrant of the abdominal wall. A perineal incision is made around the anus; and cephalad dissection is then performed through the anococcygeal ligament and levator ani muscles until the pelvis is entered. The specimen is then withdrawn through the perineal wound, and the anterior dissection is completed. The perineal and abdominal wounds are closed. Complications are frequent following APR, including sexual dysfunction such as impotence and retrograde ejaculation, neurogenic bladder, wound infection, atelectasis, pneumonia, postoperative bowel obstruction, urinary tract infection, and delayed healing of the perineal wound. Deep venous thrombosis prophylaxis helps reduce the incidence of deep venous thrombosis and potentially life-threatening pulmonary embolism. A commonly used regimen includes subcutaneously injected heparin (5000 units bid) and sequential compression devices wrapped around the patients' legs.

F. *Postoperative Therapy*

As stated earlier, transmural penetration and lymph node metastases are risk factors for recurrence of cancer. For patients with these adverse factors, the NIH issued a consensus statement declaring that postoperative radiation therapy and chemotherapy should be given.[9] The benefits of this treatment are reduced local recurrence rates and enhanced survival.[30–33] Most physicians comply with these recommendations, although concern lingers regarding treatment toxicity and its effect on bowel function. Furthermore, the validity of the studies that support the consensus statement have been questioned because of high local recurrence rates (up to 28%) noted in the patient groups undergoing surgery alone (control group). These rates have far exceeded the recurrence rates reported by Heald and others who practice TME, raising the question that the benefit seen with postoperative adjuvant therapy was because of improperly performed surgery. Standard postoperative radiation protocols employ 45–50 Gy at 180 cGy/day. Chemotherapy consists of 5-FU regimens for 6 months. There is no additional benefit gained by adding methyl-CCNU as the initial studies suggested; and this agent, in fact, increases toxicity and the potential for chemotherapy-related leukemias.

Conclusions

Unlike colon cancer, the treatment of rectal cancer has evolved considerably, aided by new diagnostic modalities such as ultrasonography and by new treatment strategies employing preoperative adjuvant therapy. Following curative treatment, a universally accepted follow-up program does not exist; in fact, the utility of such a program has been questioned. Intuitively, it makes sense that patients should be followed closely for local and distant failure with periodic serum carcinoembryonic antigen determinations, digital rectal examinations, endoscopy, and CT scans in selected instances. Rectal ultrasonography can be used to monitor local excision sites and perianastomotic tissue. If recurrence is detected early enough, salvage surgery can be considered.

References

1. Saclarides TJ, Bhattacharyya AK, Britton-Kuzel C, Szeluga D. Predicting lymph node metastases in rectal cancer. Dis Colon Rectum 1994;37:52–57.
2. Romano G, de Rosa P, Vallone G, et al. Intrarectal ultrasound and computed tomography in the pre- and postoperative assessment of patients with rectal cancer. Br J Surg 1985;72:S117–S119.
3. Rifkin MD, McGlynn ET, Marks G. Endorectal sonographic prospective staging of rectal cancer. Scand J Gastroenterol 1986;123:S99–S103.
4. Beynon J. An evaluation of the role of rectal endosonography in rectal cancer. Ann R Coll Surg Engl 1989;71:131–139.
5. Starck M, Bohe M, Fork FT, et al. Endoluminal ultrasound and low-field magnetic resonance imaging are superior to clinical examination in the preoperative staging of rectal cancer. Eur J Surg 1995;161:841–845.
6. Koruth NM, Krukowski ZH, Youngson GG, et al. Intraoperative colonic irrigation in the management of left-sided large bowel emergencies. Br J Surg 1985;72:708–711.
7. Pollock AV, Playforth MJ, Evans M. Perioperative lavage of the obstructed left colon to allow safe primary anastomosis. Dis Colon Rectum 1987; 30:171–173.
8. Dohmoto M, Hunergein M, Schlag PM. Palliative endoscopic therapy of rectal carcinoma. Eur J Cancer 1996;32A:25–29.
9. NIH Consensus Conference. Adjuvant therapy for patients with colon and rectal cancer. JAMA 1990;264:1444–1450.
10. Stockholm Colorectal Cancer Study Group. Randomized study on preoperative radiotherapy in rectal carcinoma. Ann Surg Oncol 1996;3: 419–420.
11. Swedish Rectal Cancer Trial. Improved survival with preoperative radiotherapy in resectable rectal cancer. N Engl J Med 1997;336:980–987.
12. Hyams DM, Mamounas EP, Petrelli N, et al. A clinical trial to evaluate the worth of preoperative multimodality therapy in patients with operable carcinoma of the rectum: a progress report of National Surgical Adjuvant Breast and Bowel Project Protocol R-03. Dis Colon Rectum 1997;40: 131–139.
13. Grann A, Minsky BD, Cohen AM, et al. Preliminary results of preoperative 5-fluorouracil, low-dose leucovorin, and concurrent radiation therapy for clinically resectable T3 cancer. Dis Colon Rectum 1997;40: 515–522.
14. Videtic GM, Fisher BJ, Perera FE, et al. Preoperative radiation with concurrent 5-fluorouracil infusion for locally advanced unresectable rectal cancer. Int J Radiat Oncol Biol Phys 1998;42:319–324.
15. Kaminsky-Forrett MC, Conroy T, Luporsi E, et al. Prognostic implications of downstaging following preoperative radiation therapy for operable T3-T4 rectal cancer. Int J Radiat Oncol Biol Phys 1998;42:935–941.
16. Berger C, de Muret A, Garaud P, et al. Preoperative radiotherapy (RT) for rectal cancer: predictive factors of tumor downstaging and residual tumor cell density (RTCD): prognostic implications. Int J Radiat Biol Phys 1997; 37:619–627.
17. Saclarides TJ. Transanal endoscopic microsurgery (TEM): a single surgeon's experience. Arch Surg 1998;133:595–599.
18. Bleday R, Breen E, Jessup JM, Burgess A, Sentovich SM, Steele G Jr. Prospective evaluation of local excision for small rectal cancers. Dis Colon Rectum 1997;40:388–392.
19. Wagman R, Minsky BD, Cohen AM, Saltz L, Paty PB, Guillem JG. Conservative management of rectal cancer with local excision and postoperative adjuvant therapy. Int J Radiat Oncol Biol Phys 1999;44:841–846.
20. Lezoche E, Guerrieri M, Paganini AM, Feliciotti F. Transanal endoscopic microsurgical excision of irradiated and nonirradiated rectal cancer: a 5-year experience. Surg Laparosc, Endosc Percutan Tech 1998;8:249–256.
21. Gerard JP, Baulieux J, Francois Y, et al. The role of radiotherapy in the conservative treatment of rectal carcinoma—the Lyon experience. Acta Oncol 1998;37:253–258.
22. Birnbaum EH, Ogunbiyi OA, Gagliardi G, et al. Selection criteria for treatment of rectal cancer with combined external and endocavitary radiation. Dis Colon Rectum 1999;42:727–733.
23. Heald RJ, Husband EM, Ryall RD. The mesorectum in rectal cancer surgery—the clue to pelvic recurrence? Br J Surg 1982;69:613.
24. Heald RJ, Ryall RD. Recurrence and survival after total mesorectal excision for rectal cancer. Lancet 1986;1479–1482.
25. Reynolds JV, Joyce WP, Dolan J, et al. Pathological evidence in support of total mesorectal excision in the management of rectal cancer. Br J Surg 1996;83:1112–1115.
26. Scott N, Jackson P, Al-Jaberi T, et al. Total mesorectal excision and local recurrence: a study of tumour spread in the mesorectum distal to rectal cancer. Br J Surg 1995;82:1031–1033.
27. Arbman G, Nilsson E, Hallbook O, Sjodahl R. Local recurrence following total mesorectal excision for rectal cancer. Br J Surg 1996;83: 375–379.
28. Lazorthes F, Chiotasso P, Gamagami RA, et al. Late clinical outcome in a randomized prospective comparison of colonic J pouch and straight coloanal anastomosis. Br J Surg 1997;84:1449–1451.

29. Joo J, Latulippe JF, Alabaz O, et al. How long does the functional superiority of colonic J pouch to straight coloanal anastomosis persist after low anterior resection [abstract]? Dis Colon Rectum 1997;40:A23.
30. Fisher B, Wolmark N, Rockette HE. Postoperative adjuvant chemotheraphy or radiation therapy for rectal cancer: results from NSABP protocol R01. J Natl Cancer Inst 1988;80:21–29.
31. Krook JE, Moertel CG, Gunderson LL, et al. Effective surgical adjuvant therapy for high risk rectal cancer. N Engl J Med 1991;324:709–715.
32. Gastrointestinal Tumor Study Group. Prolongation of the disease free interval in surgically treated rectal cancer. N Engl J Med 1985;312:1465–1472.
33. O'Connell MJ, Martenson JA, Weiand HS, et al. Improving adjuvant therapy for rectal cancer by combining protracted infusion fluorouracil with radiation therapy after curative surgery. N Engl J Med 1994;331:551.

CHAPTER 40

Cancer of the Appendix

JOHN V. TAYLOR
SUSAN GALANDIUK

A. Presumed Appendicitis

Primary malignancies of the vermiform appendix are uncommon. Patients may present with symptoms suggestive of acute appendicitis,[1,2] or the tumor may be discovered incidentally during an unrelated operation.[3,4] The presence of an appendiceal tumor therefore is rarely known preoperatively; furthermore, the correct diagnosis is made intraoperatively in only about 30% of patients undergoing surgery for presumed appendicitis.[5] When the operative findings are unclear, frozen section is recommended so the appropriate operative procedure can be performed immediately.[4,6–8] Otherwise, definitive surgery is delayed until histologic examination of the resected appendix discloses the presence of a cancer.

There are four histologic types of appendiceal cancer[3,4,9]: neuroendocrine (carcinoid) tumors (85%), mucinous cystadenocarcinoma (8%), colonic-type adenocarcinoma (4%), and adenocarcinoid tumors (2%).[4] The remaining 1% include such rare neoplasms as lymphosarcoma and paraganglioma, among others. Distinction among these types is important because each has its own clinical features and outcomes.

B. Carcinoids

Carcinoid tumors of the appendix account for 50% of gastrointestinal neuroendocrine tumors and are the most common appendiceal malignancy.[2,3,10–13] They are found in approximately 0.5% of appendectomy specimens.[2,3,9,10,14] The presence of carcinoid-type symptoms usually indicates advanced disease.[11] Even though most act in a benign fashion, these tumors have the potential to invade, metastasize, and produce vasoactive substances.[4,10,12,14] Metastases from appendiceal carcinoids are rare, occurring in fewer than 5% of cases.[2] When they involve the liver, they may contribute to the carcinoid syndrome,[11] producing diarrhea and flushing.

The most important factor when determining the proper treatment of appendiceal carcinoids is the size of the tumor.[1–4,9,10,14] Size should be determined before the specimen is placed in tissue fixatives because formaldehyde-treated, paraffin-embedded tissue shrinks approximately 33%.[2,9] Approximately

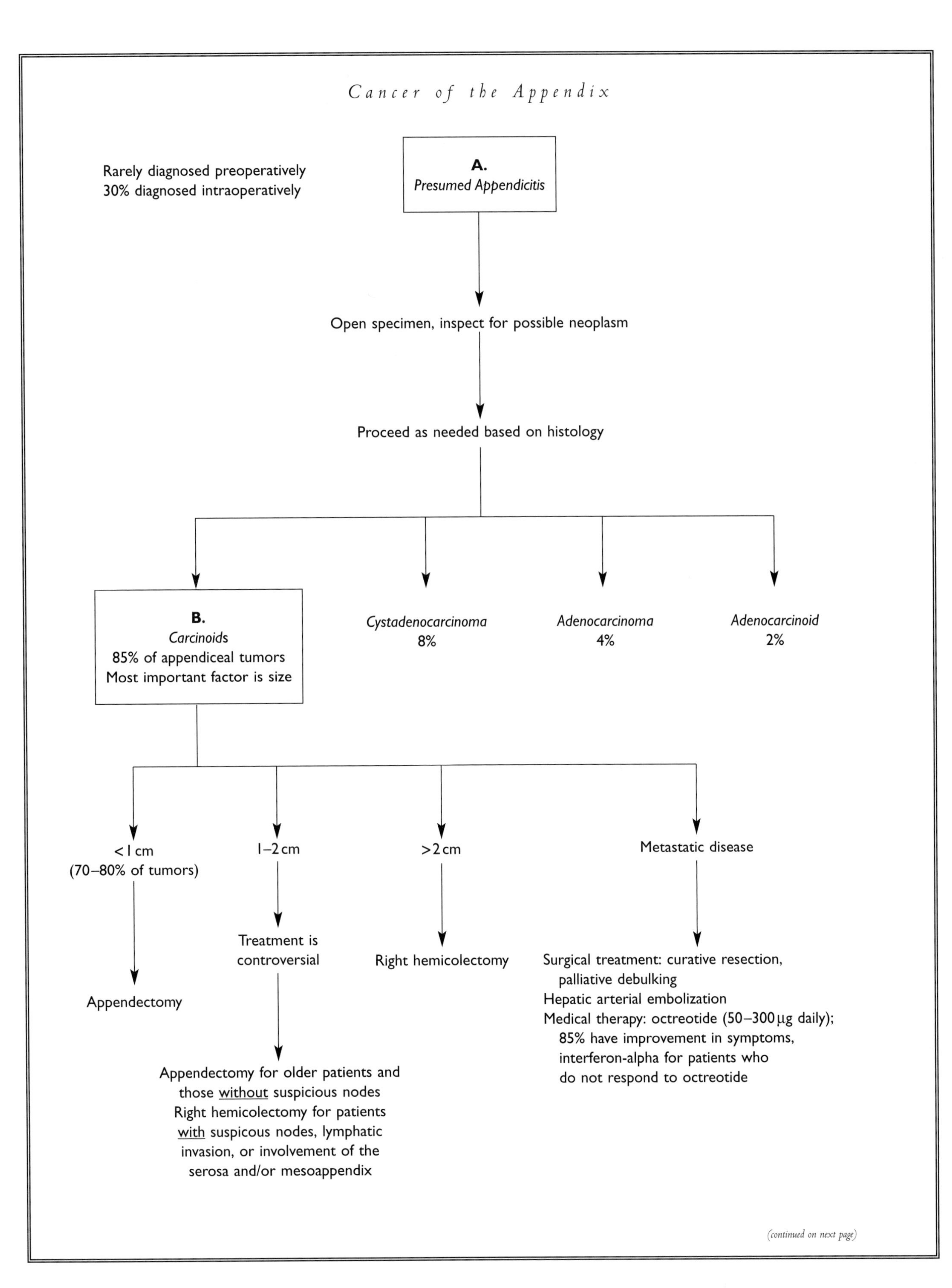

(continued on next page)

Cancer of the Appendix (continued)

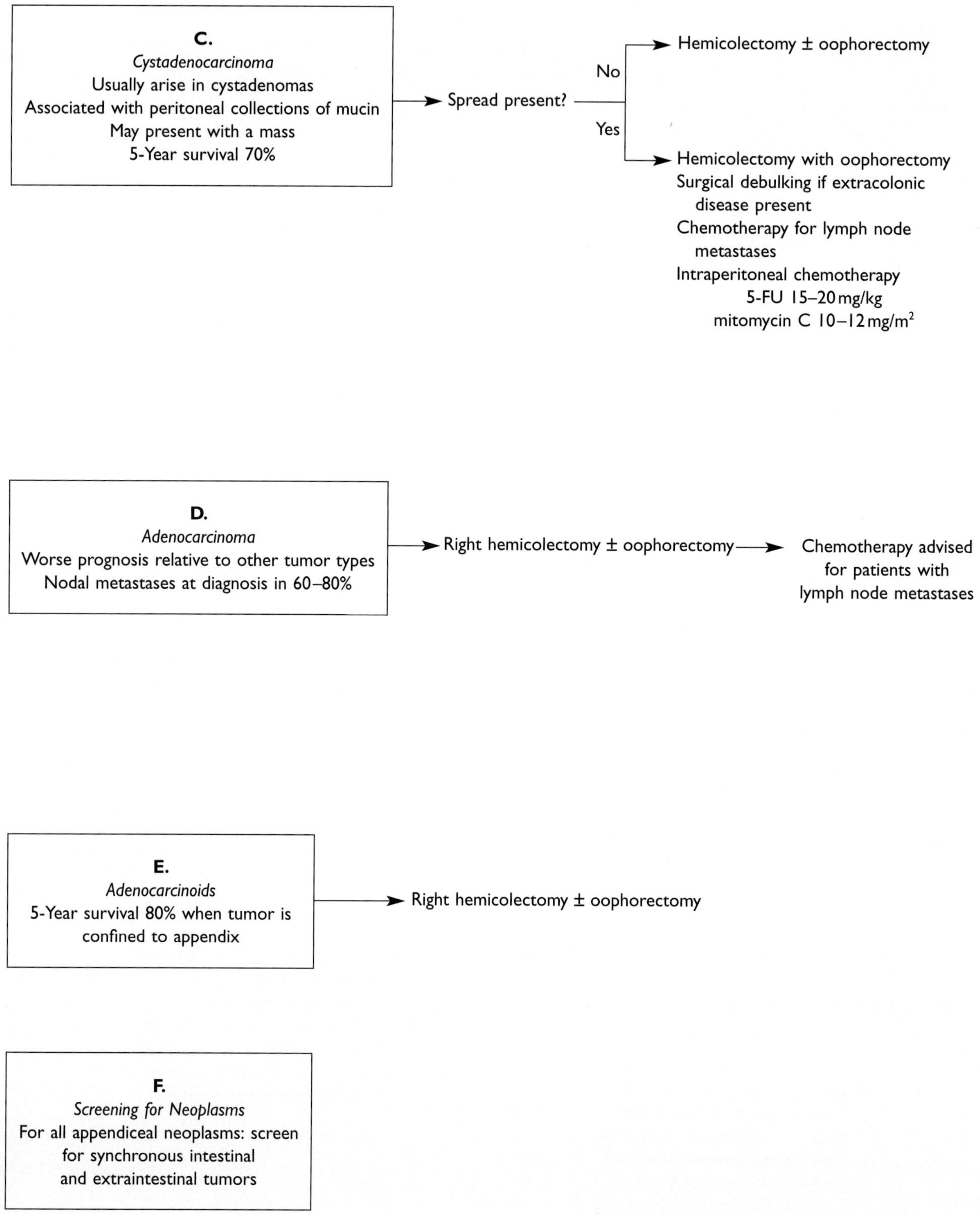

C.
Cystadenocarcinoma
Usually arise in cystadenomas
Associated with peritoneal collections of mucin
May present with a mass
5-Year survival 70%

→ Spread present?
- No → Hemicolectomy ± oophorectomy
- Yes → Hemicolectomy with oophorectomy
  - Surgical debulking if extracolonic disease present
  - Chemotherapy for lymph node metastases
  - Intraperitoneal chemotherapy
    - 5-FU 15–20 mg/kg
    - mitomycin C 10–12 mg/m^2

D.
Adenocarcinoma
Worse prognosis relative to other tumor types
Nodal metastases at diagnosis in 60–80%

→ Right hemicolectomy ± oophorectomy → Chemotherapy advised for patients with lymph node metastases

E.
Adenocarcinoids
5-Year survival 80% when tumor is confined to appendix

→ Right hemicolectomy ± oophorectomy

F.
Screening for Neoplasms
For all appendiceal neoplasms: screen for synchronous intestinal and extraintestinal tumors

70–80% of tumors are <1 cm in diameter and are found toward the tip of the appendix.[1,4,9,14] At this size, recurrence or metastases following appendectomy is rare, and appendectomy alone is considered adequate treatment.[2,4,12,14,15]

For carcinoid tumors 1–2 cm in diameter, the correct treatment remains controversial. Even at this size, metastases are infrequent, occurring in fewer than 1% of patients.[12] Appendectomy alone is considered adequate treatment provided metastatic lymph nodes are not detected at the time of surgery.[2,3,11,14] In a long-term study of 150 patients with appendiceal carcinoids up to 2 cm treated with appendectomy alone, Moertel et al.[14] found no evidence of recurrence despite lymphatic and serosal invasion (median follow-up more than 26 years). If one extrapolates these results to tumors even smaller, the rationale for conservative treatment seems justified. A more aggressive approach has been recommended for younger patients, with hemicolectomy being performed after invasion of the lymphatics, serosa, or mesoappendix.[1,4,9,12] In the elderly a conservative approach is appropriate because the time span of the disease may be longer than the life expectancy of the patient.[2,3,11,12,14,15] Obviously, right hemicolectomy is advisable if appendectomy alone cannot excise all gross disease regardless of patient age (i.e., if the base of the appendix and the cecal wall are involved).[1,12,15] In several reports, local excision of the cecal wall was adequate, provided the margins of resection were clear.[2,3,4,9,11]

For tumors >2 cm in diameter the incidence of nodal metastases is much higher (approximately 30%),[12] so right hemicolectomy is generally advised. Moertel et al.,[14] however, indicated that appendectomy alone may be curative, provided there is no gross evidence of spread at the initial operation. For elderly patients and those with several co-morbid illnesses, which put the patient at greater operative risk, a conservative approach has been advocated, but this is controversial.[3] If one compares the morbidity of appendectomy versus colectomy, there is little difference with respect to anesthetic risk and minimal increase in operating time; and the potential oncologic benefit must be considered. For patients with palpable mesenteric nodes suggestive of metastatic cancer, hemicolectomy is advised.[1,3,15]

Few patients with appendiceal carcinoids develop liver metastases. Most carcinoid hepatic metastases originate from sites other than the appendix.[11,15–17] If it is unresectable, metastatic disease is treated with palliative measures to control distressing symptoms[16,18–20] such as abdominal pain, mechanical obstruction, gut ischemia, or the flushing and diarrhea associated with the carcinoid syndrome. Some patients with accessible metastases are suitable for curative resection. McEntee et al.[21] found that 85% of patients undergoing curative surgery were free of tumor recurrence after a mean follow-up of 20 months. Even for patients in whom a cure is not possible, there is still a role for surgical intervention, as significant symptomatic relief can be obtained following palliative resection[11,16,21,22] provided 90% of the tumor bulk can be removed.[21,23] Palliative resection may also be associated with a survival benefit.[21,22] Cryosurgical ablation of liver metastases is a promising method for palliative control.[19]

Hepatic transplantation is another surgical option.[1] Although experience with transplantation for the treatment of secondary tumors of all types is disappointing because of a high incidence of early recurrence,[18] neuroendocrine tumors are considered an acceptable indication for transplantation because of their slow growth and longer patient survival compared to other tumor types. However, its benefits have yet to be shown over other forms of treatment.[16]

Another method of reducing tumor bulk is hepatic artery embolization, which reduces blood flow to the metastases.[9,11,16,22,23] Embolization has been shown to cause objective tumor regression in approximately 60% of patients; the mean duration of relief, however, is only 4–6 months, increasing to 18 months with the addition of chemotherapy.[18]

Management of the symptoms of carcinoid syndrome is also possible using long-acting somatostatin analogues,[9] particularly ocetreotide[24] (50–300 μg daily[20]). This therapy is now considered a mainstay of treatment for symptomatic relief of the carcinoid syndrome,[11] producing improvement in 85% of cases.[24] Fifty percent of patients experience stabilization of their disease, although the response is often not maintained and progression may occur.[1,20] Interferon-α has been used; although the results of clinical trials are variable,[24] it is recommended for patients who do not respond or whose disease progresses despite octreotide therapy.[1]

Cytotoxic chemotherapy is generally not used outside of controlled studies because of its frequent toxicity and poor response rates,[11,16,24] but regimens that combine embolization, intraarterial chemotherapy, and octreotide are encouraging. Even though these regimens may have more side effects,[16] refinement of the protocols may reduce those effects while achieving the desired result.[18]

C. *Cystadenocarcinoma*

Cystadenocarcinomas are usually well differentiated, progress slowly compared to the colonic-type adenocarcinomas,[1,5] have a 5-year survival rate of 70%,[4,9,25] and nearly always arise in preexisting cystadenomas.[26] Both have mucus-secreting epithelium[26] with varying degrees of atypia, mitoses, and papillary configuration.[9] Malignancy is determined by signs of invasion or the presence of epithelial cells in peritoneal collections of mucin.[9]

This tumor is often diagnosed preoperatively,[9] as many patients present with an abdominal mass.[4,27] Computed tomography may show a mass with near-water density and partly calcified walls.[4] Fifty percent of patients have intraperitoneal metastases when symptoms first occur; lymphatic or hematogenous spread is unusual.[5]

Right hemicolectomy is performed for all lesions when a malignancy is suspected.[25,27] Schlatter et al.[28] proposed appendectomy only for well differentiated lesions with clear margins of resection based on a retrospective review of 23 cases of localized disease that did not recur following appendectomy. However, a large review of 47 patients describe a survival benefit of right hemicolectomy over appendectomy (5-year survivals of 73% vs. 44%) presumably because of secondary tumor deposits in the mesentery.[5,6] In patients with peritoneal involvement, resection should be combined with aggressive debulking[4,29] and oophorectomy, as the ovaries are a common site of recurrence.[4] Systemic chemotherapy does not appear to improve survival. Intraperitoneal chemotherapy may be of some benefit,[25,29] but its use is not widespread. Sugarbaker and Jablonski[29] studied 130 patients with appendiceal cancer who had a combined approach of aggressive cytoreductive surgery and intraperitoneal chemotherapy consisting of 5-fluorouracil (5-FU) at 15–20 mg/kg combined with mitomycin C at 10–12 mg/m^2 during the early postoperative phase. They noted, however, that optimal results appeared in patients with less aggressive tumors and a low volume of residual disease following resection. Patients with large-volume, high-grade disease are not good candidates for intraperitoneal chemotherapy because high morbidity and mortality rates are expected with minimal survival benefit.

D. Adenocarcinoma

When histologic studies reveal colonic-type adenocarcinoma, the overall prognosis is significantly worse than for other cell types.[9] The tumor, in general, acts similarly to colonic adenocarcinoma, with the prognosis related to Dukes' stage.[1,30] The appendix has areas of incomplete muscular coats, so lymphatic spread to the ileocolic nodes[28] tends to be an early event,[5,25] often without involvement of the serosa.[8] Most patients therefore tend to present late in the disease course, with 60–80% of patients having clinical signs of metastases at the time of diagnosis.[6,25,28]

Because of this early pattern of lymphatic spread, right hemicolectomy is the preferred treatment to remove the regional lymph nodes, stage the extent of disease, and determine the need for chemotherapy.[6,27,31] Most tumors are found after histologic examination of an appendectomy specimen, so hemicolectomy is often performed as a secondary procedure after the initial operation.[9] As with cystadenocarcinoma of the appendix, intraperitoneal metastases may be found in the ovaries[25,32]; therefore synchronous oophorectomy has been recommended for postmenopausal women.[5] If lymph node metastases are confirmed histologically, 5-FU-based chemotherapy regimens are advised once the patient recovers from surgery. Although regimens may vary from center to center, most tend to include 5-FU and levamisole.[9] As with cystadenocarcinomas, the role of intraperitoneal chemotherapy has yet to be established. Sugarbaker and Jablonski[29] also showed it may be of potential benefit for patients with colonic-type adenocarcinoma of the appendix with peritoneal involvement, although the same indications apply (i.e., low grade malignancy with little residual disease following resection).

E. Adenocarcinoids

Adenocarcinoid tumors are unusual in that they have features of both carcinoid tumors and adenocarcinomas in terms of structure and behavior, with a prognosis intermediate between the two.[1] It has been hypothesized that they arise from a dual cell origin or from crypt base stem cells.[4–9] These tumors are, however, distinguishable enough to be classified as a distinct pathologic entity.[33,34] Prediction of their behavior is difficult because tumor size bears no relation to the risk of metastases.[9,34] Even small tumors that are not visible at gross inspection of the appendix may metastasize. A favored site of spread is the ovary. When a patient has a Krukenberg tumor with no obvious source, an appendectomy should be performed to avoid overlooking a small adenocarcinoid tumor.[9]

Because the behavior of this tumor is not well understood, treatment involves a right hemicolectomy with oophorectomy.[4,9,13] Bak and Asschenfeldt[33] reported that hemicolectomy was necessary only if the tumor showed moderate to severe atypia, a mitotic count of more than two mitoses per high-powered field, or spread beyond the appendix. Five-year survival is 80% provided the tumor is localized to the appendix.[4,9]

F. Screening for Neoplasms

Following the discovery of any neoplasm of the appendix (benign or malignant), it is necessary to screen for synchronous and metachronous neoplasia[1,9,27] at intraintestinal and extraintestinal sites.[25] Nitecki et al.[5] reported a second primary malignancy, either at the time of surgery or developing subsequently, in 35% of their series, with 50% of these lesions occurring outside the gastrointestinal tract, most frequently in the breast, uterus, prostate, or ovary.

References

1. Deans GT, Spence RA. Neoplastic lesions of the appendix. Br J Surg 1995;82:299–306.
2. Anderson JR, Wilson BG. Carcinoid tumors of the appendix. Br J Surg 1985;72:545–546.
3. Roggo A, Wood WC, Ottinger LW. Carcinoid tumors of the appendix. Ann Surg 1993;217:358–390.

4. Rutledge RH, Alexander JW. Primary appendiceal malignancies: rare but important. Surgery 1992;111:244–250.
5. Nitecki SS, Wolff BG, Shclinkert R, et al. The natural history of surgically treated primary adenocarcinoma of the appendix. Ann Surg 1994;219: 51–57.
6. Harris GJ, Urdaneta LF, Mitros FA. Adenocarcinoma of the vermiform appendix. J Surg Oncol 1990;44:218–224.
7. Lane IF, Snook SJ. Surgical management of adenocarcinoma of the appendix. Br J Clin Pract 1984;38:233–235.
8. Ben-Aaron U, Shperber J, Halevy A, et al. Primary adenocarcinoma of the appendix: report of five cases and review of the literature. J Surg Oncol 1987;36:113–115.
9. Rutledge RH. Primary appendiceal malignancies. In: Morris PJ, Malt RA (eds) Oxford Textbook of Surgery. Oxford: Oxford University Press, 1994: 1117–1120.
10. Wackym PA, Gray GF Jr. Tumors of the appendix. II. The spectrum of carcinoid. South Med J 1984;77:288–291.
11. Loftus JP, van Heerden JA. Surgical management of gastrointestinal carcinoid tumors. Adv Surg 1995;28:317–336.
12. Stinner B, Kisker O, Zielke A, et al. Surgical management for carcinoid tumors of small bowel, appendix, colon, and rectum. World J Surg 1996;20: 183–188.
13. Gouzi JL, Laigneau P, Flamant Y, et al. Indications for right hemicolectomy in carcinoid tumors of the appendix. Surg Gynecol Obstet 1993;176: 543–547.
14. Moertel CG, Weiland LH, Nagorney DM, et al. Carcinoid tumor of the appendix: treatment and prognosis. N Engl J Med 1987;317:1699–1701.
15. Rothmund M, Kisker O. Surgical treatment of carcinoid tumors of the small bowel, appendix, colon, and rectum. Digestion 1994;55(suppl 3): 86–91.
16. Ahlman H, Westberg G, Wangberg B, et al. Treatment of liver metastases of carcinoid tumors. World J Surg 1996;20:196–202.
17. Makridis C, Rastad J, Oberg K, et al. Progression of metastases and symptom improvement from laparotomy in midgut carcinoid tumors. World J Surg 1996;20:900–907.
18. Diaco DS, Hajarizadeh H, Mueller CR, et al. Treatment of metastatic carcinoid tumors using multimodality therapy of octreotide acetate, intraarterial chemotherapy, and hepatic arterial chemoembolization. Am J Surg 1995;169:523–528.
19. Johnson LB, Krebs T, Wong-You-Cheong J, et al. Cryosurgical debulking of unresectable liver metastases for palliation of carcinoid syndrome. Surgery 1997;121:468–470.
20. Wangberg B, Westberg G, Tylen U, et al. Survival of patients with disseminated midgut carcincoid tumors after aggressive tumor reduction. World J Surg 1996;20:892–899.
21. McEntee GP, Nagorney DM, Kvols LK, et al. Cytoreductive hepatic surgery for neuroendocrine tumors. Surgery 1990;108:1091–1096.
22. Soreide O, Berstad T, Bakka A, et al. Surgical treatment as a principle in patients with advanced abdominal carcinoid tumors. Surgery 1992;111: 48–54.
23. Foster JH, Lundy J. Pathology of liver metastases. Curr Probl Surg 1981; 18:157–202.
24. Arnold R. Medical treatment of metastasizing carcinoid tumors. World J Surg 1996;20:203–207.
25. Cartina R, McCormick J, Kolm P, et al. Management and prognosis of adenocarcinoma of the appendix. Dis Colon Rectum 1995;38:848 –852.
26. Wackym PA, Gray GF Jr. Tumors of the appendix. II. Neoplastic and nonneoplastic mucoceles. South Med J 1984;77:283–291.
27. Gattuso P, Reddy V, Kathuria S, et al. Primary adenocarcinoma of the appendix: a review. Mil Med 1990;155:343–345.
28. Schlatter MG, McKone TK, Schloten DJ, et al. Primary appendiceal adenocarcinoma. Am Surg 1987;53:434–447.
29. Sugarbaker PH, Jablonski KA. Prognostic features of 51 colorectal and 130 appendiceal cancer patients with peritoneal carcinomatosis treated by cytoreductive surgery and intraperitoneal chemotherapy. Ann Surg 1995; 221:124–132.
30. Ferro M, Anthony PP. Adenocarcinoma of the appendix. Dis Colon Rectum 1985;28:457–459.
31. Gilhome RW, Johnstone DH, Clark J, Kyle J. Primary adenocarcinoma of the vermiform appendix: report of a series of 10 cases and review of the literature. Br J Surg 1984;71:553–555.
32. Conte CC, Petrelli NJ, Stulc J, Herrera L, Mittel A. Adenocarcinoma of the appendix. Surg Gynecol Obstet 1988;166:451–453.
33. Bak M, Asschenfeldt P. Adenocarcinoid of the vermiform appendix: a clinicopathologic study of 20 cases. Dis Colon Rectum 1988;31:605–612.
34. Burke AP, Sobin LH, Federspiel BH, Shekitka KM, Helwig EB. Goblet cell carcinoids and related tumors of the vermiform appendix. Am J Clin Pathol 1990;94:27–35.

CHAPTER 41

Anal Cancer

THEODORE J. SACLARIDES

A. Epidemiology and Etiology

Cancers of the anal canal and perianal region are distinctly uncommon neoplasms, comprising only 1–2% of all large bowel tumors. Anal cancer differs from colorectal cancer in that there are no predisposing or inherited genetic risk factors; moreover, a long line of successive DNA mutations have not been conclusively identified, there is definite evidence of a viral cause, and it is primarily treated nonsurgically except in the earliest cases. The significant impact of irradiation and chemotherapy on these cancers is well known and almost universally accepted, and it is not the intention of this author to review the historical evolution of the treatment of anal cancer. Rather, current management recommendations are discussed, as are ongoing controversial issues.

The anatomy of the anus and anal canal is generally well understood, but the classification of tumors arising within this area has been confusing and inconsistent. The World Health Organization and the American Joint Committee on Cancer have agreed on a classification system that has helped standardize terminology and management.[1,2] According to their definition, the anal canal extends along the length of the internal sphincter; its upper border is located at the top of the anorectal ring in the vicinity of the puborectalis muscle, and the lower border is at the end of the internal sphincter muscle. In this region can be found variable epithelium, ranging from columnar epithelium above the transition zone to the transitional epithelium found between the dentate line and the tops of the columns of Morgagni, to nonkeratinized squamous epithelium below the dentate line to the anal verge. Within this area can be found squamous cell cancers, transitional cell or cloacogenic cancers, and adenocarcinomas; there is no clear anatomic boundary separating these tumor histologies. The anal verge begins at the point where the skin contains appendages such as hair follicles and sebaceous glands and extends for a circumferential distance of 5 cm externally. Anal verge tumors are similar to primary skin cancers located elsewhere on the body and are treated in a similar fashion. Using this classification system, approximately 85% of anal neoplasms arise within the anal canal. Most are squamous cell cancers; and with the exception of melanoma, the treatment and prognosis of anal canal cancers are independent of histology.

Anal Cancer

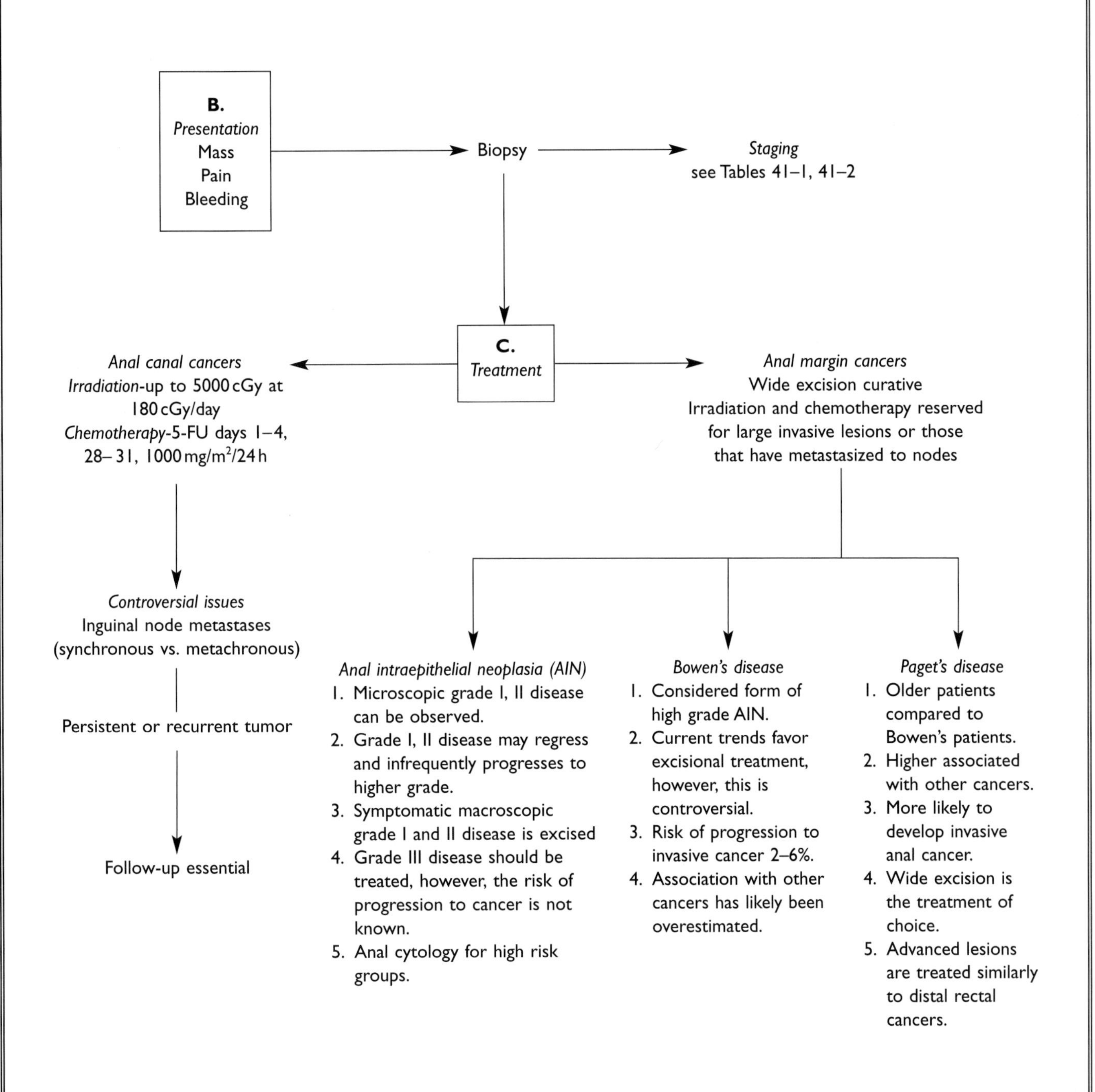

A.
Epidemiology and Etiology
1–2% of large bowel malignancies
Parallels seen with cervical cancer
Multifactorial etiology including HPV and HIV infection, immunosuppression
Screening programs for high risk groups
B.
Presentation
Mass
Pain
Bleeding
Biopsy
Staging
see Tables 41–1, 41–2
C.
Treatment
Anal canal cancers
Irradiation-up to 5000 cGy at 180 cGy/day
Chemotherapy-5-FU days 1–4, 28–31, 1000 mg/m²/24 h
Controversial issues
Inguinal node metastases (synchronous vs. metachronous)
Persistent or recurrent tumor
Follow-up essential
Anal margin cancers
Wide excision curative
Irradiation and chemotherapy reserved for large invasive lesions or those that have metastasized to nodes
Anal intraepithelial neoplasia (AIN)
1. Microscopic grade I, II disease can be observed.
2. Grade I, II disease may regress and infrequently progresses to higher grade.
3. Symptomatic macroscopic grade I and II disease is excised
4. Grade III disease should be treated, however, the risk of progression to cancer is not known.
5. Anal cytology for high risk groups.
Bowen's disease
1. Considered form of high grade AIN.
2. Current trends favor excisional treatment, however, this is controversial.
3. Risk of progression to invasive cancer 2–6%.
4. Association with other cancers has likely been overestimated.
Paget's disease
1. Older patients compared to Bowen's patients.
2. Higher associated with other cancers.
3. More likely to develop invasive anal cancer.
4. Wide excision is the treatment of choice.
5. Advanced lesions are treated similarly to distal rectal cancers.

Anal cancer is most commonly found between the age of 55 and 65, although it can be diagnosed in both older and younger patients. When subgroups of patients have been studied, it has been noted that there is an increasing incidence in men younger than 45 years. Other age groups have not shown a comparable increase. There has been a shift in gender as well; formerly thought to be a disease of elderly women, anal cancer now occurs more commonly in men in the United States.

Most patients present with symptoms of a mass, bleeding, or pain. Vague symptoms may predate the discovery of the cancer by quite a long time, and it is not uncommon for these symptoms to be overlooked by both the patient and the treating physician, who may attribute them to hemorrhoids. Any anal canal or perianal lesion that cannot be attributed to common anorectal conditions such as hemorrhoids, fistulas, or warts must be biopsied. The inguinal regions should be inspected, as approximately 15% of patients have groin metastases at presentation. In addition, at initial diagnosis approximately 10% of patients have disease extension into the rectovaginal septum, and 10–15% have metastases to the liver, lungs, or bone.

The cause of anal cancer is multifactorial; and although high risk patients have been identified, many factors must act in concert to induce carcinogenesis. Many parallels have been noted between anal and cervical cancer with respect to pathogenesis.

1. Infection with human papilloma virus (HPV) predisposes to anogenital warts and, potentially, anal and cervical cancer, particularly when types 16 and 18 are involved.

2. The prevalence of HPV type 16 in squamous cell carcinomas varies geographically, the highest incidence having been noted in California.

3. Infection with HPV type 16 is associated with the development of high grade anal intraepithelial neoplasia (AIN). The incidence of AIN is higher in homosexual men with HPV infection than in heterosexual men with HPV infection.

4. Infections with HPV types 6 and 11 are not associated with the development of cancer; instead they are associated with condyloma and low-grade AIN.

5. Cervical intraepithelial neoplasia (CIN) and AIN frequently coexist in women with a history of HPV type 16 infection.

6. HPV infection alone is not enough to cause cancer. There is evidence to suggest that in some HPV cases there is inactivation of the *p53* tumor suppressor gene product. In other HPV cases, there is an association of prior infection with herpes simplex type 1 virus, *Chlamydia trachomatis*, and the human immunodeficiency virus (HIV). Infection with herpes simplex, *Chlamydia*, and gonorrhea confer an increased risk of anal cancer even in the absence of antecedent HPV infection.

7. Immunosuppressed renal transplant patients have a 100-fold increase in anogenital tumors.

8. Infection with HIV alone may not confer an increased risk of cancer. Anal cancer in HIV-positive patients who contracted the virus through intravenous drug abuse is rarely seen.[3–7]

Between 1966 and 1981 a 500% increase in the number of patients afflicted with HPV was noted. Approximately 2 million to 3 million cases are noted each year. More than 60 types have been described. Type 6 and 11 are not incorporated into host DNA and give rise to anogenital warts and low-grade AIN. Types 16 and 18 have been extensively studied and are incorporated into host DNA and consequently are associated with anal cancer and high-grade AIN. Types 30, 42, 44, 51, and 54 are also associated with cancer.[3]

The parallels seen with cervical cancer and the benefit found with cervical Papanicolaou smear screening have led to speculation that perhaps anal screening programs could reduce the incidence and mortality from anal cancer. Anal cytology is a means of identifying precancerous conditions and consequently the patients who should be followed more closely. Easily performed in the outpatient setting, anal cytology is obtained by inserting a tongue depressor or brush into the anal canal. An adequate sample is obtained by rotating the instrument circumferentially and then immediately transferring the sample to a glass slide, which is promptly placed in alcohol. Patients with abnormal cytology are further assessed with anoscopy and application of topical 3% acetic acid. Abnormal or raised areas identified in this fashion should be biopsied.

Low-grade AIN identified by cytology and confirmed with biopsy may be simply observed, as many of these lesions spontaneously regress or rarely progress to more virulent forms of neoplasia. Follow-up is advised, although the interval between examinations is not universally accepted. High-grade AIN confirmed with biopsy generally requires treatment with excision.

Screening should be considered for the following groups of patients: (1) any patient who has previously had abnormal anal cytology; (2) HIV-negative men who practice anal-receptive intercourse; (3) HIV-positive men with CD4 counts less than 500; (4) women with high-grade CIN; and (5) HIV-positive women with CD4 counts less than 500. It is generally believed that annual screening is appropriate for these high risk patients. Screening should be performed more frequently in cases where cytology suggests an abnormality but biopsies are negative.[8]

B. *Presentation*

As stated above, most lesions are associated with symptoms of a mass, pain, or bleeding. Extension of the tumor into the sphincter produces constant, unrelenting pain. Despite the fact that most anal cancers are visible or are within reach of the examining finger, up to one-half of lesions have invaded the sphincter at presentation and up to 15% have already metastasized to inguinal lymph nodes. These cancers are hard, irregular, and usually ulcerated. Any abnormal mass in the anal canal or the anal verge must be biopsied. If office examination cannot exactly determine the location, extent, and penetration of the tumor into surrounding structures, an examination under anesthesia is warranted. Intraluminal ultrasonography may be useful for assessing the degree of sphincter involvement, thereby helping to determine which patients are potential candidates for local excision. Abnormal inguinal lymph nodes should be assessed with fine-needle aspiration.

Staging systems follow the TNM classification and permit comparison of similar patient groups (Tables 41–1, 41–2). With regard to anal cancer, these systems are limited in their usefulness for several reasons: (1) accurate pretreatment evaluation with ultrasonography is not universally available, so precise knowledge about the depth of penetration and lymph nodes is usually lacking; (2) first-line therapy consists of irradiation and chemotherapy, which cause anatomic distortion of the tumor; (3) surgical excision of the tumor and regional lymphatics is infrequently performed, so staging is done without knowledge of the histology.

TABLE 41–1.
AJCC definition of TNM and stage grouping for anal canal cancer

Primary Tumor (T)

TX	Primary tumor cannot be assessed
T0	No evidence of primary tumor
Tis	Carcinoma *in situ*
T1	Tumor 2 cm or less in greatest dimension
T2	Tumor more than 2 cm but not more than 5 cm in greatest dimension
T3	Tumor more than 5 cm in greatest dimension
T4	Tumor of any size invades adjacent organ(s): e.g., vagina, urethra, bladder (involvement of sphineter muscle[s] alone is not classified as T4)

Regional Lymph Nodes (N)

NX	Regional lymph nodes cannot be assessed
N0	No regional lymph node metastasis
N1	Metastatics in perirectal lymph node(s)
N2	Metastasis in unilateral internal iliac and/or inguinal lymph node(s)
N3	Metastasis in perirectal and inguinal lymph nodes and/or bilateral internal iliac and/or inguinal lymph nodes

Distant Metastasis (M)

MX	Distant metastasis cannot be assessed
M0	No distant metastasis
M1	Distant metastasis

Stage	*T*	*N*	M
0	Tis	N0	M0
I	T1	N0	M0
II	T2	N0	M0
	T3	N0	M0
IIIA	T1	N1	M0
	T2	N1	M0
	T3	N1	M0
	T4	N0	M0
IIIB	T4	N1	M0
	Any T	N2	M0
	Any T	N3	M0
IV	Any T	Any N	M1

SOURCE: Used with permission of the American Joint Committee on Cancer (AJCC®), Chicago, IL. The original source for this material is the AJCC® Cancer Staging Manual, 5th edition (1997) published by Lippincott Williams & Wilkins Publishers, Philadelphia, PA.

TABLE 41–2.
AJCC definition of TNM and stage grouping for perianal cancer

Primary Tumor (T)

T1–3	Same as for anal canal tumors
T4	Deep extradermal structures (e.g., cartilage, skeletal muscle, bone)

Regional Lymph Nodes (N)

NX	Regional lymph nodes cannot be assessed
N0	No evidence of lymph node metastasis
N1	Regional lymph node metastases

Distant Metastasis (M)

MX	Distant metastasis cannot be assessed
M0	No evidence of distant metastasis
M1	Distant metastases

Stage Grouping

Stage	*T*	*N*	M
0	Tis	N0	M0
I	T1	N0	M0
II	T2–3	N0	M0
III	T4	N0	M0
	any T	N1	M0
IV	any T	any N	M1

SOURCE: Used with permission of the American Joint Committee on Cancer (AJCC®), Chicago, IL. The original source for this material is the AJCC® Cancer Staging Manual, 5th edition (1997) published by Lippincott Williams & Wilkins Publishers, Philadelphia, PA.

C. *Treatment*

Management of anal cancer is discussed by location: anal canal versus anal margin. It is not the mission of this chapter to present a historical review of the evolution of treatment. However, this work would not be complete without mentioning the efforts of Norman Nigro, who was instrumental in establishing combined irradiation and chemotherapy as the primary form of treatment of anal canal cancers. The role of the surgeon has been greatly reduced from the time when abdominoperineal resection was the standard of care. Currently, the surgeon performs biopsies to establish the diagnosis, obtains tissue following the completion of treatment, performs radical surgery for patients who have failed irradiation and chemotherapy, and performs local excision for patients who are acceptable candidates for this approach.

Anal Canal Cancers

Local excision of anal lesions should be reserved for well differentiated, distally located cancers <2 cm in greatest dimension. If a tumor is penetrating the sphincter muscle, local excision should not be considered. Ultrasonography may help make this distinction. When lesions are properly selected, high cure rates can be expected, although close follow-up is mandatory to detect recurrences at an early, potentially salvageable stage.

For deeply invasive or larger anal canal cancers, the standard of care has been to treat them with combined irradiation and chemotherapy. Abdominoperineal resection is indicated only for patients who cannot tolerate combined therapy or who cannot receive radiation because of prior exposure at tissue tolerance limits. Radiation alone has been considered and compared to radiation plus chemotherapy in several studies. One randomized study showed that the addition of 5-fluorouracil (5-FU) and mitomycin-C to radiation significantly improved outcome compared to that seen after radiation alone.[9] Papillon and Montbarbon used interstitial implants in addition to external irradiation and found that the results were improved by the addition of chemotherapy.[10]

Nigro's work, supported by the work mentioned above, has therefore established the standard of care. Nigro's original protocol was as follows: External radiation, 3000 cGy, was delivered to the primary tumor and the pelvic and inguinal lymph nodes at a rate of 200 cGy/day. On day 1 a 4-day infusion of 5-FU 1000 mg/m^2/24 hr was begun and repeated beginning on day 28 for another 4 days. Mitomycin-C, 15 mg/m^2, was given on day 1. Of the 104 patients treated, 24 underwent proctectomy; and of these, 22 had no residual tumor. Altogether, 62 patients had biopsy of the scar only, and the results were negative in 61. Overall, the treatment was well tolerated, with only five patients developing toxicity that required hospitalization. The 5-year survival was 83%.[11] Higher doses of radiation are administered currently, approaching 5000 cGy, but chemotherapy doses have remained essentially the same. These higher radiation doses have yielded higher 5-year local control rates than the dose originally described in Nigro's protocol. Local recurrence and 5-year survival rates vary among reports but are approximately 10–20% and 80–90%, respectively.[12] Complications of irradiation include proctitis, cystitis, perianal irritation, anal fibrosis, anal radionecrosis, rectovaginal fistula, and incontinence. The likelihood of retaining continence following combined-modality therapy is generally 80–90%.

Two *controversial areas* merit discussion: management of inguinal node metastases and persistent or recurrent cancer following combined treatment. Prophylactic node dissection for the clinically negative groin is no longer advised because of the morbidity of the procedure and the unclear survival benefit provided. The clinically negative groin should undergo prophylactic irradiation, as it seems to reduce the likelihood of subsequent inguinal failure (15–25% vs. 3%).[13] Suspicious groin nodes at presentation should be sampled with fine-needle aspirations. If positive for metastases, the treatment generally is unchanged (i.e., combined chemoradiation); however, knowledge of metastatic disease at presentation may influence surveillance methods and intervals. Groin dissection for *synchronous* inguinal metastases is not advised, as combined-modality treatment successfully controls the primary tumor and its draining lymphatic basins. *Metachronous* inguinal node metastases carry a more favorable prognosis than their synchronous counterpart; but because these areas may have already reached their tolerance limits with respect to radiation, groin dissection with or without chemotherapy is the preferred treatment.

After chemoradiation is completed, the usual practice has been to biopsy the tumor site/scar after approximately 6 weeks. Alternatively, observation has been advocated, reserving biopsy for situations where a visible abnormality is present. Endorectal ultrasonography may assist in surveillance of the anus and perianal region. If persistent cancer is found shortly after the completion of chemoradiation, salvage abdominoperineal resection is considered the best treatment, although additional radiation may be considered provided there is a safe margin to permit treatment. If recurrent cancer is diagnosed at a time far removed from the initial treatment, the extent of disease should be determined with computed tomography (CT) scans. Although most failures are confined to the pelvis, some patients have disease at distant sites. In the absence of nonpelvic disease, salvage abdominoperineal resection should be performed. The outcome is guarded, although favorable results can be expected provided the tumor is mobile and not adherent to the lateral pelvic side walls.[14]

The most common sites for metastatic disease are the liver, lung, and bone. Once distant disease occurs, median survival is approximately 9 months. A variety of chemotherapeutic regimens have been used in these instances, but a regimen consisting of 5-FU and cisplatin is the most promising.

Anal Margin Cancers

Although anal margin cancers are external and easily noticeable by the patient and treating physician, there is frequently a delay in diagnosis. Symptoms of pain, bleeding, or a mass may be attributable to hemorrhoids. Local excision is appropriate treatment, particularly for in situ cancers or small (3–4 cm) well differentiated, superficially invasive lesions. If necessary, rotational flaps may be used for wound closure following excision of large tumors. Deeply invasive or large lesions and certainly those that have metastasized to the inguinal lymph nodes should be treated with chemotherapy and radiation (up to 70 Gy).

Anal Intraepithelial Neoplasia Anal intraepithelial neoplasia is defined as the presence of cellular and nuclear abnormalities in the perianal and anal epithelium without a breech of the epithelial basement membrane. There has been a threefold increase in AIN since 1959. It is found in up to 50% of HIV-positive patients, up to 45% of women with high grade genital intraepithelial neoplasia or cancer, and 25% of kidney transplant patients. It is generally thought that AIN may be a precursor of squamous cell carcinoma. The risk is determined by the degree of grade of abnormalities present. AIN is therefore classified as grade I, II, or III based on the histologic appearance. AIN is probably caused by human papilloma virus (HPV) infection, HIV infection, or both acting synergistically. HPV 16 has been identified in 56–86% of patients with squamous cell carcinoma and AIN and is more commonly found in grade III AIN than in lower grade AIN. AIN is commonly found in young men who practice anal-receptive intercourse and in 30–55% of HIV-positive men, in contrast to 4.7% of HIV-negative men.[15,16] The likelihood that AIN progresses to invasive cancer is not known with certainty; this risk is probably influenced by grade and patient-related risk factors. High-grade AIN has a natural history similar to that of high-grade CIN and consequently warrants aggressive intervention. It is generally thought that incidentally found microscopic evidence of AIN, such as in a hemorrhoidectomy specimen, does not progress to invasive squamous cell carcinoma.

The use of screening programs has been mentioned. The goal is to realize a reduction in incidence and mortality analogous to the effects of Papanicolaou smears for cervical cancers. A total of 169 HIV-positive and 164 HIV-negative homosexual men were enrolled in a program of anal cytology and surveillance. Of the HIV-positive men who had normal cytology at the onset of the study (32%), 50% subsequently developed AIN during the next 2 years, and 20% progressed to high-grade AIN. Of those HIV-positive men who had low-grade AIN at the onset (36%), 62% progressed to high-grade AIN and 5% regressed. In contrast, among the HIV-negative patients who had normal baseline cytology (74%), 17% progressed to AIN and 8% to high-grade AIN. Of the HIV-negative men who had low-grade AIN at the onset, 36% progressed to high-grade AIN and 50% regressed. The risk of progression in the HIV-positive group was increased according to the CD4 count (the risk was highest with a CD4 count <200) and if multiple HPV types were present. On the basis of these results, the authors concluded that annual screening with cytology should be implemented for high risk HIV-positive patients (CD4 count <500), whereas screening may be performed every 2 years for HIV-positive patients with CD4 counts >500. This approach is based on the absence of a grossly visible lesion. If a raised suspicious lesion is present, biopsy is indicated regardless of HIV status.[16]

Microscopic evidence of AIN (no visible lesion present) may be simply observed. AIN grade I or II found in a macroscopic lesion using cytology should be confirmed with biopsy. Treatment is conservative unless the patient has symptoms of itching, pain, or bleeding. This approach is based on the knowledge that regression may occur, and some of the lesions may be caused by HPV 6 and 11; however, close follow-up is needed with repetitive cytology especially in the high risk patient in whom progression of AIN may occur as noted above. AIN grade III should be treated; options include CO_2 laser or cryosurgery ablation or surgical excision. The latter is generally preferred. Small wounds may be closed primarily or allowed to close by secondary healing; large wounds may require the use of rotational flaps.

Bowen's Disease Bowen's disease is an intraepithelial squamous cell carcinoma named after John Bowen, who first described this condition in 1912. It was first thought that this disease was associated with the presence or subsequent development of internal malignancies or invasive cancer of the skin. This contention has been challenged and not substantiated in recent reports;[17] however, all would agree that Bowen's disease probably imparts an increased risk of developing invasive cancer in the skin affected by Bowen's disease. If left untreated, approximately 2–6% of cases progress to invasive squamous cell cancer. Patients present with nonspecific complaints such as burning, itching, and bleeding. Physical examination may reveal raised, scaly, irregular, red plaques with a gross appearance similar to that of other cutaneous conditions such as leukoplakia, eczema, or dermatitis. Any lesion that does not regress or respond to conservative measures should be biopsied and assessed by an experienced pathologist.

Bowen's disease is histologically recognizable by the presence of large atypical cells with large haloed hyperchromatic nuclei (bowenoid cells). Periodic acid-Schiff (PAS) staining is negative. Bowen's disease may represent the most advanced state of AIN and as such should be treated because of the risk of its progressing to invasive cancer. In fact, because some patients also have vulvar Bowen's disease, anal warts, and cervical or vulvar dysplasia, there may be a causative role of HPV in Bowen's disease. Bowen's disease is associated with HPV 16 and 18; in fact, HPV 16 has been found in 60–80% of patients.[18,19]

Mapping the perianal region has been advocated when planning treatment and is carried out by obtaining 2- to 3-mm sections from all four quadrants of the perineum and the anal canal. Once the extent of disease is known, a wide excision is planned using intraoperative frozen sections to verify the completeness of the excision. Small wounds created can be closed primarily; large defects may require split-thickness skin grafting or rotational flap closure. Follow-up is essential, but the exact means by which to do so is controversial. Obviously, any new lesion detected during the follow-up period should be biopsied. Some advocate random biopsies at the edge of skin grafts or rotational flaps. Recurrence rates of up to 30% have been noted, and most recurrences can be treated with reexcision. In a study from the Mayo Clinic, a 23% recurrence rate was noted if the excision was based on intraoperative frozen section assessment of the margins versus a recurrence rate of 53% if the excision was based on obtaining grossly negative visible margins.[18]

Many would argue that Bowen's disease should not be treated and that observation alone is sufficient. The reasons for this approach are the low incidence of invasive squamous cell carcinoma noted, our inability to eradicate HPV in the entire field, and the high recurrence rates noted even after wide excision.

PAGET'S DISEASE Paget's disease was first described in 1874 as a cutaneous disorder of the nipple. The first perianal case of Paget's disease was reported in 1893. Paget's cells contain sialomucin, which stains positive with PAS, helping to distinguish this entity from Bowen's disease. In contrast to Bowen's disease, patients with Paget's disease are older (66 vs. 48 years old), have a higher incidence of internal malignancies (50% vs. 5%), and are more likely to have or develop an invasive anal cancer (50% vs. 2–6%).[19] Once the diagnosis has been established with biopsy, a thorough examination of the colon, rectum, and anus is essential to rule out an underlying malignancy. Wide excision is the treatment of choice provided the lesion is superficial. In invasive cancer and those instances where there is an associated adenocarcinoma of the anal canal, abdominoperineal resection is the preferred treatment. The use of adjuvant irradiation and chemotherapy follows the same principles as outlined for rectal cancer (see Chapter 39).

Conclusions

Most invasive cancer of the anal canal are squamous cell carcinomas. With the exception of melanoma, the other histologic variants (cloacogenic, basaloid) are treated similarly to squamous cell cancer: with irradiation and chemotherapy. Local excision may be considered for small superficial lesions, but suitable tumors are infrequently encountered. The role of the surgeon is to obtain a tissue sample for diagnosis at presentation, assess for residual disease at the completion of treatment, and perform abdominoperineal resection for persistent or recurrent cancer. Synchronous inguinal lymph node metastases have a poor affect on prognosis; combined treatment is still the preferred therapy. Metachronous inguinal lymph node metastases are usually treated with groin dissection because radiation therapy at the limit of tissue tolerance has already been applied. Invasive cancers of the anal margin are treated with local excision.

Noninvasive perianal cancers include Bowen's disease, Paget's disease, and AIN associated with HPV infection and immunosuppression. Regarding *Bowen's disease*, the risk of progression to invasive cancer is approximately 2–6%, and the association with underlying malignancies has probably been overestimated in the past. Although wide local excision has been advocated as the preferred treatment, simple observation has also been proposed because of the low likelihood of developing squamous cell cancer, high recurrence rates following excisional therapy, and our inability to eradicate HPV infection in the entire at-risk field. *Paget's disease* has a higher risk of invasive cancer and a stronger association with cancer of the colon, rectum, and anus. Here wide excision is the preferred treatment.

The treatment of *AIN* is evolving. Low-grade microscopic AIN found in hemorrhoidectomy specimens may be observed, and follow-up is important. Grade I and II AIN found in macroscopic lesions may be treated conservatively unless the lesion causes symptoms of itching, pain, or bleeding. The natural history of these lesions is unclear, as regression may occur and nonmalignant HPV 6 and 11 may be the cause. Again, close follow-up is needed especially in high risk patients where progression to higher grade AIN may occur (homosexual men, positive HIV status, immunosuppression). Grade III AIN should be treated surgically with wide excision. Screening with anal cytology has been proposed for high risk groups. The exact risk of progression to invasive anal cancer remains to be determined.

References

1. Jass JR, Sobin LH. Histologic Typing of Intestinal Tumors, World Health Organization, 2nd ed. New York: Springer, 1989;32–33, 41–46.
2. Beahrs OH, Henson DE, Hutter RVP, Kenedy BJ. Manual for Staging of Cancer, American Joint Committee on Cancer, 4th ed. Philadelphia: Lippincott, 1992;83–87, 137–139.
3. Saclarides TJ, Klem D. Genetic alterations and virology of anal cancer. Semin Colon Rectal Surg 1995;6:131–124.
4. Palmer JG, Scholefield JH, Coates PJ, et al. Anal cancer and human papilloma viruses. Dis Clon Rectum 1989;32:1016–1022.
5. Shroyer KR, Kim JG, Manos MM, Greer CE, Pearlman NW, Franklin WA. Papillomavirus found in anorectal squamous carcinoma, not in colon adenocarcinoma. Arch Surg 1992;127:741–744.
6. Noffsinger A, Witte D, Fenoglio-Preiser CM. The relationship of human papillomavirus to anorectal neoplasia. Cancer 1992;70:1276–1287.
7. Deans GT, McAleer JA, Spence RAJ. Malignant anal tumors. Br J Surg 1994;81:500–508.
8. Palefsky JM. Rising incidence of anal cancer in HIV-positive patients: implications for the colorectal surgeon. Perspect Colon Rectal Surg 1994;7: 115–131.

9. Cummings BJ, Keane TJ, O'Sullivan B, Wong ES, Cotton CN. Epidermoid anal cancer: treatment by radiation alone or by radiation and 5-fluorouracil with and without mitomycin C. Int J Radiat Oncol Biol Phys 1991;21: 1115–1125.
10. Papillon J, Montbarbon JF. Epidermoid carcinoma of the anal canal: a series of 276 cases. Dis Colon Rectum 1987;30:324–333.
11. Nigro ND. Multidisciplinary management of cancer of the anus. World J Surg 1987;11:446–451.
12. Myerson RJ, Shapiro SJ, Lacey D, et al. Carcinoma of the anal canal. Am J Clin Oncol 1995;18:32–39.
13. Cummings BJ, Thomas GM, Keane TJ. Primary radiation therapy in the treatment of anal canal carcinoma. Dis Colon Rectum 1982;25:778–782.
14. Longo WE, Vernava AM, Wade TP, Coplin MA, Virgo KS, Johnson FE. Recurrent squamous cell carcinoma of the anal canal: predictors of initial treatment failure and results of salvage therapy. Ann Surg 1994;220:40–49.
15. Goldie SJ, Kuntz KM, Weinstein MC, Freedberg KA. Welton ML, Palefsky JM. The clinical effectiveness and cost-effectiveness of screening for anal squamous intraepithelial lesions in homosexual and bisexual HIV-positive men. JAMA 1999;281:1822–1829.
16. Palefsky JM, Holly EA, Hogeboom CJ, et al. Virologic, immunologic, and clinical parameters in the incidence and progression of anal squamous intraepithelial lesions in HIV-positive and HIV-negative homosexual men. J Acquir Immune Defic Syndr Hum Retrovirol 1998;17:314–319.
17. Marfing TC, Abel ME, Gallagher DM. Perianal Bowen's disease and associated malignancies: results of a survey. Dis Colon Rectum 1987;82: 470–474.
18. Sarmineto J, Wolff BG, Burgart LJ, Frizell FA, Ilstrup DM. Perianal Bowen's disease: associated tumors, human papillomavirus, surgery, and other controversies. Dis Colon Rectum 1997;40:912–918.
19. Clark RK, Schaldenbrand JD, Fowler JJ, Schuler JM, Lampman RM. Perianal Bowen's disease and anal intraepithelial neoplasia: review of the literature. Dis Colon Rectum 1999;42:945–951.

Section 7

Sarcomas

CHAPTER 42

Retroperitoneal Sarcomas

GEOFFREY A. PORTER
BARRY W. FEIG

A. Epidemiology and Etiology

Soft tissue sarcoma is rare, with an incidence of approximately 7000 cases per year in the United States. Of these, approximately 15% (600 cases) are retroperitoneal in location.[1,2] The peak incidence of these tumors is at about 60 years of age, with most cases scan during the fifth and sixth decades of life.[3] Risk factors for the development of any sarcoma also apply to retroperitoneal sarcomas and include specific genetic disorders: Li Fraumeni syndrome, Von Recklinghausen's disease (neurofibromatosis) and Gardner syndrome. A history of abdominal or pelvic irradiation is a specific known risk factor for this tumor.[4]

Liposarcoma and leiomyosarcoma are the two most common types of retroperitoneal sarcoma. Table 42–1 shows the various histologic subtypes and their incidence based on the cumulative experience of several large series over the past 25 years.[5–11] Other less common histologic subtypes include fibrosarcoma, malignant fibrous histiocytoma, synovial sarcoma, and unclassified sarcoma. The incidence of malignant fibrous histiocytoma is somewhat underestimated, as earlier studies did not recognize this subtype and simply classified such tumors as fibrosarcoma.

B. Presentation

The most common symptom in patients presenting with primary retroperitoneal sarcoma is abdominal pain, which is present in 40–60% of patients.[10] This pain is often nonspecific and, on average, is present 6 months prior to diagnosis. Neurologic symptoms related to direct neural involvement and compression occur in approximately 30% of patients and include paresthesia, dysesthesia, and weakness. Less common symptoms encountered are weight loss (<15%), early satiety (<10%), nausea and vomiting (<10%), and swelling or varicosities in the lower extremities (<10%).[4,8,10]

About 45–75% of patients with a retroperitoneal sarcoma have a palpable mass at presentation; and many of these patients also have increased abdominal girth.[12] The mass may vary in firmness; low-grade liposarcomas are somewhat soft, whereas higher-grade tumors are more firm. Less commonly, leg edema or testicular varicocele is present, indicating venous or lymphatic obstruction.

A.
Epidemiology and Etiology
600 New cases per year
Peak age 60 years
Risk factors
- Genetic disorders
- Abdominal or pelvic irradiation

B.
Presentation
Palpable mass in 45–75%
Abdominal pain in 40–60%
Neurologic dysfunction in 30% (paresthesias, dysesthesias, weakness)
Weight loss in < 15%
Early satiety in < 10%
Nausea, vomiting in < 10%
Testicular varicocele
Leg swelling

C.
Evaluation
History and physical examination
Laboratory tests including β-hCG, α-fetoprotein
Testicular ultrasonography

Helical CT is the investigational test of choice

D.
Treatment

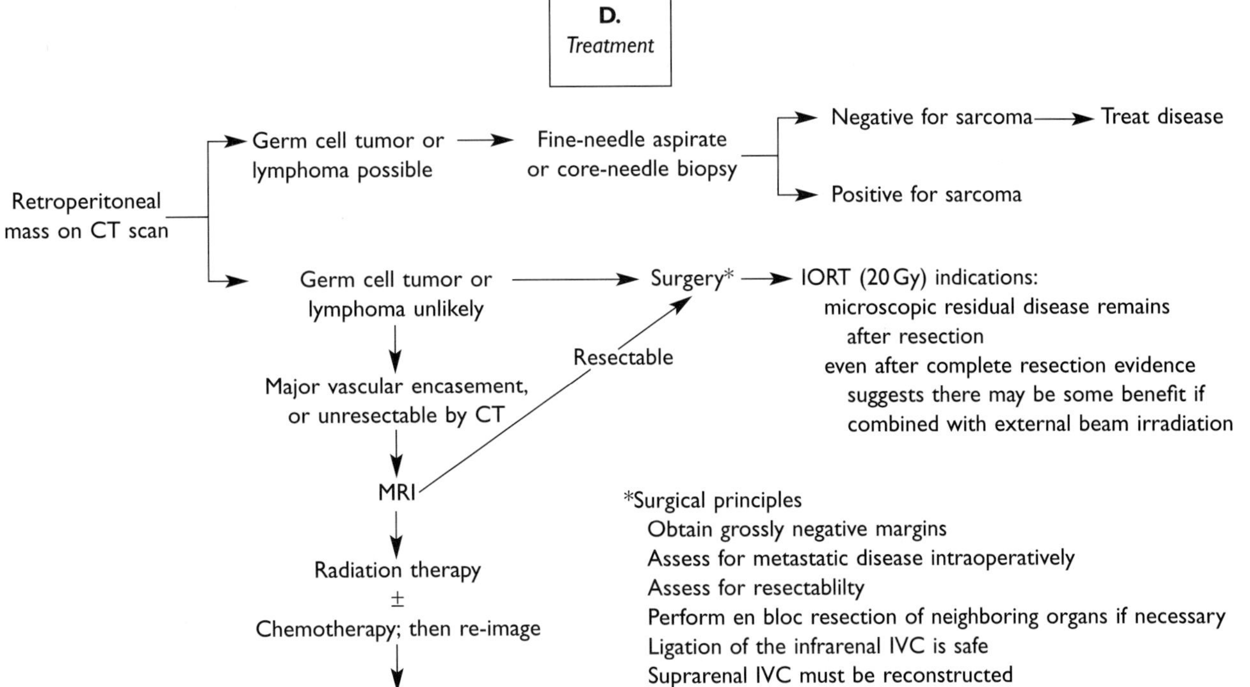

TABLE 42–1.
Histologic subtypes in 1111 patients with retroperitoneal sarcoma

Sarcoma subtype	No.	%
Liposarcoma	350	31.5
Leiomyosarcoma	315	28.4
Fibrosarcoma	114	10.3
Malignant fibrous histiocytoma	101	9.1
MPNT/neurogenic sarcoma	57	5.1
Hemangiopericytoma/angiosarcoma	25	2.3
Other	149	13.4

MPNT, malignant peripheral nerve tumor.
SOURCE: Data from references 5–11.

C. Evaluation

The differential diagnosis of a retroperitoneal mass is shown in Table 42–2. A thorough medical history and physical examination combined with high quality helical computed tomography (CT) scans of the abdomen and pelvis usually distinguish retroperitoneal sarcomas from the other lesions noted in Table 42–2. β-Human chorionic gonadotropin and α-fetoprotein levels and testicular ultrasonography may be helpful for determining the presence of a germ cell neoplasm. In some cases a hematologic workup for lymphoma is required.

If a significant likelihood exists that a retroperitoneal mass is lymphoma or a germ cell tumor after initial evaluation, preoperative tissue sampling of the mass is required. The optimal sampling technique is CT-guided fine-needle aspiration (FNA) or, if FNA is inadequate, a core-needle biopsy. An open incisional biopsy is reserved for the few cases in which FNA and core-needle biopsy are inconclusive. Tissue sampling is also required if consideration is given to preoperative adjuvant therapy. The histologic diagnosis is not required prior to surgery other than to rule out a germ cell neoplasm or lymphoma, or when neoadjuvant therapy is contemplated.

TABLE 42–2.
Differential diagnosis of a retroperitoneal mass

Benign mass
Lymphangioma
Lipoma/fibroma
Leiomyoma
Adrenal adenoma
Nephrogenic cyst
Retroperitoneal cyst
Pheochromocytoma
Hematoma
Malignant mass
Sarcoma
Germ cell neoplasm
Lymphoma
Extension of primary tumor
Renal
Adrenal
Colon
Pancreatic

High-quality helical CT of the abdomen and pelvis with enteric and intravenous administration of contrast medium remains the radiologic investigation of choice. The purpose of these scans is fourfold: (1) to establish the retroperitoneal origin of the tumor; (2) to assess the degree of necrosis; (3) to establish bilateral renal function (as up to 33% of patients may undergo nephrectomy); and (4) to evaluate the extent of disease. Magnetic resonance imaging (MRI) has the advantage of improved tumor delineation and reconstruction in sagittal, coronal, and transaxial planes. T1-weighted images show the relation of the tumor to other solid organs, such as the liver, kidneys, and pancreas; and T2-weighted images allow better differentiation between tumor and muscle or bone. Additionally, MRI delineates vascular involvement accurately and thus has largely eliminated the need for angiography in the preoperative workup of retroperitoneal sarcomas. Finally, MRI may show intratumoral changes following neoadjuvant therapy indicating tumor response.[13]

Despite these reported advantages, no study has shown an objective benefit to the routine use of MRI over CT for evaluating retroperitoneal sarcoma. Thus, owing to availability and cost, CT remains the diagnostic procedure of choice, with MRI reserved for cases in which major vascular involvement is suspected or resectability is questionable on CT scan.

The workup for metastatic disease should always include chest radiography; CT scans of the chest are performed when chest radiography is abnormal, the patient has a high-grade lesion, or a potentially disabling operation is needed to extirpate the primary tumor. There has been recent interest in using positron emission tomography (PET) to evaluate retroperitoneal sarcomas, particularly for locally recurrent and metastatic disease. Although preliminary studies are encouraging, the high cost and limited availability of the PET scanners restrict their use; thus at present PET must be considered investigational.[14,15]

The system currently used for *staging* retroperitoneal sarcomas, the same one used for staging extremity sarcomas, is the one proposed by the American Joint Committee on Cancer (AJCC).[16] Unfortunately, it is a suboptimal system, as most retroperitoneal tumors (>90%) are >5 cm in diameter and other well documented prognostic factors are not included in the AJCC system. Alternative staging approaches that employ known prognostic factors have been proposed.[4,17] The ability of a single staging system to predict prognosis equally well for both extremity and retroperitoneal sarcomas is questionable, implying that separate or modified staging systems may be required.

D. Treatment

Surgery

As with extremity sarcomas, the primary treatment of retroperitoneal sarcomas is surgical. There is no doubt that the best long-term outcomes are associated with margin-free resections. Thus the goal of any potentially curative operation is en bloc resection of the tumor with a rim of normal tissue.

Surgery for retroperitoneal sarcomas is accomplished through a midline incision; alternatively, a chevron-shaped incision is used for upper abdominal tumors. A thoracoabdominal incision is occasionally necessary for extensive tumors involving the left or right upper quadrant. Once the incision is made, an evaluation is done to detect the presence of sarcomatosis or evidence of hematogenous metastases, which appears most commonly in the liver. Next, tumor resectability is assessed. The most common reasons for aborting the operation are extensive mesenteric involvement, nerve root involvement, peritoneal sarcomatosis, and liver metastases. En bloc resection of the surrounding organ or organs is often required (53–83% of cases).[10,18–21] The kidneys and adrenal glands are the most commonly resected organs (46%), followed by the colon (24%), pancreas (15%), and spleen (10%).[18] Although retroperitoneal sarcomas rarely invade surrounding organs, the intense desmoplastic reaction surrounding these tumors makes assessment of the margins difficult; therefore the surgeon opts to resect neighboring structures rather than risk positive margins.[22] No study has documented that en bloc organ resection is an independent negative prognostic factor; however, the ability to resect a retroperitoneal sarcoma completely diminishes as the number of organs involved increases.

Inferior vena cava (IVC) involvement merits special mention. The infrarenal IVC can be resected and ligated with little morbidity. In the case of suprarenal IVC involvement, resection with primary repair or, if necessary, interposition grafting is performed.[23] Because fewer than 5% of patients with retroperitoneal sarcoma have lymphatic involvement, extensive lymphadenectomy is not indicated.

Two particular surgical situations deserve special attention: palliative resection and local recurrence. Palliative surgery, in which a gross margin of tumor remains, is associated with survival comparable to that of patients who undergo biopsy alone.[5,18] Carefully selected patients, particularly those with urinary obstruction, gastrointestinal obstruction, disabling pain, or those with low-grade lipomatous tumors may benefit from debulking surgery.[12]

There is no doubt that the presence of local recurrence portends a lower survival rate in certain patients. However, among 61 patients with recurrent retroperitoneal sarcoma who underwent resection at Memorial Sloan-Kettering Cancer Center, 35 (57%) underwent subsequent complete resection.[5] These patients had a significantly improved survival rate compared with patients who underwent incomplete resection (60% vs. 18% five-year disease-specific survival, $p < 0.01$). This suggests that there is a subset of patients with locally recurrent retroperitoneal sarcoma who have favorable biology and whose disease may be cured by re-resection.

Adjuvant Therapy

There is ample evidence that adjuvant *radiation therapy* reduces the likelihood of local recurrence of extremity sarcomas.[24–27] Evidence supporting the use of adjuvant radiation therapy for retroperitoneal sarcomas is less convincing. Some retrospective studies have suggested that there is benefit to using adjuvant external beam radiation therapy (EBRT) after gross complete resection,[28–30] whereas others have found no such benefit.[18,19] To date, there have been no randomized prospective trials comparing surgery alone with surgery plus EBRT (either preoperative or postoperative). Any potential benefit from adjuvant preoperative or postoperative EBRT must be balanced against the significant short- and long-term toxicity of EBRT.[31,32] Thus EBRT should be used as adjuvant therapy only in a clinical trial or in an attempt to convert an unresectable retroperitoneal sarcoma to a resectable tumor.

The results of combining postoperative EBRT with intraoperative radiation therapy (IORT) have been more encouraging. In the only randomized clinical trial of radiation therapy for retroperitoneal sarcoma, 35 patients received either IORT (20 Gy) plus low-dose postoperative EBRT (35–40 Gy) or high-dose postoperative EBRT (50–55 Gy) alone.[33] A portion of the patients in both arms of this study received adjuvant chemotherapy consisting of doxorubicin, cyclophosphamide, and methotrexate. All patients underwent a gross complete resection. Although this small study showed no significant difference in overall survival, local recurrence was significantly lower in the patients in the IORT arm (6/15 vs. 16/20, $p < 0.05$). In addition, there was a significantly lower incidence of radiation-induced enteritis in the patients who received IORT. Several nonrandomized studies have also suggested that there is a benefit from IORT, particularly for patients with microscopic residual disease.[12,34]

As with radiation therapy, much of the literature examining and advocating *chemotherapy* for sarcoma has focused on extremity tumors.[35,36] Although most of the randomized clinical trials of adjuvant chemotherapy for sarcoma (most of the patients with extremity tumors) have not shown a significant survival advantage, a meta-analysis of 15 such studies found

TABLE 42–3.
Resectability, local recurrence, and survival in patients presenting with nonmetastatic retroperitoneal sarcoma

Study	Year	No.	Resectability (%)	Local recurrence at 5 years (%)	5-year survival (%)
Lewis[5]	1998	397	74	41	54
Alvarenga[10]	1991	91	31	46	29
Singer[9]	1995	83	NR	NR	58

NR, not reported.

significantly improved disease-free 10-year survival rates for patients receiving adjuvant chemotherapy.[37] Unfortunately, many of these studies did not use the currently accepted combination of doxorubicin- and ifosfamide-based regimens.

Several retrospective studies of postoperative adjuvant chemotherapy for retroperitoneal sarcomas have shown no benefit;[38,39] in fact, in one study a significantly poorer survival rate was noted in the patients who received chemotherapy.[9] Furthermore, in a small prospective randomized clinical trial conducted by the U.S. National Cancer Institute, 15 patients were randomized to undergo resection with or without adjuvant chemotherapy. A trend toward a *lower* 2-year survival rate was seen in the chemotherapy arm (47% vs. 100%, $p = 0.06$).[32]

Neoadjuvant chemotherapy with doxorubicin and ifosfamide-based regimens is presently being investigated.[1] Neoadjuvant treatment offers the advantage of providing information regarding tumor response both radiographically and histologically and thus may aid in identifying patients with the greatest likelihood of benefiting from *postoperative* chemotherapy. However, the significance of the response to neoadjuvant therapy in terms of survival remains unclear.

In summary, no randomized clinical trials of reasonable size have examined the role of adjuvant or neoadjuvant chemotherapy for retroperitoneal sarcomas. Further clinical trials, preferably multicenter phase III studies, are required to define that role.

Outcomes

Outcomes from several large series of patients with primary retroperitoneal sarcomas are summarized in Table 42–3. The largest of these studies, which is also the largest single-institution series, was reported by Lewis et al.[5] from Memorial Sloan-Kettering Cancer Center.

In this study of 500 patients, the median survival was 72 months for patients who presented with primary disease, 28 months for those who presented with locally recurrent disease, and 10 months for those with metastases. Multivariate analysis for disease-specific survival showed that unresectable disease [relative risk (RR) = 4.7, $p = 0.001$], incomplete resection (RR = 4.0, $p = 0.001$), and high-grade histology (RR = 3.2, $p = 0.001$) were independent prognostic factors for disease-specific death. Moreover, there was no significant survival difference between patients with unresectable disease and those who underwent a grossly incomplete resection. It was only in an analysis of a subgroup of 231 patients with primary retroperitoneal sarcoma that tumor size >10 cm (RR = 2.0, $p = 0.04$) and microscopically positive margins (RR = 1.9, $p = 0.03$) predicted disease-specific death by multivariate analysis.

The importance of a grossly negative margin is unarguable. However, the importance of a microscopically negative margin is somewhat more confusing. First, a *true* microscopically negative margin is almost impossible to ascertain given the size of most retroperitoneal sarcomas and the consequent extensive margin sampling that would be involved. Furthermore, a microscopically positive but grossly negative surgical margin has an associated survival rate of approximately 50%, which is clearly better than that in patients with gross disease remaining after surgery.[9] Thus, we suspect that the microscopic margin status may be more a surrogate marker of tumor biology than a simple mechanical marker of the extent of tumor resection.

Conclusions

Retroperitoneal sarcomas comprise a rare, heterogeneous group of neoplasms. Routine workup should include the medical history, a physical examination, and helical CT of the abdomen and pelvis with selective use of MRI and preoperative tissue sampling. The primary treatment is complete surgical resection with a rim of normal tissue. The role of adjuvant therapy is evolving and at present should not be used outside the investigational setting.

References

1. Clark JA, Tepper JE. Role of radiation therapy in retroperitoneal sarcomas. Oncology 1996;10:1867–1872.

2. Boring CC, Squires TS, Tong T, Montgomery S. Cancer statistics, 1994. CA Cancer J Clin 1994;44:7–26.
3. James T, Adams M. Abdominal wall, omentum, mesentery and retroperitoneum. In: Schwartz SI (ed) Principles of Surgery. New York: McGraw-Hill, 1994;1511–1516.
4. Conlon KC, Brennan MF. Soft tissue sarcoma. In: Murphy, Lawrence, Lenhard (eds) Clinical Oncology. Atlanta: American Cancer Society, 1996; 436–450.
5. Lewis JJ, Leung D, Woodruff JM, Brennan MF. Retroperitoneal sarcoma: analysis of 500 patients treated and followed at a single institution. Ann Surg 1998;228:355–365.
6. Cody HS, Turnbull AD, Fortner JG, Hajdu SI. The continuing challenge of retroperitoneal sarcomas. Cancer 1981;47:2148–2152.
7. Storm FK, Eilber FR, Mira J, Morton DL. Retroperitoneal sarcoma: a reappraisal of treatment. J Surg Oncol 1981;17:1–17.
8. Kilkenny JW, Bland KI, Copeland EM. Retroperitoneal sarcoma: the University of Florida experience. J Am Coll Surg 1996;182:329–339.
9. Singer S, Corson J, Demetri GD, et al. Prognostic factors predictive of survival for truncal and retroperitoneal soft tissue sarcoma. Ann Surg 1995;221:185–195.
10. Alvarenga JC, Ball ABS, Fisher C, et al. Limitations of surgery in the treatment of retroperitoneal sarcoma. Br J Surg 1991;78:912–916.
11. Karakousis CD, Gerstenbluth R, Kontzoglou K, Driscoll D. Retroperitoneal sarcomas and their management. Arch Surg 1995;130:1105–1109.
12. Brennan MF, Casper EF, Harrison LB. Soft tissue sarcoma. In: Devita VT, Hellman S, Rosenberg RA (eds) Cancer: Principles and Practice of Oncology. Philadelphia: Lippincott-Raven, 1997;1769–1788.
13. Varma DG, Jackson EF, Pollock RE, Benjamin RS. Soft tissue sarcoma of the extremities: MR appearance of post treatment changes and local recurrences. Magn Reson Imaging Clin N Am 1995;3:695–712.
14. Kole AC, Nieweg OE, Van Ginkel RJ, et al. Detection of local recurrence of soft tissue sarcoma with positron emission tomography using [^{10}F]fluorodeoxyglucose. Ann Surg Oncol 1997;4:57–63.
15. Miraldi F, Adler LP, Faulhaber P. PET imaging in soft tissue sarcomas. Cancer Treat Res 1997;91:51–64.
16. Beahrs OH, Henson DE, Hutter RVP, Kennedy BJ (eds) American Joint Committee on Cancer Manual for Staging of Cancer, 5th ed. Philadelphia: Lippincott, 1997;149–156.
17. Gaynor JJ, Tan CC, Casper ES, et al. Refinement of clinicopathologic staging for localized soft tissue sarcoma of the extremity: a study of 423 adults. J Clin Oncol 1992;10:1317–1329.
18. Jaques DP, Coit DG, Hajdu SI, Brennan AF. Management of primary and recurrent soft tissue sarcoma of the retroperitoneum. Ann Surg 1990; 212:51–59.
19. McGrath PC, Neifeld JP, Lawrence W Jr, et al. Improved survival following complete excision of retroperitoneal sarcomas. Ann Surg 1984;200: 200–204.
20. Dalton RR, Donohue JH, Mucha P Jr, et al. Management of retroperitoneal sarcomas. Surgery 1989;106:725–733.
21. Senio G, Tenchini P, Nifosi F, Jacono C. Surgical strategy for primary retroperitoneal tumors. Br J Surg 1989;76:385–389.
22. Russo P, Kim Y, Ravindram S, et al. Nephrectomy during operative management of retroperitoneal sarcoma. Ann Surg Oncol 1997;4:421–424.
23. Mingoli A, Sapienza P, Cavallaro A, et al. The effect of extent of caval resection in the treatment of inferior vena cava leiomyosarcoma. Anticancer Res 1997;17:3877–3881.
24. Barkley HT Jr, Martin RG, Romsdahl MM, et al. Treatment of soft tissue sarcoma by preoperative irradiation and conservative surgical resection. Int J Radiat Oncol Biol Phys 1988;14:693–700.
25. Brant TA, Parsons JT, Marcus RB Jr, et al. Preoperative irradiation for soft tissue sarcomas of the trunk and extremities in adults. Int J Radiat Oncol Biol Phys 1990;19:899–906.
26. Suit HD, Mankin HJ, Schiller AL. Results of treatment of sarcoma of soft tissue radiation and surgery at Massachusetts General Hospital. Cancer Treat Symp 1985;3:33–36.
27. Suit HD, Mankin HJ, Wood W, et al. Preoperative, intraoperative, and postoperative radiation in the treatment of primary soft tissue sarcoma. Cancer 1985;55:2659–2669.
28. Bose B. Primary malignant retroperitoneal tumors: analysis of 30 cases. Can J Surg 1979;22:215–221.
29. Harrison LB, Gutierrez E, Fisher JJ. Retroperitoneal sarcoma: the Yale experience and a review of the literature. J Surg Oncol 1986;32:159–165.
30. Cody HS, Turnbull AD, Fortner JG, et al. The continuing challenge of retroperitoneal sarcomas. Cancer 1981;47:2147–2154.
31. Sondak VK, Robertson JM, Sussman JJ, et al. Preoperative idoxuridine and radiation for large soft tissue sarcomas: clinical results with five year follow up. Ann Surg Oncol 1998;5:106–112.
32. Glenn J, Sindelar WF, Kinsella T. Results of multimodality therapy of resectable soft tissue sarcomas of the retroperitoneum. Surgery 1985;97: 316–325.
33. Sindelar WF, Kinsella TJ, Chen PW, et al. Intraoperative electron beam radiotherapy in retroperitoneal sarcomas: results of a prospective randomized clinical trial. Arch Surg 1993;128:402–407.
34. Willet CG, Suit HD, Tepper JE, et al. Intraoperative electron beam radiation therapy for retroperitoneal soft tissue sarcoma. Cancer 1991; 68:278–284.
35. Bui NB, Maree D, Coindree JM, et al. First results of a prospective randomized study of CYVADIC adjuvant chemotherapy in adults with operable high risk soft tissue sarcoma. Proc Am Soc Clin Oncol 1989;8: 318.
36. Picci P, Bacci G, Gherlizoni F, et al. Results of randomized trial for the treatment of localized soft tissue tumors of the extremities in adult patients. In: Ryan JR, Baher LO (eds) Recent Concepts in Sarcoma Treatment. Amsterdom: Kluwer, 1988;144–148.
37. Sarcoma Meta-Analysis Collaboration. Adjuvant chemotherapy for localized resectable soft-tissue sarcoma of adults: meta-analysis of individual data. Lancet 1997;350:1647–1654.
38. Karakousis CP, Velez AF, Gerstenbluth R, et al. Resectability and survival in retroperitoneal sarcomas. Ann Surg Oncol 1996;3:150–158.
39. Trojani M, Contesso G, Coindre JM, et al. Soft-tissue sarcomas of adults; study of pathological prognostic variables and definition of histopathological grading system. Int J Cancer 1984;33:37–42.

CHAPTER 43

Extremity Soft Tissue Sarcomas

DANIEL M. LABOW
MURRAY F. BRENNAN

Soft tissue sarcoma is a rare malignancy affecting 5000–6000 people per year in the United States. It represents 1% of adult (age >16 years) malignancies and 15% of pediatric cancers. This malignancy can occur in any part of the body, though approximately 50% of all soft-tissue sarcomas present in an extremity (Fig. 43–1). Although some progress in the treatment of soft tissue sarcoma has been made, overall survival by stage has remained relatively constant for this disease since the early 1980s. The heterogeneous histologic and biologic nature of soft tissue sarcoma, combined with its rarity, has made it difficult for any single institution to acquire cases for protocols designed to improve treatment and survival. As a result, there is some variation in the treatment of soft tissue sarcoma from one institution to another. This chapter provides a background of the disease and focuses on an algorithmic approach to the management of extremity soft tissue sarcoma in the adult population.

A. History and Physical Examination

Unfortunately, there is often a significant delay in the diagnosis of extremity soft tissue sarcoma. Clear physical signs such as pain, skin color, or texture changes are rarely present in this disease, making early diagnosis difficult. Sarcoma can present in both upper and lower extremities, though there is a predominance for the latter. In general, any mass that is >5 cm or has undergone rapid growth or change in appearance should be investigated definitively.[1] A typical lesion presents as a painless mass on the anterior thigh, though 33% of patients complain of pain at the time of diagnosis.[2] Once the mass is identified, a careful examination is needed to estimate how deeply the lesion penetrates, how many muscle groups and compartments are involved, and if there is neurovascular involvement. In general, there are no other physical findings that make one suspect sarcoma. Inguinal or axillary lymph nodes may be palpable, though this is rarely due to metastasis because lymphatic spread is uncommon. Texture is important; whereas lipomas are usually soft and well demarcated, a firm mass or a mass of irregular margins should increase the suspicion for sarcoma. The differential diagnosis includes lipoma, posttraumatic hematoma, myositis ossificans, or other benign tumors of the extremity such as schwannoma or fibroma.

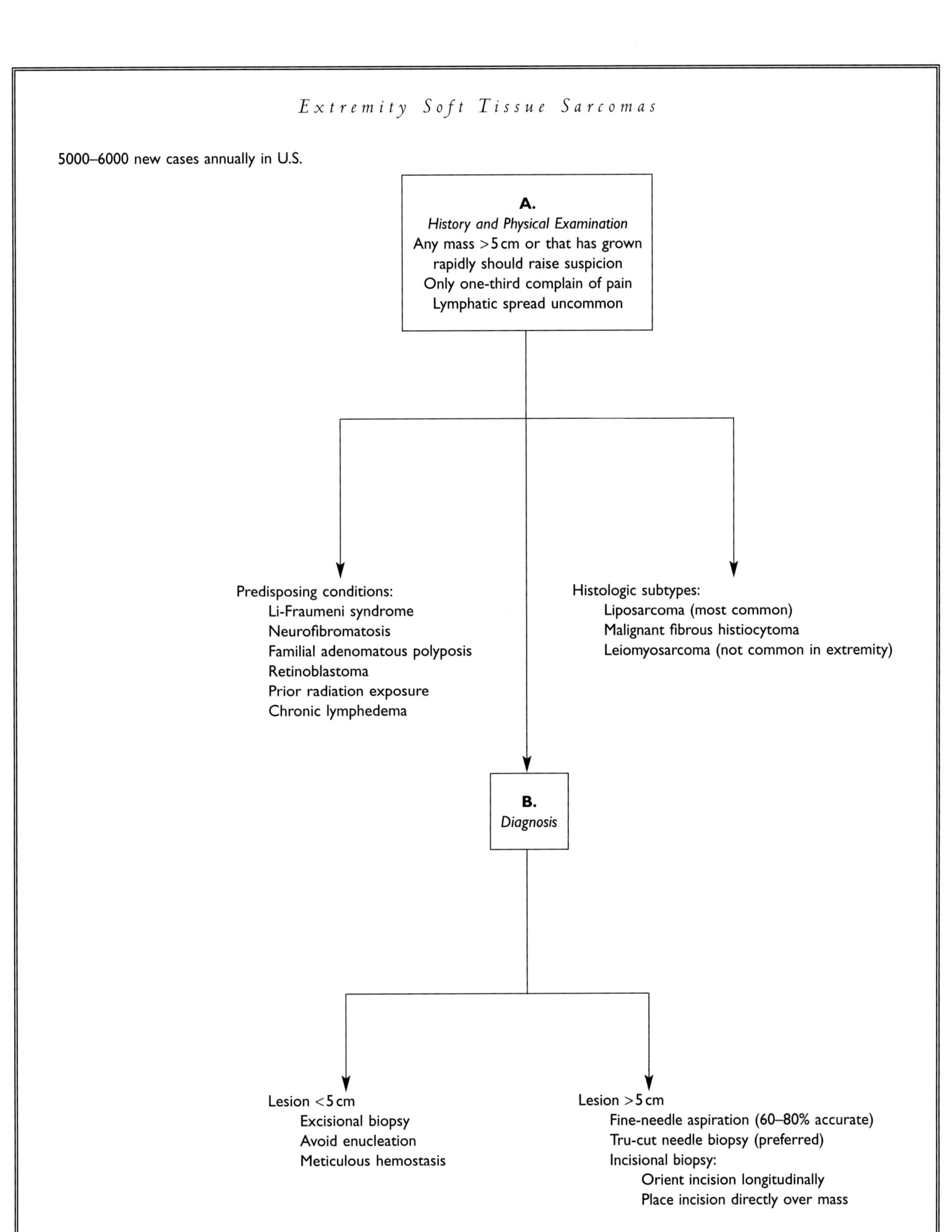

(continued on next page)

Extremity Soft Tissue Sarcomas (continued)

C.
Extent of Disease
Work-up needed

D.
Treatment

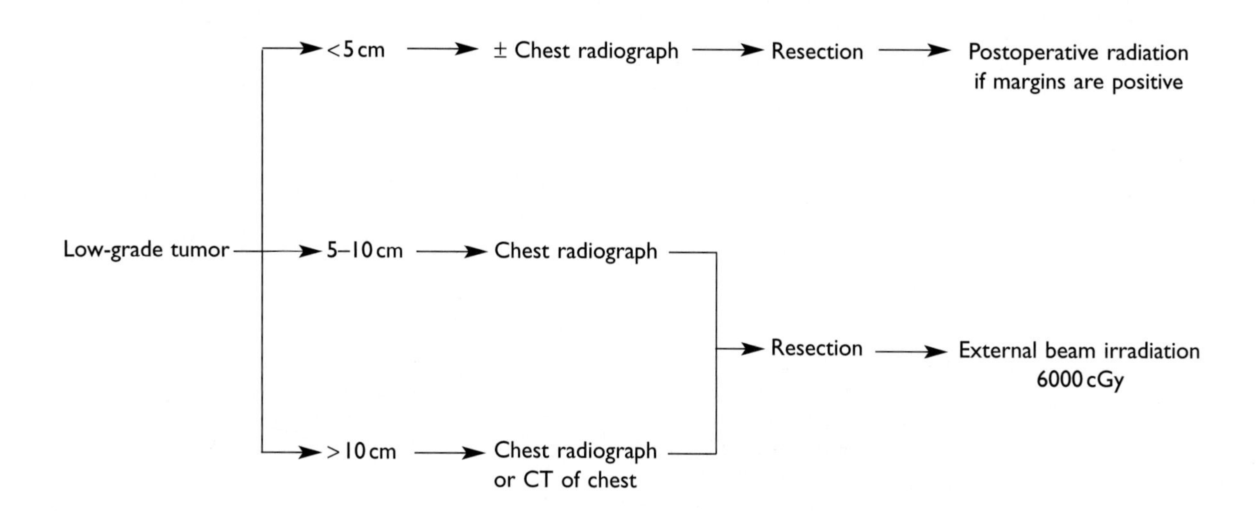

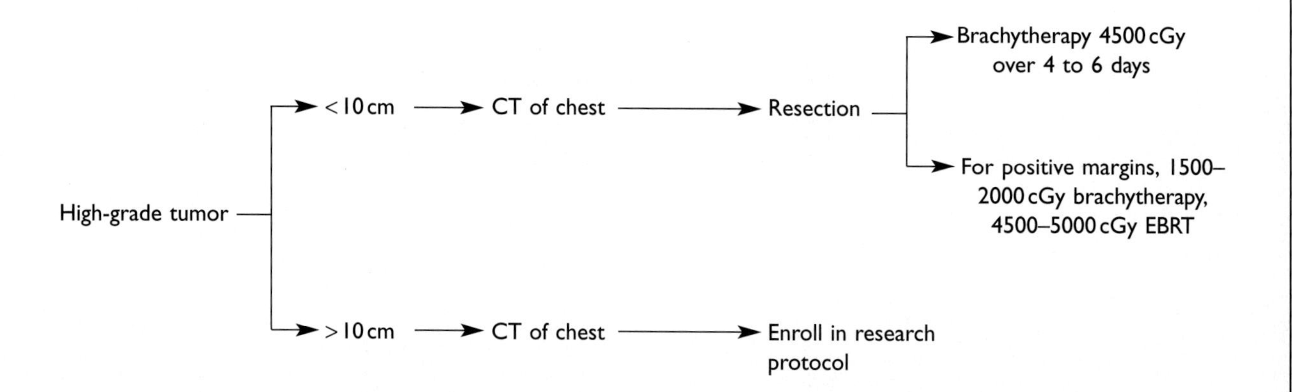

Goals of treatment for resectable disease:
- Complete removal with negative margins
- Maximal preservation of function
- Remove prior biopsy scar en bloc
- Postoperative irradiation reduces recurrence

Unresectable lesions or tumors: associated with widely disseminated disease: treat with primary irradiation 6500 cGy

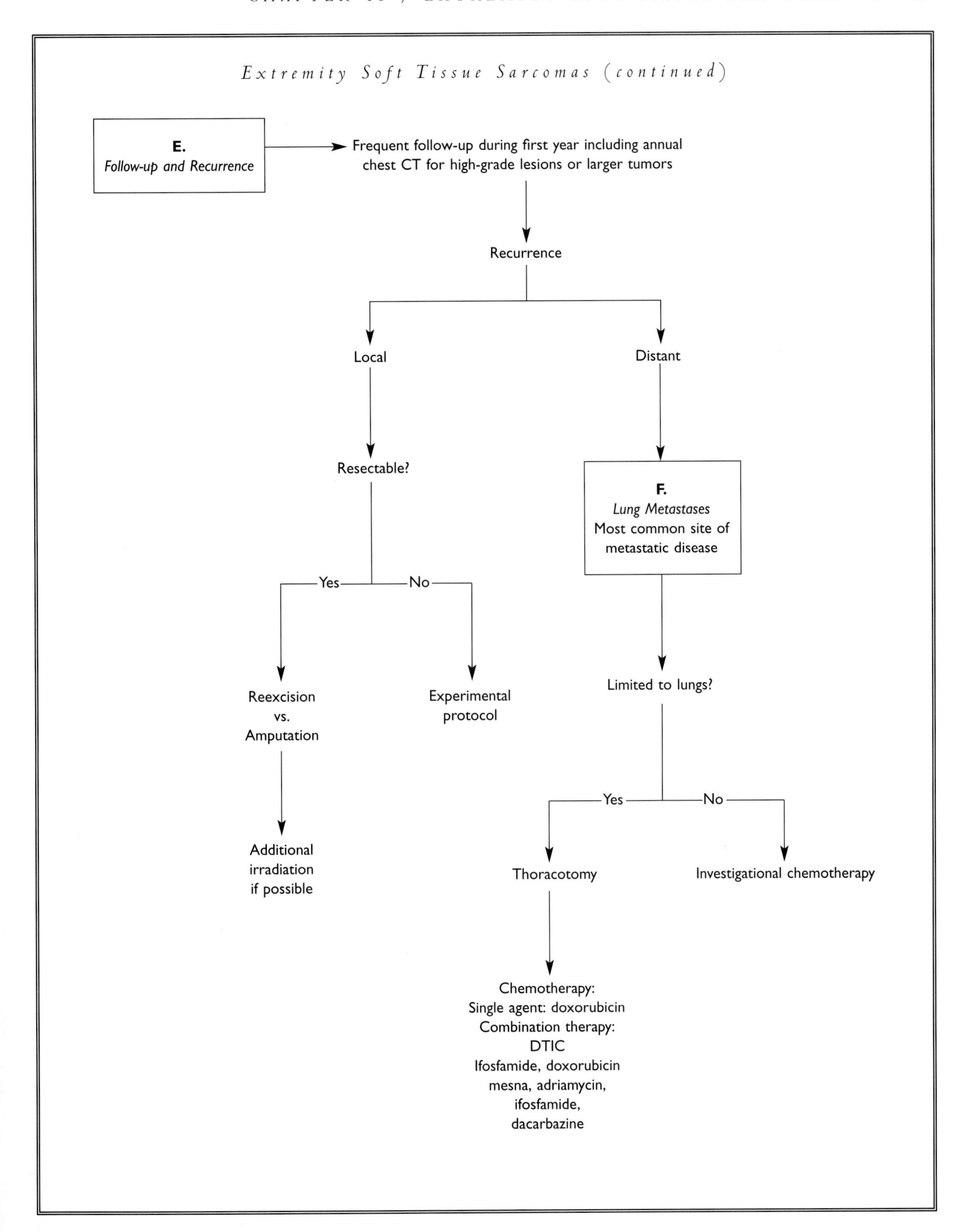
Extremity Soft Tissue Sarcomas (continued)
E.
Follow-up and Recurrence
Frequent follow-up during first year including annual chest CT for high-grade lesions or larger tumors
Recurrence
Local
Distant
Resectable?
F.
Lung Metastases
Most common site of metastatic disease
Yes
No
Reexcision vs. Amputation
Experimental protocol
Limited to lungs?
Additional irradiation if possible
Yes
No
Thoracotomy
Investigational chemotherapy
Chemotherapy:
Single agent: doxorubicin
Combination therapy:
DTIC
Ifosfamide, doxorubicin
mesna, adriamycin,
ifosfamide,
dacarbazine

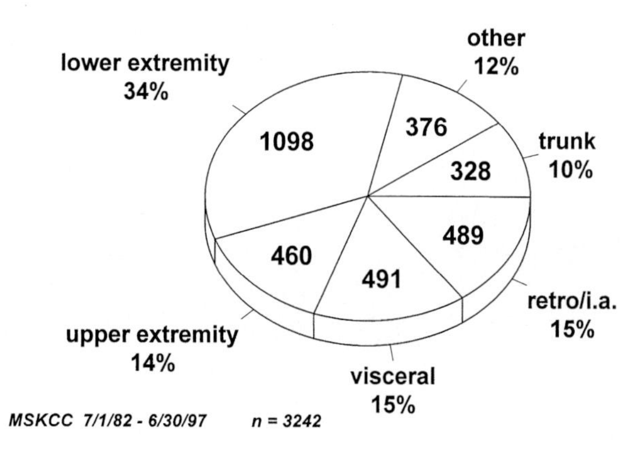

FIGURE 43–1
Distribution of soft tissue sarcomas by site at Memorial Sloan-Kettering Cancer Center (MSKCC).

In addition to a thorough physical examination, a careful history should be obtained to evaluate the patient for both familial and environmental risk factors. It should be understood, though, that an etiologic factor is rarely identified. Some have suggested that trauma or chronic inflammation in an extremity is associated with the development of sarcoma,[3] but this has not been proven. It is more likely that trauma to the extremity merely draws attention to the site of a preexisting lesion. The Li-Fraumeni syndrome, a familial germline mutation in the *p53* gene, has been linked to the development of soft tissue sarcoma and other malignancies.[4–7] Other familial risk factors associated with this disease are neurofibromatosis, familial adenomatous polyposis syndrome, and retinoblastoma. A history of radiation exposure (ortho- or megavoltage) for treatment of a prior malignancy, especially irradiation for lymphomas, increases the risk of developing extremity soft tissue sarcoma.[8,9] Finally, patients with chronic lymphedema (secondary to surgery, irradiation, or parasitic infection) are also at risk for developing this disease. First described by Stewart and Treves,[10] a typical patient is one who has undergone treatment for breast cancer with a modified radical mastectomy and usually irradiation, developed postoperative chronic lymphedema, and presents 10–20 years later with lymphangiosarcoma of the extremity.

B. Diagnosis

Once a thorough history is obtained, a physical examination is performed, and a suspicious mass is identified, a definitive diagnosis should be made expeditiously. A trial performed at Memorial Sloan-Kettering Cancer Center (MSKCC) examined the Tru-Cut biopsy as a method for diagnosing soft tissue sarcoma in 60 patients.[11] This study found a 95% accuracy rate for diagnosis. Thus for suitable lesions and with an experienced pathologist, it is an effective method for obtaining a definitive diagnosis. Fine-needle aspiration (FNA) has been shown to be accurate only 60–80% of the time[12,13] and thus is not a valid diagnostic method.

If the lesion under investigation is small (<5 cm), an excisional biopsy should be performed, serving as both a diagnostic and therapeutic procedure. If the lesion is large, a Tru-Cut (or if nondiagnostic, an incisional) biopsy is the procedure of choice. For lesions of any size, the biopsy should be performed with the definitive resection in mind.[14] Simple enucleation of a small lesion is inadequate, as it likely compromises the margins.[15] If this procedure is done and the diagnosis of soft tissue sarcoma is established, reexcision with adequate margins is essential. For incisional biopsies, the incision should be oriented longitudinally over the lesion at its most superficial location. This establishes a diagnosis with the least invasive approach. Meticulous hemostasis is vital, as any tracking of blood along tissue planes can lead to dissemination of malignant cells, necessitating a more extensive and potentially morbid resection.[14]

Once an adequate tissue specimen is obtained and the diagnosis of sarcoma is established, the histologic origin of the lesion should be identified. This can be difficult, particularly in poorly differentiated tumors, and one cannot overstate the importance of an experienced, reliable pathologist. Electron microscopy and immunohistochemistry are often employed to help establish the histogenesis of the tumor. Special immunohistochemical staining for proteins such as vimentin, S-100, desmin, factor VIII, keratin, myoglobin, and actin help establish the histopathology.[16] Genetic translocation has been identified as a diagnostic tool for patients with synovial sarcoma and other lesions.[17,18] It should be recognized that these stains become less reliable as the degree of differentiation decreases.

Overall, the three most common subtypes of soft tissue sarcoma are liposarcoma, malignant fibrous histiocytoma (MFH), and leiomyosarcoma. Among extremity soft tissue sarcomas, liposarcoma and MFH predominate. The histologic grade is determined by mitotic index, cellularity, presence of necrosis, and degree of nuclear anaplasia.[19] Each of these elements helps determine the biologic behavior of the tumor and contributes to the staging and prognosis of soft tissue sarcoma.

C. Extent of Disease

Once a tissue diagnosis of soft tissue sarcoma is established and the histology and grade of the tumor are determined, the extent of disease must be defined to plan the subsequent course of treatment. In general, for lesions >5 cm, a computed tomography[2] (CT) scan or magnetic resonance image[20] (MRI) of the involved extremity is adequate. Though more expensive than CT, MRI is preferred as it provides better resolution of each muscle group, the level of extension of the tumor, and excellent definition of neural and vascular elements. Some recent studies have

TABLE 43–1.
AJCC definition of stage grouping for soft tissue sarcoma

Stage I				
A (Low grade, small, superficial and deep)	G1-2,	T1a-1b,	N0,	M0
B (Low grade, large, superficial)	G1-2,	T2a,	N0,	M0
Stage II				
A (Low grade, large, deep)	G1-2,	T2b,	N0,	M0
B (High grade, small, superficial, deep)	G3-4,	T1a-1b,	N0,	M0
C (High grade, large, superficial)	G3-4,	T2a,	N0,	M0
Stage III				
(High grade, large, deep)	G3-4,	T2b,	N0,	M0
Stage IV				
(any metastasis)	any G,	any T,	N1,	M0
	any G,	any T,	N0,	M0

SOURCE: Used with the permission of the American Joint Committee on Cancer (AJCC®), Chicago, IL. The original source for this material is the AJCC® Cancer Staging Manual, 5th edition (1997) published by Lippincott Williams & Wilkins Publishers, Philadelphia, PA.

evaluated positron emission tomography (PET) scanning,[21,22] ^{31}P-magnetic resonance spectroscopy,[23] and gallium nuclide scintigraphy[24,25] for determining the metabolic activity of the tumor and its response to therapy or for localizing the tumor. These techniques remain experimental in the diagnosis and treatment of soft tissue sarcoma.

The current staging system (Table 43–1) incorporates the histologic grade of the tumor, the size of the primary tumor, and the presence or absence of metastases. The grade of a tumor should be thought of as one point along a continuum and not an absolute value. Numerous grading systems are available, which have confused therapeutic planning somewhat. At MSKCC we believe that categorizing grades I and II as low grade and grades III and IV as high grade has simplified our treatment plan, making it more practical and feasible for both patient and physician. In general, low-grade lesions have a small risk for metastases (<15%), whereas high-grade tumors have a higher rate of metastases (>50%). The fact that large tumors have greater risk of long-term recurrence has raised the issue of addressing size as an important, independent factor with regard to staging soft tissue sarcomas.[26] This notion is also supported by the fact that small (<5 cm) high-grade lesions are often cured by surgery alone with a small risk of developing metastatic disease. These observations led to reevaluation of the American Joint Committee on Cancer (AJCC) staging system, which is reflected in the most current system where size and grade together determine the stage of a patient.[27]

The search for the presence of any local or distant metastases completes the extent of disease evaluation and staging process. The lungs are the sole first site of metastases in 78% of patients[28] with extremity soft tissue sarcoma. Lymph node metastases occur in fewer than 3% of patients,[29] so extensive evaluation of the lesion's draining lymphatic basins is not essential. These facts guide the remainder of the preoperative workup. For small low-grade tumors, the risk of metastases to the lung is low. Therefore preoperative chest radiography is the only other potential study needed to complete the preoperative workup for these patients, though it is optional. A chest radiograph is needed for intermediate-size lesions (5–10 cm), and chest CT scans are mandatory for low-grade large tumors (>10 cm) to rule out synchronous pulmonary metastases.

The possibility of pulmonary metastases significantly increases with high-grade tumors, so more extensive examination of the lungs is indicated. As with low-grade lesions, a logical progression follows from small to large tumors, with chest radiography being adequate for high-grade tumors <5 cm in size, whereas a chest CT scan is needed for tumors 5–10 cm and is routinely utilized for tumors >10 cm.

Once a tissue diagnosis is made and the preoperative workup is complete, a clinical stage for each patient is determined. A cohesive treatment plan can then be formulated.

D. *Treatment*

Surgery remains the mainstay of treatment for an extremity soft tissue sarcoma. In the past, primary amputation was the most common surgical procedure, leading to significant morbidity. A prospective, randomized study comparing limb-sparing surgery plus irradiation to primary amputation for primary, localized extremity soft tissue sarcoma was performed at the U.S. National Cancer Institute (NCI).[30] This study showed no difference in the local recurrence rate or overall survival for these two modes of therapy. This led to transition from amputation to limb-sparing surgery with irradiation for more than 90% of patients with an extremity soft tissue sarcoma.[31] Amputation is generally reserved for tumors not resectable by other means yet have not metastasized to distant sites. Usually such lesions are large, low-grade tumors that have caused significant functional and cosmetic deformity.

The surgical principles that guide conservative resection are removal of the entire tumor with negative margins and maximal preservation of function. In general, a 2- to 3-cm margin is needed to encompass local, microscopic spread not evident at the time of resection (Fig. 43–2). If the patient has had a previous incisional biopsy, the scar should be removed en bloc with the remainder of the tumor. There are no data showing improved long-term survival or local recurrence when resection of an entire muscle group or compartment is performed compared with local, nonanatomic resection with adequate margins.

Radiation therapy is used as both primary and adjuvant therapy in the treatment of soft tissue sarcoma. Primary external therapy with high-dose radiation (>6500 cGy) has local control rates of 30–60%[32,33] and is usually reserved for unresectable or

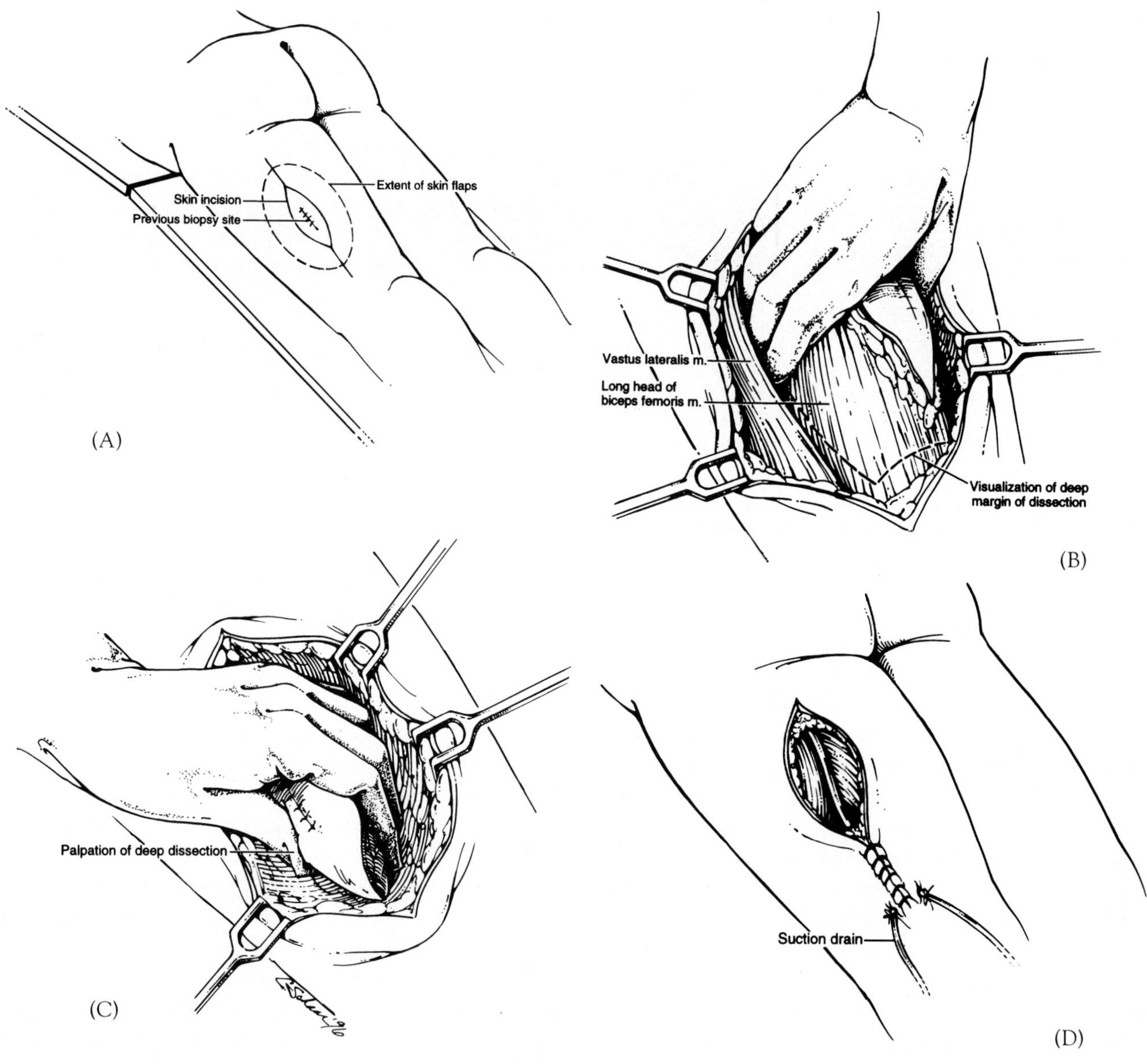

FIGURE 43–2
Surgical resection of a soft tissue sarcoma (here in the posterior thigh). The surgical objective is complete removal of the tumor with negative margins and maximal preservation of function. The incision (A) should be centered over the tumor and include complete removal of the previous biopsy site. Skin flaps are developed around the tumor to enable palpation of the deeper tissues surrounding the tumor. The surrounding muscle and connective tissue (B) are visualized, and resection is performed nonanatomically around the tumor guided by palpation (C). This is achieved by maintaining a visual three-dimensional image and preserving a 2- to 3-cm margin of normal tissue around the tumor as well as any vital neurovascular structures. Suction drains are always placed before closure, (D), taking care to place the exit site close to the wound. This approach facilitates easier re-resection in the event of subsequent local recurrence. (From ref. 14, with permission)

locally recurrent tumors associated with metastatic disease. It may also be considered for patients who are unfit for surgery. As an adjuvant treatment, radiation therapy in the form of external beam irradiation (EBRT) or brachytherapy has effectively reduced local recurrence following surgery.[34,35] The technical aspects of EBRT have been debated. Although some consider it essential to include surgical scars and drain sites in the radiation field, others are less compelled to do so. Nearly all agree that irradiation of the entire circumference of the extremity should be avoided, as it can lead to severe edema. At least one-third of the circumference should be spared. In contrast to external beam radiation, brachytherapy treats only the tumor bed with a 1- to 2-cm margin. Administered through after-loading catheters placed at the time of resection, treatment lasts only 4–6 days; patients therefore leave the hospital having completed all sarcoma-directed therapy and are more likely to return to full

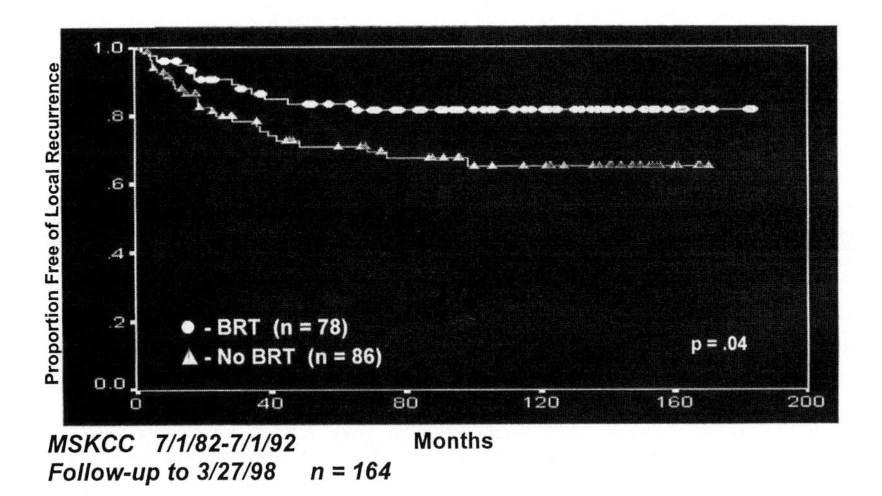

FIGURE 43–3
Soft tissue sarcoma of the extremity/trunk. Local recurrence-free survival for brachytherapy (BRT) versus no BRT at MSKCC.

activity sooner. The brachytherapy catheters are placed at 1 cm intervals, the wound is closed over the catheters with a drain in place, and the radioactive isotope is loaded on the 6th day.

When radiation is given preoperatively, the theoretic advantages include reducing tumor size to permit a more conservative surgical resection and reducing local recurrence rates. In these instances, local recurrence rates are 5–17%[34–38] and are thus comparable to recurrence rates after utilizing postoperative irradiation. The major disadvantage is the detrimental effect radiation has on wound healing.[34] It is not clear if preoperative irradiation is better than postoperative treatment, and it is unlikely that a randomized prospective study will be performed to answer this question.

More commonly, radiation therapy is administered perioperatively as brachytherapy (4500 cGy) or postoperatively as EBRT (6000 cGy). Studies of EBRT after surgical resection have reported local recurrence rates of 8–20%,[39–42] which is an improvement over recurrence rates seen without irradiation. Brachytherapy has been investigated as a possible adjuvant therapy for soft tissue sarcoma. A prospective, randomized study comparing patients treated with resection and adjuvant brachytherapy versus patients without further therapy was performed at MSKCC.[43,44] This study found a local recurrence rate of 18% for the brachytherapy arm versus 33% for the group receiving no further treatment (Fig. 43–3). The decrease in high-grade tumor recurrence was responsible for this difference after further analysis of the data. At the 5-year follow-up there was no significant difference in the incidence of distant metastasis or disease-specific survival[35,44] (Fig. 43–4).

In general, adjuvant chemotherapy has not proven to be effective in the neoadjuvant or adjuvant setting. Some studies suggest an improvement in disease-free and overall survival[45,46]

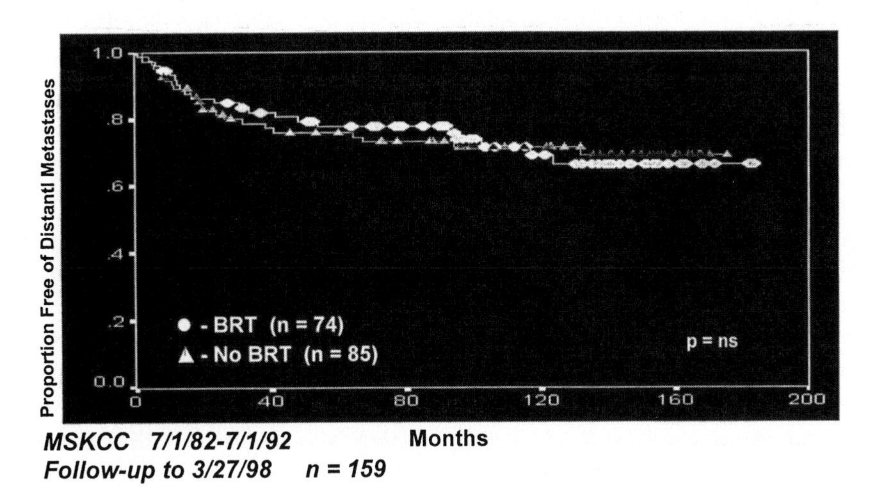

FIGURE 43–4
Soft tissue sarcoma of the extremity/trunk (excluding desmoids). Distant metastases-free survival for BRT vs. no BRT at MSKCC.

when chemotherapy is administered before definitive surgery and radiation therapy. A number of randomized, prospective trials studying adjuvant postoperative chemotherapy have shown no significant improvement.[47–49] Additionally, a trial comparing intraarterial chemotherapy versus intravenous chemotherapy showed no significant improvement in the treatment of this disease.[50] A meta-analysis examining localized, resectable soft tissue sarcoma using individual patient data from multiple trials did find some improvement in the survival in patients treated with adjuvant chemotherapy,[51] though the benefit was less than 5%. Although there may be some benefit for adjuvant chemotherapy for high-grade lesions, no clear standard has emerged from the studies done so far. The rarity of this disease makes it difficult to study the benefit of chemotherapy effectively. A large, multiinstitutional study may be the only way to enroll enough patients to answer this question definitively. Therefore based on all of the above data, we believe that any patient who receives chemotherapy for extremity soft tissue sarcoma should be enrolled in an experimental protocol until a clearer understanding of chemotherapy's role in the treatment regimen of this disease emerges.

Based on the role of each treatment modality described above, a logical approach to the treatment of this disease is as follows. For *low-grade tumors* >5 cm or between 5 and 10 cm, surgical resection is the primary treatment and usually suffices as adequate therapy, although postoperative EBRT can be considered for intermediate-size tumors. For low-grade tumors >10 cm, preoperative radiation therapy can reduce the size of the lesion, facilitate a less morbid surgical resection, and reduce the incidence of local recurrence; therefore it should be considered for large, low-grade lesions. In most centers, however, radiation is given postoperatively as EBRT to patients with low-grade tumors >10 cm or with positive margins after surgical resection regardless of tumor size.

Not surprisingly, there is greater variability in the treatment of *high-grade tumors*. As discussed earlier, surgery remains the first line of therapy for tumors <10 cm. Adjuvant treatment with EBRT or brachytherapy is important for these high-grade tumors and should be given to each patient. Most centers use brachytherapy perioperatively following complete excision of high-grade lesions, achieving local control rates in excess of 90%. If the margins of resection are positive, local control is compromised; treatment for these patients includes both brachytherapy and EBRT. The combination can improve local control to 90%. For tumors >10 cm, the prognosis is poor and experimental protocols are needed to help determine optimum treatment and to maximize control and survival rates. In these cases, neoadjuvant chemotherapy, EBRT, or both should be considered when devising the treatment regimen. Again, it is our belief that patients in this category should be enrolled in an investigational study because no clear optimal treatment exists at this time.

E. Follow-up and Recurrence

Soft tissue sarcoma of the extremity recurs in approximately one-third of all patients, including those with high- and low-grade tumors of all sizes, with a median disease-free interval of 18 months.[52] If the site of recurrence is local, the presentation is usually as a solitary, firm nodule along the incision or as multiple nodules in close proximity to the original primary site of the tumor. For extremity sarcoma, distant metastases occur first in the lung almost exclusively, with extrathoracic metastases emerging later in the presence of widely disseminated disease.[28]

Recurrence is usually discovered during routine postoperative follow-up. After resection of an extremity sarcoma, a patient should be followed at frequent intervals, especially for the first postoperative year. Each follow-up visit should include a thorough history and physical examination with particular attention paid to the site of the previous resection. For low-grade tumors, the risk of pulmonary metastases is low; therefore a careful history and physical examination should suffice, provided the patient is asymptomatic. For high-grade tumors, the risk of local or distant recurrence (or both) is greater, so a more intensive follow-up regimen is warranted. It should include a thoracic CT scan every year for the first 5 years after operation. If the patient is symptomatic or presents with signs of metastases, a definitive investigation should be performed expeditiously to identify possible recurrence.

Isolated local recurrence should be treated with resection; limb amputation is sometimes the only surgical option, but as with primary disease every effort should be made to preserve the affected limb. For low-grade recurrent sarcomas, complete resection offers long-term survival rates comparable to those found after complete resection of primary disease. Adjuvant radiation therapy should be considered even if it was previously used to treat the primary tumor. It can be in the form of EBRT or brachytherapy. One study showed that limb salvage was possible when treating local recurrence with resection and brachytherapy.[53] Chemotherapy has had minimal success but can be considered as part of a protocol. A final option to allow limb salvage is regional limb perfusion. A variety of agents and techniques have been examined, including hyperthermia, cisplatin, tumor necrosis factor-α, interferon-γ, and melphalan, with significant responses reported,[54,55] though the role for this therapy in the treatment of this disease remains to be defined.

The significance of local recurrence remains controversial. Several studies that showed decreased rates of local recurrence did not show any difference in overall survival.[43,56] A review of the MSKCC experience with 805 patients with primary extremity soft tissue sarcoma found local recurrence to be a strong predictor for the development of metastases and disease-specific death.[57]

F. Lung Metastases

Soft tissue sarcoma of the extremity metastasizes almost exclusively to the lung. In most cases the pulmonary nodules are asymptomatic and are discovered by routine follow-up chest radiography or CT scan. Extrathoracic metastases are rarely the sole site of disease but, rather are found as part of widespread disseminated disease. When evaluating a patient with primary or recurrent extremity sarcoma, a bone scan or head CT scan is not necessary if the lungs are free of metastatic disease.

If metastatic spread of the disease is limited to the lungs, the current treatment of choice is thoracotomy with wedge resection of all pulmonary nodules. There is no benefit from formal lobectomy or lymph node dissection. Bilateral lesions can be resected at one operation via a bilateral thoracotomy ("clamshell" approach) or with staged thoracotomies. At MSKCC, 28 patients underwent resection of their metastatic osteosarcoma and achieved an overall 5-year survival of 32%[58]; there were no long-term survivors if surgery was not done. This finding has been supported by a number of subsequent studies.[28,59,60] The benefits achieved by pulmonary metastasectomy seem to be limited to cases where all pulmonary nodules can be resected[28,59] and when there are three or fewer nodules to be removed.[60] Repeat thoracotomy can be performed with reasonable expectations. A study done at the NCI found that nearly three-fourths of patients were able to undergo repeat thoracotomy with a median postoperative survival of 25 months.[61]

Chemotherapy is often employed as another mode of therapy for the treatment of recurrent disease either in combination with surgery or alone if the recurrence is unresectable. As with primary tumors, chemotherapy has yielded minimal success to date, and all patients undergoing such treatment should be enrolled in an experimental protocol. A wide variety of chemotherapeutic agents, alone and in combination, have been investigated. The most active single agent is doxorubicin[62] with a response rate of approximately 25%. A variety of combinations have been used, including dacarbazine (DTIC),[63] ifosfamide and doxorubicin,[64,65] and more recently MAID (mesna/adriamycin/ifosfamide/dacarbazine).[66] Response rates vary between 25% and 47%. Unfortunately, there has been little impact on overall survival regardless of the chemotherapeutic regimen employed, and further studies are needed to find more effective agents to treat this disease. Recently, a Phase I trial employing isolated lung perfusion to treat unresectable pulmonary metastases was completed at MSKCC.[67] It is unclear at this time whether this method affects survival from unresectable metastatic soft tissue sarcoma to the lung.

Specific Histologic Subtypes

Soft tissue sarcomas, as described previously, are rare neoplasms comprised of a diverse group of histologic subtypes. This chapter has focused on how to diagnose and treat the more important histologic subtypes. Though not an exhaustive list, a brief discussion of some of the less frequently encountered diagnoses that may be encountered is warranted.

Desmoid fibrosarcomas ("*desmoids*") are rare lesions arising from the musculoaponeurotic tissues in the body. They behave as low-grade, locally invasive tumors. Pathologic distinction between these lesions and malignant fibrosarcomas and fibromatoses can be difficult, with significant discrepancies among pathologists.[68] Most desmoids are found in the abdominal wall and often occur in pregnant women, though a significant subclass of these tumors arise in the extremity. There is a strong association between Gardner's syndrome and desmoid tumors, first described by Smith in 1958.[69] Other etiologic factors include elevated levels of estrogen[70] and a history of trauma.[71]

In general, surgery is the primary mode of therapy for desmoids, with principles similar to those for resection of other extremity soft tissue sarcomas. These tumors tend to grow in a slow, locally invasive manner, and thus adequate wide, local excision at the initial operation is essential to reduce local recurrence.[72] Surgery alone is often effective if negative microscopic margins are obtained. Radiation therapy, with a more limited role, is employed when resection margins are positive or in conjunction with surgery to allow limb-sparing surgical resection. A variety of chemotherapeutic regimens have been examined including steroids, vincristine/actinomycin D/cyclophosphamide combination therapy and tamoxifen. At present, it is unclear what role chemotherapy may play in the treatment of desmoids. Caution should be exercised with intraabdominal desmoids associated with Gardner syndrome as rapid growth can occur following attempts at resection. For this reason, treatment with nonoperative means should be attempted first and can be accomplished with cytotoxic chemotherapy (adriamycin), antiestrogen therapy, or both.

Extraskeletal Ewing's sarcoma is a rare tumor that differs from its more common bony counterpart in that it is usually located axially and does not originate from bone. It was recognized as a distinct entity only during the late 1970s. It usually presents as a rapidly growing, painful mass in the paravertebral, intercostal, or pelvic girdle regions. There is often periosteal involvement and occasionally frank bony invasion. These facts add to the difficulty of distinguishing this tumor from Ewing's sarcoma of bone.

Extraskeletal Ewing's sarcoma is usually an anaplastic tumor and consequently has a poor prognosis. In one series of 37 cases, 22 patients died of their disease 1 month to 14 years after diagnosis.[73] In general, a multidisciplinary approach to treatment is best. In a series of three patients, successful treatment by wide surgical resection, Ewing's sarcoma of bone chemotherapy regimens, and radiation therapy in the range of 4000–8400 cGy was reported.[74] The long-term risk of radiation-induced sarcoma should be noted for these patients.

Alveolar soft part sarcomas comprise another rare class of soft tissue neoplasms that usually present in the lower extremity of young adults. The histologic origin is unclear, though certain studies suggest skeletal muscle as the site of origin.[75] The 5-year survival is approximately 60%. Recommended therapy includes limb-sparing surgical resection, irradiation, systemic chemotherapy, or a combination of these modalities. Extreme care should be taken at the time of resection, as these tumors are often quite vascular and blood loss can be substantial.

Conclusions

Soft tissue sarcoma is a rare malignancy that accounts for approximately 6000 cases per year in the United States. Surgical resection is the primary mode of therapy, and in many cases no further therapy is required. Local recurrence is best controlled with surgical resection and adjuvant radiation therapy in the form of EBRT or brachytherapy. Numerous trials of various chemotherapy regimens, mainly doxorubicin-based, have been performed. It is unclear at this time what role chemotherapy has in the treatment of this disease, and all potential patients should be enrolled in investigational studies.

Approximately one-third of patients have locally recurrent disease with a median disease-free interval of 18 months. Treatment for local recurrence involves reexcision and usually adjuvant radiation therapy, with results approaching those for treatment of the primary lesion if complete resection can be attained. Metastatic disease occurs primarily in the lungs alone. Resection of isolated pulmonary lesions can be undertaken with 3-year survival rates of 20–30%. Nonresectable pulmonary metastasis or extrapulmonary metastatic disease has a poor prognosis, and these patients should be treated with investigational chemotherapeutic regimens.

References

1. Brennan MF. Management of extremity soft-tissue sarcoma. Am J Surg 1989;158:71–78.
2. Lawrence WJ, Donegan WL, Natarajan N, et al. Adult soft tissue sarcomas: a pattern of care survey of the American College of Surgeons. Ann Surg 1987;25:349–359.
3. Brand KG. Foreign body induced sarcomas. In: Becker FF (ed) Cancer. New York: Plenum, 1975;485–489.
4. Li FP, Fraumeni JF. Soft-tissue sarcomas, breast cancer, and other neoplasms: a familial syndrome? Ann Intern Med 1969;71:747–752.
5. Li FP, Fraumeni JF, Mulvihill JJ, et al. A cancer family syndrome in twenty-four kindreds. Cancer Res 1988;48:5358–5362.
6. Sorensen SA, Mulvihill JJ, Nielsen A. Long-term follow-up of Von Recklinghausen neurofibromatosis: survival and malignant neoplasms. N Engl J Med 1986;314:1010–1015.
7. Barken D, Wright E, Nguyen K. Gene for Von Recklinghausen neurofibromatosis is in the pericentromeric region of chromosome 17. Science 1987;236:1100–1102.
8. Robinson E, Neugut AI, Wylie P. Clinical aspects of postirradiation sarcomas. J Natl Cancer Inst 1988;80:233–240.
9. Davidson T, Westbury G, Harmer CL. Radiation-induced soft-tissue sarcoma. Br J Surg 1986;73:308–309.
10. Stewart FW, Treves N. Lymphangiosarcoma in post mastectomy lymphedema: a report of six cases of elephantiasis chirugica. Cancer 1948;1:64–68.
11. Heslin MJ, Lewis JJ, Woodruff JM, Brennan MF. Core needle biopsy for the diagnosis of extremity soft tissue sarcoma. Ann Surg Oncol 1997;4:421–431.
12. Kissen MW, Fisher C, Webb AJ, et al. Value of fine needle aspiration cytology in the diagnosis of soft tissue tumors: a preliminary study on the excised specimens. Br J Surg 1987;74:479–480.
13. Akerman M, Idvall I, Rydholm A. Cytodiagnosis of soft tissue tumors and tumor-like conditions by means of fine needle aspiration biopsy. Arch Orthop Trauma Surg 1980;96:61–67.
14. Brennan MF, Lewis JJ. Soft tissue sarcomas. Curr Probl Surg 1996;33:819–872.
15. Bowden L, Booher RJ. The principles and techniques of resection of soft parts for sarcomas. Surgery 1958;44:963–977.
16. Brooks JJ. Immunohistochemistry in sarcomas. In: Ryan JR, Baker LO (eds) Recent Concepts in Sarcoma Treatment. Boston: Kluwer, 1988;48–73.
17. Kawai A, Woodruff JM, Healey JH, et al. SYT-SSX gene fusion as a determinant of morphology and prognosis in synovial sarcoma. Nat Genet 1998;338:153–160.
18. Ladanyi M. The emerging molecular genetics of sarcoma translocations. Diagn Mol Pathol 1995;4:162–173.
19. Hadju SI. Differential diagnosis of soft tissue and bone tumors. Philadelphia: Lea & Febiger, 1986:402–404.
20. Demas BE, Heelan RT, Lane J, et al. Soft-tissue sarcomas of the extremities: comparison of MR and CT in determining extent of disease. AJR Am J Roentgenol 1988;150:615–620.
21. Kern KA, Brunetti A, Norton JA, et al. Metabolic imaging of human extremity musculoskeletal tumors by PET. J Nucl Med 1988;29:181–186.
22. Adler LP, Blair HF, Makley JT, et al. Noninvasive grading of musculoskeletal tumors using PET. J Nucl Med 1991;32:1508–1512.
23. Shinkwin MA, Lenkinski RE, Daly JM, et al. Integrated magnetic resonance imaging and phosphorus spectroscopy of soft tissue tumors. Cancer 1991;67:1849–1858.
24. Schwartz HS, Jones CK. The effect of gallium scintigraphy in detecting malignant soft tissue neoplasms. Ann Surg 1992;215:78–82.
25. Southee AE, Kaplan WD, Jochelson MS, et al. Gallium imaging in metastatic and recurrent soft-tissue sarcoma. J Nucl Med 1992;33:1594–1599.
26. Geer RJ, Woodruff JM, Casper ES, et al. Management of small soft-tissue sarcoma of the extremity in adults. Arch Surg 1992;127:1285–1289.
27. Fleming ID, Cooper JS, Henson DE, et al. Soft tissue sarcoma. In: AJCC Cancer Staging Manual. Philadelphia: Lippincott Williams & Wilkins, 1997:149–156.
28. Gadd MA, Casper ES, Woodruff JM, et al. Development and treatment of pulmonary metastases in adult patients with extremity soft tissue sarcoma. Ann Surg 1993;218:705–712.
29. Fong Y, Coit DG, Woodruff JM, et al. Lymph node metastases from soft tissue sarcoma in adults: analysis of data from a prospective database of 1772 sarcoma patients. Ann Surg 1993;217:72–77.
30. Rosenberg SA, Tepper J, Glatstein E, et al. The treatment of soft-tissue sarcomas of the extremities: prospective randomized evaluations of limb-sparing surgery plus radiation therapy in the management of sarcoma of the soft tissues. Ann Surg 1982;196:305–315.
31. Lewis JJ, Brennan MF. Soft tissue sarcomas. In: Sabiston DC (ed) The Biological Basis of Modern Surgical Practice. Philadelphia: Saunders, 1996;528–534.
32. Lindberg RD. Soft tissue sarcoma. In: Fletcher CD (ed) Textbook of Radiotherapy. Philadelphia: Lea & Febiger, 1980:922–942.
33. Tepper JE, Suit HD. Radiation alone for sarcoma of soft tissue. Cancer 1985;56:475–479.
34. Suit HD, Mankin HJ, Schiller AL. Results of treatment of sarcoma of soft

tissue by radiation and surgery at Massachusetts General Hospital. Cancer Treat Symp 1985;3:33–47.

35. Pisters PW, Leung DH, Woodruff J, et al. Analysis of prognostic factors in 1041 patients with localized soft tissue sarcoma of the extremities. J Clin Oncol 1996;14:1679–1689.
36. Enneking WF, McAuliffe JA. Adjunctive preoperative radiation therapy in treatment of soft tissue sarcomas: a preliminary report. Cancer Treat Symp 1985;3:37–42.
37. Brant TA, Parsons JT, Marcus RBJ, et al. Preoperative irradiation for soft tissue sarcomas of the trunk and extremities in adults. Int J Radiat Oncol Biol Phys 1990;19:899–906.
38. Barkley HT, Martin RG, Romsdahl MM, et al. Treatment of soft tissue sarcomas by preoperative irradiation and conservative surgical resection. Int J Radiat Oncol Biol Phys 1988;14:693–699.
39. Lindberg RD, Martin RG, Romsdahl MM, et al. Conservation surgery and postoperative radiotherapy in 300 adults with soft-tissue sarcomas. Cancer 1981;47:2391–2397.
40. Potter DA, Glenn J, Kinsella T, et al. Patterns of recurrence in patients with high-grade soft-tissue sarcomas. J Clin Oncol 1985;3:353–366.
41. Leibel SA, Tranbaugh RF, Wara WM, et al. Soft-tissue sarcomas of the extremities: survival and patterns of failure with conservative surgery and postoperative irradiation compared to surgery alone. Cancer 1982; 50:1076–1083.
42. Suit HD, Mankin HJ, Wood W, et al. Preoperative, intraoperative, and postoperative radiation in the treatment of primary soft tissue sarcoma. Cancer 1985;55:2659–2667.
43. Brennan MF, Hilaris B, Shiu MH, et al. Local recurrence in adult soft tissue sarcoma: a randomized trial of brachytherapy. Arch Surg 1987;122: 1289–1293.
44. Pisters PW, Harrison LB, Leung DH, et al. Long-term results of a prospective randomized trial of adjuvant brachytherapy in soft tissue sarcoma. J Clin Oncol 1996;14:859–868
45. Casper ES, Gaynor JJ, Harrison LB, et al. Preoperative and postoperative adjuvant chemotherapy for adults with high-grade soft tissue sarcoma. Cancer 1994;73:1644–1651.
46. Pezzi CM, Pollack RE, Evans HL, et al. Preoperative chemotherapy for so-ft-tissue sarcoma of the extremities. Ann Surg 1990;211:476–481.
47. Ravaud A, Nguyen BB, Coindre JM, et al. Adjuvant chemotherapy with CyVADIC in high-grade soft tissue sarcoma: a randomized prospective trial. In: Salmon S (ed) Adjuvant Therapy of Cancer. Philadelphia: Saunders, 1990:556–566.
48. Gherlinzoni F, Bacci G, Picci P, et al. A randomized trial for the treatment of high-grade soft-tissue sarcomas of the extremities: preliminary observations. J Clin Oncol 1986;4:552–558.
49. Rosenberg SA, Tepper J, Glatstein E, et al. Prospective randomized evaluation of adjuvant chemotherapy in adults with soft tissue sarcomas of the extremities. Cancer 1983;52:424–434.
50. Eilber FR, Guilano JF, Huth JF, et al. Intravenous (IV) vs. intraarterial (IA) adriamycin, 2800r radiation and surgical excision for extremity soft tissue sarcomas: a randomized prospective trial, abstracted. Proc Am Soc Clin Oncol 1990;9:309.
51. Anonymous. Adjuvant chemotherapy for localized resectable soft tissue sarcoma for adults: a meta-analysis of individual patient data. Lancet 1997;350:1647–1654.
52. Brennan MF, Casper ES, Harrison LB, et al. The role of multimodality therapy in soft tissue sarcomas. Ann Surg 1991;214:328–336.
53. Nori D, Schupak K, Shiu MH, et al. Role of brachytherapy in recurrence extremity sarcoma in patients treated with prior surgery and irradiation. Int J Radiat Oncol Biol Phys 1991;20:1229–1233.
54. Lienard D, Ewalenko P, Delmotte JJ, et al. High-dose recombinant tumor necrosis factor alpha in combination with interferon gamma and melphalan in isolation perfusion of limbs for melanoma and sarcoma. J Clin Oncol 1992;10:52–60.
55. Pommier RF, Moseley HS, Cohen J, et al. Pharmacokinetics, toxicity, and short-term results of cisplatin hyperthermic isolated limb perfusion for soft-tissue sarcoma and melanoma of the extremities. Am J Surg 1988;155:667–671.
56. Yang JC, Rosenberg SA. Surgery for adult patients with soft tissue sarcomas. Surgery 1990;65:1727–1729.
57. Lewis JJ, Leung D, Heslin MJ, et al. The association of local recurrence with subsequent survival in extremity soft tissue sarcoma. J Clin Oncol 1997;15:646–652.
58. Martini N, Huvos AG, Mike V, et al. Multiple pulmonary resections in the treatment of osteogenic sarcoma. Ann Thorac Surg 1971;12:271–280.
59. Verazin GT, Warneke JA, Driscoll DL, et al. Resection of lung metastases from soft-tissue sarcomas: a multivariate analysis. Arch Surg 1992; 127:1407–1411.
60. Casson AG, Putnam JB, Natarajan G, et al. Five-year survival after pulmonary metastasectomy for adult soft tissue sarcoma. Cancer 1992;69: 662–668.
61. Pogrebniak HW, Roth JA, Steinberg SM, et al. Reoperative pulmonary resection in patients with metastatic soft tissue sarcoma. Ann Thorac Surg 1991;52:197–203.
62. Schoenfeld DA, Rosenbaum C, Horton J, et al. A comparison of adriamycin versus vincristine and adriamycin, and cyclophosphamide for advanced sarcoma. Cancer 1982;50:2757–2762.
63. Gottlieb JA, Benjamin RS, Baker LH, et al. Role of DTIC (NSC-123127) in the chemotherapy of sarcomas. Cancer Treat Rep 1976;60:199–203.
64. Wiltshaw E, Westbury G, Harmer C, et al. Ifosfamide plus mesna with and without adriamycin in soft tissue sarcoma. Cancer Chemother Pharmacol 1986;18:S10–S12.
65. Schutte J, Mouridsen HT, Stewart W, et al. Ifosfamide plus doxorubicin in previously untreated patients with advanced soft tissue sarcoma: the EORTC Soft Tissue and Bone Sarcoma Group. Eur J Cancer 1990;26: 558–561.
66. Elias A, Ryan L, Sulkes A, et al. Response to mesna, doxorubicin, ifosfamide, and dacarbazine in 108 patients with metastatic or unresectable sarcoma and no prior chemotherapy. J Clin Oncol 1989;7:1208–1216.
67. Burt ME, Liu D, Abolhoda A, et al. Isolated long perfusion with unresectable metastases from sarcoma: a phase I trial. Ann Thorac Surg 2000; 69(5):1542–1549.
68. Fine G, Hadju SI, Morton DL, et al. Soft tissue sarcomas: classification and treatment (a symposium). Pathol Annu 1982;17:155–195.
69. Smith WG. Multiple polyposis, Gardner's syndrome and desmoid tumors. Dis Colon Rectum 1958;1:323–332.
70. Hayry P, Reitamo JJ, Totterman S, et al. The desmoid tumor. II. Analysis of factors possibly contributing to the etiology and growth behavior. Am J Clin Pathol 1982;77:674–680.
71. Geschickter GF, Lewis D. Tumors of connective tissue. Am J Cancer 1935;25:630–655.
72. Posner MC, Shiu MH, Newsome JL, et al. The desmoid tumor: not a benign disease. Arch Surg 1989;124:191–196.
73. Angerwall L, Enzinger FM. Extraskeletal neoplasm resembling Ewing's sarcoma. Cancer 1975;36:240–251.
74. Gillespie JJ, Roth LM, Wells ER, et al. Extraskeletal Ewing's sarcoma. Am J Surg Pathol 1979;3:99–108.
75. Ordonez NG, Ro JY, Mackay B. Alveolar soft part sarcoma: an ultrastructural and immunocytochemical investigation of its histogenesis. Cancer 1989;63:1721–1736.

Section 8

Bone Cancers

Chapter 44

Osteogenic Sarcoma

STEVEN GITELIS
ALEXANDER A. GREEN
JOHN R. CHARTERS

A. Introduction

Osteogenic sarcoma is the most common primary bone malignancy; approximately 500–1000 tumors are diagnosed in the United States each year. The World Health Organization (WHO) defines osteosarcoma as "a malignant tumor characterized by the direct formation of bone or osteoid by the proliferating tumor cells."[1] This tumor affects males more than females (6:4), and most occur (58%) during the second decade of life.

Osteosarcoma is typically divided into conventional and osteosarcoma variants.[1,2] This distinction is important because it affects prognosis and management. The osteosarcoma variants include parosteal osteosarcoma, periosteal osteosarcoma, low-grade medullary osteosarcoma, small cell osteosarcoma, telangiectatic osteosarcoma, and secondary osteosarcoma.[1,2] The secondary osteosarcomas include osteosarcoma secondary to Paget's disease and postradiation osteosarcoma.

B. Presentation

Most conventional osteosarcomas occur about the knee including the lower end of the femur and upper end of the tibia. Other common sites include the humerus and upper end of the femur.[1,2] The typical clinical presentation is unremitting and progressive limb pain, which is constant and usually requires analgesics. In addition, some patients present with a mass or limb enlargement. When the knee joint is involved a flexion/contracture of the knee occurs, and there is frequently loss of function. Some patients present with a pathologic fracture secondary to bone weakness created by the tumor.

C. Diagnosis

The radiologic presentation of an osteosarcoma is characteristic, and a diagnosis can often be made based on the initial radiograph. Radiographically (Fig. 44–1), a conventional osteosarcoma involves the medullary space and destroys bone, creating an osteolytic defect. Ninety percent of osteosarcomas are

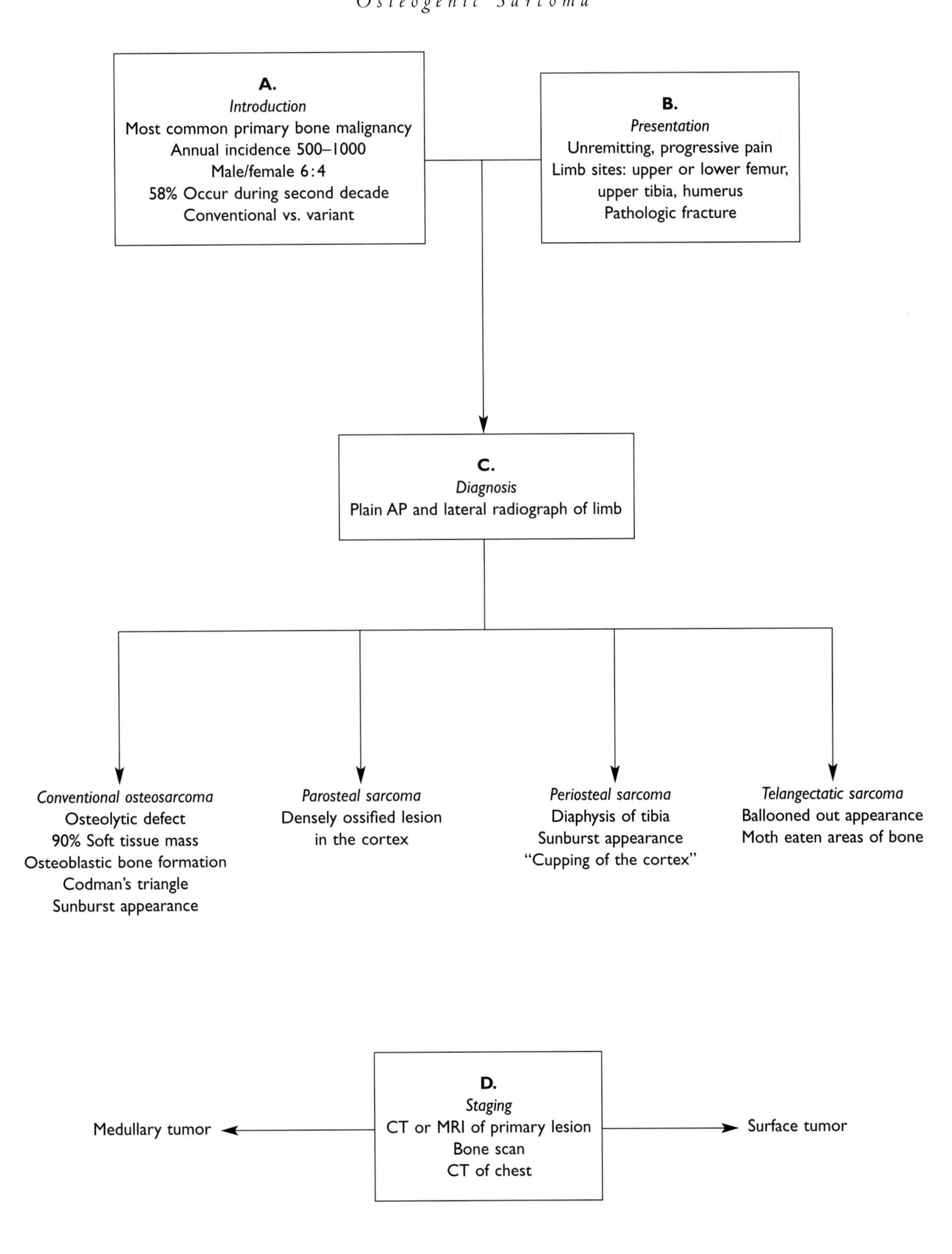

(continued on next page)

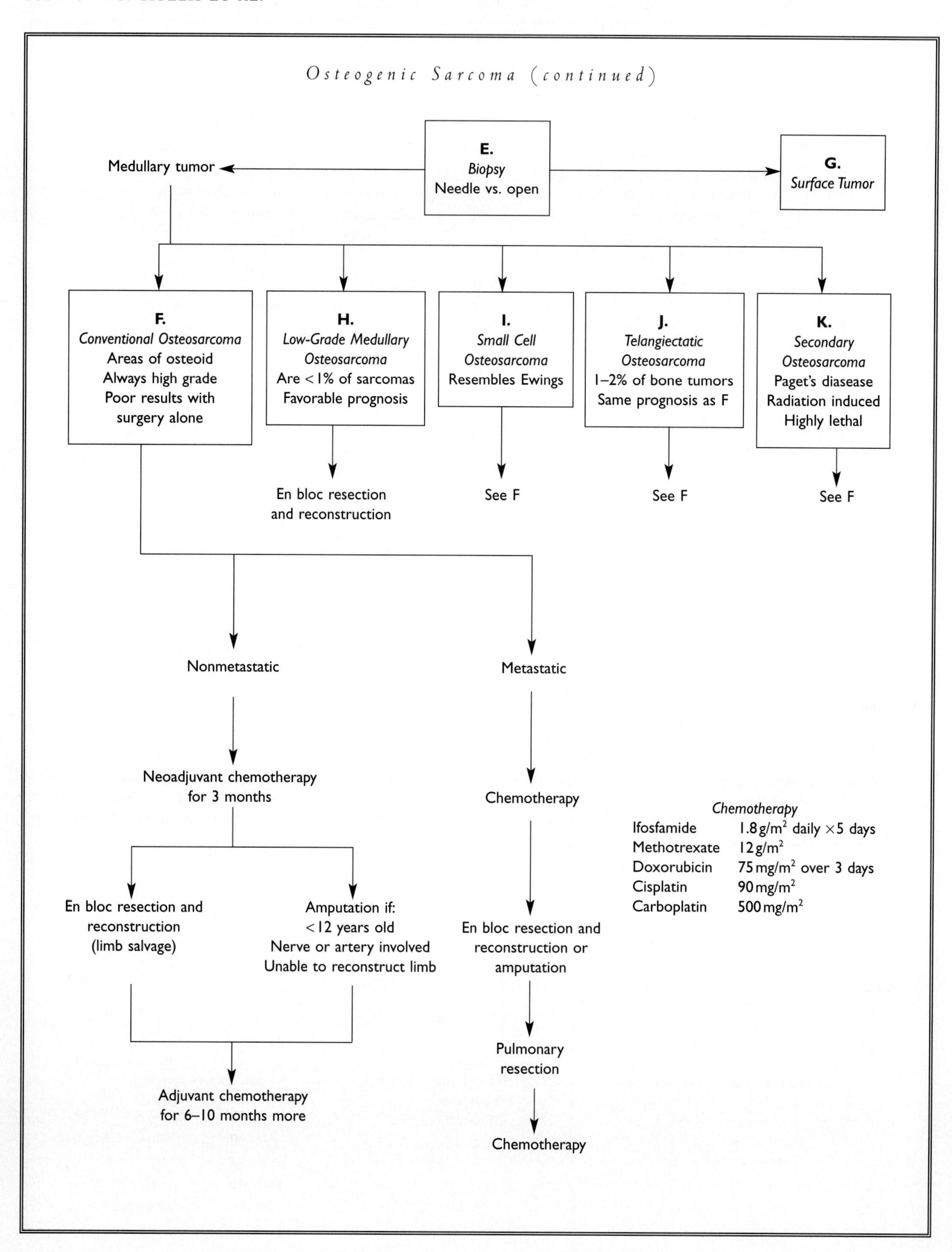

Osteogenic Sarcoma (continued)
E.
Biopsy
Needle vs. open
Medullary tumor
G.
Surface Tumor
F.
Conventional Osteosarcoma
Areas of osteoid
Always high grade
Poor results with
surgery alone
H.
Low-Grade Medullary
Osteosarcoma
Are <1% of sarcomas
Favorable prognosis
I.
Small Cell
Osteosarcoma
Resembles Ewings
J.
Telangiectatic
Osteosarcoma
1–2% of bone tumors
Same prognosis as F
K.
Secondary
Osteosarcoma
Paget's diasease
Radiation induced
Highly lethal
En bloc resection
and reconstruction
See F
See F
See F
Nonmetastatic
Metastatic
Neoadjuvant chemotherapy
for 3 months
Chemotherapy
En bloc resection and
reconstruction
(limb salvage)
Amputation if:
<12 years old
Nerve or artery involved
Unable to reconstruct limb
En bloc resection and
reconstruction or
amputation
Pulmonary
resection
Adjuvant chemotherapy
for 6–10 months more
Chemotherapy
Chemotherapy
Ifosfamide 1.8 g/m2 daily ×5 days
Methotrexate 12 g/m2
Doxorubicin 75 mg/m2 over 3 days
Cisplatin 90 mg/m2
Carboplatin 500 mg/m2

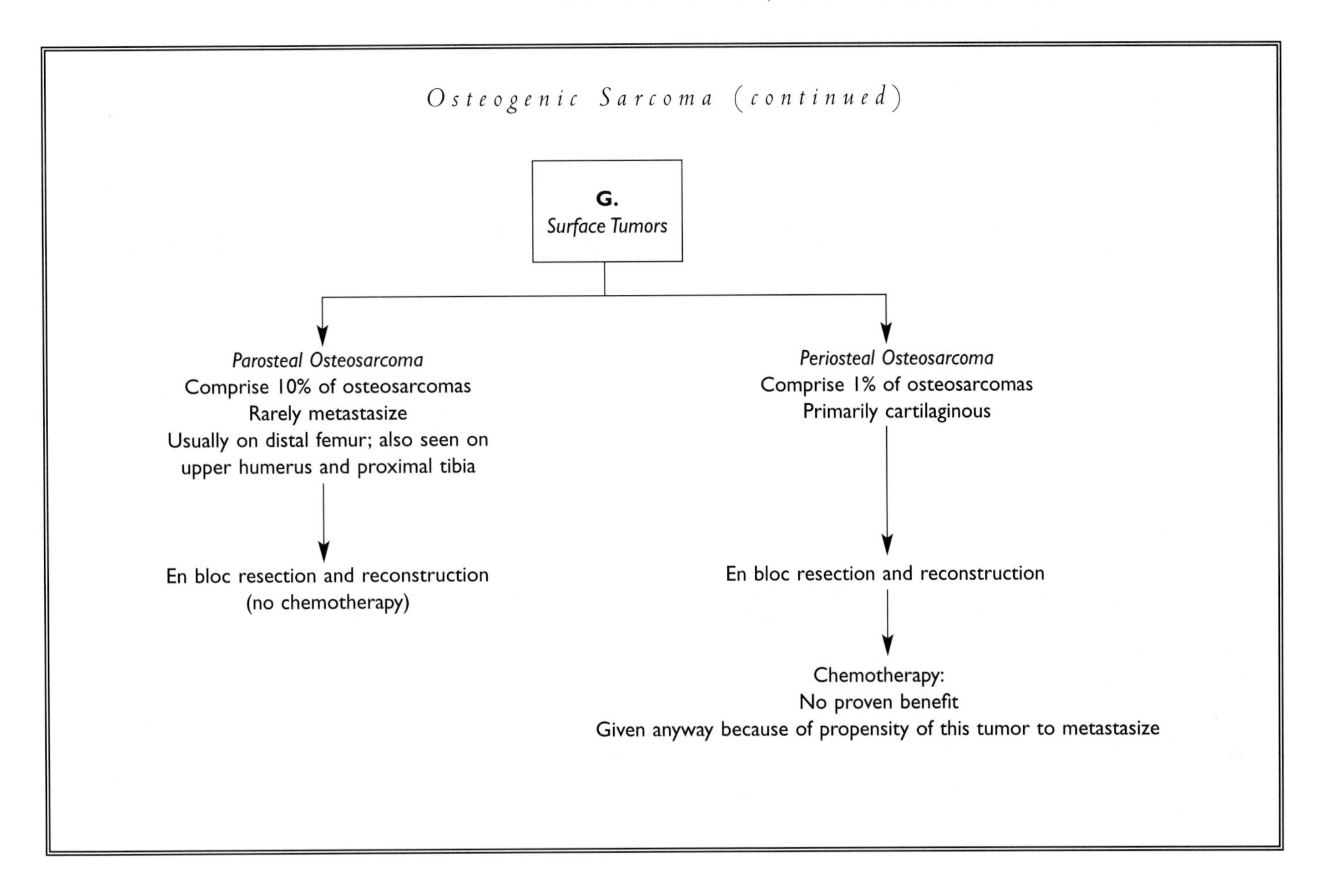

associated with a soft tissue mass that sometimes can be seen on plain radiographs but are better imaged with computed tomography (CT) or magnetic resonance image (MRI) scans.[3] In addition to osteolysis, osteosarcoma is frequently associated with osteoblastic bone formation, which appear's radiographically as areas of dense bone formation in the osteolytic defect. As the tumor breaks out of the bone and lifts the periosteum, two well described radiographie features become evident: (1) Codman's triangle, which represents bone formation as a result of periosteal lifting; or (2) a sunburst, which is perpendicular formation of bone as a result of soft tissue extension of the tumor. When the tumor occurs in proximity to a joint, invasion can occur along ligament attachments. Rarely, an osteosarcoma invades the articular cartilage or the growth plate.[4] Although most osteosarcomas occur in the metaphysis of a long bone, some affect the mid-shaft or diaphysis.

D. Staging

The next step in patient management is staging. Osteosarcoma is a highly malignant tumor that is both locally aggressive and potentially metastatic. Clinical trials have demonstrated that as many as 80% of osteosarcomas at presentation have evidence of either macro- or micrometastatic disease. The most common site of involvement with metastatic disease is the lungs, manifesting within the first year after surgery. Other bones are involved on occasion. Staging should consist of a technetium-99 diphosphonate bone scan to determine whether the tumor is monostotic or polyostotic. In addition, a chest radiograph and a CT scan of the lungs are obtained to determine if there is evidence of metastatic disease.

E. Biopsy

Once staging is complete, a biopsy is performed using a needle or an open technique. The latter provides more tissue for diagnosis but must be done carefully to avoid complications. Incisional biopsies should be via longitudinal incisions, preferably *through* muscle, avoiding anatomic planes. This approach preserves these planes for subsequent definitive treatment/excision. Moreover, the biopsy must be carefully placed so the specimen can be removed en bloc with the bone at the time of definitive surgery. The biopsy is usually limited to the soft tissue component of the tumor.

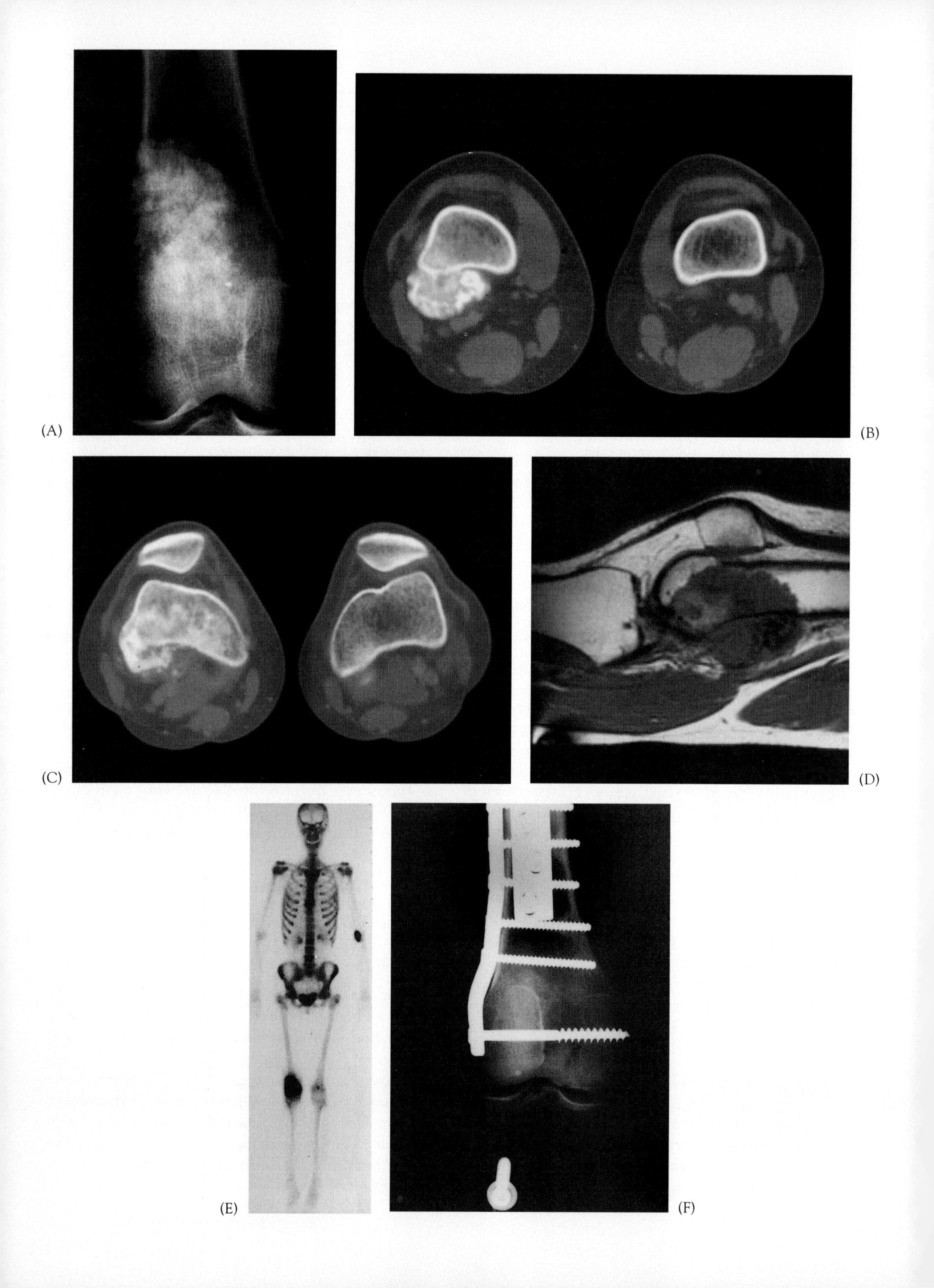
(A)
(B)
(C)
(D)
(E)
(F)

TABLE 44–1.
Enneking staging system for osteosarcoma

Stage IA	Low grade intracompartmental
Stage IB	Low grade extracompartmental
Stage IIA	High grade intracompartmental
Stage IIB	High grade extracompartmental
Stage III	Metastatic

SOURCE: Enneking WF, Spanier SS, Goodman MA. A system for the surgical staging of musculoskeletal sarcoma. Clin Orthop 1980;153:106. Used with permission.

F. Conventional Osteosarcoma

The pathologic features of a conventional osteosarcoma are those of a high-grade spindle cell malignancy with areas of osteoid.[1,2] It is the latter feature that is an absolute requirement for the diagnosis of osteosarcoma. The tumor can be fibroblastic, chondroblastic, or osteoblastic, distinctions that currently are not important in terms of prognosis. The Enneking staging system (Table 44–1) is most commonly used for osteosarcoma; it takes into account the grade of the tumor, whether it is contained in the bone, and the presence or absence of metastases.[5] A conventional osteosarcoma is always high grade histologically, and most extend outside the bone (stage IIB).[3] Ten percent of osteosarcomas are contained within the bone (IIA). Metastatic osteosarcoma is stage III.

Because surgery alone provides 5-year survival rates of less than 20%, current treatment of osteosarcoma consists of neoadjuvant chemotherapy followed by surgical removal of the primary disease.[6–11] The addition of chemotherapy has improved relapse-free and overall survival. Chemotherapy is continued for a period of up to 9 months following surgery, and regimens typically consist of combinations of four or five intravenously administered drugs such as doxorubicin, methotrexate, ifosfamide, cisplatin, or carboplatin. No standard length of therapy has been established, although all clinical trials administer treatment for approximately 1 year.

After 3 months a decision is made regarding surgical removal of the tumor. Follow-up studies such as MRI are done to determine the intramedullary extent of the tumor and to detect "skip" metastases.[12,13] The primary surgical objective is to obtain negative margins following resection, which amounts to removing the tumor en bloc with a cuff of normal tissue completely encircling the tumor. Most of the time this can be accomplished by limb salvage (Fig. 44–2).[14] Limb salvage has become particularly popular owing to advancements in reconstruction. Patients not amenable to limb salvage include patients under the age of 12 years where growth creates a significant obstacle. Other contraindications for limb salvage include involvement of a major nerve and artery and an inability to reconstruct the limb adequately after tumor removal. Successful limb reconstruction can be performed in most patients with the use of allografts, modular oncology prosthetics, and vascularized bone grafts. These reconstructive procedures must be individualized based on the age of the patient, functional demands, and desire.

Once the tumor is removed, it is analyzed by the pathologist to determine the effectiveness of the preoperative chemotherapy. Patients whose tumors demonstrate a significant degree of necrosis are treated with the same regimen, whereas poor responders are treated with a modified approach consisting of different drugs or intensified doses of the same medications. Postoperative chemotherapy is delivered for approximately 9 months. Patients are then followed closely with both extremity imaging and imaging of the lungs. If pulmonary metastases occur, they are treated aggressively with thoracotomy and resection, which has been shown to improve survival. For synchronous pulmonary metastases, preoperative chemotherapy is given followed by resection of both the primary bone sarcoma and the pulmonary metastases by thoracotomy or sternotomy. Chemotherapy is then resumed after thoracotomy. Deaths from osteosarcoma usually result from uncontrolled pulmonary metastases. When local failure occurs, amputation is required. The reported 5-year survival for conventional osteosarcoma is 60% to 70%.[8]

G. Surface Tumors

Parosteal Osteosarcoma

Parosteal osteosarcoma is a variant of osteosarcoma that differs in both treatment and prognosis. The WHO defines parosteal osteosarcoma as a distinctive malignant type of osteosarcoma characterized by having its origin on the external surface of a bone and a high degree of structural differentiation.[1] These

FIGURE 44–1
(A) A 22-year-old woman had osteosarcoma involving the right distal femur. Note the malignant bone formation. (B) Computed tomography (CT) scan of the right and left femur. Bone-forming mass is evident on the surface of the right femur. (C) CT scan reveals tumor involving the medullary bone. (D) Magnetic resonance image. The signal abnormality demonstrates the tumor, which involves bone and soft tissue. (E) Technetium bone scan shows intense activity in the right distal femur. (F) Postoperative radiograph. The right distal femur has been resected and reconstructed with an allograft.

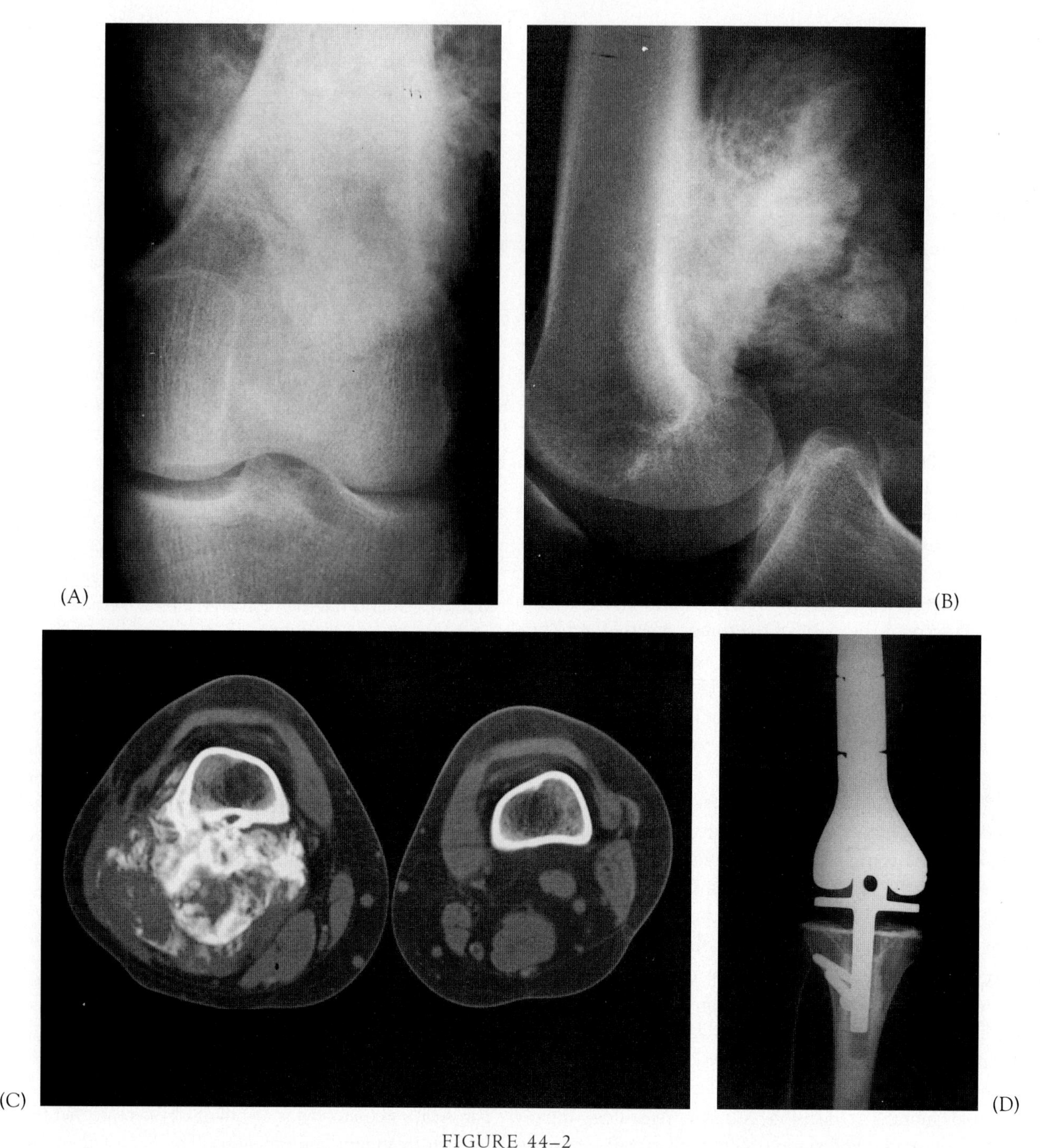

FIGURE 44–2
(A, B) This 24-year-old woman has an osteosarcoma involving the right distal femur. (C) CT scan shows it to be a surface tumor without medullary involvement. Biopsy revealed a high-grade surface osteosarcoma. (D) Postoperative radiograph after resection of the right distal femur and prosthetic reconstruction.

tumors are relatively slow-growing and have a better prognosis than a conventional osteosarcoma.[15] Parosteal osteosarcoma is far less common than conventional osteosarcoma and accounts for 10% of all osteosarcomas. It typically occurs in patients more than 20 years of age with the third and fourth decades being the most common age at presentation.[16,17] Most parosteal osteosarcomas occur on the surface of the lower end of the femur posteriorly (Fig. 44–3). Other common sites include the upper end of the humerus and upper end of the tibia. Radiographically, a parosteal osteosarcoma is a densely ossified surface tumor located on the cortex of the involved bone. Although a cleft may be visible between the tumor and the cortex in some areas, there is always a site of attachment to the cortex, which differentiates it from myositis ossificans. The tumor is frequently lobulated.

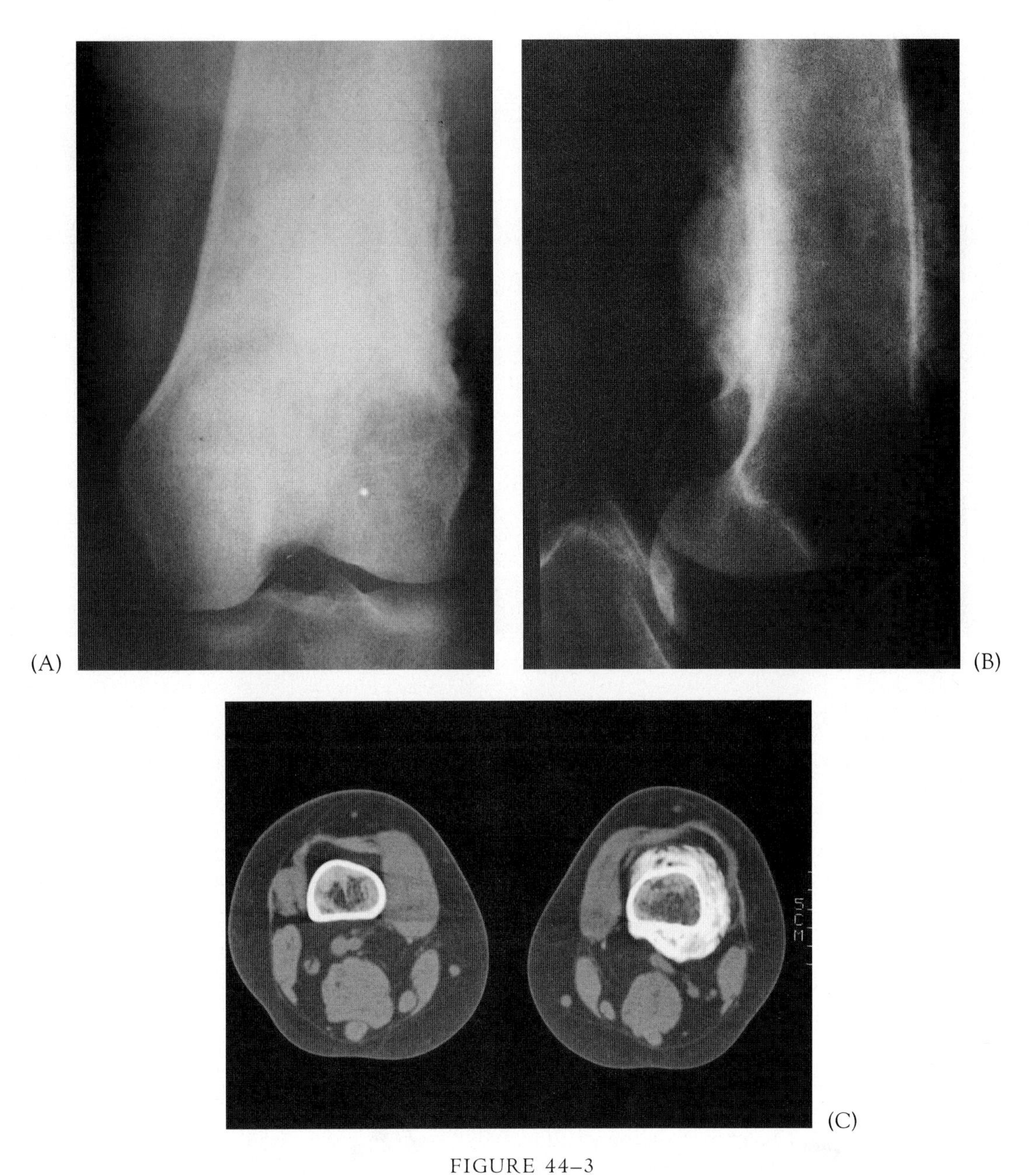

(A) (B) (C)

FIGURE 44–3
(A, B) This 30-year-old woman has an osteosarcoma involving the left distal femur. (C) CT scan shows that the tumor involves the surface of the femur. Biopsy revealed a parosteal osteosarcoma.

A small percentage of parosteal osteosarcomas invade the medullary space.[18] Pathologically, this tumor consists of a low-grade spindle cell sarcoma that resembles a fibrosarcoma but, in addition, has well differentiated bone formation. It typically has a zonal phenomenon. The most immature portions of this tumor are toward its surface, whereas centrally the tumor tends to be far more mature.

Unlike conventional osteosarcomas, management of a parosteal sarcoma is entirely surgical.[19] Chemotherapy is generally not required, as these tumors rarely metastasize. Complete surgical removal of the tumor with wide margins is adequate. The prognosis for a parosteal osteosarcoma is good, but patients must still be followed closely for local relapse and the rare metastasis.

Periosteal Osteosarcoma

The periosteal osteosarcoma accounts for approximately 1% of all osteosarcomas.[20–22] This tumor is primarily cartilaginous and has the appearance of a chondrosarcoma, but there are areas of

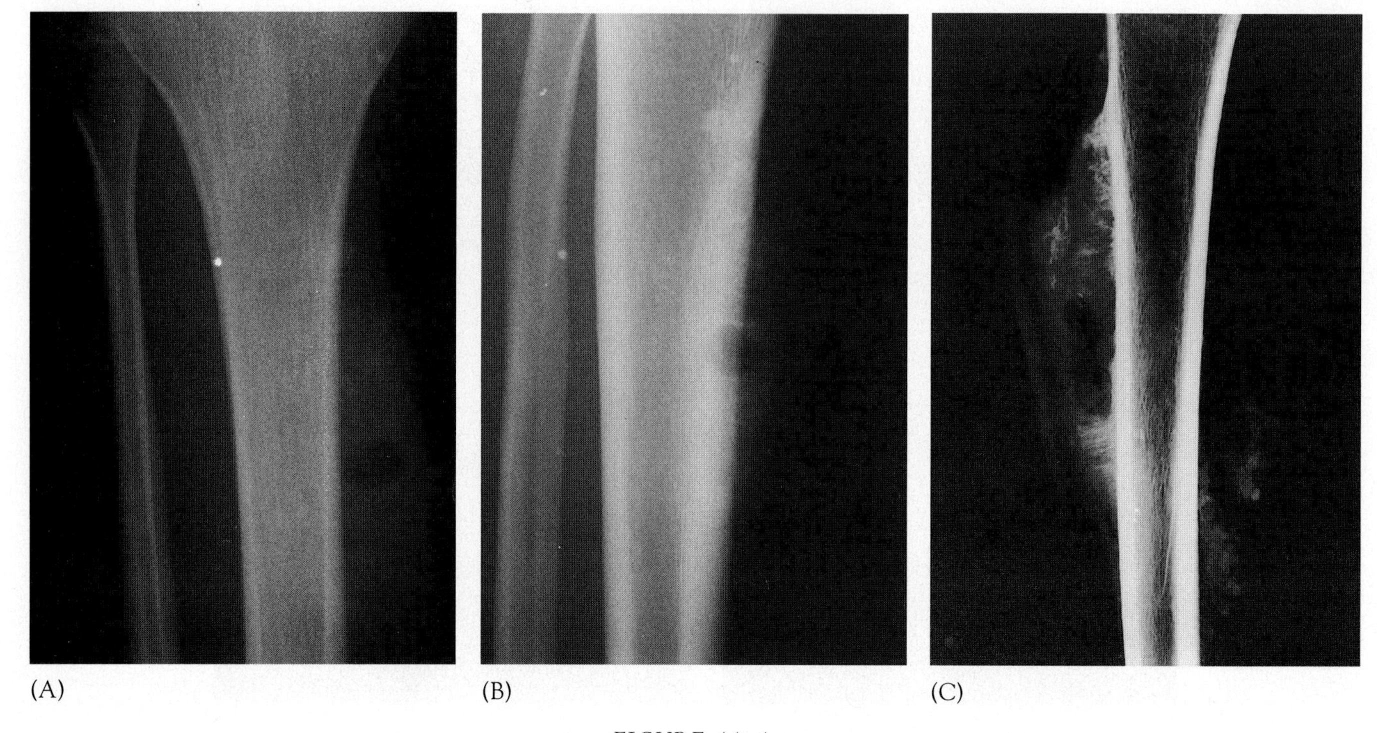

FIGURE 44–4
(A, B) This 22-year-old woman has a periosteal osteosarcoma of the tibia. (C) The specimen radiograph shows a surface tumor with "cupping" and calcification.

malignant cells forming osteoid within the tumor. The name periosteal implies that it is a surface osteosarcoma similar to parosteal osteosarcoma; the difference is that this tumor involves the diaphysis of the tibia and radiographically has a sunburst-type appearance next to the cortical bone (Fig. 44–4). The cortex may have a "cupping" appearance, which is a scalloped-out indentation of the bone. Treatment of this variant is surgical, with en bloc removal of the tumor with a wide margin, which is usually successful in local control of the tumor. Its behavior, however, is slightly more aggressive than that of a parosteal osteosarcoma. Although chemotherapy has not been proven to be an effective adjunct, some patients are treated because of the risk of metastatic disease. Patients must be followed after surgery with chest radiographs and CT scans of the lungs to rule out metastatic disease.

H. Low-Grade Medullary Osteosarcoma

Low-grade medullary osteosarcoma is a rare variant of osteosarcoma (1%) with a distinctly favorable prognosis.[23–26] This well differentiated tumor is composed of fibrous tissue with malignant cells forming bone. The latter, however, lacks atypia or other features of high-grade malignancy. In fact, the bone formation in a well differentiated osteosarcoma can resemble fibrous dysplasia. It occurs in older patients and typically has a protracted history of pain. These tumors can involve almost any bone but favor the metaphysis of the distal femur (Fig. 44–5). Treatment of this tumor is wide en bloc resection followed by reconstruction. Chemotherapy is not used, and metastatic disease is distinctly uncommon.

I. Small Cell Osteosarcoma

The small cell osteosarcoma is a high-grade, bone-forming, round cell malignancy.[27–31] The tumor resembles Ewing's sarcoma; what distinguishes it from this tumor are areas of malignant cells forming osteoid. It is an extremely rare tumor, and there are no large series of patients in the literature. The few patients who have been reported have shown a significant risk of metastatic disease. For this reason, most authors recommend chemotherapy; in addition, local disease must be treated aggressively with wide en bloc resection followed by reconstruction. This tumor, like other aggressive forms of osteosarcoma, must be followed carefully for metastatic disease after surgery.

J. Telangiectatic Osteosarcoma

Telangiectatic osteosarcoma, a high-grade variant of osteosarcoma, accounts for 1–2% of all osteosarcomas.[32–35] Some authors have reported that the incidence of this tumor exceeds 10%. Its most distinguishing features are its ballooned-out appearance on

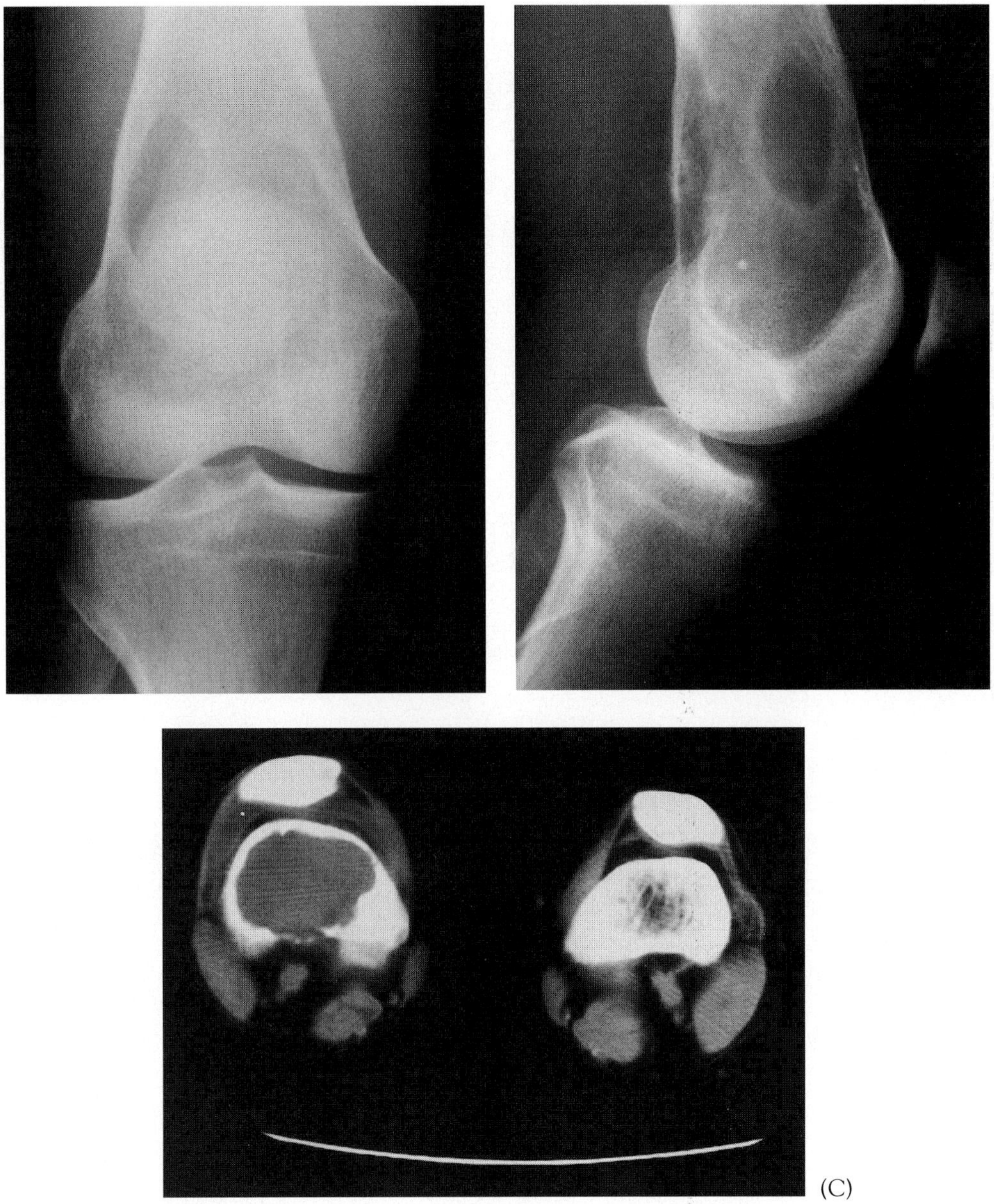

(A)

(B)

(C)

FIGURE 44–5
(A, B) This 26-year-old patient has low-grade medullary osteosarcoma of the right distal femur. (C) CT scan shows the lytic nature of the tumor without obvious bone formation.

radiographs and lakes of blood seen histologically. Mixed with these lakes of blood are areas of high-grade malignant cells forming osteoid. Radiographically, in addition, are areas of moth-eaten bone destruction (Fig. 44–6). It occurs at the same age as a conventional osteosarcoma and involves the same sites. The tumor can be challenging diagnostically, as many benign tumors have a ballooned-out appearance; therefore it is important to look for high-grade malignant tissue forming osteoid, which defines the aggressiveness of this tumor. Telangiectatic osteosarcoma historically was thought to have a poor prognosis, but with modern chemotherapy its prognosis is the same as that for conventional osteosarcoma.

K. Secondary Osteosarcoma

Osteosarcoma can occur as a secondary lesion. It has been reported as a complication of Paget's disease, which is a metabolic bone disease characterized by osteolytic or osteosclerotic bone formation. Paget's disease occurs in older individuals, may be associated with fractures,[36–38] and may cause deformity of bone and other problems such as cardiac failure. Its most devastating complication is a Paget's osteosarcoma. This secondary malignancy is extremely aggressive and highly lethal. It is reported to occur in approximately 1% of patients with Paget's disease. It can occur in any bone, and its clinical hallmark is the develop-

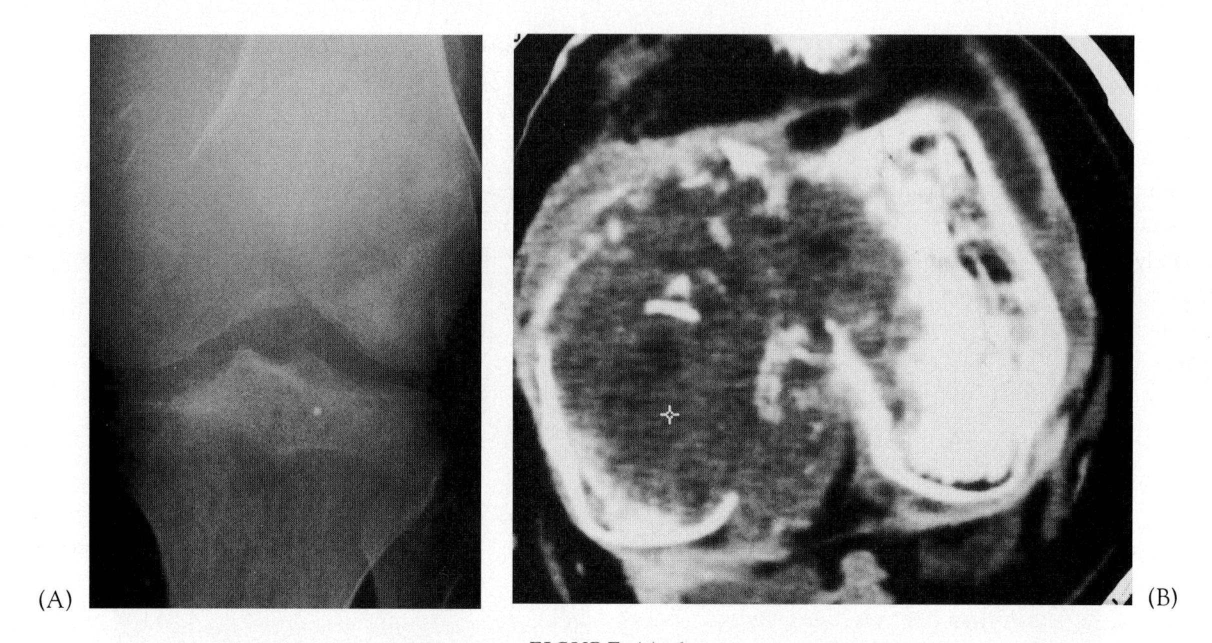

(A) (B)

FIGURE 44–6
(A) Telangiectatic osteosarcoma of the left distal femur. (B) CT scan shows that the distal femur has expanded.

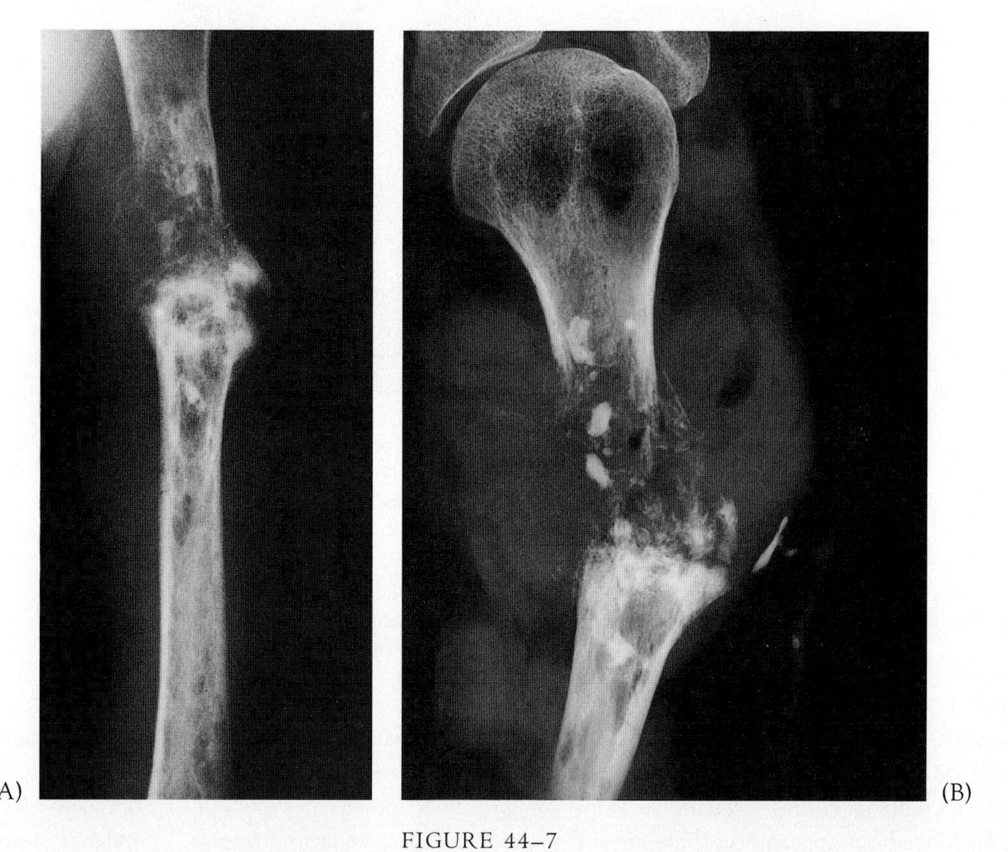

(A) (B)

FIGURE 44–7
(A) A 30-year-old woman has a postradiation osteosarcoma of the left humerus. (B) Specimen radiograph shows bone destruction and a pathologic fracture.

ment of intractable pain and frequently a soft tissue mass in a patient with known Paget's disease. Rapid elevation of the alkaline phosphatase level is another feature. Despite aggressive treatment with surgery and chemotherapy, it is invariably fatal. Similarly, postradiation osteosarcoma is a highly lethal condition (Fig. 44–7) that develops usually after a latency period of approximately 10 years. Histologically, the tumor has areas of high-grade spindle cell malignancy associated with bone formation. Despite aggressive therapy, these patients are at significant risk for metastatic disease. The use of chemotherapy is recommended along with aggressive surgical removal of the tumor.

Conclusions

The treatment and prognosis of osteosarcoma has improved in recent years as a result of better imaging of the tumor and aggressive chemotherapy. Other than the secondary osteosarcomas, the outcome is generally favorable. Patients are not only surviving longer with a higher cure rate but are retaining their limbs. Improvement in implants is allowing better functional recovery and a more normal life.

References

1. Schajowicz F. Osteosarcoma. In: Schajowicz F (ed) Tumors and Tumor-like Lesions of Bone, 2nd ed. Berlin: Springer, 1994:71–141.
2. Unni KK. Osteosarcoma of bone. In: Unni KK (ed) Bone Tumors. New York: Churchill Livingstone, 1989:107.
3. Glasser DB, Lane JM. Stage IIB osteogenic sarcoma. Clin Orthop 1991; 270:29.
4. Enneking WF, Kagan A. Transepiphyseal extension of osteosarcoma: incidence, mechanism and implications. Cancer 1978;41:1526–1537.
5. Enneking WF. Staging musculoskeletal tumors. In: Enneking WF (ed) Musculoskeletal Tumor Surgery. Ner York: Churchill Livingstone, 1983:69–123.
6. Rosen G, Marcove RC, Caparros B, et al. Primary osteogenic sarcoma: the rationale for preoperative chemotherapy and delayed surgery. Cancer 1979; 43:2163–2177.
7. Rosen G, Caparros B, Huvos AG, et al. Preoperative chemotherapy for osteogenic sarcoma: selection of postoperative adjuvant chemotherapy based on the response of the primary tumor to preoperative chemotherapy. Cancer 1982;49:1221–1230.
8. Bacci G, Picci P, Pignatti G, et al. Neoadjuvant chemotherapy for nonmetastatic osteosarcoma of the extremities. Clin Orthop 1991; 279:87.
9. Gorrin AM, Anderson JW. Experience with multiagent chemotherapy for osteosarcoma. Clin Orthop 1991;270:22.
10. Link MP, Goorin AM, Miser AS, et al. The effect of adjuvant chemotherapy on relapse-free survival in patients with osteosarcoma of the extremity. N Engl J Med 1986:1600–1606.
11. Link MP, Goorin AM, Horowitz M, et al. Adjuvant chemotherapy of high-grade osteosarcoma of the extremity: updated results of the multi-institution osteosarcoma study. Clin Orthop 1991;270:8.
12. Enneking WF, Kagan A. The implications of "skip" metastases of osteosarcoma. Clin Orthop 1975;111:33–41.
13. Enneking WF, Kagan A. "Skip" metastases in osteosarcoma. Cancer 1975;36:2192–2205.
14. Simon MA. Limb salvage for osteosarcoma: current concepts, review. J Bone Joint Surg Am 1988;70:307.
15. Campanacci M, Picci P, Gherlinzoni F, et al. Parosteal osteosarcoma. J Bone Joint Surg Br 1984;55:313–321.
16. Raymond AK. Surface osteosarcoma. Clin Orthop 1991;270:140.
17. Campanacci M, Picci P, Gherlinzoni F, et al. Parosteal osteosarcoma. J Bone Joint Surg Br 1984;55:313.
18. Picci P, Campanacci M, Bacci G, et al. Medullary involvement in parosteal osteosarcoma: a case report. J Bone Joint Surg Am 1987;69:131–136.
19. Enneking WF, Springfield D, Gross M. The surgical treatment of parosteal osteosarcoma in long bones. J Bone Joint Surg Am 1985;67:125–135.
20. Bertoni F, Boriani S, Laus M, et al. Periosteal chondrosarcoma and periosteal osteosarcoma: two distinct entities. J Bone Joint Surg Br 1982;64:370–376.
21. Hall R, Robinson L, Malawer M, et al. Periosteal osteosarcoma. Cancer 1985;55:165–171.
22. Unni KK, Dahlin DC, Beabout JW. Periosteal osteogenic sarcoma. Cancer 1976;37:2476–2485.
23. Unni KK, Dahlin DC, McLeod RA, et al. Intraosseous well-differentiated osteosarcoma. Cancer 1977;40:1337–1347.
24. Kurt AM, Unni KK, McLeod RA, et al. Low-grade intraosseous osteosarcoma. Cancer 1990;5:1418–1428.
25. Mirra JM. Malignant tumors. Osteosarcoma: intra-medullary variants. In: Mirra J (ed) Bone Tumors Clinical, Radiologic and Pathologic Correlations. Vol 1. Malvern, PA: Lea & Febiger, 1989:248.
26. Bertoni F, Bacchini P, Fabbri N, et al. Osteosarcoma: low-grade intraosseous-type osteosarcoma, histologically resembling parosteal osteosarcoma, fibrous dysplasia, and desmoplastic fibroma. Cancer 1993;71:338.
27. Ayala AG, Ro JY, Raymond AK, et al. Small cell osteosarcoma: a clinicopathologic study of 27 cases. Cancer 1989;64:2162–2173.
28. Bertoni F, Present D, Bacchini P, et al. The Istituto Rizzoli experience with small cell osteosarcoma. Cancer 1989;64:2591–2599.
29. Edeiken J, Raymond AK, Ayala AG, et al. Small cell osteosarcoma. Skeletal Radiol 1987;15:521–628.
30. Sim FH, Unni KK, Beabout JW, et al. Osteosarcoma with small cells stimulating Ewing's tumor. J Bone Joint Surg Am 1979;61:207–215.
31. Sim FH, Unni KK, Beabout JW. Osteosarcoma with small cells simulating Ewing's tumor. J Bone Joint Surg Am 1979;61:207.
32. Huvos AG, Rosen G, Bretsky SS, et al. Telangiectatic osteogenic sarcoma: a clinicopathologic study of 124 patients. Cancer 1982;49:1679–1689.
33. Rosen G, Huvos AG, Marcove R, et al. Telangiectatic osteogenic sarcoma: improved survival with combination chemotherapy. Clin Orthop 1986;207: 164–173.
34. Mervak TR, Unni KK, Pritchard DJ, et al. Telangiectatic osteosarcoma. Clin Orthop 1991;270:135.
35. Pignatti G, Bacci G, Picci P, et al. Telangiectatic osteogenic sarcoma of the extremities: results in 17 patients treated with neoadjuvant chemotherapy. Clin Orthop 1991;270:99.
36. Huvos AG. Osteogenic sarcoma of bones and soft tissues in older persons: a clinicopathologic analysis of 117 patients older than 60 years. Cancer 1986;57:1442–1449.
37. Huvos AG, Butler A, Bretsky SS. Osteogenic sarcoma associated with Paget's disease of bone: a clinicopathologic study of 65 patients. Cancer 1983;52:1489–1495.
38. Schajowicz F, Santini Araujo E, Berenstein M. Sarcoma complicating Paget's disease of bone: a clinicopathologic study of 62 cases. J Bone Joint Surg Br 1983;65:299–307.

CHAPTER 45

Ewing's Sarcoma Family of Tumors

EDWARD F. HOLLINGER
EDWARD H. KOLB

In 1921 James Ewing described a malignant primary bone tumor that, unlike osteogenic sarcoma, was sensitive to irradiation.[1] It was characterized by anaplastic, small round cells closely associated with blood vessels and occurred most often in the diaphysis of long bones. Ewing hypothesized that this tumor was of vascular endothelial origin, calling it a "diffuse endothelioma of bone." Others suggested that it originated from primitive mesenchymal cells. Recent cytogenetic and immunohistochemical studies have confirmed a neural crest origin for Ewing's sarcoma and suggested a spectrum of related malignancies, often termed "Ewing's sarcoma family of tumors" (ESFT). Currently ESFT is defined to include several tumors, all originating from primitive neuroectoderm but with varying degrees of differentiation.[2,3] The least differentiated are classic Ewing's sarcoma (ES), a primary tumor of bone, and extraosseous Ewing's sarcoma (EES), which originates in soft tissues. Atypical Ewing's sarcoma, which can occur in either bone or soft tissue, has additional neural features. Finally, peripheral primitive neuroectodermal tumors (PPNETs), including peripheral neuroepithelioma, adult neuroblastoma, and malignant small cell tumor of the thoracopulmonary region (Askin tumor), represent the most well differentiated members of the ES family.

One of the unifying features of ESFT malignancies is the presence of characteristic genetic translations. The t(11,22) translocation, seen in more than 90% of ESFT malignancies, recombines the *EWS* gene on chromosome 22 and the *FLI-1* gene (which codes for a family of DNA-binding transcription activators) on chromosome 11. Related translocations such as t(21,22) and t(7,22) are less frequent in ESFT lesions. These recombinations produce aberrant proteins that presumably result in inappropriate DNA transcription, yielding an ESFT malignancy.[4]

A. Epidemiology

Ewing's family tumors are second only to osteogenic sarcoma as the most common malignant bone tumors of childhood and adolescence. Overall they represent the fourth most common malignant tumors of bone, occurring in the United States at a rate of about three cases per million white children less

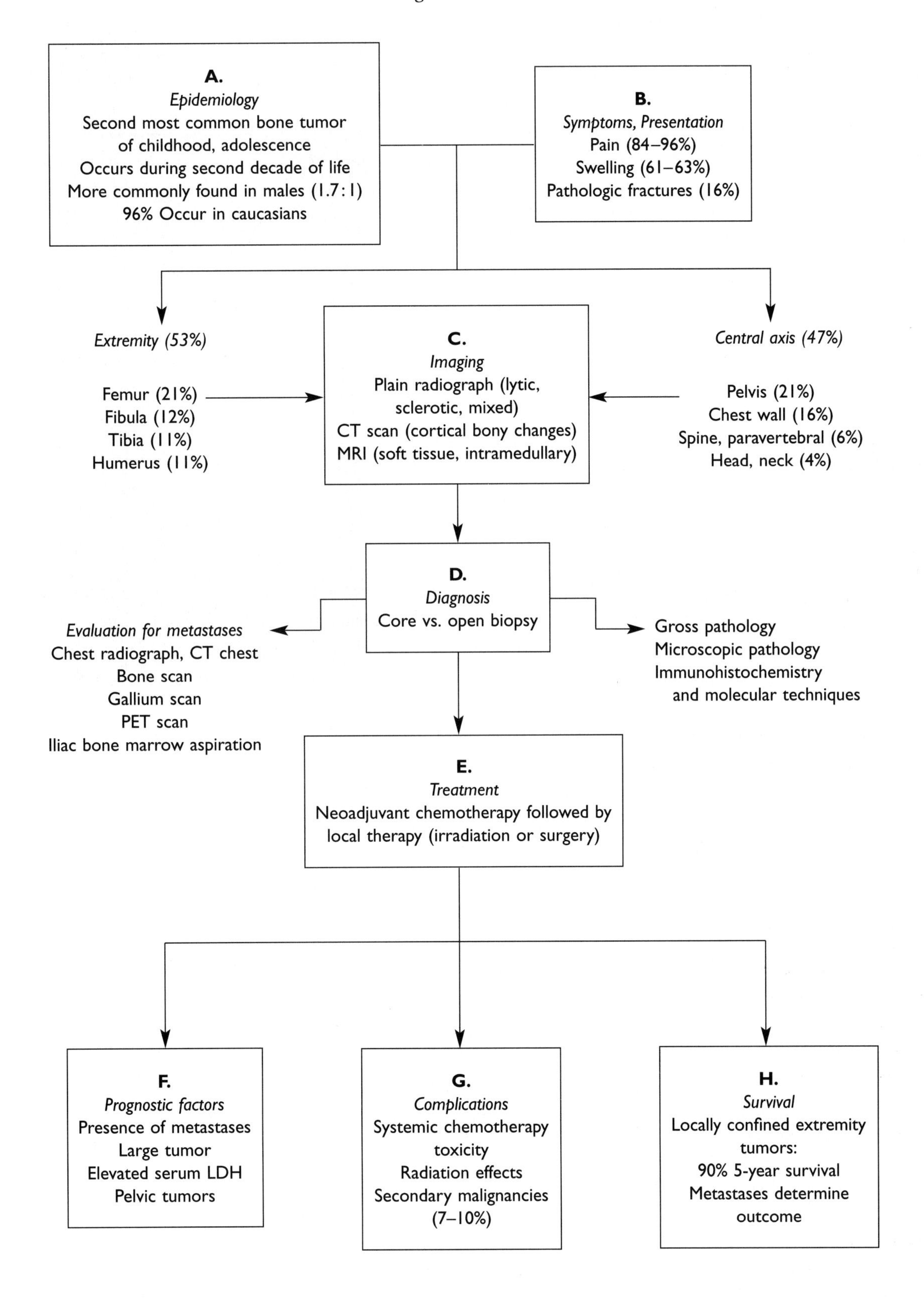
Ewings's Sarcoma
A.
Epidemiology
Second most common bone tumor
of childhood, adolescence
Occurs during second decade of life
More commonly found in males (1.7:1)
96% Occur in caucasians
B.
Symptoms, Presentation
Pain (84–96%)
Swelling (61–63%)
Pathologic fractures (16%)
Extremity (53%)
Femur (21%)
Fibula (12%)
Tibia (11%)
Humerus (11%)
C.
Imaging
Plain radiograph (lytic,
sclerotic, mixed)
CT scan (cortical bony changes)
MRI (soft tissue, intramedullary)
Central axis (47%)
Pelvis (21%)
Chest wall (16%)
Spine, paravertebral (6%)
Head, neck (4%)
D.
Diagnosis
Core vs. open biopsy
Evaluation for metastases
Chest radiograph, CT chest
Bone scan
Gallium scan
PET scan
Iliac bone marrow aspiration
Gross pathology
Microscopic pathology
Immunohistochemistry
and molecular techniques
E.
Treatment
Neoadjuvant chemotherapy followed by
local therapy (irradiation or surgery)
F.
Prognostic factors
Presence of metastases
Large tumor
Elevated serum LDH
Pelvic tumors
G.
Complications
Systemic chemotherapy
toxicity
Radiation effects
Secondary malignancies
(7–10%)
H.
Survival
Locally confined extremity
tumors:
90% 5-year survival
Metastases determine
outcome

than 15 years of age. Several recent studies encompassing 1505 patients with ESFT including ES (87%), EES (8%), and PPNET (5%) provide some insight into the epidemiology.[5] ESFT malignancies occur most commonly during the second decade of life (64%) and less commonly during the first (27%) or third (9%), although tumors may occur in children as young as 5 months or in older adults. They occur more frequently in males (1.7 : 1), with most being seen in white patients (96%); they are rare in African-Americans (1.8%) or other nonwhite races (2.2%). ESFT malignancies are not commonly associated with congenital diseases or familial cancers, and their incidence in siblings is low. Finally, ESFT lesions usually do not occur as a second malignancy.

B. *Symptoms, Presentation*

Ewing's sarcoma can present with local or constitutional symptoms. Local symptoms include pain (84–96%), swelling (61–63%), and pathologic fractures (16%). Fever is the most common systemic symptom (21–28%).[6] Back pain and paraplegia are unusual initial presentations of ESFT (about 1–3%) but require immediate evaluation because untreated spinal cord compression resulting from primary or metastatic disease may cause irreversible neurologic damage. Necrosis in an osseous tumor can cause local hyperemia, warmth, and swelling, which in concert with constitutional symptoms may suggest a diagnosis of osteomyelitis.[7] Extraosseous lesions most frequently present as palpable masses (75%) often with local pain (66%). A long delay between the onset of symptoms and a definitive diagnosis is common, especially with pelvic tumors. In one study the mean treatment delay for Ewing's sarcoma was nearly 10 months.[8] Delay is more common when tumor pain is intermittent (68% of cases in one study) or when no palpable mass is present.

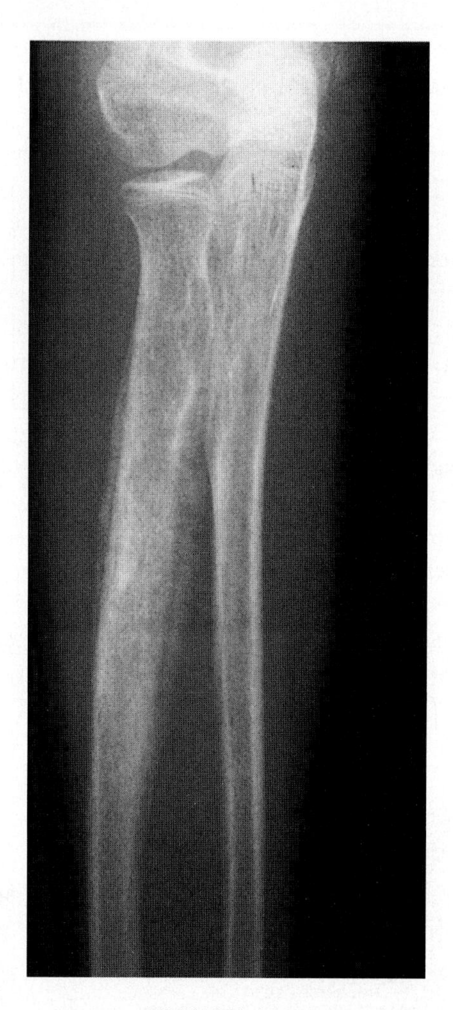

FIGURE 45–1
Ewing's sarcoma of the radius. There is permeative destruction of the cortex of the proximal one-half of the bone with an extensive "spiculated" perpendicular periosteal reaction.

C. *Imaging*

The evaluation and staging of patients with ESFT malignancies focuses on careful characterization of the primary site and a search for metastatic disease. No specific serologic tumor markers are currently available. The erythrocyte sedimentation rate (ESR) may be elevated (about 50% of patients), and the lactate dehydrogenase (LDH) level should be measured because increases are associated with a worse prognosis.[9] In the future, molecular techniques may be available to assist with the serologic diagnosis. For the present, however, evaluation of patients with ESFT is primarily by imaging and biopsy.

Unlike osteosarcoma, which predominantly develops in long bones, Ewing's family malignancies can develop at almost any site. In a recent compilation, the primary ESFT lesion occurred in an extremity in 53% of cases and the central axis in the remainder. Central axis tumors occurred most frequently in the pelvis (45%), chest wall (34%), spine or paravertebral region (12%), or the head and neck (9%). Extremity tumors were nearly evenly split between distal (52%) and proximal (48%) locations.[5] The lower extremity is more commonly involved than the upper, with most tumors occurring in the femur (21% of all tumors), fibula (12%), tibia (11%), or humerus (11%).[6] In long bones Ewing's sarcoma usually develops in the diaphysis rather than at the epiphysis, the typical location for osteosarcoma. PPNETs usually occur in the central axis (74%), most often in or around the chest (60%).

Local disease should be evaluated with plain radiographs of the involved site and with tomographic techniques.[10] Plain-film radiographs of Ewing's sarcoma of cylindrical bones often reveal a lytic or mixed lytic and sclerotic lesion of the diaphysis, sometimes with periosteal or trabecular reactive bone formation. Several patterns of periosteal reaction are possible. Lesions with rapid intermittent growth may form multiple thin shells of ossification oriented parallel to the shaft of the bone, yielding a lamellated "onion skin" appearance. Those that grow more continuously display a perpendicular periosteal reaction with a spiculated "hair on end" appearance of ossified Sharpey's fibers (Fig. 45–1). Finally, ossification along a flap of elevated periosteum creates a Codman's triangle when viewed tangentially on a radiograph (Fig. 45–2). Lesions of flat bones such as the pelvis can present as geographic lytic or mixed lytic and sclerotic lesions (Fig. 45–3). However, a wide variety of imaging findings are possible, and "classic" presentations are the exception rather than the rule. Computed tomography (CT) and magnetic resonance imaging (MRI) provide complementary information about the extent of local disease (Fig. 45–2). CT scans best demonstrate cortical bony changes, whereas MRI is more sensitive for assessing soft tissue and medullary involvement. Bone marrow involvement is best assessed from T1-weighted MRI sequences, and soft tissues are usually better defined on intermediate (proton density) or T2-weighted images.[11] Finally, angiography may be useful for delineating the vascular anatomy prior to any surgical intervention.

D. *Diagnosis: Biopsy*

Biopsy of the primary tumor should be undertaken with careful consideration to several factors. Fine-needle aspiration generally does not obtain sufficient tissue for histologic evaluation, so core or open biopsy is preferred. The biopsy site must be chosen with consideration for potential resection incision sites or irradiation fields. Furthermore, biopsy sites in poorly vascularized tissues are at higher risk for injury following irradiation or chemotherapy. Biopsy techniques and sites must also be chosen carefully to minimize compromise of underlying bone stability with the accompanying increased risk of pathologic fractures. Finally, open biopsy should be conducted with attention to minimizing contamination of adjacent tissues or compartments. In one study 4.5% of patients underwent unnecessary amputations, and 8.5% had adverse outcomes because poor biopsy techniques were

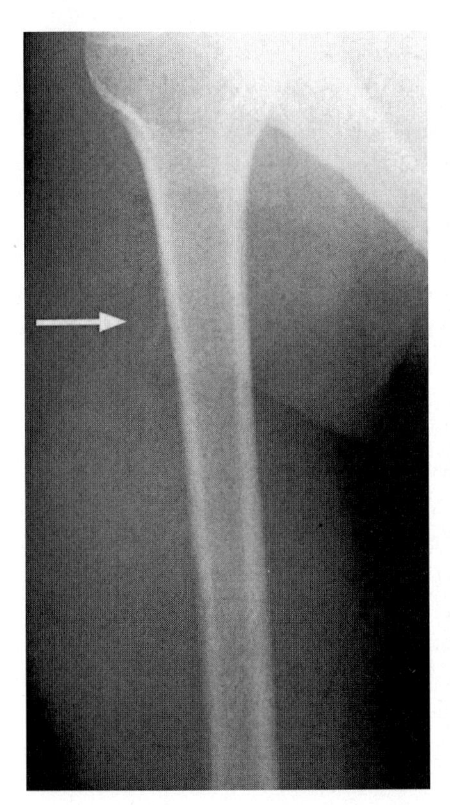

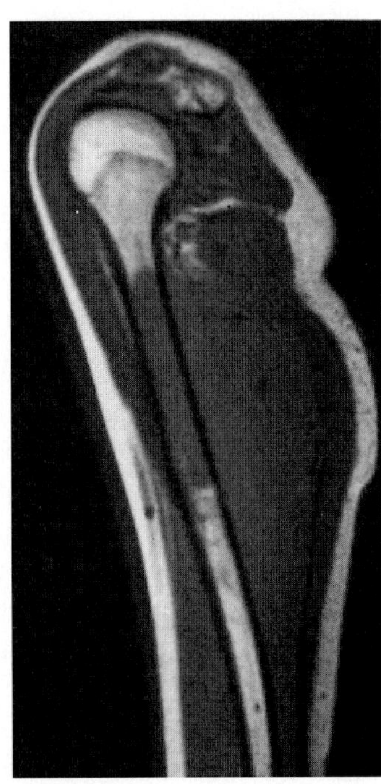

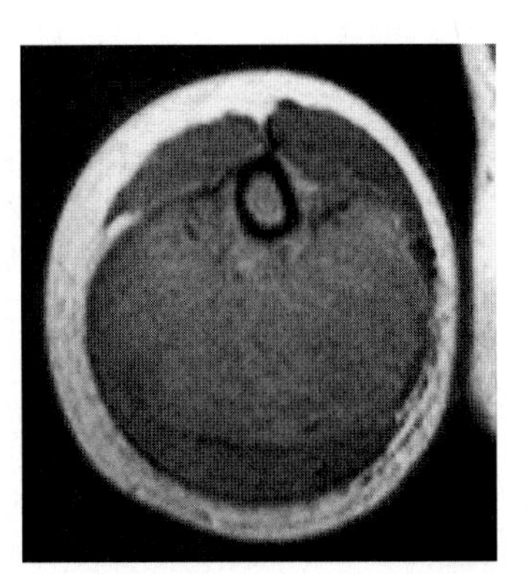

FIGURE 45–2

Ewing's sarcoma of the humerus. Plane film radiograph (left) demonstrates a thin rim of periosteal elevation (Codman's triangle) along the posterior aspect of the proximal humerus (arrow), slight thinning of the cortex, and surrounding increased soft tissue density. The longitudinal T1-weighted magnetic resonance image (middle) demonstrates an extensive signal void in the medullary cavity, and the proton-density transaxial magnetic resonance image (right) shows a surrounding large soft tissue mass.

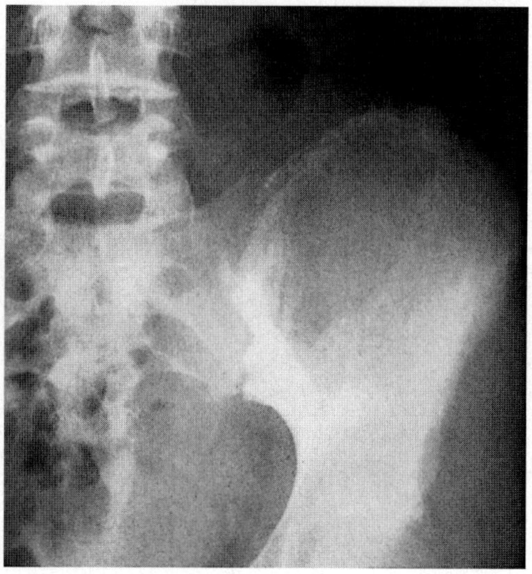

FIGURE 45–3
Ewing's sarcoma of the pelvis. A large "geographic" lytic lesion of the left ileum is seen extending to but not involving the sacroiliac joint. Note destruction of the cortical rim of the superior aspect of the ileum.

used.[12] This led the authors to recommend that the surgeon who is to perform the definitive procedure also conduct the biopsy, as biopsy-related problems occurred more frequently when the biopsy was performed at a referring institution rather than the treatment center.

Gross Pathology

The ESFT lesions are composed of firm, gray-white soft tissue that has a glistening, wet appearance when sectioned. Tumors originating from bone may extend through the cortex to form an accompanying soft tissue component, and often diffusely involve the marrow cavity. Likewise, primary soft tissue lesions such as extraosseous Ewing's sarcoma may invade adjacent bony structures and often are more friable on sectioning. In both cases tumor necrosis can result in hemorrhagic or cystic regions in the tumor.

Microscopic Pathology

The ESFT lesions are members of a group of neoplasms composed of small, round, blue cells. Other "small round cell" tumors include non-Hodgkin's lymphoma, neuroblastoma, and rhabdomyosarcoma. On light microscopy ESFT lesions exhibit increased mitotic activity, often with focal regions of tumor hemorrhage and necrosis. Classic undifferentiated Ewing's sarcoma is composed of broad sheets of small round cells with scant cytoplasm and homogeneous round basophilic nuclei. Cells are tightly packed with little intervening extracelluar matrix, but islands of fine fibrovascular septa containing small-caliber blood vessels may be seen. Periodic acid-Schiff (PAS) staining of classic Ewing's sarcoma cells demonstrates abundant glycogen after alcohol fixation but usually not after formalin fixation. Tumors usually invade adjacent tissues by compression, resulting in "pushing" margins at the tumor borders. Atypical Ewing's sarcoma shows somewhat larger cells with more prominent nuclear heterochromatin and nucleoli. The cells are arranged in sheets or nests often with some intervening collagen matrix and usually contain less glycogen than classic Ewing's cells. Infiltrative margins are more commonly seen with atypical Ewing's sarcoma.

The PPNETs are the most well differentiated of the ESFT malignancies, and often demonstrate neural phenotypic features. Microscopically, PPNET cells have more abundant cytoplasm and may have neurite-like cytoplasmic processes containing neurofilaments or microtubules. The cells are arranged in organoid, alveolar, or lobular patterns and may comprise Flexner-type rosettes (gland-like structures) or Homer-Wright pseudorosettes (annuli of cells around a central collection of eosinophilic fibrils) more typical of neural tumors. However, mature neural elements such as ganglion cells or nerve fascicles are not seen.[5,13]

Immunohistochemical and Molecular Techniques

Often ESFT malignancies cannot be differentiated from other small round cell tumors strictly on the basis of microscopic findings. Several other techniques can be applied to strengthen the diagnosis. The HBA-71 (CD99) and 12E7 antibodies recognize cell surface antigens expressed in more than 90% of ESFT malignancies, forming the basis for the "Ewing's stain."[14] More well differentiated ESFT lesions such as PPNETs may be identified by neural markers such as S-100 and neuron-specific enolase. The presence of other markers such as leukocyte common antigen (lymphoma) or desmin and muscle actin (rhabdomyosarcoma), suggests alternative tumor types. Thus a panel of markers can be used to identify the tumor morphology more definitively. Molecular assays such as the reverse transcriptase-polymerase chain reaction (RT-PCR) can look for characteristic translocations in tumor tissue even when traditional histopathologic techniques are equivocal.[4] These assays are beginning to be employed to diagnose ESFT and to distinguish ESFT lesions from other sarcomas; they may supplant other testing in the future.

Prior to the advent of systemic chemotherapy, distant failure rates in excess of 80% following radical amputation were observed. This suggests that most patients with ESFT malignancies have at least micrometastases when diagnosed; on average, about 25% of patients have clinically overt metastases at the time of diagnosis. Metastasis occurs primarily by the hematogenous route, usually to the lung (38%), bone (31%), and bone marrow (11%).[15] Metastasis to the central nervous system, lymph nodes, or liver is much less common. Extraosseous Ewing's sarcoma may spread directly to adjacent structures, including intraabdominal viscera; and chest wall tumors can invade the pleural space, causing pleural effusions.

Evaluating for Metastasis

Imaging for metastatic disease should also be conducted at the time of the initial diagnosis. Chest radiography and CT should be used to identify pulmonary metastases. Radionuclide techniques may be useful for evaluating local disease but are most helpful when screening for distant metastases. Bone scans with technetium-99m methylene diphosphonate (MDP) can demonstrate reactive bone formation surrounding metastatic lesions. Ewing's sarcoma also avidly accumulates gallium-67 citrate. Finally, positron emission tomography with 18-fluorodeoxyglucose (FDG) may be useful for evaluating primary tumors and metastases and their response to therapy.[16] A biopsy of bone marrow distant to the primary tumor should be undertaken to evaluate for metastatic disease. Bilateral iliac bone marrow aspiration has been suggested for this purpose.

E. Treatment

There is no generally accepted staging system for ESFT malignancies, although treatment protocols are often delineated based on the presence or absence of metastatic disease and the location of the primary tumor. Treatment of ESFT malignancies focuses on local control using surgery, radiotherapy, or both, as well as systemic chemotherapy to treat occult or overt metastatic disease. Patients with ESFT malignancies should be treated with protocols specifically designed for these diseases. In general, after thorough evaluation, treatment begins with intense neoadjuvant chemotherapy that treats metastatic disease and usually reduces local tumor volume. Local therapy can then be attempted with surgery or radiotherapy (or both).[17] PPNET responds to the same chemotherapeutic agents used to treat ES, but outcomes are generally poorer.[18] Optimal therapy for ESFT lesions remains the subject of significant research.

Radiotherapy or surgery alone is associated with high failure rates, and significant survival benefits are seen when systemic chemotherapy is added. The most commonly used chemotherapeutic agents include vincristine, dactinomycin, cyclophosphamide, and doxorubicin. Specific doses and treatment schedules are largely dictated by local protocols and the occurrence of side effects, especially neutropenia. Studies have also demonstrated benefit when ifosfamide and etoposide are added for patients with localized bone tumors.[19]

The relative roles of surgery and radiotherapy in achieving local control continue to be debated. Several studies have suggested that surgery with chemotherapy yields better local control or better survival than radiotherapy plus chemotherapy.[18,20] Not all analyses support this conclusion. It is generally agreed that tumors of dispensable bones such as the clavicles, fibula, ribs, or small bones of the hands or feet should be resected. Large lesions that fail to respond to induction chemotherapy or lesions that persist after chemotherapy and local radiotherapy are also candidates for surgical salvage. In young patients, lesions near the epiphysis may be more amenable to surgery than radiotherapy because of the significant growth and functional deficits associated with epiphyseal irradiation. The specific choice of surgical procedure is based on tumor location and size, with careful consideration given to achieving complete tumor eradication and maximizing postoperative function. Although earlier studies suggested that surgical resection margins should be based on tumor size at diagnosis, recent protocols generally define complete resection based on tumor margins after induction chemotherapy. Complete resection (radical or wide margins) is associated with lower relapse rates than incomplete resection (marginal or intralesional margins) even when combined with radiotherapy.[21,22] If radiotherapy is to be combined with surgery, postoperative irradiation may be preferred because of the lower incidence of surgical complications.[23]

Radiation therapy has also been applied for local treatment of ESFT malignancies. Traditionally, the entire medullary cavity of the involved bone was included for at least part of the treatment. However, several studies have suggested that tailored irradiation fields encompassing less than the whole bone can be just as effective.[24] Common practice is to use initial doses of 40–55 Gy with an additional 10–15 Gy to the boost volume, for a total tumor dose of 50–65 Gy. A conventional radiotherapy schedule (1.8–2.0Gy/fraction once a day, 5 days a week) is typically used, although other schedules are under investigation.

F. Prognostic Factors

Several prognostic factors for ESFT lesions have been identified. The presence of metastatic disease, large tumor volume (>8cm longest diameter in some studies), elevated serum LDH, hypoalbuminemia, and patient age older than 17 years at diagnosis have been associated with poorer prognoses in various studies.[19,25] Pelvic tumors have worse outcomes than tumors in other locations, although this may stem from the fact that pelvic tumors are often relatively large at the time of diagnosis. Extraosseous ESFT lesions may have a worse prognosis than primary bone lesions.[26] Finally, good radiologic and pathologic responses of the tumor to induction chemotherapy are associated with more favorable outcomes.[19] The prognosis for patients with recurrent disease is poor, with the length of survival depending on the extent and site of recurrence, the aggressiveness of the tumor, previous therapy, and time to failure.

G. Complications

The most significant complications following therapy for ESFT malignancies are systemic toxicity associated with chemotherapy, local effects of irradiation, and late complications. The most serious late complication is the development of secondary malignancies, which occurs in 7–10% of patients treated for ESFT.[27,28] This risk is considered significant enough to warrant long-term screening for survivors of ESFT malignancies.

H. Survival

Introduction of neoadjuvant systemic chemotherapy along with local tumor control has drastically improved outcomes associated with ESFT malignancies from the 5–10% five-year survival seen 25 years ago. The presence of metastatic disease at diagnosis remains the most important predictor of long-term survival. Patients with localized extremity tumors without metastases have been shown to have 5-year actuarial and metastasis-free survivals of 90% and 48%, respectively.[29] Overall, long-term survivals of 50–70% are generally reported. However, if clinical imaging at diagnosis demonstrates metastatic disease, long-term survival decreases to less than 30% at 4 years.[30]

References

1. Ewing J. Diffuse endothelioma of bone. Proc NY Pathol Soc 1921;21:17.
2. Kovar H. Ewing's sarcoma and peripheral primitive neuroectodermal tumors after their genetic union. Curr Opin Oncol 1998;10:334–342.
3. Granowetter L. Ewing's sarcoma and extracranial primitive neuroectodermal tumors. Curr Opin Oncol 1996;8:305–310.
4. Kovar H, Aryee D, Zoubek A. The Ewing family of tumors and the search for the Achilles' heel. Curr Opin Oncol 1999;11:275–284.
5. Horowitz ME, Malawer MM, Woo SY, Hicks MJ. Ewing's sarcoma family of tumors: Ewing's sarcoma of bone and soft tissue and the peripheral primitive neuroectodermal tumors. In: Pizzo PA, Poplack DG (eds) Principles and Practice of Pediatric Oncology. Philadelphia: Lippincott-Raven, 1997: 831–863.
6. Kissane JM, Askin FB, Foulkes M, Stratton LB, Shirley SF. Ewing's sarcoma of bone: clinicopathologic aspects of 303 cases from the Intergroup Ewing's Sarcoma Study. Hum Pathol 1983;14:773–779.
7. Durbin M, Randall RL, James M, Sudilovsky D, Zoger S. Ewing's sarcoma masquerading as osteomyelitis. Clin Orthop 1998;357:176–185.
8. Sneppen O, Hansen LM. Presenting symptoms and treatment delay in osteosarcoma and Ewing's sarcoma. Acta Radiol Oncol 1984;23:159–162.
9. Bacci G, Ferrari S, Longhi A, et al. Prognostic significance of serum LDH in Ewing's sarcoma of bone. Oncol Rep 1999;6:807–811.
10. Fletcher BD. Imaging pediatric bone sarcomas: diagnosis and treatment-related issues. Radiol Clin North Am 1997;35:1477–1494.
11. Boyko OB, Cory DA, Cohen MD, Provisor A, Mirkin D, DeRosa GP. MR imaging of osteogenic and Ewing's sarcoma. AJR Am J Roentgenol 1987; 148:317–322.
12. Mankin HJ, Lange TA, Spanier SS. The hazards of biopsy in patients with malignant primary bone and soft-tissue tumors. J Bone Joint Surg Am 1982;64:1121–1127.
13. Dehner LP. Primitive neuroectodermal tumor and Ewing's sarcoma. Am J Surg Pathol 1993;17:1–13.
14. Ushigome S, Shimoda T, Takaki K, et al. Immunocytochemical and ultrastructural studies of the histogenesis of Ewing's sarcoma and putatively related tumors. Cancer 1989;64:52–62.
15. Cangir A, Vietti TJ, Gehan EA, et al. Ewing's sarcoma metastatic at diagnosis: results and comparisons of two intergroup Ewing's sarcoma studies. Cancer 1990;66:887–893.
16. Jones DN, McCowage GB, Sostman HD, et al. Monitoring of neoadjuvant therapy response of soft-tissue and musculoskeletal sarcoma using fluorine-18-FDG PET. J Nucl Med 1996;37:1438–1444.
17. Bacci G, Picci P, Mercuri M, et al. Predictive factors of histological response to primary chemotherapy in Ewing's sarcoma. Acta Oncol 1998;37: 671–676.
18. Kimber C, Michalski A, Spitz L, Pierro A. Primitive neuroectodermal tumours: anatomic location, extent of surgery, and outcome. J Pediatr Surg 1998;33:39–41.
19. Grier HE. The Ewing family of tumors: Ewing's sarcoma and primitive neuroectodermal tumors. Pediatr Clin North Am 1997;44:991–1004.
20. Givens SS, Woo SY, Huang LY, et al. Non-metastatic Ewing's sarcoma: twenty years of experience suggests that surgery is a prime factor for successful multimodality therapy. Int J Oncol 1999;14:1039–1043.
21. Sabanathan S, Shah R, Mearns AJ. Surgical treatment of primary malignant chest wall tumours. Eur J Cardiothorac Surg 1997;11:1011–1016.
22. Ozaki T, Hillmann A, Hoffmann C, et al. Significance of surgical margin on the prognosis of patients with Ewing's sarcoma: a report from the Cooperative Ewing's Sarcoma Study. Cancer 1996;78:892–900.
23. Hillmann A, Ozaki T, Rube C, et al. Surgical complications after preoperative irradiation of Ewing's sarcoma. J Cancer Res Clin Oncol 1997; 123:57–62.
24. Donaldson SS, Torrey M, Link MP, et al. A multidisciplinary study investigating radiotherapy in Ewing's sarcoma: end results of POG: 8346. Int J Radiat Oncol Biol Phys 1998;42:125–135.

25. Aparicio J, Munarriz B, Pastor M, et al. Long-term follow-up and prognostic factors in Ewing's sarcoma: a multivariate analysis of 116 patients from a single institution. Oncology 1998;55:20–26.
26. Baldini EH, Demetri GD, Fletcher CD, Foran J, Marcus KC, Singer S. Adults with Ewing's sarcoma/primitive neuroectodermal tumor: adverse effect of older age and primary extraosseous disease on outcome. Ann Surg 1999;230:79–86.
27. Kuttesch JF Jr, Wexler LH, Marcus RB, et al. Second malignancies after Ewing's sarcoma: radiation dose-dependency of secondary sarcomas. J Clin Oncol 1996;14:2818–2825.
28. Novakovic B, Fears TR, Horowitz ME, Tucker MA, Wexler LH. Late effects of therapy in survivors of Ewing's sarcoma family tumors. J Pediatr Hematol Oncol 1997;19:220–225.
29. Elomaa I, Blomqvist C, Saeter G, et al. Chemotherapy in Ewing's sarcoma: the Scandinavian Sarcoma Group experience. Acta Orthop Scand Suppl 1999;285:69–73.
30. Paulussen M, Ahrens S, Burdach S, et al. Primary metastatic (stage IV) Ewing tumor: survival analysis of 171 patients from the EICESS studies; European Intergroup Cooperative Ewing Sarcoma Studies. Ann Oncol 1998;9:275–281.

CHAPTER 46

Osseous Metastases

MICHAEL J. HEJNA

The survival of patients with osseous metastases has improved over the past several years owing to advances in the understanding of tumor cell biology and refinement of treatment protocols. For example, 50% of patients with breast cancer metastatic to bone survive 35 months after the development of osseous lesions.[1] With the increased life expectancy of patients with bony metastases has come a greater need to address the problems associated with these lesions, namely pain and pathologic fracture. Either can result in significant functional loss with an attendant decrease in the quality of life. The primary objectives of orthopedic management are to reduce pain, prevent pathologic fracture, provide stability when fractures occur, and protect vital structures, particularly the neural elements. Rapid return of function is paramount in patients undergoing surgery for metastatic disease of the skeletal system.

Skeletal metastases occur most frequently in the axial skeleton and proximal segments of the appendicular skeleton.[2] Management of skeletal metastases involves (1) establishing the diagnosis, (2) assessing the impact of the lesion(s) on the patient's quality of life, and (3) applying available orthopedic techniques and devices when appropriate. Devices used for surgical management of osseous metastases are either identical to or slight modifications of those used in the nonpathologic setting. The surgeon must be cognizant of the biologic and biomechanical factors affecting the individual patient and lesion.

A. Diagnosis

The diagnosis of osseous metastases should be clearly established prior to considering surgical management. Frequently, the patient presents with bone pain and a history of metastatic cancer. The surgeon should thoroughly review the medical history and any imaging studies performed during the course of the initial workup or subsequent surveillance. Radiographs of the symptomatic region should be evaluated for evidence of bony destruction. A bone scan should be obtained to confirm the presence of a destructive process and to evaluate for the presence of additional lesions that may affect the surgical plan. Biopsy is not necessary if the patient has documented bony metastases, in which case surgical stabilization can be performed if indicated by the mechanical and clinical circumstances.

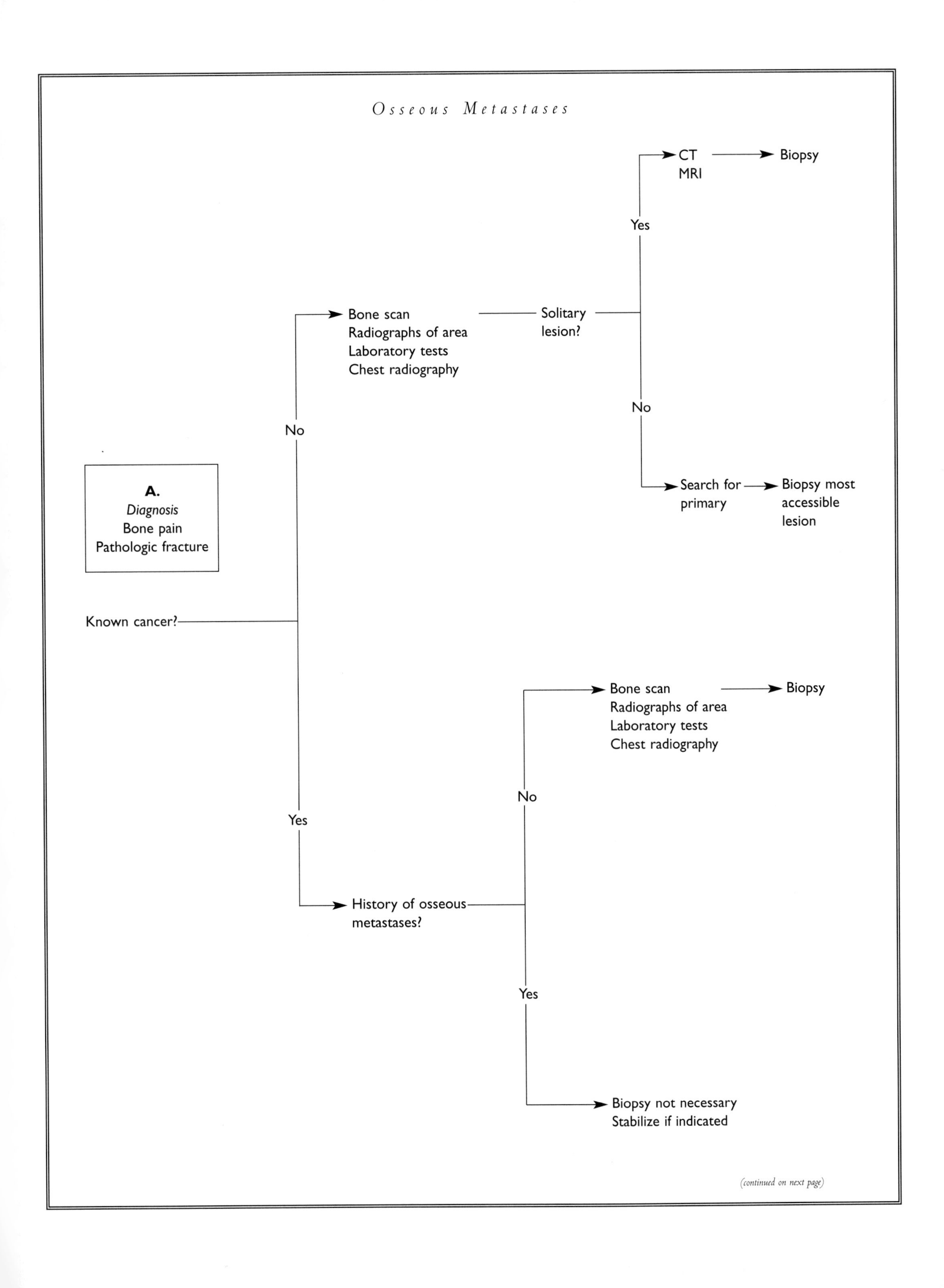

(continued on next page)

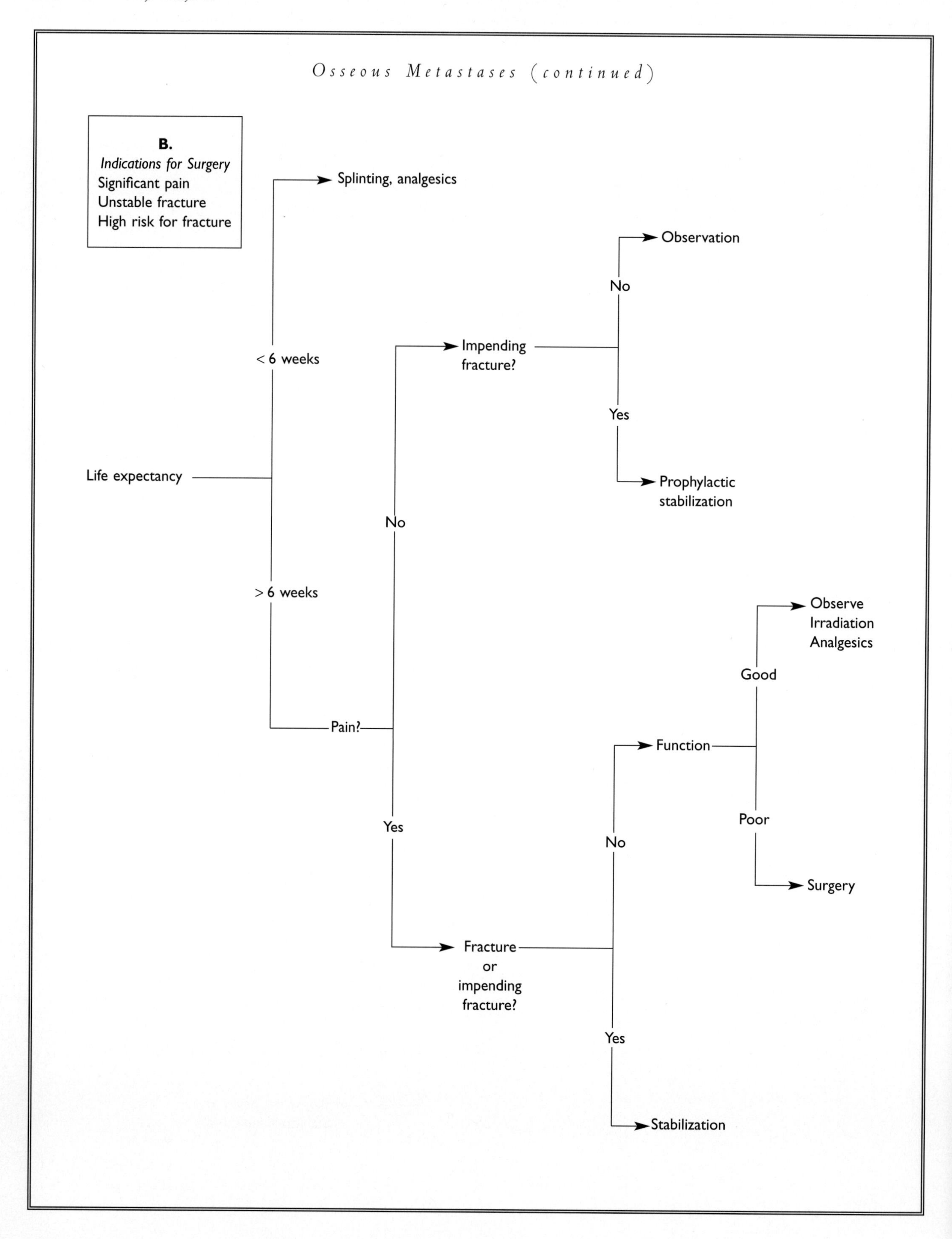
Osseous Metastases (continued)
B.
Indications for Surgery
Significant pain
Unstable fracture
High risk for fracture
Life expectancy
< 6 weeks
Splinting, analgesics
> 6 weeks
Pain?
No
Impending fracture?
No
Observation
Yes
Prophylactic stabilization
Yes
Fracture or impending fracture?
No
Function
Good
Observe
Irradiation
Analgesics
Poor
Surgery
Yes
Stabilization

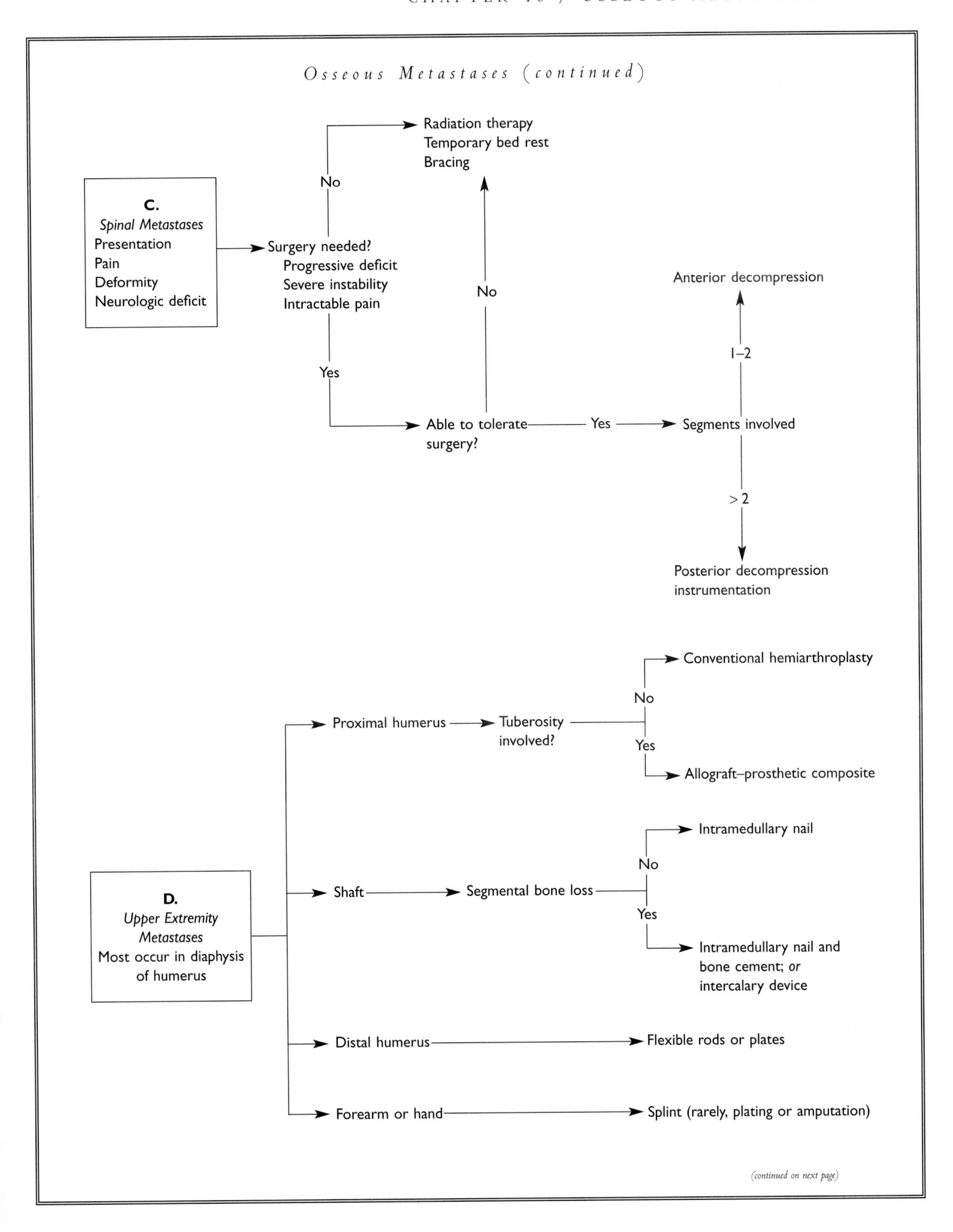

(continued on next page)

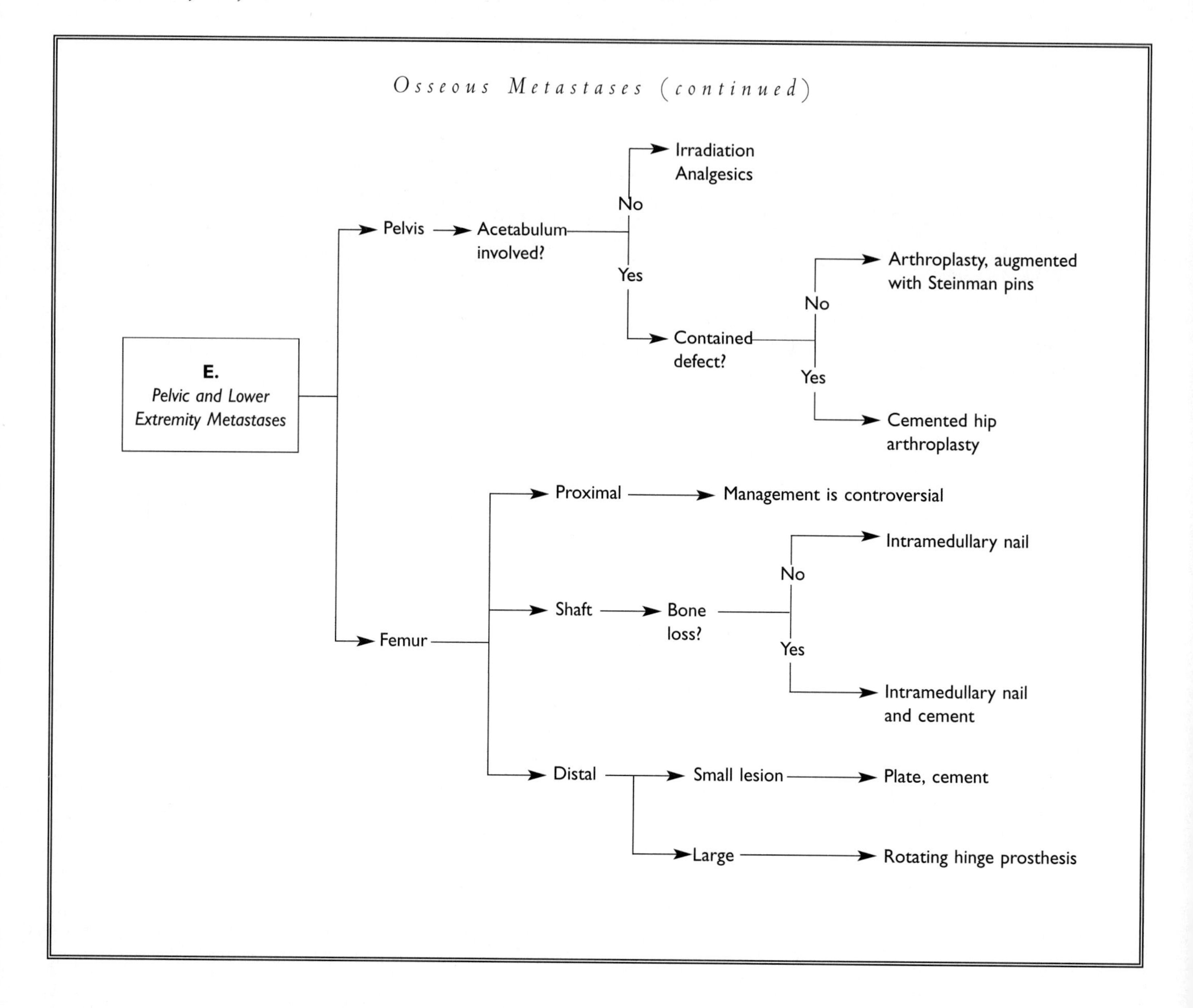

Less frequently, the patient presents with a history of malignancy but no known metastatic disease. The patient may have musculoskeletal pain or a fracture in this clinical setting, and the diagnosis must be confirmed histologically prior to surgical treatment. The workup should be coordinated with the internist and medical oncologist. Occasionally, the history of cancer is relatively remote, and the patient may believe that he or she is cured of the disease or that the disease is in remission. The emotional response of the patient to being informed of the potential diagnosis of metastatic cancer should not be underestimated.

As stated, the skeletal evaluation should include a bone scan. Radiographs should be obtained of areas demonstrating increased uptake of radionuclide. Additional local imaging may be necessary to determine the degree of bone destruction and extent of intramedullary or soft tissue extension. Chest radiography should be performed, as should laboratory tests. The most accessible lesion, skeletal or nonskeletal, should be biopsied to confirm the diagnosis of metastasis. Orthopedic management according to the principles outlined below is then planned.

Occasionally, the patient presents with a destructive bone lesion or pathologic fracture with no history of a prior malignancy. Thorough evaluation of the patient is necessary and obtaining a histologic diagnosis is mandatory prior to operative orthopedic management. Primary bone sarcoma must be clearly ruled out, as the surgical management differs substantially from that of osseous metastases. Inappropriate initial management of a primary bone sarcoma may preclude limb salvage surgery and may jeopardize survival.

The most common sites of origin of skeletal metastases are breast, lung, thyroid, kidney, and prostate.[2] Suspected bony metastases can be biopsied by percutaneous or open means. If the cortex has been completely eroded by the tumor, needle biopsy is generally sufficient and is usually performed under computed tomography (CT) guidance. If needle aspiration is not possible or fails to provide the diagnosis, open biopsy is indicated. If multiple lesions are present, the lesion that can be biopsied with the lowest morbidity is selected. The surgical approach is through an overlying muscle rather than through intermuscular planes, thereby facilitating resection of a single muscle group should the lesion be found to be a primary bone sarcoma. The cortex is opened using a drill, small trephine, or burr under fluoroscopic guidance. Histologic evaluation with frozen section should be performed; if the diagnosis is clear by frozen section, stabilization can be performed immediately. If the diagnosis is unclear, stabilization should be delayed to prevent dissemination of a potentially resectable tumor. Meticulous hemostasis should be obtained.

B. *Indications for Surgery*

The decision to recommend surgery for metastatic bone disease is multifactorial and involves input from the patient, patient's family, internist, medical oncologist, radiation oncologist, and orthopedic surgeon. Of primary importance is the anticipated survival of the patient. Surgery is generally not indicated for patients with an anticipated survival of less than 6–8 weeks. This time period may be adjusted slightly depending on the surgical morbidity and length of recovery for the procedure in question and on the risks of nonoperative management. Closed nailing of a long bone to prevent fracture through a metastatic focus may be indicated even with a relatively short life expectancy, whereas reconstruction for a symptomatic acetabular lesion may not be indicated unless the prognosis for survival is otherwise good.

The severity of symptoms is a major determinant when treating osseous metastases. Pain due to metastatic lesions of the skeleton may be severe and may significantly affect the quality of life. Surgical treatment is occasionally indicated to relieve symptoms even if there is relatively little risk of an impending fracture (e.g., lesions of the acetabulum). If the lesion does not pose a significant risk of fracture and symptoms can be alleviated by radiotherapy or the use of analgesics, nonoperative orthopedic management is indicated.

The decision to perform an orthopedic procedure for osseous metastases must involve consideration of the patient's medical status. The presence of metastases to other organs and their impact on the patient's ability to tolerate anesthesia should be carefully assessed. Neutropenia, electrolyte abnormalities, coagulopathy, and significant anemia should be corrected if possible to minimize the risk of perioperative complications. Patient and family wishes must be respected in the decision-making process. The acceptance of surgical risk, additional hospital stay, postoperative discomfort, extent of rehabilitation, and cost must be weighed against the burden of chronic pain and functional limitation.

The orthopedic implications of the metastatic focus are extremely important in the decision to undertake operative treatment. If a fracture has occurred, its stability should be determined. Shaft fractures of the femur are extremely unstable and require surgical management in nearly all ambulatory patients. Compression fractures of the vertebrae, in contrast, are generally stable and usually can be treated with observation or bracing.

If fracture has not occurred, the risk of fracture must be assessed. Femoral shaft lesions more than 2.5 cm in diameter or more than 50% of the diameter of the bone are at high risk for fracture and should be stabilized.[3,4] These criteria may be adjusted depending on the quality of bone, thickness of the cortex, and presence of additional lesions. Determining the fracture risk is quite difficult in some locations; large interobserver differences have been noted for evaluating fracture risk for lesions of the proximal femur, for example.[5] Certain fractures present difficult treatment problems, and therefore prevention is desirable (e.g., subtrochanteric fracture of the femur). Consideration should be given to stabilization for small lesions in these locations (see specific anatomic algorithms).

Lesions in weight-bearing locations require more aggressive management than those of non-weight-bearing regions. The impact of reduced weight-bearing by the upper extremities should be carefully assessed and not underestimated. Patients with lower extremity disorders that affect their ability to ambulate (metastatic disease, degenerative joint disease, neurologic dysfunction) may depend increasingly on the upper extremities for support. A reduction in upper extremity function may render the patient wheelchair-bound, which in turn may lead to requirement of a full-time caregiver.

Involvement of joints and the effect on joint function by the disease and its treatment should be assessed. Joint replacement for lesions involving the proximal femur may provide rapid relief of symptoms and return of function. Prosthetic implants are now available for reconstructing extensive portions of the proximal and distal femur. The advantages of using joint prostheses must be weighed against longer operating times, greater blood loss, and greater potential for perioperative and late morbidity.

The degree of bone loss affects the ability to achieve mechanical stability. Orthopedic fracture implants generally are load-sharing devices that experience fatigue failure if unsupported by bone. In the nonpathologic fracture setting, fracture healing usually occurs before the implant fails. Often the patient's postoperative management is tailored to reduce the likelihood of implant failure prior to fracture healing. This may be accomplished, for example, by maintaining partial weight-bearing with crutches until the fracture heals. The patient with osseous metastases presents several major problems with respect to the biomechanical performance of fracture implants. First, fracture healing is less rapid and less predictable than in the nonpathologic setting. This is due to the presence of tumor and may be further impaired by poor nutritional status and treatment of the tumor with radiation. Second, the ability of most cancer patients to tolerate and adhere to weight-bearing restrictions is poor. Finally, the need for rapid return to function to maximize quality of life is great. Fracture implants for osseous metastases must be selected to accommodate more immediate function. Large implants and implants not dependent on bone healing (e.g., joint prostheses) are utilized when possible. Often the implant must be modified or augmented with bone cement.

C. *Spinal Metastases*

Patients with metastatic disease of the spine may present with pain, deformity, a neurologic deficit, or a combination of these problems. Nonoperative treatment with radiation therapy, temporary bed rest, or bracing results in improvement in most cases.[6] Indications for surgical intervention are progressive neurologic deficit, intractable pain, and significant spinal instability.[7] Pathologic burst fractures in which there are fragments of bone in the spinal canal are most likely to result in a neurologic deficit refractory to conservative care.

Most commonly, metastases to the spine involve the vertebral body. Collapse of the anterior and middle columns may lead to retropulsion of fragments into the spinal canal and kyphotic deformity. Decompression of the spinal canal by laminectomy alone further destabilizes the spine and is therefore contraindicated. Anterior spinal decompression and stabilization is performed for involvement of up to two consecutive vertebrae. Use of allograft bone or a prosthetic device to restore the anterior and middle columns is necessary. This may require a thoracotomy or retroperitoneal exposure, depending on the levels involved. Longer segments requiring stabilization (three or more vertebrae) are treated with posterior instrumentation and fusion. The ability of the patient to tolerate surgery of this magnitude and the relatively lengthy recuperative period must be carefully considered.

D. *Upper Extremity*

The majority of osseous metastases of the upper extremity occur in the *diaphysis of the humerus*. Pathologic fractures are common. The use of an intramedullary nail with proximal and distal locking is recommended for most shaft fractures.[8] It provides for rotational and axial stability and protects the entire shaft against fracture should additional lesions develop. Shoulder pain following insertion of a humeral nail is common and has led many orthopedic surgeons to treat traumatic shaft fractures of the humerus with plates. In the patient with osseous metastases, the advantages of reduced operating time, surgical dissection, and blood loss outweigh the potential for chronic shoulder pain. Augmentation of the device with methacrylate may be necessary when there is significant segmental bone loss. Care must be taken to avoid injury to the radial nerve which courses posterior to the shaft at its midpoint. The nerve may be injured by trauma or by heat produced during exothermic curing of the methacrylate cement.

Intercalary implants may also be used to treat segmental defects of the humerus. The intercalary device consists of a body with a diameter approximating that of the humeral shaft and with a stem designed for intramedullary placement at each end. The construct is modular so bodies and stems of appropriate length can be selected. The stems are cemented into the proximal and distal segments of the humerus. Because the surgery is of significantly greater magnitude than intramedullary nailing, use of the intercalary device is reserved for cases of failed internal fixation or extensive bone destruction and tumors for which radiotherapy is not likely to be effective.[9]

Lesions of the proximal humerus are generally treated with hemiarthroplasty. If there is destruction of the tuberosities, rotator cuff function is poor. Patients should be counseled that forward elevation and abduction is generally less than 90°. For extensive destruction of the proximal humerus, allograft–prosthesis composite reconstruction is indicated. The long-stem prosthetic humeral implant is first cemented into an allograft segment of the proximal humerus. The protruding portion of the stem of the prosthesis is then cemented into the remaining distal portion of the native humerus followed by the rotator cuff tendons of the allograft being sutured to those of the patient, which minimizes the chance of subluxation or dislocation of the humeral head.

Pathologic fractures of the distal humerus are difficult to manage owing to the complexity of the elbow joint and the limited amount of bone available for attachment of the implant. Rush rods and other flexible intramedullary devices are generally used to treat these fractures. External support (bracing) is usually required to provide additional stability.

E. *Pelvis and Lower Extremity*

Metastatic lesions of the pelvis and lower extremity are a common cause of pain and loss of quality of life. A wide range of surgical implants and techniques are available. Surgery provides the greatest stability and symptomatic relief with the lowest possible morbidity, and quickest return of function. *Pelvic lesions other than those of the acetabulum do not require surgical treatment.* Lesions of the iliac wing, pubis and ischium are generally treated with radiotherapy and analgesics. Acetabular lesions are amenable to treatment by total hip arthroplasty. In contained defects in which the acetabular walls are intact, the lesion is debulked by intralesional curettage after dislocation of the hip. The acetabulum is then prepared to accept a cemented acetabular component. The component is cemented in place as in conventional cemented hip arthroplasty.

Uncontained lesions of the acetabulum require additional support for the cement and acetabular component. It is provided by Steinman pins, which are drilled into the ilium from within the bony acetabulum.[8] The acetabular component is then cemented in place, incorporating the Steinman pins as reinforcing bars in the cement. The femoral head is replaced out of necessity to provide congruity with the prosthetic acetabulum. This procedure requires extensive exposure and poses significant risk to the sciatic nerve and iliac vessels.

There are no clear guidelines for stabilizing the proximal femur in the presence of osseous metastases without fracture. Interobserver agreement is poor for assessing the fracture risk of lesions of the femoral head, neck, and intertrochanteric region.[5] Surgical treatment should be undertaken if pain is poorly controlled, the patient is unable to ambulate, or there is significant fracture risk in the surgeon's judgment. Lesions confined to the femoral head and neck are treated with conventional hip replacement. If the lesion extends to the intertrochanteric region, a calcar-replacement device is utilized. For lesions extending to the subtrochanteric region, a proximal femoral replacement device is required.

Isolated lesions of the intertrochanteric region are treated by stabilization with a compression screw-side plate device. The lesion is curetted through a drill hole in the lateral cortex of the femur. Liquid cement is then injected into the bone, and the device is cemented prior to curing of the cement.

Isolated lesions of the subtrochanteric region and shaft are generally better delineated on radiographs owing to the involvement of cortical bone. Lesions more than 2.5 cm in length or more than 50% of the diameter of the bone should be treated with prophylactic intramedullary nailing. Stabilization of smaller lesions, particularly in the subtrochanteric region, may be considered, as this is an area of extremely high mechanical stress. Full-length radiographs of the shaft of the femur should be obtained and a bone scan carefully examined for coexisting lesions of the distal femur that might preclude distal locking of the nail. The distal end of the nail should not lie at or near a metastatic focus, as the resultant stress-riser predisposes to fracture.

Metastatic lesions of the distal femur are uncommon. The difficulty of assessing fracture risk in the metaphyseal bone of the proximal femur apply to the distal femur as well. Small lesions may be treated with conventional fracture devices supplemented with methacrylate cement. Larger lesions extending to the articular surface should be treated with a rotating hinge-type distal femoral replacement prosthesis that allows removal of as much bone as necessary. Conventional knee replacement implants have little role in the management of metastatic disease as they preserve all but a small amount of subchondral bone.

Metastases to the distal portions of the upper and lower extremities are rare. These lesions should be managed with radiotherapy, casting or bracing, or both A dysfunctional limb with osseous metastasis is rarely amputated.

Pathologic fractures of the proximal femur require surgical treatment to alleviate pain and allow ambulation. The exception is the patient with an expected survival of less than 4–6 weeks. The type of implant depends on the location of the fracture and is the same as described for an impending fracture. Occasionally, a custom device such as a long-stem prosthesis with holes for distal locking is required.

In all cases of surgical management of osseous metastases, avoiding complications is paramount. Postoperative irradiation and chemotherapy, if indicated, should be postponed for 2–3 weeks to allow soft tissue healing. Perioperative antibiotics should be employed and wounds carefully monitored for signs of infection, particularly in the neutropenic patient. Complications requiring additional hospitalization and treatment are particularly significant for patients with limited life expectancy.

Summary

Orthopaedic care of the patient with osseous metastases requires thorough evaluation of the patient and careful assessment of the orthopaedic implications of the skeletal lesion or lesions. The diagnosis must be clearly established prior to surgical treatment. Both the physician and patient must have a clear understanding of the goals of surgery. With effective orthopaedic management patients with skeletal metastases can experience significant improvement in their function and quality of life.

References

1. Yamashita K, Koyama H, Inaji H. Prognostic significance of bone metastasis from breast cancer. Clin Orthop 1995;312:89–94.
2. Frassica F, Sim F. Pathogenesis and prognosis. In: Sim F (ed) Diagnosis and Management of Metastatic Bone Disease: A Multidisciplinary Approach. New York: Raven, 1988:1–6.
3. Beals R, Lawton G, Snell W. Prophylactic internal fixation of the femur in metastatic breast cancer. Cancer 1971;28:1350–1354.
4. Parrish F, Murray J. Surgical treatment for secondary neoplastic fractures: a retrospective study of ninety six patients. J Bone Joint Surg Am 1970;52:665–686.
5. Hipp J, Springfield D, Hayes W. Predicting pathologic fracture risk in the management of metastatic bone defects. Clin Orthop 1995;312:120–135.
6. Harrington K. Metastatic tumors of the spine: diagnosis and treatment. J Am Acad Orthop Surg 1993;1:76–86.
7. Hosono N, Yonenobu K, Fuji T, et al. Orthopaedic management of spinal metastases. Clin Orthop 1995;312:148–159.
8. Harrington K. Orthopaedic management of extremity and pelvic lesions. Clin Orthop 1995;312:136–147.
9. Sim F, Frassica F, Chao Y. Orthopaedic management using new devices and prostheses. Clin Orthop 1995;312:160–172.

SECTION  9

Genitourinary Cancers

CHAPTER 47

Cancer of the Bladder

JAMES M. KOZLOWSKI
NORM SMITH

A. *Epidemiology and Etiology*

The urothelial "system" is the transitional cell-lined urinary conduit that includes the renal calyx, pelvis, ureter, bladder, and proximal urethra. Consequently, more than 90% of the malignancies arising within this "system" are transitional cell carcinomas. Because it serves as a reservoir and is thus subject to more prolonged contact with the initiators, promoters, and propagators of carcinogenesis, bladder involvement vastly exceeds that of the ureter and renal pelvis (50:3:1, respectively). Bladder cancers are typified by the field cancerization concept, which implies a predisposition to multifocality and recurrence rates of 50–75%. Despite this well recognized trend toward polychronotropism, molecular studies have confirmed the uniclonal origin of most bladder cancers.[1–3]

Approximately 54,000 new bladder cancers are diagnosed annually in the United States, and this neoplasm accounts for about 12,000 cancer-related deaths.[4] These tumors are more common in men than in women (2–3:1), are more common in Caucasians than in African-Americans (2:1), and have a peak incidence during the mid-sixth decade. Bladder cancer represents the fourth most common cancer in men and the eighth most common cancer in women.[4]

Acknowledged risk factors include cigarette smoking; occupational exposure to aryl amines (particularly 4-aminobiphenyl)[5]; urinary tract inflammation associated with chronic infection (*Schistosoma haematobium*), indwelling catheters, and stones[6]; prolonged cyclophosphamide exposure[7]; and phenacetin abuse. Balkin nephropathy and hereditary nonpolyposis colon cancer (HNPCC) predispose to upper tract disease.[8] Individual susceptibility to these and other provocative factors appears to be determined by such factors as the polymorphic expression of the *N*-acetyltransferase (*NAT*) and *S*-transferase M1 (*GSTM1*) genes.[9]

B. *Natural History*

As stated previously, most bladder cancers are transitional cell carcinomas (90%). Squamous cell carcinomas (8–9%) tend to develop in a background of chronic inflammation and infection. Pure adenocarcinomas (1–2%) generally originate as solitary tumors from the trigone or bladder dome, with

Bladder Cancer

A.
Epidemiology and Etiology
54,200 New cases per year
12,100 Annual deaths
Men > women
Caucasians > African-Americans
Peak sixth decade
Risk factors: exposure to aryl amines; chronic infection; stones; catheters; hereditary colon cancer

B.
Natural History
90% Transitional cell, 8–9% squamous cell, 1–2% adenocarcinoma
75% Superficial (muscle spared); of these, 15–25% progress and invade
25% Invasive; of these, 50% have metastases

C.
Presentation
Hematuria
Imitative voiding symptoms

D.
Diagnosis
Imaging studies mandatory: intravenous pyelography (study of choice), US, CT scan (obtain before transurethral resection)
Cystoscopy: initially can be performed in office; if TURBT is planned, perform in operating room; obtain urine culture and cytology

E.
Staging
Second cystoscopy may be needed

(continued on next page)

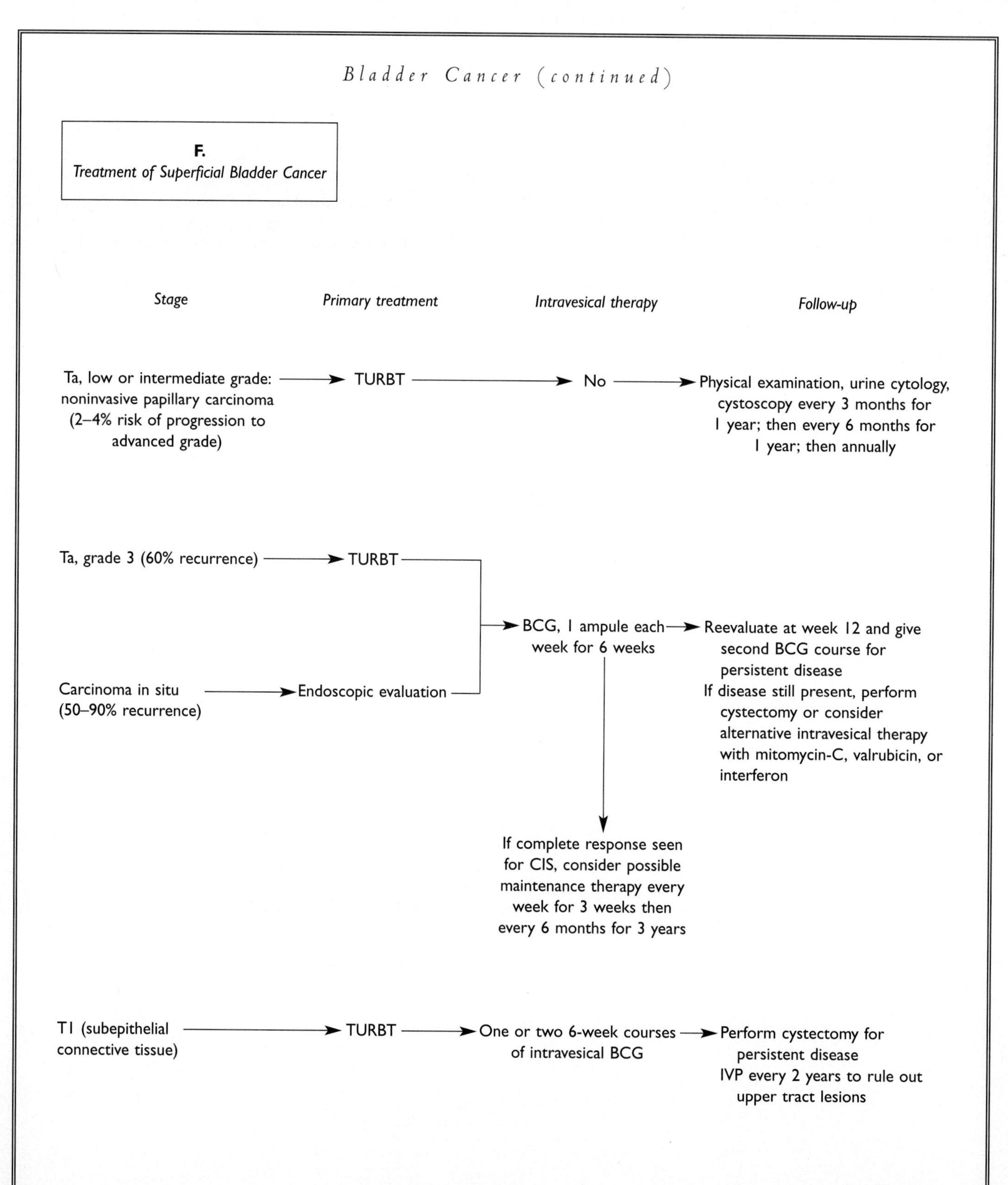
Bladder Cancer (continued)
F.
Treatment of Superficial Bladder Cancer
Stage
Primary treatment
Intravesical therapy
Follow-up
Ta, low or intermediate grade: noninvasive papillary carcinoma (2–4% risk of progression to advanced grade)
TURBT
No
Physical examination, urine cytology, cystoscopy every 3 months for 1 year; then every 6 months for 1 year; then annually
Ta, grade 3 (60% recurrence)
TURBT
BCG, 1 ampule each week for 6 weeks
Reevaluate at week 12 and give second BCG course for persistent disease
If disease still present, perform cystectomy or consider alternative intravesical therapy with mitomycin-C, valrubicin, or interferon
Carcinoma in situ (50–90% recurrence)
Endoscopic evaluation
If complete response seen for CIS, consider possible maintenance therapy every week for 3 weeks then every 6 months for 3 years
T1 (subepithelial connective tissue)
TURBT
One or two 6-week courses of intravesical BCG
Perform cystectomy for persistent disease
IVP every 2 years to rule out upper tract lesions

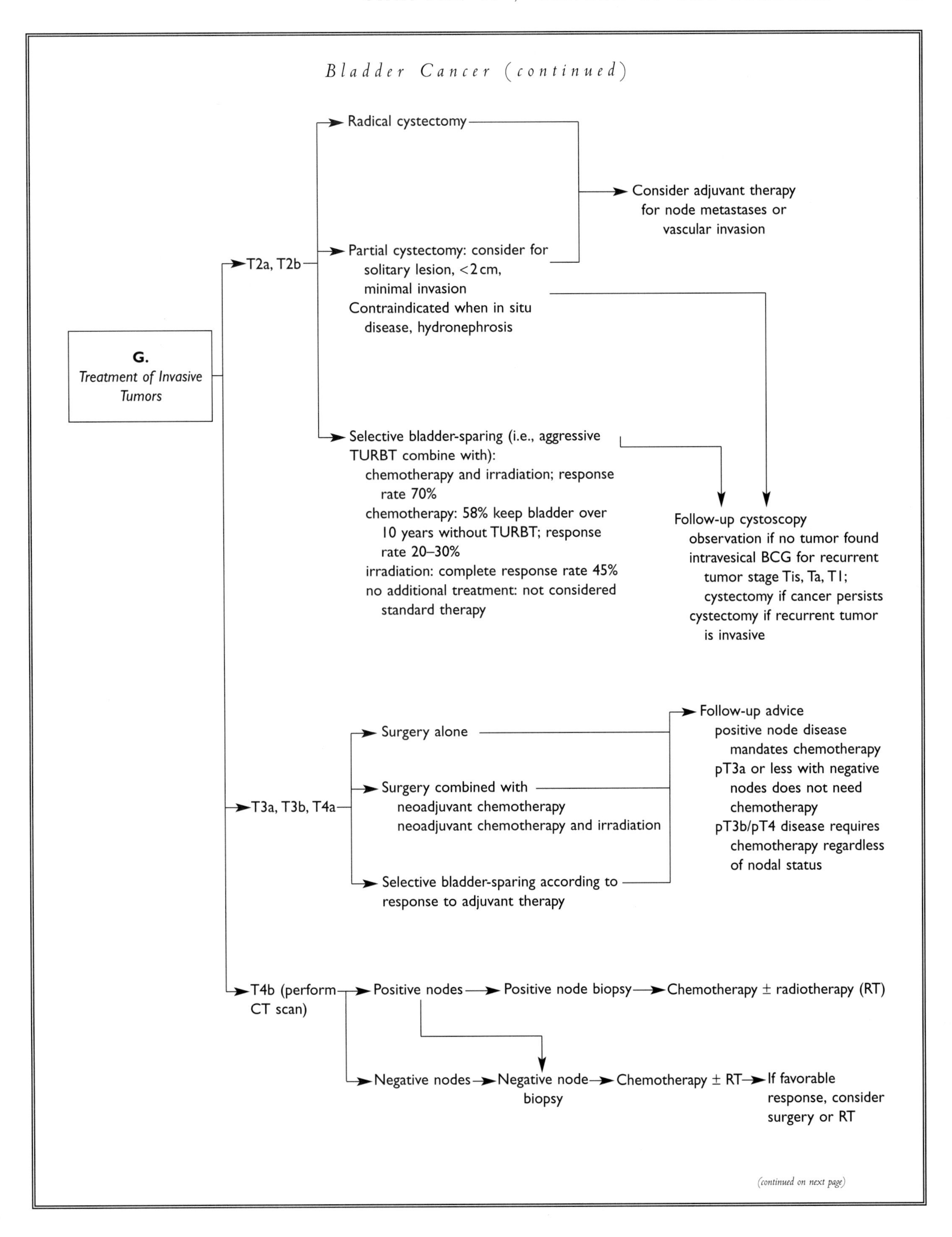

(continued on next page)

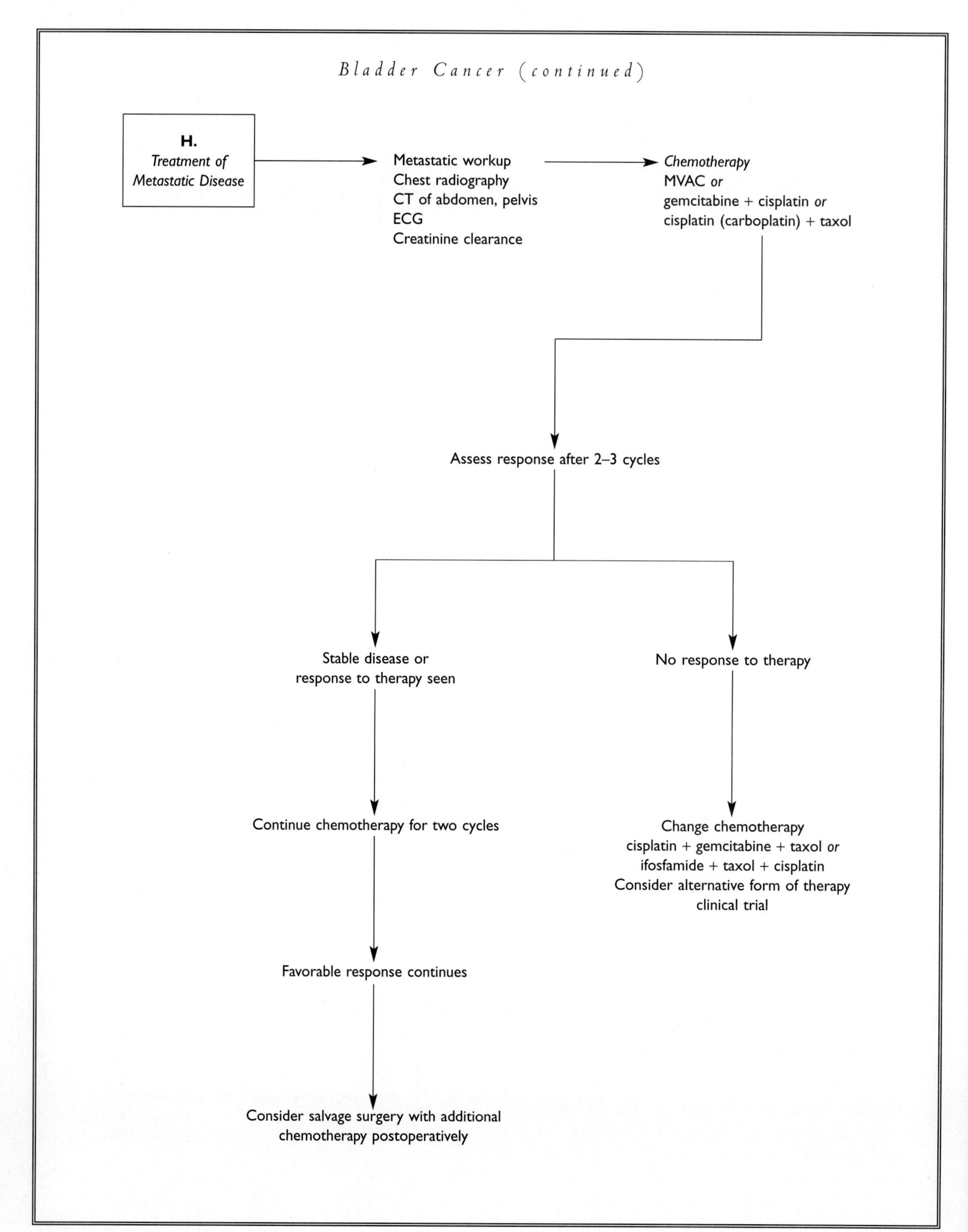
Bladder Cancer (continued)
H.
Treatment of
Metastatic Disease
Metastatic workup
Chest radiography
CT of abdomen, pelvis
ECG
Creatinine clearance
Chemotherapy
MVAC or
gemcitabine + cisplatin or
cisplatin (carboplatin) + taxol
Assess response after 2–3 cycles
Stable disease or
response to therapy seen
No response to therapy
Continue chemotherapy for two cycles
Change chemotherapy
cisplatin + gemcitabine + taxol or
ifosfamide + taxol + cisplatin
Consider alternative form of therapy
clinical trial
Favorable response continues
Consider salvage surgery with additional
chemotherapy postoperatively

the latter reflecting malignant degeneration of the urachal remnant.

About 75% of bladder cancers are "superficial," which implies that the true muscular wall of the bladder (tunica muscularis propria) is not involved. An additional 25% of cases are "invasive" at initial presentation. With respect to the latter, 50% of the patients have occult metastases and ultimately succumb to the disease process. Of note, only 15–25% of superficial cancers progress to a muscle-invasive variant. It is the current perception that superficial and invasive tumors represent biologically distinct neoplasms that differ with respect to many phenotypes. The latter includes the preferential expression of distinct angiogenic pathways (superficial tumors: vascular endothelial growth factor; invasive tumors: thymidine phosphorylase).[10]

Confined to the Mucosa

Most superficial bladder tumors are mucosa-confined papillary neoplasms of low to intermediate grade (60%). Pure carcinoma in situ (CIS) is seen in 10% of cases, is generally diffuse, and is typified by irritative voiding symptoms. CIS may be seen with 30–70% of exophytic bladder tumors, and its presence renders progression to muscle-invasive disease much more likely (42–83%). Virtually all CIS lesions are high grade (grade III) and exhibit DNA aneuploidy.

Invasion of the Lamina Propria

Tumors that invade the lamina propria (T1) account for 30% of superficial cancers. Indeed, T1 tumors represent a unique subset of "superficial disease"; approximately 25–30% progress to muscle-invasive disease, and 7–10% have metastasized to the pelvic nodes at presentation. The potential volatility of T1 lesions has prompted an attempt at pathologic microstaging. PT1a is defined as tumor extension superficial to the muscularis mucosa–vascular plexus level; pT1b represents extension within that interface, and pT1c represents extension beyond this boundary.[11] The latter represents penetration into the lamina propria of >1.5 mm. The potential importance of such microstaging is validated by observations that a combination of pT1c and CIS increases the risk of progression by a factor of 27 compared with the absence of pT1c and CIS.[11]

Invasion of Muscularis

Muscle-invasive tumors involve the tunica muscularis propria and beyond (T2–T4). Involvement of intramural lymphatic and vascular channels is characteristic of these tumors, which are generally grade III neoplasms. It is of note that virtually all squamous cell carcinomas and adenocarcinomas are muscle-invasive. The current American Joint Committee on Cancer (AJCC) staging classifications are summarized in Table 47–1.

TABLE 47–1.
AJCC definition of TNM and stage grouping for bladder cancer

Primary Tumor (T)

TX	Primary tumor cannot be assessed
T0	No evidence of primary tumor
Ta	Noninvasive papillary carcinoma
Tis	Carcinoma *in situ*: "flat tumor"
T1	Tumor invades subepithelial connective tissue
T2	Tumor invades muscle
T2a	Tumor invades superficial muscle (inner half)
T2b	Tumor invades deep muscle (outer half)
T3	Tumor invades perivesical tissue
T3a	Microscopically
T3b	Macroscopically (extravesical mass)
T4	Tumor invades any of the following: prostate, uterus, vagina, pelvic wall, abdominal wall
T4a	Tumor invades prostate uterus, vagina
T4b	Tumor invades pelvic wall, abdominal wall

Regional Lymph Nodes (N)

Regional lymph nodes are those within the true pelvis; all others are distant lymph nodes.

NX	Regional lymph nodes cannot be assessed
N0	No regional lymph node metastasis
N1	Metastasis in a single lymph node, 2 cm or less in greatest dimension
N2	Metastasis in a single lymph node, more than 2 cm but not more than 5 cm in greatest dimension; or multiple lymph nodes, none more than 5 cm in greatest dimension.
N3	Metastasis in a lymph node more than 5 cm in greatest dimension

Distant Metastasis (M)

MX	Distant metastasis cannot be assessed
M0	No distant metastasis
M1	Distant metastasis

Stage Grouping

Stage	*T*	*N*	M
0a	Ta	N0	M0
0is	Tis	N0	M0
I	T1	N0	M0
II	T2a	N0	M0
	T2b	N0	M0
III	T3a	N0	M0
	T3b	N0	M0
	T4a	N0	M0
IV	T4b	N0	M0
	Any T	N1	M0
	Any T	N2	M0
	Any T	N3	M0
	Any T	Any N	M1

SOURCE: Used with the permission of the American Joint Committee on Cancer (AJCC®), Chicago, IL. The original source for this material is the AJCC® Cancer Staging Manual, 5th edition (1997) published by Lippincott Williams & Wilkins Publishers, Philadelphia, PA.

Molecular studies have provided a number of useful insights. Nearly all superficial tumors exhibit 9q deletions compared to fewer than one-half of muscle-invasive tumors.[12] Molecular phenotypes that predispose to disease progression include DNA aneuploidy, high S-phase activity, 11p deletions, increased expression of epidermal growth factor receptor and its ligands (epidermal growth factor and transforming growth factor-α)[13] and loss of heterozygosity at 17p. The latter is particularly important because it represents the locus for the *p53* tumor suppressor gene. Normal or wild-type p53 is an important cell cycle regulator that modulates traversing the G_1–S interface. Indeed, overexpression of mutated *p53* ($\geq$20%) in the tumor cell nuclei detected by immunohistochemical methods constitutes a significant independent predictor of disease recurrence and overall survival.[14]

C. Presentation

Hematuria is the most common symptom at presentation and can be identified in about 75% of patients. The degree of hematuria is not related to tumor volume or stage.[15] Gross hematuria is classically of the "total, painless" variety. Irritative or "infection-like" symptoms such as urgency and severe dysuria are noted in 30% of cases. Indeed, these symptoms are the presentation hallmark of carcinoma in situ, which provokes an intense inflammatory reaction within the bladder wall. Tumors involving the ureter or upper collecting system may cause flank pain or be associated with a palpable mass. The latter may be secondary to hydronephrosis, expansive tumor growth, or both. Finally, some patients present with symptoms referable to locally advanced or metastatic disease. With respect to the latter, the potential target sites include deep pelvic/upper retroperitoneal lymph nodes, lung, liver, bone, and brain.

D. Diagnosis

A thorough history and complete physical examination are mandatory. In addition, urinalysis, complete blood count, and serum chemistries should be performed. In most instances urine is also submitted for culture and sensitivity testing. Voided urine cytologic examination is recommended despite its poor sensitivity for low-grade transitional cell carcinomas. The urinary cytology is typically positive in patients with multifocal carcinoma in situ given the high-grade nature of this neoplasm and its proclivity for poor cell-to-cell attachment.

All patients require endoscopic evaluation of the lower urinary tract (cystoscopy) and ureterorenoscopy is required if imaging studies suggest an upper tract abnormality. Cystoscopy permits visual inspection of the entire lower tract "field." All tumor-bearing areas are either resected to visual completion [i.e., transurethral resection of a bladder tumor (TURBT)] or appropriately sampled to establish a histologic diagnosis. Whether the problem is unifocal or multifocal is determined, and the presence/absence of tunica muscularis propria involvement is documented. Fluorescence endoscopy with δ-aminolevulinic acid may improve bladder tumor detection rates. Random biopsies are performed judiciously to avoid iatrogenic tumor implantation. After the bladder is rendered visually disease-free, bladder washing may be a useful adjunct. This procedure involves mechanical exfoliation of the urothelial lining and often obviates the need for multiple bladder biopsies. The pelvis should be examined under anesthesia (EUA) to rule out fixation of the bladder to the bony parietes or adjacent viscera. Finally, the intravesical instillation of mitomycin-C: (40 mg/40 cc sterile water) for 30–60 minutes following TURBT may decrease iatrogenic seeding.

Appropriate imaging studies of the urinary tract are mandatory. When not contraindicated, intravenous pyelography (IVP) is the imaging study of choice.[16] Typically, urothelial cancer presents as a "filling defect" that may involve both lower and upper tracts. The differential diagnosis of such "filling defects" includes tumor, stone, blood clot, sloughed papilla, fungus ball, urothelial inflammation with edema, and "pseudotumors" created by overlying vessels and adjacent segments of bowel. Alternative imaging strategies might include ultrasonography or noncontrast computed tomography (CT) imaging in concert with retrograde pyelography performed at the time of endoscopic evaluation. In general, CT and magnetic resonance imaging (MRI) are not used for the initial evaluation of these patients. If the IVP strongly suggests the possibility of bladder cancer, it is desirable to undertake CT imaging prior to endoscopic resection, as resection may create a distortion artifact.

The general lack of sensitivity of urinary cytology to detect bladder cancer (particularly low-grade tumors) has served as the impetus to identify more sensitive markers of bladder cancer that can be identified in voided urine specimens.[17] The latter include assays for the following: human complement (H) factor (BTA STAT/TRAK Tests)[18]; nuclear matrix protein NMP 22[19]; telomerase[20]; fibrinogen/fibrin degradation products (Accu-Dx and AuraTek FDP)[21]; and tumor-associated hyaluronidase and hyaluronic acid.[22] Each of these assays has demonstrated some degree of enhanced sensitivity for detecting urothelial cancers, but their ultimate application to individual patients awaits clarification. A comparative analysis of these new markers documented that urinary telomerase has the highest combination of sensitivity (70%) and specificity (99%).[23] Other approaches with potential utility include the analysis of nuclear shape/DNA content; urothelium-associated cytokeratins (8, 18, 20); and urinary angiogenic peptides (VEGF).

E. Staging

The most recent AJCC staging system is summarized in Table 47–1. Tumors that do not involve the tunica muscularis propria are designated "superficial bladder cancers." As stated previously, tumors involving the lamina propria (T1) represent a unique subset of superficial cancers. Further subsetting of this group (T1a–c) has been described. Repeat endoscopic resection should be considered for T1 lesions to rule out a staging error (i.e., T2–T3), which occurs in about one-third of patients with residual disease following the second-look TURBT. In general, additional diagnostic imaging for staging purposes is not required in patients with unequivocally superficial disease.

Involvement of the tunica muscularis propria defines "muscle-invasive" disease. These patients should also be considered for a "second look" endoscopic procedure that would permit additional sampling of the tumor base. Approximately 10% of patients are rendered pathologically disease-free (stage P0) with such an approach. All patients with invasive disease require additional diagnostic imaging. A chest radiograph is usually sufficient to evaluate the lungs (if negative). Any abnormality on the chest radiograph should prompt CT imaging. All patients require abdominal/pelvic CT imaging (with infusion). MR imaging of the pelvis is used selectively. Bone scans and imaging of the central nervous system are required only when involvement of those sites is strongly suspected because of symptoms. An assessment of differential renal function (MAG-3 renal scan) is prudent in patients with upper tract involvement due to intrinsic disease or lower tract obstruction. Detection of significant hydronephrosis should prompt a consideration of retrograde or antegrade decompression (with placement of double-J ureteral stents) prior to embarking on a definitive course of therapy.

F. *Treatment of Superficial Bladder Cancer*

Ta, G1 or G2 Lesions

Noninvasive, papillary (Ta) tumors of low to intermediate grade (G1, G2) are associated with a low risk of progression to a more advanced stage (2–4%). Consequently, TURBT without intravesical therapy constitutes appropriate management. Given the fact that these tumors have a high likelihood of recurrence (50–75%), appropriate surveillance is required. The latter consists of physical examination, urine cytology, and repeat cystoscopy at 3-month intervals for the first year, at 6-month intervals for the second year, and yearly for a lifetime.[16] Disease recurrence mandates reversion to 3-month surveillance intervals and should prompt a trial of intravesical therapy [usually bacillus Calmette-Guérin (BCG)].

Ta, G3 or Tis Lesions

The likelihood of recurrence increases with disease multiplicity and tumor size. Ta G3 lesions are associated with a 60% probability of recurrence and a moderate probability of disease progression. Similarly, primary Tis lesions are all high grade, have recurrence rates of 50–90%, and are associated with a high probability of tumor progression (42–83%).[16] Standard therapy for these lesions should consist of thorough endoscopic evaluation (Tis) or resection (TaG3), followed by full-dose BCG immunotherapy. The latter constitutes the "gold standard" and involves topical instillation of one ampule of BCG in solution on a weekly basis for 6 weeks. This is generally followed by a 6-week rest, with full reevaluation at week 12. Persistent disease at that point generally prompts a second 6-week course of therapy.[15,24,25] Durable (but not infinite) complete responses can be achieved in about 70% of patients.[26] The use of high-dose antioxidant vitamins may also be beneficial.[27] Maintenance BCG instillations (3 weekly treatments every 6 months for 3 years) may prolong treatment efficacy.[28] Other potentially useful treatment adjuncts include: increased fluid consumption; short course use of COX-2 inhibitors; aged garlic extract; and selective use of quinolone antibiotics.

Patients who fail to achieve a complete response following a second 6-week course of BCG (particularly if p53-positive) should be considered for cystectomy.[29,30] In selected cases consideration can be given to the use of alternative intravesical agents, including mitomycin-C (40 mg/40 cc saline),[31] valrubicin (800 mg/75 ml saline),[32] or interferon (50×10^6 units ± BCG).[33] If the latter approach is chosen and fails, the patient should proceed promptly to cystectomy. The utility of photodynamic therapy in the management of treatment-refractory Tis is considered investigational.[34] This general management strategy is also appropriate for patients with transitional cell carcinoma associated with mucosal (but not stromal) involvement of the prostatic urethra.[35]

T1 Lesions

The T1 tumors constitute a unique subset of superficial bladder cancer. These lesions are frequently understaged, an observation that has prompted the recommendation for endoscopic reevaluation and repeat resection of the old tumor site to exclude involvement of the tunica muscularis propria. High risk groups in the T1 disease category include G3 or multifocal lesions, T1b–c subsets, tumors associated with vascular invasion, and p53-positive lesions that recur following BCG therapy.[36–39] In general, T1 lesions are treated with one or two 6-week courses of intravesical BCG. Patients with persistent disease should be considered for prompt cystectomy. Alternative topical therapies are generally ineffective and consume valuable biologic time.

The use of intravesical BCG has profoundly influenced the management of recurrent superficial bladder cancer. Patients treated with TURBT and BCG exhibit a 10-year progression-free rate of about 62% and a 10-year disease-specific survival rate of approximately 75%.[40,41] Most tumors recur or progress within the first 5 years.[42] Despite these favorable outcomes, whether BCG treatments actually prevent disease progression remains conjectural.

The use of upper tract imaging (IVP) in patients with superficial bladder cancer who have achieved a complete response must be individualized. The reported incidence of subsequent carcinoma of the ureter or renal pelvis in such patients is about 2.2%. For that reason, annual excretory urography may not be necessary in low risk subsets (Ta, G1,2).[43] Conversely, upper tract involvement approaching 20% has been reported in high risk groups. For that reason, performance of an IVP every 1–2 years is desirable in patients with Tis and T1 disease.[44]

G. *Treatment of Invasive Tumors*

The "gold standard" treatment for muscle-invasive bladder cancer is *aggressive* surgical therapy, consisting of a thorough abdominal and pelvic exploration, wide-field resection of the deep pelvic lymph nodes, and anterior pelvic exenteration. In the absence of urethral involvement, consideration can be given to urethral (male) and urethral/vaginal (female) preservation. Use of the Multifire Endo-GIA 30 stapler expedites bladder pedicle division during radical cystectomy.[45] The neurovascular bundles can be preserved in selected male patients without compromising local recurrence rates and with the expectation that sexual function is preserved in approximately 40–50% of cases.[46]

Urinary diversion alternatives include (1) a standard ileal conduit, (2) construction of a continent urinary reservoir requiring intermittent catheterization (Indiana pouch),[47] or (3) creation of an orthotopic neobladder.[48–50] The latter is best suited for highly motivated and compliant patients who are willing to accept the potential complications of this diversion option (incontinence, retention)[51] and who are at low statistical risk for local disease recurrence.

Contemporary radical cystectomy is associated with a postoperative mortality rate of about 1.8%. Five-year survival rates of 75% for stage pT1, 63% for stage pT2, 50% for stage pT3a, 15% for stage pT3b, and 21% for stage pT4 disease have been observed. The overall actuarial 5-year survival rate is about 55%.[52] In male patients contiguous and noncontiguous involvement of the prostate is associated with 5-year survival rates of 6% and 37%, respectively. Although lymph node involvement is associated with a poor prognosis, patients with minimal nodal involvement (N1) and otherwise organ-confined disease (p0–p3a) exhibit a 5-year survival rate of approximately 58%. In contrast, nodal involvement in patients with non-organ-confined disease is associated with a 5-year survival rate of only 22%.[53,54]

Patients with tumors that are pT3a or less (without nodal involvement) are considered to be at low risk and do not generally require adjuvant chemotherapy. Tumors that are pT3b/pT4 (without nodal involvement) or any pT with nodal involvement (or vascular invasion) have a greater than 50% risk of systemic relapse and should be considered for platinum-based chemotherapy administered in the neoadjuvant and/or adjuvant setting.[16,55–57] The latter might involve the standard four-drug regimen designated MVAC (methotrexate/vinblastine/adriamycin/cisplatin) or one of the newer two-drug regimens such as cisplatin (or carboplatin)/taxol or cisplatin/gemcitabine. Studies have begun to stratify patients on the basis of p53 status and have observed that tumors with more than 20% positive cells appear to be at higher risk for systemic relapse.[14] Unfortunately, tumors that floridly express mutated *p53* tend to be more refractory to systemic therapy.

Alternatives to radical cystectomy include *bladder sparing options*. Selected patients with pT2/pT3a tumors can be considered for bladder-sparing surgical approaches such as *partial cystectomy*, which is feasible in 5–10% of cases. This approach requires a thorough clinical evaluation and documentation of a unifocal (rather than multifocal) abnormality generally located in the dome or lateral walls. Involvement of the trigonal complex and bladder neck are relative contraindications. A 2 cm disease-free margin must be attainable.

Another bladder-sparing surgical option involves performance of *repeat, aggressive TURBT*, which is predicated on the observation that about 10% of cystectomy patients have no residual tumor (P0). This approach is used in cases when the lesion is solitary, less than 2 cm in size, and has only minimally invaded the tunica muscularis propria.[58,59] Contraindications include in situ disease, a palpable mass, and associated hydronephrosis. Use of electrovaporization,[60] a surgical laser (Nd:YAG, holmium), or both are useful adjuncts to standard electrocautery.

Neoadjuvant platinum-based chemotherapy following bladder-sparing surgery has been used to treat patients with T2-3 N0 M0 neoplasms. About 58% of those patients who achieve a disease-free status after systemic chemotherapy preserve their bladders for up to 10 years with bladder-sparing surgery.[58] Not unexpectedly, patients whose tumors exhibit *p53* overexpression are less likely to respond to neoadjuvant chemotherapy. Indeed, long-term survival has been observed in about 41% of patients with *p53* overexpression versus 77% in whom *p53* was not overexpressed.[60,61]

Radiation therapy alone, chemotherapy alone, and chemotherapy plus radiation are alternative treatments to surgery, however, results are poor. These modalities should be used in conjunction with TURBT if one is searching for an alternative to cystectomy. In concert with a complete TURBT, radiation therapy can achieve a clinical complete response rate of approximately 45%. These disappointing results suggest that this approach should be considered only in patients who are unsuitable for more potentially effective therapies. Similarly, platinum-based chemotherapy alone has a clinical complete response rate of only 20–30%. This approach must be used in concert with bladder-sparing surgery or radiation in order to achieve durable responses.[62]

TURBT plus chemoradiotherapy can achieve a clinical complete response rate of about 70%.[63] The concurrent use of cisplatin and radiotherapy (60Gy)[64,65] appears to achieve results in near parity to those reported following two cycles of CMV (cisplatin, methotrexate, vinblastine) induction followed by concurrent use of Cisplatin plus radiotherapy (65Gy).[66,67] In each case, however, over 25% of patients develop new superficial or invasive disease requiring the use of intravesical and surgical therapy, respectively. As a result, the 5-year overall survival rate with an intact functioning bladder is about 43%.

Treatment of local relapse after these bladder-sparing approaches is generally based upon the extent of disease at the time of relapse and the form of antecedent treatment rendered. Superficial disease (Tis, Ta, or T1) is generally managed with intravesical BCG therapy. Persistent disease within the bladder following BCG should prompt salvage cystectomy. A positive cytology without evidence of disease in the bladder warrants evaluation of the upper tracts and the prostatic urethra. Radical cystectomy should also be performed in those patients with persistent or recurrent invasive disease. Salvage chemotherapy would only be considered in those patients deemed unsuitable for aggressive surgical therapy.[16]

Patients with unresectable disease (fixed bladder mass) or those with multiple positive nodes documented prior to laparotomy should be considered for systemic chemotherapy alone or chemotherapy with radiation (± hyperthermia). Salvage surgery can be considered in patients who have achieved satisfactory downstaging, particularly those in whom the pre-chemotherapy sites of disease are restricted to the bladder and pelvis or regional lymph nodes.

H. *The Treatment of Metastatic Disease*

Patients who present with metastatic disease (or those who develop metastases following treatment) should undergo the detailed staging workup described previously. In addition, they may require an assessment of cardiac and renal function. The optimal chemotherapy regimen depends on the presence/absence of medical co-morbidities, as well as evaluation of the patient's risk classification. "Good risk" patients are defined as those with a good performance level; an absence of cardiac, pulmonary, and skeletal involvement, and the presence of normal alkaline phosphatase and lactic dehydrogenase levels. "Poor-risk" patients are deficient in these areas and may also have demonstrated previous intolerance to multiple-agent chemotherapy. Another adverse factor is the presence of non-transitional cell cancer.[16]

Metastatic transitional cell carcinoma is a chemotherapy-responsive malignancy, and MVAC has been considered the "gold standard". The MVAC regimen has been associated with overall response rates of 40–70%, with 20–30% of patients achieving a complete response. Despite this high response rate, the median survival time for responders is 9–12 months, and only 3–11% of patients achieve long-term survival.[68] Less toxic regimens that appear to achieve equivalent results include CMV,[16,69] ITP (ifosfamide/taxol/cisplatin),[70] cisplatin (carboplatin)/taxol,[71,72] cisplatin/gemcitabine,[73] and cisplatin, taxol, plus gemcitabine.

Patients with metastatic disease are generally reevaluated after two or three cycles of a given chemotherapy regimen. For patients whose disease responds or remains stable, treatment is continued for two more cycles. Salvage surgery may be an option for patients who have a significant response and a previously unresectable primary tumor. Surgery may also be a viable option in individuals who exhibit a solitary site of extravesical disease following intensive chemotherapy. Two additional cycles of chemotherapy are administered following resection. In general, six cycles of a particular regimen would be considered maximum therapy, depending on the response. An alternative regimen should be considered in patients who do not exhibit a significant response after two or three cycles of first-line therapy or in those who experience significant treatment-related morbidity.[16]

Treatment of Upper Tract Disease

A detailed discussion of upper tract urothelial carcinoma and its management are beyond the scope of this chapter. Nonetheless, a brief commentary is relevant to the previous discussion. Patients with upper tract tumors (calyces, pelvis, ureters) have a 30–50% chance of developing bladder cancer during their lifetimes. Conversely, patients with lower tract disease (bladder) have a 2–3% chance of upper tract involvement. Most upper tract tumors are transitional cell carcinomas. They may present with gross (total) hematuria, flank pain, or a palpable mass (secondary to the tumor or hydronephrosis). The initial evaluation scheme is identical to that already described for bladder cancer. In addition, ureterorenoscopy is required. The staging workup for upper tract tumors is virtually identical to that described for evaluation of muscle-invasive bladder cancer.

Treatment options are contingent on the level of involvement and tumor stage. Tumors confined to the lower ureter are generally treated by distal ureterectomy and reimplantation of a healthy ureter into a mobilized segment of bladder (psoas hitch with or without a Boari flap). Tumors of the mid-ureter may be amenable to resection and end-to-end anastomosis. Cancers involving the proximal ureter and upper collecting system are most often treated with a radical nephroureterectomy (open, hand-assisted laparoscopic, complete laparoscopic). Excision of the entire ureter (including the cuff of the bladder) is important to avoid tumor recurrence in the defunctionalized stump (20–30% risk). The presence of a solitary kidney or markedly impaired global renal function may prompt consideration of kidney-sparing treatment. The latter generally involves percutaneous renal surgery (fulguration, electrovaporization, laser treatment) followed by antegrade instillation of BCG. This approach can be effective in patients with relatively low volume/grade involvement of the upper tract. Upper tract urothelial cancers metastasize to regional lymph nodes, lung, liver, bone, brain, and other sites. Metastatic disease is approached in a manner virtually identical to that described for bladder cancer. The overall response rates are also equivalent.

References

1. Pycha A, Mian C, Hofbauer J, et al. Multifocality of transitional cell carcinoma results from genetic instability of entire transitional epithelium. Urology 1999;53:92–97.
2. Sidransky D, Frost P, Von Eschenbach A, Oyasu R, Preisinger AC, Vogelstein V. Clonal origin of bladder cancer. N Engl J Med 1992;326:759–761.
3. Chern H-D, Becich MJ, Persad RA, et al. Clonal analysis of human recurrent superficial bladder cancer by immunohistochemistry of P53 and retinoblastoma proteins. J Urol 1996;156:1846–1849.
4. Landis SH, Murray T, Bolden S, Wingo PA. Cancer statistics, 1999. Cancer 1999;49:8–31.
5. Vineis P. Epidemiological models of carcinogenesis: the example of bladder cancer. Cancer Epidemiol Biomarkers Prev 1992;1:149–153.
6. Navon JD, Soliman H, Khonsari F, Ahlering T. Screening cystoscopy and survival of spinal cord injured patients with squamous cell cancer of the bladder. J Urol 1997;157:2109–2111.
7. Fernandes ET, Manivel JC, Reddy PK, Ercole CJ. Cyclophosphamide associated bladder cancer: a highly aggressive disease: Analysis of 12 cases. J Urol 1996;156:1931–1933.
8. Sijmons RH, Kiemeney LA, Witjes JA, Vasen HF. Urinary tract cancer and hereditary nonpolyposis colorectal cancer: Risks and screening options. J Urol 1998;160:466–470.
9. Grossman HB, Tex WA, Moncrief D. Superficial bladder cancer: Decreasing the risk of recurrence. Oncology 1996;10:1617.
10. O'Brien T, Cranston D, Fuggle S, Bicknell R, Harris AL. Different angiogenic pathways characterize superficial and invasive bladder cancer. Cancer Res 1995;55:510–513.
11. Smits G, Schaafsma E, Kiemeney L, Caris C, Debruyne F, Witjes JA. Microstaging of pT1 transitional cell carcinoma of the bladder: Identification of subgroups with distinct risks of progression. Urol 1998;52:1009–1013.
12. Kroft SH, Oyasu R. Urinary bladder cancer: Mechanisms of development and progression. Laboratory Invest 1994;71:158–174.
13. Smith K, Fennelly JA, Neal DE, Hall RR, Harris AL. Characterization and quantitation of the epidermal growth factor receptor in invasive and superficial bladder tumors. Cancer Res 1989;49:5810–5815.
14. Esrig D, Elmajian D, Groshen S, et al. Accumulation of nuclear p53 and tumor progression in bladder cancer. N Engl J Med 1994;331:1259–1264.
15. Lamm DL. Bladder cancer: twenty years of progress and the challenges that remain. Cancer 1998;48:263–284.
16. Scher H, Bahnson R, Cohen S, et al. NCCN urothelial cancer practice guidelines. Oncology 1998;12:225–271.
17. Konety BR, Getzengerg RH. Urine based markers of urological malignancy. J Urol 2001;165:600–611.
18. Sharody MF, DeVere White RW, Soloway MS, et al. Results of a multicenter trial using the BTA test to monitor for and diagnose recurrent bladder cancer. J Urol 1995;154:379–384.
19. Soloway MS, Briggman JV, Carpinito GA, et al. Use of a new tumor marker, urinary NMP22, in the detection of occult or rapidly recurring transitional cell carcinoma of the urinary tract following surgical treatment. J Urol 1996;156:363–367.
20. Lin Y, Miyamoto H, Fujinami K, et al. Telomerase activity in human bladder cancer. Clin Cancer Res 1996;2:929–932.
21. Johnston B, Morales A, Emerson L, Lundie M. Rapid detection of bladder cancer: a comparative study of point of care tests. J Urol 1997;158: 2098–2101.
22. Lokeshwar VB, Obek C, Soloway MS, Block NL. Tumor-associated hyaluronic acid: A new sensitive and specific urine marker for bladder cancer. J Urol 1997;57:773–777.
23. Ramakumar S, Bhuiyan J, Besse JA, et al. Comparison of screening methods in the detection of bladder cancer. J Urol 1999;161:388–384.
24. Hudson MA, Herr HW. Carcinoma in situ of the bladder. J Urol 1995;153:564–572.
25. Coplen DE, Marcus MD, Myers JA, Ratliff TL, Catalona WJ. Long-term followup of patients treated with 1 or 2, 6-week courses of intravesical bacillus Calmette-Guérin: analysis of possible predictors of response free of tumor. J Urol 1990;144:652–665.
26. Nadler RB, Catalona WJ, Hudson MA, et al. Durability of the tumor-free response for intravesical bacillus Calmette-Guérin therapy. J Urol 1994;152:367–373.
27. Lamm DL, Riggs DR, Shriver JS, van Gilder PF, Rach JF, DeHaven JI. Megadose vitamins in bladder cancer: a double-blind clinical trial. J Urol 1994;151:21–26.
28. Lamm DL. BCG immunotherapy for transitional-cell carcinoma in situ of the bladder. Oncology 1995;9:947–965.
29. Lacombe L, Dalbagni G, Zhang Z-E, et al. Overexpression of p53 protein in a high-risk population of patients with superficial bladder cancer before and after bacillus Calmette-Guérin therapy: correlation to clinical outcome. Clin Onc 1997;14:2646–2642.
30. Sarkis AS, Dalbagni G, Cordon-Cardo C, et al. Association of p53 nuclear overexpression and tumor progression in carcinoma in situ of the bladder. J Urol 1994;152:388–382.
31. Lundholm C, Norlen BJ, Ekman P, et al. A randomized prospective study comparing long-term intravesical instillations of mitomycin C and bacillus Calmette-Guérin in patients with superficial bladder carcinoma. J Urol 1996;156:372–376.
32. Greenberg RE, Bahnson RR, Wood D, et al. Initial report on intravesical administration of N-trifluoroacetyladriamycin-14-valerate (AD 32) to patients with refractory superficial transitional cell carcinoma of the urinary bladder. Urology 1997;49:471–475.
33. Belldegrun AS, Franklin JF, O'Donnell MA, et al. Superficial bladder cancer: the role of interferon-alpha. J Urol 1998;159:1793–1801.
34. Nseyo UO, Shumaker B, Klein EA, et al. Photodynamic therapy using porfimer sodium as an alternative to cystectomy in patients with refractory transitional cell carcinoma in situ of the bladder. J Urol 1998;160:39–44.
35. Hillyard RW Jr, Ladaga L, Schellhammer PF. Superficial transitional cell carcinoma of the bladder associated with mucosal involvement of the prostatic urethra: results of treatment with intravesical bacillus Calmette-Guérin. J Urol 1988;139:290–293.
36. Hermann GG, Horn T, Steven K. The influence of the level of lamina propria invasion and the prevalence of p53 nuclear accumulation on survival in stage T1 transitional cell bladder cancer. J Urol 1998;159:91–94.
37. Holmang S, Hedelin H, Anderstrom C, Holmberg E, Johansson SL. The importance of the depth of invasion of stage T1 bladder carcinoma: a prospective cohort study. J Urol 1997;157:800–804.

38. Hurle R, Losa A, Ranieri A, Graziotti P, Lembo A. Low dose pasteur bacillus Calmette-Guérin regimen in stage T1, grade 3 bladder cancer therapy. J Urol 1996;156:1602–1605.
39. Zhang GK, Uke ET, Sharer WC, Borkon WD, Bernstein SM. Reassessment of conservative management for stage T1N0M0 transitional cell carcinoma of the bladder. J Urol 1996;155:1907–1909.
40. Herr HW, Schwalb DM, Zhang Z-F, et al. Intravesical bacillus Calmette-Guérin therapy prevents tumor progression and death from superficial bladder cancer: ten-year follow-up of a prospective randomized trial. J Clin Oncol 1995;13:1404–1408.
41. Herr HW, Laudone VP, Badalament RA, et al. Bacillus Calmette-Guérin therapy alters the progression of superficial bladder cancer. J Clin Oncol 1998;6:1450–1455.
42. Herr HW, Wartinger DD, Fair WR, Oettgen HF. Bacillus Calmette-Guérin therapy for superficial bladder cancer: a 10-year followup. J Urol 1992;147:1020–1023.
43. Holmang S, Hedelin H, Anderstrom C, Holmberg E, Johansson SL. Long-term followup of a bladder carcinoma cohort: routine followup urography is not necessary. J Urol 1998;160:45–48.
44. Herr HW. Extravesical tumor relapse in patients with superficial bladder tumors. J Clin Oncol 1998;16:1099–1102.
45. Yamashita T, Muraishi O, Umeda S, Matsushita T. Radical cystectomy using endoscopic stapling devices: preliminary experience with a simple and reliable technique. J Urol 1997;157:263–265.
46. Schoenberg MP, Walsh PC, Breazeale DR, Marshall FF, Mostin JL, Brendler CB. Local recurrence and survival following nerve sparing radical cystoprostatectomy for bladder cancer: 10-year followup. J Urol 1996;155:490–494.
47. Mills RD, Studer UE. Potential metabolic complications of continent urinary diversion. Contemp Urol 2001;May:110–114.
48. Hautmann RE, de Petriconi R, Gottfried H-W, Kleinschmidt K, Mattes R, Paiss T. The ileal neobladder: complications and functional results in 363 patients after 11 years of followup. J Urol 1999;161:422–428.
49. Schoenberg M, Hortopan S, Schlossberg L, Marshall FF. Anatomical anterior exenteration with urethral and vaginal preservation: illustrated surgical method. J Urol 1998;161:569–572.
50. Shimogaki H, Okada H, Fujisawa M, et al. Long-term experience with orthotopic reconstruction of the lower urinary tract in women. J Urol 1999;161:573–577.
51. Hautmann RE, Paiss T, de Petriconi R. The ileal neobladder in women: 9 years of experience with 18 patients. J Urol 1996;155:76–81.
52. Pagano F, Bassi P, Galetti TP, et al. Results of contemporary radical cystectomy for invasive bladder cancer: a clinicopathological study with an emphasis on the inadequacy of the tumor, nodes and metastases classification. J Urol 1991;145:45–50.
53. Vieweg J, Gschwend JE, Herr HW, Fair WR. Pelvic lymph node dissection can be curative in patients with node positive bladder cancer. J Urol 1999;161:449–454.
54. Vieweg J, Gschwend JE, Herr HW, Fair WR. The impact of primary stage on survival in patients with lymph node positive bladder cancer. J Urol 1999;161:72–76.
55. Logothetis CJ, Johnson DE, Chong C, et al. Adjuvant chemotherapy of bladder cancer: a preliminary report. J Urol 1988;139:1207–1211.
56. Skinner DG, Dahiels JR, Russell CA, et al. The role of adjuvant chemotherapy following cystectomy for invasive bladder cancer: a prospective comparative trial. J Urol 1991;145:459–464; discussion 464–467.
57. Stockle M, Meyenburg W, Wellek S, et al. Advanced bladder cancer (stages pT3b, pT4a, pN1 and pN2): improved survival after radical cystectomy and 3 adjuvant cycles of chemotherapy. Results of a controlled prospective study. J Urol 1992;148:302–307.
58. Herr HW, Bajorin DF, Scher HI. Neoadjuvant chemotherapy and bladder-sparing surgery for invasive bladder cancer: ten-year outcome. J Clin Oncol 1998;16(4):1298–1301.
59. Solsona E, Iborra I, Ricos JV, Monros JL, Casanova J, Calabuig C. Feasibility of transurethral resection for muscle infiltrating carcinoma of the bladder: long-term followup of a prospective study. J Urol 1998;159:95–99.
60. McKiernan JM, Kaplan SA, Santarosa RP, Te AE, Sawczuk IS. Transurethral electrovaporization of bladder cancer. Urology 1996;48:207–210.
61. Sarkis AS, Bajorin DF, Reuter VE, et al. Prognostic value of p53 nuclear overexpression in patients with invasive bladder cancer treated with neoadjuvant MVAC. J Clin Oncol 1995;13(6):1384–1390.
62. Herr HW, Bajorin DF, Scher HI, Cordon-Cardo C, Reuter VE. Can p53 help select patients with invasive bladder cancer for bladder preservation? J Urol 1999;161:20–23.
63. McCaffrey JA, Bajorin DF, Scher HI, Bosl GJ. Combined-modality therapy for bladder cancer. Oncology 1997;11(suppl 9):18–26.
64. Tester W, Caplan R, Heaney J, et al. Neoadjuvant combined modality program with selective organ preservation for invasive bladder cancer: results of radiation therapy oncology group phase II trial 8802. J Clin Oncol 1996;14:119–126.
65. Chauvet B, Brewer Y, Felix-Faure C, Davin J-L, Choquenet C, Reboul F. Concurrent cisplatin and radiotherapy for patients with muscle invasive bladder cancer who are not candidates for radical cystectomy. J Urol 1996;156:1258–1262.
66. Shipley WU, Winter KA, Kaufman DS, et al. Phase III trial of neoadjuvant chemotherapy in patients with invasive bladder cancer treated with selective bladder preservation by combined radiation therapy and chemotherapy: initial results of radiation therapy oncology group 89–3. J Clin Oncol 1998;16:3576–3583.
67. Kaufman DS, Shipley WU, Griffin PP, et al. Selective bladder preservation by combination treatment of invasive bladder cancer. N Engl J Med 1993;329:1377–1382.
68. Kachnic LA, Kaufman DS, Heney NM, et al. Bladder preservation by combined modality therapy for invasive bladder cancer. J Clin Oncol 1997;15:1022–1029.
69. Saxman SB, Propert KJ, Einhorn LH, et al. Long-term follow-up of a phase III intergroup study of cisplatin alone or in combination with methrotrexate, vinblastine, and doxorubicin in patients with metastatic urothelial carcinoma: a cooperative group study. J Clin Oncol 1997;15: 2564–2569.
70. Bajorin DF, McCaffrey JA, Hilton S, et al. Treatment of patients with transitional-cell carcinoma of the urothelial tract with ifosfamide, paclitaxel, and cisplatin: a phase II trial. J Clin Oncol 1998;16:2722–2727.
71. Sengelov L, Kamby C, Lund B, Engelholm SA. Docetaxel and cisplatin in metastatic urothelial cancer: a phase II study. J Clin Oncol 1998;16:3392–3397.
72. Vaughn DJ, Malkowicz SB, Zoltick B, et al. Paclitaxel plus carboplatin in advanced carcinoma of the urothelium: an active and tolerable outpatient regimen. J Clin Oncol 1998;16:255–260.
73. Bergman AM, Ruiz van Haperen VW, Veerman G, Kuiper CM, Peters GJ. Synergistic interaction between cisplatin and gemcitabine in vitro. Clin Cancer Res 1996;2:521–530.

CHAPTER 48

Cancer of the Kidney

PAUL RUSSO

A. Epidemiology and Etiology

In 2000 it was estimated that there were 31,900 new cases of kidney cancer diagnosed in the United States, leading to 12,000 deaths. Renal cell carcinoma (RCC) accounts for 2–3% of all adult malignancies and 2.3% of all deaths in the United States due to cancer. Factors implicated in its development include cigarette smoking, exposure to petroleum products, obesity, diuretic use, cadmium exposure, and ionizing radiation. Data from the Connecticut Tumor Registry collected between 1935 and 1989 shows an increase in incidence from 0.7/100,000 to 4.2/100,000 females and 1.6/100,000 to 9.6/100,000 males. Improvements in radiologic imaging techniques such as ultrasonography, computed tomography (CT) scanning, and magnetic resonance imaging (MRI) have found an increasing number of incidental renal tumors; the overall percentage of such has risen from 10–15% to 50–70%. These imaging techniques have also effectively excluded masses of the kidney (e.g., cysts, fat-containing angiomyolipomas) from operation that were formerly explored and resected. Today, fewer than 5% of patients present with the classic triad of hematuria, flank pain, and a renal mass. Approximately 25% of renal cancer patients present with locally advanced or metastatic disease. A strong family history can be elicited in approximately 5% of cases of RCC.

Investigative efforts into the genetic aspects of familial RCC, beginning initially with von Hippel-Lindau (VHL) disease, followed by familial RCC and hereditary papillary renal cell carcinoma (HPRC), have identified germline mutations involving chromosome 3p (VHL, sporadic RCC), defects not found in HPRC. Molecular genetic analysis of other histologic subtypes of RCC, such as chromophobe, papillary, collecting duct, and the usually benign oncocytoma, has uncovered a variety of chromosomal defects unique to a given subtype. Emerging from this work is the impression that renal cell carcinoma is in fact a *group* of tumors, each with unique genetic abnormalities. Malignant behavior varies, ranging from the most potentially aggressive conventional clear cell carcinoma, to the intermediate papillary RCC and chromophobe RCC, to the almost completely benign oncocytoma. Ultimately, histology must be incorporated in the staging systems for RCC.

Renal Cancer

A.
Epidemiology and Etiology
30,000 New cases/year
Risk factors: cigarette smoking, petroleum products, obesity, diuretic use, cadmium exposure, ionizing radiation
10% Present with hematuria, flank pain, a mass
20% Present with locally advanced or metastatic disease
5% Strong family history

↓

B.
Differential Diagnosis
90% Renal cortical neoplasm
10% Complex cyst, sarcoma, metastasis
Benign neoplasm

↓

C.
Diagnosis, Staging
Chest radiograph, CT scan
MRI to evaluate vascular involvement

Poor Prognostic Features:
- Nodal involvement
- Size > 10 cm
- Sarcomatoid features
- Elevated ESR
- Weight loss
- Hypercalcemia

(continued on next page)

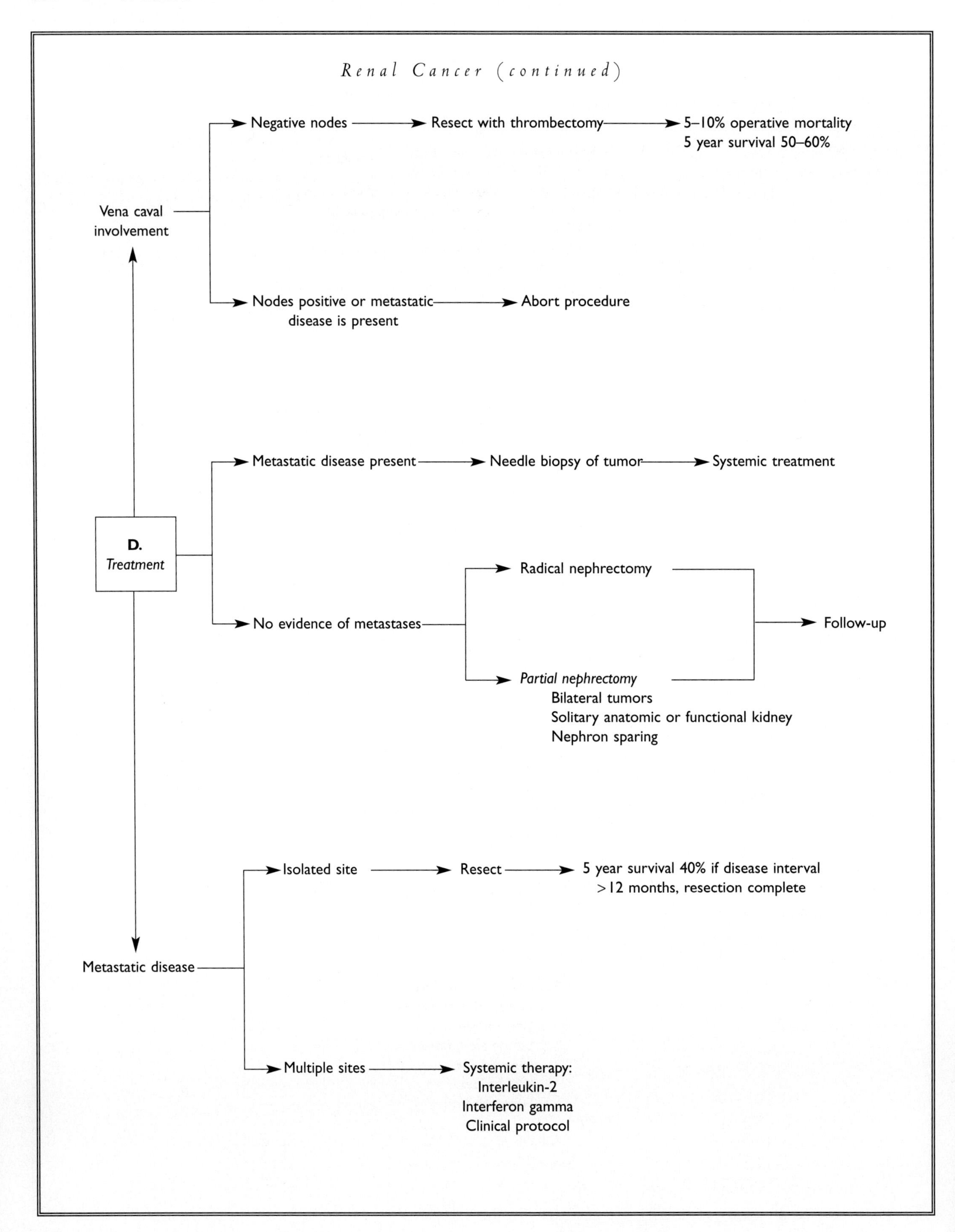
Renal Cancer (continued)
Vena caval involvement
Negative nodes
Resect with thrombectomy
5–10% operative mortality
5 year survival 50–60%
Nodes positive or metastatic disease is present
Abort procedure
D. Treatment
Metastatic disease present
Needle biopsy of tumor
Systemic treatment
No evidence of metastases
Radical nephrectomy
Partial nephrectomy
Bilateral tumors
Solitary anatomic or functional kidney
Nephron sparing
Follow-up
Metastatic disease
Isolated site
Resect
5 year survival 40% if disease interval >12 months, resection complete
Multiple sites
Systemic therapy:
Interleukin-2
Interferon gamma
Clinical protocol

B. Differential Diagnosis

The differential diagnosis of a renal mass includes a benign cyst (simple or complex), pseudo-tumors (column of Bertin), angiomyolipoma, renal cortical tumor, sarcoma, metastatic tumor, vascular abnormality, urothelial carcinoma, and lymphoma. A metastatic tumor presenting as an isolated mass in the kidney is rare. Similarly, although renal involvement by lymphoma is common, it is very rare for a solid, isolated renal mass to be a primary lymphoma (in the absence of lymphoma elsewhere). Renal sarcomas are rare tumors with a poor prognosis and a natural history similar to that of retroperitoneal sarcomas. Prognosis is determined by grade (high or low) and size (<5 cm or ≥5 cm). Most sarcomas are high grade and reach massive proportions prior to symptomatic presentation. Despite complete resection, there are few long-term survivors.

Tumors discovered during abdominal imaging by CT scan, MRI, or ultrasonography have similar histologic grade, DNA ploidy, and histopathologic appearance when compared to larger, symptomatic tumors. Overall, when treated by radical or more recently partial nephrectomy (nephron-sparing surgery), these tumors have an excellent overall prognosis, with a long-term survival of 90–95%.

C. Presentation, Staging

Symptomatic RCC is associated with hematuria, weight loss, and flank pain as well as a wide array of paraneoplastic systemic symptoms including anemia, polycythemia, hypercalcemia, fever, and malaise. The physical examination is performed with special attention to supraclavicular nodes, abdominal bruits, lower extremity edema, and subcutaneous nodules that often involve unusual sites such as the vegina, penis, and digits. Laboratory evaluation should include a complete blond count (CBC), serum calcium assay, liver function tests (LFTs), and serum creatinine assay.

Evaluation of the extent of disease should include a chest radiograph and abdominal CT scan, with and without intravenous contrast. If a nodule is observed on the chest radiograph, chest CT is performed. The T stage can be correctly predicted by an abdominal CT scan in more than 80% of cases. Bone scanning is not recommended in the absence of symptoms and in the presence of normal alkaline phosphatase and serum calcium levels. If the CT scan raises the possibility of renal vein involvement extending into the inferior vena cava, abdominal MRI is done to determine the uppermost extent of the tumor thrombus. Preoperative arteriography is restricted to the unusual case of a centrally located RCC where nephron-sparing surgery is planned. CT of the brain is performed only for the symptomatic patient.

There are two staging systems for RCC: the Robson and TNM classifications (Table 48–1). At Memorial Sloan Kettering Cancer Center (MSKCC) we employ the latter because of the greater detail provided concerning the extent of venous [renal vein, inferior vena cava (IVC)] and regional nodal involvement. Tumors confined to Gerota's fascia are associated with long-term survival rates of 80% or more. Involvement of perinephric fat (T3a) decreases long-term survival to 60%. Pre-

TABLE 48–1.
AJCC definition of TNM, stage grouping, and histopathologic grading for kidney cancer

Primary Tumor (T)

TX	Primary tumor cannot be assessed
T0	No evidence of primary tumor
T1	Tumor 7 cm or less in greatest dimension limited to the kidney
T2	Tumor more than 7 cm in greatest dimension limited to the kidney
T3	Tumor extends into major veins or invades adrenal gland or perinephric tissues but not beyond Gerota's fascia
T3a	Tumor invades adrenal gland or perinephric tissues but not beyond Gerota's fascia
T3b	Tumor grossly extends into renal vein(s) or vena cava below diaphragm
T3c	Tumor grossly extends into vena cava above the diaphragm
T4	Tumor invades beyond Gerota's fascia

Regional Lymph Nodes (N)*

NX	Regional lymph nodes cannot be assessed
N0	No regional lymph node metastasis
N1	Metastasis in a single regional lymph node
N2	Metastasis in more than one regional lymph node

**Laterality does not affect the N classification.*

Distant Metastasis (M)

MX	Distant metastasis cannot be assessed
M0	No distant metastasis
M1	Distant metastasis

Histopathologic Grading (G)

GX	Grade cannot be assessed
G1	Well differentiated
G2	Moderately differentiated
G3–4	Poorly differentiated or undifferentiated

Stage Grouping

Stage	T	N	M
I	T1	N0	M0
II	T2	N0	M0
III	T1	N1	M0
	T2	N1	M0
	T3a	N0	M0
	T3a	N1	M0
	T3b	N0	M0
	T3b	N1	M0
	T3c	N0	M0
	T3c	N1	M0
	T4	N0	M0
IV	T4	Any N	M0
	Any T	N2	M0
	Any T	Any N	M1

SOURCE: Used with the permission of the American Joint Committee on Cancer (AJCC®), Chicago, IL. The original source for this material is the AJCC® Cancer Staging Manual, 5th edition (1997) published by Lippincott Williams & Wilkins Publishers, Philadelphia, PA.

cipitous decreases in long-term survival occur with any nodal involvement (N1–N4) (<20%). Although imaging studies often reveal enlarged regional nodes, approximately 50% of them are inflammatory, 50 operative exploration should not be denied based on this finding alone. In highly selected patients with isolated metastases at presentation (M1), resection of the primary and metastatic tumor translates into long-term disease-free survival in up to 30% of cases. Whether this approach reflects a therapeutic effect of surgical resection or the uncertain and often protracted natural history of RCC is not known. Other adverse prognostic indicators, usually associated with locally advanced or metastatic tumors, include tumor size larger than 10 cm, sarcomatoid features (which can arise from any of the above described histologic subtypes), elevated erythrocyte sedimentation rate (ESR), weight loss, and hypercalcemia.

A unique clinical situation is bilateral RCC, which is found in 5% of renal cancer patients. Most (80%) patients present with synchronous tumors; in those presenting with metachronous lesions, intervals of up to 30 years have been documented between tumors, again illustrating the long and often unpredictable natural history of this disease. Therapeutic strategies for patients with bilateral RCC have two goals: eradication of all local tumor and preservation of enough renal function to avoid dialysis. To that end, combinations of partial and radical nephrectomy are used, depending on the location and size of the index tumors. The presence of adverse prognostic features that enhance the likelihood of metastatic disease (regional nodal metastases or sarcomatoid histology) may delay surgery for the second tumor during which time there is a careful search for metastatic disease.

D. *Treatment*

Surgical resection is currently the only curative therapy for renal cancer. Radical nephrectomy, popularized during the 1960s by Robson to include removal of perirenal fat, regional lymph nodes, and the ipsilateral adrenal gland, remains the standard operation for treating this disease. However, clinical research has led to changes in the standard surgical approach to RCC, including the following.

1. Restriction of adrenalectomy to large tumors involving the entire kidney or its upper pole

2. Assessment of the need for and extent of regional lymphadenectomy, particularly in cases of incidental detection of RCC

3. Wide application of partial nephrectomy in cases of tumor in a solitary kidney or bilateral renal tumors and in the strategy termed "nephron-sparing" (partial nephrectomy to resect small renal tumors in the presence of a contralateral kidney that is normal)

4. Aggressive surgical resection of RCC with involvement of the inferior vena cava and right atrium

5. Selective surgical resection of metastatic disease

Ipsilateral Adrenalectomy

Ipsilateral adrenal gland involvement occurs in approximately 4% of patients undergoing radical nephrectomy. In most instances adrenal involvement occurs in association with large, poorly differentiated primary tumors with regional extension and lymph node metastases. In this modern era of incidental renal tumor detection, adrenal involvement is expected to decline further. Adrenal involvement with RCC may be a result of direct extension, regional lymph nodal encasement, or metastatic deposits. For patients with adrenal involvement the overall prognosis remains poor despite adrenalectomy and is similar to that of patients with regional nodal disease. Adrenalectomy can be reserved for those whose preoperative studies are suspicious for involvement as well as for patients with large primary tumors, particularly if the upper pole is involved.

Regional Lymphadenectomy

Enlargement of the regional lymph nodes detected on preoperative imaging studies such as the CT scan may be the result of tumor involvement, again common in large, poorly differentiated tumors; or it may be an inflammatory response to the primary tumor. Adenopathy alone, in the absence of other obvious sites of metastatic disease, should not deter one from exploration and resection of the tumor and regional nodes. In the era of the incidental renal tumor, it is expected that regional lymph node involvement will become increasingly uncommon. In addition, enhanced detection of systemic disease may reduce the number of laparotomies and the number of patients found to have regional node metastases. Regional node dissection at the time of radical nephrectomy provides important prognostic information, but there is little evidence that a therapeutic effect is gained. Because the lymphatic network is vast, tumor cells may bypass local nodes and drain into the cisterna chyli, and hematogenous metastases may occur. Node dissection should encompass an area 4–6 cm above and below the renal vessels in addition to the lymphatics posterior to the aorta and vena cava. Among the 10–15% of patients undergoing radical nephrectomy and regional node dissection who are found to have metastatic nodal disease, progression to disseminated disease usually occurs within 1 year. In the absence of effective adjunctive systemic therapy for metastatic renal cancer, it is still recommended that node dissection be done in the hope that disease is restricted to the involved node alone. The finding of metastatic nodal disease also can provide entry into poor prognostic clinical research protocols.

Partial Nephrectomy

Accepted indications for partial nephrectomy to treat RCC include situations in which standard radical nephrectomy would render the patient functionally anephric, requiring dialysis. Absolute indications for partial nephrectomy are the presence of (1) bilateral tumors and (2) cancer in a solitary anatomic or functional kidney. Relative indications include a contralateral kidney threatened by disease such as hypertension or diabetes mellitus. A functioning renal remnant of at least 20% is needed to maintain adequate renal function off dialysis. With careful case selection, local disease recurrence following partial nephrectomy is less than 4%.

The above-described increase in incidental tumors augmented by improvements in preoperative imaging modalities has encouraged the concept of elective partial nephrectomy or *nephron-sparing surgery*. Evidence from a number of major centers in the United States and Europe has demonstrated that in carefully selected patients with small tumors (<4cm in diameter) survival rates are not significantly different from those of patients treated by radical nephrectomy. Concerns relative to tumor multicentricity can be addressed at the time of operation by intraoperative ultrasonography and careful inspection of the entire kidney. Combined experience now suggests that local recurrence rates are as low as 1–3% in patients treated with nephron-sparing surgery. These results, coupled with enhanced understanding of the graded malignant potential of renal tumors, ranging from the more benign oncocytoma, to the intermediate-risk papillary and chromophobe tumors, to the most potentially aggressive conventional clear cell carcinoma, further motivates urologic oncologists to consider nephron-sparing approaches whenever possible.

RCC Involvement of the Vena Cava Renal cell carcinoma has a propensity to invade the renal vein and inferior vena cava, occasionally reaching the right atrium and right ventricle but not necessarily metastasizing in the process. In the absence of detectable metastases by preoperative imaging or intraoperative assessment, approximately one-half of patients whose tumors extend into the vena cava can achieve prolonged survival after complete resection and extraction of the tumor thrombus. Prognostic factors of importance in these cases include the status of the regional lymph nodes, the presence of metastatic disease, and whether the thrombus is free-floating in the vena cava or invading the vena caval wall. Median survival for patients with regional metastatic nodal disease is less than 10 months; thus preoperative documentation of such disease should discourage attempted surgical resection. Tumors of high grade, including those with sarcomatoid features, are more likely to invade the wall of the vena cava. Complete tumor resection with an intact thrombus and without node metastases is associated with 5-year survival rates in the range of 50–60%.

Depending on the extent of tumor extension in the vena cava, resection of tumor and thrombus may require specialized techniques of venovenous bypass and cardiopulmonary bypass with or without circulatory arrest. In these cases the urologic surgeon should work closely with a cardiovascular surgical team. Despite advances in perioperative support for these challenging operations, perioperative mortality remains in the 5–10% range; hence these operations should be undertaken only at centers with substantial experience.

Surgical Resection of Metastatic Disease
Renal cell carcinomas may present with limited metastatic disease or evolve into a state of limited metastatic disease following prior surgical treatment. Because RCCs may have an unpredictable natural history and systemic treatments are generally ineffective, the case for complete surgical resection of limited metastatic disease is currently being made in many centers. In reported series on the surgical management of limited metastatic disease, important, uncontrolled selection factors include the site and number of metastatic foci, the ability to resect a metastasis completely, co-morbid medical conditions, and the disease-free interval. Currently, patients with a long disease-free interval (>12 months) and a completely resected single site of metastatic disease (i.e., lung), can achieve a 5-year survival rate in the range of 40%. Other indications for resection of metastatic disease in RCCs include resection of isolated local recurrence and palliative resection of symptomatic brain and skeletal metastases. Nephrectomy is contraindicated for the intended purpose of inducing spontaneous tumor metastasis regression, as there is a lack of evidence that this real phenomenon (<1%) is actually induced by resecting the primary tumor. There are reports of spontaneous regression of metastatic disease sites in the absence of nephrectomy.

Recommendations for Follow-up After Resection of Localized Disease

After resection of localized RCC, 20–30% of patients develop metastatic disease at a median of 15–18 months, with 85%

of relapses occurring within 3 years. Lung metastasis is the most common site of distant recurrence, ultimately occurring in 50–60% of patients who develop metastases. Because adjuvant treatment trials have been unsuccessful to date, careful observation remains the standard of care after operation. The intensity of follow-up depends on the stage of the primary tumor and includes the history and physical examination, chest radiography, CBC, and LFTs every 4–6 months for the first 2 years. For patients with localized tumors, additional imaging studies may be considered, such as bone and brain scans or symptom-directed CT scans of the abdomen and chest. Patients treated by partial nephrectomy for required or elective indications should undergo annual ultrasonography or CT imaging of the kidney for early detection of a recurrent or metachronous tumor. With an increased understanding of the various histologic subtypes and their metastatic potentials, follow-up for the less aggressive forms of RCC, such as the chromophobe, papillary, and oncocytoma, can be tailored to occur at greater intervals than that of the conventional clear cell carcinomas.

Systemic Therapy for Advanced Local or Metastatic Disease

Despite the careful study of chemotherapeutic agents, hormonal therapies, and biologic response modifiers, alone or in combination, in more than 200 clinical trials, locally advanced or metastatic RCC remains resistant to systemic therapy. Although excitement has been generated by a number of biologically active agents, particularly interferon and interleukin-2, when clinical trials are carefully controlled and responses are defined as a *complete response* (complete disappearance of all tumor) or a *partial response* (more than 50% reduction in measurable tumor burden) no single agent, alone or in combination, has achieved an overall response rate of more than 20% with durable responses of 5% or less. These findings, when coupled with the often unpredictable natural history of RCC (e.g., lengthy periods of stable disease, rare spontaneous regression) make a search for effective therapies imperative. Active clinical and basic research in this area continues.

Suggested Readings

Grimaldi G, Reuter VE, Russo P. Bilateral non-famialial renal cell carcinoma. Ann Surg Oncol 1998;5:548–552.

Herrlinger JA, Schrott KM, Schot G, Sigel A. What are the benefits of extended dissection of the regional lymph nodes in the therapy of renal cell carcinoma? J Urol 1991;146:1224–1227.

Kattan MW, Reuter V, Motzer RJ, Katz J, Russo P. A postoperative prognostic nomogram for renal cell. J Urol 2001;166:63–67.

Kavolius JP, Mastorakos MD, Pavlovich C, Russo P, Burt ME, Brady MS. Resection of metastatic renal cell carcinoma. J Clin Oncol 1998;16:2261–2266.

Lee CT, Katz J, Shi W, Thaler HT, Reuter VE, Russo P. Surgical management of renal tumors 4 cm or less in a contemporary cohort. J Urol 2000;73:730–736.

Libertino JA, Zinman L, Watkins E. Long term results of resection of renal cell carcinoma with extension in the inferior vena cava. J Urol 1987;137:21–24.

Licht MR, Novick AC. Nephron sparing surgery for renal cell carcinoma. J Urol 1993;149:1–7.

Linehan WM, Lerman MI, Zbar B. Identification of the von Hippel-Lindau (VHL) gene: its role in renal cancer. JAMA 1995;273:564–570.

Minasian LM, Motzer RJ, Gluck L, Mazumdar M, Vlais V, Krown SE. Interferon alfa-2a in patients with advanced renal cell carcinoma: treatment results and survival in 159 patients with long term follow up. J Clin Oncol 1993;11:1368–1375.

Motzer R, Russo P. Systemic therapy for renal cell carcinoma. J Urol 2000;163:408–417.

Motzer RJ, Bander NH, Nanus DM. Renal cell carcinoma. N Engl J Med 1996;335:865–875.

Motzer RJ, Madhu M, Bacik J, Russo P, Berg WJ, Metz EM. Effect of cytokine therapy on survival for patients with advanced renal cell carcinoma. J Clin Oncol 2000;18:1928–1935.

Motzer RJ, Russo P, Nanus DM, Berg WJ. Renal cell carcinoma. Current Problems in Cancer 1997;21:187–232.

Motzer RJ, Schwartz L, Law TM, et al. Interferon alfa-2a and 13 cis-retinoic acid in renal cell carcinoma: antitumor activity in a phase 2 trial and interactions in vitro. J Clin Oncol 1995;13:1950–1957.

Novick AC, Streem S, Montie JE, Pontes JE, Siegel S, Montague D, Goormastic M. Conservative surgery for renal cell carcinoma: a single center experience with 100 patients. J Urol 1989;141:835.

Perez-Ordonez B, Hamed G, Campbell S, et al. Renal oncocytoma: a clinicopathological study of 70 cases. Am J Surg Pathol 1997;21:871–883.

Rabbani F, Grimaldi G, Russo P. Multiple primary malignancies in renal cell carcinoma. J Urol 1998;160:1255–1259.

Rabbani F, Reuter VR, Katz J, Russo P. Second primary malignancies associated with renal cell carcinoma: Influence of histologic type. Urology 2000; 56:399–403.

Rabbani F, Russo P. Lack of association between renal cell carcinoma and non-Hodgkin's lymphoma. Urology 1999;54:28–32.

Robson CJ, Churchill BM, Anderson W. The results of radical nephrectomy for renal cell carcinoma. J Urol 1969;101:297–301.

Rosenberg SA, Lotze MT, Muul LM, et al. A progress report on the treatment of 157 patients with advanced cancer using lymphokine activated killer cells and interleukin-2 or high dose interleukin-2 alone. N Engl J Med 1987;316:889–897.

Russo P. Evolving understanding and surgical management of renal cortical tumors. Mayo Clinic Proceedings 2000;75:1233–1235.

Russo P. Renal cell carcinoma: presentation, staging, and surgical treatment. Seminars in Oncology 2000;27:160–176.

Sadock DS, Seftl AD, Resnick MI. A new protocol for follow up of renal cell carcinoma based on pathological stage. J Urol 1995;154:28–31.

Sagalowsky AI, Kadesky KT, Ewalt DM, Kennedy TJ. Factors influencing adrenal metastasis in renal cell carcinoma. J Urol 1994;151:1118–1124.

Silver DA, Morash C, Brenner P, Campbell S, Russo P. Pathological findings at the time of nephrectomy for renal mass. Ann Surg Oncol 1997;4:570–574.

Smith SJ, Bosniak MA, Megibow AJ, et al. Renal cell carcinoma: earlier discovery and increased detection. Radiology 1989;170:699–703.

Thrasher JB, Robertson JE, Paulson DF. Expanding indications for conservative renal surgery in renal cell carcinoma. Urology 1994;43:160–168.

Yagoda A, Petrylak D, Thompson S. Cytotoxic chemotherapy for advanced renal cell carcinoma. Urol Clin North Am 1993;20:303–321.

CHAPTER 49

Prostate Cancer

ERNST W. LISEK IV
LEV ELTERMAN
CHARLES F. McKIEL, JR.
JEROME HOEKSEMA

A. *Epidemiology*

Prostate carcinoma is the most common malignancy in men; an estimated 184,500 new cases were diagnosed in 1998, which is 15,000 more than the number of new breast cancers in women.[1] Prostate cancer is second only to lung cancer in death rates, with an annual projected 39,200 deaths (19% of all cancer deaths).[1] The lifetime probability of prostate cancer in the United States is roughly 1 : 5.[1] Prostate cancer rates doubled between 1976 and 1994, and the mortality increased by 20%.[2] This increase is attributed to improved detection and greater patient awareness.

B. *Risk Factors*

Age seems to be the strongest risk factor associated with prostate cancer. The age-adjusted incidence rates per 100,000 in 1990 were 45.2 for men ages 50–55, 337.5 for ages 60–64, and 1000 for men older than 65.[2] Autopsy studies show that 70–90% of men age 80–90 years have histologic evidence of prostate carcinoma.[3] Prostate cancer rates increase with age more than any other malignancy.

Heredity plays an important role in prostate cancer. The occurrence of cancer is categorized as *sporadic* (randomly occurring in the population), *familial* (unpredictable clustering of disease in families), and *hereditary* (strong clustering in individual families and earlier onset).[4] An individual with a first-degree relative with prostate cancer has an increased risk of 2.0- to 2.41-fold.[4,5] If age at the time of prostate cancer diagnosis is taken into consideration, the relative risk increases sevenfold for men whose first-degree relatives had their cancer diagnosed before age 50.[4] Therefore a positive family history of prostate cancer should initiate appropriate screening and counseling.

The incidence of cancer-related deaths is 9.4% for African-Americans and 3.7% for Asians and Pacific Islanders.[1] From 1986 to 1993, the 5-year cancer survival rates differed significantly between Whites and African-Americans: 90% and 75%, respectively.[1] During 1992–1995 Norway had the leading age-adjusted death rates, with 23.8 prostate cancer-related deaths per 100,000 population; the United States ranked 11th, with 17.3 deaths per 100,000; the lowest incidence was in Uzbekistan (1.4).[1]

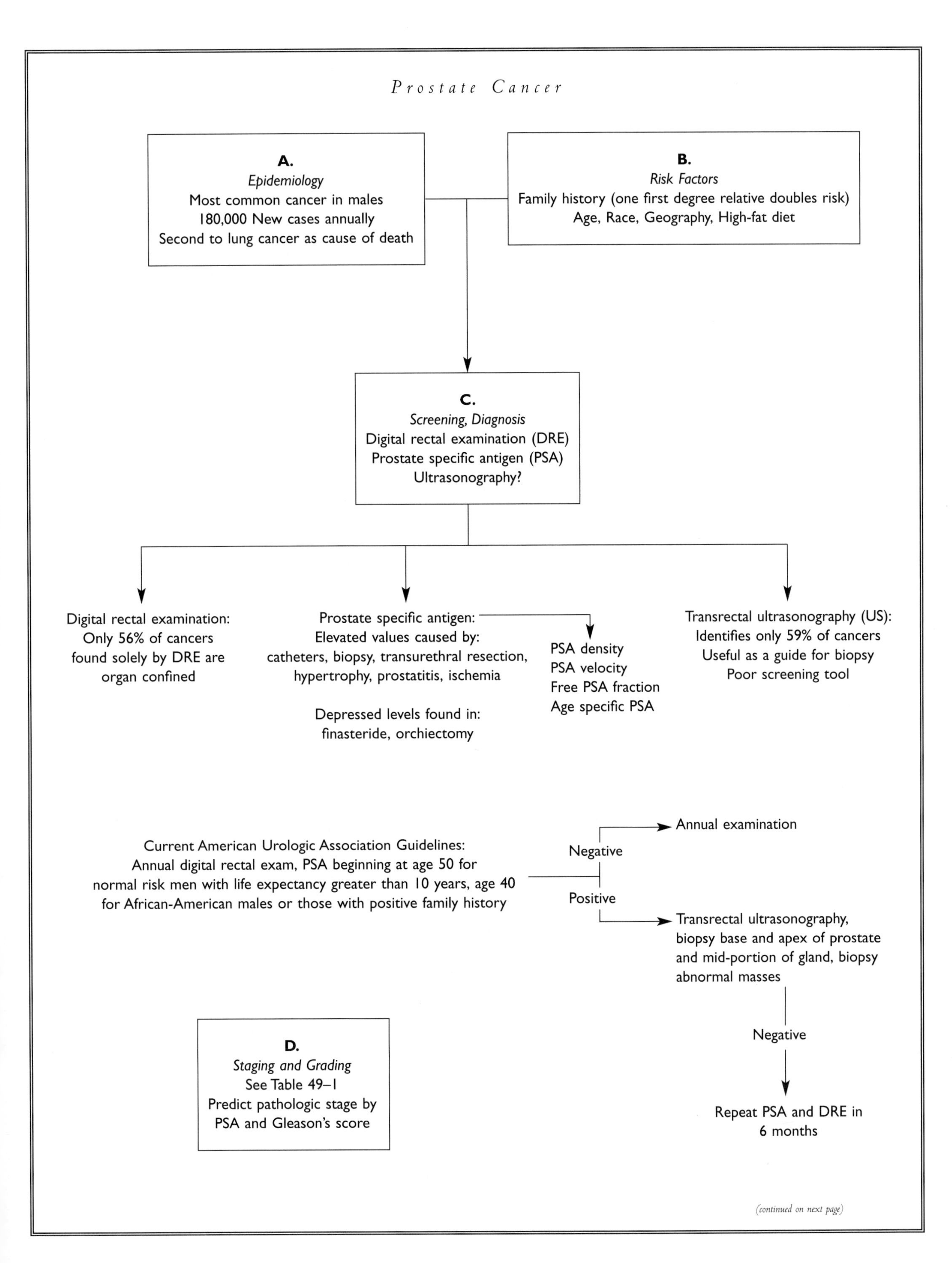
Prostate Cancer
A.
Epidemiology
Most common cancer in males
180,000 New cases annually
Second to lung cancer as cause of death
B.
Risk Factors
Family history (one first degree relative doubles risk)
Age, Race, Geography, High-fat diet
C.
Screening, Diagnosis
Digital rectal examination (DRE)
Prostate specific antigen (PSA)
Ultrasonography?
Digital rectal examination:
Only 56% of cancers
found solely by DRE are
organ confined
Prostate specific antigen:
Elevated values caused by:
catheters, biopsy, transurethral resection,
hypertrophy, prostatitis, ischemia
Depressed levels found in:
finasteride, orchiectomy
PSA density
PSA velocity
Free PSA fraction
Age specific PSA
Transrectal ultrasonography (US):
Identifies only 59% of cancers
Useful as a guide for biopsy
Poor screening tool
Current American Urologic Association Guidelines:
Annual digital rectal exam, PSA beginning at age 50 for
normal risk men with life expectancy greater than 10 years, age 40
for African-American males or those with positive family history
Negative
Annual examination
Positive
Transrectal ultrasonography,
biopsy base and apex of prostate
and mid-portion of gland, biopsy
abnormal masses
Negative
Repeat PSA and DRE in
6 months
D.
Staging and Grading
See Table 49–1
Predict pathologic stage by
PSA and Gleason's score
(continued on next page)

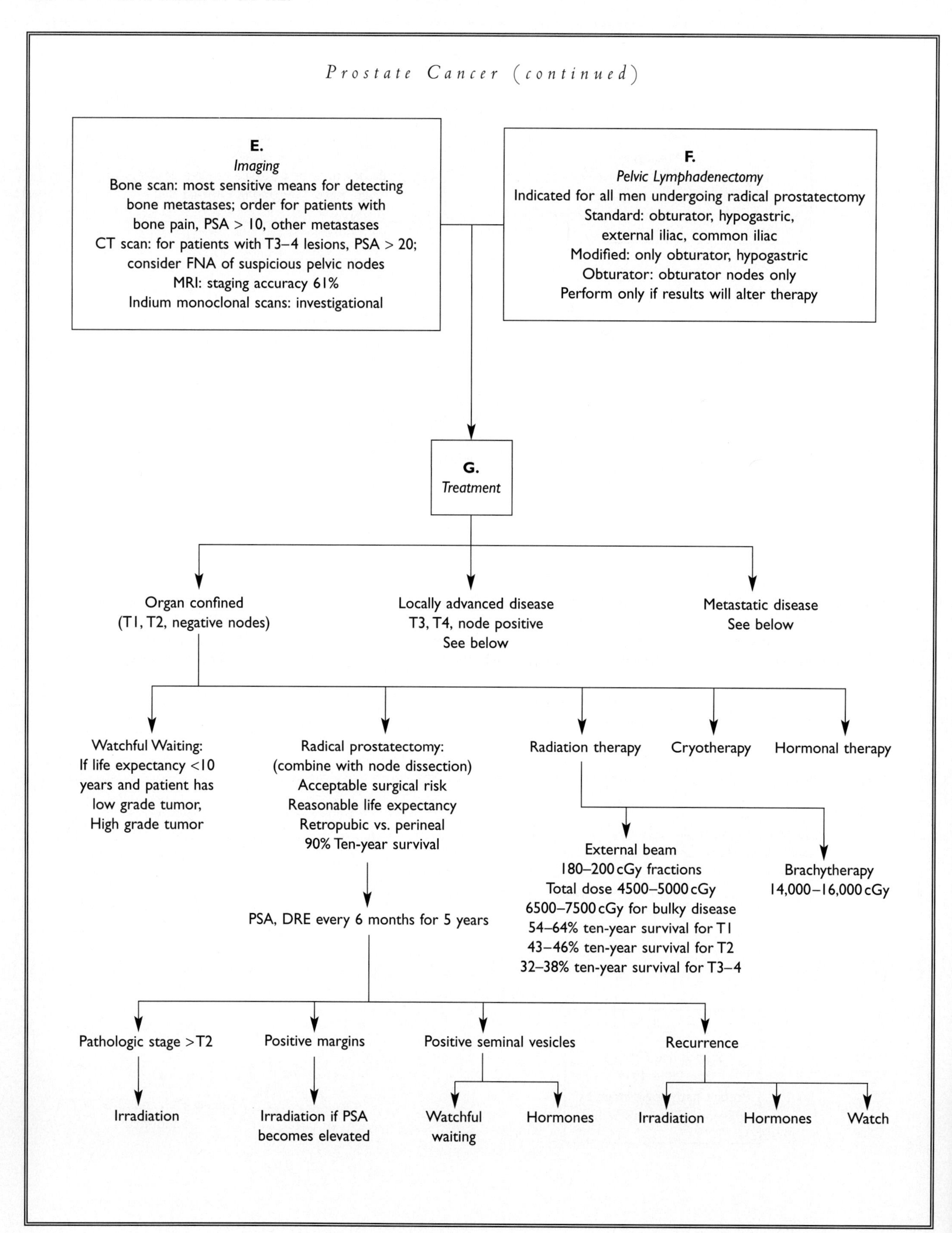

Prostate Cancer (continued)
E.
Imaging
Bone scan: most sensitive means for detecting bone metastases; order for patients with bone pain, PSA > 10, other metastases
CT scan: for patients with T3–4 lesions, PSA > 20; consider FNA of suspicious pelvic nodes
MRI: staging accuracy 61%
Indium monoclonal scans: investigational
F.
Pelvic Lymphadenectomy
Indicated for all men undergoing radical prostatectomy
Standard: obturator, hypogastric, external iliac, common iliac
Modified: only obturator, hypogastric
Obturator: obturator nodes only
Perform only if results will alter therapy
G.
Treatment
Organ confined (T1, T2, negative nodes)
Locally advanced disease T3, T4, node positive See below
Metastatic disease See below
Watchful Waiting: If life expectancy <10 years and patient has low grade tumor, High grade tumor
Radical prostatectomy: (combine with node dissection) Acceptable surgical risk Reasonable life expectancy Retropubic vs. perineal 90% Ten-year survival
Radiation therapy
Cryotherapy
Hormonal therapy
External beam 180–200 cGy fractions Total dose 4500–5000 cGy 6500–7500 cGy for bulky disease 54–64% ten-year survival for T1 43–46% ten-year survival for T2 32–38% ten-year survival for T3–4
Brachytherapy 14,000–16,000 cGy
PSA, DRE every 6 months for 5 years
Pathologic stage >T2
Positive margins
Positive seminal vesicles
Recurrence
Irradiation
Irradiation if PSA becomes elevated
Watchful waiting
Hormones
Irradiation
Hormones
Watch

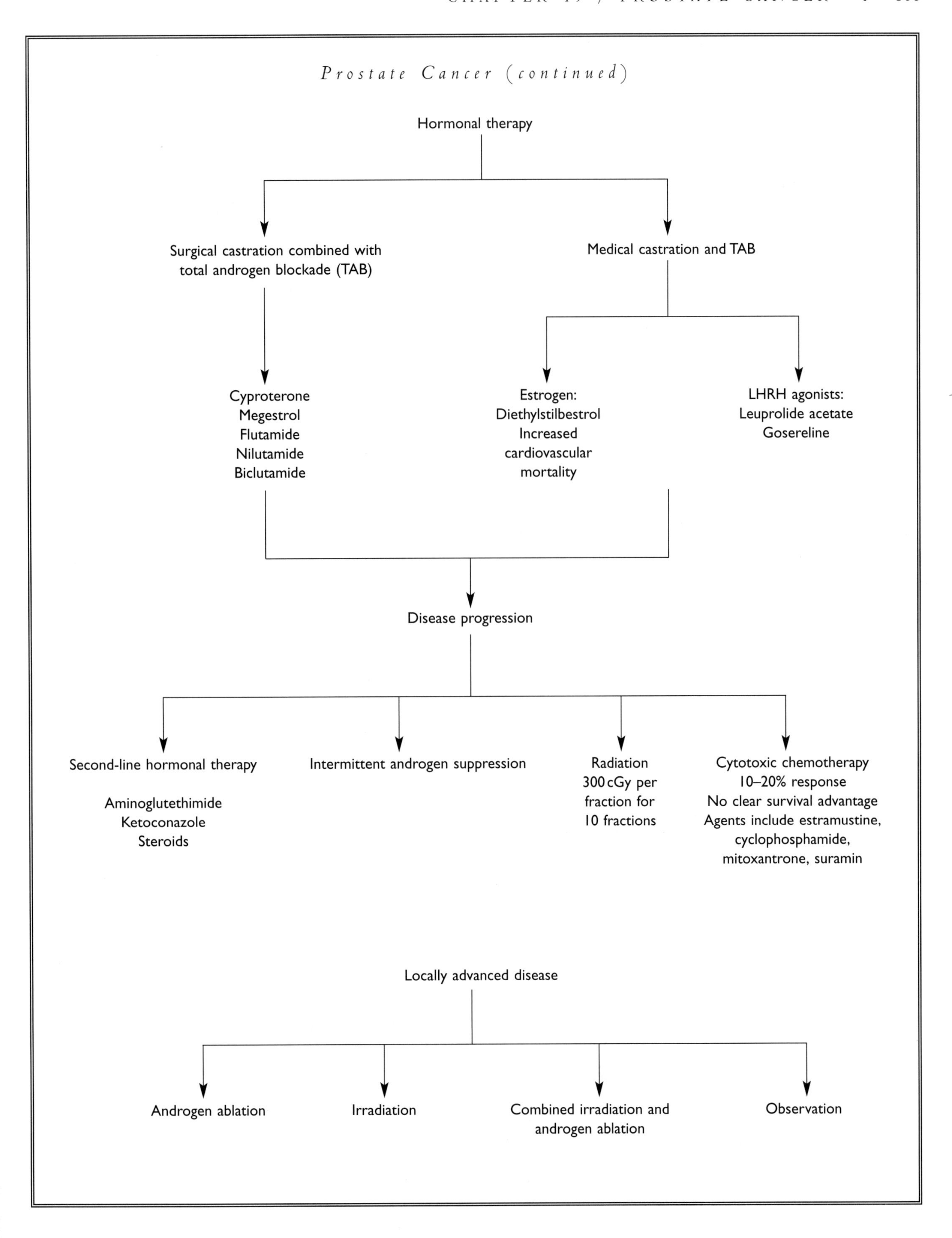
Prostate Cancer (continued)
Hormonal therapy
Surgical castration combined with total androgen blockade (TAB)
Medical castration and TAB
Cyproterone
Megestrol
Flutamide
Nilutamide
Biclutamide
Estrogen:
Diethylstilbestrol
Increased cardiovascular mortality
LHRH agonists:
Leuprolide acetate
Gosereline
Disease progression
Second-line hormonal therapy
Aminoglutethimide
Ketoconazole
Steroids
Intermittent androgen suppression
Radiation
300 cGy per fraction for 10 fractions
Cytotoxic chemotherapy
10–20% response
No clear survival advantage
Agents include estramustine, cyclophosphamide, mitoxantrone, suramin
Locally advanced disease
Androgen ablation
Irradiation
Combined irradiation and androgen ablation
Observation

This difference may be explained by several factors including genetic predisposition, environment, diet, and accepted medical practices.

Diet has been implicated and may account for some of the differences in incidence between racial groups, socioeconomic groups, and geographic sites. There is a positive association between fat intake and prostate cancer risk;[6] diets rich in fruits and vegetables seem to have a protective effect.[6] *Obesity* increases the risk of prostate cancer death twofold.[6] Conflicting reports have appeared regarding *hormones* and their influence on prostate cancer; it has been established that eunuchs, prepubertal castrates, and men with congenital abnormal androgen metabolism do not develop prostate cancer.

C. Screening and Diagnosis

Localized prostate cancer usually causes no symptoms. Voiding difficulty, irritative urinary complaints, hematuria, and erectile dysfunction may be symptoms of locally advanced or invasive cancer, whereas bone pain is a manifestation of metastatic disease. Although bladder outlet obstruction is often present, these symptoms are usually caused by coincidental benign prostatic hyperplasia, which is common in this age group. Early detection of potentially curable disease necessitates evaluating asymptomatic men at risk. Currently, digital rectal examination (DRE), prostate-specific antigen (PSA), and transrectal ultrasound (TRUS)—directed prostate biopsy are considered the primary screening modalities. The serum PSA level, however, remains the single best screening test.

Serum PSA

Prostate-specific antigen, a serine protease produced by the columnar cells of the prostate glandular epithelium, serves as a liquefying agent in seminal fluid.[7] PSA levels in the bloodstream correspond to about one-millionth of that in semen due to the barriers offered by the normal basement membrane, acinar basal cells, and stromal cells. Intact barriers in benign prostatic hyperplasia (BPH) maintain blood secretion rates of 0.3 ng/ml/g of tissue, whereas the distorted architecture of cancer tissue causes secretion rates of 3.5 ng/ml/g.[8] Serum PSA levels therefore increase in proportion to the amount of cancer. Normal levels are less than 4.0 ng/ml, but PSA elevations above 4.0 ng/ml do not always indicate the presence of cancer. In most screening studies the positive predictive value of a PSA level ≥4.0 ng/ml was approximately 32%.[9] PSA elevation is considered to have the strongest association with prostate cancer of all the screening techniques.

Prostate manipulations, such as inserting a urethral indwelling catheter, prostate biopsy, and transurethral resection of the prostate have been shown to increase serum PSA levels.[8,10,11] Other conditions that elevate serum PSA are BPH, prostatitis, acute urinary retention, and prostatic infarction or ischemia.[12–15] Because the half-life of PSA in the bloodstream is 3.2 days, it has been recommended that PSA be measured no earlier than 2–3 weeks following resolution of the condition or manipulation of the gland. DREs, TRUS, prostatic massage, and ejaculation have not been shown to influence the serum PSA levels significantly.[15,16]

Normal prostatic glandular tissue and adenocarcinoma cells are sensitive to the hormonal milieu. Prostate-directed treatment such as finasteride (Proscar), hormonal manipulations, and orchiectomy lead to decreased serum PSA levels. Finasteride has been shown to decrease PSA levels by 50% over a 12-month period; therefore if after finasteride therapy a significant drop in PSA levels is not seen, the presence of occult prostate cancer should be considered.[17]

To improve its predictive value, several PSA indices have been investigated.

1. *PSA density*. In 1992 Benson et al.[18] proposed using PSA density, defined as the serum PSA/prostate volume ratio, as a means of predicting BPH or cancer. This technique requires TRUS assessment of volume. Values above 0.15 ng/ml/g are abnormal, and the utility of this measurement is controversial. At present, PSA density is not considered a routine test.

2. *PSA velocity*. Carter et al. in 1992[19] suggested, based on a longitudinal study, that an increase in serum PSA of more than 0.75 ng/ml/year strongly correlates with the presence of prostate cancer. They recommended obtaining three PSA readings over a 2-year period. PSA velocity appears to be a promising adjunct to standard PSA determination, but more studies are necessary to validate this technique.

3. *PSA fraction*. In the bloodstream, PSA exists as *unbound (free)* molecules, molecules bound to *α_1-antichymotrypsin* (PSA-ACT complex), and molecules bound to *α_2-macroglobulin* (PSA-AMG complex). α_2-Macroglobulin covers PSA's antigenic determinants and renders this complex "invisible" to immunoassays. Oesterling et al.[20] suggested that a *free/total PSA* ratio less than 0.15 (15%) was associated with a significantly higher risk of having prostate cancer irrespective of age. This index improves the specificity of PSA determinations without a significant loss in sensitivity. Studies are under way to determine its usefulness.

4. *Age-specific PSA*. As mentioned above, the serum PSA level is dependent on prostate glandular volume and BPH, both of which become more prevalent with advancing age.

This results in a gradual increase of mean serum PSA levels with age. Age-specific reference PSA ranges were introduced in an effort to detect early cancers in younger men and to reduce the negative biopsy rate in older men. For men ages 40–49 and 50–59 years, the PSA cutoff values were lowered to 2.4 and 3.8 ng/ml, respectively, and raised to 5.6 and 6.9 ng/ml for men ages 60–69 and 70–79 years, respectively.[21] Use of age-adjusted PSA ranges may improve the selection of patients for prostate biopsy.

Digital Rectal Examination

The DRE is important in the detection of prostate cancer and should be performed with particular attention to prostate size, firmness, asymmetry, irregularities, and nodules. The positive predictive value of a DRE in screening population is currently 21%.[9] DRE tends to miss small prostate masses, and interpretation is examiner-dependent. Only 56% of cancers discovered by DRE alone are organ-confined and therefore potentially curable.[9] However, combining DRE with PSA significantly increases the sensitivity of screening, detecting 78% of prostate cancers in the organ-confined stage. Patients with abnormal DRE findings should undergo a prostate biopsy.

The goal of prostate cancer screening is to identify low-stage prostate cancer in asymptomatic men; and the ability of widespread prostate cancer screening programs to accomplish this is debatable. Opponents cite the lack of specificity and sensitivity of PSA determinations and digital rectal examinations, the unproven efficacy or necessity of treating low-stage prostate cancer, and concern over the cost of screening and treatment. Screening proponents note that effective local therapy—radical prostatectomy and irradiation—are best applied to the lowest-stage cancers. By targeting men who are at risk by virtue of their age, race, and family history and who are likely to benefit from cancer therapy based on their longevity, screening may be effectively implemented in appropriate patients. The American Urological Association (AUA) recommends screening for (1) men over 50 years of age or (2) men over 40 years of age with risk factors, including those of African descent.[22] Currently, screening consists of yearly DRE and serum PSA determinations. Elderly patients or patients in poor overall health with an estimated life expectancy under 10 years are usually excluded from screening. Although early cancers are more likely to be found with screening programs, a survival advantage to screening has not been established, and studies are in progress to address this very issue.

Ultrasonography

Transrectal ultrasonography is one of the best modalities for visualizing the prostate and seminal vesicles, but its usefulness for diagnosing prostate cancer is limited by its lack of specificity and sensitivity. Only 59% of tumors can be identified on TRUS.[23] However, it is invaluable for guiding prostate biopsies and determining prostatic volume. Cancerous lesions in the peripheral and central zones appear hypoechoic, but only 32.5% of all hypoechoic lesions are cancerous, and up to 39% of cancers are isoechoic.[24–26] Therefore the positive predictive value of hypoechoic lesions for TRUS for the presence of carcinoma in the peripheral zone is only 41%, making TURS a poor screening tool.[25]

The prostate is divided into four zones according to histology and embryologic origin of each portion of the gland.[27] The urethra divides the prostate into the anterior fibromuscular stroma and posterior glandular tissue; the former does not contain glandular tissue and therefore does not give rise to adenocarcinoma.[28] The peripheral zone is the most posterior part of the prostate and is adjacent to the rectum. It gives rise to 68% of prostatic carcinomas.[28] Anterior to it lies the central zone, where only 8% of carcinomas arise.[28] The transition zone surrounds the urethra proximal to the verumontanum. It is enlarged in the presence of BPH and gives rise to 24% of prostate cancers.[28] On TRUS images, the peripheral and central zones are isoechoic, and the transition zone is slightly hypoechoic.

A TRUS-guided biopsy of the prostate is indicated for patients with suspicious DREs or elevated serum PSA levels. Some recommend using PSA indexes, such as age-specific ranges, to decrease the rate of negative biopsies and to find early stages of cancer in young patients.[29] TRUS-guided prostate biopsy is a well tolerated office procedure that does not usually require sedation or local anesthetic. Patients are advised to stop nonsteroidal antiinflammatory agents (NSAIDs) and other anticoagulation medication if medically possible. Patients with artificial joints and artificial heart valves and men who are at risk for bacterial endocarditis are given appropriate antibiotic prophylaxis. Others receive oral quinolone prior to the procedure and 1 day following the biopsy. A Fleet enema is usually given 1 hour prior to the procedure. A 7 MH rectal ultrasound probe is used to identify suspicious areas, determine prostatic size, and guide the biopsy needle. An 18-gauge core biopsy needle powered by a spring-loaded biopsy gun is used to obtain the tissue sample. Patients with an elevated PSA and no identifiable abnormalities on DRE or TRUS undergo biopsy of the prostatic base, mid-prostate, and apex on each side, constituting *sextant* biopsies. Suspicious areas on DRE or TRUS are biopsied in addition to the described regions. Digital pressure usually stops bleeding after the biopsy.

Use of quinolone antibiotic prophylaxis and the biopsy gun have significantly reduced the complications of bleeding and infection. Currently, the overall complication rates are 2.1–2.4%.[30,31] Postoperative fever occurs in 0.6–0.8%, and rectal

TABLE 49–1.
AJCC definition of TNM for prostate cancer

Primary Tumor (T)

TX	Primary tumor cannot be assessed
T0	No evidence of primary tumor
T1	Clinically inapparent tumor not palpable or visible by imaging
T1a	Tumor incidental histological finding in 5% or less of tissue resected
T1b	Tumor incidental histological finding in more than 5% of tissue resected
T1c	Tumor identified by needle biopsy (e.g., because of elevated PSA)
T2	Tumor confined within prostate*
T2a	Tumor involves one lobe
T2b	Tumor involves both lobes
T3	Tumor extends through the prostatic capsule**
T3a	Extracapsular extension (unilateral or bilateral)
T3b	Tumor invades seminal vesicle(s)
T4	Tumor is fixed or invades adjacent structures other than seminal vesicles: bladder neck, external sphincter, rectum, levator muscles, and/or pelvic wall

*Tumor found in one or both lobes by needle biopsy, but not palpable or reliably visible by imaging, is classified as T1c.
**Invasion into the prostatic apex or into (but not beyond) the prostatic capsule is not classified as T3, but as T2.

Regional Lymph Nodes (N)

NX	Regional lymph nodes cannot be assessed
N0	No regional lymph node metastasis
N1	Metastasis in regional lymph node or nodes

Distant Metastasis (M)***

MX	Distant metastasis cannot be assessed
M0	No distant metastasis
M1	Distant metastasis
M1a	Nonregional lymph node(s)
M1b	Bone(s)
M1c	Other site(s)

***When more than one site of metastasis is present, the most advanced category is used. pM1c is most advanced.

SOURCE: Used with permission of the American Joint Committee on Cancer (AJCC®), Chicago, IL. The original source for this material is the AJCC® Cancer Staging Manual, 5th edition (1997) published by Lippincott Williams & Wilkins Publishers, Philadelphia, PA.

mucosal bleeding is seen in 0.6–1.2%, mostly in patients taking NSAIDs.[30,31] Other complications include hematuria and urinary tract infections.

D. *Staging and Grading*

Adenocarcinoma is the predominant histologic type of prostate cancer; other types include squamous carcinoma, sarcomas, carcinosarcomas, and primary prostatic lymphomas. These types are rare and are omitted from the following discussion.

There are several prostate cancer staging systems. The Whitmore-Jewett classification, introduced in 1956 and later modified in 1975, was a widely used system.[32] The TNM classification is now the preferred *clinical* staging system. The final version of this system was adapted in 1997 and is summarized in Table 49–1.[33] Clinical staging relies on DRE, serum markers, tumor markers, tumor grade, and imaging modalities.

The *pathologic* stage is determined by examining the prostatectomy specimen for extracapsular involvement, tumor extension into surrounding structures, and regional lymph nodes. Pathologically, prostate cancer is classified as organ-confined (cancer confined within the prostatic capsule); capsular penetration (extension into the periprostatic tissue, excluding seminal vesicles); seminal vesicle involvement; and pelvic lymph node involvement. Pathologic stage correlates closely with the prognosis. Men with organ-confined disease (T1, T2) are the best candidates for radical local therapy; therefore identifying these men *before treatment* is of paramount importance. Predicting pathologic stage before surgery uses serum markers and histologic grading scores of the biopsy specimens.

PSA Staging

Serum PSA levels correlate with advancing pathologic and clinical stage.[34] In a study of 4133 patients who underwent radical prostatectomy, the probability of organ-confined disease decreased linearly with increasing preoperative serum PSA level.[34] Men with PSA levels less than 4.0 ng/ml had a 64% probability of having organ-confined disease and only a 1% chance of pelvic lymph node involvement. In contrast, men with PSA levels higher than 50 ng/ml had only a 9% chance of having organ-confined disease and 27% probability of having pelvic lymph nodes involved with a tumor.

Prostatic Acid Phosphatase Staging

Prostatic acid phosphatase (PAP) is a serum marker that was widely used prior to the PSA era. PAP is not prostate-specific, though elevated levels in the blood correlate with the presence of metastatic disease. Men with abnormal PAP values have a greater than 80% chance of having extraprostatic disease.[35] Normal PAP levels are not as useful for predicting the absence of extraprostatic disease. With the advent of PSA testing, PAP determinations do not add substantial information and do not affect clinical decision-making.

Gleason Score

The Gleason histologic grading system for prostate cancer[36] is currently most widely used; it correlates closely with pathologic extent of disease. The Gleason system is based on architectural tumor patterns scored 1 to 5, with 5 being the least differentiated pattern. The Gleason sum or score represents the addition of Gleason grades from the first and second most predominant patterns present. Men with a Gleason score of less than 5 have less than a 1% chance of having regional lymph node involvement at the time of prostatectomy, whereas a Gleason score of 8–10 carries a 20% risk of "positive" lymph nodes and an 83% risk of extraprostatic extension.[34]

Predicting Stage

The combined use of DRE, serum PSA level, and Gleason score of the biopsy specimen can predict the extent of cancer. Partin et al. reported a multivariant analysis of 4133 men who had undergone radical prostatectomy for localized disease,[34] establishing tables that predict the probability of organ-confined disease, capsular penetration, seminal vesicle involvement, and lymph node involvement (Table 49–2). Knowledge of these data is crucial when counseling patients and making treatment decisions.

E. Imaging Studies

Imaging studies include the radionuclide bone scan, computed tomography (CT), magnetic resonance imaging (MRI), and radioimmunologic scanning.

Bone Scan

Bone scintigraphy, shown to be the most sensitive test for identifying bony metastases,[37] is superior to a skeletal survey and alkaline and acid phosphatase levels. False-negative results occur in less than 1%, and sensitivity approaches 100%. The likelihood of positive findings correlates well with the serum PSA level and is low for patients with PSA levels less than 10 ng/ml.[38] Some therefore recommend reserving bone scanning for patients with bone pain, a PSA level higher than 10 ng/ml, or evidence of other metastases.[39]

CT Imaging

Computed tomography imaging has limited application for staging prostate cancer. Pelvic lymph nodes may have micrometastatic disease that escapes CT detection; CT imaging relies on an enlarged node size (>1.0 cm) to be considered suspicious for metastatic disease. Consequently, the sensitivity of pelvic CT ranges from 27% to 75%, and specificity from 66% to 100%.[40,41] CT-guided fine-needle aspiration is sometimes used to enhance the accuracy of nodal staging. CT imaging is indicated for patients with serum PSA levels above 20 ng/ml who are willing to undergo percutaneous aspiration of suspicious nodes and are not likely to undergo staging lymphadenectomy.

Magnetic Resonance Imaging

Magnetic resonance imaging is used to assess the local extent of prostate cancer. The MRI criteria for extraprostatic extension include capsular disruption by direct tumor extension, obliteration of the normal periprostatic fat planes, and indistinct or irregular prostatic margins. Overall staging accuracy is 61%.[42] Use of an endorectal coil does not seem to enhance accuracy and is considered investigational.[42] MRI has not demonstrated any superiority over TRUS for staging accuracy.[43]

Radioimmunologic Scanning

Radioimmunologic scanning with indium-111-labeled CYT-356 antibody is now being investigated. CYT-356 antibody

TABLE 49–2.
Gleason prediction of pathologic stage of prostate cancer

Gleason	PSA 0–4.0 ng/ml, by clinical stage							PSA 4.1–10.0 ng/ml, by clinical stage							PSA 10.1–20.0 ng/ml, by clinical stage							PSA > 20.0 ng/ml, by clinical stage						
score	T1a	T1b	T1c	T2a	T2b	T2c	T3a	T1a	T1b	T1c	T2a	T2b	T2c	T3a	T1a	T1b	T1c	T2a	T2b	T2c	T3a	T1a	T1b	T1c	T2a	T2b	T2c	T3a
Organ-confined disease																												
2–4	90	80	89	81	72	77	—	84	70	83	71	61	66	43	76	58	75	60	48	53	—	—	38	58	41	29	—	—
5	82	66	81	68	57	62	40	72	53	71	55	43	49	27	61	40	60	43	32	36	18	—	23	40	26	17	19	8
6	78	61	78	64	52	57	35	67	47	67	51	38	43	23	—	33	55	38	26	31	14	—	17	35	22	13	15	6
7	—	43	63	47	34	38	19	49	29	49	33	22	25	11	33	17	35	22	13	15	6	—	—	18	10	5	6	2
8–10	—	31	52	36	24	27	—	35	18	37	23	14	15	6	—	9	23	14	7	8	3	—	3	10	5	3	3	1
Established capsular penetration																												
2–4	9	19	10	18	25	21	—	14	27	15	26	35	29	44	20	36	22	35	43	37	—	—	47	34	48	52	—	—
5	17	32	18	30	40	34	51	25	42	27	41	50	43	57	33	50	35	50	57	51	59	—	57	78	60	61	55	54
6	19	35	21	34	43	37	53	27	44	30	44	52	46	57	—	49	38	52	57	50	54	—	51	49	60	57	51	46
7	—	44	31	45	51	45	52	36	48	40	52	54	48	48	38	46	45	55	51	45	40	—	—	46	51	43	37	29
8–10	—	43	34	47	48	41	—	34	42	40	49	46	40	34	—	33	50	46	38	33	26	—	24	34	37	28	23	17
Seminal vesicle involvement																												
2–4	0	1	1	1	2	2	—	1	2	1	2	4	5	10	2	4	2	4	7	8	—	—	9	7	10	14	—	—
5	1	2	1	2	3	3	7	2	3	2	3	5	6	12	3	5	3	5	8	9	15	—	10	9	11	15	19	26
6	1	2	1	2	3	4	7	2	3	2	3	5	6	11	—	4	4	5	7	9	14	—	8	8	10	13	17	21
7	—	6	4	6	10	12	19	6	9	8	10	15	18	26	8	11	12	14	18	22	28	—	—	22	24	27	32	36
8–10	—	11	9	12	17	21	—	10	15	15	19	24	28	35	—	15	20	22	25	30	34	—	20	31	33	33	38	40
Lymph node involvement																												
2–4	0	0	0	0	0	0	—	0	1	0	0	1	1	1	0	2	0	1	1	1	—	—	4	1	1	3	—	—
5	0	1	0	0	1	1	2	1	2	0	1	2	2	3	3	5	1	2	4	4	7	—	10	3	3	7	7	11
6	1	2	0	1	2	2	5	3	5	1	2	4	4	9	—	13	3	4	10	10	18	—	23	7	8	16	17	26
7	—	6	1	2	5	5	9	8	12	3	4	9	9	15	18	24	8	9	17	18	26	—	—	14	14	25	25	32
8–10	—	14	4	5	10	10	—	18	23	8	9	16	17	24	—	40	16	17	29	29	37	—	51	24	24	36	35	42

PSA, prostate-specific assay; DRE, digital rectal examination.
The numbers indicate the probability of a respective pathologic stage, given the combination of serum PSA, Gleason score, and DRE.
—, insufficient data.
SOURCE: Data from Partin et al.[34]

recognizes a prostate-specific membrane antigen located intracellularly. Preliminary reports suggest that this technique may detect pelvic lymph node metastases more accurately than CT or MRI.[44] Other reports state that radioimmunologic scanning may be helpful for localizing cancer recurrence in patients with a rising PSA level after radical prostatectomy.[45] The results of this test are promising, but the technique remains investigational and should be used only in carefully selected patients.

F. Pelvic Lymphadenectomy

Pelvic lymph node dissection is the best means of confirming metastases to the pelvic lymph nodes; it can be performed via a traditional open approach through a low midline incision as a separate procedure or at the time of radical prostatectomy. Lymphadenectomies have been performed via a laparoscopic approach, or a 6 cm minilaparotomy incision. All of the techniques have comparable yield and are selected according to the surgeon's experience and the patient's preference. Pelvic lymphadenectomy is classified as standard (removal of obturator, hypogastric, external iliac, and common iliac nodes), extended (standard lymphadenectomy plus removal of presciatic and presacral nodes), modified (removal of obturator and hypogastric nodes only), and obturator (removal of obturator lymph nodes only). The extent of lymphadenectomy correlates with the complication rate, and both standard and modified lymphadenectomy appear to be reasonable options. Obturator lymphadenectomy may under-stage the lesion.

Pelvic lymphadenectomy is a staging tool and confers no therapeutic benefit to patients so treated. Therefore it should be performed only if its results will alter future therapy. Although some contend that it may not be necessary for patients with stage T2b disease if the Gleason score is less than 5 and the PSA is less than 4.0 ng/ml, some patients who meet these criteria are found to have nodal micrometastatic disease. Because the morbidity of node dissection is low, lymphadenectomy is generally indicated for all men undergoing radical prostatectomy. This is especially so for patients with a PSA level higher than 10 ng/ml, a Gleason score higher than 6, and clinical stage T2c or higher.[46]

G. Treatment

Watchful Waiting

Because prostate cancer grows slowly, especially in its early stages, studies of the efficacy of various therapies (including no treatment) for organ-confined disease must have follow-up in excess of 10 years before differences become significant. Patients in poor health may be observed without treatment until disease progression or symptoms occur. Such management has been termed "watchful waiting." Patients with low-grade tumors have 10-year mortality rates of 9–13%, which is comparable to that of age-matched controls.[47,48] Studies evaluating the treatment benefit in quality-adjusted years indicate that men age 60–65 with poorly differentiated tumors have a treatment benefit of 3.86 and 2.68 quality-adjusted years, respectively. Based on these data, the authors consider patients with a life expectancy of less than 10 years and a low-grade tumor as candidates for watchful waiting.[49] Patients with high-grade tumors may also be candidates for watchful waiting because it is unlikely their disease can be controlled.[50]

Radical Prostatectomy

Radical prostatectomy is indicated for organ-confined prostate cancer (stage T1–T2) in patients of acceptable surgical risk and reasonable life expectancy. Poor surgical candidates or patients with a short life expectancy should receive alternative therapy (irradiation or androgen deprivation). As previously stated, radical prostatectomy may be done independently of pelvic lymphadenectomy, or they may be performed at one sitting, in which case node dissection with frozen section analysis of the nodes is done first. If the analysis reveals nodal metastases, prostatectomy is sometimes deferred because of the notion that radical local treatment adds little to survival. This practice has been challenged by several centers that proceed with prostatectomy even in the presence of nodal disease, citing improved survival when hormonal therapy is given early during the postoperative period.

The prostate is located in the true pelvis cephalad to the membranous urethra, is attached to the symphysis pubis anteriorly by the paired puboprostatic ligaments, and is bounded posteriorly be Denonvillier's fascia and the rectum. The prostate and seminal vesicles are surrounded by the inner layer (stratum) of the pelvic fascia. The inferior vesical artery is the main arterial supply of the prostate, and venous drainage consists of lateral venous plexus draining into the internal iliac vein. The superficial branch of the dorsal vein of the penis courses between the puboprostatic ligaments on the anterior of the prostate and can be a source of significant blood loss if not ligated.[51] Neurovascular bundles run dorsolaterally along the prostate capsule and contain the autonomic innervation of the corpora cavernosum necessary for potency.[52]

Radical retropubic prostatectomy begins with an infraumbilical midline incision to gain extraperitoneal access to the pelvis. The puboprostatic ligaments are divided, and the dorsal venous complex is ligated. Dissection and excision of the prostate and seminal vesicles follows, with the prostatic capsule and Denonvillier's fascia left intact. The remaining urethral stump and bladder neck are reanastomosed. This retropubic approach allows access to the pelvis for staging dissection of pelvic lymph nodes. Patients with preoperative potency who have no induration or nodularity at the apex or dorsolateral aspects of the prostate and are not at high risk for extraprostatic disease are candidates for a nerve-sparing or anatomic radical retropubic prostatectomy where the neurovascular bundles are preserved.

The *radical perineal prostatectomy* is another approach via a transverse perineal incision for resecting the prostate and seminal vesicles. The advantage of this approach is avoidance of a lower abdominal incision, an advantage in obese patients. Patients who cannot be placed in the exaggerated lithotomy position are not suitable candidates for this approach. Because the approach does not provide access to the pelvic lymph nodes, an additional procedure is required to perform node dissection. In general, surgeon familiarity typically governs the approach selection for a radical prostatectomy.

In a report by Zincke et al., survival rates were 90% and 82% at 10 and 15 years, respectively, for 3170 men following radical prostatectomy. Recurrence-free survival rates of 72% and 61% were 10 and 15 years, respectively.[53] Some studies have reported that 70% of patients with organ-confined disease have undetectable PSA 10 years after prostatectomy by actuarial analysis.[54] Radical prostatectomy is capable of providing long-term cancer-free survival over an extended period of time. It is not clear if radiation therapy is capable of doing the same.

Mortality rates for radical prostatectomy are less than 1%,[55] rectal injury occurs in less than 1%, and transfusion rates range from 5.0% to 11.5%.[53,56] Total incontinence rates under 2% have been reported,[54] with stress incontinence occurring in 5–8% of patients.[53,54] Impotence is dependent on age and surgical technique; erectile function was preserved in 75% of men age 50–60 years and 25% of men older than 70 years.[57]

Margin-positive disease occurs most commonly at apical, rectal, posterolateral, and bladder neck margins.[58] It is thought by some that a positive urethral margin is typically due to a pathologic artifact from the urethra retracting into the prostate. Radiation therapy to the prostatic bed in positive margin disease is reserved for patients with a rising PSA level after initially undetectable PSA.[59] Patients with positive seminal vesicle involvement have a greater risk of progression to metastatic disease; such patients may undergo watchful waiting or be treated with hormonal therapy.[60]

Preoperative androgen deprivation therapy has been used for patients with stage T1, T2, or T3 disease in an effort to reduce the incidence of positive margins and to down-stage tumors. However, only 35% of patients with T3 *clinical* disease treated in this fashion have histologic organ-confined disease, which seems to indicate that preoperative androgen deprivation therapy does not down-stage clinical T3 tumors.[61] Studies evaluating its role in organ-confined clinical disease (T1, T2) have demonstrated a decrease in the rate of positive margins but have not demonstrated a reduction in PSA recurrence over radical prostatectomy alone.[61] Positive margins appear to be a sentinel event, signaling the statistical probability of disseminated disease. Establishing negative margins with neoadjuvant hormonal therapy does not appear to change the fact that disseminated disease is still likely.

Radiation Therapy

Radiation therapy has been used as primary treatment of clinical stage T1–T3 disease, for local recurrence after radical prostatectomy, and for palliation of painful bony metastasis. For *external beam radiation therapy*, daily doses of 180–200 cGy are given to a total dose of 4500–5000 cGy for treatment of micrometastases and 6500–7500 cGy for treatment of bulky disease.[62] In the United States the mean 10-year survival is 54–64% for T1 tumors, 43–46% for T2 tumors, and 32–38% for T3 and T4 patients.[63] Cause-specific 15-year survival rates up to 75% have been reported in patients with T1N0 and T2N0 disease.[64] Long-term complications include incontinence in 0.9%, hematuria in 5.1%, and rectal bleeding in 5.4%.[65] Neoadjuvant androgen suppression using a luteinizing hormone-releasing hormone (LHRH) agonist and an antiandrogen has been used in conjunction with radiotherapy for locally advanced (T3) tumors. Progression-free survival was 36% at 5 years for patients treated in this fashion compared to 15% for irradiation alone.[66] To date, there has been no significant improvement in survival demonstrated in patients treated with neoadjuvant androgen suppression.[63] Conformal radiation therapy using three-dimensional treatment planning reduces bladder and rectal exposure by 14%, thereby decreasing complication rates and allowing dose escalation to 7900 cGy.[67,68] Long-term data are required to assess the efficacy of this technique.

Adjuvant radiation therapy following radical prostatectomy is indicated for patients with pathologic T3 disease. No survival advantage has been noted, although doses of 4500–6400 cGy have lowered the rate of local recurrence.[69] Further studies are in progress evaluating postoperative irradiation for locally advanced tumors.

Radioactive seed implantation, *brachytherapy*, has been used for primary treatment of organ-confined prostate cancer. Iodine-125 and palladium-103 seeds are implanted by a perineal percutaneous approach under transrectal ultrasound guidance. Placement and dosimetry are planned based on pretreatment CT or ultrasonographic images. Doses of 14,000–16,000 cGy are typically delivered. Although long-term data are lacking, 79% of patients with T1 or T2 disease had PSA levels less than 0.5 ng/ml at 7 years using iodine-125 implants.[70]

Following prostatectomy or primary radiation therapy, serum PSA levels are measured to detect early recurrence that is potentially salvageable. The prognosis of radiation-resistant prostate cancer is poor, with the 5-year disease-free survival only 30%. In the absence of distant disease, these men may be treated with salvage prostatectomy. Alternatively, hormonal therapy may be considered.

Radiotherapy in the form of *external beam irradiation and radioisotopes* has been used as a palliative measure to treat painful bone metastases; 83% of patients have noted at least partial pain relief after palliative therapy.[71] Doses of 300 cGy in 10 treatments is typically administered.[62] Spinal cord compression secondary to vertebral bony metastasis is an emergency and requires immediate radiotherapy. Radiotherapy is contraindicated in cases of malignant fractures, which should be surgically repaired and then treated with hormonal therapy.[62]

Strontium-89 is a radioisotope absorbed by osteoblastic metastases. Patients treated with this radioisotope have had fewer occurrences of new pain sites and a decreased need for further radiotherapy compared to patients treated with palliative external beam irradiation only.[72,73]

Cryotherapy

Cryosurgery of the prostate has been performed as a primary treatment of organ-confined prostate cancer as well as salvage therapy for local recurrence after external beam radiation therapy. The procedure is performed using a transperineal percutaneous approach under transrectal ultrasound guidance. Ultrasonography is used to place the cryoprobes accurately and to ensure that the prostate is adequately frozen without including the rectum in the iceball. Two freeze–thaw cycles are performed with the probes in the same position. The probes are then retracted slightly to treat any apical tissue not included in the first cycle. Rates of biopsy-proven residual cancer 3–6 months after cryotherapy range from 7.7% to 23.0%, with 33% of patients having a PSA less than 0.2 ng/ml at 1 year.[74,75] Complications include urinary obstruction secondary to necrotic prostate tissue (3–30%), urinary incontinence (2–27%), and rates of impotence as high as 86%.[76–78] Complication rates tend to increase in series where intraoperative urethral warming was inconsistent and for patients undergoing salvage cryotherapy. Long-term survival data are not yet available.

Hormonal Therapy

The effect of androgens on prostate cancer was first reported by Huggins and Hodges in 1941.[79] 5α-Dihydrotestosterone, converted from testosterone in the prostatic epithelial cell or plasma, binds with the androgen receptor within the prostatic cell resulting in activation of the genes controlling cell division. Withdrawal or blockade of the androgen receptor then results in apoptosis or cell death.[80] The main role of androgen deprivation therapy currently is in the treatment of metastatic prostatic cancer.

Surgical castration (bilateral orchiectomy) causes a 90–95% drop in serum testosterone levels.[81] Orchiectomy avoids the need to adjust medication doses based on a patient's metabolic state and the cardiovascular complications seen with high-dose estrogen therapy.

Medical castration consists of treatment with estrogens or, more commonly, LHRH agonists (leuprolide acetate 7.5 mg SC monthly, goserelin 3.5 mg monthly). The constant level of these agonists result in down-regulation of pituitary receptors controlling the release of luteinizing hormone, thereby dropping testicular androgen production. Because of the initial stimulating activity of LHRH agonists on testosterone production, patients may note an acute increase in bony pain of metastatic disease, termed "flare syndrome." To prevent this syndrome, an antiandrogen is administered for the first 1–3 weeks of LHRH agonist therapy. Antiandrogens block androgens at the prostate tissue level. Both forms of castration have similar side effects, including impotence, loss of libido, hot flashes, bone density loss, and memory deficits. Both forms result in a median survival of 2.5 years from the treatment of symptomatic metastases and in some cases as much as a 5-year survival advantage over placebo.[82–84] Estrogen therapy such as diethylstilbestrol, though as effective, has fallen out of favor because of an increase in cardiovascular mortality in the early clinical trials.[85]

Despite significant drops in serum testosterone levels with castration, intraprostatic androgen levels may be 25% of precastration levels secondary to androgens synthesized by the adrenal gland.[86] As a result, an antiandrogen must be added to medical or surgical castration for *total androgen blockade* (*TAB*). Steroidal (cyproterone, megestrol acetate) and, more commonly, pure antiandrogens (flutamide, nilutamide, bicalutamide) are used to bind cellular androgen receptors competitively. Though an increase in progression-free and overall survival has been reported in patients undergoing TAB, a more recent meta-analysis of 22 randomized trials found no difference in survival between *TAB* and *castration* alone.[87–89] Several studies are under way to evaluate the optimal timing of androgen deprivation therapy initiation and the use of antiandrogen monotherapy.[90,91]

Despite all advances made in androgen deprivation therapy, metastatic prostate carcinoma eventually progresses typically 18–24 months after diagnosis of metastasis. This progression is termed "hormone-refractory" or "androgen-independent disease" and is thought to be the result of an alteration or mutation of the androgen receptor gene or its expression.[80] The resulting cell lines no longer undergo apoptosis with androgen deprivation therapy. Several researchers have suggested that intermittent androgen suppression (IAS) allows these cell lines to regain their androgen sensitivity and potential for apoptosis with androgen deprivation. IAS has been shown to increase the time to endocrine resistance in certain prostate cancer cell lines and may delay the onset of hormone-refractory prostate cancer.[92] Patients undergoing *IAS* are taken off androgen suppression and are restarted only after symptoms return or the PSA level rises to a certain level. No clear survival advantage has been demonstrated in early studies, but clinical trials continue. Preliminary results indicate that patients tolerate the therapy well with few side effects and may return to sexual activity.[93]

Antiandrogens may eventually contribute to the growth of hormone-refractory prostate cancer. In vitro studies have supported this hypothesis by demonstrating prostatic cell growth when antiandrogens have been bound to androgen receptors in certain prostate cancer cell lines.[94] Approximately 20% of patients with hormone-refractory prostate cancer being treated with TAB have a drop in their PSA levels when the antiandrogen is discontinued. This syndrome is called "antiandrogen withdrawal syndrome" and lasts 3.5–5.0 months.[95] Antiandrogen withdrawal is considered by many the first therapeutic intervention in patients on TAB with evidence of hormone-refractory prostate cancer.

Patients who progress after antiandrogen withdrawal may respond to second-line hormonal therapy. This response is thought to be due to persistent hormone-sensitive receptors and hormone-sensitive cells in hormone-refractory prostate cancer. Blockade of adrenal androgen synthesis with aminoglutethimide, ketoconazole, and corticosteroids has resulted in a decreased PSA level in 22–80% of patients with hormone-refractory prostate cancer.[95] These results are short-lived; and at the present time there is no cure for hormone-refractory prostate cancer.

Cytotoxic Chemotherapy

Patients who fail second-line hormonal therapy or who are symptomatic with hormone-refractory prostate cancer may be considered for an experimental trial of cytotoxic chemotherapy or palliative radiotherapy. Median survival rates are 6–12 months after relapse of hormone-refractory prostate cancer.[96] Though trials using chemotherapy have not clearly demonstrated survival over 1 year, clinical trials continue to evaluate agents. Only 10–20% of patients have a response (decreased pain or symptoms) to conventional cytotoxic chemotherapeutic agents.[97] The focus has shifted to combination therapy. Estramustine, an estradiol molecule linked to nitrogen mustard, undergoes conversion to estrone, allowing it to enter the prostate. In 50–61% of patients treated with estramustine in combination with another agent (etoposide, paclitaxel, vinblastine, vinorelbine), the PSA level dropped by 50%.[96] Cyclophosphamide (100 mg/m^2/day PO × 14 days) is popular owing to its low cost and mild toxicity; 60% of patients noted alleviation of their tumor-associated symptoms.[98] An anthraquinone derivative, mitoxantrone (14 mg/m^2 IV every 21 days), in combination with hydrocortisone decreased the PSA level by 50% in 33% of patients compared to 18% in patients taking hydrocortisone alone.[99] Suramin, a polysulfonated naphthylurea, and topotecan, a reversible inhibitor of topoisomerase, are currently being evaluated.[100] At present, no clear survival advantage has been shown with any of the chemotherapeutic agents in metastatic prostate cancer.

References

1. Landis SH, Murray T, Bolden D, et al. Cancer statistics, 1998. CA Cancer J Clin 1998;48:6–29.
2. Haas GP, Sark WA. Epidemiology of prostate cancer. CA Cancer J Clin 1997;47:273–287.
3. Guileyardo JM, Johnson WD, Welsh RA, et al. Prevalence of latent prostate carcinoma in two U.S. populations. J Natl Cancer Inst 1980;65:311–316.
4. Carter BS, Bova GS, Beaty TH, et al. Hereditary prostate cancer: epidemiologic and clinical features. J Urol 1993;150:797–802.
5. Spitz MR, Currier RD, Fueger JJ, et al. Familial patterns of prostate cancer: a case control analysis. J Urol 1991;146:1305–1307.
6. Whittemore AS, Kolonel LN, Wu AH, et al. Prostate cancer relation to diet, physical activity, and body size in blacks, whites, and Asians in the United States and Canada. J Natl Cancer Inst 1995;87:652–661.
7. Lilja H. A kallikrein-like serine protease in prostatic fluid cleaves the predominant seminal vesicle protein. J Clin Invest 1985;76:1899–1903.
8. Stamey TA, Young N, Hay AR, et al. Prostate-specific antigen as a serum marker for adenocarcinoma of the prostate. N Engl J Med 1987;317:909–916.
9. Catalona WJ, Richie JP, Amann FR, et al. Comparison of digital rectal examination and serum prostate specific antigen in the early detection of prostate cancer: results of a multicenter clinical trial of 6630 men. J Urol 1994;151:1283–1290.
10. Oesterling JE, Rice DC, Glensky WJ, Bergstralh EJ. Effect of cystoscopy, prostate biopsy, and transurethral resection of the prostate on serum prostate specific antigen concentration. Urology 1993;42:276–282.
11. Batislam E, Arik AI, Karakoc A, et al. Effect of transurethral indwelling catheter on serum prostate-specific antigen level in benign prostatic hyperplasia. Urology 1997;49:50–54.
12. Ercole CJ, Lange PH, Mathisen M, et al. Prostatic specific antigen and prostatic acid phosphatase in the monitoring and staging of patients with prostatic cancer. J Urol 1987;138:1181–1184.
13. Seamonds B, Yang N, Anderson K, et al. Evaluation of prostate specific antigen and prostatic acid phosphatase as prostate cancer markers. Urology 1986;28:472–479.

14. Armitage TG, Cooper EH, Newling DW, et al. The value of the measurement of serum prostatic specific antigen in patients with benign prostatic hyperplasia and untreated prostate cancer. Br J Urol 1988;62: 584–589.
15. Juan JJ, Coplen DE, Petros JA, et al. Effects of rectal examination, prostatic massage, ultrasonography, and needle biopsy on serum prostate specific antigen levels. J Urol 1992;148:810–814.
16. Heidenreich A, Vorreuther R, Neubauer S, et al. The influence of ejaculation on serum levels of prostate specific antigen. J Urol 1997;157: 209–211.
17. Guess HA, Heyse JF, Gormley GJ, et al. Effect of finasteride on serum PSA concentration in men with benign prostatic hyperplasia: results from the North American phase III clinical trial. Urol Clin North Am 1993; 20:627–636.
18. Benson MC, Whang IS, Olsson CA, et al. The use of prostate specific antigen density to enhance the predictive value of intermediate levels of serum prostate specific antigen. J Urol 1992;147:817–821.
19. Carter HB, Pearson JD, Metter EJ, et al. Longitudinal evaluation of prostate-specific antigen levels in men with and without prostate disease. JAMA 1992;267:2215–2220.
20. Oesterling JE, Jacobsen SJ, Kllee GG, et al. Free, complexed, and total serum prostate specific antigen: the establishment of appropriate reference ranges for the concentrations and ratios. J Urol 1995;154: 1090–1095.
21. DeAntoni EP. Age-specific reference ranges for PSA in the detection of prostate cancer. Oncology 1997;11:475–485.
22. Early Detection of Prostate Cancer. Policy Statements. American Urological Association, Baltimore Maryland, 1997:63.
23. Rifkin MD, Zerhouni EA, Gatsonis CA, et al. Comparison of magnetic resonance imaging and ultrasonography in staging early prostate cancer: results of a multi-institutional cooperative trial. N Engl J Med 1990; 323:621–626.
24. Lee F, Gray JM, McLeary RD, et al. Prostatic evaluation by transrectal sonography: criteria for diagnosis of early carcinoma. Radiology 1986; 168:389–394.
25. Lee F, Torp-Pedersen ST, McLeary RD. Transrectal ultrasound diagnosis of prostate cancer. Urol Clin North Am 1989;16:663–673.
26. Shinohara K, Wheeler TM, Scardino PT. The appearance of prostate cancer on transrectal ultrasonography: correlation of imaging and pathological examination. J Urol 1989;142:76–82.
27. McNeal JE. Regional morphology and pathology of the prostate. Am J Clin Pathol 1968;49:347–357.
28. McNeal JE, Redwine EA, Freiha FS, et al. Zonal distribution of prostatic adenocarcinoma: correlation with histologic pattern and direction of spread. Am J Surg Pathol 1988;12:897–906.
29. Oesterling J, Cooner W, Jacobsen S, et al. Influence of patients' age on the serum PSA concentration: an important clinical observation. Urol Clin North Am 1993;20:671–680.
30. Desmond PM, Clark J, Thompsom IM, et al. Morbidity with contemporary prostate biopsy. J Urol 1993;15:1425–1426.
31. Hodge KK, McNeal JE, Stamey TA. Ultrasound guided transrectal core biopsies to the palpably abnormal prostate. J Urol 1989;144:66–70.
32. Jewett HJ. The present status of radical prostatectomy for stages A and B prostatic cancer. Urol Clin North Am 1975;2:105–124.
33. American Joint Committee on Care. AJCC Staging Manual, 5th ed. Philadelphia: Lippincott, 1997.
34. Partin AW, Kattan MW, Subong EN, et al. Combination of prostate-specific antigen, clinical stage, and Gleason score to predict pathological stage of localized prostate cancer. JAMA 1997;277:1445–1451.
35. Oesterling JE, Brendler CB, Epstein JI, et al. Correlation of clinical stage, serum prostatic acid phosphatase and preoperative Gleason grade with final pathological stage in 275 patients with clinically localized adenocarcinoma of the prostate. J Urol 1987;138:92–98.
36. Gleason DF, VACURG. Histological grading and clinical staging of prostatic carcinoma. In: Tannenbaum M (ed) Urologic Pathology: The Prostate. Philadelphia: Lea & Febiger, 1977:171–197.
37. Schaffer D, Pendergrass HP. Comparison of enzyme, clinical, radiographic, and radionuclide methods of detecting bone metastases from carcinoma of the prostate. Radiology 1976;121:431–434.
38. Chybowski FM, Keller JJL, Bergstralh EJ, et al. Predicting radionuclide bone scan findings in patients with newly diagnosed, untreated prostate cancer: prostate specific antigen is superior to other clinical parameters. J Urol 1991;145:313–318.
39. Oesterling JE. Using PSA to eliminate the staging radionuclide bone scan: significant economic implications. Urol Clin North Am 1993;20: 705–711.
40. Walsh JE, Amendola MA, Konerding KR, et al. Computed tomographic detection of pelvic and inguinal lymph-node metastases from primary and recurrent pelvic malignant disease. Radiology 1980;137:157–166.
41. Emory TH, Reinke DB, Hill AL, et al. Use of CT to reduce understaging in prostatic cancer: comparison with conventional staging techniques. AJR Am J Roentgenol 1983;141:351–354.
42. Tempany CM, Zhou X, Zrhouni EA, et al. Staging of prostate cancer: results of radiology diagnostic oncology group project comparison of three techniques. Radiology 1994;192:47–54.
43. Vapnek JM, Hricak H, Shinohara K, et al. Staging accuracy of magnetic resonance imaging versus transrectal ultrasound in stages A and B prostatic cancer. Urol Int 1994;53:1535–1538.
44. Babaian RJ, Sayer J, Podoloff DA, et al. Radioimmunoscintigraphy of pelvic lymph nodes with (111) indium-labeled monoclonal antibody CYT-356. J Urol 1994;152:1954–1955.
45. Kahn D, Williams RD, Seldin DW, et al. Radioimmunoscintigraphy with 111 indium labeled CYT-356 for detection of occult prostate cancer recurrence. J Urol 1994;152:1490–1495.
46. Wolf JS, Andriole GL. The selection of patients for cross-sectional imaging and pelvic lymphadenectomy before radical prostatectomy. AUA Update Ser 1997:114–119.
47. Albertsen P, Fryback DG, Storer BE, et al. Long-term survival after conservative treatment of clinically localized prostate cancer. JAMA 1995; 274:626–631.
48. Chodak GW, Thisted RA, Gerber GS, et al. Results of conservative management of clinically localized prostate cancer. N Engl J Med 1994; 330:242–248.
49. Kattan M, Beck JB, Miles BJ, Scardino PT. Reexamination of the decision analysis for clinically localized prostate cancer: age and grade comparisons [abstract 646]. J Urol 1995;153:390A.
50. Partin AW, Pound CR, Clemens JQ, et al. Serum PSA after anatomic radical prostatectomy: the Johns Hopkins experience after 10 years. Urol Clin North Am 1993;20:713–725.
51. Reiner WG, Walsh PC. An anatomical approach to the surgical management of the dorsal vein and Santorini's plexus during radical retropubic surgery. J Urol 1979;121:198–200.
52. Walsh PC, Donker PJ. Impotence following radical prostatectomy: insight into etiology and prevention. J Urol 1982;128:492–497.
53. Zincke H, Oesterling JE, Blute ML, et al. Long-term (15 years) results after radical prostatectomy for clinically localized (stage T2c or lower) prostate cancer. J Urol 1994;152:1850–1857.
54. Walsh PC, Partin AW, Epstein JI. Cancer control and quality of life following anatomical radical retropubic prostatectomy: results at 10 years. J Urol 1994;152:1831–1836.
55. Murphy GP, Mettlin C, Menck H, et al. National patterns of prostate cancer treatment by radical prostatectomy: results of a survey by the

American College of Surgeons Commission on Cancer. J Urol 1994; 152(suppl):1817–1819.

56. Andriole GL, Smith DS, Rao G, et al. Early complications of contemporary anatomical radical retropubic prostatectomy. J Urol 1994;152: 1858–1860.
57. Quinlan DM, Epstein JI, Carter BS, et al. Sexual function following radical prostatectomy: influence of preservation of neurovascular bundles. J Urol 1991;145:998–1002.
58. Rosen MA, Goldstone L, Lapin S, et al. Frequency and location of extracapsular extension and positive surgical margins in radical prostatectomy specimens. J Urol 1992;148:331–337.
59. McCarthy JF, Catalona WJ, Hudson M. Effect of radiation therapy on detectable serum prostate specific antigen levels following radical prostatectomy: early vs. delayed treatment. J Urol 1994;151;1575–1578.
60. Middleton RG, Smith JA, Meltzer RB, et al. Patient survival and local recurrence rate following radical prostatectomy for prostatic carcinoma. J Urol 1986;136:422–424.
61. Cookson MS, Fair WR. Neoadjuvant androgen deprivation therapy and radical prostatectomy for clinically localized prostate cancer. AUA Update 1997;16:lesson 13.
62. Porter AT, Littrup P, Grignon D, et al. Radiotherapy and cryotherapy for prostate cancer. In: Walsh PC, Retic AB, Stamey TA, et al (eds) Campbell's Urology, 7th ed. Philadelphia: Saunders, 1998:2605–2626.
63. Hanks GE. Long-term control of prostate cancer with radiation. Urol Clin North Am 1996;23:605–616.
64. Lee RJ, Sause WT. Surgically staged patients with prostatic carcinoma treated with definitive radiotherapy—15 year results. Urology 1994;43: 640–644.
65. Shipley WU, Zietman AL, Hanks GE, et al. Treatment related sequelae following external beam radiation for prostate cancer: a review with an update in patients with stages T1 and T2 tumor. J Urol 1994;152: 1799–1805.
66. Pilepich MV, Krall JM, Al-Sarraf M, et al. Androgen deprivation with radiation therapy compared with radiation therapy alone for locally advanced prostatic carcinoma: a randomized comparative trial of the Radiation Therapy Oncology Group. Urology 1995;45:616–623.
67. Soffen EM, Hanks GE, Hunt MA, et al. Conformal static field radiation therapy treatment of early prostate cancer versus non-conformal techniques: a reduction in acute morbidity. Int J Radiat Oncol Biol Phys 1992;24:485–488.
68. Hanks GE. Conformal radiation in prostate cancer: reduced morbidity with hope of increased local control [editorial]. Int J Radiat Oncol Biol Phys 1993;25:377–378.
69. Forman JD, Velasco J. Therapeutic radiation in patients with a rising post-prostatectomy PSA level. Oncology 1998;12:33–39.
70. Ragde H, Blasko JC, Grimm PD, et al. Interstitial iodine-125 radiation without adjuvant therapy in the treatment of clinically localized prostate carcinoma. Cancer 1997;80:442–453.
71. Tong D, Gillick L, Hendrickson FR. The palliation of symptomatic osseous metastases: final results of the Radiation Therapy Oncology Group. Cancer 1982;50:893–899.
72. Porter AT, McEwan AJB, Powe JE, et al. Results of a randomized phase III trial to evaluate the efficacy of strontium-89 adjuvant to local field external beam irradiation in the management of endocrine resistant metastatic prostate cancer. Int J Radiat Oncol Biol Phys 1993;25:805–813.
73. Quilty PM, Kirk D, Bolger JJ, et al. A comparison of the palliative effects of strontium-89 and external beam radiotherapy in metastatic prostate cancer. Radiother Oncol 1994;31:33–40.
74. Connolly JA, Shinohara K, Presti JC, Carroll PR. Should cryosurgery be considered a therapeutic option in localized prostate cancer? Urol Clin North Am 1996;23:623–631.
75. Coogan CL, McKiel CF. Percutaneous cryoablation of the prostate: preliminary results after 95 procedures. J Urol 1995;154:1813–1817.
76. Bahn DK, Lee F, Solomon MH, et al. Prostate cancer: ultrasound-guided percutaneous cryoablation. Radiology 1995;194:551–556.
77. Shinohara K, Carroll PR. Improved results of cryosurgical ablation of the prostate. J Urol 1995;153:627A.
78. Cox RL, Crawford ED. Complications of cryosurgical ablation of the prostate to treat localized adenocarcinoma of the prostate. Urology 1995; 45:932–935.
79. Huggins C, Hodges CV. The effect of castration, of oestrogen and of androgen injection on serum phosphatases in metastatic carcinoma of the prostate. Cancer Res 1941;1:942.
80. Galbraith SM, Duchesne GM. Androgens and prostate cancer: biology, pathology and hormonal therapy. Eur J Cancer 1997;33:545–554.
81. Grayhack JT, Keeler TC, Kozlowski JM. Carcinoma of the prostate: hormonal therapy. Cancer 1987;60(suppl):589–601.
82. Byar DP, Corle DK. Hormone therapy for prostate cancer: results of the VACURG studies: consensus development conference on the management of clinically localized prostate cancer. Natl Cancer Inst Monogr 1988;7:165–170.
83. Parmar H, Phillips RH, Lightman SL, et al. Randomized controlled study of orchidectomy vs long acting D-trp-6-LHRH microcapsules in advanced prostatic carcinoma. Lancet 1985;2:1201–1205.
84. Emmett JL, Greene LF, Papantoniou A. Endocrine therapy in carcinoma of the prostate gland: 10-year survival studies. J Urol 1960;83:471–484.
85. Mellinger GT. Treatment and survival of patients with cancer of the prostate: the Veterans Administration Co-operative Urological Research Group. Surg Gynecol Obstet 1967;124:1011–1017.
86. Geller J. Basis for hormonal management of advanced prostate cancer. Cancer 1993;71:1039–1045.
87. Crawford ED, Eisenberger MA, Mcleod DG, et al. A controlled trial of leuprolide with and without flutamide in prostatic carcinoma. N Engl J Med 1989;321:419–424.
88. Denis LJ, Carneiro de Moura JL, Bono A, et al. Goserelin acetate and flutamide versus bilateral orchiectomy: a phase III EORTC trial (30853). Urology 1993;42:119–130.
89. Prostate Cancer Trialists' Collaborative Group: Maximum androgen blockade in advanced prostate cancer: an overview of 22 randomized trials with 3283 deaths in 5710 patients. Lancet 1995;346:265–269.
90. Denis L, Murphy GP. Overview of phase III trials on combined androgen treatment in patients with metastatic prostate cancer. Cancer 1993; 72:3888–3895.
91. Chodak G, Sharifi R, Kasimis B, et al. Single-agent therapy with bicalutamide: a comparison with medical or surgical castration in the treatment of advanced prostate cancer. Urology 1995;46:849–855.
92. Gleave M, Bruchovsky N, Bowden M, et al. Intermittent androgen suppression prolongs time to androgen independent procession in the LNCaP prostate tumor model. J Urol 1994;151:457A.
93. Goldenberg SL, Bruchovsky N, Gleave ME, et al. Intermittent androgen suppression in the treatment of prostate cancer: a preliminary report. Urology 1995;45:839–845.
94. Scher HI, Kelly WK. Flutamide withdrawal syndrome: its impact on clinical trials in hormone-refractory prostate cancer. J Clin Oncol 1993;11: 1566–1572.
95. Small EJ, Vogelzang NJ. Second-line hormonal therapy for advanced prostate cancer: a shifting paradigm. J Clin Oncol 1997;15:382–388.

96. Waselenko JK, Dawson NA. Management of progressive metastatic prostate cancer. Oncology 1997;11:1551–1560.
97. Raghavan D, Koczwara B, Javle M. Evolving strategies of cytotoxic chemotherapy for advanced prostate cancer. Eur J Cancer 1997;33:566–574.
98. Raghavan D, Cox K, Pearson BS, et al. Oral cyclophosphamide for the management of hormone-refractory prostate cancer. Br J Urol 1993; 72:625–628.
99. Kantoff PW, Conaway M, Winer E, et al. Hydrocortisone with and without mitoxantrone in patients with hormone-refractory prostate cancer: preliminary results from a prospective randomized Cancer and Leukemia Group B (9182) comparing chemotherapy to best supportive care [abstract 2013]. Proc Am Soc Clin Oncol 1996;14:1748.
100. Eisenberger M, Reyno L, Sinibaldi V, et al. The experience with suramin in advanced prostate cancer. Cancer 1995;75(suppl):1927–1934.

CHAPTER 50

Evaluation of the Scrotal Mass

THOMAS G. MATKOV
CHRISTOPHER L. COOGAN

A. Introduction

The presentation of a patient with a scrotal mass is an issue of immediate concern. Although most cases have a benign cause, prompt investigation into this complaint can potentially identify early-stage malignant tumors. Presentation may be delayed secondary to patient embarrassment or social prejudices. When presented with this complaint, however, the physician should pursue the evaluation in a meticulous fashion, without delay.

B. History

A careful history is one of the most important initial steps in the evaluation, as it may direct assessment and treatment. The duration of clinical symptoms and a history of trauma are important historical points. Trauma may heighten the patient's awareness of his scrotum, leading to the discovery of a preexisting scrotal mass.[1] Previous urologic or inguinal surgery or a history of a urinary tract infection (UTI), sexually transmitted disease (STD), or epididymitis should be ascertained. The age of the patient can be a determining factor in the differential diagnosis. The presence or absence of pain as well as its onset, quality, and intensity should be determined. Pain originating in other areas should be investigated, as visceral pain may be referred to the testicles.[2] Constitutional symptoms such as abdominal pain, nausea, vomiting, fever, chills, dysuria, or hematuria can point to specific diagnoses.

C. Physical Examination

The physical examination requires an understanding of the normal anatomy of the scrotum and its contents. Knowledge of the layers of the scrotal wall, their embryologic origin, and associated structures is essential to understanding the pathophysiology of scrotal masses (Fig. 50–1). The scrotal skin is hair-bearing and densely populated with sweat and sebaceous glands. Dartos' layer is composed of fascia and smooth muscle and is contiguous with Colles' and Scarpa's fascia. The external spermatic fascia arises from the external oblique fascia. The internal spermatic fascia is the inferior continuation of the transversalis fascia. Between the external and internal spermatic fascia is the cremaster muscle and fascia arising from the internal oblique muscle. Deep to the internal spermatic fascia are the parietal and visceral layers of the tunica vaginalis, which are formed as the testes pass through the peritoneum on their

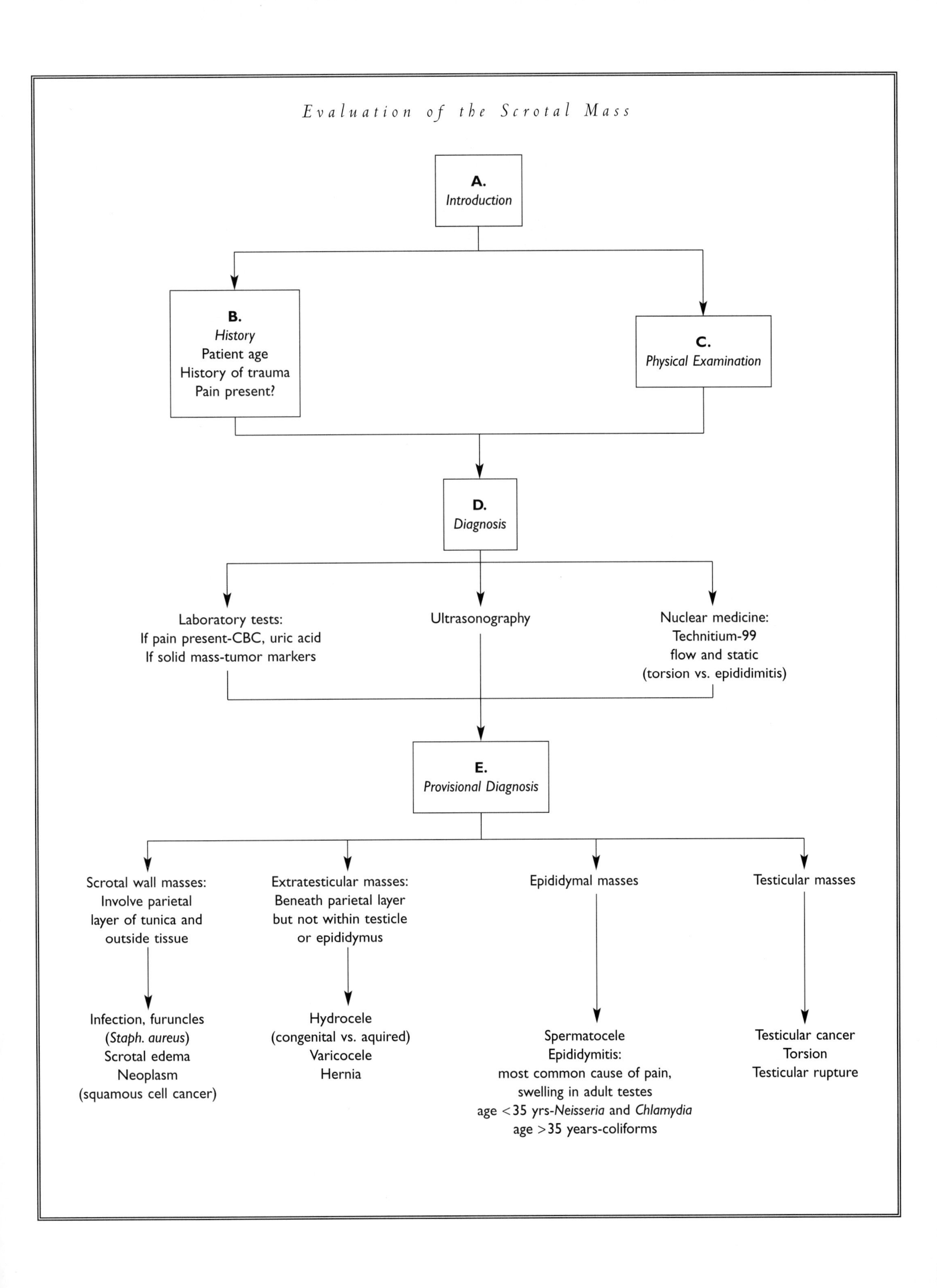

Evaluation of the Scrotal Mass
A.
Introduction
B.
History
Patient age
History of trauma
Pain present?
C.
Physical Examination
D.
Diagnosis
Laboratory tests:
If pain present-CBC, uric acid
If solid mass-tumor markers
Ultrasonography
Nuclear medicine:
Technitium-99
flow and static
(torsion vs. epididimitis)
E.
Provisional Diagnosis
Scrotal wall masses:
Involve parietal
layer of tunica and
outside tissue
Extratesticular masses:
Beneath parietal layer
but not within testicle
or epididymus
Epididymal masses
Testicular masses
Infection, furuncles
(Staph. aureus)
Scrotal edema
Neoplasm
(squamous cell cancer)
Hydrocele
(congenital vs. aquired)
Varicocele
Hernia
Spermatocele
Epididymitis:
most common cause of pain,
swelling in adult testes
age <35 yrs-Neisseria and Chlamydia
age >35 years-coliforms
Testicular cancer
Torsion
Testicular rupture

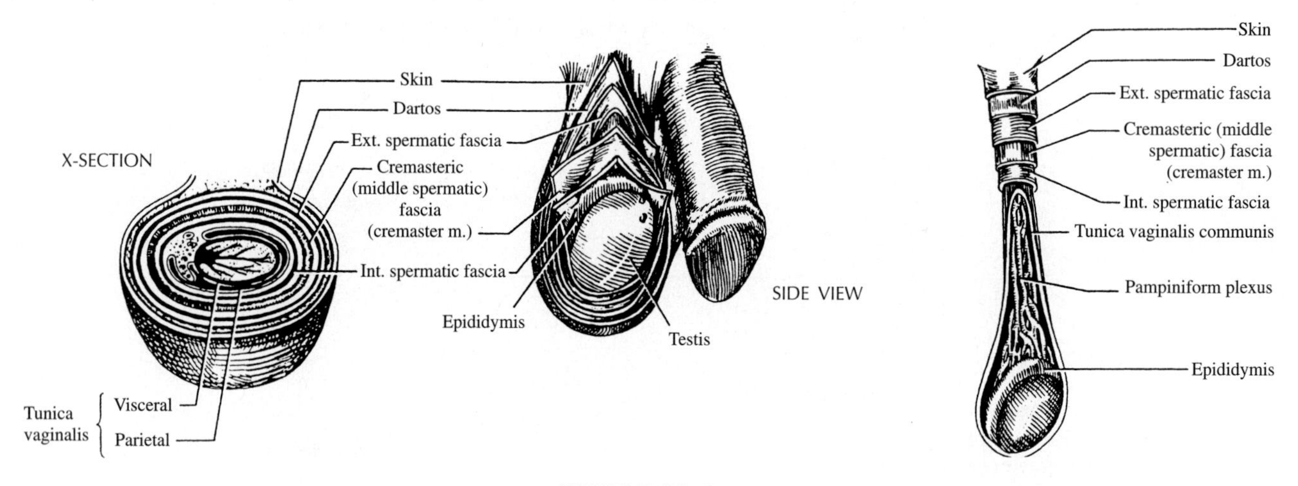

FIGURE 50–1
Scrotum and its layers. (From Pansky B. Review of Gross Anatomy, 6th ed. New York: McGraw-Hill, 1997;483, with permission.)

descent into the scrotum. The scrotum is separated by a midline septum, confining each side's contents to its own hemiscrotum.[1]

The normal testis is 4–6 cm in length and approximately 3 cm in both width and depth. A tough capsule is comprised of the visceral layer of the tunica vaginalis and the tunica albuginea. The epididymis lies posterior to the testicle and can be palpated as a distinct entity, comprised of the head, body, and tail. The spermatic cord can be palpated superiorly, extending into the external inguinal ring. The vas deferens, with a diameter of approximately 3 mm, can be palpated as a firm, cord-like structure.

Physical examination of the scrotum begins with the patient standing in a relaxed fashion in front of the seated examiner. On inspection of the scrotal skin, any dermatologic abnormalities should be noted. Palpation of the testicles should be carried out in a systematic fashion, with examination of the unaffected side first. The testicle should be gently grasped in one hand, with the surface of the testicle and epididymis examined with the fingertips of both hands or between the thumb and finger of one hand. Examination for hernia can be performed by gently inserting the index finger into the scrotum and entering the external inguinal ring. The patient should then be instructed to bear down (Valsalva maneuver); a hernia may be felt as a bulge against the tip of the finger. The spermatic cord should also be examined during the Valsalva maneuver, as it may reveal a varicocele. Transillumination of any scrotal masses may distinguish between cystic or solid masses: The former transilluminate, whereas the latter do not.[1,3,4] Diagnostic studies such as laboratory tests and radiographic examinations are indicated based on the history and physical examination.

D. *Diagnosis*

Laboratory Evaluation

If pain is the primary feature and epididymitis, orchitis, torsion, and incarcerated hernia are possible diagnoses, a complete blood count (CBC) and urinalysis with culture are indicated. Patients with solid testicular masses should have serum tumor marker assays: α-fetoprotein (AFP), human chorionic gonadotropin (hCG), lactic dehydrogenase (LDH). AFP (half-life 5–7 days) and hCG (half-life 24–36 hours) are glycoproteins produced in certain testicular cancers, and baseline determinations are important to follow the results of therapy. LDH is a cellular enzyme that is nonspecific, but there appears to be a relation between LDH levels and tumor burden.[1]

Scrotal Ultrasonography

Ultrasonography (US) is invaluable when evaluating scrotal contents. Bree and Hoang have referred to scrotal US as the first and only imaging examination necessary.[5] US is carried out with the patient in the supine position, with a towel supporting the scrotum and the penis elevated onto the abdomen. Scrotal US should be performed with high frequency transducers (5–10 MHz) and color Doppler capabilities to study arterial and venous flow.[4–6] Sonographically, the normal testicle has uniform, medium-level homogeneous echogenicity. The epididymis is isoechoic or slightly hyperechoic to the testicle (Fig. 50–2). Scrotal US is most effective and reliable for determining testicular from paratesticular lesions, and it is also utilized for differentiating testicular torsion from epididymoorchitis.[5]

Radionuclide Scanning

Technetium-99 (^{99m}Tc) radionuclide scanning of the scrotum has also been advocated, usually for the patient with scrotal pain. In this situation this test is highly sensitive and specific for differentiating between torsion and epididymitis[4,6] (Fig. 50–3). The usual dose of technetium is 20 mCi for adults; a reduced dose is used in children based on the patient's weight. The patient is placed on the examination table with the penis supported suprapubically

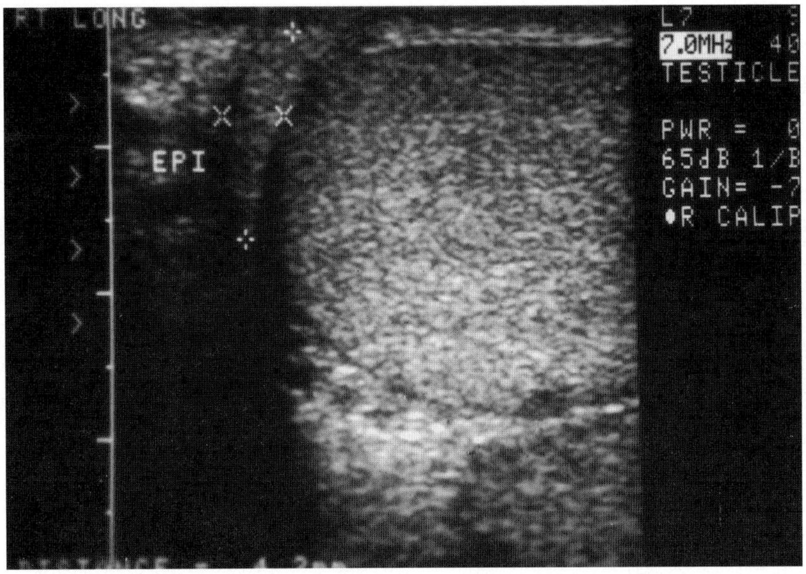

FIGURE 50–2
Normal ultrasound scan of the testis. The head of the epididymis is seen at the superior aspect of the testicle and displays similar echogenicity.

and the scrotum elevated with a sling. Flow and static studies should be obtained. Examination of the normal scrotum should reveal no abnormal vascular flow patterns, with static images demonstrating symmetric tissue activity in the testes.[4]

E. *Provisional Diagnosis*

Masses of Scrotal Wall

Masses of the scrotal wall are confined within the layers of the scrotum (i.e., between the skin and the parietal layer of the tunica vaginalis). The testes, epididymides, and spermatic cords are normal in such instances.

Infections

Infections of the scrotum can present as painful scrotal masses. Furuncles, also referred to as boils, may appear on any hair-bearing area of the body. Lesions may grow rapidly, up to 3 cm in size. Treatment involves antibiotic coverage for *Staphylococcus aureus* as well as incision and drainage of any fluctuant areas.[7] Fournier's gangrene is a form of necrotizing fasciitis of the genital and anorectal regions and may present with scrotal inflammation or cellulitis. Lesions are characteristically painful, red, and warm quickly progressing to necrotic lesions capable of causing profound sepsis. Treatment consists of wide débridement and intravenous antibiotics[7,8] effective against a polymicrobial infection.

Scrotal Edema

Scrotal edema may be present in any patient who has diffuse anasarca. This includes, but is not limited to, patients with extensive surgery, volume overload, and renal or liver failure. Treatment consists of aggressive skin care to prevent breakdown and elevating the scrotum to improve lymphatic drainage.[7]

Neoplasms of the Scrotal Wall

Malignancies of the scrotal skin are rare. The most common type is squamous cell carcinoma (SCC). Percival Potts first described the disease in 1775 in chimney sweeps, which earned the disease

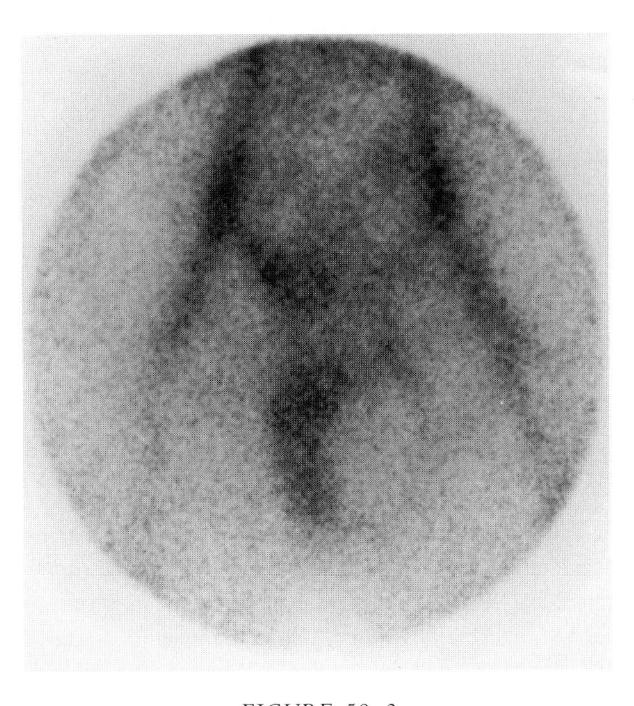

FIGURE 50–3
Radionuclide scan of the scrotum shows lack of perfusion to the right testis, which is diagnostic of acute testicular torsion.

the name of "Potts' disease" or "chimney sweep disease." SCC presents as a painless, slowly growing nodule of the scrotal wall. Advanced disease is often ulcerated and painful. Treatment is wide local excision of the primary lesion with 2 cm margins.[7,9,10] Inguinal lymphadenectomy is traditionally reserved for patients with proven metastatic disease; prophylactic groin dissection is controversial and not widely practiced.[11]

Extratesticular Masses

Extratesticular scrotal masses are those that lie underneath the parietal layer of the tunica vaginalis but not within the testicle or epididymis.

Hydrocele

Hydroceles are collections of fluid between the parietal and visceral layers of the tunica vaginalis.[4,12] They occur in all age groups and may be classified as congenital (communicating) or acquired (noncommunicating). *Congenital* hydroceles are generally found in the pediatric population and are almost always associated with an inguinal hernia.[1,4,12,13] They result from a patent processus vaginalis, thereby establishing a communication between the hydrocele and the peritoneal cavity. Pediatric hydroceles are repaired by high ligation of the hernia sac, similar to a pediatric hernia repair.[12,13] *Acquired* hydroceles are idiopathic or secondary. Idiopathic hydroceles are the result of lymphatic obstruction that interferes with normal transudate uptake, causing accumulation of fluid. The etiology is not known. Secondary hydroceles are caused by trauma, tumor, infections, or other inflammatory processes. They may also occur in the postoperative setting, especially after varicocele ligation or renal transplantation.[12]

Hydroceles are generally nontender, chronic masses of the scrotum. A thorough testicular examination, should be performed to evaluate the causes of a secondary hydrocele. If the testicular examination is abnormal or the size of the hydrocele precludes an adequate testicular examination, scrotal US is indicated.[4] Treatment of idiopathic hydroceles is generally not necessary unless the patient experiences discomfort or embarrassment. Aspiration and sclerotherapy are associated with high recurrence rates or infection. Traditionally, treatment of a symptomatic hydrocele is hydrocelectomy.[13]

Varicocele

A varicocele arises from abnormally dilated veins of the pampiniform plexus of the testis. Its incidence in the general population is approximately 15%.[1,2,13,14] The incidence in the infertile man is somewhat higher (35–40%) owing to the deleterious effect of varicoceles on seminal fluid variables.[13] Varicoceles are usually asymptomatic; in large cases, however, symptoms may include testicular pain and atrophy. Varicoceles are more common on the left, which is thought to be secondary to venous drainage of the left testicle into the left renal vein. The acute onset of a varicocele warrants further investigation, as it may signify proximal obstruction of the vein by a neoplasm.[13]

On physical examination, the characteristic finding is a scrotum that contains a "bag of worms." The examination should be performed with the patient in the standing position, both with and without the Valsalva maneuver. Ultrasonography is useful for diagnosing a varicocele, particularly with color duplex sonography, which has improved both the sensitivity and specificity of the diagnosis. Treatment should be reserved for patients who present with pain, testicular atrophy, or infertility that cannot be attributed to other causes. The treatment of choice is varicocelectomy, with multiple approaches described (laparoscopic, inguinal, subinguinal, retroperitoneal, microscopic).[12,13]

Hernia

Hernias can also present as scrotal masses. They are more common in infants, especially if born prematurely. Indirect hernias are caused by failure of the processus vaginalis to obliterate. Repair is indicated once the child is able to tolerate anesthesia. Elderly patients may also present with large inguinal hernias, which may extend into the scrotum. These hernias may contain fat, small or large bowel, or bladder and should be repaired. Physical examination may reveal a large scrotal mass that does not transilluminate, within which bowel sounds are occasionally detected. No radiologic investigation is usually indicated unless the hernia makes an adequate testicular examination impossible.

Epididymal Masses

Masses of the epididymis are generally benign. These lesions may be further subdivided into painless and painful masses. They are discussed in detail below.

Spermatocele

Spermatoceles are cystic dilations of the epididymis, rete testis, or efferent ducts and contain dead spermatozoa.[13] They are generally located in the head of the epididymis. On physical examination they are tense, well circumscribed, cystic lesions that transilluminate. Surgical intervention is rarely necessary unless there is associated unremitting pain.

Epididymitis

The most common cause of testicular pain and swelling in the adult male is epididymitis. In young men (less than 35 years old) the disease is often the result of STDs, with the most common pathogens being *Neisseria gonorrhoeae* and *Chlamydia trachomatis*. In men over 35 years old, the most common pathogens are coliforms. Epididymitis is thought to result from retrograde ascent of urethral pathogens via the ejaculatory duct and vas deferens to the epididymis. Most patients with epididymitis have coexisting infection of the testicle, which is then termed epididymoorchitis.[3]

Patients presenting with epididymitis generally have a 1- to 2-day history of increasing scrotal pain and swelling and may have dysuria and frequency, as well as urethral discharge. A history of low-grade fever is often elicited. Physical examination reveals a painful, swollen hemiscrotum with a tender, inflamed epididymis and testicle. The pain is relieved by lifting the scrotum over the symphysis pubis (Prehn's sign). Urinalysis usually reveals pyuria, and a CBC generally is significant for mild leukocytosis. Both US and testicular scintigraphy are valuable for evaluating the patient with testicular pain, especially when the history and physical examination are nondiagnostic. Treatment of the bacterial infection is generally directed toward broad-spectrum coverage of the usual organisms. Fluoroquinolone therapy for 10–14 days is generally sufficient treatment.[3] Trimethoprim/sulfamethoxazole or its equivalent has also proven to be efficacious. The younger patient with epididymitis requires follow-up with a urologist for a careful testicular examination after resolution of the infection; the older patient requires urologic evaluation to further evaluate his lower urinary tract.

Testicular Masses

Testicular masses, depending on their presentation, may be subdivided into benign and malignant causes.

Testicular Cancer Testicular cancer represents the most common cause of malignancy in males between the ages of 15 and 35. The usual presenting symptom is a painless mass in one testicle. Acute pain is infrequently the presenting symptom (approximately 10%); when present, it is usually due to epididymitis or hemorrhage within the tumor. Urgent scrotal US is indicated in all patients who have a mass arising from the testicle. See Chapter 51 for further management.

Torsion Although many entities can present with acute scrotal swelling, testicular torsion is the single diagnosis that must either be ruled out in the emergency room or the patient taken to the operating room. Torsion is most common in adolescents but has been described in all age groups. Two types of torsion have been described: extravaginal and intravaginal. Extravaginal torsion is seen almost exclusively in newborns; it occurs when the entire spermatic cord, tunica vaginalis, and testis rotate on itself.[1] The testicle is almost always necrotic or atrophic at presentation. Patients commonly present at birth with a scrotal mass or discolored scrotum, often without evidence of distress. Treatment of extravaginal torsion is nonemergent orchiectomy, with contralateral orchiopexy still considered controversial.

Intravaginal torsion occurs secondary to the absence of fixation of the testicle by the gubernaculum testis. This is the so-called "bell-clapper deformity," which predisposes the patient to torsion. The patient usually presents with unremitting, sudden onset of testicular pain and occasionally with nausea and vomiting. In an adolescent, acute pain and testicular swelling should be considered torsion until proven otherwise.[1,13] Physical examination reveals an asymmetric scrotum that is painful and tender, with the characteristic high, horizontally riding testicle (Brunzel's sign). Elevation of testis does not relieve the pain (negative Prehn's sign), and the cremasteric reflex is absent.[4] Acutely, the CBC is normal and urinalysis is negative for pyuria, helping to distinguish this entity from epididymitis. Color duplex US or testicular scintigraphy may each confirm the diagnosis, but scrotal exploration should not be delayed if the diagnosis is suspected, as the testicle may be viable for only 4–6 hours after the onset of symptoms. At exploration, if viable testis is encountered it should be affixed to the scrotal wall (orchiopexy) to prevent recurrence. Orchiopexy should also be performed on the contralateral side for intravaginal torsion, as there is a propensity for the deformity to be bilateral.[12–14]

Testicular Rupture Testicular rupture can result from blunt or penetrating injury to the scrotum. Rupture occurs secondary to disruption of the tunica albuginea. The patient's history should suggest the diagnosis, with the physical examination revealing a variable amount of hematoma with indistinct borders of the testis and epididymis. Scrotal imaging is helpful for the diagnosis but has a high false-negative rate. Scrotal exploration should not be delayed on the basis of a negative radiologic procedure in the face of a strongly suggestive history and physical examination.

Treatment is surgical exploration with débridement of injured tissue and closure of the tunica albuginea. A drain should be placed and broad-spectrum antibiotics given for at least 1 week.[1]

References

1. Walsh PC. Campbell's Urology, 7th ed. Philadelphia: Saunders, 1997.
2. McGee S. Referred scrotal pain: case reports and review. J Gen Intern Med 1993;8:694–701.
3. Gillenwater JY, Grayhack JT, Howards SS, Duckett JW. Adult and Pediatric Urology, 3rd ed. St. Louis: Mosby, 1996.
4. Hricak H, Hamm B, Kim B. Imaging of the Scrotum: Textbook and Atlas. New York: Raven, 1995.
5. Bree RL, Hoang DT. Scrotal ultrasound. Radiol Clin North Am 1996; 34:1183–1205.
6. Pollack HM. Clinical Urography. Philadelphia: Saunders, 1990.
7. Fitzpatrick TB, Eisen AZ, Wolff K, Freedberg IM, Austen KF. Dermatology in Clinical Medicine, 4th ed. New York: McGraw-Hill, 1993.
8. Hejase MJ, Simonin JE, Bihrle R, Coogan CL. Genital Fournier's gangrene: experience with 38 patients. Urology 1996;47:734–739.
9. Lowe FC. Squamous cell carcinoma of the scrotum. J Urol 1983;130: 423–427.
10. Raghavan D, Scher HI, Leibel SA, Lange P. Principles and Practice of Genitourinary Oncology. Philadelphia: Lippincott-Raven, 1997.
11. Crawford ED, Das S. Current Genitourinary Cancer Surgery. Baltimore: Williams & Wilkins, 1997.
12. Droller MJ. Surgical Management of Urologic Disease: An Anatomic Approach. St. Louis: Mosby, 1992.
13. Marshall FF. Textbook of Operative Urology. Philadelphia: Saunders, 1996.
14. Rabinowitz R, Hulbert WC Jr. Acute scrotal swelling. Urol Clin North Am 1995;22:101–105.

CHAPTER 51

Testicular Tumors

BEJAN FAKOURI
CHRISTOPHER L. COOGAN

A. Epidemiology and Etiology

Testicular cancer is a relatively rare malignancy with an annual incidence of approximately 4.5 cases per 100,000.[1] This number increased from a previously reported incidence of 2.88 cases per year per 100,000 men in the U.S. army between 1940 and 1947.[1] Despite its rare occurrence, testicular cancer is the most common malignancy in males between 15 and 35 years of age.[1] Remarkable strides in surgical, chemotherapeutic, and radiation treatment during the twentieth century greatly improved cure rates. In 1970 the mortality rate was approximately 90%; now the cure rate is higher than 90% with the use of multimodal therapy.[1] Accurate diagnosis and staging with radiographic, surgical, and histologic means are of utmost importance; and distinguishing between seminomatous and nonseminomatous histology is the key to stratifying lesions into the proper treatment modalities. Most cancers arise from the germinal elements of the testicle (90–95%); the remaining cases arise from nongerminal elements, including gonadal stroma, mesenchymal structures, and ducts.[2]

The incidence of testicular cancer is increasing in the United States. White men in the United States and western Europe have the highest incidence, in contrast to Asians, Africans, and North Americans of African descent.[1] Seminoma is the most common histologic type and has a peak incidence at age 35–39 years.[3] Nonseminomatous germ cell testicular tumors, including embryonal carcinoma, teratocarcinoma, and choriocarcinoma, occur more commonly in the 20- to 30-year age range. Spermatocytic seminoma occurs in older men, typically over age 50. Yolk sac tumors are the most common tumors of infants.[2] Malignant testicular lymphomas and metastatic lesions to the testis typically occur in men over age 50.

Several factors are associated with the development of testicular cancer. A history of a cryptorchid (undescended) testis has been found in up to 10% of patients. Approximately 5% of cases occur in patients previously treated for cancer of the contralateral testicle.[1] Trauma has long been implicated in cases of testicular cancer, but it is now thought that a traumatic event simply focuses attention on a scrotum already harboring a tumor.[2] Hormonal factors such as diethylstilbestrol exposure in utero have been implicated, but studies are conflicting.[1] Genetic factors have also been implicated in the

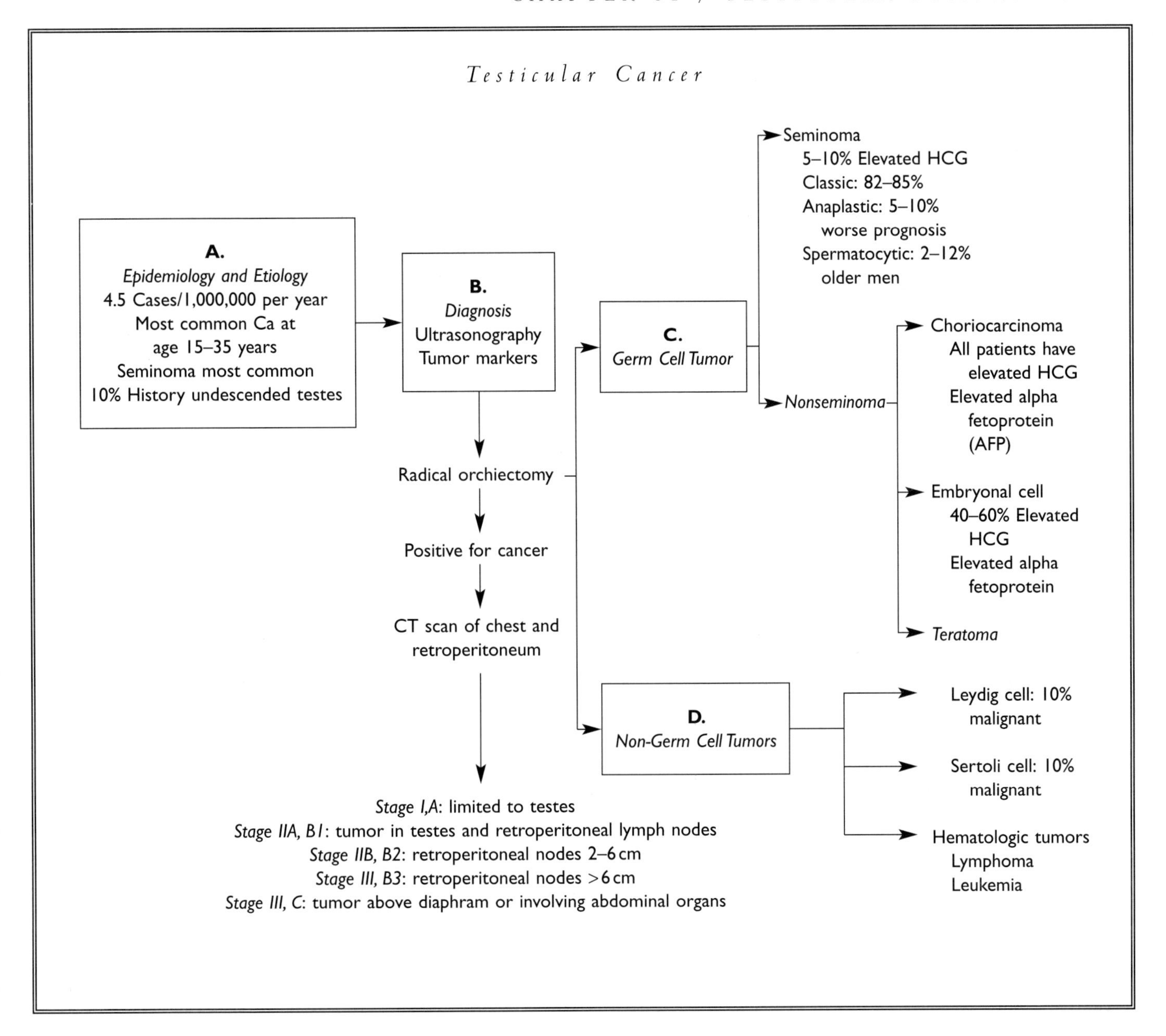

development of testicular cancer, as up to 5% of cases have been found to occur bilaterally and occasionally in families. Isochromosomal deletions on the short arm of chromosome 12 have been found in many patients with both seminoma and nonseminomatous germ cell tumors.[4]

B. Diagnosis

Any firm mass in the testicle should be considered a tumor until proven otherwise. The most common presentation is a painless mass. The differential diagnosis includes epididymitis, orchitis, torsion, hydrocele, spermatocele, varicocele, or a hernia.[1] There is often a delay of several months between detection of the mass and the time at which the patient seeks medical attention. Approximately 10% of patients present with metastatic disease, such as a supraclavicular neck mass, lung nodules, retroperitoneal metastases, central or peripheral nerve involvement, or unilateral or bilateral iliac vein or vena caval obstruction or thrombosis.[2]

Physical examination of the testicles begins with palpation of the unaffected testicle and epididymis first. The testicle should be homogeneous in texture and freely movable. The involved side should next be assessed for consistency, mobility, tenderness, inhomogeneity, and involvement of the epididymis, spermatic cord, or scrotum. Ultrasound examination of the scrotum is mandatory in patients with a testicular mass and is highly accurate in the diagnosis of testicular cancer.[5] Once the presence of an intratesticular mass is confirmed, serum tumor markers are obtained and the patient is prepared for a radical orchiectomy.

Scrotal exploration and radical orchiectomy through an inguinal approach must be performed if a lesion is suspicious.

Following orchiectomy and once a diagnosis of cancer is established, a computed tomography (CT) scan of the abdomen and pelvis is performed to assess the retroperitoneum. CT scan of the chest is the most sensitive method for identifying pulmonary metastases.[6] Scan results are then used to render a *clinical* stage. The Indiana University testicular cancer clinical staging system is one that has been commonly adopted.[7]

Stage A or I	tumor limited to the testis alone
Stage B1 or IIA	tumor of the testis and retroperitoneal lymph nodes
Stage B2 or IIB	tumor of retroperitoneal lymph nodes 2–6 cm in greatest dimension by CT
Stage B3 or IIC	tumor of retroperitoneal lymph nodes >6 cm in greatest dimension by CT
Stage C or III	tumor above the diaphragm or involving abdominal solid organs

Tumor markers are often elevated in patients with testicular tumors. Measurement of serum levels is important for diagnosis and staging, assessing the response to therapy, and detecting relapse of the cancer. Human chorionic gonadotropin (hCG) is a 38,000-kDa glycoprotein that is frequently elevated in patients with germ cell tumors. The hCG is produced by syncytiotrophoblastic cells; it has a half-life of 24–36 hours and is produced in all patients with choriocarcinoma and 40–60% of all patients with embryonal carcinoma. Approximately 5–10% of patients with a pure seminoma have elevated hCG levels.[2] α-Fetoprotein (AFP) is a 70,000-kDa single-chain glycoprotein produced by yolk sac and fetal liver. The half-life of AFP ranges from 5–7 days. An elevated AFP level indicates the presence of a nonseminomatous germ cell tumor.[1] Levels of these markers should normalize in accordance with their half-lives after complete removal of the offending tumor. Subsequent elevation may herald recurrent disease. Serum lactate dehydrogenase (LDH) has also been found to be elevated in up to 60% of nonseminomatous germ cell tumors.[8]

Radical Orchiectomy

Orchiectomy is performed through an inguinal incision. The external inguinal ring is opened, and the spermatic cord is isolated and doubly occluded with a Penrose drain to prevent venous outflow and tumor dissemination. The testicle is delivered from the scrotum and freed from its gubernaculum. The testicle and epididymis are then grossly inspected. If there is any suspicion of malignancy, the testicle is removed. The spermatic cord is transected and suture-ligated.

Most tumors spread via lymphatics, although some spread hematogenously. The primary lymphatic drainage of the *right* testicle is the interaortocaval lymph node basin and subsequently the precaval, preaortic, and paracaval lymph nodes. Once the interaortocaval nodes are involved, there tends to be spread from the right to the left side and the left paraaortic area.[2] The *left* side's primary drainage site is the left paraaortic nodal basin just below the left renal vein and subsequently the preaortic nodes. Inguinal metastases can occur when the tunica albuginea has been violated. Distant spread most commonly is to the lungs. Visceral metastases may occur in the liver, brain, or bone.[2]

The *histologic* classification of testicular tumors determines which therapy should be employed. Although many tumors consist of a mixture of tumor types, a rough classification of germ cell tumors into seminomatous or nonseminomatous type is helpful. If a tumor contains both seminomatous and nonseminomatous elements, it is considered a nonseminoma. Additionally, within the grouping of nonseminomas, there are several nonseminomatous elements.

Three subtypes of pure seminoma have been identified: classic, anaplastic, and spermatocytic. *Classic seminoma* accounts for 82–85% of seminomas, most often occurring in patients during their third decade of life.[2] The classic type is relatively slow-growing. *Anaplastic seminoma* occurs in the same age range, accounts for 5–10% of seminomas, and is characterized by high mitotic activity, a high rate of local invasion, an increased rate of metastatic spread, and a high rate of hCG production. Up to 30% of men dying of testicular cancer have the anaplastic form, despite its low incidence.[2] *Spermatocytic seminoma* accounts for 2–12% of seminomas and typically occurs in older men. These tumors have low metastatic potential, and orchiectomy is usually adequate.[3]

Nonseminomatous germ cell tumors present with metastases in 50–70% of the cases, in contrast to 20–30% of patients with seminomas.[2] Histologically, nonseminomas have a variety of patterns. *Embryonal carcinomas* generally present as small irregular masses involving the tunica vaginalis, with areas of hemorrhage and necrosis. Embryonal tumors have a higher relapse rate following therapy owing to their predilection for hematogenous spread.[9] *Pure choriocarcinoma* may appear as a palpable nodule, and histologically it contains syncytiotrophoblasts and cytotrophoblasts. Thus both AFP and hCG may be elevated in these patients. *Teratoma* consists of more than one germ cell layer in various stages of maturation and differentiation. "Mature" elements resemble benign structures derived from ectoderm, endoderm, and mesoderm. "Immature" elements resemble undifferentiated primitive tissues from each of the three germ cell layers. Grossly they are large and inhomogeneous in consistency. *Yolk sac tumors* are the most common testis tumor in infants and children. In adults, yolk sac elements are often present with other cell types and account for the characteristics production of AFP with this cell type.[2]

C. Germ Cell Tumors

Seminoma

Seminoma is the most common histologic type of testis tumor, accounting for approximately 60–65% of all germ cell tumors of the tests. Seminoma usually presents with low-stage disease; approximately 75% of patients are diagnosed with clinical stage I.[2] Seminoma is a radiosensitive tumor, and a more than 95% survival rate should be expected with low-stage disease.[2]

Patients with *stage I disease* can be given 25–35 Gy of radiation directed to the periaortic and ipsilateral pelvic lymph nodes in 20 daily fractions over 4 weeks. The in-field control rate is close to 100% with radiation therapy.[2] Patients predisposed to relapse are those with invasion of the tunica albuginea or anaplastic histology. Patients with relapse should be treated with platinum-based combined chemotherapy (see below). The 5- and 10-year survival rates for stage I seminoma are 99% and 92%, respectively.[3] Alternatively, observation alone following orchiectomy has been proposed for stage I disease; however, 15% of these patients subsequently fail in the retroperitoneum. Therefore observation is not without risk and should be undertaken with caution. These patients are closely monitored with serial chest radiographs, abdominal and pelvic CT scans, and tumor markers. If the cancer recurs, these patients are treated with retroperitoneal irradiation or chemotherapy.[3]

Stage II disease is measured by the diameter of the largest retroperitoneal mass. *Stage IIA* disease is the most common presentation for patients with seminoma metastases. These patients have traditionally been treated with radiation therapy to their paraaortic and pelvic lymph nodes using a regimen similar to that for patients with stage I disease. Patients with stage IIA disease have survival rates above 90%.[2]

Patients with extensive disease, *stage IIB* (nodes 2–6 cm in dimension), may be treated with irradiation or chemotherapy. Radiation doses of 25 Gy are applied to the entire treatment zone with boosts of 10 Gy to the involved nodes.[3] Persistent retroperitoneal masses following irradiation often encase the great vessels. This desmoplastic reaction makes surgical resection technically difficult. Persistent retroperitoneal disease after irradiation is difficult to cure, and patients usually require salvage chemotherapy.[8] The overall disease-free survival for patients with stage IIB disease or greater treated with abdominal irradiation is only 50%.[2] Therefore cisplatin-based chemotherapy combined with bleomycin and etoposide has emerged as an improved modality capable of achieving cure rates of approximately 90%.[3] These patients are assessed after treatment with repeat CT scans of the retroperitoneum to evaluate the status of their metastases.

Patients with *high stage II disease* (IIC, IIB—controversial) and *stage III disease* should be treated primarily with chemotherapy. It is unclear how to manage persistent retroperitoneal disease following chemotherapy. These masses may contain fibrotic tissue, necrotic tumor, or viable cancer. Recent guidelines suggest surveillance for residual masses <3 cm and surgical resection for masses >3 cm.[10] If residual cancer is discovered during resection, the patient should receive radiation therapy or further chemotherapy.[10]

Nonseminoma

Nonseminomatous germ cell tumors frequently follow a less favorable course. Depending on referral patterns, 50–70% of patients with nonseminoma present with metastatic disease.[2] As with seminoma, the most common sites of metastasis are the retroperitoneal lymph nodes.[2] Embryonal carcinoma accounts for 20–25% of nonseminomatous testicular cancers, teratocarcinoma 25–30%, teratoma 5–10%, and choriocarcinoma 1%.[11] According to Mostofi approximately 40% of tumors have more than one histologic type present.[11]

Accurate staging is of paramount importance with nonseminomatous tumors, as the prognosis and the chemotherapy and surgical options vary according to stage. Clinical staging is similar to that for patients with seminoma. Tumor markers (AFP, hCG) are obtained before and after orchiectomy. CT scans of the abdomen, pelvis, and chest are done to assess for metastatic disease. These scans can detect metastatic lesions in the retroperitoneum <2 cm in diameter, although 30% of patients are understaged by CT (confirmed by subsequent retroperitoneal lymph node dissection).[7] Elevated hCG levels are found in 40–60% of patients with nonseminomatous germ cell tumors; and approximately 70% of yolk sac and embryonal germ cell tumors have elevated AFP levels.[8] The presence of persistently elevated tumor marker levels or levels decreasing less than expected (calculated by their half-lives following orchiectomy) suggests the possibility of residual disease. Overall, nonseminomatous germ cell cancer has a cure rate of approximately 80% for all stages and should approach 100% for low-stage disease.[9]

Treatment of *clinical stage I* nonseminomatous testis cancer is controversial. Patients are offered retroperitoneal lymph node dissection (RPLND) or surveillance. A failure rate of 30% can be expected with the latter. Identification of appropriate patients for surgery is based on tumor size, histology, fertility issues, patient preference, cost, and patient compliance for follow-up.

Metastatic sites for nonseminomatous germ cell cancer are usually the interaortal caval region on the right and the

Seminoma

Treatment following radical orchiectomy;
retroperitoneal staging done with CT scanning

Clinical Stage

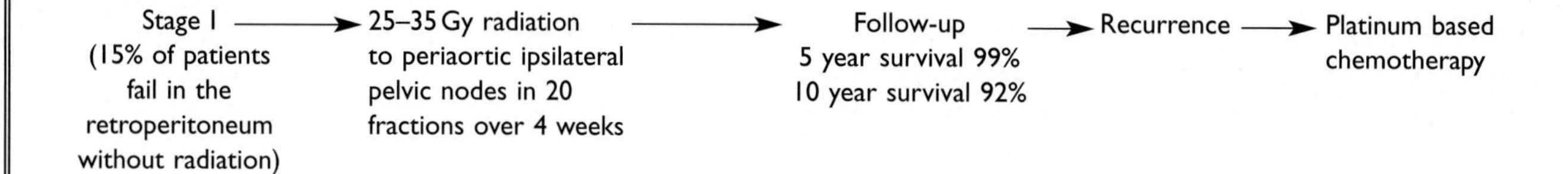

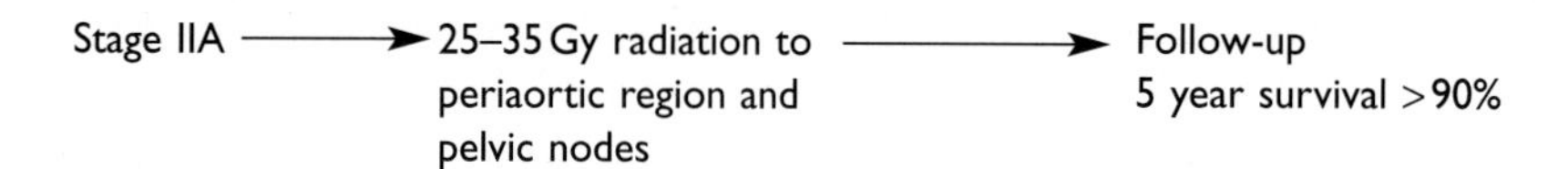

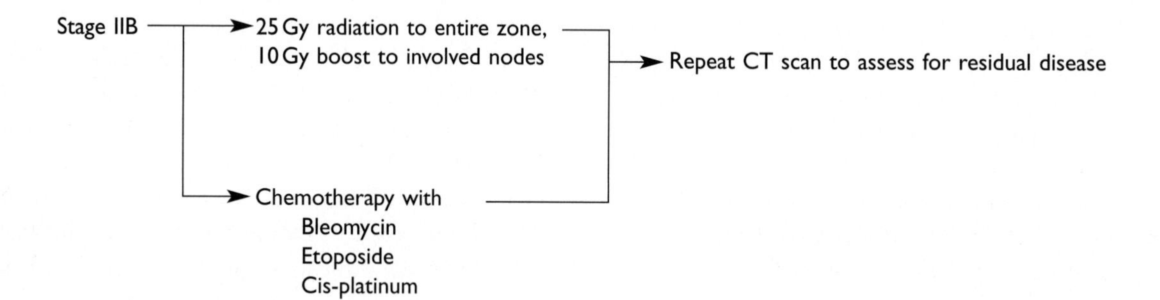

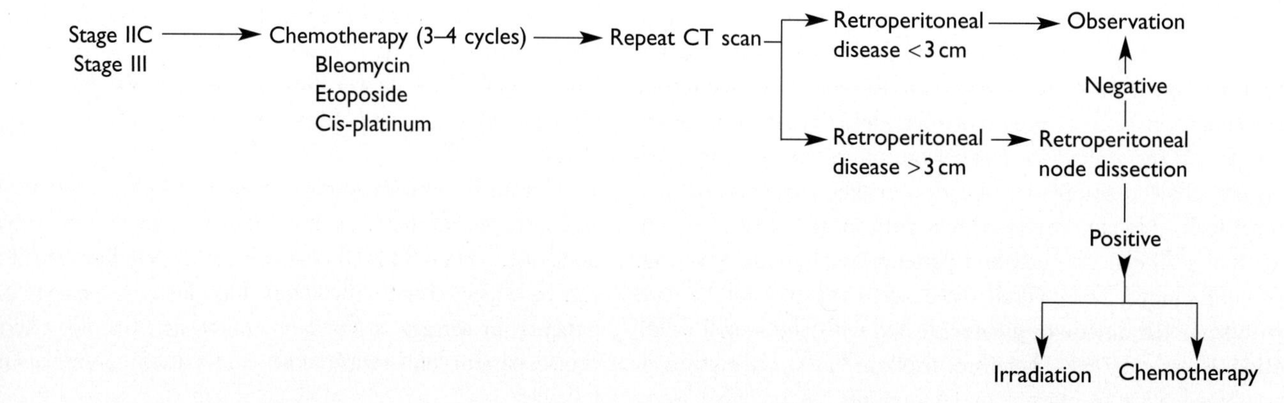

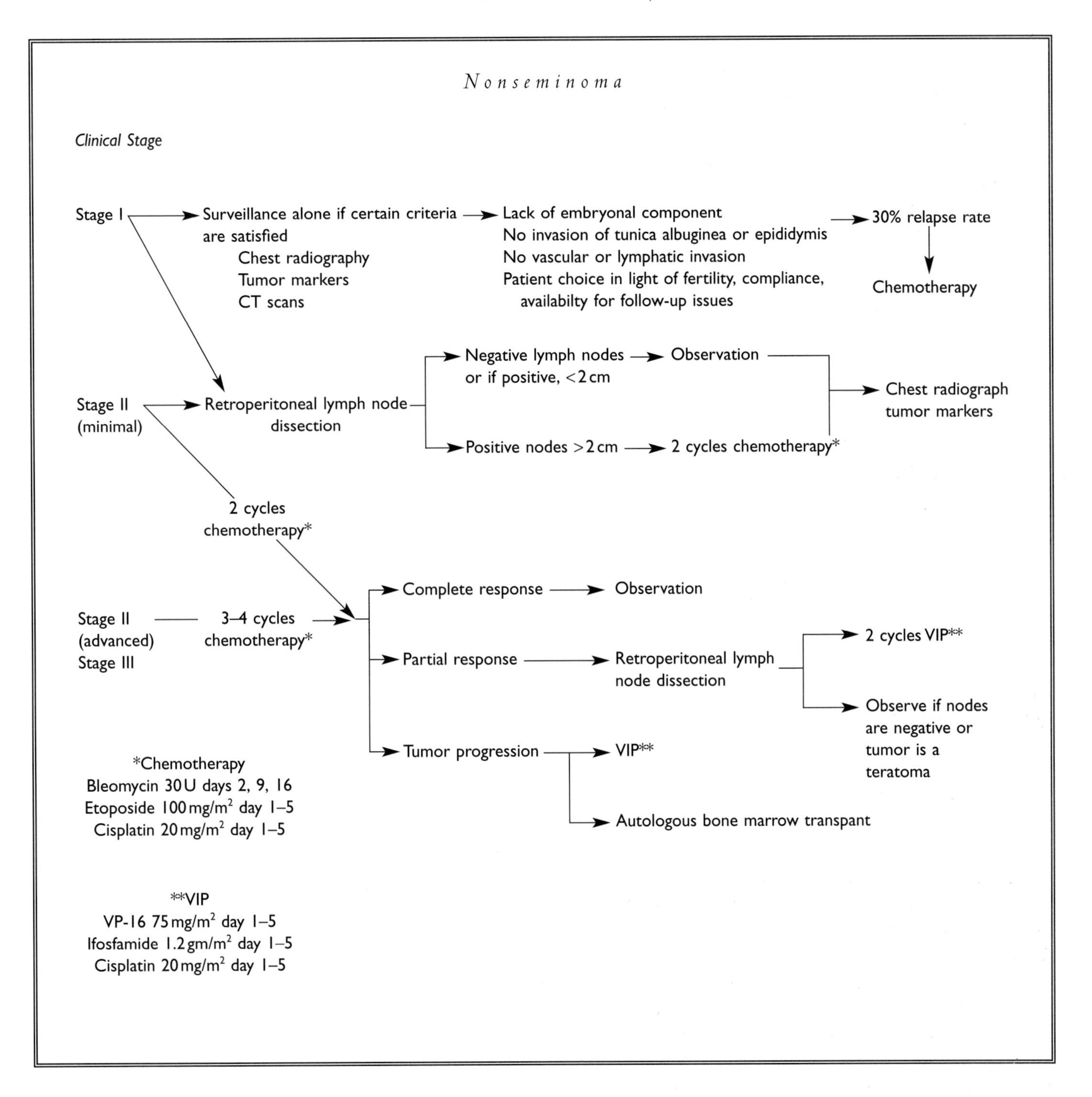

paraaortic and preaortic nodes on the left. Metastases localize first in the retroperitoneum in 90% of cases. There is a 99.6% cure rate for pathologically confirmed stage I disease with RPLND alone.[9] If a recurrence does happen, it usually does so during the first 2 years of therapy, and there is a high cure rate with administration of chemotherapy.[9]

Patients with low-stage disease who undergo RPLND must be followed diligently with chest radiographs, tumor markers, and physical examinations every 1–2 months for the first year and then every 2–3 months for the next year. After 2 years patients are followed every 6 months or yearly for 5 years, then annually. Relapse usually occurs in the lumgs or the retroperitoneum or patients may have elevated serum tumor markers without evidence of clinically or radiographically demonstrable disease.

Surgical Considerations RPLND has evolved through the years with modifications in technique to decrease morbidity. Mortality for the procedure is now less than 1%; the morbidity is 5–25% and consists primarily of atelectasis, pneumonitis, ileus, lymphocele, pancreatitis, small bowel obstruction,

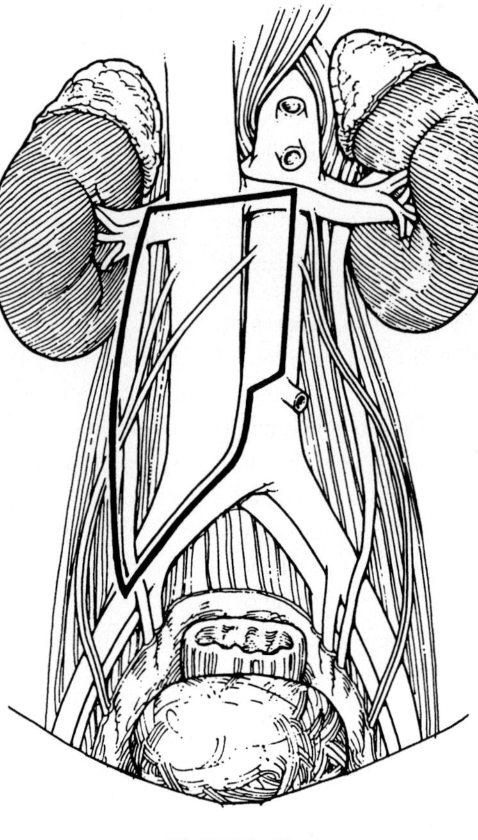

FIGURE 51–1
Right modified nerve-sparing retroperitoneal lymph node dissection (RPLND) template. (From Coogan and Rowland, with permission.[1])

and wound infection.[12,13] A major complication of the procedure is interruption of the sympathetically mediated nerves originating from L1–4, which traverse the retroperitoneum and control seminal emission. However, modifications of the surgical boundaries described by Donohue during the 1980s have made maintenance of ejaculation a possibility for patients undergoing RPLND.[14]

The modified RPLND is performed through a midline incision from the xiphoid to the pubic symphysis. The retroperitoneum is grossly palpated to evaluate for metastatic disease. High volume disease mandates abandonment of the modified technique and performance of a full bilateral lymphadenectomy. A *right*-sided dissection is performed by incising the posterior peritoneum from the cecum to the ligament of Treitz (Fig. 51–1). The root of the small bowel is dissected off the retroperitoneum, and the inferior mesenteric vein is divided. A self-retaining retractor is generally used to retract the bowel once the retroperitoneum is entered. The boundaries for the *right*-sided dissection involve the bilateral renal hilar areas superiorly. The dissection on the right is carried to the junction of the right common iliac artery and the right ureter. The lymphadenectomy is initiated by splitting and rolling the lymphatic tissue medially from the left renal vein down to the origin of the inferior mesenteric artery on the anterior surface of the aorta. The anterior surface of the vena cava is then freed of nodal tissue with the origin of the right spermatic vein identified and divided. The lymphatics overlying the cava are rolled medially, and the lumbar veins coming off the cava posteriorly are identified and divided. Prior to dividing them, the efferent sympathetic fibers are identified and preserved. These fibers usually pass superior to the lumber veins. The lumbar arteries medially on the aorta are also divided. The interaortocaval and right paracaval lymphatic tissues are then dissected off the posterior body wall. The right gonadal vein is dissected distally to the internal ring and sent off as a separate specimen.

Exposure for *left*-sided dissections is obtained by incising the posterior peritoneum lateral to the left colon, and the left colon and mesocolon are elevated off the retroperitoneum and retracted medially. The splenocolic ligament must be incised to protect the spleen from injury. The left-sided efferent fibers are next identified by dissecting a condensation of the fibers at the left common iliac artery and then dissecting the fibers proximally. The origin of the left gonadal vein is identified and divided from the renal vein and dissected distally to the internal ring. The lateral border of the dissection is the left ureter. The lymphatic tissue medial to this ureter is dissected free. This tissue is dissected off the psoas muscle, exposing the sympathetic chain. The posterior lumbar arteries arising from the aorta are divided. The lymphatic tissue is then freed and divided from the left side of the aorta. Finally, interaortocaval tissue and upper preaortic lymphatic tissue is taken to complete the dissection as described above using the "split and roll" technique. The medial border is the lateral border of the inferior vena cava.

The dissection on the left is carried down the left ureter to the level of the inferior mesenteric artery (Fig. 51–2). Both sympathetic side chains are preserved, and the ipsilateral spermatic vessels are removed.

SURVEILLANCE Because 70% of stage I patients who undergo RPLND have histologically negative nodes and 5–10% experience recurrent cancer outside the retroperitoneum, consideration has been given to avoiding RPLND and simply observing the patient. If relapse does occur (30% probability), effective chemotherapy is available. Surveillance consists of physical examination, chest radiography, and tumor marker assays performed once a month for the first year, every 2 months for the second year, and every 3–6 months thereafter. CT scanning of the retroperitoneum should be performed approximately every 2–3 months for the first 2 years and every 6 months thereafter. Surveillance is recommended for at least 5–10 years.

Pathologic staging of the orchiectomy specimen is useful when deciding whether the patient should be observed or undergo RPLND. Favorable prognostic factors include lack of an embryonal component, lack of invasion of the tunica albuginea and epididymis, and lack of vascular or lymphatic invasion

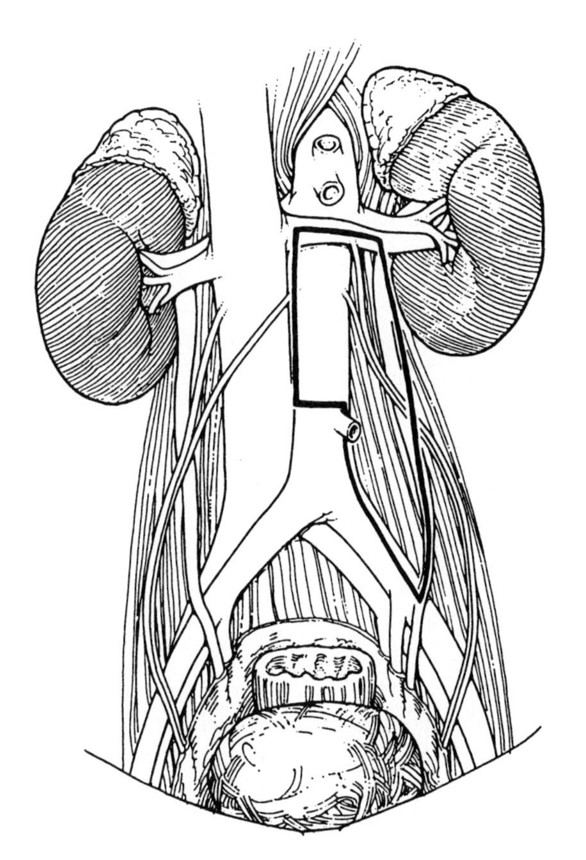

FIGURE 51–2
Left modified nerve-sparing RPLND template. (From Coogan and Rowland, with permission.[1])

in the orchiectomy specimen.[15] The relapse rate in nontreated patients with stage I disease is about 30% for the combined data from several large series.[2] Those who relapse do so at a higher stage 80% of the time and do not respond as well to chemotherapy as patients who undergo RPLND at the onset.[2] These patients also have a higher death rate when they do relapse.

Patients with *low volume stage II*, nonseminomatous germ cell tumors may be treated with RPLND or chemotherapy. RPLND is capable of eradicating resectable disease in more than 65% of patients with stage II tumors.[16] Patients who are found to have multiple positive lymph nodes in the retroperitoneum are usually treated with chemotherapy, but selected cases may undergo surveillance.

Patients with *high stage II* clinical disease (stage IIB) should undergo chemotherapy as the first line of therapy with three or four cycles of bleomycin (30 units on treatment days 2, 9, 16), etoposide (VP-16) (100 mg/m^2 on days 1–5), and cisplatin (20 mg/m^2 on days 1–5).[2] Six weeks after completion of chemotherapy, residual retroperitoneal disease should be treated with RPLND. Pathologic examination may reveal fibrosis (40%), teratoma (40%), or residual cancer (20%).[17] If cancer is confirmed following RPLND, adjuvant chemotherapy consisting of VP-16 (75 mg/m^2 on days 1–5), ifosfamide (1.2 g/m^2 on days 1–5), and cisplatin (20 mg/m^2 on days 1–5) may be given.[2] Patients with complete resection of viable malignant tumor followed by two courses of salvage chemotherapy have been reported to produce a 70% disease-free rate without additional therapy.[17] Without salvage chemotherapy a significant percentage of resected tumors recur, usually in the lungs.

Chemotherapy has evolved over the past 30 years into a successful first-line therapy for patients with *stage III disease*. Currently, three or four cycles of bleomycin/etoposide/platinum (BEP) should be administered.[2] Cisplatin-based chemotherapy effectively cures approximately 70% of patients with disseminated germ cell tumors.[2] Tumor markers should be followed in these patients and residual masses surgically excised (RPLND) once the markers normalize. Patients who have residual cancer in the resected specimen should receive salvage chemotherapy [vinblastine/ifosfamide/cisplatin (VIP)]. Additionally, patients who fail to respond to initial chemotherapy should have second-line chemotherapy consisting of VIP. Third-line chemotherapy has not yet been clearly delineated. A high-dose carboblatin-based chemotherapy regimen and bone-marrow are frequently used.

The surgical approach for patients with residual disease after chemotherapy includes a full bilateral RPLND (Fig. 51–3). A

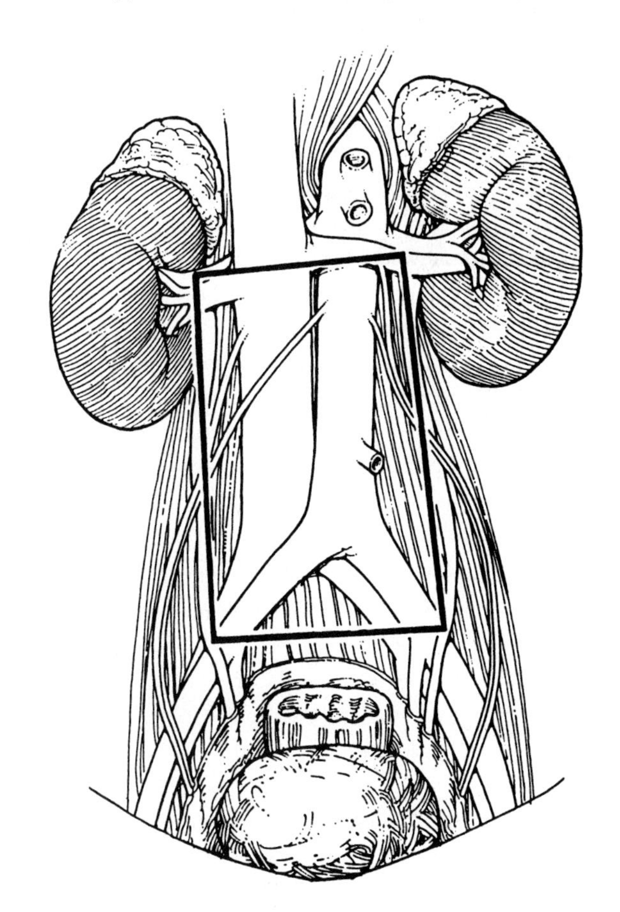

FIGURE 51–3
Template for full bilateral RPLND. (From Coogan and Rowland, with permission.[1])

midline approach is recommended with full small bowel mobilization on the superior mesenteric artery and ligation of the inferior mesenteric artery. The fibrotic mass in the retroperitoneum usually encompasses the aorta, vena cava, or both. The ureters should be dissected free from any neighboring fibrosis and the inferior vena cava cleared of disease. Lumbar arteries and veins should be divided. It is also essential to examine the retrocrural space on preoperative CT scans for nodes in this area. It is of note that patients undergoing postchemotherapy lymph node dissection require meticulous fluid management intraoperatively and postoperatively owing to their predilection for bleomycin-induced pulmonary toxicity.

D. Non-Germ Cell Tumors

Stromal tumors account for 5–10% of testicular tumors.[2] They usually appear as hypoechoic lesions on ultrasonography; and hCG and AFP levels typically are not elevated. Tissue is needed to confirm the diagnosis.

Leydig Cell Tumors

Leydig cell tumors are the most common sex cord-mesenchyme lesions, accounting for 1–3% of all testicular cancers. The age range is vast, and they can occur in prepubertal boys and men aged 20–60. The etiology of these tumors is unknown, and they are not associated with cryptorchidism. About 10% of these tumors are of a malignant nature, and there is no reliable way to differentiate benign from malignant except on the basis of histologic examination. Clinically, prepubertal boys present with precocious puberty, which must be differentiated from congenital adrenocortical hyperplasia, which produces the same signs and symptoms. Adults usually present with an endocrinologic imbalance and a palpable testicular mass. Patients may present with feminizing features including impotence, decreased libido, and gynecomastia.[2] Histologically, the characteristic feature of Leydig cell tumors are Reinke's crystals, which are cigar-shaped cytoplasmic inclusions.[10] Radical orchiectomy is adequate therapy in most cases, as 90% are benign. CT evaluation of the retroperitoneal nodes is warranted. RPLND should be performed when there is evidence of retroperitoneal metastases.[2]

Sertoli Cell Tumors

Sertoli cell tumors, which can occur in any age group, account for fewer than 1% of all testis tumors. The size range at presentation can vary, and 10% of these tumors are malignant.[2] Clinically, gynecomastia is present 20% of the time and tends to be more indicative of malignant lesions.[18] Again, confirmation of diagnosis and malignancy can be accomplished only with radical orchiectomy. Pathologically, structures known as Call-Exner bodies, which consist of secretory material, are present.[10] Malignancy is confirmed only by the presence of metastases. RPLND should be performed when there is evidence of retroperitoneal metastases.[2]

Hematologic Tumors

Lymphoma accounts for approximately 5% of all testicular tumors and is the most common secondary neoplasm of the testis.[2] Lymphoma represents 50% of testicular cancers in men over age 65, and more than 80% of all testicular lymphomas are seen in men over age 50.[18] Most commonly, patients present with a unilateral, painless mass. Fifty percent of testicular lymphomas are bilateral, with 10% occurring simultaneously. All varieties of lymphoma can present in the testicle, with the histiocytic type of non-Hodgkin's lymphoma occurring most commonly. Retroperitoneal imaging should be carried out to determine the extent of disease. The prognosis for lymphoma involving the testes is generally poor but is related to the stage at presentation.

The testicle is a prime site of acute lymphocytic *leukemia* relapse in boys. A biopsy is essential to establish the diagnosis. Testicular irradiation of 1200 cGy over a 6- to 8-day period is needed to eradicate the disease in the testes.[2]

Conclusions

Although testicular cancer is a relatively rare malignancy, it is the most common cancer in males between 15 and 35 years of age. Its incidence is increasing in the United States. Once noted to be a highly lethal disease, cure rates in excess of 90% have been reached because of advances in multimodal therapy.

Any firm mass in the testicle must be managed without delay. Ultrasonography of the scrotum is mandatory for these patients; and if an intratesticular mass is confirmed, serum tumor markers should be assayed. The patient is then prepared for a radical orchiectomy through an inguinal approach. Once a diagnosis of cancer is established, clinical staging is performed with a CT scan. Treatment strategies are determined by clinical stage and histology.

References

1. Coogan C, Rowland R. Testis tumors: diagnosis and staging. In: Oesterling J, Richie J (eds) Urologic Oncology. Philadelphia: Saunders, 1997:457–465.
2. Richie JP. Neoplasms of the testis. In: Walsh P, Retik A, Vaughn E, Wein A (eds) Campbell's Urology, 7th ed. Philadelphia: Saunders, 1998: 2411–2452.
3. Jewett M, Khakpour G, Gospodarowicz M. Seminoma: management and prognosis. In: Oesterling J, Richie J (eds) Urologic Oncology. Philadelphia: Saunders, 1997:466–480.

4. Sagalowsky AI. Current considerations in the diagnosis and initial treatment of testicular cancer. Compr Ther 1994;20:688–694.
5. Richie JP, Burnholz J, Garnick MB. Ultrasonography as a diagnostic adjunct for the evaluation of masses in the scrotum. Surg Gynecol Obstet 1982; 254:695.
6. Husband J. Advances in tumor imaging. In: Horwich A (ed) Testicular Cancer: Investigation and Management. London: Chapman & Hall, 1991:15.
7. Rowland RG, Foster RS, Donohue JP. Scrotum and testis. In: Gillenwater JY, Grayhack JT, Howards SS, Duckett JW (eds) Adult and Pediatric Urology, 3rd ed. St. Louis: Mosby, 1996:1917–1949.
8. Sarosdy M. Testicular cancer: an overview. In: Crawford ED, Das S (eds) Current Genitourinary Cancer Surgery. Philadelphia: Lea & Febiger, 1990:306.
9. Richie JP. Nonseminomatous germ cell tumors: management and prognosis. In: Oesterling J, Richie J (eds) Urologic Oncology. Philadelphia: Saunders, 1997:481–495.
10. Motzer R, Bosl G, Heelan R, et al. Residual mass: an indication for further therapy in patients with advanced seminoma following system chemotherapy. J Clin Oncol 1987;5:1064–1070.
11. Mostofi FK. Testicular tumors: epidemiologic, etiologic and pathologic features. Cancer 1973;32:1186.
12. Baniel J, Foster RS, Rowland RG, et al. Complications of primary retroperitoneal lymph node dissection. J Urol 1994;152:424–427.
13. Foster RS, Donohue JP, Bihrle R. Retroperitoneal lymphadenectomy. In: Marshall F (ed) Operative Urology. Philadelphia: Saunders, 1996: 365–372.
14. Donohue JP, Thornhill JA, Foster RS, et al. Retroperitoneal lymphadenecotomy for clinical stage A testis cancer (1965–1989): modifications of technique and impact on ejaculation. J Urol 1993;149: 237–243.
15. Raghaven D, Peckham MJ, Heyderman E, et al. Prognostic factors in clinical stage I nonseminomatous germ-cell tumors of the testis. Br J Cancer 1982;45:167.
16. Donohue JP, Thornhill JA, Foster RS, Bihrle R, Rowland RG, Einhorn LH. The role of retroperitoneal lymphadenectomy in clinical stage B testis cancer: the Indiana University experience (1965 to 1989). J Urol 1995; 153:85–89.
17. Fox EP, Weathers TS, Williams SD, et al. Outcome analysis for patients with persistent nonteratomatous germ cell tumor in postchemotherapy retroperitoneal lymph node dissections. J Clin Oncol 1993;11:1294–1299.
18. Klein EA, Levin HS. Non-germ cell tumors of the testis. In: Oesterling J, Richie J (eds) Urologic Oncology. Philadelphia: Saunders, 1997:496–514.

Section 10

Gynecologic Cancers

Chapter 52

Endometrial Cancer

SHARMILA MAKHIJA
RICHARD BARAKAT

A. Epidemiology

Endometrial cancer is the most common type of female genital cancer in the United States, with an estimated 36,100 new cases and 6300 deaths per year. Its prevalence is 5 cases per 1000 asymptomatic women over 45 years of age, and it is seen primarily in postmenopausal women. The peak incidence occurs at age 60. Only women with the following high risk factors benefit from screening [endometrial sampling, transvaginal ultrasonography (TVUS)]: age over 40 years with abnormal uterine bleeding, massive obesity, history of endometrial hyperplasia, or unopposed estrogen or tamoxifen use.

B. Screening

Regarding screening one must keep in mind that among asymptomatic women over age 45 the prevalence for endometrial cancer is low (5/1000 subjects), and there is no noninvasive, inexpensive, cost-effective, highly predictive test for asymptomatic patients. Endometrial sampling and ultrasonography can be used for diagnosis, but they are not acceptable screening tools for the average-risk, asymptomatic woman. Cervical cytology is abnormal in fewer than half of the endometrial cancers. Endometrial sampling can be performed in the office setting but may be hampered by the presence of fibroids or cervical stenosis. TVUS detects changes in endometrial thickness; and a value of 5 mm is used to determine abnormally thick endometrial tissue. Thickness may be altered by exogenous hormones. In general, therefore, only high risk individuals benefit from screening with sampling and ultrasonography.

C. Presentation

The most common presenting sign of endometrial cancer is abnormal uterine bleeding. Symptomatic patients should undergo an office endometrial biopsy; most (85%) have an adequate tissue sample, revealing benign tissue. Of these, 90% become asymptomatic and require only an annual gynecologic follow-up; the remaining 10% have persistent bleeding 30 days or more beyond the initial biopsy. These

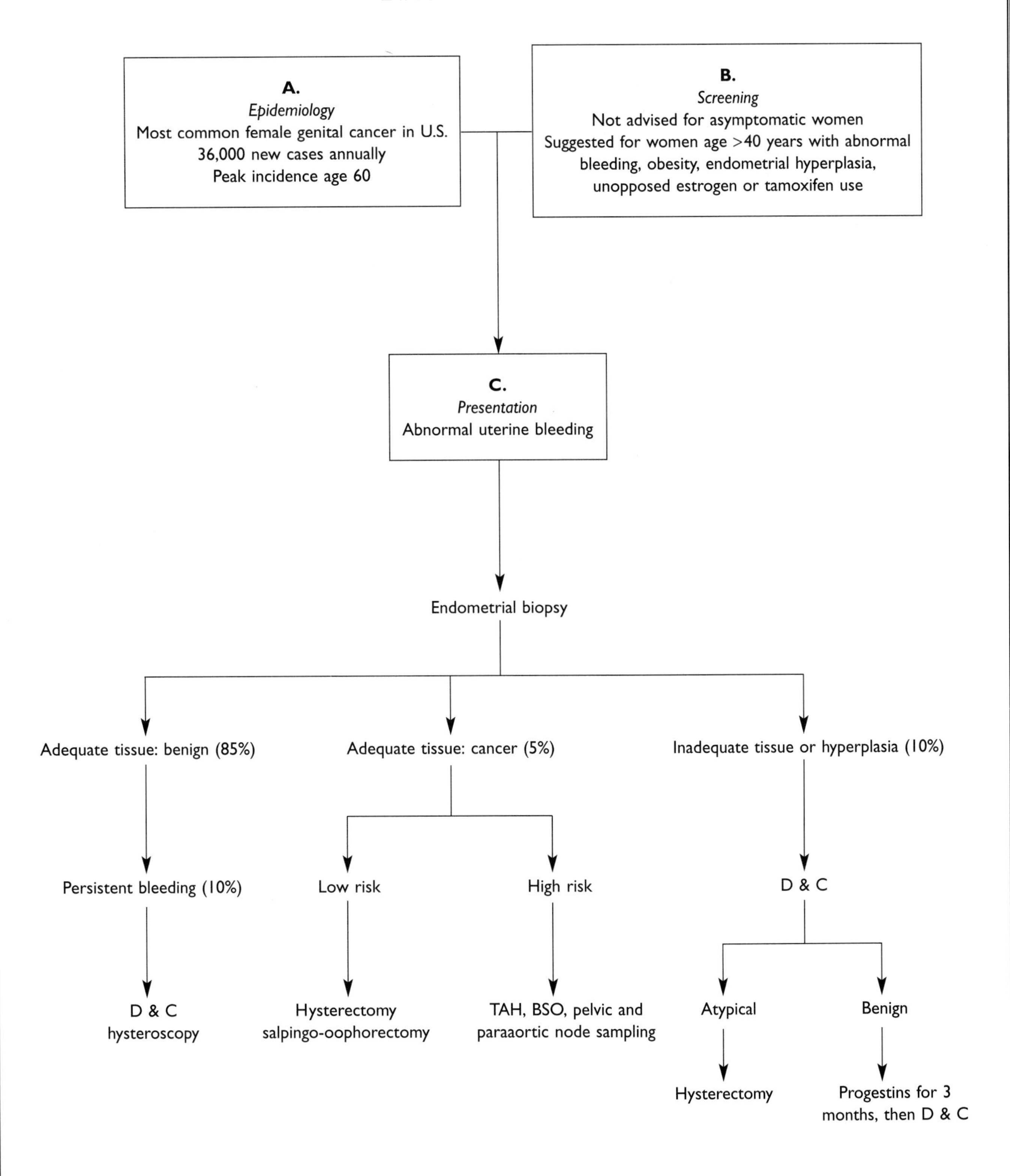

(continued on next page)

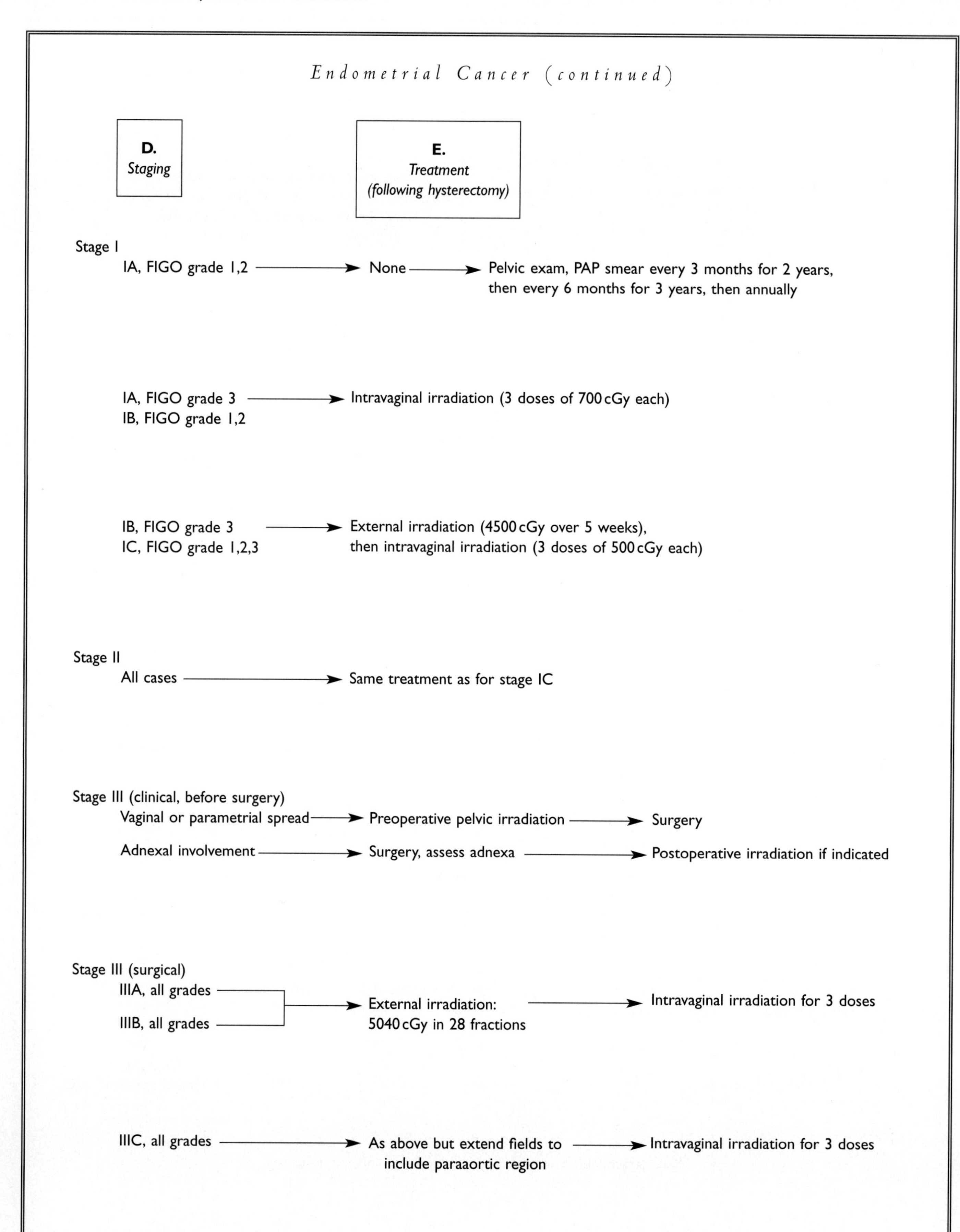
Endometrial Cancer (continued)
D. Staging
E. Treatment (following hysterectomy)
Stage I
IA, FIGO grade 1,2
None
Pelvic exam, PAP smear every 3 months for 2 years, then every 6 months for 3 years, then annually
IA, FIGO grade 3
IB, FIGO grade 1,2
Intravaginal irradiation (3 doses of 700 cGy each)
IB, FIGO grade 3
IC, FIGO grade 1,2,3
External irradiation (4500 cGy over 5 weeks), then intravaginal irradiation (3 doses of 500 cGy each)
Stage II
All cases
Same treatment as for stage IC
Stage III (clinical, before surgery)
Vaginal or parametrial spread
Preoperative pelvic irradiation
Surgery
Adnexal involvement
Surgery, assess adnexa
Postoperative irradiation if indicated
Stage III (surgical)
IIIA, all grades
IIIB, all grades
External irradiation: 5040 cGy in 28 fractions
Intravaginal irradiation for 3 doses
IIIC, all grades
As above but extend fields to include paraaortic region
Intravaginal irradiation for 3 doses

Endometrial Cancer (continued)

Stage IV (clinical stage)

- IV A → External beam irradiation
- IV B → External beam irradiation

Stage IV (surgical stage, grade 2,3)

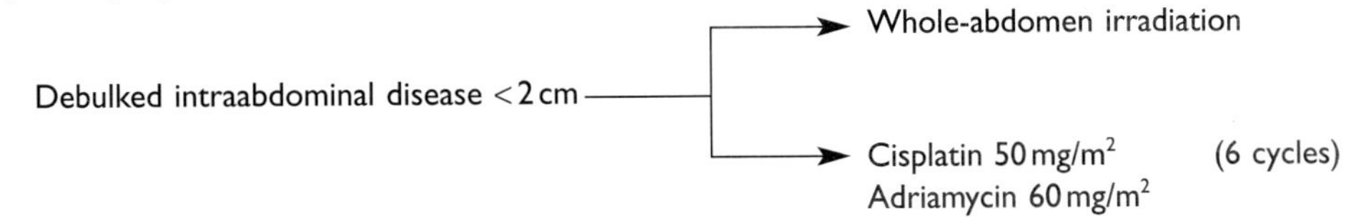

- Debulked intraabdominal disease <2 cm → Whole-abdomen irradiation
- Debulked intraabdominal disease <2 cm → Cisplatin 50 mg/m^2, Adriamycin 60 mg/m^2 (6 cycles)
- Debulked intraabdominal disease >2 cm → Chemotherapy as above; Follow CT scans, CA-125; Consider more chemotherapy or second laparotomy

Stage IV (surgical stage, grade 1)

- No extraabdominal disease → Progestins
- Extraabdominal disease present → Chemotherapy with cisplatin and Adriamycin vs. progestins

Recurrent disease, prior surgery and irradiation

- FIGO grade 1,2 → Progestins
- FIGO grade 2,3 → Cisplatin, adriamycin
- (both) → Consider exenteration for small, isolated recurrence

Recurrent disease, prior surgery only

- Abdominal and pelvic disease → Whole-abdomen radiation therapy (WART)
- Pelvis only → Preoperative irradiation (5000 cGY), surgery
- Vaginal disease → Combined external and intravaginal irradiation

patients require formal dilatation and curettage (D&C) with hysteroscopy. About 10% of patients undergoing office endometrial biopsy have either inadequate tissue sampling or evidence of hyperplasia and therefore require formal D&C with hysteroscopy. Only 5% of patients have cancer diagnosed by the initial office biopsy. Most patients (80%) undergoing curettage have a benign etiology for the bleeding, and 20% have evidence of either hyperplasia or carcinoma requiring treatment.

Of patients with inadequate tissue sampling or hyperplasia, 40% have benign findings following D&C and should continue with annual follow-ups. Those with *atypical hyperplasia* are at risk for progression to cancer and are best managed with hysterectomy. Alternatively, they may be treated medically if they wish to preserve fertility. Patients whose biopsies reveal *hyperplasia without atypia* may be managed medically with a 3-month course of progestins followed by short-term follow-up including formal curettage. The hyperplasia is reversed in 60% of these patients, and 35% may require an additional course of progestins. The 5% who progress to cancer require treatment.

Most of the patients (95%) with endometrial cancer are treated surgically. Following a preoperative evaluation that includes chest radiography, electrocardiography (ECG), and routine blood work, the low risk patient (see below) undergoes a hysterectomy with bilateral salpingo-oophorectomy and pelvic washing for cytology. The omentum, liver, peritoneal surfaces, cul-de-sac, and adnexa are palpated through a lower midline incision, as are the paraaortic nodes. Although this procedure is most commonly performed abdominally, approximately 25% of patients are candidates for a laparoscopically assisted approach. Extended surgical staging for high risk patients includes sampling of retroperitoneal lymph nodes from the pelvic and paraaortic regions. High risk patients are those with suspicious pelvic or paraaortic nodes, grossly positive adnexae, deep (>50%) myometrial invasion on frozen section, histopathologic grade 3 lesions, or lesions with high risk histology, including papillary, serous, and clear cell cancers. Approximately 5% of patients are found to have extrauterine metastases at the time of surgery; for these patients an effort should be made to remove all gross disease. This usually involves performing an omentectomy and tumor debulking.

D. Staging

The International Federation of Gynecology and Obstetrics set forth the currently used staging system, which is based on histopathologic factors and surgical findings (Table 52–1). These variables also determine if adjuvant therapy is necessary.

Preoperatively, the physical examination and results of fractional curettage are vitally important. In most cases (>75%) there is no clinical evidence of extrauterine involvement, and for these patients the required preoperative staging studies are

TABLE 52–1.
FIGO staging system for endometrial cancer

Stage	*Grade*	*Description*
IA	G1,2,3	Tumor limited to endometrium
IB	G1,2,3	Invasion to less than one-half the myometrium
IC	G1,2,3	Invasion to more than one-half the myometrium
IIA	G1,2,3	Endocervical gland involvement only
IIB	G1,2,3	Cervical stromal invasion
IIIA	G1,2,3	Tumor invades serosa and/or adnexa, and/or positive peritoneal cytology
IIIB	G1,2,3	Vaginal metastases
IIIC	G1,2,3	Metastases to pelvic and/or paraaortic lymph nodes
IVA	G1,2,3	Tumor invasion of bladder and/or bowel mucosa
IVB		Distant metastases including intraabdominal and/or inguinal lymph nodes

Histopathology: degree of differentiation
Carcinoma of the corpus should be classified (or graded) according to the degree of histologic differentiation, as follows.
- G1 ≤5% of a nonsquamous or nonmorular solid growth pattern
- G2 6–50% of nonsquamous cell or nonmorular solid growth pattern
- G3 >50% of a nonsquamous cell or nonmorular solid growth pattern

Notes on pathologic grading
1. Notable nuclear atypia, inappropriate for the architectural grade, raises the grade of a grade 1 or 2 tumor by 1.
2. Nuclear grading takes precedence for serous adenocarcinomas, clear cell adenocarcinomas, and squamous carcinomas.
3. Adenocarcinomas with squamous differentiation are graded according to the nuclear grade of the glandular component.

Rules related to staging
1. Because corpus cancer is now staged surgically, procedures previously used for determination of stage are no longer applicable, such as the findings from fractional D&C to differentiate between stage I and stage II.
2. It is appreciated that there may be a small number of patients with corpus cancer who are treated primarily with radiation therapy. If that is the case, the clinical staging adopted by FIGO in 1971 would still apply, but the designation of the staging system would be noted.
3. Ideally, the width of the myometrium is measured along with the width of tumor invasion.

SOURCE: International Federation of Gynecology and Obstetrics. Annual report on the results of treatment in gynecologic cancer. Int J Gynaecol Obstet 1989;28:189–190. Reproduced with permission.

chest radiography, serum chemistries, and a serum CA-125 assay. High risk histology (poor differentiation, papillary serous, clear cell sarcoma), abnormal blood tests (elevated CA-125, liver function tests), and clinical evidence of extrauterine disease mandates a computed tomography (CT) scan or magnetic resonance imaging (MRI). Hysteroscopy is indicated if the extent of involvement cannot be determined by the usual means.

E. Treatment

Once the endometrial cancer has been diagnosed, surgical staging followed by adjuvant therapy (if needed) is the accepted regimen. Alternatively, preoperative irradiation with brachytherapy or external beam radiation followed by surgery can be applied, with the results equally as good. However, a possible disadvantage is the overtreatment of patients with early, superficial disease.

Regarding treatment for advanced-stage tumors, decisions are often based on the clinical staging (i.e., information obtained from the physical examination and radiographic tests). In contrast, for earlier lesions surgical staging is often performed first, and the need for postoperative radiation therapy is determined by tumor grade, depth of invasion, lymphovascular invasion, and nodal status. The following recommendations are for general treatment by tumor stage.

Stage I Lesions

The need for adjuvant posthysterectomy radiation therapy for patients whose tumor is confined to the uterine corpus (stage I) is determined by FIGO grade and depth of invasion. Patients with *stage* IA, FIGO *grade 1 and* 2 tumors (limited to the endometrium) have a 95–100% likelihood of being cured by surgery alone, and therefore no further therapy is indicated. Follow-up should include a pelvic examination and a Papanicolaou (Pap) smear every 3 months for 2 years, every 6 months for the following 3 years, and annually thereafter. Patients with *stage IA, FIGO grade 3* and *stage IB, FIGO grade 1 and 2* tumors (invading less than one-half of the myometrium) have a 10–15% chance of local or regional failure; the risk of vaginal failure alone constitutes two-thirds of this risk. Therefore, vaginal cuff irradiation is used as the sole adjuvant therapy in this setting. Vaginal cuff irradiation is generally administered utilizing the high-dose-rate remote afterloader. This procedure is performed on an outpatient basis with three brief visits 2 weeks apart. Generally, a dose of 700 cGy is prescribed at a depth of 0.5 cm from the vaginal mucosa. The total dose of 2100 cGy delivered is considered the biologic equivalent of approximately 5000 cGy. For *stage IB, FIGO grade 3* and *stage IC, FIGO grades 1–3* tumors (invasion of more than one-half of the myometrium) pelvic irradiation *and* intravaginal irradiation are indicated. Generally, the external-beam portion of the treatment begins 3–6 weeks after hysterectomy. A simulation is performed, and treatment is carefully planned. At the time of simulation, a radiopaque marker is placed in the patient's vagina, small bowel contrast material is administered, and a small rectal tube is placed to opacify the rectum. Custom cerroband shielding is employed in all four fields, and for each patient a custom dosimetry plan is devised prior to starting therapy. It is customary to deliver a total dose of 4500 cGy in 25 fractions on consecutive days over 5 weeks. At the completion of treatment, the patient undergoes intravaginal irradiation at a reduced dose compared to that administered for stage IB, grade 1, 2 disease (in consideration of the radiation already administered via external beam). Usually, 500 cGy is prescribed at 0.5 cm on three occasions, which is the biologic equivalent of 3000 cGy. Follow-up includes a pelvic examination every 6 months for 3 years. Pap smears can be performed annually thereafter, but their utility is questionable. Approximately 25% of these tumors recur: 75% of them are at distant sites, with the remainder being local recurrences. Almost half of the local recurrences can be salvaged with further surgery; the others are treated as though metastatic disease is present (discussed below).

Stage II Lesions (Endocervical Gland Involvement or Invasion of the Cervical Stroma)

Patients with clinically normal cervixes but microscopic involvement found on endocervical curettage are treated in a fashion similar to that for patients with stage IC disease. Pelvic and aortic node dissection may be performed more often in these instances. If the cervical stroma is involved, whole pelvic irradiation and intracavitary irradiation are given in a manner similar to that for stage IC disease.

Stage III Lesions

Treatment is determined by the pattern of disease and differs according to serosal, adnexal, or nodal involvement. Treatment also differs according to whether staging was done clinically or surgically. For example, patients with *clinical* stage II disease by virtue of vaginal or parametrial spread are treated with pelvic radiation therapy followed by surgery if the disease appears resectable. If vaginal metastases or direct extension are present at the time of diagnosis, a variety of radiotherapeutic interventions are available. Depending on the other surgical/pathologic findings, a combination of external-beam radiation therapy plus intravaginal brachytherapy may be employed. In the setting of gross vaginal metastasis the dose of intravaginal brachytherapy would almost certainly be higher, and in this case the external-beam portion of the treatment would probably be altered at approximately 4000 cGy, at which point a midline block would be inserted so when the vaginal tissues are brought to a higher dose using brachytherapy the tolerance of the bladder and rectum are generally not exceeded. Patients with *clinical* stage III disease by virtue of adnexal involvement should undergo surgery without preoperative irradiation to determine the nature of the adnexal mass, surgically stage the extent of disease, and perform cytoreductive surgery. If resectable, hysterectomy is performed at this time as well. If a patient has stage III disease on the basis of *surgical* staging, treatment is similar to that for patients with stage IC disease. In these instances, pelvic irradiation may be brought to a total dose of 5040 cGy in 28 fractions. Extended-field irradiation is employed for positive paraaortic nodes. Generally, this therapy is delivered utilizing a four-field technique that requires a CT scan for accurate localization of the kidneys. The fields are treated simultaneously with one isocenter, and dosimetry is performed at several levels in the field to ensure homogeneity of the prescribed dose. Depending on the findings in the pelvis, a total dose of 4500–5040 cGy is delivered in 25 fractions to the paraaortic lymph nodes; intravaginal radiation is then administered as well.

Clinical Stage IV Lesions

Stage IVA tumors (invasion of bladder or bowel mucosa) are rare, and therapy is directed at relieving local symptoms. A radical course of radiation therapy can be given as an alternative to exenterative surgery. A Memorial applicator might be used in an effort to eradicate the intrauterine portion of the tumor. Alternatively, a Syed-Neblett template-type implant could be utilized under laparoscopic guidance to attempt to encompass any tumor that remains after the external-beam portion of radiation. For a large tumor conventional treatment consists of a total dose of 4000 cGy utilizing a four-field technique, subsequently switching to an anteroposterior/posteroanterior technique. A midline block is used to shield the bladder and rectum. An intravaginal implant is then utilized for the brachytherapy portion to deliver a higher central dose, thereby not exceeding the tolerance of the bladder or rectum. In this setting, the potential for a local complication must be accepted if the likelihood of control is considered reasonable. For patients with *stage IVB* disease (distant metastases including intraabdominal or inguinal lymph node metastases, or both), irradiation is used as a palliative modality. Under most circumstances a dose of 3000 cGy in 10 fractions is considered sufficient to ensure relief of symptoms during the limited survival of these patients.

Surgical Stage IV Lesions

Following surgery, patients found to have *stage IV FIGO grade 2, 3* disease whose tumors are surgically debulked to less than 2 cm remaining cancer can undergo whole-abdomen radiation therapy (WART) or combination chemotherapy. Chemotherapy consists of cisplatin 50 mg/m^2 and Adriamycin 60 mg/m^2 for six cycles. Measurable tumor is followed radiographically and by serum CA-125 levels; and treatment is continued for another six cycles if there has been a favorable response to treatment. Occasionally, a second-look laparotomy is performed to resect residual disease. Patients with grade 1 or estrogen receptor/progesterone receptor (ER/PR)-positive tumors should receive progestins first unless there is a clinical need to gain control of the tumor more rapidly than is possible using hormones, in which case chemotherapy is given. Progestins used include medroxyprogesterone acetate 50–100 mg three times a day or megestrol acetate 80 mg two or three times daily. If residual tumor measures >2 cm, WART is not an option, and combination chemotherapy for FIGO grade 2–3 is recommended.

For stage IV, FIGO grade 2, 3 disease involving the liver or sites outside the abdominal cavity (e.g., supraclavicular lymph nodes), patients should be treated with systemic chemotherapy alone. If such patients have FIGO grade 1 tumors, they should first receive progestin unless more rapid control is clinically indicated.

Recurrent Disease

Recurrent grade 1 tumors (biopsy performed to exclude dedifferentiation) treated with prior surgery and irradiation should be treated with progestins. Grade 2, 3 tumors are treated with combined chemotherapy. Exenterative surgery, however, should be considered in selective cases especially if the disease-free interval is more than 1–2 years and the recurrence is isolated. If resectability is borderline and radiation was not previously given, patients may receive preoperative radiation up to approximately 5000 cGy followed by surgery in 2 weeks, with a dose of intraoperative radiation or a permanent interstitial implant considered for the tumor bed. If recurrence involves the abdomen and pelvis and radiation was not given previously, WART is an option.

Recurrence involving only the vagina can be associated with a favorable prognosis. These patients are treated with whole-pelvis radiation to a total dose of 4000 cGy in 20 fractions. A midline block is then placed, and the remainder of the pelvis is brought to 4600–5000 cGy. The vaginal tissues are boosted utilizing a high-dose-rate remote afterloader, a low-dose-rate custom cylinder, or an interstitial implant. The inguinal lymph nodes are at risk if there is lower-third vaginal involvement, and they are treated as part of the external-beam portion and brought to a total dose of 4500 cGy.

If positive peritoneal cytology is the only adverse risk factor and the patient would otherwise be treated with intravaginal radiation alone, she may be treated with colloidal ^{32}P (approximately 15 mCi) in addition to intravaginal radiation therapy or with progestins in addition to intravaginal irradiation. If there are other adverse findings indicating that radiation to the pelvic or paraaortic region (or both) is indicated, WART may be employed.

Conclusions

There is no cost-effective screening program for asymptomatic patients, although high risk patients should be evaluated with ultrasonography and endometrial sampling. High risk factors are patients over 40 years of age with abnormal uterine bleeding, massively obese patients, a history of hyperplasia, and a history of unopposed use of estrogen or tamoxifen. Women with abnormal uterine bleeding should undergo endometrial biopsy; those with persistent bleeding, inadequate samples, or hyperplasia should undergo D&C and hysteroscopy.

Once a cancer is diagnosed, the treatment is initially surgical for most patients. Staging is performed using the FIGO system, which is based on surgical findings and pathology reports. FIGO stage and tumor grade determine the need for postoperative adjuvant therapy as well as the irradiation technique if it is used. A clinical stage can be assigned for advanced disease, and for such patients irradiation may be used as an alternative to surgery for the initial treatment. Recurrent disease is treated with surgery, irradiation, chemotherapy, or progestins depending on the site of recurrence and method of treating the primary disease.

Suggested Reading

Hoskins WJ, Perez CA, Young RC (eds) Principles and Practice of Gynecologic Oncology, 2nd ed. Philadelphia: Lippincott-Raven, 1997.

Morrow CP, Curtin JP (eds) Gynecologic Cancer Surgery. New York: Churchill Livingstone, 1996.

Society of Gynecologic Oncology. Practice guidelines: uterine-corpus-endometrial cancer. Oncology 1998;12:122–126.

Chapter 53

Cervical Cancer

NADEEM R. ABU-RUSTUM

A. Epidemiology and Etiology

Cervical cancer is the third most common gynecologic malignancy in the United States following endometrial and ovarian cancer. It is estimated that 13,700 new cases and 4900 cancer-related deaths occurred in 1998.[1] The peak age is during the late forties, with almost half of the cases diagnosed in women under age 35. Cervical cancer remains a major cause of morbidity and mortality in developing countries, although, the incidence of invasive cervical cancer in industrialized countries has dramatically decreased since the introduction and popularization of cervical screening cytology techniques [Papanicolaou (Pap) smear] during the latter half of the twentieth century. Several risk factors have been associated with the development of cervical carcinoma, including advanced age, low socioeconomic class, limited access to screening, early coitarche, large number of sexual partners, genital human papilloma virus (HPV) infection, smoking, and immunodeficiency states including human immunodeficiency virus (HIV) infection.[2]

B. Diagnosis

Patients may present with abnormal vaginal bleeding or discharge, although many are asymptomatic and their cancer is detected only during routine screening. Pelvic pain, lower extremity edema or deep venous thrombosis, and obstructive renal failure are less common presentations and are associated with advanced disease.

Although invasive cervical cancer may be suspected after inspection and palpation of the cervix, histologic confirmation is essential before proceeding with definitive therapy. If a patient is referred for management of a newly diagnosed cervical cancer, the outside biopsy material should be carefully reviewed and the diagnosis confirmed prior to commencing with treatment. Colposcopy with directed cervical biopsy is commonly recommended for the initial evaluation of abnormal or suspicious Pap smears; it is safe and generally well tolerated by most women. Although vaginal bleeding may occur from the biopsy site, it can usually be controlled with gentle pressure and application of topical silver

Cervical Cancer

A.
Epidemiology and Etiology

Gynecologic cancers—order of frequency
- Endometrial
- Ovarian
- Cervical

Risk factors
- Poor socioeconomic status
- Poor access to screening
- Early coitarche
- Multiple sex partners
- Infection with human papilloma virus
- Immunodeficiency syndrome

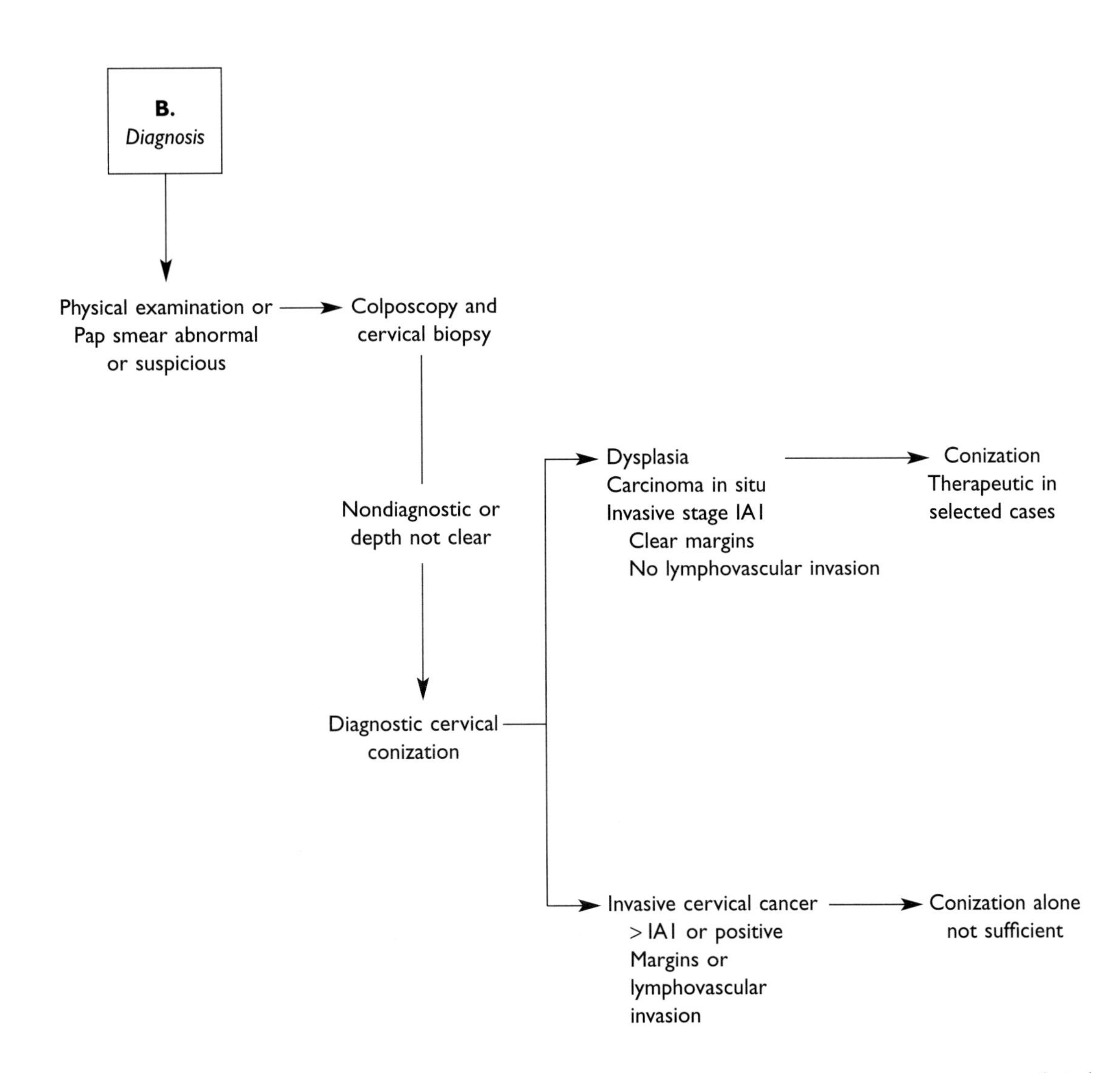

(continued on next page)

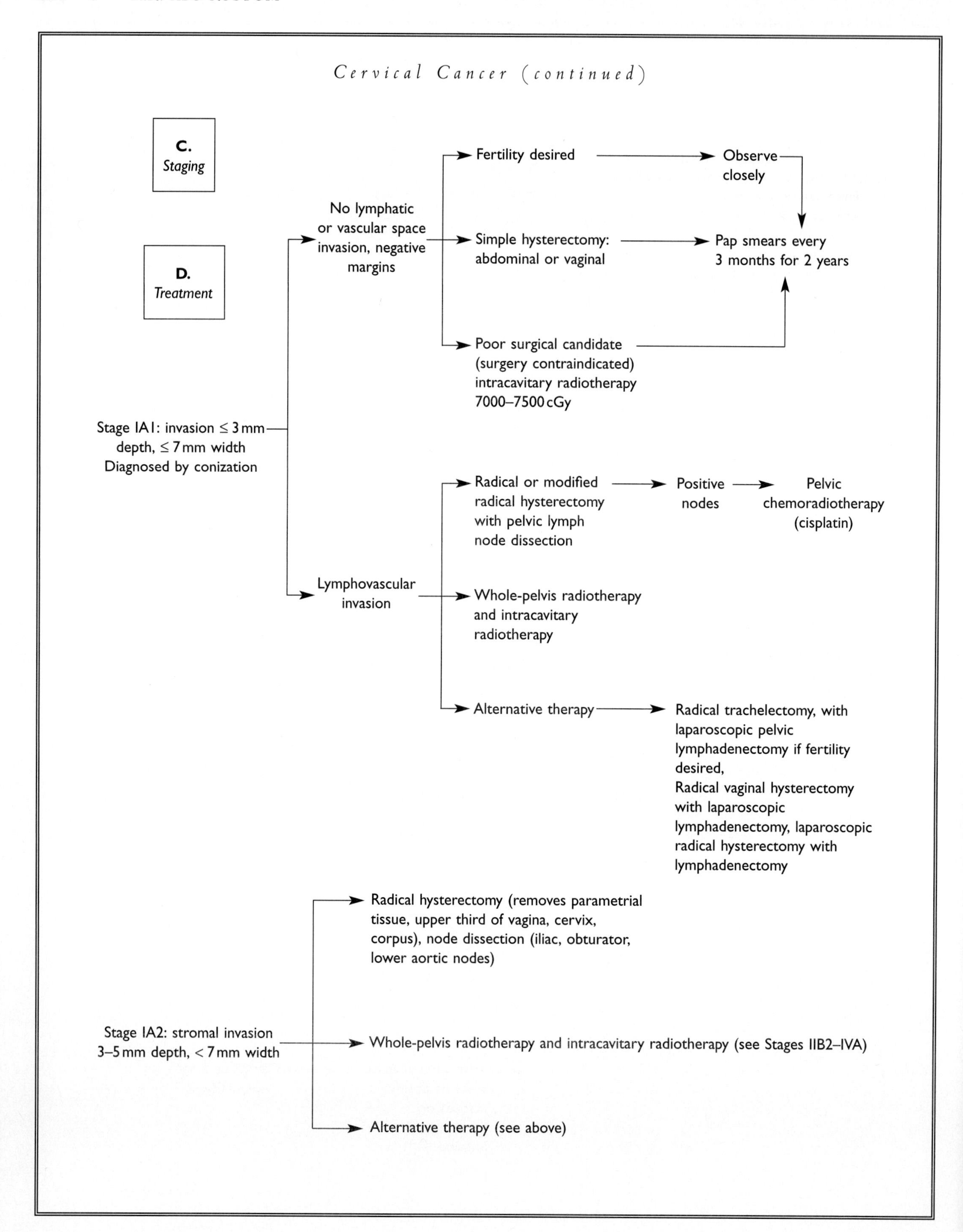
Cervical Cancer (continued)
C.
Staging
D.
Treatment
Stage IA1: invasion ≤ 3 mm depth, ≤ 7 mm width
Diagnosed by conization
No lymphatic or vascular space invasion, negative margins
Fertility desired
Observe closely
Simple hysterectomy: abdominal or vaginal
Pap smears every 3 months for 2 years
Poor surgical candidate (surgery contraindicated) intracavitary radiotherapy 7000–7500 cGy
Lymphovascular invasion
Radical or modified radical hysterectomy with pelvic lymph node dissection
Positive nodes
Pelvic chemoradiotherapy (cisplatin)
Whole-pelvis radiotherapy and intracavitary radiotherapy
Alternative therapy
Radical trachelectomy, with laparoscopic pelvic lymphadenectomy if fertility desired,
Radical vaginal hysterectomy with laparoscopic lymphadenectomy, laparoscopic radical hysterectomy with lymphadenectomy
Stage IA2: stromal invasion 3–5 mm depth, < 7 mm width
Radical hysterectomy (removes parametrial tissue, upper third of vagina, cervix, corpus), node dissection (iliac, obturator, lower aortic nodes)
Whole-pelvis radiotherapy and intracavitary radiotherapy (see Stages IIB2–IVA)
Alternative therapy (see above)

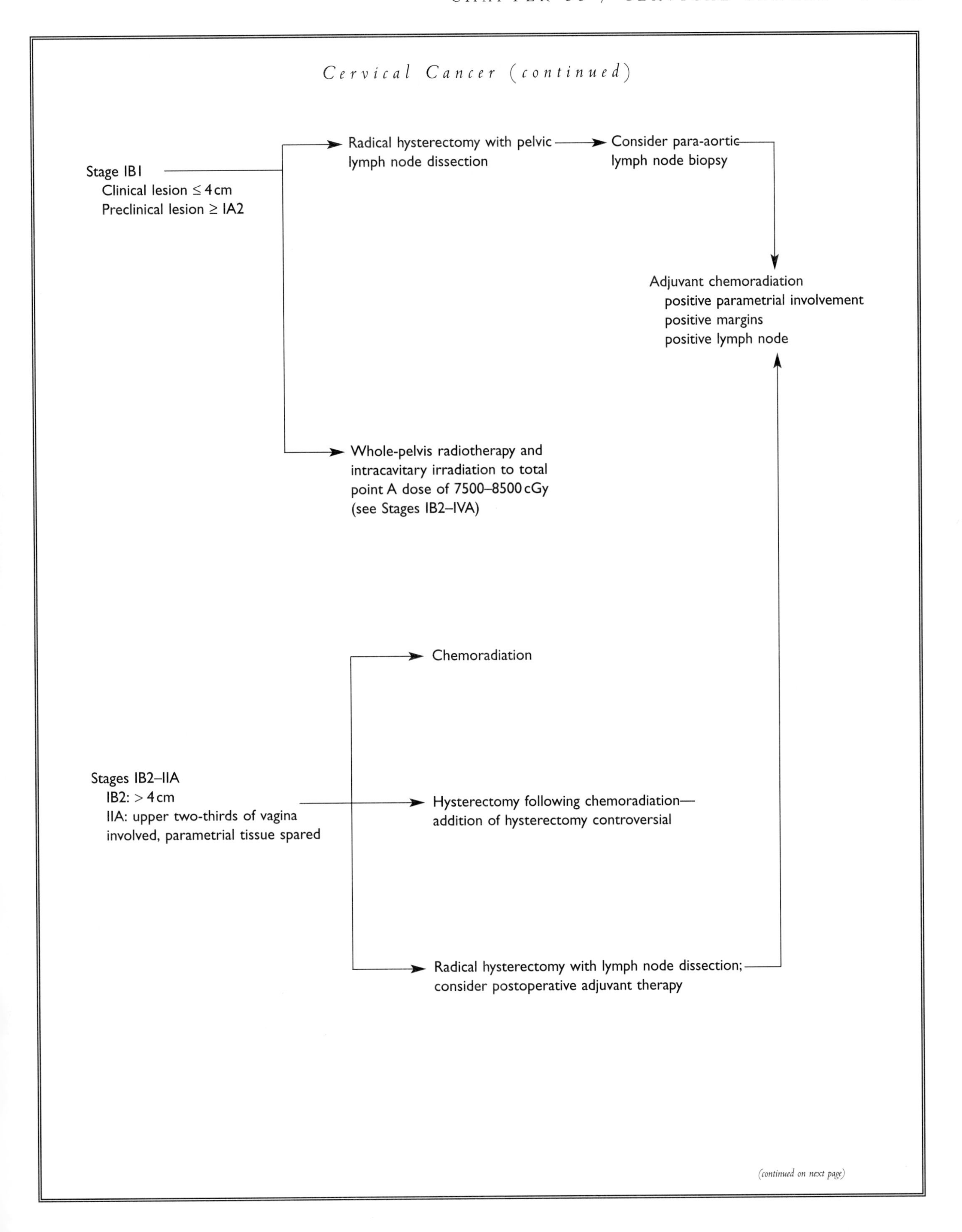

(continued on next page)

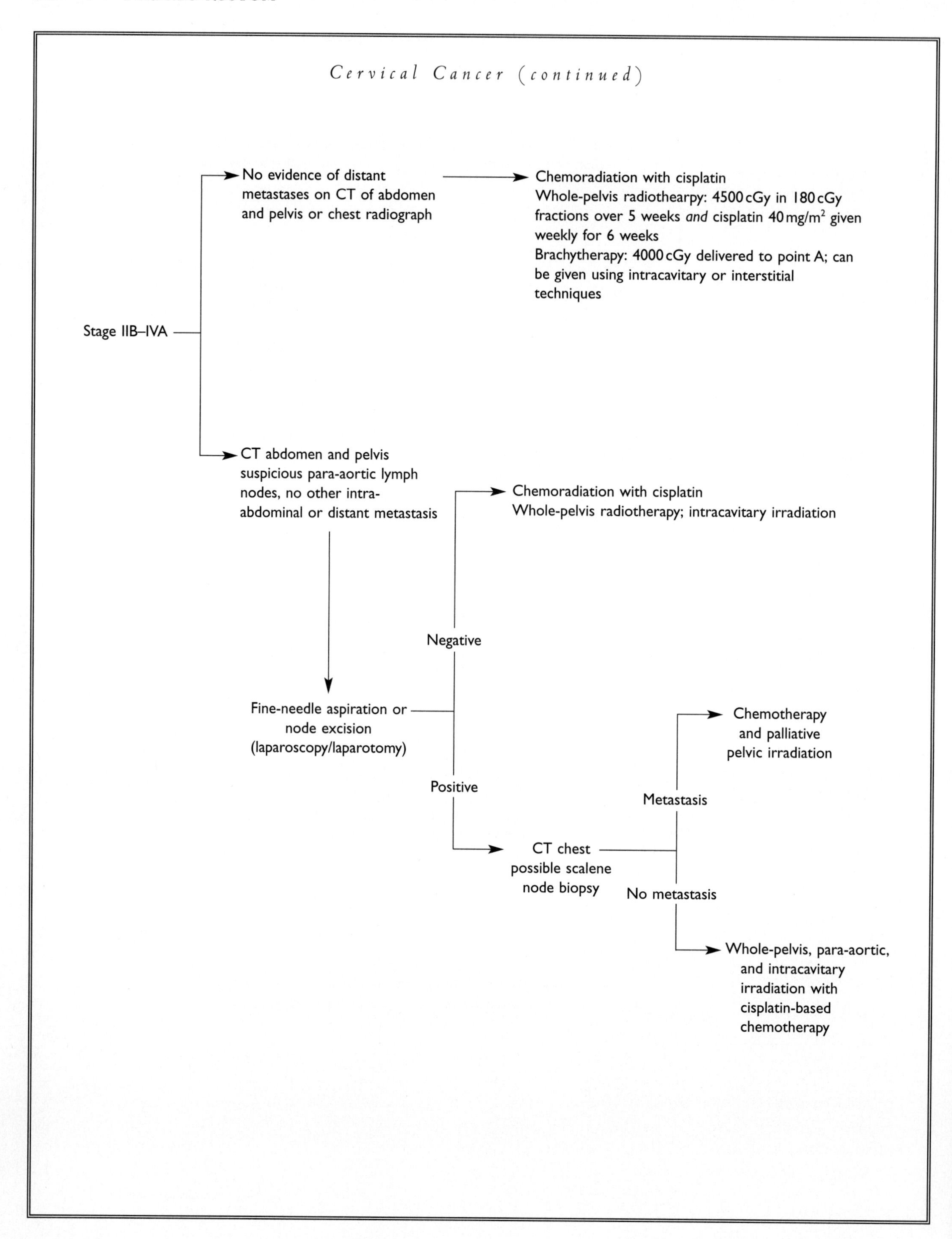
Cervical Cancer (continued)
Stage IIB–IVA
No evidence of distant metastases on CT of abdomen and pelvis or chest radiograph
Chemoradiation with cisplatin
Whole-pelvis radiothearpy: 4500 cGy in 180 cGy fractions over 5 weeks and cisplatin 40 mg/m2 given weekly for 6 weeks
Brachytherapy: 4000 cGy delivered to point A; can be given using intracavitary or interstitial techniques
CT abdomen and pelvis suspicious para-aortic lymph nodes, no other intra-abdominal or distant metastasis
Chemoradiation with cisplatin
Whole-pelvis radiotherapy; intracavitary irradiation
Negative
Fine-needle aspiration or node excision (laparoscopy/laparotomy)
Positive
Chemotherapy and palliative pelvic irradiation
Metastasis
CT chest possible scalene node biopsy
No metastasis
Whole-pelvis, para-aortic, and intracavitary irradiation with cisplatin-based chemotherapy

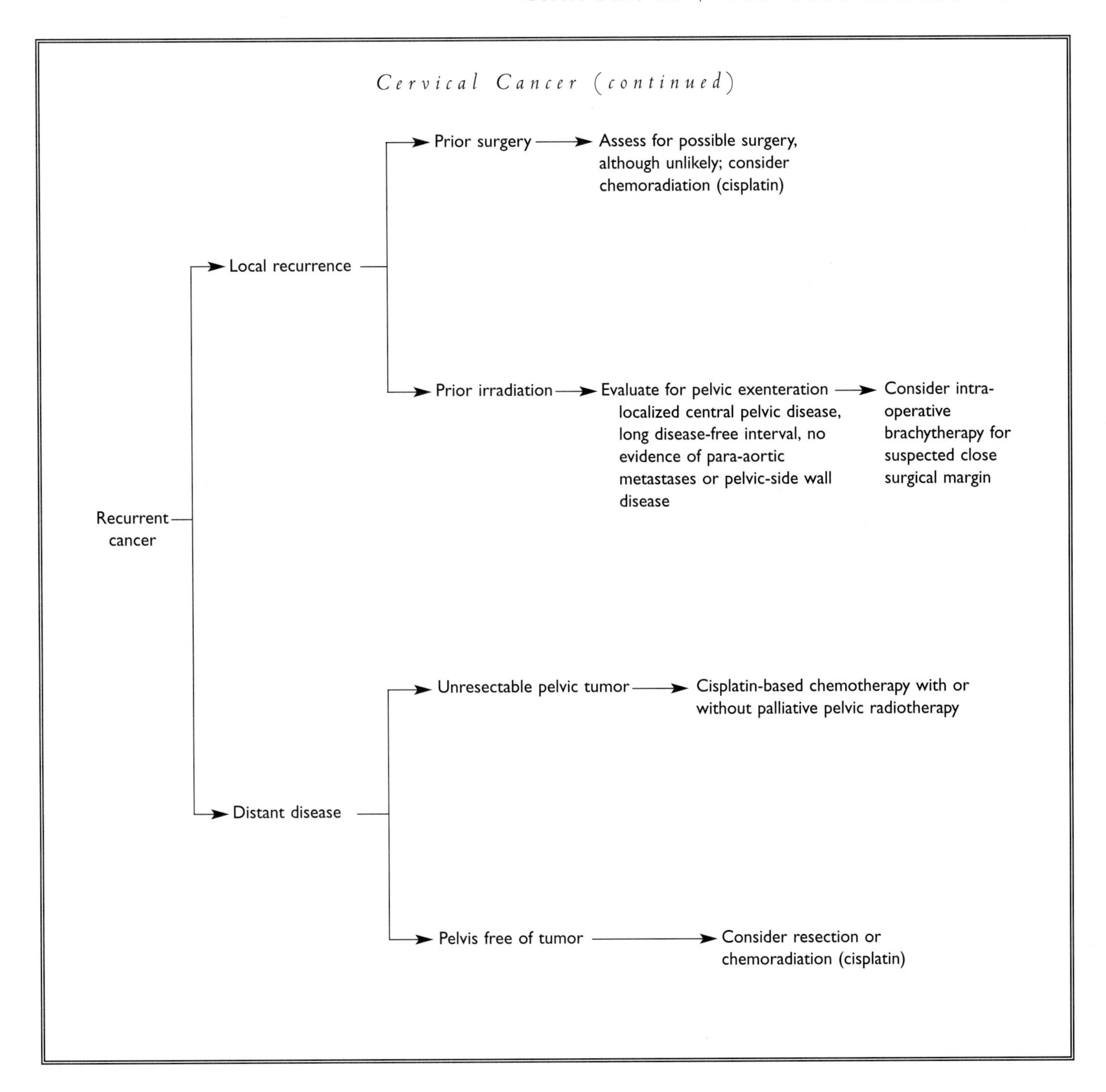

nitrate or ferric subsulfate (Monsel's solution). Excessive bleeding that requires vaginal packing and hospitalization or transfusion is rare.

If a carcinoma is suspected but the biopsy was not diagnostic, or if cancer was seen but the degree of invasion could not be reliably determined, a diagnostic cervical conization is necessary. Diagnostic conization is also therapeutic if the histology shows only dysplasia, squamous-cell carcinoma in situ, or invasive squamous-cell carcinoma stage IA1, with negative margins and no lymphovascular invasion. For more invasive squamous-cell cancers, conization alone is not sufficient treatment. Diagnostic cervical conization is crucial for accurate staging of preclinical, early invasive cervical cancer [International Federation of Gynecology and Obstetrics (FIGO) stages IA1, IA2, and preclinical IB1 lesions] where the management options and recommendations vary depending on the depth of penetration and size of these early lesions. Women with squamous-cell carcinoma stage IA1 may be candidates for more conservative treatment (therapeutic conization) compared to those with preclinical (no gross tumor) stage IB1 disease; the differentia-

TABLE 53–1.
1995 FIGO clinical staging for cervical cancer

Stage	Definition
0	Carcinoma in situ
I	Confined to the cervix (disregard corpus extension)
IA1	Stromal invasion ≤3 mm (depth), ≤7 mm (width)
IA2	Stromal invasion >3 mm, ≤5 mm (depth), ≤7 mm (width)
IB1	Clinical lesion ≤4 cm or preclinical lesion >IA2
IB2	Clinical lesion >4 cm
II	Tumor extends beyond the cervix but not to the pelvic wall or lower third of vagina
IIA	Vaginal involvement limited to upper two-thirds, no parametrial involvement
IIB	Parametrial involvement
III	Extension to pelvic wall or lower third of vagina or hydronephrosis related to tumor
IIIA	Vaginal invasion to lower third, no extension to pelvic wall
IIIB	Extension to pelvic wall or hydronephrosis related to tumor
IV	Bladder or rectal mucosal invasion or extension beyond the true pelvis
IVA	Mucosal invasion of the bladder or rectum
IVB	Distant metastasis

tion between these two stages is usually not feasible without diagnostic cervical conization.

C. Staging

Cervical carcinoma is clinically staged according to the 1995 FIGO classification (Table 53–1). The staging procedures allowed by FIGO and generally practiced by most physicians include physical examination, cervical biopsy, cervical conization (for subclinical tumors), chest radiography, intravenous pyelography, cystoscopy, and proctoscopy. The latter three procedures have relatively low yield, are less important in patients with stage IA1–IB1 disease, and may be omitted based on physician discretion. Other staging procedures allowed by FIGO include barium enema, which is reserved for symptomatic patients or those with locally advanced disease (stage III–IVA). Computed tomography (CT), ultrasonmography, magnetic resonance imaging (MRI), and lymphangiography may be used to evaluate tumor spread, and the information obtained from these tests may modify the treatment plan. Pretreatment CT with oral and intravenous contrast is frequently done in patients with stage IB2–IV tumors, where the risk of regional and distant metastasis is increased. Suspicious lesions noted on imaging studies usually require histologic evaluation with fine-needle aspiration or biopsy, particularly if the results would alter the initial treatment plan. HIV testing should be offered to all women diagnosed with cervical cancer, especially young women.[3] The diagnosis of HIV infection generally does not alter the oncologic treatment plan but does allow identification of subjects who may benefit from antiretroviral therapy, which may ultimately improve survival.

D. Treatment

The standard treatment strategies for invasive cervical cancer are radical surgery, radiotherapy and chemoradiation. Radiotherapy can be utilized for all stages of cervical cancer with certain modifications in dosimetry and technique. Each patient must be evaluated individually and a treatment scheme tailored to achieve the best outcome with the least morbidity.

Stage IA1 Lesions

The surgical options for stage IA1 disease (≤3 mm depth of stromal invasion and ≤7 mm width) depend on several factors, including the desire for future fertility, histology, lymphatic or vascular invasion, and cone margin status. Women with evidence of lymphatic or vascular invasion may be at increased risk for metastasis, and the treatment should be modified to address this issue.[3–5] Simple hysterectomy or cervical conization with negative margins (in patients desiring fertility) are adequate therapy for stage IA1 squamous-cell lesions with no lymphatic or vascular invasion[6]; however, if such invasion is present, a modified radical hysterectomy or radical hysterectomy with pelvic lymphadenectomy, or radical trachelectomy with laparoscopic pelvic lymphadenectomy should be considered.[3] If surgical therapy is contraindicated, selected patients with stage IA cervical cancer at low risk for nodal metastases (<3 mm stromal invasion and no lymphatic or vascular invasion) may be treated with intracavitary radiation therapy alone for a total dose of 7000–7500 cGy to point A, an imaginary point located 2 cm superior and 2 cm lateral to the external cervical os.

Stage IA2 Lesions

Women with cervical stromal invasion >3 mm and <5 mm in depth or 7 mm in width (stage IA2) should be offered radical hysterectomy with pelvic lymphadenectomy or, alternatively, radiotherapy (whole-pelvis and intracavitary). This should be regardless of lymphatic or vascular invasion, as the risk of metastasis is increased when the depth of stromal invasion exceeds 3 mm. Radical vaginal hysterectomy with laparoscopic pelvic lymphadenectomy, radical transvaginal trachelectomy (removal of the cervix) with laparoscopic pelvic lymphadenectomy, and laparoscopic radical hysterectomy with laparoscopic pelvic lymphadenectomy may be alternatives for patients with early cervical cancer and are becoming more popular in the United States. The main technical differences between the various surgical approaches to early cervical cancer are summarized in Table 53–2.[7–9]

Treatment of *invasive cervical adenocarcinoma*, which constitutes approximately 20% of all cervical cancers, is essentially similar to that of squamous-cell carcinomas. The management of *adenocarcinoma in situ* in women who desire future fertility may be more challenging than its squamous-cell counterpart, as several retrospective reports have indicated that conservative therapy with cervical conization leaves residual cancer in 30–40% of patients even if negative surgical margins were obtained. Nevertheless, conization is the appropriate initial step for documenting in situ or invasive disease. For the former, simple hysterectomy may be the safest treatment; conservative therapy should be undertaken only with caution.[10–12] Patients with the latter are best treated with radical hysterectomy and pelvic lymphadenectomy (abdominal, vaginal, or laparoscopic) or radiotherapy. Radical vaginal trachelectomy with laparoscopic pelvic lymphadenectomy may be suitable on selected patients, who desire fertility. Unlike microinvasive squamous carcinoma, the diagnosis of a microinvasive cervical adenocarcinoma remains controversial, and no universally agreed upon pathologic criteria are available to establish the diagnosis. Therefore, cervical adenocarcinoma with any stromal invasion is usually treated with radical hysterectomy and pelvic lymphadenectomy or definitive radiation therapy. Some maintain, however, that microinvasive adenocarcinoma of the cervix is a clinicopathologic entity that appears to have the same prognosis and should be treated in the same way as its squamous-cell counterpart.[13]

Stage IB1 Lesions

Stage IB cervical cancer is categorized into two subgroups: IB1 (≤4 cm) and IB2 (>4 cm). Stage IB1 disease can be adequately treated, with comparable cure rates, using radical hysterectomy and pelvic lymphadenectomy or definitive radiotherapy. Advantages of surgery include allowing exploration of the abdomen and pelvis to exclude metastasis, shorter overall treatment duration, preservation of ovarian function in premenopausal women, preservation of vaginal pliability and lubrication, limited injury to normal tissue, and less risk of bowel fistulas and disturbances in intestinal function. Furthermore, if

TABLE 53–2.
Surgical approaches to early-stage cervical cancer

Tissue	Cervical conization	Total agdominal/vaginal hysterectomy	Modified radical hysterectomy	Radical abdominal hysterectomy	Radical vaginal trachelectomy	Radical vaginal hysterectomy
Cervix	Partially removed	Completely removed	Completely removed	Completely removed	Most removed	Completely removed
Corpus	Preserved	Completely removed	Completely removed	Completely removed	Preserved	Completely removed
Adnexa	Preserved	Preserved	Preserved	Preserved	Preserved	Preserved
Parametria and paracolpos	Preserved	Preserved	Removed at level of ureter	Removed lateral to ureter	Partially removed	Removed at level of ureter
Uterine vessels	Preserved	Ligated at level of internal os	Ligated at level of ureter	Ligated at origin from hypogastric	Preserved	Ligated at level of ureter
Uterosacral ligaments	Preserved	Ligated at uterus	Ligated midway to rectum	Ligated near rectum	Partially removed	Partially removed
Vaginal cuff	Preserved	Removed <1 cm	Removed 1–2 cm	Removed ≥2 cm	Removed 1–2 cm	Removed ≥2 cm

complications such as urinary tract fistulas occur as a result of treatment, corrective surgery is more easily performed in nonirradiated tissue without the need for diversion. Moreover, surgery can be utilized in a variety of conditions where radiotherapy may not be indicated, such as pyometra, presence of an adnexal mass, pelvic prolapse, altered vaginal anatomy, history of severe pelvic adhesions, inflammatory bowel disease, pelvic inflammatory disease, and presence of a pelvic kidney.[8] Surgical approaches for early cervical cancer other than the classic radical abdominal hysterectomy, include laparoscopic radical hysterectomy with pelvic lymphadenectomy, vaginal radical hysterectomy with laparoscopic pelvic lymph node dissection, and radical trachelectomy with laparoscopic pelvic lymphadenectomy for selected patients who desire preservation of fertility.[14–19]

On the other hand, radiotherapy may be used in almost all women; it is associated with less direct mortality and usually less risk of urinary tract injury. Intracavitary radiation therapy (ICRT) for stage IB cervical cancer is performed with a technique similar to that used for more advanced lesions, using a tandem and two colpostats (Fletcher or Henshkie). The tandem is a metallic hollow curved rod that is inserted into the cervical os to the fundus and the colpostats or ovoids are two metallic rods, each with a cavity at the tip for radioactive sources, placed on either side of the tandem. Cesium-137 is then loaded in the tandem and two colpostats for brachytherapy. Intracavitary irradiation treats central pelvic disease, whereas external-beam irradiation treats the primary tumor and its locoregional draining lymphatic tissue. The combination is associated with better local control and survival than is seen with external beam radiation alone. Interstitial implants are not indicated for stage I lesions. The timing and insertion is similar to that for advanced lesions; however, the total dose provided by ICRT may be modified based on tumor size and frequently is less than that for more advanced and bulky lesions with a total dose ranging from 7500 to 8500 cGy to point A.

Stage IB2–IIA Lesions

Tumor size and volume of early-stage cervical cancers appear to be independent prognostic factors in several retrospective studies,[20,21] and prospective randomized trials are currently being conducted nationally and internationally to identify the best treatment modality for women with bulky early-stage cervical cancer (>4 cm, stage IB2–IIA). The best treatment modality for these early-stage bulky tumors remains to be determined, as these tumors are associated with a higher risk for local and distant metastasis and recurrence. Currently, neoadjuvant induction chemotherapy followed by radical hysterectomy and pelvic chemoradiotherapy for selected patients is being investigated. The optimal treatment strategy with the best therapeutic index will hopefully become clear after more data are available from current clinical trials.

The Gynecologic Oncology Group completed a study of women with bulky stage IB tumors (≥4 cm in diameter). Patients were randomized to radiation alone or in combination with cisplatin; all subjects subsequently underwent hysterectomy. Irradiation consisted of both external-beam and intracavitary irradiation, reaching a dose of 75 cGy to point A (cervical parametrium) and 55 cGy to the lateral pelvis. Cisplatin (40 mg/m^2 weekly for six doses) was given during external irradiation. Hysterectomy was done 3–6 weeks after irradiation. In the preoperative combined treatment group, the progression-free survival and overall survival rates were significantly higher, although there were more hematologic and gastrointestinal side effects. In addition, more patients in the combined group had no detectable cancer in the hysterectomy specimens (52% vs. 41%, $p = 0.04$).[22] The role of hysterectomy following adjuvant therapy is controversial, and many contend that eliminating hysterectomy from the two treatment arms above would not have adversely affected survival for patients with bulky IB disease (>4 cm). The current trend is to combine radiotherapy with cisplatin-based chemotherapy for women with stage IB2–IVA disease. For patients with stage I or II disease, hysterectomy has the benefit of preserving ovarian and vaginal function and completing treatment over a shorter period of time; postoperative adjuvant therapy is given under certain instances.[23]

Stage IIB–IVA Lesions

Women with stage IIB–IVA (Table 53–1) cervical cancer are initially treated with definitive *chemoradiotherapy*; surgical resection of these locally advanced tumors usually requires extended radical or ultraradical resection of adjacent organs to secure negative margins; it is rarely if ever indicated as the initial treatment. Radiotherapy consists of a combination of external-beam therapy (teletherapy) followed by brachytherapy. Teletherapy usually delivers approximately 4500 cGy to the pelvis in 180 cGy daily fractions 5 days per week over 5 weeks to cover the primary tumor and its draining pelvic lymphatics. Brachytherapy, which is usually given in one of two forms, intracavitary or interstitial, usually follows teletherapy; this practice permits more central tumor mass reduction and, hopefully, normal reproductive organ anatomy for easier insertion of the implants and better tumor dosimetry. Intracavitary applicators with a tandem and two colpostats or ovoids (Fletcher or Henshkie) are most commonly utilized; however, interstitial implants (Syed-Neblett template) may be indicated for selected patients with more locally advanced tumors. Brachytherapy usually delivers an additional 4000 cGy to point A in one or two applications at 1- to 2-week intervals; in addition, parametrial boosts with external radiotherapy may be given as indicated. The complete course of radiotherapy is preferably completed within 8 weeks. The total dose prescribed varies depending on the tumor stage and size, but it usually ranges from 8500 to 9000 cGy total dose to point A, keeping the bladder and rectal dose limited to radiation tolerance. The availability of outpatient high-dose-rate brachytherapy may eliminate the need for hospitalization to deliver low-dose-rate brachytherapy, as is traditionally employed.[24] Concomitant platinum-based chemotherapy with radiotherapy is generally well tolerated by most patients and has been shown to improve survival. Subsequently, it has become the standard of care in the United States.

Three studies from the Gynecologic Oncology Group deserve mention. Morris et al. studied women with stage IIB–IVA disease or stage IB or IIA disease with tumors >5 cm or positive pelvic lymph nodes. The women were randomized to groups undergoing pelvic and para-aortic irradiation or pelvic irradiation and a fluorouracil/cisplatin regimen. The radiation dose was 45 cGy. Chemotherapy was given on days 1–5 and 22–26. One or two applications of intracavitary radiation and a third cycle of chemotherapy were given. The 5-year survival was better (73% vs. 58%, $p = 0.004$) for the combined-therapy group.[25] In another study, women with stage IIB–IVA disease received external beam radiation and were also randomized into one of three chemotherapy arms.

1. Cisplatin 40 mg/m^2 per week for 6 weeks, *or*
2. Cisplatin 50 mg/m^2 on days 1 and 29 followed by 5-fluorouracil (5-Fu) 4 g/m^2 on days 1, 29 *and* hydroxyurea 2 g/m^2 twice weekly for 6 weeks
3. Hydroxyurea 3 g/m^2 twice weekly for 6 weeks

The group receiving hydroxyurea alone had a lower rate of progression-free survival and a lower overall survival rate.[26] The survival advantage of cisplatin-based chemoradiation in stage IIB–IVA cervical carcinoma was further confirmed by another large, randomized Gynecologic Oncology Group–Southwest Oncology Group trial.[27]

Concerning the role of oophorectomy during radical hysterectomy for cervical cancer, Sutton et al. in a Gynecologic Oncology Group study reported on the incidence of ovarian metastases in 990 patients with stage IB cervical carcinoma. Ovarian metastases were noted in 4 of 770 (0.5%) patients with squamous cell carcinoma and 2 of 121 (1.7%) with adenocarcinoma ($p = 0.19$).[28] No patients with adenosquamous carcinoma or other histology had ovarian metastases. These data suggest no increase in occult ovarian metastasis in nonsquamous cell cervical cancers, and ovarian preservation is commonly performed in women younger than 40 years where there is no gross ovarian abnormality and no obvious extracervical metastasis at the time of radical hysterectomy.

Recurrence

Recurrent cervical cancer usually carries a poor prognosis, as no effective salvage therapy is generally available. Ultraradical pelvic surgery (pelvic exenteration) and radiotherapy may salvage some patients with isolated pelvic recurrences following primary irradiation or surgery, respectively. In addition, patients with isolated distant metastasis in the lung or liver may be candidates for surgical resection provided the pelvis is tumor-free. Unfortunately, many patients with recurrent disease have unresectable cancer in a previously irradiated pelvis or have combined locoregional and distant metastases; these patients are usually treated with salvage cisplatin-based systemic chemotherapy but have a poor overall outcome.

Optimal candidates for pelvic exenteration are women who (1) were previously treated with definitive pelvic irradiation and have a small (<3 cm) localized central pelvic recurrence; (2) have a relatively long disease-free interval (>1 year); and (3) are medically and psychologically fit to undergo major pelvic surgery. Permanent urinary and fecal diversion are usually needed.[29,30] Preoperative evaluation may include CT scans of the abdomen, pelvis, and chest; and some physicians recommend scalene lymph node sampling. An exenteration is undertaken only if there is no evidence of distant disease. At the time of exploration, a thorough inspection for intraabdominal metastasis is performed, and a paraaortic lymph node biopsy specimen is sent for frozen section analysis, as are biopsy specimens of any enlarged pelvic lymph nodes. The paravesical and pararectal spaces are opened, and tumor fixation to the pelvicside wall is assessed. If intra-abdominal, retroperitoneal, or pelvic-wall metastases are noted, the procedure is abandoned, as these patients tend to have poor survival and should be spared a potentially highly morbid procedure. On the other hand, pelvic exenteration may provide a 5-year survival rate of approximately 30–50% in selected women with recurrent cervical cancer who successfully undergo the operation.[29,31] Laparoscopy may provide an alternative to laparotomy for initial assessment of resectability, and it may spare some patients (50%) laparotomy if distant disease is identified. Selected patients are candidates for anterior or posterior exenteration rather than total pelvic exenteration; the decision is usually made intraoperatively. Table 53–3 summarizes the surgical approaches for management of centrally recurrent cervical cancer. Continent urinary diversion with a colonic reservoir and neovaginal reconstruction with myocutaneous flaps provide some patients with improved quality of life after pelvic exenteration. Low rectal reanastomosis following radical pelvic radiotherapy is associated with a high anastomosis leak rate; and, if performed, temporary proximal intestinal diversion may be of benefit.[30]

As our knowledge and skills for treating cervical cancer improve, we should continue to seek the most effective and least

TABLE 53–3.
Surgical approaches to centrally recurrent cervical cancer in the pelvis

Tissue removed	Anterior exenteration	Posterior exenteration	Total exenteration
Bladder	Removed	Preserved	Removed
Vagina	Removed	Removed	Removed
Uterus	Removed	Removed	Removed
Adnexa	Removed	Removed	Removed
Parametria and paracolpos	Removed	Removed	Removed
Rectum	Preserved	Removed	Removed

morbid treatment modality, and our focus should remain on primary prevention. A proven and cost-effective screening tool (Pap smear) has been available for decades; and if it is made available on a regular basis to all women, advanced invasive disease may become one of the rarest malignancies in humans.

Conclusions

Cervical cancer is one of the more common pelvic malignancies, and fortunately the death rate has dropped substantially because of early diagnosis (Pap smear screening). Stage IA1 (<3 mm invasion) is rarely associated with lymph node metastases and therefore may be treated conservatively in the appropriate candidate with excellent control rates. Higher-stage disease (up to IIA) can be treated with surgery or irradiation with comparable cure rates. Surgery consists of radical hysterectomy (i.e., removal of cervix, corpus parametrial tissues, upper third of the vagina) and node dissection of the iliac, obturator, and lower aortic regions. Surgery may be accomplished abdominally, vaginally, or laparoscopically. Stage IA2–IIA can also be treated with primary irradiation or chemoradiation consisting of intracavitary irradiation *and* external beam irradiation of the whole pelvis. For patients with stage IIB and higher disease, surgery is rarely performed initially. Rather, external beam irradiation *and* either interstitial or intracavitary irradiation are applied concomitantly with cisplatin-based chemotherapy. Following treatment, patients with cervical cancer should have close follow-up on a regular basis. Most persistant or recurrent disease will manifest in the first 2 years after completion of therapy. Follow-up includes cytologic studies and biopsy of abnormal areas every 3 months the first 2 years, then every 6 months for 5 years, then every 6–12 months thereafter.

References

1. Landis SH, Murray T, Bolden S, Wingo PA. Annual report on estimated new cancer cases by sex, United States 1998. CA Cancer J Clin 1998; 48:10–14.
2. Jones WB, Shingleton HM, Russell AH, et al. Patterns of care for invasive cervical cancer: results of a national survey of 1984 and 1990. Cancer 1995;76:1934–1947.
3. Society of Gynecologic Oncology. Clinical practice guidelines: cervical cancer. Oncology 1998;12:134–138.
4. Benedet JL, Anderson GH. Stage IA carcinoma of the cervix revisited. Obstet Gynecol 1996;87:1052–1059.
5. Ostor AG. Studies on 200 cases of early squamous cell carcinoma of the cervix. Int J Gynecol Pathol 1993;12:193–207.
6. Morris M, Mitchell MF, Silva EG, Copeland LJ, Gershenson DM. Cervical conization as definitive therapy for early invasive squamous carcinoma of the cervix. Gynecol Oncol 1993;51:193–196.
7. Morrow CP, Curtin JP. Surgery for cervical neoplasia. In: Gynecologic Cancer Surgery. New York: Churchill Livingstone, 1996;451–568.
8. DiSaia PJ. Surgical aspects of cervical carcinoma. Cancer 1981;48:548–559.
9. Piver SM, Rutledge F, Smith JP. Five classes of extended hysterectomy for women with cervical cancer. Obstet Gynecol 1974;44:265–272.
10. Wolf JK, Levenback C, Malpica A, Morris M, Burke T, Mitchell MF. Adenocarcinoma in situ of the cervix: significance of cone biopsy margins. Obstet Gynecol 1996;88:82–86.
11. Poynor EA, Barakat RR, Hoskins WJ. Management and follow-up of patients with adenocarcinoma in situ of the uterine cervix. Gynecol Oncol 1995;57:158–164.
12. Im DD, Duska LR, Rosenshein NB. Adequacy of conization margins in adenocarcinoma in situ of the cervix as a predictor of residual disease. Gynecol Oncol 1995;59:179–182.
13. Ostor A, Rome R, Quinn M. Microinvasive adenocarcinoma of the cervix: a clinicopathologic study of 77 women. Obstet Gynecol 1997;89:88–93.
14. Spirtos NM, Schlaerth JB, Kimball RE, Leiphart VM, Ballon SC. Laparoscopic radical hysterectomy (type III) with aortic and pelvic lymphadenectomy. Am J Obstet Gynecol 1996;174:1763–1767; discussion 1767–1768.
15. Renaud MC, Plante M, Roy M. Combined laparoscopic and vaginal radical surgery in cervical cancer. Gynecol Oncol 2000;79:59–63.
16. Roy M, Plante M, Renaud MC, Tetu B. Vaginal radical hysterectomy versus abdominal radical hysterectomy in the treatment of early-stage cervical cancer. Gynecol Oncol 1996;62:336–339.
17. Schneider A, Possover M, Kamprath S, Endisch U, Krause N, Noschel H. Laparoscopy-assisted radical vaginal hysterectomy modified according to Schauta-Stoeckel. Obstet Gynecol 1996;88:1057–1060.
18. Querleu D. Laparoscopically assisted radical vaginal hysterectomy. Gynecol Oncol 1993;51:248–254.
19. Dargent D, Martin X, Sacchetoni A, Mathevet P. Laparoscopic vaginal radical trachelectomy: a treatment to preserve the fertility of cervical carcinoma patients. Cancer 2000;88:1877–1882.

20. Hoskins WJ. Prognostic factors for risk of recurrence in stage Ib and IIa cervical cancer. Baillieres Clin Obstet Gynaecol 1988;2:817–828.
21. Dargent D, Frobert L, Beau G. V factor (tumor volume) and T factor (FIGO classification) in the assessment of cervix cancer prognosis: the risk of lymph node spread. Gynecol Oncol 1985;22:15–22.
22. Keys HM, Bundy BN, Stehman FB, Muderspach LI, Chafe WE, Suggs CL 3rd, et al. Cisplatin, radiation, and adjuvant hysterectomy compared with radiation and adjuvant hysterectomy for bulky stage IB cervical carcinoma. N Engl J Med 1999;340:1154–1161.
23. Peters WA 3rd, Liu PY, Barrett RJ 2nd, Stock RJ, Monk BJ, Berek JS, et al. Concurrent chemotherapy and pelvic radiation therapy compared with pelvic radiation therapy alone as adjuvant therapy after radical surgery in high-risk early-stage cancer of the cervix. J Clin Oncol 2000;18:1606–1613.
24. Stehman FB, Perez CA, Kurman RJ, Thigpen JT. Uterine cervix. In: Hoskins WJ, Perez CA, Young RC (eds) Principles and Practice of Gynecologic Oncology, 2nd ed. Philadelphia: Lippincott-Raven, 1997;785–858.
25. Morris M, Eifel PJ, Lu J, Grigsby PW, Levenback C, Stevens RE, et al. Pelvic radiation with concurrent chemotherapy compared with pelvic and para-aortic radiation for high-risk cervical cancer. N Engl J Med 1999;340: 1137–1143.
26. Rose PG, Bundy BN, Watkins EB, Thigpen JT, Deppe G, Maiman MA, et al. Concurrent cisplatin-based radiotherapy and chemotherapy for locally advanced cervical cancer. N Engl J Med 1999;340:1144–1153.
27. Whitney CW, Sause W, Bundy BN, Malfetano JH, Hannigan EV, Fowler WC Jr, Clarke-Pears et al. Randomized comparison of fluorouracil plus cisplatin versus hydroxyurea as an adjunct to radiation therapy in stage IIB–IVA carcinoma of the cervix with negative para-aortic lymph nodes: a Gynecologic Oncology Group and Southwest Oncology Group study. J Clin Oncol 1999;17:1339–1348.
28. Sutton GP, Bundy BN, Delgado G, et al. Ovarian metastasis in stage IB carcinoma of the cervix: a Gynecologic Oncology Group study. Am J Obstet Gynecol 1992;166:50–53.
29. Barber HRK. Relative prognostic significance of preoperative and operative findings in pelvic exenteration. Surg Clin North Am 1969;49:431–447.
30. Shingleton HM, Soong SJ, Gelder MS, Hatch KD, Baker VV, Austin JM. Clinical and histopathologic factors predicting recurrence and survival after pelvic exenteration for cancer of the cervix. Obstet Gynecol 1989;73: 1027–1034.
31. Curtin JP, Hoskins WJ. Pelvic exenteration for gynecologic cancers. Surg Oncol Clin N Am 1994;3:267–276.

CHAPTER 54

Ovarian Cancer

ROBERTO ANGIOLI
SCOTT COHEN
HERVY E. AVERETTE

A. Epidemiology

Ovarian cancer is the fourth most frequent cause of cancer deaths in women (5% of all cancer deaths). The estimated number of new cases worldwide is more than 160,000 annually.[1] In the United States more than 25,000 new cases of ovarian cancer and more than 14,000 deaths attributable to this disease are reported each year.[2] Moreover, the lifetime risk of developing ovarian cancer is 1–2%.[3]

The incidence varies with age, geographic distribution, and ethnicity, increasing with age and peaking during the eighth decade. The incidence in women younger than 20 years of age is less than 1 per 100,000, increasing to 59 per 100,000 at age 75–79 years.[4] The incidence also varies among countries; and, with the exception of Japan, higher rates are reported in developed countries. In North America the age-adjusted incidence rate is 15.8 per 100,000 compared to a rate of 6.6 per 100,000 in Japan. Northern European countries show a much higher incidence (18.9 per 100,000) than southern European countries (10.8 per 100,000). In contrast, a lower incidence is found in the northern regions of South America compared to the southern regions.[1] Finally, the incidence is higher in white women: The average incidence in black women is 10 per 100,000 compared to a 13–15 per 100,000 in white women.

B. Pathogenesis

There are no known causes of ovarian cancer, but several factors have been identified that may increase the risk of developing this disease. They include diet, environment, hormones, and oncogenes. A small number of ovarian cancer patients have a genetic predisposition.

DIET

Several dietary factors have been associated with an increased risk of ovarian cancer. A diet high in meat and animal fat has been implicated as a risk factor.[3,4] Populations with a high lactose consumption to transferase activity (L/T) ratio also have a higher incidence of ovarian cancer.[5] Furthermore,

Ovarian Cancer

A.
Epidemiology
Fourth leading cause of cancer deaths in women
Lifetime risk 1–2%
25,000 Annual cases in U.S.
Incidence varies with age, geography, race

B.
Pathogenesis
Diet: high meat, animal fat
Environment: asbestos, talc, radiation, rubella, mumps, influenza
Hormones: incessant ovulation
Oncogenes: c-*myc*, H-*ras*, K-*ras* *erb*-B2, *p53*
Heredity: family history of breast or ovarian cancer; *BRCA1* and *BRCA2* mutation

C.
Presentation
Usually diagnosed at advanced age
Can have abdominal distension and pain

D.
Diagnosis
US with abdominal CT
Consider UGI/LGI series and IVP if symptoms warrant

E.
Screening
No effective methods

F.
Staging
FIGO system (see Table 54–1)
Surgical staging based on intraoperative findings

G.
Malignant Epithelial Tumors
Serous: most common
Mucinous: 5–10% bilateral
Endometrial: 10% have endometriosis
Clear cell: 5–10% bilateral, 25% endometriosis
Brenner and transitional

(continued on next page)

Ovarian Cancer (continued)

H.
Borderline Tumors
Comprise 10–15% of epithelial cancers
Treat surgically
Recurrences require reoperation

I.
Pseudomyxoma Peritonei
Mucinous appendiceal or ovarian (more common) tumor

J.
Germ Cell Tumors
Most common in young women
Dysgerminoma: most common, radiosensitive, LDH
Endodermal sinus tumor: age 20–30, α-fetoprotein (AFP)
Immature teratoma: AFP, LDH, CA-125
Embryonal carcinoma: age 15, hCG, AFP
Polyembryoma: AFP, hCG, human placental lactogen
Choriocarcinoma: hCG
Management: consider unilateral surgery for young patients
Complete staging needed
All nondysgerminomas receive postoperative chemotherapy except stage IA, grade 1 tumors

K.
Sex Cord Stromal Neoplasms
Granulosa-stroma cell tumors: occur perimenopausally in adults; 80% of juvenile patients have sexual precocity
Thecoma-fibroma: Meigs syndrome (ascites, hydrothorax, ovarian fibroma)
Sertoli-Leydig cell tumors: masculinizing
Sex cord with annular tubules: associated Peutz–Jeghers syndrome
Gynandroblastoma
Management: surgery as for epithelial tumors; conservative therapy for premenopausal women desiring childbearing; chemotherapy regimen not standard

Ovarian Cancer (continued)

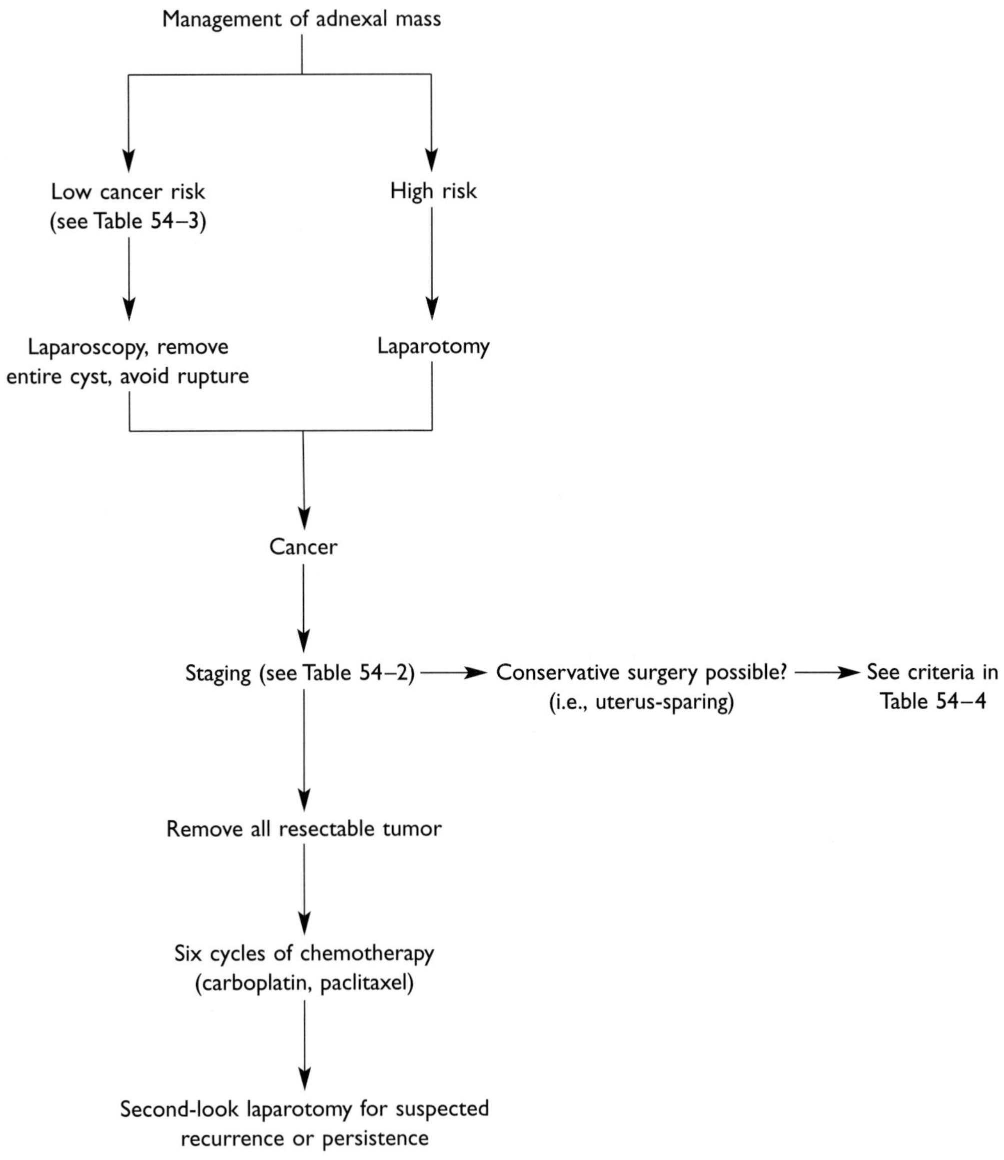

Management of adnexal mass

Low cancer risk (see Table 54–3) → Laparoscopy, remove entire cyst, avoid rupture

High risk → Laparotomy

→ Cancer

→ Staging (see Table 54–2) → Conservative surgery possible? (i.e., uterus-sparing) → See criteria in Table 54–4

→ Remove all resectable tumor

→ Six cycles of chemotherapy (carboplatin, paclitaxel)

→ Second-look laparotomy for suspected recurrence or persistence

L.
Follow-Up
CA-125
Pelvic examinations
CT of pelvis
(Frequency depends on interval since diagnosis; see text)

some studies have suggested that the risk is increased with high coffee and tobacco use, but these data are controversial.

Environmental Factors

Exposure to asbestos and talc (hydrous magnesium trisilicate), which is used as dusting powder on diaphragms, may lead to an increased risk due to the passage of these components through the vagina to the ovary.[6] Ionizing radiation and common viruses such as rubella, mumps, and influenza have also been associated with an increased risk of acquiring ovarian cancer, but the data are conflicting.

Hormonal Factors

Hormones may be a contributing factor. The Ovarian Patient Care Study has proposed that incessant ovulation may play a role in the development of ovarian cancer.[7] Oral contraceptives, which contain combinations of estrogen and progesterone, act to block ovulation by interfering with the pulsatile release of follicle-stimulating hormone (FSH) and luteinizing hormone (LH). Consequently, several studies have shown that oral contraceptive use may decrease a person's risk by 30–60%. Similarly, it appears that any factor that decreases ovulation also decreases a patient's risk. These factors include multiparity, older age at first menstruation, and early menopause.

Oncogenes

Sporadic epithelial ovarian cancer is associated with multiple and complex karyotypic abnormalities. The most commonly identified chromosomal abnormalities are found on chromosomes 1 and 11. Certain oncogenes may have a role in the etiology and progression of ovarian cancer; the most commonly associated oncogenes are c-*myc*, H-*ras*, Ki-*ras* and *erbB2*.[8] A mutation in the *p53* gene, which codes for a tumor suppressor protein, is also commonly found in ovarian cancer (up to 62% of patients)[9]; this gene mutation is associated with a worse prognosis.

Hereditary Ovarian Cancer

It has been noted that women with a family history of breast or ovarian cancer are at increased risk for these cancers. The use of genetic sequencing techniques has enabled researchers to decipher patterns of genetic information contained in DNA and to use this information to link specific genetic defects to genetic disease. Several syndromes of hereditary ovarian cancer have been identified, including breast-ovarian cancer syndrome, site-specific ovarian cancer syndrome, and hereditary nonpolyposis colorectal cancer (HNPCC).

The *breast-ovarian syndrome* has a high probability of linkage to gene mutations on *BRCA1* and *BRCA2*. The American Society of Clinical Oncologists has identified families with the highest likelihood of having mutations as families with more than two breast cancers and one or more ovarian cancers diagnosed at any age; families with more than three breast cancers diagnosed before age 50; or families with sister pairs with either two breast cancers, two ovarian cancers, or a breast and ovarian cancer.[10] In the presence of a *BRCA1* mutation and a family history of cancer, the risk of developing ovarian cancer can be more than 60%. The incidence of a *BRCA1* mutation in the general population is about 1 in 800 and increases to 1 in 100 for persons of Eastern European Jewish descent. Studies have shown that patients with ovarian cancer and a *BRCA1* mutation have a better prognosis than a patient with sporadic ovarian cancer.

C. Presentation

The clinical presentation of ovarian cancer follows a specific pattern that is directly related to the size and growth of the tumor. Unfortunately, most ovarian cancer patients are not diagnosed until the cancer is at an advanced stage. Early-stage ovarian cancer is often asymptomatic and therefore difficult to diagnose unless an adnexal mass is palpated during routine pelvic examination. As the tumor grows it compresses adjacent pelvic structures, producing symptoms of urinary frequency, pelvic pressure, bloating, constipation, and abdominal discomfort. In some instances the patient even complains of dyspareunia. When the ovarian mass exceeds 12–15 cm in the adult, the pelvis no longer can accommodate the mass. At this point, the patient may notice an increase in abdominal girth, weight gain, and ascites. Abdominal distension and abdominal pain are the two most common presenting symptoms of ovarian cancer. These symptoms, as well as the presence of ascites or abnormal vaginal bleeding, should trigger a workup for ovarian cancer.

D. Diagnosis

The diagnostic workup for ovarian cancer includes a thorough history and physical examination, pregnancy testing, pelvic ultrasonography, chest radiography, and serum CA-125 assay. The physician must be aware of the wide range of diseases that may present with symptomatology similar to that of ovarian cancer. Ultrasonography is the most frequently used diagnostic tool in the presence of an adnexal mass palpated on physical examination. Morphologic characteristics on ultrasonography such as wall thickness, inner wall structure, characteristics of septae, the character of fluid contents, and echogenicity suggest the presence or absence of malignancy. Based on the ovarian Patient Care Evaluation Study, ultrasonography and CT of the abdomen should be considered routine tests during the assessment workup for ovarian cancer. These tests can identify specific characteristics of the tumor, the presence of ascites, and metastasis to the liver, spleen, omentum, or lymph nodes.[7]

Other tests may assist with the diagnosis. A chest radiograph should be routinely examined to rule out the possibility of metastatic disease. A barium enema, upper gastrointestinal (GI) series or intravenous pyelography (IVP) are undertaken if symptoms suggest involvement of these systems. Color Doppler imaging is occasionally used to study the blood flow of adnexal masses, but its use is still controversial. The use of magnetic resonance imaging (MRI) has not been shown to be superior to the CT scan.

E. Screening/Prevention

Because ovarian cancer often presents in the later stages of the disease, screening may be useful for identifying early cases. The most widely studied screening methods are pelvic examination, ultrasonography, and CA-125 determinations. Unfortunately, no individual screening method has been shown to be overwhelmingly effective.

Vaginal ultrasonography has been used in recent years, but in a study of 1000 asymptomatic women age 40 years and older an abnormality rate of 3.1% was reported, of which only one case of ovarian cancer was identified.[11] Serum CA-125 levels are neither specific nor sensitive. The combination of ultrasonography and CA-125 assay is highly specific but has a low positive predictive value and sensitivity. In a study of 22,000 women with a CA-125 level higher than 30 U/ml who underwent an ultrasound examination, the specificity for detecting ovarian cancer was 99.9%, the sensitivity was less than 80%, and the positive predictive value for early-stage cancer was only 9.8%.[12] Other cancer markers commonly used to detect ovarian cancer include α-fetoprotein (AFP) in endodermal sinus tumors, embryonal cell carcinomas, or mixed germ cell tumors; human chorionic gonadotropin (hCG) in ovarian choriocarcinoma and potentially dysgerminoma; and CA 19-9 and carcinoembryonic antigen (CEA) in mucinous ovarian carcinoma.

Unfortunately, preliminary studies have shown that the most common ovarian cancer screening methods have a high false-positive rate, which can lead to an unacceptably high rate of negative laparotomies. As a result, the 1994 NIH Consensus Conference concluded that there is no effective method for screening and detecting early ovarian cancer.[13] Furthermore, there are few alternative options for preventing it, especially in the high risk groups. Currently, preventive measures for high risk patients include prophylactic oophorectomy. This procedure may significantly reduce the incidence of ovarian carcinoma, but the psychosocial, medical, and legal implications of such a procedure are still widely debated.

F. Staging

Ovarian cancer is staged surgically according to the International Federation of Gynecology and Obstetrics (FIGO) method of staging (Table 54–1). Accurate staging is fundamental when determining a patient's prognosis and treatment options. To stage a tumor accurately, certain steps must be followed, especially for early-stage disease (Table 54–2). First, the abdomen should be entered through a vertical midline incision from the umbilicus down to the pubic symphysis to obtain adequate exposure. The incision is often extended superiorly when the presence of cancer is confirmed. After opening, the next step is to remove the ascites and send the fluid for cytologic evaluation. If there is no ascites or the amount is minimal, peritoneal washing must be performed. Next, all abdominopelvic viscera should be evaluated. In the absence of a grossly positive extrapelvic tumor, the surgery should include omentectomy and peritoneal biopsies of the right and left diaphragm, right and left colic gutter, right and left pelvis, anterior and posterior pelvic peritoneum, and pelvic and paraaortic lymph nodes.

G. Malignant Epithelial Tumor

Most ovarian tumors are of epithelial origin. Malignant epithelial tumors, which account for 85% of all ovarian cancers, are classified as serous, mucinous, endometrioid, transitional, clear cell, or a combination of the above. In about 15% of cases the cells are poorly differentiated and the tumor cannot be classified according to the cell type.

Histology

Serous Type Serous carcinoma is the most common cancer of the ovary, representing about 50% of all ovarian epithelial cancers. The tumor presents with bilateral ovarian involvement in 30% of cases and is most commonly identified in advanced stages. The tumor mass is usually partially cystic and partially solid, and psammoma bodies are found in 30% of the cases.

Mucinous Type Mucinous carcinoma tends to be larger than the serous type and is more often diagnosed at an earlier stage. Fifty percent of the cases are diagnosed at stage I or II, and the tumor is bilateral in 5–10% of cases. Grossly, the tumor appears multilocular with a solid component. The liquid of the cystic component is either gelatinous or watery. Microscopically, the cell layer is similar to the endocervical or intestinal epithelium.

Endometrioid Type Endometrioid ovarian cancer is found in association with endometriosis in 10% of patients and with endometrial cancer in 15–30%. In general, however, ovarian cancer is associated with endometrial cancer in fewer

TABLE 54–1.
FIGO staging of ovarian carcinoma

Stage	Description
I	growth limited to the ovary(ies)
IA	growth limited to one ovary; no ascites, no external excrescences, capsule intact
IB	growth limited to both ovaries; no ascites, no external excrescences, capsule intact
IC	tumor extent of either stage IA or IB but with malignant ascites or positive peritoneal washings, capsular excrescences, or tumor rupture
II	pelvic metastasis/extension of tumor
IIA	metastasis/extension to the uterus and/or tubes
IIB	metastasis/extension to other pelvic tissues
IIC	tumor extent either stage IIA or IIB but with malignant ascites or positive peritoneal washings, capsular excrescences, or tumor rupture
III	tumor metastasis outside the pelvis to involve peritoneal surfaces or retroperitoneal/inguinal lymph nodes
IIIA	tumor grossly confined to the pelvis but with histologically proven metastasis to peritoneal surfaces
IIIB	grossly apparent peritoneal metastasis, <2 cm in largest diameter
IIIC	grossly apparent peritoneal metastasis, >2 cm in largest diameter, and/or positive retroperitoneal or inguinal lymph nodes
IV	distant or hepatic parenchymal metastasis

NOTE: For ascites to result in classification of stage IC or IIC, cytology must contain malignant cells. Metastasis to the serosa of the liver without parenchymal involvement is classified as stage III disease. For pleural effusion to result in classification IV, cytology must contain malignant cells.

than 5% of cases. About 15% of stage I tumors appear bilaterally. These tumors have a cystic component that is usually filled with mucoid or chocolate material. Microscopically, endometrioid ovarian cancer and endometrial cancer are indistinguishable. Identification of an endometrioid tumor by histology is considered a favorable independent prognostic factor. These patients usually have a better outcome than patients with tumors of mucinous or serous histology.[14]

TABLE 54–2.
Surgical procedure to stage early ovarian cancer

Vertical incision*
Evaluation of all abdomino-pelvic viscera
Peritoneal washings
Peritoneal biopsies
Total abdominal hysterectomy and bilateral salpingo-oophorectomy**
Omentectomy
Pelvic and para-aortic lymph node sampling

* Laparoscopy is an alternative.
** Young patient desiring future childbearing with unilateral tumor can be staged with preservation of the healthy ovary and the uterus.

TABLE 54–3.
Indications for laparoscopic management of adnexal masses

Unilateral simple cystic mass, <8 cm diameter
No ascites
Young age
Normal CA-125 (<35 U/ml)
No family history of ovarian cancer
No evidence of metastatic disease

CLEAR CELL TYPE The clear cell type of ovarian tumor makes up 2–5% of all ovarian cancers. More than 50% of patients with clear cell ovarian cancer are diagnosed at stage I, and of these 5–10% present with bilateral ovarian involvement. Twenty-five percent of the cases are associated with endometriosis compared to 8% for all ovarian cancers. Microscopically, hobnail cells with a clear, glycogen-filled cytoplasm characterize clear cell ovarian cancer.

BRENNER AND TRANSITIONAL CELLS Brenner tumors are believed to arise from mesothelial cells through transitional cell metaplasia. These tumors are usually benign but can present as borderline or malignant tumors. Transitional cell carcinoma, a second urothelial cancer, in contrast to the Brenner tumor, lacks the presence of a cancer precursor.[15] Transitional cell tumors are more aggressive than the Brenner malignant tumor but are highly sensitive to chemotherapy.

MANAGEMENT

EARLY DISEASE Laparoscopic surgery for management of adnexal masses should be limited to patients with a low risk of cancer; the accepted indications are summarized in Table 54–3. Even when the risk of cancer is low, it is advisable to remove the entire cyst without rupture. In fact, the incidence of malignant cysts in a patient believed to have benign pathology preoperatively is 0.04–3.70%.[16] Management of an ovarian cyst by aspiration is contraindicated for various reasons. First, even in the case of benign pathology, the incidence of a recurrent cyst is high. Second, cytology has a poor negative predictive value.[17] Finally, the risk of tumor spread in the event of a malignancy is high.

Conservative surgery for ovarian cancer can be performed in selected patients and consists of preservation of the uterus and contralateral ovary. These patients should have low risk cancer, which includes stage IA, with well or moderately differentiated histology. Even when conservative surgery is performed, the lesion must be fully staged, as outlined in Table 54–2. Table 54–4 summarizes the indications for conservative surgery of ovarian cancer.

ADVANCED DISEASE Management of advanced ovarian cancer includes removal of all resectable tumor and chemotherapy. Griffith[18] showed that patients whose residual tumor was <1.5 cm after cytoreductive surgery fared better and had a better prognosis than patients with larger residual tumor, regardless of initial tumor dimension. These data have been confirmed numerous times.

Following the initial surgery, patients with advanced stages are usually treated with six cycles of chemotherapy. After surgery and chemotherapy a second-look laparotomy can be performed for patients with suspected tumor recurrence or persistence and for patients undergoing investigational studies. The concept of "interval debulking," although relatively new, has been intro-

TABLE 54–4.
Criteria for conservative surgery for ovarian cancer

Premenopausal woman desiring future childbearing
Unilateral tumor
Stage IA
Well or moderately differentiated histology
Adequate staging
Close follow-up available with tumor markers and ultrasonography

duced to manage advanced ovarian cancer that was unresectable at the initial surgery. Patients whose initial cytoreduction was suboptimal undergo "interval debulking" following three or four cycles of chemotherapy; the outcome is improved in these instances.[19]

Chemotherapy

Epithelial ovarian cancer is highly sensitive to chemotherapy, and cisplatin has been considered for many years to be the most active drug. Initially, chemotherapy was administered as a single agent, the most frequently used drugs have been alkalating agents such as melphalan, cyclophosphamide, chlorambucil, thiotepa, and platinum-based agents. Anthracyclines such as doxorubicin and other agents including hexamethylmelamine have also been used. It has been shown that multiagent therapy containing platinum is superior to single agent therapy alone. Platinum and cyclophosphamide were initially found to be the most effective combination; doxorubicin was added but was discontinued because of minimal improvement and higher toxicity.

Many treatment regimens have been introduced. McGuire et al. showed that platinum 75 mg/m^2 IV plus paclitaxel (Taxol) 135 mg/m^2 IV (24-hour infusion) is superior to platinum 75 mg/m^2 IV plus cyclophosphamide 750 mg/m^2 IV in patients with suboptimal debulking (>1 cm residual tumor).[20] Carboplatin has been shown to have equivalent antitumor activity but fewer side effects than cisplatin. Most institutions are presently using carboplatin in combination with Taxol instead of cisplatin as first line chemotherapy in patients with ovarian cancer.

One method of administering chemotherapy is to place the agents directly into the peritoneum. Intraperitoneal chemotherapy achieves high intraperitoneal concentrations of the drug without reaching toxic systemic levels. The use of intraperitoneal chemotherapy is presently limited to cases with minimal residual tumor, as the drug penetrates the tumor only a few millimeters.

Radiotherapy

The use of radiotherapy is limited because of its toxicity to the abdominal organs. Ovarian cancer spreads to the intraperitoneal abdominopelvic cavity and the retroperitoneum; therefore the treatment would have to include all the abdominopelvic organs. Intraperitoneal radioactive isotopes and whole-abdomen irradiation were used in the past but are, at best, equivalent to chemotherapy, with a high incidence of severe complications. Nevertheless, some authors report good long-term survival in patients with small-volume residual disease.[21] Presently, the use of radiation to treat ovarian cancer is limited to highly selected cases and clinical trials.

H. Borderline Tumors

Borderline tumors, also called tumors with low malignant potential, are a distinct entity; and each of the histologic types described above can present in a borderline form. Borderline tumors are characterized by proliferating activity and nuclear abnormalities, but they lack infiltrative destructive growth. Borderline tumors account for 10–15% of epithelial ovarian cancers. Most occur during the reproductive age, and most are found at an early stage. The mucinous type can be complicated by pseudomyxoma peritonei, as described below. Excellent survival is reported for all stages.

Borderline tumors are managed surgically, as their slow growth rate renders them poorly sensitive to chemotherapy. Early stages can be completely cured by initial surgery. Advanced stages tend to recur, especially if there is residual tumor after debulking. Recurrent tumors are managed surgically. Most deaths are due to complications such as bowel obstruction, bowel perforation, malabsorption, or short bowel syndrome due to multiple resections. Young patients with early-stage disease can be treated by conservative surgery with subsequent contralateral oophorectomy after childbearing.

I. Pseudomyxoma Peritonei

Pseudomyxoma peritonei is characterized by filling of the peritoneal cavity with gelatinous tumor deposits that may be partially free or partially attached to the peritoneal surface. It is associated with mucinous ovarian or appendiceal tumors. Most cases are associated with low malignant potential ovarian tumors. Survival is related to the degree of malignancy of the primary tumor, the initial stage, and the resectability of the tumor at the time of diagnosis.

J. Germ Cell Tumors

Approximately 15–20% of all primary ovarian neoplasms are germ cell tumors. They are most commonly found in young women, with a mean age of 19 years. Nearly 60–75% of malignant germ cell tumors are stage I at diagnosis, which is in great contrast to most ovarian malignancies, which present in advanced stages. Germ cell tumors have also been associated with a familial occurrence. Malignant germ cell tumors can be divided into dysgerminomas, endodermal sinus tumors, immature teratomas, embryonal carcinomas, polyembryonas, and choriocarcinomas. The most commonly used tumor markers to follow these patients are serum CA-125, serum lactate dehydrogenase (LDH), serum AFP, and serum hCG.

Histology

Dysgerminoma Dysgerminoma is the most common germ cell tumor, accounting for 40% of cases. This malignancy is rare in women older than 35 years of age, with 75% occurring during the early reproductive years. The tumors are usually found on routine physical examination and may appear lobulated, solid, or soft and firm. Serum LDH is a useful tumor marker for dysgerminomas, with the LDH levels sometimes rising higher than is seen with epithelial ovarian malignancies. The overall 5-year survival for a pure dysgerminoma at stage Ia is nearly 95%, but the recurrence rate approaches 15%.

Endodermal Sinus Tumors Endodermal sinus tumor (EST) is one of the most malignant tumors arising from the ovary. Most occur in women around age 20 and are confined to one ovary at the time of diagnosis. Grossly, these tumors appear smooth and shiny, with a distinct microscopic appearance consisting of a reticular growth pattern, intracellular and extracellular hyaline droplets, and Schiller-Duval bodies. AFP can be detected in most patients with this type of tumor.

Immature Teratoma About 20% of germ cell tumors are immature teratomas that contain tissue of a normal embryo. The tumors are usually cystic-solid with components of all three germ layers. AFP, LDH, and CA-125 have been reliable tumor markers for the immature teratoma. The outcome of patients with this tumor is based on the degree of differentiation at the time of diagnosis, the stage of the disease, and the presence of other malignant elements, such as an EST. The immature teratoma can undergo spontaneous maturation, which usually follows the initial diagnosis. It presents as a nodule of glial tissue that is often associated with ascites, called gliomatosis peritonei.

Embryonal Carcinoma The embryonal carcinoma appears in girls or women slightly younger than those with other ovarian malignancies; the mean age at appearance is 15 years. It is composed of embryonal cells, embryonal bodies, and syncytiotrophoblastic giant cells; and it produces both hCG and AFP.

Polyembryona A germ cell tumor, the polyembryoma is rare. It is composed of embryoid bodies in various stages of presomite development. The tumor may present with increased levels of AFP, hCG, and human placental lactogen.

Choriocarcinoma Choriocarcinoma is a rare germ cell tumor that usually appears in a mixed form. The tumor also produces hCG, which may help in the diagnosis, treatment, and follow-up of patients. It does not respond to chemotherapy as well as does gestational choriocarcinoma.

Management

Germ cell tumors are managed surgically regardless of the histologic type. Germ cell tumors in general occur in young patients and are usually unilateral. The surgical treatment is therefore unilateral salpingo-oophorectomy unless the tumor has spread beyond the ovary (Table 54–4). If a cystic structure is seen in the contralateral ovary, cystectomy is recommended. Usually the contralateral cyst is a benign dermoid. We recommend complete staging for the patient even if the tumor is confined to one ovary. The histology of the germ cell tumor plays an important role in postoperative therapy. The dysgerminomas are sensitive to radiation, whereas the nondysgerminomatous germ cell tumors are more sensitive to chemotherapy. All patients with nondysgerminomatous germ cell malignancies are candidates for postoperative chemotherapy, with the exception of stage IA grade 1 tumors. The most commonly used combinations of chemotherapy are bleomycin/etoposide/cisplatin (BEP); vincristine/actinomycin D/Cytoxan (VAC); and etoposide/ifosfamide/cisplatin (VIP). Of these regimens, BEP is the treatment that currently has produced the best results. Dysgerminomas are radiosensitive, but BEP chemotherapy is also widely used with these tumors and has produced good results.[22]

K. *Sex Cord Stromal Neoplasms*

Sex cord tumors account for 5% of ovarian neoplasms. These tumors originate from specialized gonadal stroma and usually maintain hormone production capability. The high level of estrogen production increases the risk of endometrial cancer in these patients. The sex cord stromal neoplasms are classified according to their differentiation toward ovarian follicles (granulosa-stroma cell tumor), Leydig cells (Sertoli-Leydig cell tumor), testicular tubules (sex cord tumor with annular tubules, or SCTAT), and adrenal cortical cells (gynandroblastomas).

Histology

Granulosa-Stroma Cell Tumor Granulosa-stroma cell tumors are composed of granulosa and theca cells. The most frequent forms of these tumors are the adult-type granulosa cell tumor (95%) and the juvenile granulosa cell tumor (5%). The adult form occurs mainly during the perimenopausal period and manifests with nonspecific abdominal symptoms such as abdominal distension and pain. About 10% of cases present with hemoperitoneum due to acute rupture. Endocrine manifestations are present in 75% of the cases; 50% of the patients have associated endometrial hyperplasia or a polyp, and 5–15% of the patients have concomitant endometrial cancer. Most cases (90%) are diagnosed at stage I, with fewer than 5% presenting bilaterally. The juvenile granulosa cell tumor is usually unilateral and is associated with sexual precocity in 80% of the cases.

Thecomas-Fibromas Thecomas-fibromas are tumors composed of fibroblasts, theca cells, or a combination of the two cell types. Most of the tumors are benign, but malignant thecomas and ovarian fibrosarcomas have been reported. The presence of ascites and a hydrothorax with an ovarian fibroma is a condition known as *Meigs syndrome*.

Sertoli-Leydig Cell Tumors Sertoli-Leydig cell tumors (SLCTs), also known as androblastomas, are typically masculinizing neoplasms, although high estrogen production is also present. SLCTs are classified based on their degree of differentiation.[23] The degree of differentiation and the stage are the main prognostic factors. Pure Leydig cell tumors are almost always benign. The most common form of SLCT is the arrhenoblastoma, which contains Sertoli cells, Leydig cells, and tissue similar to fetal testis.

Sex Cord Tumor with Annular Tubules Sex cord tumors with annular tubules (SCTATs) are associated with Peutz-Jeghers syndrome in one-third of patients. These tumors are usually benign and 15% of the time are also associated with adenoma malignum of the cervix.

Gynandroblastoma Gynandroblastoma is a rare entity. It contains granulosa cell elements associated with tubules and Leydig cells characteristic of the arrhenoblastoma.

Management

Granulosa cell tumors are treated surgically, similar to epithelial-type tumors. Conservative treatment is performed in premenopausal women if childbearing is not completed. There is little evidence that adjunctive therapy is effective in completely resected tumors, although both irradiation and chemotherapy have been used. Recurrent and advanced cancers have a poor prognosis and are usually treated with chemotherapy, although a standard regimen has not been established. The juvenile-type granulosa cell tumor has a good prognosis when confined to one ovary and can be treated with tumor excision (cystectomy) alone.

L. Follow-up

Follow-up care for a patient treated for ovarian cancer includes serial CA-125 measurements, pelvic examinations, chest radiography, and CT scans. During chemotherapy, a CA-125 assay is usually performed every month. Pelvic examination is also performed every month, and a CT scan is obtained after the third and the last (sixth) cycle of chemotherapy. Progressive or persistent disease is managed with surgery or a change in the chemotherapy regimen.

Most recurrences appear within 2 years following a complete response to surgery and chemotherapy. As a result, it is suggested that patients be followed every 3 months during the first 2 years. If the test results have been negative for 2 years, the patient can increase the time between visits to every 6 months. A rectovaginal examination should be performed at each visit. The CA-125 assay is initially performed every month to follow the efficacy of chemotherapy but then can be obtained every 3–6 months. CT scans should be done once a year. Chest radiography is performed every 6–12 months. Suspicion of a recurrence by physical examination or a rise in the CA-125 level warrants radiologic examination and even surgical exploration to detect the presence of a recurrent tumor.

Other tumor markers may be useful for detecting sex cord stromal tumors and tracking tumor progression. Such markers include testosterone, inhibin, AFP, and estradiol levels. Other useful markers for germ cell tumors are hCG, LDH, and AFP.

References

1. Parkin DM, Pisani P, Ferlay J. Estimates of the worldwide incidence of eighteen major cancers in 1985. Int J Cancer 1993;54:594–606.
2. CA Cancer J Clin 1998;48:6–29.
3. Piver MS, Baker TR, Piedmonte M, Sandecki AM. Epidemiology and etiology of ovarian cancer. Semin Oncol 1991;18:177–185.
4. Greene MH, Clark JW, Blayney DW. The epidemiology of ovarian cancer. Semin Oncol 1984;11:209–226.
5. Cramer DW, Harlow BL, Willett WC, et al. Galactose consumption and metabolism in relation to the risk of ovarian cancer. Lancet 1989;2:66–71.
6. Cramer DW, Welch WR, Scully RE, Wojciechowski CA. Ovarian cancer and talc: a case control study. Cancer 1982;50:372–376.
7. Averette HE, Hoskins WJ, Nguyen HN, Boike G, Flessa HC, Chmiel JS. National Survey of ovarian carcinoma. I. A Patient Care Evaluation Study of the American College of Surgeons. Cancer 71;4(suppl):1629–1638.
8. Perez RP, Godwin AK, Hamilton TC, Ozols RF. Ovarian cancer biology. Semin Oncol 1991;18:186–204.
9. Hartmann LC, Podratz KC, Keeney GL, et al. Prognostic significance of p53 immunostaining in epithelial ovarian cancer. J Clin Oncol 1994;12: 64–69.
10. Statement of the American Society of Clinical Oncology: genetic testing for cancer susceptibility. J Clin Oncol 1996;5:1730–1736.
11. van Nagell JR Jr, Higgins RV, Donaldson ES, et al. Transvaginal sonography as a screening method for ovarian cancer: a report of the first 1000 cases screened. Cancer 1990; 65:573–577.
12. Jacobs I, Davies AP, Bridges J, et al. Prevalence screening for ovarian cancer in postmenopausal women by CA-125 measurement and ultrasonography. BMJ 1993;306:1030–1034.
13. Kramer BS, Gohagan J, Prorok PC. NIH consensus 1994 screening. Gynecol Oncol 1994;55:S20–S21.
14. Kline RC, Wharton JT, Atkinson EN, Burke TW, Gershenson DM, Edwards CL. Endometrioid carcinoma of the ovary: retrospective review of 145 cases. Gynecol Oncol 1990;39:337–346.
15. Austin RM, Norris HJ. Malignant Brenner tumor and transitional cell carcinoma of the ovary: a comparison. Int J Gynecol Pathol 1987;6:29–39.
16. Crawford RAF, Shepherd JH. Epithelial ovarian cancer: chemotherapy and other postoperative therapy. In: Shingleton HM, Fowler WC, Jordan JA, Lawrence WD (eds) Gynecologic Oncology: Current Diagnosis and Treatment. London: Saunders, 1966;203–214.
17. Nicklin JL, Van Eijkeren M, Athanasatos P, Wain GV, Hacker NF. A comparison of ovarian cyst aspirate cytology and histology: the case against aspiration of cystic pelvic masses. Aust NZ J Obstet Gynaecol 1994;34:546–549.
18. Griffith CT. Surgical resection of tumor bulk in the primary treatment of ovarian carcinoma. Natl Cancer Inst Monogr 1975;42:101–104.

19. van der Berg MEL, van Lent M, Kobierska A, et al. The effect of debulking surgery after induction chemotherapy on the prognosis in advanced ovarian cancer. N Engl J Med 1993;332:629–634.
20. McGuire WP, Hoskins WJ, Brady MF, et al. Cyclophosphamide and cisplatin compared with paclitaxel and cisplatin in patients with stage III and stage IV ovarian cancer. N Engl J Med 1996;334:1–6.
21. Thomas GM, Dembo AJ. Integrating radiation therapy into the management of ovarian cancer. Cancer 1993;71:1710–1718.
22. Gershenson DM, Morris M, Cangir A, et al. Treatment of malignant germ cell tumors of the ovary with bleomycin, etoposide, and cisplatin. J Clin Oncol 1990;8:751–720.
23. Young RH, Scully RE. Ovarian Sertoli-Leydig cell tumors: a clinicopathological analysis of 207 cases. Am J Surg Pathol 1985;9:8543–8569.

Section 11

Pediatric Tumors

Chapter 55

Wilms' Tumor

ANDREW M. DAVIDOFF

In 1956 Farber introduced systemic chemotherapy to supplement surgery and radiation therapy and in 1964 reported an 89% survival rate among 53 cases. Because of the rarity of this tumor, further clinical investigation was limited until establishment of the National Wilms' Tumor Study (NWTS) in 1969. It represented a cooperative effort among several groups treating patients in a clearly defined manner so statistically relevant comparisons of treatment variations could be made. Four trials have been completed, with NWTS—V currently open. The basic goal of each successive NWTS trial has been to maintain a high cure rate while reducing the intensity and duration of therapy based on stage and histologic evaluation. The NWTS has served as a prototype for other collaborative studies of childhood tumors.

A. Epidemiology

Wilms' tumor is the most common intraabdominal cancer of childhood. It represents approximately 6% of all pediatric cancers and accounts for more than 95% of all tumors of the kidney in the pediatric age group.[1] In the United States, there is an annual incidence of eight cases per million children less than 15 years of age with the total incidence estimated at about 350 cases per year.[2] Approximately 75% of the cases occur in children less than five years of age with a peak incidence at two to three of age.[3]

Classic Wilms' tumor has a triphasic histologic appearance, the three cell types being stromal, epithelial, and blastemal. All three elements are not required simultaneously, however, to diagnose Wilms' tumor. The neoplastic cells can often be seen forming primitive tubules and glomeruli. There are two distinct hisopathologic categories (favorable and unfavorable) which correlated with prognosis.[4] The *unfavorable* histological group includes Wilms' tumors with anaplasia (marked cytological atypia) and two distinct renal tumors with sarcomatous stroma, clear cell sarcoma of the kidney (CCSK), and malignant rhabdoid tumor of the kidney.[4] The remainder are considered to have favorable histology. Anaplasia is present in approximately 5% of Wilms' tumors and is more common in older children, reaching a peak at approximately five years of age.[5] This histopathologic variant is also more frequent in African-American than in Caucasian patients.

The eponym Wilms' tumor was adopted for nephroblastoma following the classic monogram by Max Wilms in 1899 in which he described seven cases of malignant mixed tissue tumors of the kidney

Wilms' Tumor

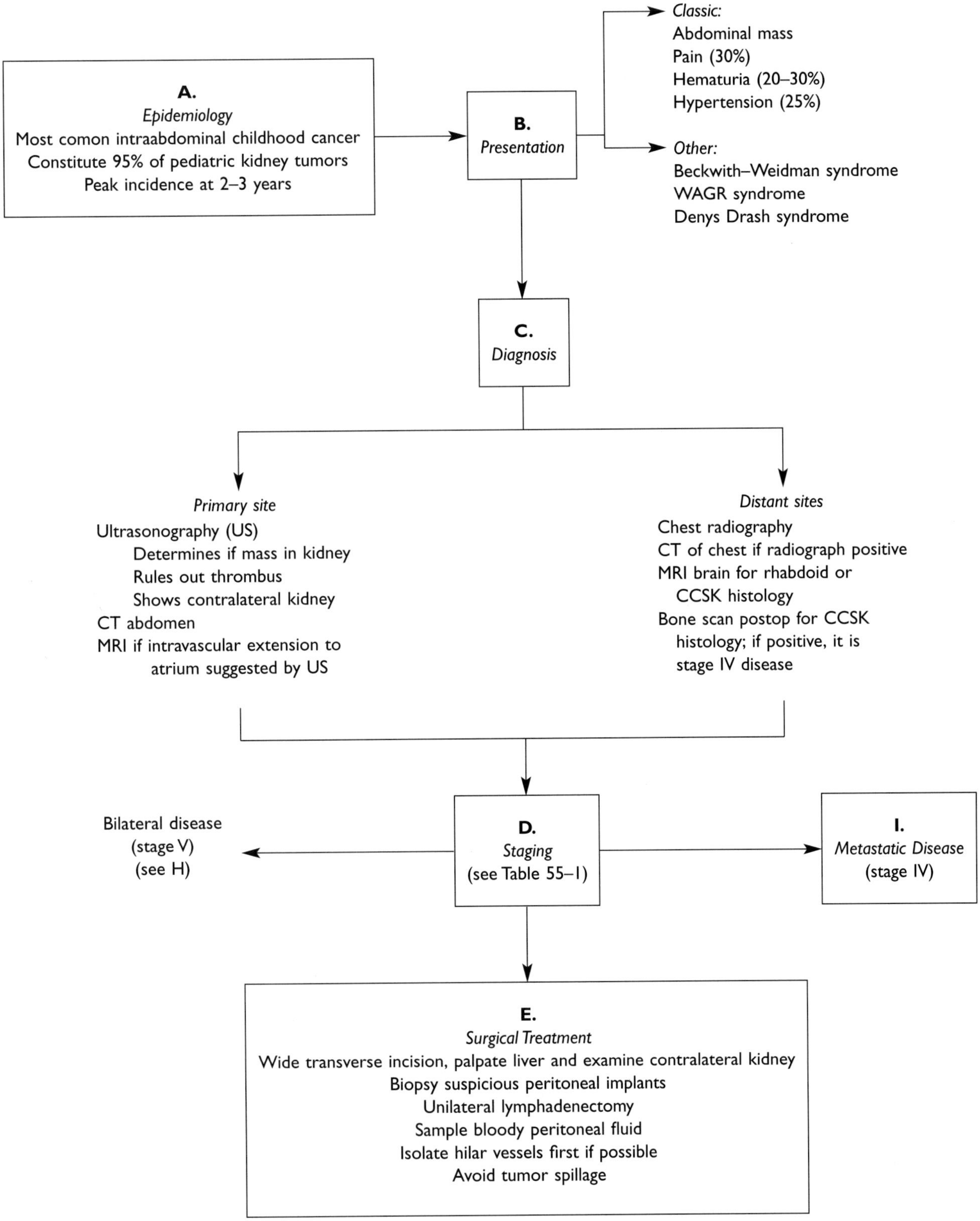

A.
Epidemiology
Most comon intraabdominal childhood cancer
Constitute 95% of pediatric kidney tumors
Peak incidence at 2–3 years

B.
Presentation

Classic:
Abdominal mass
Pain (30%)
Hematuria (20–30%)
Hypertension (25%)

Other:
Beckwith–Weidman syndrome
WAGR syndrome
Denys Drash syndrome

C.
Diagnosis

Primary site
Ultrasonography (US)
- Determines if mass in kidney
- Rules out thrombus
- Shows contralateral kidney

CT abdomen
MRI if intravascular extension to atrium suggested by US

Distant sites
Chest radiography
CT of chest if radiograph positive
MRI brain for rhabdoid or CCSK histology
Bone scan postop for CCSK histology; if positive, it is stage IV disease

D.
Staging
(see Table 55–1)

Bilateral disease
(stage V)
(see H)

I.
Metastatic Disease
(stage IV)

E.
Surgical Treatment
Wide transverse incision, palpate liver and examine contralateral kidney
Biopsy suspicious peritoneal implants
Unilateral lymphadenectomy
Sample bloody peritoneal fluid
Isolate hilar vessels first if possible
Avoid tumor spillage

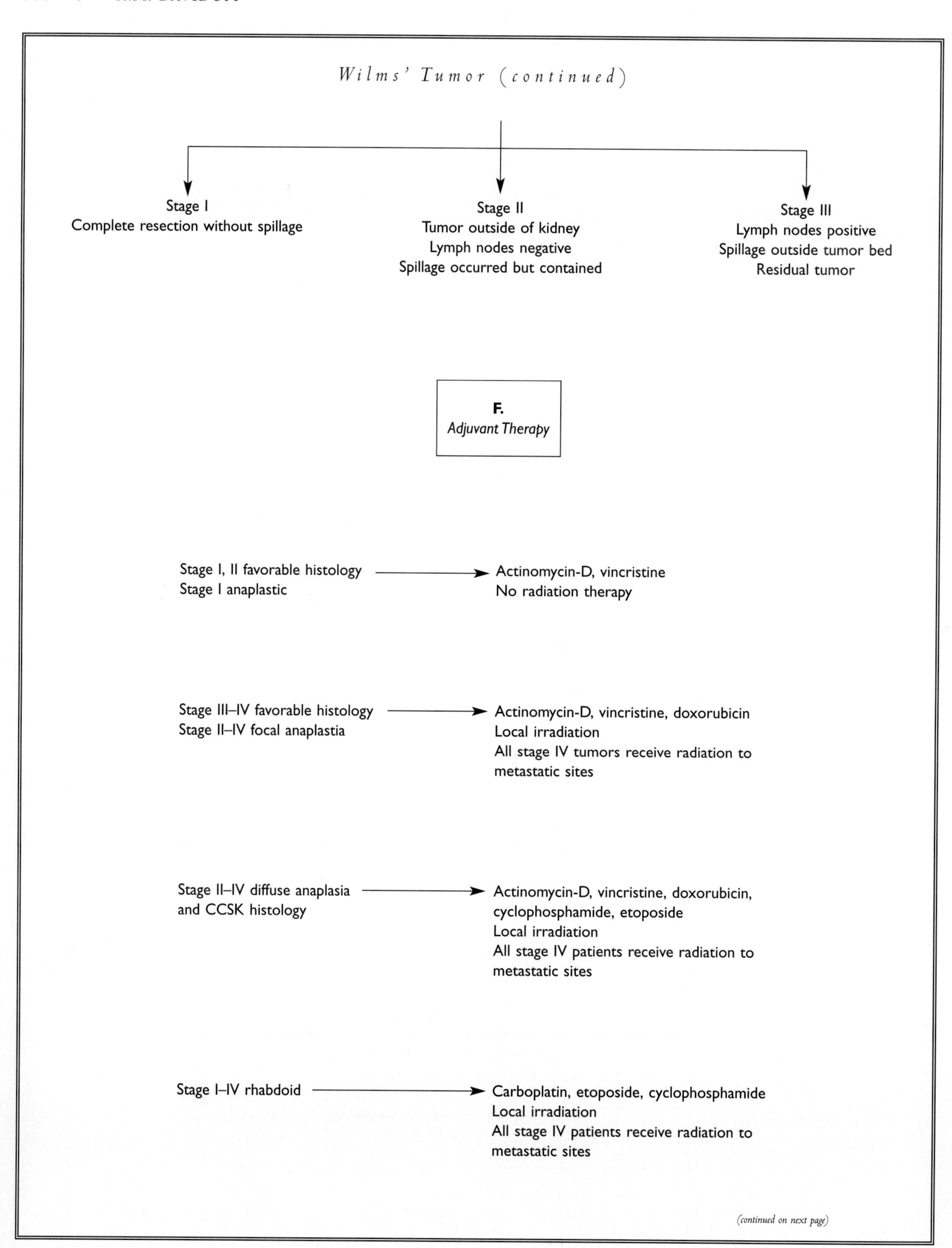

(continued on next page)

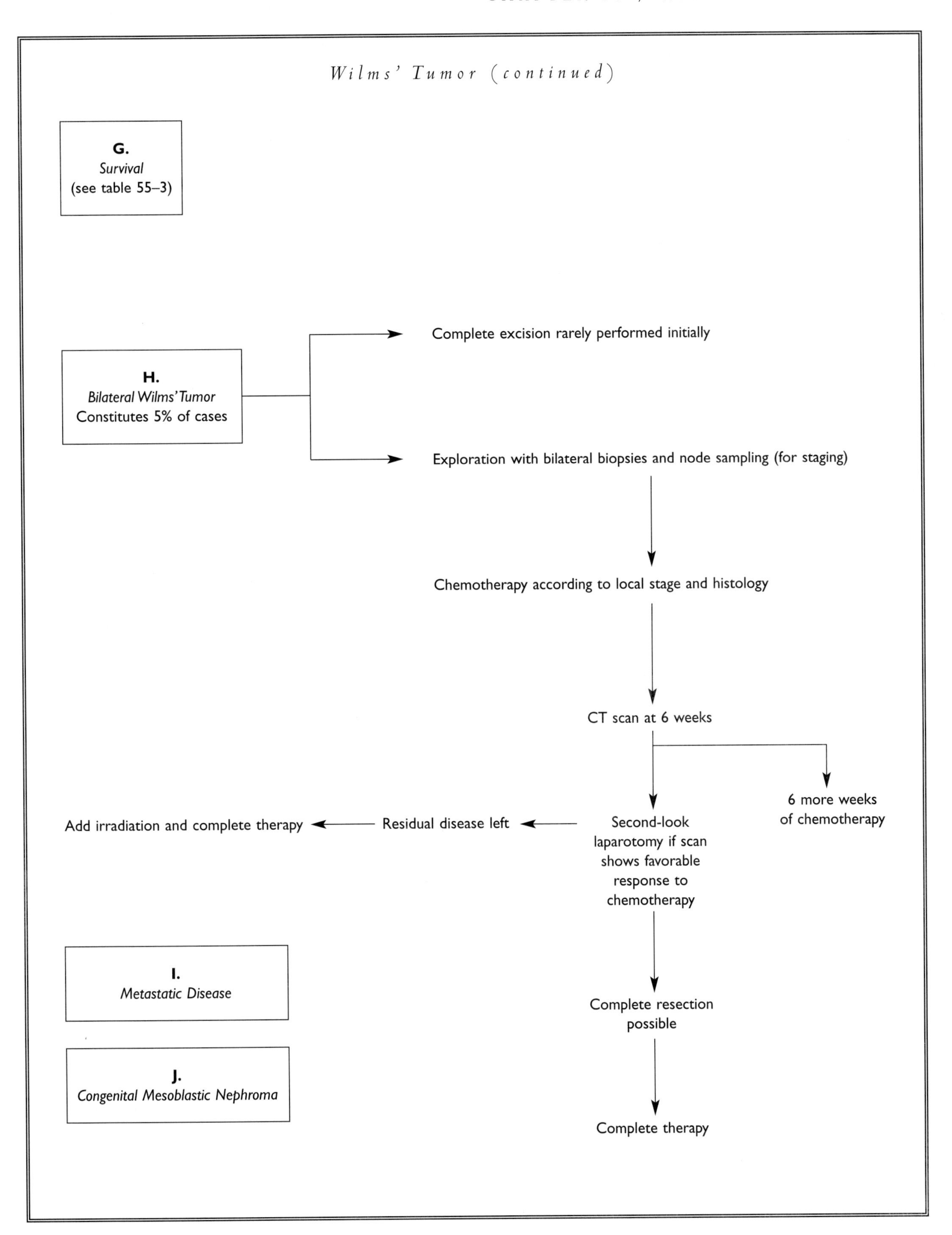
Wilms' Tumor (continued)
G.
Survival
(see table 55–3)
H.
Bilateral Wilms' Tumor
Constitutes 5% of cases
Complete excision rarely performed initially
Exploration with bilateral biopsies and node sampling (for staging)
Chemotherapy according to local stage and histology
CT scan at 6 weeks
Second-look laparotomy if scan shows favorable response to chemotherapy
6 more weeks of chemotherapy
Residual disease left
Add irradiation and complete therapy
Complete resection possible
Complete therapy
I.
Metastatic Disease
J.
Congenital Mesoblastic Nephroma

in children. The first successful nephrectomy for Wilms' tumors was performed in 1877 but it was not until the early 1900s that surgery became effective therapy for this tumor. In 1941, Ladd and Gross, utilizing a transabdominal approach, reported a survival of 24%. When radiation was given after surgery, Gross and Neuhauser noted an increased survival up to 47% in 1950.

B. Presentation

Children with Wilms' tumor typically present with an asymptomatic abdominal mass. It is not uncommon for the tumor to be discovered by a parent while bathing the child or by a relative who notices a protuberant abdomen. Associated signs and symptoms such as malaise, pain, and either microscopic or gross hematuria are found in approximately 20–30% of the children. Hypertension presumably due to increased renin activity is present in approximately 25% of children with Wilms' tumor. Occasionally a child presents with a rapidly enlarging abdominal mass, anemia, hypertension, pain, and fever. These children usually have a subcapsular hemorrhage in the tumor that leads to these symptoms.

Although most Wilms' tumors are sporadic, others occur as part of a number of clinical syndromes and are therefore potentially detectable with screening programs. The *Beckwith-Weidmann syndrome* consists of a number of abnormalities that include macroglossia, macrosomia, hypoglycemia, visceromegaly, and omphalocele in addition to a predisposition to a number of tumors, most commonly Wilms' tumor. Patients with the rare congenital *WAGR syndrome* have aniridia, genitourinary malformations, and mental retardation as well as Wilms' tumor. Another syndrome associated with Wilms' tumor is *Denys-Drash syndrome*. Patients with this syndrome have severe genitourinary abnormalities (e.g., male pseudohermaphroditism) and renal failure secondary to progressive, diffuse glomerular nephropathy; 50–90% of these patients develop Wilms' tumor.

C. Diagnosis

The workup of a child with a suspected Wilms' tumor should proceed in a systematic fashion. The differential diagnosis primarily includes Wilms' tumor and neuroblastoma; and as such, imaging studies should be limited to those necessary to establish the presence of an intrarenal lesion.[6] Usually this distinction is relatively easy, as a Wilms' tumor is intrarenal and causes a characteristic intrinsic abnormality of the urinary collecting system. Neuroblastomas arise within the adrenal gland or the paravertebral sympathetic ganglia, and these masses displace rather than distort the kidney. Benign conditions included in the differential diagnosis are multicystic kidneys, obstructive uropathy, and renal carbuncles. Wilms' tumor presenting as an abdominal mass on the left side must be distinguished from an enlarged spleen.

Real-time ultrasonography can determine whether the mass is intrarenal or extrarenal and whether it is cystic or solid in consistency. Ultrasonography can also determine the presence and extent of thrombus within the renal vein or inferior vena cava. Although ultrasonography also determines the presence of a contralateral kidney, an intravenous pyelogram (IVP) or CT scan is necessary to determine its function. Echocardiography should be performed if there is any suggestion of a tumor thrombus extending into the right atrium.

Computed tomography (CT) scans should be performed if the surgeon believes that added information is required before proceeding with surgery. Patients who present with abdominal pain, for example, often have late-stage disease, usually due to tumor rupture. This subset of patients should undergo an abdominal CT scan to determine the resectability of the tumor (Fig. 55–1). Magnetic resonance imaging (MRI) can also provide further information but is frequently not helpful unless there is suspected intravascular extension of tumor, in which case MRI is probably the most sensitive imaging study available at the present time.

Because the lungs are a frequent site of metastatic disease, posteroanterior and lateral chest radiographs should be obtained. CT scans of the chest are not indicated in patients with a negative chest radiograph, as small nodules detected on CT scan are usually benign. Because of this the NWTS recommends that treatment decisions be based on the local stage of the tumor as determined at operation in patients whose pulmonary lesions were detected only by CT scan (negative chest radiograph). If

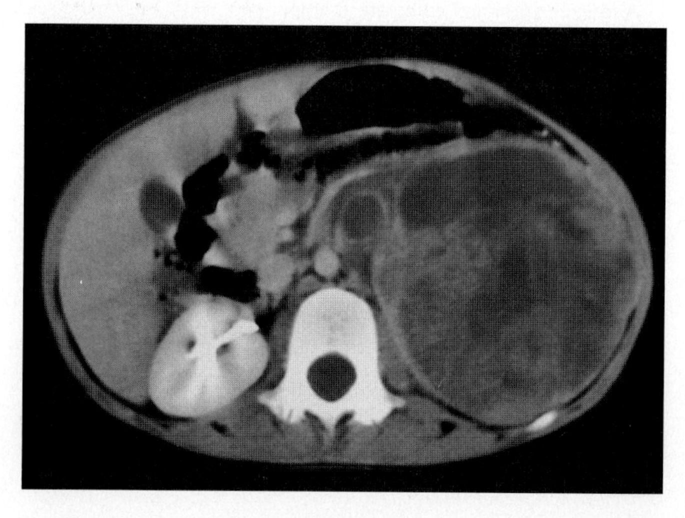

FIGURE 55–1
Computed tomography scan showing a large Wilms' tumor arising in the left kidney.

the tumor histology is rhabdoid or CCSK, MRI of the brain should be performed postoperatively and a skeletal survey or bone scan carried out.

D. Staging

Accurate staging of patients with Wilms' tumor is imperative, and the staging system developed by the NWTS (Table 55–1) has received wide acceptance in the United States. Thorough abdominal exploration should be carried out because the presence of disease beyond the kidney significantly affects therapy and the prognosis. The liver and contralateral kidney should be carefully investigated. The presence of peritoneal implants or bloody peritoneal fluid and the presence or absence of enlarged lymph nodes should be noted. Careful lymph node sampling is important, as the presence of nodal involvement along the periaortic or inferior vena caval lymph node chain is associated with an increased incidence of tumor relapse and a poorer prognosis. Because a review of lymph node sampling by the NWTS demonstrated a false-negative rate of 31% and a false-positive rate of 18%, even clinically negative lymph nodes along the aorta and inferior vena cava should be carefully sampled as well as any suspicious lymph nodes detected at the time of the resection.

TABLE 55–1.
NWTS—4 staging system

Stage	Criteria
I	Tumor limited to kidney and completely excised. Surface of the renal capsule is intact. Tumor was not ruptured before or during removal. There is no residual tumor apparent beyond the margins of excision.
II	Tumor extends beyond the kidney but is completely excised. There is regional extension of the tumor (i.e., penetration through the outer surface of the renal capsule into perirenal soft tissues). Vessels outside the kidney substance are infiltrated or contain tumor thrombus. The tumor may have been biopsied, or there has been local spillage of tumor limited to the flank. There is no residual tumor apparent at or beyond the margins of excision.
III	Residual nonhematogenous tumor is confined to the abdomen. Any one or more of the following occur. 1. Lymph nodes on biopsy are found to be involved in the hilus, the periaortic chains or beyond. 2. There has been diffuse peritoneal contamination by tumor (e.g., by spillage of tumor beyond the flank before or during surgery) or by tumor growth that has penetrated the peritoneal surface. 3. Implants are found on the peritoneal surfaces. 4. Tumor extends beyond the surgical margins microscopically or grossly. 5. Tumor is not completely resectable because of local infiltration into vital structures.
IV	Hematogenous metastases are present. Deposits are beyond stage III (i.e., lung, liver, bone, brain).
V	Bilateral renal involvement is seen at diagnosis. An attempt is made to stage each side according to the above criteria on the basis of extent of disease prior to biopsy.

NWTS, National Wilms' Tumor Study.

Treatment

E. Surgical Treatment

The role of surgery in the therapy of Wilms' tumor is paramount, as a meticulous, well performed procedure accurately determines stage and subsequent therapy. A poorly performed procedure can lead to inadequate therapy if patients are not appropriately staged or to unnecessarily intensive therapy if operative spill of the tumor occurs or resection of the primary tumor is incomplete. The main responsibility of the surgeon is to remove the primary tumor completely, without spillage, and to accurately assess the extent to which the tumor has spread. A radical nephrectomy should be carried out through a generous transverse, transperitoneal incision; a thoracic extension may be necessary but has been associated with a higher complication rate. Any suspicious lesions that may represent metastases should be biopsied. The contralateral kidney should be visualized and palpated to rule out bilateral involvement prior to resection of the primary tumor if technically feasible. Unsuspected small foci of tumor in the contralateral kidney have been reported even in patients with negative imaging studies.

The hilar vessels should be isolated prior to mobilizing the primary tumor if possible. However, initial ligation of the hilar vessels should not be pursued if technically difficult or dangerous, as major vascular injury to the superior mesenteric artery, celiac vessels, and aorta have been reported. This complication has been seen especially with large left-sided tumors and is preventable if the tumor is adequately mobilized before ligation of the renal artery and vein. Lymph node sampling is imperative, as mentioned previously, and any involved or suspicious lymph nodes should be excised. Titanium clips should be used to mark the tumor bed. Biopsy of the primary tumor should not be carried out prior to removal, and a meticulous dissection to avoid rupture of the tumor capsule with spillage of tumor cells is imperative. Because staging is affected by the degree of spillage if it occurs, careful control of the extent of contamination is important. Localizing the spillage to the tumor bed allows a stage II classification rather than stage III in patients with diffuse peritoneal spillage. This distinction is extremely important, as stage III patients require total-abdomen irradiation and addition of doxorubicin to the chemotherapy regimen. During tumor resection the ureter is ligated and divided as low as possible, but complete removal of the ureter down to the bladder is not necessary.

Wilms' tumors rarely invade surrounding structures but frequently adhere to adjacent organs. If the tumor cannot be cleanly separated from adjacent structures, the tumor with surrounding structures can be excised in continuity if the surgeon believes that all tumor tissue can be completely removed. Because patients with a small volume of residual disease (stage III) respond well to chemotherapy and an increased incidence of complications has been associated with tumor resections that include adjacent structures, radical resection is indicated only if all of the tumor can be removed. This issue of resecting adjacent organs is an important one in light of the intensity of therapy required for stage III tumors.

Preoperative tumor rupture is sometimes encountered, and bloody peritoneal fluid should be considered a sign of major spillage in the peritoneal cavity. Rupture posteriorly without hemorrhage or hematoma is classified as stage II (provided all gross disease is removed without spillage); but when a hematoma occurs in association with operative rupture, microscopic residual disease is assumed (stage III). In the case of hepatic invasion, part of the liver along with the primary tumor can usually be resected. A formal hepatectomy is rarely indicated.

Vena caval and intraatrial extension of Wilms' tumor occurs in approximately 4% of patients. Survival does not appear to be affected, and the prognosis is comparable stage by stage to that for children without intravascular involvement. Thrombus should be identified prior to operation, which is usually possible utilizing real-time ultrasonography, echocardiography, and possibly MRI scanning. Surgical excision of the primary tumor and thrombus is recommended when technically feasible. An intraabdominal approach is sufficient for infrahepatic lesions, with extraction of the caval thrombus after proximal and distal control of the vena cava is obtained. Use of a Fogarty or Foley catheter balloon may be required. Patients with free-floating thrombi that are easily removed are classified as having stage II disease, but those with thrombi that either invade the vessel or are markedly adherent to the vessel wall are classified as stage III. Exposure of the inferior vena cava (IVC) as it enters the atrium can be obtained through a thoracoabdominal incision or through the membranous portion of the diaphragm. The IVC is isolated and occluded at the atrium, and the tumor thrombus is removed through an infrahepatic incision in the vena cava. Patients with atrial extension of a tumor thrombus require cardiopulmonary bypass for thrombus removal. A midline abdominal incision with a median sternotomy can be used. Alternatively, strong consideration should be given to use of preoperative chemotherapy, as discussed below.

F. Adjuvant Therapy

The roles for chemotherapy and radiation therapy have evolved based on results of the NWTS trials. The first NWTS showed that postoperative abdominal radiotherapy was not necessary for children who are less that 2 years of age with tumors limited to the kidney that were completely resected. In addition, the combination of vincristine and actinomycin D was shown to be more effective for treating children with tumors that extend beyond the kidney than either drug alone. The second NWTS demonstrated that 6 months of combination chemotherapy with vincristine and actinomycin D was effective treatment for children with tumors limited to the kidney that were completely resected; none of these children underwent abdominal irradiation. The addition of doxorubicin to the combination of vincristine and actinomycin D improved the relapse-free survival of other patients. The separation of Wilms' tumor into distinct histopathologic categories based on prognosis was used to stratify patients in the third NWTS.[7] The fourth NWTS examined the utility of dose-intensive scheduling to reduce the duration of therapy.[8] Based on the results of these trials, a single-arm therapeutic trial has been defined for the fifth NWTS (Table 55–2). The goal of this trial is to evaluate the prognostic value of certain biologic markers in Wilms' tumor. This information, such as loss of heterozygosity of 16q or 1p, or increased DNA content, can then be used to further stratify patients in future therapy trials.[9]

Radiation therapy is administered to the tumor bed for all rhabdoid and clear cell sarcoma tumors as well as stage II–IV

TABLE 55–2.
Protocol for National Wilms' Tumor Study—5

Stage of tumor	Radiotherapy (local)	Chemotherapy
Stage I, II, FH, and stage I anaplastic	None	Pulse-intensive AMD plus VCR (18 weeks)
Stage III, IV FH, and stage II–IV focal anaplastic	Yes[a]	Pulse-intensive AMD, VCR, and DOX (24 weeks)
Stage II–IV diffuse anaplasia and CCSK	Yes[a]	Regimen I[b]
Stage I–IV rhabdoid tumor of the kidney	Yes[a]	Regimen RTK[c]

CCSK, clear cell carcinoma of the kidney; FH, favorable histology; AMD, actinomycin D; VCR, vincristine; DOX, doxorubicin.

[a] Stage IV FH patients are given local irradiation based on the local tumor stage. All stage IV patients receive irradiation to metastatic sites.

[b] Regimen I: AMD, VCR, DOX, cyclophosphamide, etoposide.

[c] Regimen RTK: carboplatin, etoposide, cyclophosphamide.

anaplastic tumors. Stage III favorable histology tumors also receive radiation therapy to the tumor bed. In all cases the field of irradiation is increased to include areas of adenopathy, tumor thrombus, and tumor spillage as well as sites of distant metastasis. Patients with stage IV favorable histology tumors undergo local irradiation as dictated by the local stage of the tumor.

One of the main controversies in the treatment of Wilms' tumor is whether to administer *preoperative chemotherapy* as suggested by the International Society of Pediatric Oncology (SIOP). Such therapy can complicate staging and histologic evaluation, and it can potentially lead to overtreatment or undertreatment. The dangers of undertreatment were suggested by an SIOP study that showed an increased incidence of infradiaphragmatic relapses in patients who did not receive postoperative radiation therapy. Furthermore, preoperative chemotherapy may down-stage a tumor by treating metastatic lymph nodes, which creates confusion as to the exact stage of a patient (i.e., II vs. III) and how chemotherapy and radiation should be used postoperatively. If this problem is to be avoided, radiation therapy should be given to all of these children, or the potential cardiotoxic drug doxorubicin must be added to the postoperative chemotherapy regimen. Side effects of radiation therapy are well recognized, as are the toxic side effects of the various chemotherapeutic agents.[10] In addition, the occurrence of second malignant neoplasms must be considered for individuals receiving combined-modality therapy. Another potential hazard of preoperative therapy is that the histologic appearance of the primary tumor may be altered and resemble unfavorable anaplastic histology at the time of nephrectomy, which would lead to unnecessary intensification of therapy.

Proponents of preoperative therapy suggest that the tumor is easier to resect with a decreased incidence of tumor spill and lower morbidity and mortality. However, the morbidity and mortality following tumor resection in the NWTS was extremely low, and the incidence of tumor spill should be less than 10%. In addition, local tumor spill alters therapy very little (if the spill is confined), as these patients are classified as having stage II disease according to NWTS protocols.

Another argument used for preoperative therapy is that renal units can be spared and the so-called hyperfiltration syndrome can be prevented. There is little evidence to support the concept that preoperative therapy allows partial nephrectomy in a significant number of patients treated in this manner, and the problem of hyperfiltration injury following unilateral nephrectomy in children is rare and poorly documented.

Despite the arguments given above against the use of preoperative therapy, specific patient groups can be identified who may benefit. These are patients with bilateral tumors, IVC and intraatrial involvement,[11] or massive tumors considered by the operating surgeon to be unresectable without undue risk to the patient. If preoperative therapy is considered, a needle biopsy to confirm the diagnosis of Wilms' tumor is imperative, as an error rate of 5–9% has been reported. In children with bilateral Wilms' tumor both sides must be biopsied, as the histology may be favorable on one side and unfavorable on the other.

G. Survival

The overall survival for patients with Wilms' tumors is higher than 95%. Surgery is the mainstay of treatment, although the addition and refinement of chemotherapy have had a profound effect on the improved survival rates. The most important prognostic variables are histology and stage.[12] Survival statistics based on these factors are shown in Table 55–3. Guidelines for follow-up of patients treated for Wilms' tumor are outlined in Table 55–4.

H. Bilateral Wilms' Tumors

Bilateral Wilms' tumors occur in approximately 5% of affected children. These patients tend to present at an early age and have an increased frequency of genitourinary anomalies and hemihypertrophy.[13] Despite sophisticated diagnostic techniques, the contralateral lesion is not known preoperatively in approximately one-third of patients. Unfavorable histology is seen in 10%, and there is discordant histology in a significant number of cases. Of importance is the fact that the larger tumor does not necessarily contain the unfavorable histologic type. This finding underscores the importance of biopsying both lesions prior to therapy.

The present NWTS recommendation for the treatment of bilateral Wilms' tumors stresses the importance of preserving

TABLE 55–3.
Four-year survival for patients with Wilms' tumor

Stage	Survival (%)
Favorable histology	
I	99
II	97
III	99
IV	90
Anaplastic (diffuse) histology	
I	90
II[a]	70
III[a]	56
IV[a]	17

[a] Regimen included vincristine, dactinomycin, doxorubicin and cyclophosphamide.
SOURCE: Adapted from Green et al.[5,8]

TABLE 55–4.
Imaging studies for follow-up of children with renal neoplasms of proven histology and free of metastases at diagnosis

Tumor type	Study	Schedule following primary therapy
Mesoblastic nephroma (MN)[a]	Abdominal US	q 3months × 6
Wilms' tumor/favorable histology, all patients, and stage I anaplastic disease	Chest films	6 weeks and 3 months postop; then q 3months × 5, q 6months × 3, yearly × 2
Irradiated patients only	Bony structure (e.g., LS spine ± pelvis[b])	Yearly to full growth, then q 5years indefinitely[c]
Without nephrogenic rests, stages I and II	Abdominal US	Yearly × 3
Without nephrogenic rests, stage III	Abdominal US	As for chest films
With nephrogenic rests, any stage[d]	Abdominal US	q 3months × 10 q 6months × 5, yearly × 5
Stage II and III anaplastic Wilms' tumor	Chest films	As for favorable histology
	Abdominal US	q 3months × 4: q 6months × 4
Renal cell carcinoma	Chest films	Like favorable histology
	Skeletal survey and bone scan	Like CCSK
Clear cell sarcoma (CCSK)	Brain MRI and/or opacified CT	When CCSK is established, q 6months × 10
	Skeletal survey and bone scan	As for favorable histology
	Chest films	
Rhabdoid tumor	Brain MRI and/or opacified CT	As for CCSK
	Chest films	As for favorable histology

US, ultrasonography; CT, computed tomography; MRI, magnetic resonance imaging.

[a] Data from the files of Dr. J. B. Beckwith reveal that 20 of 293 MN patients (7%) relapsed or had metastases at diagnosis; 4 of the 20 in the lungs, one of the four at diagnosis. All but one of the 19 relapses occurred within 1 year. Chest films for MN patients may be elected on a schedule such as every 3 months × 4, every 6 months × 2.

[b] To include any irradiated osseous structures.

[c] To detect second neoplasms, benign (osteochondromas) or malignant.

[d] The panelists at the first International Conference on Molecular and Clinical Genetics of Childhood Renal Tumors, Albuquerque, New Mexico, May 1992, recommended a variation: q 3months for 5 years or until age 7, whichever comes first.

SOURCE: From D'Angio et al.,[6] with permission.

renal units.[14] A transperitoneal operation is carried out, but initial nephrectomy is avoided. The histologic subtype and stage of both tumors is determined by bilateral biopsy and lymph node sampling. Wedge resection may be considered if two-thirds or more of the total renal parenchyma can be preserved. Postoperative chemotherapy with actinomycin D and vincristine is administered. The response to therapy should be evaluated approximately 6 weeks after initiating chemotherapy. A CT scan should be performed at this time to assess the reduction in tumor volume and the feasibility of partial resection. A second-look procedure can be carried out if resection is feasible. At the time of the second-look procedure, partial nephrectomy or wedge resection of the tumors should be performed so long as the margins are not compromised. If there is extensive tumor involvement precluding partial resection of one kidney, nephrectomy is performed on that side and a wedge resection performed on the contralateral kidney. If persistent tumor remains, a third-look procedure can be performed and all residual tumor removed if possible. If the third abdominal exploration confirms the presence of unresectable disease, the patient should then undergo radiation therapy to the involved areas. Bench surgery, in which the entire kidney is removed, the tumor excised, and the remaining tumor-free kidney returned to the patient, may be considered in difficult cases and can be combined with intraoperative radiation therapy. Patients with bilateral Wilms' tumor require long-term follow-up, as relapses have occurred as late as 5 years following treatment, and renal failure has been seen in approximately 5% of patients.

I. Metastatic Disease

The treatment of metastatic disease depends on the time at which metastases are diagnosed and the pathology of the primary tumor. Patients with stage IV favorable histology tumors at diagnosis have a good prognosis, whereas those with unfavorable histology and those who relapse with metastatic disease have a grave prognosis. Approximately 12% of Wilms' tumor patients have evidence of hematogenous metastases at diagnosis, and 20% of favorable histology patients relapse following therapy.

About 80% of stage IV patients have pulmonary metastases and are usually treated with combined chemotherapy and radiation therapy.[15] Pulmonary resection is rarely indicated because chemotherapy is extremely effective.

The presence of liver metastases at diagnosis should not alter the therapy of the primary tumor. As mentioned earlier, major hepatic lobectomy in conjunction with radical nephrectomy is rarely required and should be reserved for selected cases. Although the presence of liver metastases at initial diagnosis does not significantly alter the prognosis, metachronous relapse in the liver carries a grave prognosis with or without hepatic resection. If an isolated liver metastasis is detected and there is no evidence of extrahepatic disease, hepatic resection should be considered. Unfortunately, this is a rare occurrence.

J. Congenital Mesoblastic Nephroma

Congenital mesoblastic nephroma is a relatively benign tumor of infants usually less than 3 months of age. Although true Wilms' tumors do occur in infants, they are rare. The treatment of mesoblastic nephroma should be total excision using the same surgical guidelines as described for Wilms' tumor. Chemotherapy of congenital mesoblastic nephroma should be reserved for cases with incomplete resection or in which there was intraoperative rupture. The chemotherapy protocol used for these cases should follow the recommendations for favorable histology stage I Wilms' tumor.

References

1. Shochat SJ. Wilms' tumor: diagnosis and treatment in the 1990's. Semin Pediatr Surg 1993;2:59–68.
2. Li EF. Cancers in children. In: Schottenfeld D, Fraumeni JF Jr (eds) Cancer Epidemiology and Prevention. Philadelphia: Saunders, 1982;1012–1024.
3. Breslow NE, Beckwith JB. Epidemiological features of Wilms' tumor: results of the National Wilms' Tumor Study. J Natl Cancer Inst 1982;68: 429–436.
4. Beckwith JB, Palmer NF. Histopathology and prognosis of Wilms' tumor. Cancer 1978;41:1927–1948.
5. Green DM, Beckwith JB, Breslow NE, et al. Treatment of children with stages II–IV anaplastic Wilms' tumor: a report from the National Wilms Tumor Study Group. J Clin Oncol 1994;12:2126–2131.
6. D'Angio GJ, Rosenberg H, Sharples K, et al. Imaging methods for primary renal tumors of childhood: cost versus benefits. Med Pediatr Oncol 1993;21:205–213.
7. D'Angio GJ, Breslow, N, Beckwith JB, et al. Treatment of Wilms' tumor: results of the Third National Wilms' Tumor Study. Cancer 1989;64: 349–360.
8. Green DM, Breslow NE, Beckwith JB, et al. Comparison between single-dose and divided-dose administration of dactinomycin and doxorubicin for patients with Wilms' tumor: a report from the National Wilms' Tumor Study Group. J Clin Oncol 1998;16:237–245.
9. Grundy PE, Telzerow PE, Breslow N, et al. Loss of heterozygosity for chromosomes 16q and 1p in Wilms' tumors predicts an adverse outcome. Cancer Res 1994;54:2331–2333.
10. Evans AE, Norkool P, Evans MS, et al. Late effects of treatment of Wilms' tumor: a report from the National Wilms' Tumor Study. Cancer 1991; 67:331–336.
11. Ritchey ML, Kelalis PP, Haase GM, et al. Preoperative therapy for intracaval and atrial extension of Wilms' tumor. Cancer 1993;71:4104–4110.
12. Breslow NE, Sharples K, Beckwith JB, et al. Prognostic factors in nonmetastatic, favorable histology Wilms' tumor. Cancer 1991;68:2345–2353.
13. Blute ML, Kelalis PP, Offord KP, et al. Bilateral Wilms' tumor. J Urol 1987;138:968–973.
14. Horwitz JR, Ritchey ML, Moksness J, et al. Renal salvage procedures in patients with synchronous bilateral Wilms' tumors: a report from the National Wilms' Tumor Study Group. J Pediatr Surg 1996;31:1020–1025.
15. Green DM, Breslow N, Ii Y, et al. The role of the surgicla excision in the management of Wilms' tumor patients with pulmonary metastases: a report from the National Wilms' Tumor Study. J Pediatr Surg 1991;16: 728–733.

Chapter 56

Neuroblastoma

MARC L. CULLEN

A. Epidemiology

Neuroblastoma is the most common solid tumor seen during infancy. It accounts for half of all cancer cases in children less than 2 years old and has a mean age of 22 months at presentation. It represents 8–10% of all childhood malignancies and is the cause of 15% of all pediatric cancer deaths. The tumor is rare in adults, who have a worse outcome despite similar stages and therapy.[1] Neuroblastoma is a unique malignancy with biologic diversity and widely disparate prognoses. It has the highest spontaneous rate of regression and yet is metastatic in more than 50% of cases at the time of presentation.

Embryologically, neuroblastoma arises from neural crest tissue, which forms the sympathetic ganglia and adrenal medulla. Neuroblastomas, which can occur anywhere from the base of the skull to the dome of the bladder, are associated with other neurocrestopathies, such as neurofibromatoses, Hirschsprung's disease, and Ondine's curse (central hypoventilation syndrome).[2] These tumors exhibit three distinct clinical behaviors: spontaneous regression (2–5%),[3] spontaneous differentiation into a benign form, and invasive malignant behavior with lymphatic and hematogenous spread in the older child. There are three distinct histologic patterns—neuroblastoma, ganglioneuroblastoma, ganglioneuroma—reflecting a spectrum of maturation, differentiation, and clinical behavior. The combination of clinical presentation, age, stage, histology, and genetic and biologic factors determine the choice of treatment and ultimately the outcome. Despite significant improvements in care and a clearer understanding of tumor biology, the prognosis for the older child with disseminated disease remains dismal.

B. Presentation

Neuroblastoma may present with a variety of symptoms and may arise at various locations. Most are located in the abdomen and are discovered during a workup for abdominal pain or incidentally by a parent when the child bathes. Thoracic tumors may be found on a chest radiograph performed to evaluate a persistent cough. Neurologic symptoms such as weakness progressing to paraplegia may indicate

Neuroblastoma

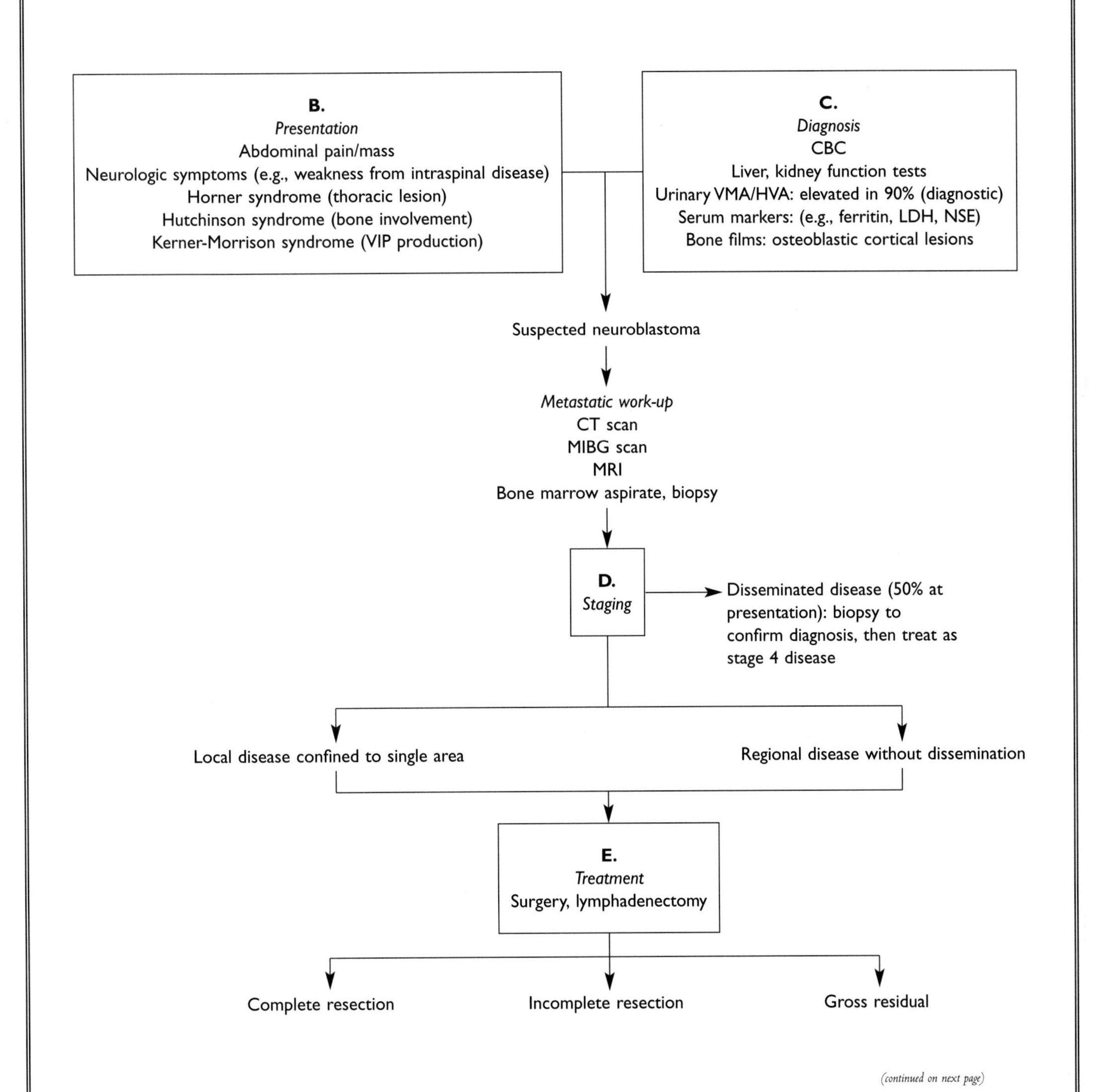

(continued on next page)

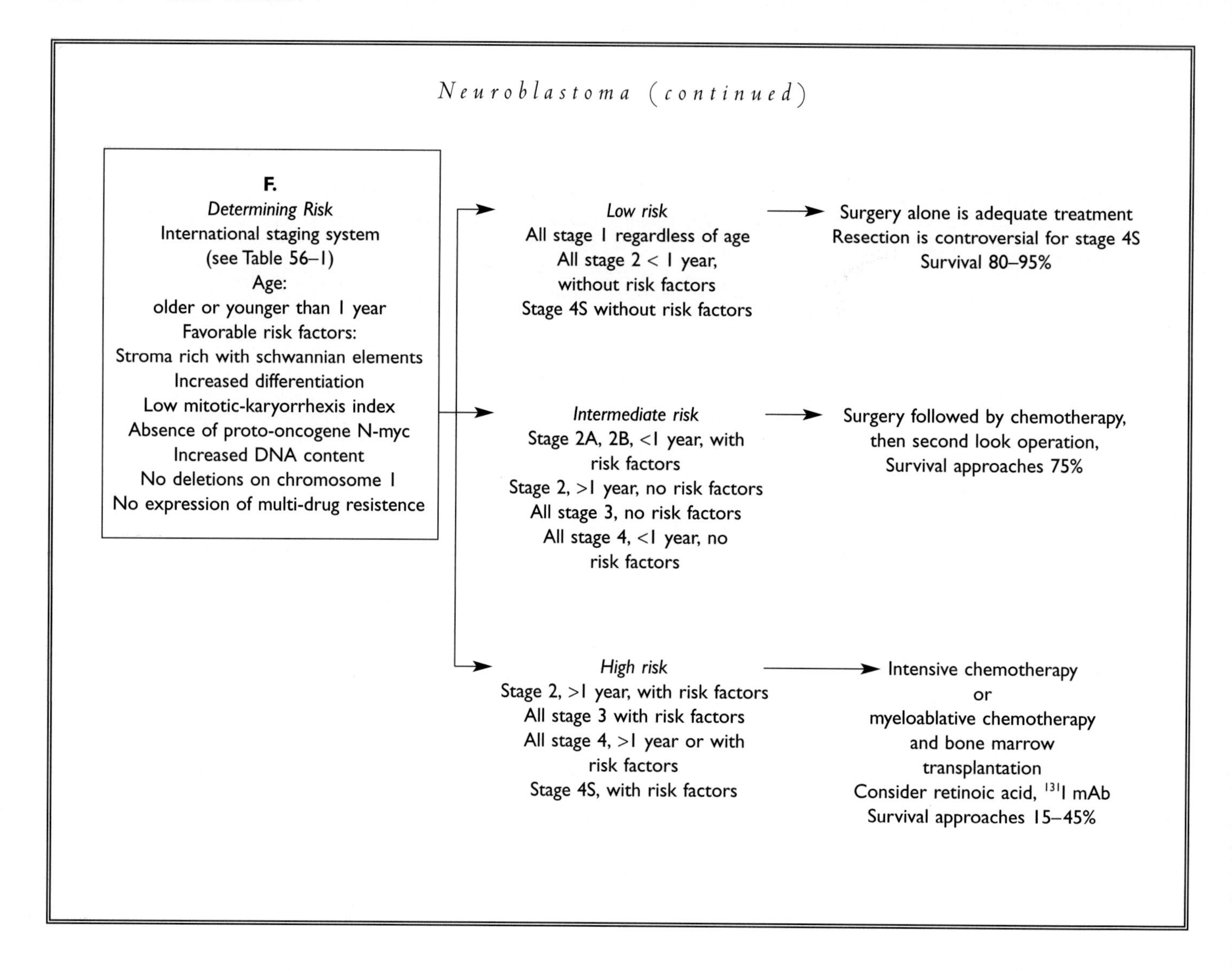

intraspinal extension of a "dumbbell" thoracic tumor causing extradural spinal cord compression. Horner syndrome (ptosis, myosis, anhidrosis) may signal the presence of a cervicothoracic mass. Changes in bowel and bladder function may result from nerve root or direct organ compression by large pelvic tumors. Rapidly enlarging abdominal tumors or massive hepatomegaly in infants may cause respiratory distress by compressing the diaphragm. Fever, bone pain, and a limp (Hutchinson syndrome) may be evidence of neuroblastoma metastatic to bone. Bluish skin and subcutaneous nodules comprise a unique pattern of metastases in infants with advanced disease. Cerebellar ataxia, myoclonic jerking motions, and darting eye movements (opsomyoclonus) require careful evaluation for neuroblastoma.[4] Watery diarrhea, dehydration, and hypokalemia (Kerner-Morrison syndrome) are associated with vasoactive intestinal peptide (VIP) production by the primary tumor.[5]

Neuroblastoma can mimic many common pediatric disorders. Cervical tumors can be confused with torticollis or infectious lymphadenopathy. "Raccoon eyes" associated with retroorbital metastases and pathologic fractures may be mistaken for abuse. Fever, anemia, and bone pain may be confused with arthritis, osteomyelitis, leukemia, or Ewing's sarcoma. Hepatomegaly may be confused with other solid tumors or glycogen storage disease. The common clinical features shared by these conditions may explain why only one-third of patients are diagnosed within the first month after symptoms appear.[6] History and physical examination including a careful neurologic examination and rectal examination should be performed. The review of systems should include a search for weight loss, malaise, genitourinary problems, gait disturbances, and diarrhea.

C. Diagnosis

Laboratory Tests

Laboratory tests include a complete blood count (CBC), and liver and renal function tests. Urinary products of catecholamine metabolism [vanillylmandelic acid/homovanillic acid) (VMA/HVA)] are found in 90% of cases and elevations 3 SD above age norms are diagnostic of neuroblastoma.[7] Radiographs may show a mass effect or calcific stippling. Cortical bone lesions can be seen on a skeletal survey. These bone lesions are osteoblastic and demonstrate increased isotopic activity by scan. An ultrasound scan can confirm the presence and character of the primary mass. Serum markers that include ferritin (>140 ng/ml), lactate dehydrogenate (LDH) (>1500 IU/L), and neuron-specific enolase (NSE) (>100 ng/ml) are nonspecific indices of tumor burden and may be used to follow the response to therapy.[8–10] Chromogranin A and G_{D2} ganglioside can be detected in 80–90% of patients' sera and correlate with disease stage and tumor burden.[11,12]

Metastatic Workup

An extent-of-disease workup is used for clinically staging a suspected neuroblastoma. Computed tomography (CT) scanning (faster and more easily available) and magnetic resonance imaging (MRI) (better for pelvis, mediastinum, and spine) are used to determine tumor location, local invasion, lymphatic enlargement, paravertebral extension, and metastatic spread. Metaiodobenzylguanidine (MIBG) scanning is both sensitive and specific for primary and metastatic disease and is better for assessing bone and soft tissue. A bone marrow evaluation including aspirate and biopsy from bilateral sites confirms metastatic disease in up to 50% of patients at the time of diagnosis.[13] Hepatic or pulmonary involvement when suspected is assessed by CT or MRI.

D. Staging

Clinical staging results in three distinct categories of disease: (1) local disease, confined to a single anatomic area without evidence of metastatic spread; (2) regional disease, with more extensive tumor without metastatic spread; and (3) disseminated disease. Fully 50% of tumors are metastatic at the time of initial diagnosis. Despite increasingly sophisticated techniques, clinical and radiologic assessment are not entirely accurate, and there is a discrepancy between clinical and surgical stage in up to 38% of cases.[14]

E. Treatment

The role of surgery is to establish an accurate diagnosis and to excise tumor when possible. Additionally, surgery must distinguish localized from disseminated disease, assess lymph nodes (25% variance between clinical and pathologic status), and provide tissue for assignment of biologic risk.[15] Total gross excision improves outcome, but when it is performed in a primary setting it should avoid sacrificing critical nerves, vessels, and organs (kidney). En bloc resections are not required for primary operations. For larger, more vascular lesions surgery may be delayed until after chemotherapy has been completed; biopsy in this instance shows the effects of therapy. Hopefully, delayed surgery renders patients with initially advanced-stage disease tumor-free. The philosophy at the time of delayed primary or secondary surgery is different; in this setting the surgical approach is more aggressive and may involve en bloc organ removal, as the ultimate resectability of the tumor determines outcome.[16]

Complications of surgery occur in 10–20% of cases.[17] These tumors are large, friable, and vascular; and they are often wrapped around adjacent vital structures, encasing vessels and nerves. Separation of the tumor from these structures may require violation of the apparent tumor capsule and dissection in or on the adventitial wall. Aggressive attempts at resection may cause injuries to systemic and mesenteric vessels. Hemorrhage, intraoperative hypotension, and death have resulted from overly aggressive resections at both primary and secondary operations. Nephrectomy incidental to en bloc resection or as a result of vascular injury has been reported.[18] Neurologic injury and paraplegia can occur as the result of devascularization of the spinal cord or from attempts at controlling dural space bleeding.[19] These complications are more common in infants, who for the most part have better survival. The incidence of surgical complications may be reduced when resection is delayed until a tumor is rendered less friable, less vascular, and more fibrotic by chemotherapy.[20]

Initial exploration completes the surgical staging, allows stratification of similar tumors into their appropriate treatment group, and provides criteria by which therapy can be adjusted to match the risk of recurrence. Accurate surgical staging also allows prognostication about outcome and comparison of clinical trials. Staging of neuroblastoma has traditionally been by three systems (Table 56–1). The Evans system emphasizes the extent of disease relative to the anatomic midline.[21] The St. Jude system emphasizes the results of surgery and lymphatic involvement.[22] The International Neuroblastoma Staging System (INSS) attempts to unify the Evans and St. Jude systems and purports to define the importance of the anatomic midline, tumor resectability, and the impact of lymph node involvement.[7] All of these systems accurately identify the patient with low-stage disease who has a high probability of survival (90%) and those with high-stage disease who have a poor prognosis despite aggressive therapy (30%). The INSS may help to discriminate among intermediate-risk patients and to direct appropriate therapy. Although surgical and pathologic staging systems endeavor to predict outcome accurately and identify optimal treatment regimens, they fall short of their goals because they are restricted to assessing the tumor primarily at a macroscopic

TABLE 56–1.
Neuroblastoma staging systems

Evans classification	St. Jude classification	INSS
Stage I: Tumor confined to the organ of origin.	*Stage A*: Complete gross resection of the primary tumor. Intracavitary lymph nodes not adherent to the primary tumor; microscopically free. Nodes adherent to the surface of or within the primary may be positive. Liver free of tumor.	*Stage 1*: Localized tumor. Complete gross excision. Ipsilateral and contralateral lymph nodes microscopically negative.
Stage II: Tumor extending beyond the organ or origin, but not crossing the midline. Regional lymph nodes on the ipsilateral side may be involved.	*Stage B*: Grossly unresected primary tumor. Nodes and liver the same as in stage A.	*Stage 2A*: Unilateral tumor with incomplete gross excision. Identifiable ipsilateral and contralateral lymph nodes microscopically negative. *Stage 2B*: Unilateral tumor with complete or incomplete gross excision. Positive ipsilateral regional lymph nodes; identifiable contralateral lymph nodes microscopically negative.
Stage III: Tumor extending beyond the midline. Regional lymph nodes may be involved bilaterally.	*Stage C*: Complete or incomplete resection of primary. Intracavitary nodes not adherent to primary; histologically positive for tumor. Liver as in stage A.	*Stage 3*: Tumor infiltrating across the midline with or without regional lymph node involvement; *or* unilateral tumor with contralateral lymph node involvement; *or* midline tumor with bilateral lymph node involvement.
Stage IV: Remote disease involving the skeleton, bone marrow, soft tissue, and distant lymph nodes.	*Stage D*: Dissemination of disease beyond intracavitary nodes (i.e., extracavitary nodes, liver, skin, bone marrow, bone).	*Stage 4*: Dissemination of tumor to bone, bone marrow, liver, distant lymph nodes, and/or other organs (except as defined for stage 4S).
Stage IV-S: As defined in stage I or II, with remote disease confined to the liver, skin, or bone marrow (without cortical bone metastases).	*Stage DS*: Infants <1 year of age with Evans' stage IV-S disease.	*Stage 4S*: Localized primary tumor as defined for stage 1 or 2 with dissemination limited to liver, skin, and/or bone marrow.

INSS, International Neuroblastoma Staging System.
SOURCE: Brodeur et al.,[7] Evans et al.,[21] and Hayes et al.[22]

level. Prediction of outcomes with neuroblastoma requires assessment of the biologic risk.

F. Determining Risk

Clinically useful assessments of biologic risk include an assessment of tumor genetics and DNA content (DNA index), oncogene products (N-*myc*), and histology (Shimada classification). Age also appears to act as an important risk modifier in higher-stage disease.

Histology

Assignment of biologic risk starts with assessing tumor histology. Favorable histology as defined by Shimada includes a nodular stroma rich with Schwannian elements, increased differentiation, and a low mitosis/karyorrhexis index (MKI) (<200).[23] The presence of a proto-oncogene known as N-*myc*, when amplified (30% of primary tumors), predicts rapid tumor progression and poor outcome.[24] DNA content assessed by flow cytometry results in two distinct patterns. Tumors with an increased DNA content (DNA index >1) exhibit a favorable response to chemotherapy and a better prognosis regardless of stage. In contrast, children with diploid tumors (DNA index = 1) have advanced-stage disease, respond poorly to chemotherapy, and have a less favorable outcome.[25] In addition to histopathology, N-*myc* amplification, and the DNA index, other predictive biologic markers have been identified. Deletions on chromosome 1 (loss of heterozygosity, or LOH) result in the absence of a suppressor gene and apparently allow malignant progression.[26] Genes coding for a multidrug resistance protein (MDRP) are associated with N-*myc* amplification and predict poor survival.[27] Nerve growth factor (NGF) and its high-affinity receptor (TRK-A) are associated with neural cellular differentiation and regression of neuroblastoma. High levels of the receptor gene are associated with a favorable outcome.[28]

Treatment According to Risk Category

Surgery remains the mainstay of therapy for low risk disease, whereas chemotherapy is the primary treatment for advanced disease. Chemotherapeutic agents commonly used are cyclophosphamide and its congener ifosamide, vincristine, doxorubicin, the epipodophyllotoxins teniposide (VM-26) and etoposide (VP-16), and the platins (cisplatin and carboplatin). These agents have been effectively used singly and in combination.[29] Multiagent therapy takes advantage of drug synergy and may prevent resistance. Induction therapy attempts to deplete tumor cells rapidly, arrest tumor growth, and prevent or impede tumor spread. A consolidation phase is given to eradicate residual tumor. Higher doses over shorter times increase the response rates but also increase complications. Intensive chemotherapy protocols have increased response rates but have not significantly changed long-term survival for advanced disease.[29,30] Protocols using intensive myeloablative chemotherapy followed by hematologic reconstitution with allogeneic or autologous marrow have increased survival to 45% for patients with disseminated disease. Bone marrow purging with filtration and anti-neuroblastoma monoclonal antibodies appears to reduce tumor cells significantly without removing hematopoietic stem cells.[31] These therapies appear to be more effective if begun before disease progression has occurred.[32]

Radiation therapy is currently used infrequently. It can be used as an alternative to chemotherapy to produce a rapid relief of symptomatic spinal cord compression. It is also used in low doses for stage IVS-in infants with hepatomegaly who have significant respiratory distress. Radiation therapy may help control regional tumor of the poor prognosis stage 3 patient over 1 year of age. It may also be used for stage IV patients as an adjunct to myeloablative therapy prior to bone marrow transplantation.[33] Tumor-specific radiotherapy using ^{125}I or ^{131}I-MIBG has been shown to produce a response rate of 30%.[34] Toxicity has been related to thrombocytopenia and appears to be more severe after bone marrow transplant.

Low Risk

The lowest risk group (INSS) includes all the stage 1 patients and all the stage 2 (2A/2B) patients without biologic risk factors (RF-negative) and the stage 4S infants who are RF-negative. The management strategy for these low risk patients is surgery and supportive care. Infants with stage 4S disease should be managed on an individual basis; resection of the primary tumor is controversial.[35,36] Many of these patients do well with supportive care alone. Severe hepatomegaly causing respiratory distress is treated with low-dose chemotherapy or radiation therapy. Three times as many infants die of therapy-related complications as die from metastatic disease.[37] Intraspinal extension, nodal metastases, and the occasional recurrence is managed by chemotherapy. Overall survival varies between 80% and 95%.

Intermediate Risk

Patients at intermediate risk include all stage 3 (INSS) patients who are RF-negative, stage 4 patients less than 1 year of age who are RF-negative, and arguably stage 2A/2B patients over 1 year of age who are RF-negative. These patients are treated with chemotherapy and second-look surgery. Radiation does not appear to add any survival benefit. Overall survival approaches 75%.

High Risk

Patients at high risk include stage 2 patients (INSS) over 1 year of age who are RF-positive, all stage 3 patients who are RF-positive, all stage 4 patients who are over 1 year of age or RF-positive, and the rare instances of stage 4S infants who are RF-positive. These patients require intensive chemotherapy or myeloablative chemotherapy and bone marrow transplantation. Surgery to control the primary tumor following chemotherapy may be beneficial.[36] The use of retinoic acid, which induces tumor differentiation following chemotherapy, appears to prolong survival significantly.[38] ^{131}I-labeled monoclonal antibodies to neuroblastoma cells followed by bone marrow transplantation has achieved a 25% response in a small series (two of eight patients).[39] The overall survival with advanced-stage, high risk disease is 15–45%.

Other Neuroblastoma Detection Methods

Antenatal ultrasonography and infant screening programs are two relatively new pathways for neuroblastoma detection. Current data from a large North American study shows that screening detects neuroblastoma with favorable characteristics that may have been destined to undergo spontaneous regression. There was no reduction in advanced-stage neuroblastoma in older children, suggesting that overall survival may not be affected by screening.[40]

Prenatal detection of neuroblastoma by ultrasonography has become more frequent.[41,42] These patients are considered to have stage 4S disease and should undergo a postnatal ultrasonography and be clinically staged. These tumors are managed conservatively so long as they remain small, show no spinal involvement, and do not cause hepatomegaly that interferes with ventilation.

Children with neuroblastoma remain a challenge to surgeons involved in their care. Staging and definitive therapy requires a carefully planned, individualized approach ranging from a simple biopsy and access device for chemotheropopy to extensive, complex resections of bulky residual disease after chemotherapy. Future challenges include refining the role of surgery in stage 4 and 4S disease, designing less toxic chemotherapy, pursuing immune-mediated tumor regression, and exploiting the biologic and genetic characteristics of the tumor to enhance suppression and differentiation. This may ultimately improve outcomes that have changed little for the patient with advanced disease.

References

1. Young JLJ, Ries LG, Silverberg E, Horm JW, Miller RW. Cancer incidence, survival, and mortality for children younger than age 15 years. Cancer 1986;58(Suppl) 601–602.
2. Stovroff M, Dykes F, Teague WG. The complete spectrum of neurocristopathy in an infant with congenital hypoventilation, Hirschsprung's disease, and neuroblastoma. J Pediatr Surg 1995;30:1218–1221.
3. Everson TC, Cole WH. Spontaneous regression of neuroblastoma. In: Everson TC, Cole WH (eds) Spontaneous Regression of Cancer. Philadelphia: Saunders, 1966:88.
4. Solomon GE, Chutorian AM. Opsoclonus and occult neuroblastoma. N Engl J Med 1968;279:475–477.
5. Mitchell CH, Sinatra FR, Crast FW, Griffin R, Sunshine P. Intractable watery diarrhea, ganglioneuroblastoma, and vasoactive intestinal peptide. J Pediatr 1976;89:593–595.
6. Wilson LM, Draper GJ. Neuroblastoma, its natural history and prognosis: a study of 487 cases. BMJ 1974;3:301–307.
7. Brodeur GM, Seeger RC, Barrett A, et al. International criteria for diagnosis, staging, and response to treatment in patients with neuroblastoma. J Clin Oncol 1988;6:1874–1881.
8. Tsuchida Y, Honna T, Iwanaka T, et al. Serial determination of serum neuron-specific enolase in patients with neuroblastoma and other pediatric tumors. J Pediatr Surg 1987;22:419–424.
9. Hann HW, Evans AE, Siegel SE, et al. Prognostic importance of serum ferritin in patients with stages III and IV neuroblastoma: the Childrens Cancer Study Group experience. Cancer Res 1985;45:2843–2848.
10. Joshi VV, Cantor AB, Brodeur GM, et al. Correlation between morphologic and other prognostic markers of neuroblastoma: a study of histologic grade, DNA index, N-myc gene copy number, and lactic dehydrogenase in patients in the Pediatric Oncology Group. Cancer 1993;71:3173–3181.
11. Hsiao RJ, Seeger RC, Yu AL, O'Connor DT. Chromogranin A in children with neuroblastoma: serum concentration parallels disease stage and predicts survival. J Clin Invest 1990;85:1555–1559.
12. Valentino L, Moss T, Olson E, Wang HJ, Elashoff R, Ladisch S. Shed tumor gangliosides and progression of human neuroblastoma. Blood 1990; 75:1564–1567.
13. Mills AE, Bird AR. Bone marrow changes in neuroblastoma. Pediatr Pathol 1986;5:225–234.
14. Foglia R, Fonkalsrud E, Feig S, Moss T. Accuracy of diagnostic imaging as determined by delayed operative intervention for advanced neuroblastoma. J Pediatr Surg 1989;24:708–711.
15. Wilson ER, Altshuler G, Smith EI, et al. Gross observation does not predict regional lymph node metastasis in the surgicopathologic staging of neuroblastoma [abstract]. Proc Am Soc Clin Oncol 1989;8:304.
16. Haase GM, Wong KY, deLorimier AA, Sather HN, Hammond GD. Improvement in survival after excision of primary tumor in stage III neuroblastoma. J Pediatr Surg 1989;24:194–200.
17. Azizkhan RG, Shaw A, Chandler JG. Surgical complications of neuroblastoma resection. Surgery 1985;97:514–517.
18. Shamberger RC, Smith EI, Joshi VV, et al. The risk of nephrectomy during local control in abdominal neuroblastoma. J Pediatr Surg 1998;33: 161–164.
19. Boglino C, Martins AG, Ciprandi G, Sousinha M, Inserra A. Spinal cord vascular injuries following surgery of advanced thoracic neuroblastoma: an unusual catastrophic complication. Med Pediatr Oncol 1999;32:349–352.
20. Berthold F, Utsch S, Holschneider AM. The impact of preoperative chemotherapy on resectability of primary tumor and complication rate in metastatic neuroblastoma. Z Kinderschir 1985;44:21.
21. Evans AE, D'Angio GJ, Randolph J. A proposed staging for children with neuroblastoma: Children's Cancer Study Group A. Cancer 1971;27: 374–378.
22. Hayes FA, Green A, Hustu HO, Kumar M. Surgicopathologic staging of neuroblastoma: prognostic significance of regional lymph node metastases. J Pediatr 1983;102:59–62.
23. Chatten J, Shimada H, Sather HN, Wong KY, Siegel SE, Hammond GD. Prognostic value of histopathology in advanced neuroblastoma: a report from the Children's Cancer Study Group. Hum Pathol 1988;19:1187–1198.
24. Seeger RC, Brodeur GM, Sather H, et al. Association of multiple copies of the N-myc oncogene with rapid progression of neuroblastomas. N Engl J Med 1985;313:1111–1116.
25. Look AT, Hayes FA, Shuster JJ, et al. Clinical relevance of tumor cell ploidy and N-myc gene amplification in childhood neuroblastoma: a Pediatric Oncology Group study. J Clin Oncol 1991:9:581–591.
26. Caron H, vanSluis P, DeKraker J, et al. Allelic loss of chromosome 1p as a predictor of unfavorable outcome in patients with neuroblastoma. N Engl J Med 1996;334:225–230.
27. Norris MD, Bordow SB, Marshall GM, Haber M. Expression of the gene for multidrug-resistance-associated protein and outcome in patients with neuroblastoma. N Engl J Med 1996;334:231–238.
28. Nakagawara A, Arima-Nakagawara M, Scavarda NJ, Azar CG, Cantor AB, Brodeur GM. Association between high levels of expression of the TRK gene and favorable outcome in human neuroblastoma. N Engl J Med 1993;328:847–854.
29. Cheung NV, Heller G. Chemotherapy dose intensity correlates strongly with response, median survival, and median progression-free survival in metastatic neuroblastoma. J Clin Oncol 1991;9:1050–1058.
30. Morgan ER, Gaynon PS, Herzog P, et al. A pilot study of "6 in 1" chemotherapy for poor prognosis neuroblastoma [abstract]. Proc Am Soc Clin Oncol 1988;7:266.
31. Seeger RC, Villablanca JG, Matthay KK, et al. Intensive chemoradiotherapy and autologous bone marrow transplantation for poor prognosis neuroblastoma. In: Evans AE, D'Angio G, Knudson AG, Seeger RC (eds) Advances in Neuroblastoma Research. New York: Wylie/Liss, 1991: 527–533.
32. Pole JG, Casper J, Elfenbein G, et al. High-dose chemoradiotherapy supported by marrow infusions for advanced neuroblastoma: a Pediatric Oncology Group study. J Clin Oncol 1991;9:152–158. Erratum. J Clin Oncol 1991;9:1094.
33. August CS, Serota FT, Koch PA, et al. Treatment of advanced neuroblastoma with supralethal chemotherapy, radiation, and allogeneic or autologous marrow reconstitution. J Clin Oncol 1984;2:609–616.

34. Voute PA, Hoefnagel CA, DeKraker J, Valdez Olmos R. Results of treatment with 131-I-MIBG in patients with neuroblastoma; future prospects. In: Evans A, D'Angio GJ, Knudson AG, Seeger RC (eds) Advances in Neuroblastoma Research. New York: Wiley/Liss, 1991;439–445.
35. Martinez DA, King DR, Ginn-Pease ME, Haase GM, Wiener ES. Resection of the primary tumor is appropriate for children with stage IV-S neuroblastoma: an analysis of 37 patients. J Pediatr Surg 1992;27:1016–1020.
36. La Quaglia MP, Kushner BH, Heller G, Bonilla MA, Lindsley KL, Cheung NK. Stage 4 neuroblastoma diagnosed at more than 1 year of age: gross total resection and clinical outcome. J Pediatr Surg 1994;29:1162–1165.
37. Evans AE, Baum E, Chard R. Do infants with stage IV-S neuroblastoma need treatment? Arch Dis Child 1981;56:271–274.
38. Villablanca JG, Khan AA, Avramis VI, et al. Phase I trial of 13-cis-retinoic acid in children with neuroblastoma following bone marrow transplantation. J Clin Oncol 1995;13:894–901.
39. Kemshead JT, Goldman A, Jones D. Therapeutic application of radiolabelled monoclonal antibody UJ13A in children with disseminated neuroblastoma: a phase I study. In: Evans AE, D'Angio G, Seeger RC (eds) Advances in Neuroblastoma Research. New York: Liss, 1985:533–534.
40. Woods WG, Tuchman M, Robison LL, et al. A population-based study of the usefulness of screening for neuroblastoma. Lancet 1996;348:1682–1687.
41. Holgersen LO, Subramanian S, Kirpekar M, Mootabar H, Marcus JR. Spontaneous resolution of antenatally diagnosed adrenal masses. J Pediatr Surg 1996;31:153–155.
42. Ho PT, Estroff JA, Kozakewich H, et al. Prenatal detection of neuroblastoma: a ten-year experience from the Dana-Farber Cancer Institute and Children's Hospital. Pediatrics 1993;92:358–364.

Chapter 57

Pediatric Hepatic Tumors

NICHOLAS C. SAENZ

Abdominal masses in children are usually discovered incidentally; the three most frequently encountered pediatric abdominal malignancies are neuroblastoma, Wilms' tumor, and tumors of the liver (half of which are malignant). Hepatoblastoma is the most common liver tumor followed by hepatocellular carcinoma.[1–3] The current overall survival for hepatoblastoma is 70%, which has risen substantially compared to 33% noted 20 years ago.[4] Chemotherapy has had a dramatic impact on survival, although surgical resection remains the mainstay of therapy and still provides the only chance of cure for both hepatoblastoma and pediatric hepatocellular carcinoma.

A. Clinical Presentation

The median patient age at diagnosis of hepatoblastoma is 1 year, and most patients are diagnosed by 18 months.[5,6] Hepatocellular carcinoma has a bimodal presentation, with the first peak incidence before the fifth year. The second peak occurs between the ages of 12 and 15.[7] Hepatoblastoma tends to occur in boys at a slightly higher ratio of 3:2.[3]

Liver tumors in children commonly present as a painless abdominal mass or generalized abdominal enlargement. As with Wilms' tumors, these children are usually asymptomatic; the masses are discovered by a parent or caregiver during bathing or dressing. Fewer than 25% of patients with hepatoblastoma present with symptoms such as anorexia, weight loss, pain, vomiting, or jaundice.[3] This is in contrast to children with neuroblastoma, who tend to present with systemic symptoms by the time the mass has become large enough to be noticeable.

B. Diagnosis

Laboratory Tests

The most important test for both diagnosis and follow-up of children with liver tumors is the serum α-fetoprotein assay, which is elevated in 80–90% of patients with hepatoblastoma[8] and 50% of patients with hepatocellular carcinoma.[9] Other laboratory tests are relatively nonspecific. Most of the children

Pediatric Hepatic Tumors

Hepatoblastoma is the most common.

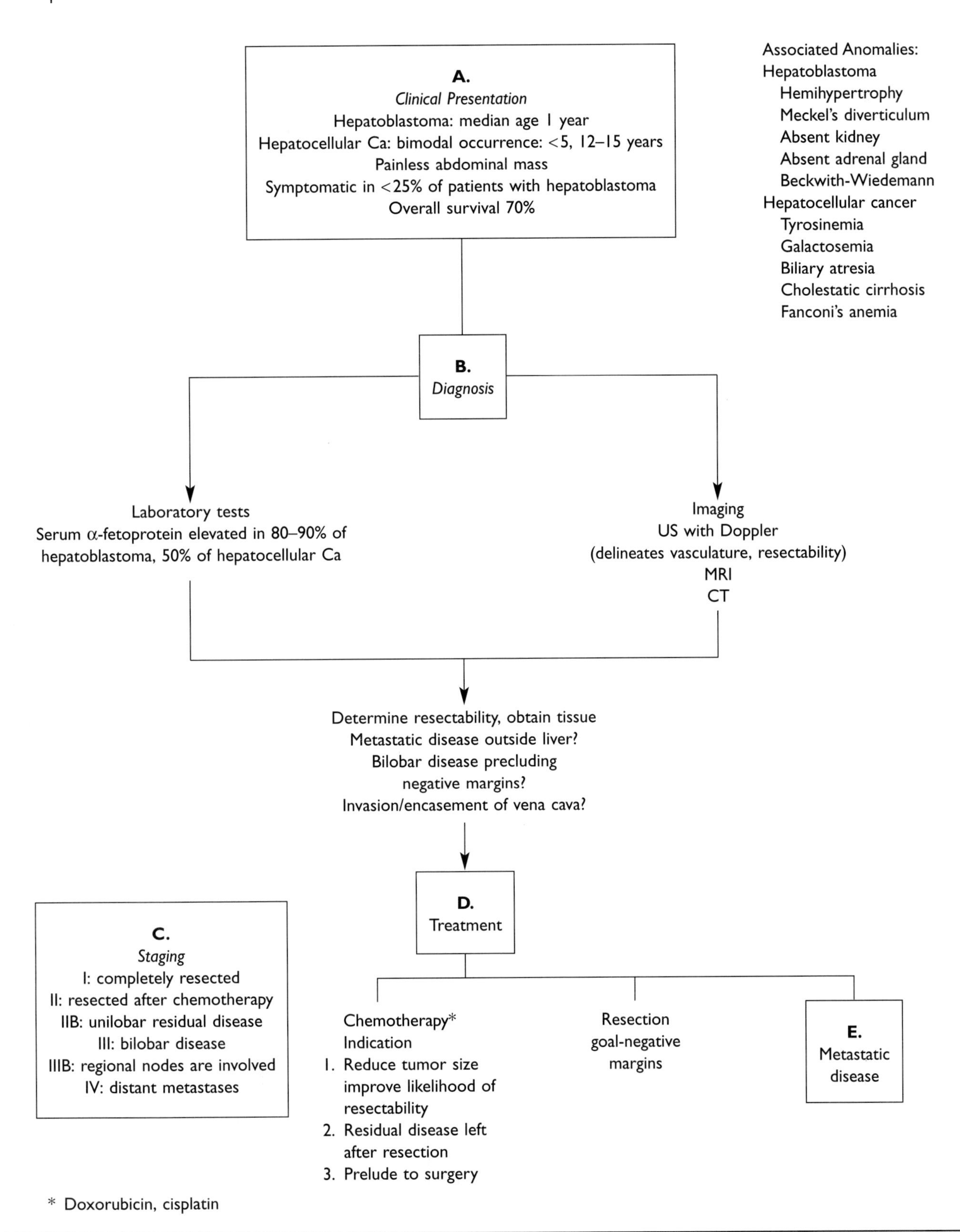

are not jaundiced and do not have an elevated liver transaminase level. Patients rendered disease-free following resection of their hepatoblastoma usually have a marked fall in the serum α-fetoprotein level; therefore it is an excellent marker for following disease recurrence and progression.

Imaging

The differential diagnosis of pediatric abdominal masses includes Wilms' tumor, neuroblastoma, and liver tumors (i.e., hepatoblastoma and hepatocellular carcinoma). Based on the physical examination alone, it may be difficult to determine the organ of origin. A large Wilms' tumor of the right kidney, a neuroblastoma primary located in the right adrenal, and a primary hepatic neoplasm may yield similar physical examinations; therefore, imaging studies should be scheduled immediately. Plain radiographs of the abdomen are likely to be nonspecific, revealing only the presence of a soft tissue mass. Calcifications are often present in neuroblastomas; they are not pathognomonic, as they are occasionally seen in hepatoblastomas (6%) and hepatic hemangiomas (12%).[10] Abdominal ultrasonography is a good screening examination to determine the organ of origin. For patients with Wilms' tumors, high quality Doppler ultrasonography is useful for ruling out tumor thrombus in the renal vein or vena cava.[11] We also routinely employ the Doppler technique prior to liver resection to delineate the hepatic vasculature in relation to the tumor, determine resectability, and determine the extent of the resection required for negative margins.

Computed tomography (CT) and magnetic resonance imaging (MRI) are excellent modalities by which to image a liver tumor and determine resectability; however, neither can accurately predict malignant or benign histology.[12] MRI with gadolinium has been shown to be more helpful for determining resectability, and it has become our imaging modality of choice.[13] However, CT of the chest and abdomen with intravenous contrast can provide useful information as well. An added attractive feature of MRI is the ability to view the tumor in more than one plane; and if MRI is combined with angiography it may help delineate the hepatic vasculature as it relates to potential dissection planes.[14]

Resectability

An area of ambiguity with respect to presentation and management is resectability. The term "unresectable" may convey different meanings depending on the anatomy and surgical expertise. For the sake of this discussion, we define a tumor as "unresectable" at presentation if there is (1) metastatic disease outside the liver; (2) bilobar disease precluding resection with negative margins; or (3) encasement or invasion of the vena cava.

Once the laboratory and imaging studies have been completed, a tissue diagnosis is needed. Tissue sampling may be easily performed by percutaneous needle biopsy with high accuracy and low morbidity without causing tumor spillage or seeding.[15–18] Needle biopsy also avoids the need for general anesthesia and the potential complications associated withextensive dissection in the right upper quadrant. Once the diagnosis is established, a treatment plan may be designed and implemented using a multidisciplinary approach involving pediatric oncologists and pediatric surgeons working together.

C. Staging

Staging is important for predicting prognosis and stratifying patients for inclusion in clinical trials. Clinical grouping after resection has become important for pediatric liver tumors and is based on the extent of the tumor and surgical resection. Patients in group I have undergone complete resection at the time of diagnosis. Patients undergoing resection after chemotherapy are assigned to group II (group IIB if there is unilobar residual disease). Patients are assigned to group III if residual bilobar disease is present and to group IIIB if regional nodes are involved. Finally, group IV includes patients with distant metastases. This is a useful staging system but suffers in that it relies on surgical exploration to complete the staging; it does not identify patients preoperatively who may benefit from neoadjuvant chemotherapy.

D. Treatment of Primary Hepatoblastoma

Chemotherapy

For patients in whom the initial resection is unlikely to yield a negative margin, several chemotherapy regimens significantly reduce tumor size, potentially rendering it resectable. These regimens are platinum-based or doxorubicin-based. In one report using preoperative continuous-infusion doxorubicin ($25\,mg/m^2$/day × 3 days) and cisplatin ($20\,mg/m^2$/day × 5 days) reduced the tumor size (as shown by CT scan) 35–95% in 22 consecutive patients. A minimum of three cycles were completed for each patient. Complete surgical excision was possible in 13 children, including 10 who had previously harbored unresectable tumors and five with pulmonary metastases.[19]

The Children's Cancer Group reported results with continuous-infusion doxorubicin and cisplatin in patients with unresectable or incompletely resected hepatoblastoma. This was a single-arm study of repeated courses of cisplatin $100\,mg/m^2$

over 4 hours followed by continuous-infusion doxorubicin 20 mg/m² for 96 hours. Courses were repeated every 3–4 weeks if the absolute neutrophil count was above 1000/μl and the platelet count was higher than 100,000/μl. Good responses to chemotherapy occurred in 25 of 26 patients with hepatoblastoma. Nine of these patients had previously undergone partial resections prior to chemotherapy and at second-look procedures had no evidence of residual disease.[20] Only one patient's tumor remained unresectable.

Similar results from a European multiinstitutional study were reported with either complete or very good partial responses in most of the children with hepatoblastoma. Cisplatin was administered in Brussels at a dose of 80 mg/m² over 24 hours and at 90 mg/m² over 6 hours in Italy. Doxorubicin was uniformly given at a dose of 60 mg/m² over 48 hours (days 2 and 3). The courses were repeated at weekly intervals, and the response was evaluated after four courses.[21]

In a Pediatric Oncology Group study, a regimen without anthracyclines was investigated to estimate the disease-free survival rate in children with grossly resected hepatoblastoma treated with cisplatin, four courses of vincristine, and fluorouracil (5-FU): cisplatin 90 mg/m² followed by four courses of cisplatin plus vincristine 1.5 mg/m² and 5-FU 600 mg/m². Sixty assessable patients with hepatoblastoma were included. Of 21 patients with stage I or II disease, 19 were free of disease (actuarial survival 90% at 5 years). Of the 31 patients with stage III disease, 24 achieved a complete remission after chemotherapy. Relatively brief exposure to chemotherapy with a nonanthracycline regimen provided excellent disease control for patients with grossly resected tumors. Of the 37 patients whose lesions were deemed initially unresectable, 29 had significant tumor reduction, and 26 went on to have complete surgical resection of the tumor; response and survival rates were comparable to regimens that contain anthracyclines.[22]

A recently published study comparing an anthracycline-based regimen with a non-anthracycline-based regimen was from the Pediatric Intergroup Hepatoblastoma study (Pediatric Cancer Group and Children's Cancer Group). The study looked at children with hepatoblastoma (all stages) and evaluated resectability after four courses of cisplatin 90 mg/m², vincristine 1.5 mg/m² on day 3, and 5-FU 600 mg/m² versus four courses of cisplatin 90 mg/m² and doxorubicin 20 mg/m²/day continuous infusion × 4 days. Overall survival and event-free survival were not significantly different for the two groups.[23]

For newly diagnosed hepatoblastomas, we favor an initial course of cisplatin, vincristine, and 5-FU with radiographic imaging after one course. If tumor progression has occurred, doxorubicin is added to the regimen and repeat imaging is performed after two or three additional courses. Resection is then performed, with the goal being microscopically negative margins. Patients then undergo postoperative chemotherapy. If their tumor was sensitive to the nonanthracycline regimen, this combination is used again postoperatively. Follow-up imaging and serum α-fetoprotein levels are monitored closely on a regular basis.

Unlike those with hepatoblastoma, only one-third of patients with hepatocellular carcinoma have resectable lesions; and of these patients, only one-third are long-term survivors. Doxorubicin-based regimens have successfully obtained partial remissions in only 16–28%.[23,24]

Resection

Resection in children follows the same principles as for liver resection in adults. The primary surgical goal in the treatment of hepatoblastoma or hepatocellular carcinoma is to achieve negative margins; the ability to do so directly affects survival. Hepatic resection in children should be performed only in institutions in which there are anesthesiologists and critical care personnel specializing in the care of children. Because many children undergoing hepatic resection have received chemotherapy prior to resection, special attention must be paid to potential sequelae that may arise as a result of the administration of these agents. For example, if the chemotherapy regimen has included anthracyclines, a preoperative echocardiogram may be necessary to assess left ventricular function.

The principles of venous and arterial access in children are similar to those for adults. Central venous access devices previously used for chemotherapy are adequate for induction of anesthesia and for maintenance fluids; however, because of their relatively small caliber and long length (and therefore high resistance), they are not adequate for rapid transfusion. Two large-bore, upper extremity lines are preferable.

Most liver tumors in children can be approached using an abdominal incision, although on rare occasions a thoracoabdominal incision is necessary. We prefer a chevron incision with a midline vertical extension to the level of the xiphoid process; a Buchwalter retractor allows upward retraction of the costal margins. Once resectability is confirmed, we proceed with mobilization of the liver. Childhood hepatoblastomas are usually located in the right lobe, and right hepatic lobectomy or trisegmentectomy is sufficient to achieve negative margins. Once the liver is mobilized, intraoperative ultrasonography is performed to assess resectability and the proximity of the tumor to the vena cava and hepatic veins. After dissecting the porta hepatis and ligating the accessory hepatic veins, which drain the right lobe directly into the vena cava, the main right hepatic vein is controlled and ligated. A Pringle maneuver is then performed with a soft rubber vessel loop, and hepatic parenchymal division is performed; blood vessels and small biliary ductules are ligated under direct vision. It is important for the surgeon to remain constantly aware of the tumor location, as a negative margin is necessary. This is best done by grasping the lesion in the left hand and fracturing the hepatic parenchyma with the right hand. After the tumor has been removed, frozen sections of adjacent hepatic parenchyma are obtained and examined to ensure that negative margins have been achieved. The raw liver edge is sealed with an argon beam coagulator. We do not routinely place transperitoneal drains. Usually these patients are transported to the pediatric intensive care unit, where they remain while intubated. Once extubated, they are transferred from the intensive care unit and are begun on a clear liquid diet once intestinal peristalsis has returned. The average hospital stay is usually 5–7 days.

E. *Treatment of Pulmonary Metastases*

Approximately 24% of hepatoblastomas present with metastatic disease, with about 10% metastasizing to lung.[25,26] Bone and regional nodes are other common metastatic sites, and on rare occasions one may detect metastases to the kidneys, the epidural space, and other areas. Although most agree that complete resection of the hepatic primary is necessary for cure, there are few data from which to infer the role of metastasectomy. There are data from reported cases of pulmonary metastasectomy for metachronous disease. These cases demonstrate that resection of pulmonary metastases is feasible and associated with significant postthoracotomy disease-free intervals.[27–29] There are no accounts, however, of the total number of patients developing metastases (only those undergoing surgery) or of a comparison to alternative therapy (i.e., chemotherapy or radiotherapy). Significant resolution of synchronous pulmonary metastases with chemotherapy alone has been noted. We therefore recommend pulmonary metastasectomy for primary hepatoblastoma in patients with significant localized disease who have shown a response but not total resolution after induction chemotherapy. The serum α-fetoprotein level can be used to detect relapse in these patients, and its determination is useful when trying to differentiate benign (scar, fungal infection) from malignant pulmonary nodules.

References

1. Young JL Jr, Miller RW. Incidence of malignant tumors in U.S. children. J Pediatr 1975;86:254–258.
2. Randolph JG, Altman RP, Arensman RM, Matlak ME, Leikin SL. Liver resection in children with hepatic neoplasms. Ann Surg 1978;187:599–605.
3. Exelby PR, Filler RM, Grosfeld JL. Liver tumors in children in the particular reference to hepatoblastoma and hepatocellular carcinoma: American Academy of Pediatrics Surgical Section Survey—1974. J Pediatr Surg 1975;10:329–337.
4. Fraumeni JF Jr, Miller RW, Hill JA. Primary carcinoma of the liver in childhood: an epidemiologic study. J Natl Cancer Inst 1968;40:1087–1099.
5. Mahour GH, Wogu GU, Siegel SE, Isaacs H. Improved survival in infants and children with primary malignant liver tumors. Am J Surg 1983;146:236–240.
6. Ishak KG, Glunz PR. Hepatoblastoma and hepatocarcinoma in infancy and childhood: report of 47 cases. Cancer 1967;20:396–422.
7. Dehner LP. Hepatic tumors in the pediatric age group: a distinctive clinical-pathologic spectrum. Perspect Pediatr Pathol 1978;4:217–268.
8. Lack EE, Neave C, Vawter GF. Hepatoblastoma: a clinical and pathologic study of 54 cases. Am J Surg Pathol 1982;6:693–705.
9. Yachnin S. The clinical significance of human alpha-fetoprotein. Ann Clin Lab Sci 1978;8:84–90.
10. Miller JH, Gates GF, Stanley P. The radiological investigation of hepatic tumors in childhood. Radiology 1977;124:451–458.
11. Ohtsuka Y, Takahashi H, Ohnuma N, Tanabe M, Yoshida H, Iwai J. Detection of tumor thrombus in children using color Doppler ultrasonography. J Pediatr Surg 1997;32:1507–1510.
12. Boechat MI, Kangarloo H, Ortega J, et al. Primary liver tumors in children: comparison of CT and MR imaging. Radiology 1988;169:727–732.
13. Finn JP, Hall-Craggs MA, Dicks-Mireaux C, et al. Primary malignant liver tumors in childhood: assessment of resectability with high-field MR and comparison with CT. Pediatr Radiol 1990;21:34–38.
14. Hubbard AM, Meyer JS, Mahboubi S. Diagnosis of liver disease in children: value of MR angiography. AJR Am J Roentgenol 1992;159:617–621.
15. Dekmezian R, Sneige N, Popok S, Ordonez NG. Fine-needle aspiration cytology of pediatric patients with primary hepatic tumors: a comparative study of two hepatoblastomas and a liver-cell carcinoma. Diagn Cytopathol 1988;4:162–168.
16. Wakely PE Jr, Silverman JF, Geisinger KR, Frable WJ. Fine needle aspiration biopsy cytology of hepatoblastoma. Mod Pathol 1990;3:688–693.
17. Bottles K, Cohen MB. An approach to fine-needle aspiration biopsy diagnosis of hepatic masses. Diagn Cytopathol 1991;7:204–210.
18. Das DK, Bhambhani S, Chachra KL, Murthy NS, Tripathi RP. Small round cell tumors of the abdomen and thorax. Role of fine needle aspiration cytologic features in the diagnosis and differential diagnosis. Acta Cytol 1997;41:1035–1047.
19. Filler RM, Ehrlich PF, Greenberg ML, Babyn PS. Preoperative chemotherapy in hepatoblastoma. Surgery 1991;110:591–596.
20. Ortega JA, Krailo MD, Haas JE, et al. Effective treatment of unresectable or metastatic hepatoblastoma with cisplatin and continuous infusion doxorubicin chemotherapy: a report from the Childrens Cancer Study Group. J Clin Oncol 1991;9:2167–2176.
21. Ninane J, Perilongo G, Stalens JP, Guglielmi M, Otte JB, Mancini A. Effectiveness and toxicity of cisplatin and doxorubicin (PLADO) in childhood hepatoblastoma and hepatocellular carcinoma: a SIOP pilot study. Med Pediatr Oncol 1991;19:199–203.
22. Reynolds M, Douglass EC, Finegold M, Cantor A, Glicksman A. Chemotherapy can convert unresectable hepatoblastoma. J Pediatr Surg 1992;27:1080–1084.
23. Melia WM, Johnson PJ, Williams R. Controlled clinical trial of doxorubicin and tamoxifen versus doxorubicin alone in hepatocellular carcinoma. Cancer Treat Rep 1987;71:1213–1216.

24. Chlebowski RT, Brzechwa-Adjukiewicz A, Cowden A, Block JB, Tong M, Chan KK. Doxorubicin (75 mg/m^2) for hepatocellular carcinoma: clinical and pharmacokinetic results. Cancer Treat Rep 1984;68:487–491.
25. Black CT, Luck SR, Musemeche CA, Andrassy RJ. Aggressive excision of pulmonary metastases is warranted in the management of childhood hepatic tumors. J Pediatr Surg 1991;26:1082–1086.
26. King DR, Ortega J, Campbell J, et al. The surgical management of children with incompletely resected hepatic cancer is facilitated by intensive chemotherapy. J Pediatr Surg 1991;26:1074–1081.
27. Lembke J, Havers W, Doetsch N, Rohm N, Sadony V. Long-term results following surgical removal of pulmonary metastases in children with malignomas. Thorac Cardiovasc Surg 1986;34(special no 2):137–139.
28. Ballantine TV, Wiseman NE, Filler RM. Assessment of pulmonary wedge resection for the treatment of lung metastases. J Pediatr Surg 1975;10:671–676.
29. Di Lorenzo M, Collin PP. Pulmonary metastases in children: results of surgical treatment. J Pediatr Surg 1988;23:762–765.

Section  12

Hematologic Malignancies

CHAPTER 58

Hodgkin's Disease

LILY L. LAI
RODERICH E. SCHWARZ

Hodgkin's disease was first described in 1832 when Thomas Hodgkin published a paper describing seven patients with primary nodal pathology. Much has changed during the intervening years with respect to improvements in diagnosis, treatment, and outcome. Although the disorder is treated with the combined modalities of chemotherapy and radiotherapy, the surgeon can play a significant role in the diagnosis and staging of the disease.

Recent data demonstrate a decrease in the incidence of new cases of Hodgkin's disease. In particular, there has been a decrease in the incidence among older patients, perhaps as a result of more accurate diagnosis of non-Hodgkin's lymphoma.[1] Of significance is the improvement in survival in recent years. The 5-year survival rate during the early 1980s was 75% in the white population and 72% in the black population. By the early 1990s the respective 5-year survival rates were 82% and 74%.[2]

A. Diagnosis

Hodgkin's disease is a lymphoproliferative disorder. The clinical presentation is usually that of unexplained, persistent lymph node enlargement that does not respond to antibiotic therapy. Pathognomonic in the histologic diagnosis of Hodgkin's disease is the Reed-Sternberg cell; these enlarged binucleated cells (or variants) are an essential component of the histopathologic diagnostic process and are thought to originate from B lymphocytes.[3] Frequently, these cells are identified amid a background of benign-appearing lymphoid cells. Also associated with the disease are the single nucleated large cells termed Hodgkin's cells. There is still some uncertainty regarding the etiology of the disease. The underlying disease mechanisms cause dysregulation of the immune system, leading to immunodeficiency. If left untreated, fewer than 5% of patients with the disease survive after 5 years.

Hodgkin's disease is classified into four histologic types: lymphocyte-predominant, nodular sclerotic, mixed cellular, and lymphocyte-depleted. Each subtype is associated with a different prognosis and treatment (Table 58–1).

Hodgkin's disease in a patient with peripheral lymphadenopathy can be diagnosed using fine-needle aspiration (FNA). The test is safe, relatively pain-free, and easily performed in the outpatient office.

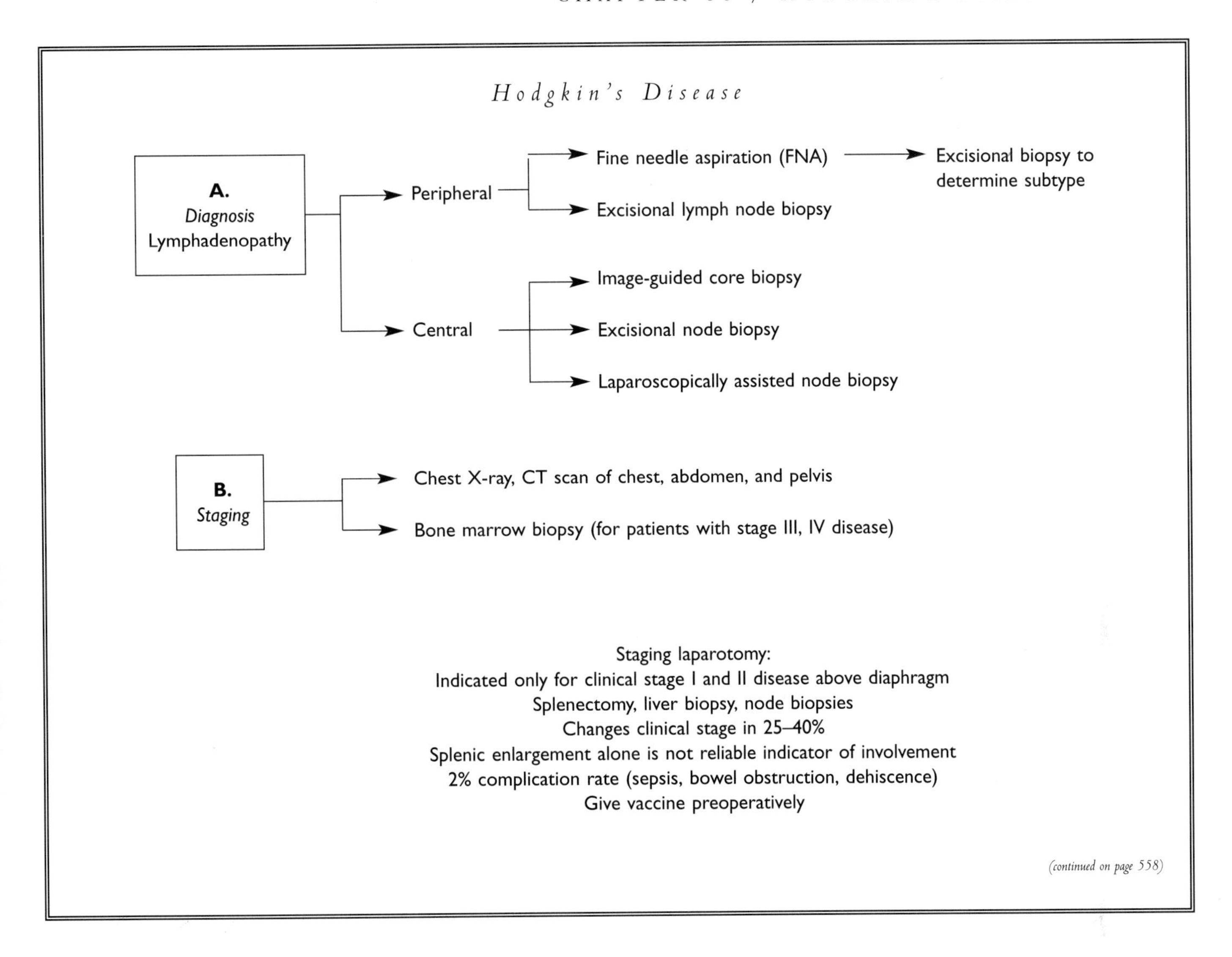

(continued on page 558)

Numerous studies have reported the accuracy of FNA to be in the range of 85–94%.[5–7] The main limitation of FNA is its ability to determine the histologic subtype (50–60% success); lymphoid architecture is generally needed to facilitate this determination. The success rate may be improved with differential cell counts[8] and immunohistochemistry,[6] although most recommend that if a diagnosis of Hodgkin's disease has been made via FNA excisional biopsy of an enlarged lymph node should be performed to subtype the disease.

Image-guided core-needle biopsy has also been used to establish the diagnosis of Hodgkin's disease. Its chief advantage is its minimal invasiveness under radiologic guidance such computed tomography (CT) scans or ultrasonography. In addition, because of the larger amount of tissue obtained with the core needle, it is possible to make a diagnosis and to subtype the disease in most cases. This form of biopsy is particularly useful in patients without peripheral lymphadenopathy or those with extranodal disease. Core-needle biopsy may also be used in patients who are poor candidates for operation. Pappa et al. reported image-guided core-needle biopsies in 96 patients.[9] A successful biopsy was defined as one that "provided sufficient information for a therapeutic decision." Included in the population described were patients who presented with new disease and those who had been treated for lymphoma previously. In recurrent cases the technique identified patients whose disease had transformed into a higher-grade histology or different subtype.

TABLE 58–1.
Subtypes of Hodgkin's disease

Subtypes	Frequency (%)	5-Year survival (%)
Lymphocyte predominance	6.7	83.9
Nodular sclerosis	51.0	82.2
Mixed cellularity	23.8	68.1
Lymphocyte depletion	5.7	36.4
Miscellaneous others	12.8	60.8
Overall	100	73.5

SOURCE: Modified from Medeiros and Greiner.[4]

The overall accuracy was 83%, and the accuracy for Hodgkin's disease was 72%.[9]

The ability to define subtypes of disease accurately by core-needle biopsy has been confirmed by other studies. Ben-Yehuda et al. reported an accuracy rate of 86% in identifying histologic subtypes in patients with Hodgkin's disease.[10] Only 4 of 29 patients required an open excisional biopsy for subtype diagnosis. The other 25 were diagnosed with image-guided core-needle biopsy only.

The gold standard for the diagnosis of Hodgkin's remains the excisional lymph node biopsy. Its advantages are its high accuracy in diagnosing malignancy and its ability to analyze intact nodal architecture. The biopsy is a simple operative procedure with low morbidity; complications include bleeding, persistent lymphatic leak, and infection. For patients with a high likelihood of lymphoma (previously identified on FNA or a history of Hodgkin's disease), nodal biopsy may be combined with placing a central venous catheter for subsequent chemotherapy.

In recent years there has been increasing use of laparoscopy for lymph node biopsy. Advances in laparoscopic technology have facilitated the location and removal of lymph nodes in the peritoneal cavity and retroperitoneum. In a report from Memorial Sloan-Kettering Cancer Center, 101 laparoscopic biopsy procedures were performed on patients with possible lymphoma.[11] The laparoscopically assisted biopsy was diagnostic in 90%, and there was adequate pathologic information obtained to initiate treatment. The population included patients with Hodgkin's disease, non-Hodgkin's lymphoma, and other neoplastic conditions.[11]

This technique may be best applied to patients with central lymphadenopathy only and those who may have failed image-guided core-needle biopsy. Disadvantages of this technique include postoperative ileus, wound infection, and the need for general anesthesia.

TABLE 58–2.
AJCC stage grouping for Hodgkin's disease

Stage	Criteria
I	Involvement of a single lymph node region (I) or localized involvement of a single extralymphatic organ or site (I_E)
II	Involvement of two or more lymph node regions on the same side of the diaphragm (II) or localized involvement of a single associated extralymphatic organ or site and its regional lymph node(s) with or without involvement of other lymph node regions on the same side of the diaphragm (II_E)
III	Involvement of lymph node regions on both sides of the diaphragm (III), which may also be accompanied by localized involvement of an associated extralymphatic organ or site (III_E), involvement of the spleen (III_S), or both (III_{E+S})
IV	Disseminated (multifocal) involvement of one or more extralymphatic organs, with or without associated lymph node involvement, or isolated extralymphatic organ involvement with distant (nonregional) nodal involvement.

Systemic symptoms: Each stage assignment is subdivided into "A" (patients without systemic symptoms) and "B" (patients with systemic symptoms) categories. The "B" designation is given to patients with (1) unexplained loss of more than 10% of body weight during the 6 months before diagnosis; (2) unexplained fever with temperatures above 38°C; and (3) drenching night sweats.

SOURCE: Used with the permission of the American Joint Committee on Cancer (AJCC®), Chicago, IL. The original source for this material is the AJCC® Cancer Staging Manual, 5th edition (1997) published by Lippincott Williams & Wilkins Publishers, Philadelphia, PA.

B. Staging

After Hodgkin's disease is diagnosed, staging is the next important step before designing the treatment. A complete history, physical examination, and laboratory studies and done, including hemoglobin, white blood cell count, erythrocyte sedimentation rate (ESR), and alkaline phosphatase assay. In addition, radiographic imaging assists in determining stage. Imaging includes chest radiography or computed tomography (CT) scans of the chest, abdomen, and pelvis (or both).[12] Other studies that have been utilized include bipedal lymphography, gallium radionuclide scans, bone scans, and now PET scans. Patients with stage III or IV disease also require bone marrow biopsies. The stage is defined by the number of involved nodal sites, whether the sites are above or below the diaphragm (or both), if the nodes are contiguous, and if the patient has general symptoms ("B" symptoms, as described in Table 58–2).

Operative staging continues to be part of the staging process, although the need for a staging laparotomy has come under scrutiny; the indications for it are limited. The improving accuracy of clinical staging with noninvasive imaging has greatly diminished the need for a staging laparotomy. In general, operative staging is needed if it is likely to change the treatment (i.e., if the pathologic stage is different from the clinical stage). For example, if a patient with clinical disease confined to one supradiaphragmatic nodal area is found to have infradiaphragmatic disease by staging laparotomy, treatment would be expanded to include chemotherapy as well as irradiation.

Operative staging is the most sensitive method for diagnosing infradiaphragmatic disease, especially splenic involvement. Clinical examination (palpation of the abdomen) and imaging are less sensitive; in fact, 25–40% of patients who undergo a staging laparotomy have their clinical stage changed as a result. Breuer et al. reported the Boston Children's Hospital experience in 1994[14] and found that of the patients who were up-staged 96%

had splenic involvement not detected on imaging. The spleen was the only site of involvement in 42% of the patients. Splenic enlargement on abdominal radiographic imaging is an unreliable indicator, as splenic involvement is found in only 50% of such cases and normal-size spleens are involved in up to 30%.[15]

A staging laparotomy includes splenectomy (with accessory spleens), removal of selected retroperitoneal lymph nodes, and liver biopsy. The abdominal nodal basins biopsied include the celiac, splenic arterial, splenic hilar, hepatic/portal, paraaortic, paracaval, and bilateral iliac lymph nodes. Areas of biopsy are commonly marked with clips. An iliac crest bone marrow biopsy should be considered if it was not performed previously. To prepare for possible subsequent treatment, an oophoropexy, operatively fixing the ovaries behind the uterus or laterally away from an irradiation field, is also performed in females of reproductive age, and clips can be used for subsequent identification. An appendectomy may be included.[15,16] Some studies have reported no significant survival differences in patients who undergo staging laparotomy compared to those who are only clinically staged.[17,18]

Long-term complications of staging laparotomy were evaluated by Jockovich et al.[19] Among 133 patients there were 10 episodes of overwhelming postsplenectomy infection in 9 patients (in 6.8% of all patients). These episodes occurred only in patients who had not been vaccinated against pneumococci prior to splenectomy. Other complications included small bowel obstruction, atelectasis, abscess formation, and wound dehiscence. No surgical deaths were reported. A pediatric patient series also reported no surgical mortality, with a morbidity rate of only 3%.[14] Because of the risk of overwhelming postsplenectomy sepsis, all patients should be vaccinated against pneumococcal, *Haemophilus*-related, and even meningococcal infections prior to the staging laparotomy.

In an attempt to decrease the morbidity associated with a staging laparotomy, several groups have used minimally invasive techniques. Laparoscopic staging, similar to other laparoscopic procedures, shortens the hospital stay, lessens postoperative pain, and shortens the duration of postoperative ileus. The ability to stage the lesion laparoscopically (i.e., retrieve lymph nodes and perform splenectomy, oophoropexy, and liver biopsy) is equivalently successful.[20,21] Although experience is limited at this time, laparoscopic staging may supplant the staging laparotomy in the future, offering the opportunity for accurate staging without some of the possible complications of open abdominal procedures. Before its use becomes routine, however, the accuracy of laparoscopic staging and its long-term clinical implications must be carefully evaluated.

Approximately 85–90% of patients with Hodgkin's disease have supradiaphragmatic disease; only a small percentage have infradiaphragmatic disease alone. Patients with infradiaphragmatic disease may not benefit from operative staging. Patients who present with clinical stage (CS) I, infradiaphragmatic disease, are rarely restaged through an operative procedure.[22] CS II patients with infradiaphragmatic disease are at high risk of relapse; treatment therefore includes a combination of chemotherapy and irradiation. Consequently, operative staging in these patients is not indicated[23] (Table 58–3). Currently, operative staging is advised only for clinical stage I and II disease above the diaphragm. The need for a staging laparotomy is further determined by the histologic subtype and the presence of favorable factors.

TABLE 58–3.
Clinical stages and possible need for staging laparotomy

Clinical stage	Possible need for staging laparotomy
Stage I	
Above the diaphragm	Yes
Below the diaphragm	No
Stage II	
Above the diaphragm	Yes
Below the diaphragm	No
Stage III	No
Stage IV	No

C. *Clinical Stage I*

Patients with clinical stage I disease, the lymphocyte-predominant subtype of Hodgkin's disease (LPHD), do not benefit from a staging laparotomy. Numerous studies have demonstrated that the final stage of patients with LPHD seldom changes after a staging laparotomy. Up-staging occurs in fewer than 10% of the patients with CS I LPHD regardless of gender or age.[14,16,24,25] The decision to perform a staging laparotomy in patients with other histologic subtypes depends on the presence of the factors enumerated below.

Favorable Factors

Studies indicate that in CS I patients without LPHD certain favorable factors are seldom associated (less than 10% of the time) with up-staging. They include female gender, nonbulky mediastinal involvement, and high cervical involvement in men. These patients are treated with radiation alone, with good results.[14,16]

Unfavorable Factors

Certain unfavorable factors in CS I patients without LPHD mandate treatment with both radiation and chemotherapy. As such, staging laparotomy is not indicated. These factors have been defined by the latest guidelines of the National

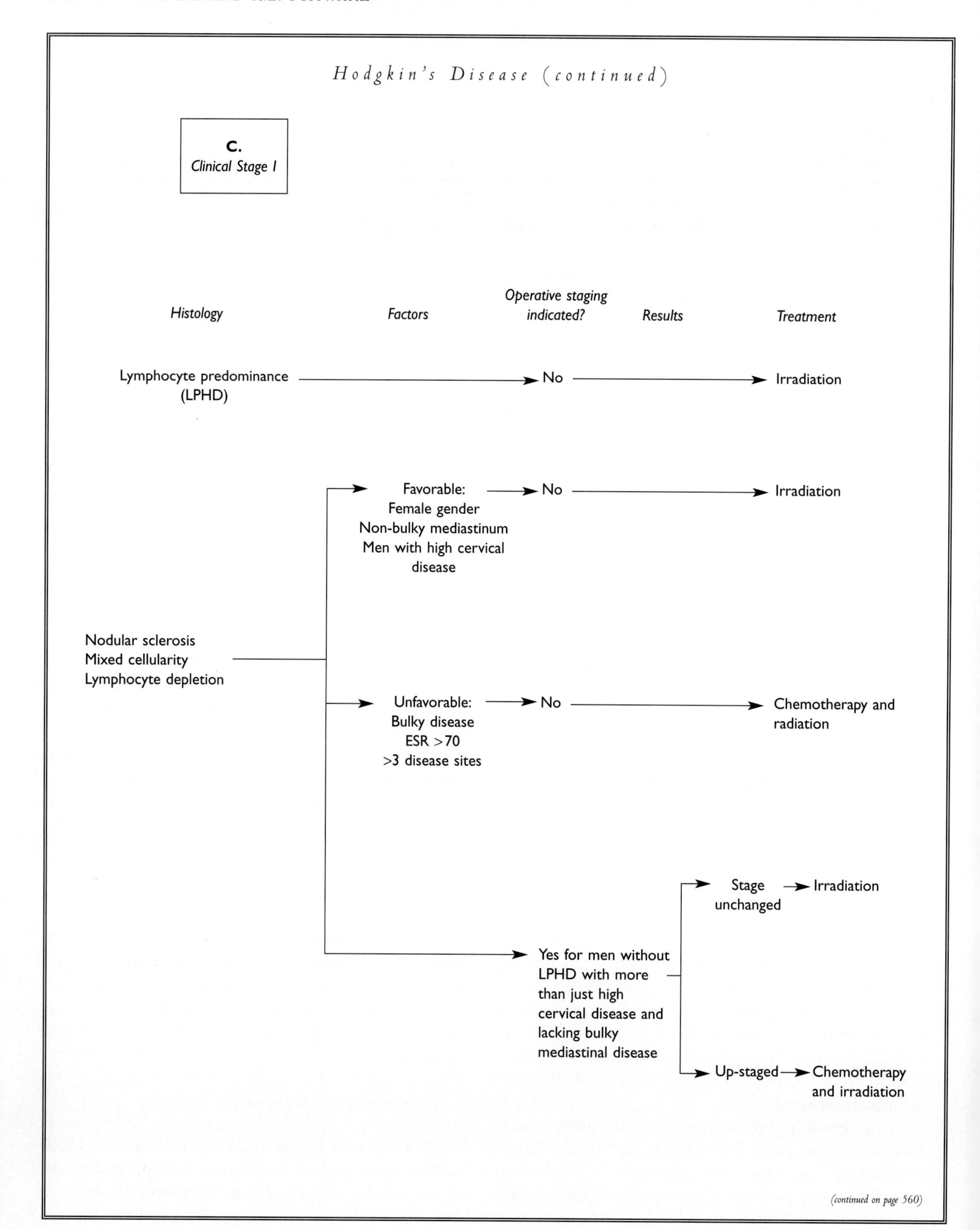

(continued on page 560)

Comprehensive Cancer Network and predict a worse outcome. Therefore systemic and local therapy are advised. These factors are bulky disease (maximum mass width/maximum intrathoracic diameter ratio higher than 1:3); any mass >10cm; ESR >70; and more than three sites of involvement.

Several studies have looked at the predictive value of "B" symptoms in determining a patient's likelihood of the lesion being up-staged with operative staging. Studies are divided regarding the prognostic value of the "B" symptoms. Some have indicated that they correlate well with infradiaphragmatic disease,[24] but this has not been confirmed in other series.[14,16]

The patient group with CS I that benefits most from operative staging (i.e., the stage changes as a result of surgical/pathologic staging and treatment is affected accordingly) consists of men who do not have the lymphocyte-predominant subtype, have more extensive disease than high cervical disease alone, or have no bulky mediastinal disease.

D. Clinical Stage II

For CS II patients with favorable factors, treatment with radiotherapy alone is possible if the staging laparotomy is normal. As in CS I patients, those with a CS II lesion with lymphocyte-predominant histology have an improved overall prognosis and should not undergo a staging laparotomy. Operative staging is indicated for patients with supradiaphragmatic disease only if the treatment would change based on the presence of favorable or unfavorable variables. One favorable scenario would be a woman less than 27 years of age with fewer than three sites of involvement. Up-staging would occur in fewer than 10% of these patients during a staging laparotomy; therefore this procedure is unnecessary and not indicated. Patients with unfavorable factors also do not benefit from a staging laparotomy. Such factors include bulky disease as defined by a maximum mass width/maximum intrathoracic diameter ratio higher than 1:3; any mass >10cm; ESR >70; involvement at more than three sites. These patients are treated with a combination of chemotherapy and radiation at the onset. As a result, operative staging does not affect treatment and is not indicated.

Treatment and Outcome

Treatment of Hodgkin's disease may entail irradiation only, irradiation and chemotherapy, or chemotherapy alone. For early disease, irradiation encompasses the nodal region involved as well as neighboring nodal stations at risk for subclinical involvement while limiting excessive radiation exposure to adjacent organs. The typical radiation dose as the sole treatment modality is 36Gy in daily fractions of 180cGy over 4 weeks, with a possible boost to the clinically affected sites.[15] Irradiation as the only treatment modality has been shown to be effective against stage I and II disease with overall survival around 80% at 10 years and a 30% relapse rate.

Radiation therapy and chemotherapy together have been shown to decrease the rate of relapse for patients with bulky stage II disease. In most series the overall survival is similar for patients who undergo combination chemoradiation compared with those who receive radiation therapy alone. Consolidation radiotherapy may be given after prior chemotherapy for advanced-stage (III and IV) Hodgkin's disease, although improved efficacy of combined treatment is still uncertain at this time.

Combination chemotherapy has markedly improved the disease-free survival and overall survival in patients with advanced Hodgkin's disease. The standard chemotherapy regimen is mechlorethamine/vincristine/procarbazine/prednisone (MOPP). Various regimens have been proposed and used with equivalent efficacy and decreased acute toxicity, including doxorubicin/bleomycin/vinblastine/dacarbazine (ABVD). The current National Comprehensive Cancer Network practice guidelines for treatment of Hodgkin's disease recommend ABVD as the first-line chemotherapy combination.[23] Following combination chemotherapy for stage III or IV Hodgkin's disease, complete responses are achieved in 70–90% of patients, but the relapse rate can be as high as 35%.[15] Surgical treatment of local relapses is generally not beneficial or indicated. Salvage radiation and high-dose chemotherapy with stem cell support are therapeutic options in this setting.

Long-term complications after potentially curative treatment of Hodgkin's disease include the development of second solid malignancies, myelodysplasia, leukemia, infertility, and cardiac or pulmonary complications. Of particular importance to the surgical oncologist is the increased risk of breast cancer (up to 35%) in women 40 years of age who underwent radiation therapy during childhood.[26] Earlier screening and closer clinical follow-up are recommended for women with a history of Hodgkin's disease treatment before adulthood.

Conclusions

The need for an accurate diagnosis and complete staging mandates that the surgeon have a clear understanding of Hodgkin's disease. The role of surgical procedure in the diagnostic and staging workup of this disease have been greatly reduced primarily to providing an adequate tissue biopsy to confirm the diagnosis, for which excisional lymph node biopsy remains the standard. Staging laparotomy is rarely performed now, as indications for the use of systemic chemotherapy have been set more liberally for patients who have features linked to higher risks for infradiaphragmatic disease, and as diagnostic imaging has become more accurate. Only patients with supradiaphragmatic stage I or II disease who do not have extremely good prognostic features (young female, lymphocyte predominance) or extremely

Hodgkin's Disease (continued)

D.
Clinical Stage II

Histology	*Factors*	*Operative staging indicated?*	*Result*	*Treatment*
Lymphocyte predominance (LPHD)		No		Irradiation*
Nodular sclerosis, Mixed cellularity, Lymphocyte depleted	Favorable: Female, < 27 years old, < 3 sites	No		Irradiation*
	Unfavorable: Bulky disease, ESR >70, >3 sites of disease	No		Chemotherapy** and irradiation
		Yes	Stage unchanged	Irradiation*
			Up-staged	Chemotherapy* and irradiation

*36 Gy in 180 cGy daily fractions over 4 weeks

**MOPP (mechlorethamine, vincristine, procarbazine, prednisone);
ABVD (doxorubicin, bleomycin, vinblastine, dacarbazine)

poor prognostic features (bulky disease) can potentially benefit from this procedure. Laparoscopic staging has been advocated by some, and laparoscopic biopsy confirmation of disease recurrences may be helpful. The surgeon must be aware of the increased risk of second malignancies in patients with a history of Hodgkin's disease and irradiation or chemoradiation.

References

1. DeVita VT, Mauch PM, Harris NL. Hodgkin's disease. In: DeVita VT, Hellman S, Rosenberg SA (eds) Cancer: Principles and Practice of Oncology, 5th ed. Philadelphia: Lippincott-Raven, 1997:2242–2284.
2. Landis SH, Murray T, Bolden S, Wingo PA. Cancer statistics, 1998. CA Cancer J Clin 1998;48:6–29.
3. Brauninger A, Hansmann ML, Strickler JG, et al. Identification of common germinal-center B-cell precursors in two patients with both Hodgkin's disease and non-Hodgkin's lymphoma. N Engl J Med 1999;340:1239–1247.
4. Medeiros LJ, Greiner TC. Hodgkin's disease. Cancer 1995;75:357–369.
5. Das DK, Gupta SK, Datta BN, Sharma SC. Fine needle aspiration cytodiagnosis of Hodgkin's disease and its subtypes. I. Scope and limitations. Acta Cytol 1990;34:329–336.
6. Fulciniti F, Vetrani A, Zeppa P, et al. Hodgkin's disease: diagnostic accuracy of fine needle aspiration; a report based on 62 consecutive cases. Cytopathology 1994;5:226–233.
7. Stewart CJ, Duncan JA, Farquharson M, Richmond J. Fine needle aspiration cytology diagnosis of malignant lymphoma and reactive lymphoid hyperplasia. J Clin Pathol 1998;51:197–203.
8. Das DK, Gupta SK. Fine needle aspiration cytodiagnosis of Hodgkin's disease and its subtypes. II. Subtyping by differential cell counts. Acta Cytol 1990;34:337–341.
9. Pappa VI, Hussain HK, Reznek RH, et al. Role of image-guided core-needle biopsy in the management of patients with lymphoma. J Clin Oncol 1996;14:2427–2430.
10. Ben-Yehuda D, Polliack A, Okon E, et al. Image-guided core-needle biopsy in malignant lymphoma: experience with 100 patients that suggests the technique is reliable. J Clin Oncol 1996;14:2431–2434.
11. Mann GB, Conlon KC, LaQuaglia M, et al. Emerging role of laparoscopy in the diagnosis of lymphoma. J Clin Oncol 1998;16:1909–1915.
12. Lister TA, Crowther D, Sutcliffe SB, et al. Report of a committee convened to discuss the evaluation and staging of patients with Hodgkin's disease: Cotswolds meeting. J Clin Oncol 1989;7:1630–1636. Erratum. J Clin Oncol 1990;8:1602.
13. AJCC. Hodgkin's disease. In: AJCC Cancer Staging Handbook, 5th ed. Philadelphia: Lippincott Williams & Wilkins, 1998;259–261.
14. Breuer CK, Tarbell NJ, Mauch PM, et al. The importance of staging laparotomy in pediatric Hodgkin's disease. J Pediatr Surg 1994;29:1085–1089.
15. Yahalom J, Straus D. Hodgkin's disease. In: Pazdur R, Coia LR, Hoskins WJ, Wagman LD (eds) Cancer Management: A Multidisciplinary Approach, 3rd ed. Melville, NY: PRR, 1999.
16. Leibenhaut MH, Hoppe RT, Efron B, et al. Prognostic indicators of laparotomy findings in clinical stage I–II supradiaphragmatic Hodgkin's disease. J Clin Oncol 1989;7:81–91.
17. Cosset JM, Henry-Amar M, Meerwaldt JH, et al. The EORTC trials for limited stage Hodgkin's disease: the EORTC Lymphoma Cooperative Group. Eur J Cancer 1992;11:1847–1850.
18. Rock DB, Murray KJ, Schultz CJ, et al. Stage I and II Hodgkin's disease in the pediatric population: long-term follow-up of patients staged predominantly clinically. Am J Clin Oncol 1996;19:174–178.
19. Jockovich M, Mendenhall NP, Sombeck MD, et al. Long-term complications of laparotomy in Hodgkin's disease. Ann Surg 1994;219:615–621.
20. Baccarani U, Carroll BJ, Hiatt JR, et al. Comparison of laparoscopic and open staging in Hodgkin disease. Arch Surg 1998;133:517–521.
21. Lefor AT, Flowers JL, Heyman MR. Laparoscopic staging of Hodgkin's disease. Surg Oncol 1993;2:217–220.
22. Mason MD, Law M, Ashley S, et al. Infradiaphragmatic Hodgkin's disease. Eur J Cancer 1992;11:1851–1852.
23. Hoppe R, Winter J. Practice guidelines: Hodgkin's disease. Presented at the National Comprehensive Cancer Network, 3rd Annual Conference, Ft. Lauderdale, FL, 1998.
24. Aragon de la Cruz G, Cardenes H, Otero J, et al. Individual risk of abdominal disease in patients with stages I and II supradiaphragmatic Hodgkin's disease: a rule index based on 341 laparotomized patients. Cancer 1989; 63:1799–1803.
25. Mauch P, Larson D, Osteen R, et al. Prognostic factors for positive surgical staging in patients with Hodgkin's disease. J Clin Oncol 1990;8:257–265.
26. Bhatia S, Robison LL, Oberlin O, et al. Breast cancer and other second neoplasms after childhood Hodgkin's disease. N Engl J Med 1996;334: 745–751.

Section  13

Oncologic Emergencies

Chapter 59

Spinal Cord Compression

CHRISTOPHER J. DEWALD

Spinal cord compression (SCC) can occur secondary to spinal trauma, congenital anomalies, primary spinal cord tumors, or tumors involving the vertebral column (benign or malignant). One of the most common causes of SCC in the adult is metastatic disease involving the spine. This chapter addresses the management of SCC due to metastatic disease, highlighting the importance of spinal stabilization if neurologic compromise is present.

Primary tumors of the spine can cause SCC. *Benign primary tumors* such as giant cell tumors or aneurysmal bone cysts may cause spinal canal compression and neural deficits.[1–3] The difficulty treating these tumors is their high recurrence rates, particularly with giant cell tumors, if complete excision is not obtained. Complete excision can be extremely difficult when trying to preserve nerve and spinal cord function. *Malignant primary tumors* can cause SCC.[2,4] Examples include Ewing's sarcoma and osteogenic sarcoma, which arise from bone marrow stem cells and can involve the spine. Chordomas are primary lesions that arise from remnants of the notochord and almost exclusively involve the spine. These malignant lesions cause SCC usually by direct aggressive extension into the spinal canal. It is often impossible to provide a truly complete radical excision of these malignant lesions because of the proximity of the neural structures, excision of which may cause significant morbidity. Thus, resections of primary malignant tumors of the spine are often marginal excisions and require adjunctive treatment, including radiation therapy and chemotherapy.

Incidence and Mechanism of Metastatic Spinal Cord Compression

By far the most common oncologic cause of SCC is metastatic disease. With improvements in cancer treatment and longer median cancer survival rates, an increasing number of patients are presenting with spinal metastases. The spinal column is the most frequent site of metastatic involvement of the skeleton, occurring in up to 70% of patients with metastatic breast cancer.[5–8] A metastatic lesion of the spine frequently causes localized spinal pain but may also be asymptomatic despite significant bony

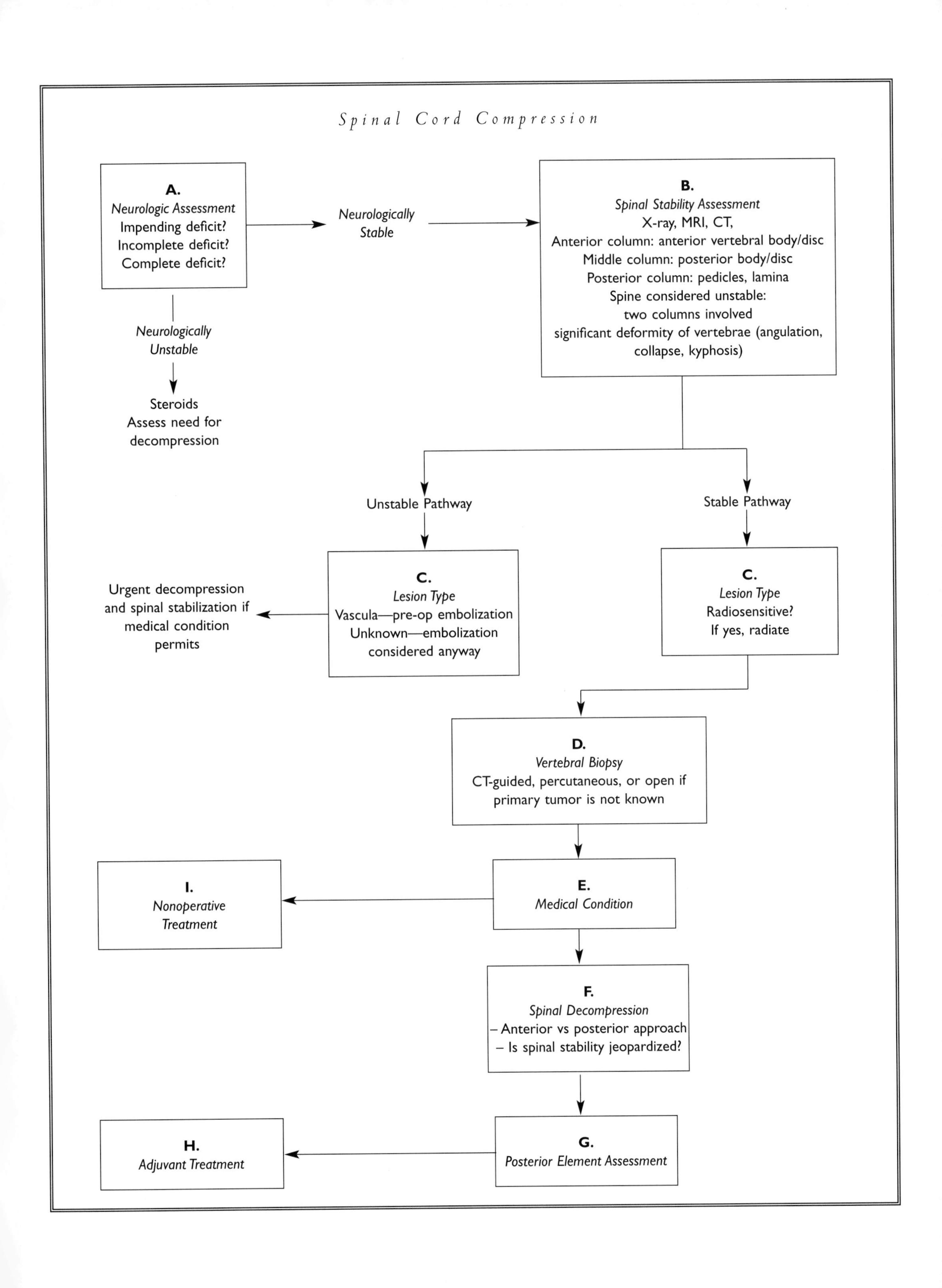
Spinal Cord Compression
A.
Neurologic Assessment
Impending deficit?
Incomplete deficit?
Complete deficit?
Neurologically Stable
B.
Spinal Stability Assessment
X-ray, MRI, CT,
Anterior column: anterior vertebral body/disc
Middle column: posterior body/disc
Posterior column: pedicles, lamina
Spine considered unstable:
two columns involved
significant deformity of vertebrae (angulation, collapse, kyphosis)
Neurologically Unstable
Steroids
Assess need for decompression
Unstable Pathway
Stable Pathway
Urgent decompression and spinal stabilization if medical condition permits
C.
Lesion Type
Vascula—pre-op embolization
Unknown—embolization considered anyway
C.
Lesion Type
Radiosensitive?
If yes, radiate
D.
Vertebral Biopsy
CT-guided, percutaneous, or open if primary tumor is not known
I.
Nonoperative Treatment
E.
Medical Condition
F.
Spinal Decompression
– Anterior vs posterior approach
– Is spinal stability jeopardized?
H.
Adjuvant Treatment
G.
Posterior Element Assessment

involvement. It has been reported that up to 80% of patients with prostatic cancer have asymptomatic spinal metastases found on postmortem examination.[5,9] Metastatic spread to the spine is thought to occur as a result of arterial emboli, direct extension, or retrograde venous flow through the retroperitoneal and vertebral venous plexus as described by Batson (Batson's plexus).[10,11]

Approximately 10–30% of patients with metastatic lesions of the spine develop SCC.[5,12–15] The median survival depends on the tumor type but decreases to 2–4 months if significant neural deficits develop.[14,16] The mechanism of SCC is pathologic vertebral fracture with retropulsion of bone into the spinal canal, direct extension of the tumor into the epidural space from the vertebral body, or a paraspinal tumor through the neuroforamina. Neurologic impairment is thought to be due to arterial ischemia of the spinal cord or venous congestion leading to localized edema and necrosis.[5,17,18]

Certain carcinomas have a higher propensity to metastsize to bone. Medical students are taught the pneumonic "PT Barnum Loves Kids" to remember which primary carcinomas metastasize to bone: prostate, thyroid, breast, lung, kidney. These tumors cause 80–90% of spinal metastases; the remainder are due to lesions of the hematopoietic system (i.e., multiple myeloma and lymphoma).[5,14,15,19,20] The latter are primary malignancies of bone marrow, which are considered metastatic disease because of multiple involved areas and their relatively common occurrence in adults. Cancellous bone constitutes most of the vertebral body and thus is often extensively involved by such malignancies (Fig. 59–1). Whether multiple lesions of these hematopoietic lesions are considered metastatic or a continuum of the primary disease in a single organ system is a matter of semantics. Standard treatment utilizes chemotherapy and irradiation, as complete surgical excision is not possible because of multicentric disease. Surgical intervention may be required when vertebral collapse, spinal instability, or neurologic deficit occurs; and it may be required even for patients with disseminated bony disease when a single level collapses causing SCC, as is commonly seen with multiple myeloma (Fig. 59–1E).

Although SCC denotes actual compression of the spinal cord by a pathologic process, lesions with the *potential* to cause SCC must be addressed. Unfortunately, it is too often the case where a known spinal lesion is neglected because there are no neurologic symptoms despite the presence of mechanical instability. A prophylactic stabilization procedure could avoid a permanent neurologic deficit or paraplegia. In addition to maintaining a patient's independence (ambulation and personal hygiene) and quality of life,[8,12,16,20–26] early stabilization of an impending paraplegic lesion can be cost-effective considering the level of care necessary for a paralyzed patient.[27,28] An impending paraplegic lesion should be treated as aggressively and perhaps even more so than a lesion responsible for an existing neurologic impairment.[10,21]

Unknown Primary Lesion

Neurologic dysfunction can be the initial symptom of a previously undiagnosed cancer. In such a case not only must the patient's neurologic status be critically evaluated, but identification of the tumor's cell type and hence determination of the patient's overall prognosis are required, as they may have a significant bearing on any proposed surgical treatment. Identification of the unknown primary malignancy must be fastidiously determined simultaneous with treatment of the neurologic impairment. Often this requires a "best guess" prior to urgent surgical decompression of the spinal canal; tissue can be obtained for histologic diagnosis at the time of the decompression. Workup of an unknown metastatic spinal lesion includes the history, physical examination, chest radiography or chest computed tomography (CT), renal ultrasonography or abdominal CT scan, bone scan, urinalysis, complete blood count (CBC), prostate-specific antigen (PSA) assay, thyroid function tests, and serum protein electrophoresis.

Clinical Examination

An appropriate history includes any history of cancer, recent or preceding back pain, significance of accompanying injury, night pain, pain lasting more than 6 weeks, or progressive pain. As the spine is the most common site for skeletal metastases, any spinal lesion in a patient over age 50 should be suspected of being a metastasis. Any patient with a history of carcinoma with continued back pain no matter how "cured" they believed they were, is considered to have a metastatic lesion until proven otherwise. Often these spinal lesions become painful with or without neurologic impairment owing to a pathologic fracture sustained after a relatively minor injury.

The physical examination includes an examination of common primary sites including a breast or prostate examination. Examination of the spine includes percussion/palpation of the spine, determination of dermatomal/sensory level via pinprick, motor examination of all muscle groups and their respective myotomes, rectal examination, deep tendon reflexes, and determination of the presence of pathologic reflexes (i.e., Babinski sign, Hoffman's sign, clonus). This examination can be challenging and often requires an orthopedic or neurosurgical consultation. It must be repeated at regular intervals to determine changes or progression.

The first step in identifying the etiology of any SCC in an adult, particularily without a history of significant trauma, is to determine the location of the lesion. Most metastatic lesions involve the thoracic and lumbar spine.[19,29,30] The cervical spine is affected less commonly but can still be the location of significant SCC.[29–31]

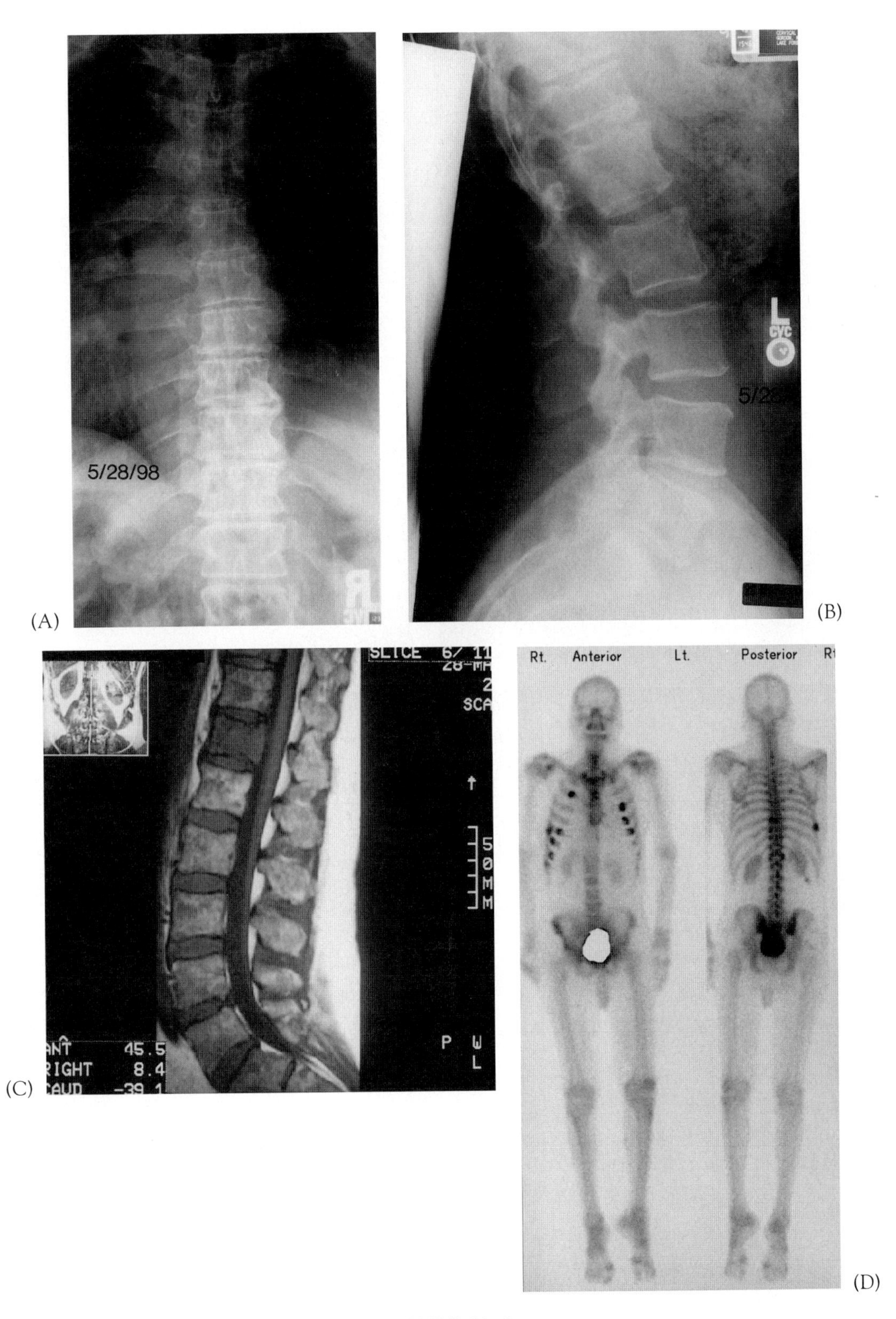

FIGURE 59–1

This 51-year-old patient has multiple myeloma. (A, B) On 5/28/98 this radiograph was obtained because of increased back pain. Note the relatively good contour of the spine in the (A) anteroposterion (AP) and (B) sagittal planes. (C) Magnetic resonance imaging (MRI) reveals significant vertebral involvement without vertebral collapse or spinal cord compression (SCC). Note the difference in vertebral body signal and amount of tumor involved in T12. Reviewing the plain radiographs again, T12 appears mildly compressed and osteopenic on the lateral radiograph. (D) Bone scans in multiple myeloma patients are relatively benign and can be negative owing to the lack of osteoblastic activity characteristic of multiple myeloma. The increased uptake in multiple ribs strongly suggests a metastatic process, although the spine has little uptake.

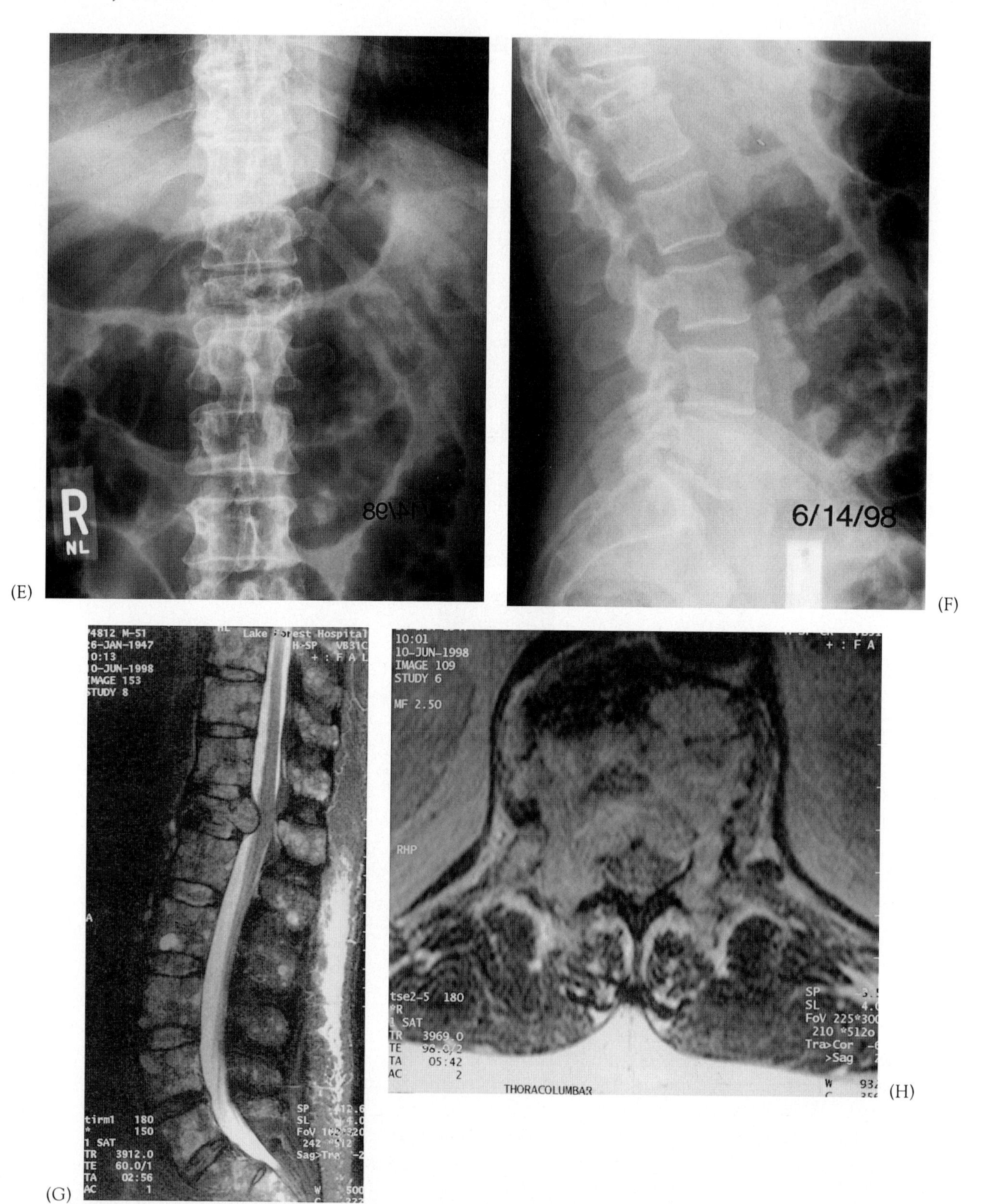

FIGURE 59–1 *Continued*

(E) Two weeks later T12 collapses and the patient develops a neurologic deficit due to the SCC from the pathologic fracture. AP view. (F) Lateral view revealing significant vertebral collapse and segmental kyphosis. (G) MRI obtained after the vertebral collapse reveals compression of the spinal cord and diffuse involvement of the remaining vertebral bodies. (H) Axial MRI reveals involvement of the vertebral body and posterior elements, as well as the severity of the neural compression.

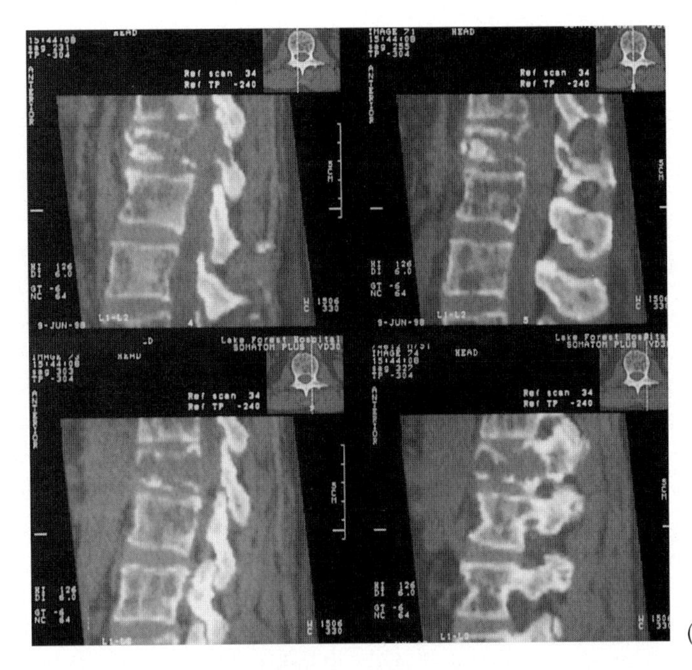

(I)

FIGURE 59–1 *Continued*
(I) Computed tomography (CT) scan with sagittal reconstructions can further define the severity of spinal column involvement. Note the pedicle involvement of the pathologic fracture compared to the vertebral levels below.

Although symptoms of SCC can be the earliest sign of metastatic disease, SCC is usually preceded by weeks to months of insidious back pain. This back pain is typically mechanical in nature, increasing with activity; but it is characteristically a slowly progressive unrelenting pain not relieved by rest or recumbency. It is this type of pain that results in the classic description of night pain. This pain pattern connotes a "red flag" warning differentiating it from the common back pain seen in most adults.

Treatment

The treatment of SCC due to metastases depends on many factors, including the presence or absence of a neurologic deficit, presence or absence of spinal instability, histologic type of the tumor, medical condition of the patient, location of the spinal lesion, expected survival of the patient, and maintenance of the patient's quality of life. Radiation therapy remains the mainstay of nonsurgical treatment; the best results have been noted in radiosensitive spinal lesions not accompanied by vertebral collapse or instability of the spine.[13,32] Radiation therapy can decrease spinal canal compression in a radiosensitive lesion, but it cannot reverse a neurologic deficit due to vertebral body collapse or kyphosis. Additionally, irradiation alone, without steroids, cannot reverse a neurologic deficit, nor does it result in improved neurologic function after acute neurologic deterioration. Chemotherapy and hormonal therapy also play a role in the nonsurgical treatments of spinal lesions, although chemotherapy ineffectively treats neurologic deterioration and is used mostly as an adjunct for systemic disease.

The goals of surgical treatment are to maintain or improve quality of life, relieve pain, maintain or restore neurologic function, and stabilize the spine. The indications for surgical intervention are a neurologic deficit due to radioresistant tumors or unstable spinal lesions, progressive neurologic spinal cord compromise, or continued or recurrent neural deficit following radiation treatments.[10,13] An additional indication is a metastatic lesion with significant involvement of the vertebral body resulting in impending vertebral body collapse and instability (Fig. 59–1A–C).

Patients with SCC have specialized needs pertaining to the neurologic deficit and its effect on ambulation. Patients are typically placed on bed rest and consequently should be started on deep venous thrombosis prophylaxis (mechanical compression boots) and decubitus precautions. The latter include not only heel protection and a special mattress but also careful daily visual examination and nursing care of the areas at risk. This is especially a concern for the paraplegic patient who has a sensory deficit. Sacral decubiti are a potential site of sepsis and patient demise. Nutrition is also a concern regarding paraparetic, paralyzed, or bedridden patients; poor nutrition can lead to wound infection, wound dehiscence, and decubitus ulcers.

Algorithm

Evaluation of a patient with SCC due to a metastatic lesion involves three nearly equal parts: (1) neurologic impairment; (2) spinal stability; and (3) tumor type. When considering the neurologic impairment a number of questions must be answered: Is the neurologic deficit complete or incomplete? Is the incomplete neurologic deficit stable or progressive? Is the patient neurologically intact but has an impending paraplegic lesion? What is the prognosis for neurologic recovery? The prognosis depends on the acuteness of the neurologic impairment. Acute development of paralysis (less than 12 hours) has a poor prognosis for neural recovery versus slowly developing neural impairment.[4,5,33] The urgency of patient evaluation and surgical intervention can vary greatly depending on the severity of the neurologic involvement. Progressive neurologic impairment, however, has the greatest need for urgent/emergent decompression.

The second area to evaluate is the stability of the spinal column. Instability of the spine is difficult to assess owing to variable definitions of instability among spinal surgeons. The most widely used definition of instability is based on the three-column description of the spine initially noted for spinal fractures.[4] The three columns are the anterior column (anterior half of the vertebral body and disc), middle column (posterior vertebral body and disc), and posterior column (posterior elements: facet joints, pedicles, lamina). If two or more columns are involved within a vertebral body it is considered unstable. As most vertebral metastases involve the vertebral body,[4,34] careful evaluation of the CT scan for metastatic involvement of the pedicles and facet joints help determine the stability of the spinal column (Fig. 59–11).

It has been postulated that spinal canal decompression via posterior laminectomy without proper spinal stability can potentiate the neurologic impairment and so was considered to be no more advantageous than irradiation alone.[6,20,35–40] Since the mid-1980s multiple studies have shown this to be false. Proper surgical decompression and instrumentation based on the location of the neural compression has resulted in much more favorable outcomes pertaining to the surgical treatment of metastatic spinal lesions.[2,8,12,21,22,24–26,29,30,41–47] Unfortunately, it is the early reports of surgical intervention for SCC not having a significant benefit over radiation therapy alone that seem to remain in the memory of many primary medical services. The result is that continued irradiation for mechanically unstable spinal lesions has been advocated. Proper spinal stability must be obtained with spinal instrumentation during spinal decompression to expect a successful outcome.

The third area of concern is the histologic tumor type, as it determines treatment and prognosis.[43] Certain lesions respond differently to nonsurgical treatment than others. Many malignant lesions are radiosensitive (e.g., lymphomas), whereas others are radioresistant (e.g., hypernephroma, sarcoma). Certain metastatic malignancies (e.g., lung cancer) have a worse prognosis with a shorter life expectancy than the much improved and relatively long survival of treated patients with metastatic breast carcinoma. The histologic type of the metastatic tumor may also have a bearing on the surgical plan; for example, renal cell carcinomas are extremely vascular lesions, and attempted excision without preoperative arterial embolization of the lesion may lead to excessive, potentially fatal blood loss.[16,48]

Thus, complete evaluation of a patient with SCC due to a metastatic lesion requires determination of (1) spinal column stability; (2) the patient's neurologic status (whether there is complete or incomplete neurologic impairment and the prognosis for neurologic recovery); and (3) the tumor type. The patient's quality of life must always be strongly considered when contemplating the best treatment method. This of course depends on the patient's overall medical condition and nutritional level.

A. Neurologic Assessment

Whether the patient has complete neurologic impairment (no motor or sensory function below the level of the SCC) or an incomplete neurologic deficit (sparing of some function of the motor/sensory systems), the patient should be started on a steroid regimen. Steroids decrease the severity of edema and inflammation associated with neural compression.[18,49] Unfortunately, the dosage and length of steroid use have not been clearly defined. The use of steroids, in combination with recumbency, in patients with neurologic impairment following SCC is the current standard of care and produces quite dramatic results in terms of returning function. Although steroid regimens vary, dexamethasone 4–10 mg given every 6 hours for 3 days up to 2 weeks is frequently used. Steroids continued for more than 2 weeks have been shown to increase complications related to wound healing and gastrointestinal bleeding.[5,38] In the presence of an unstable spinal lesion, steroids alone are not sufficient to restore or protect neurologic function.

If an impending paraplegic lesion exists in the spinal column *without neurologic deficit*, steroids are not needed. This lesion usually causes localized back pain that is mechanical in nature and present and unrelenting at rest. If a metastatic lesion is thought to be unstable or at serious risk of instability without a current neurologic deficit, the patient should be placed on bed rest and surgical intervention considered. Continued ambulation and movement across such a lesion leads to vertebral collapse and potential neurologic impairment. Again, it is imperative to provide appropriate deep venous thrombosis and decubitus precautions for any patient placed on bed rest with a spinal lesion, especially if a neurologic deficit is already present.

The first step in the SCC algorithm is to determine the patient's neurologic status and start a steroid regimen if necessary. Repeat neurologic examinations are required to determine the stability of the patient's neurologic status. If neurologic deterioration is noted in the impending paraplegic or neurologically incomplete-SCC patient, the patient is considered neurologically "unstable," and more urgent or emergent surgical decompression is required. Often the problem lies in defining a true neurologic change. It is difficult to assess changes in neurologic status when there are multiple examiners evaluating the patient. It therefore resides with the spinal surgeon to make the final decision regarding the presence and significance of neurologic deterioration. Many times a careful history reveals that the patient has been on "bed rest" for a couple of weeks due to back pain and was just noted to be unable to move the legs. Often these patients have had slow, progressive impairment of their neurologic function resulting in a paraparetic condition, making it difficult to truly decipher an acute significant neurologic change. A slowly progressive neurologic impairment has a much improved prognosis for partial neurologic recovery than an acute neurologic change (less than 12 hours).[4,5,33]

B. *Spinal Stability Assessment*

Concurrently, the spinal column and its stability must be evaluated as the second step in the algorithm. Using the three-column definition of spinal stability, if two columns are involved the spine is considered potentially unstable. Kostuik and Weinstein further defined spinal stability in pathologic lesions by subdividing the three columns into right and left halves, making a total of six divisions.[33] Lesions involving three or four divisions are considered to be at moderate risk of instability, and lesions involving five or six divisions are considered grossly unstable pathologic spinal lesions. Thus if more than three divisions of the vertebrae are involved with metastatic disease, or if significant angulation, vertebral collapse, or kyphosis exists in a spinal lesion, the spine is considered unstable. Multiple lesions can be evaluated separately but contiguous vertebral lesions are considered to be less stable. Often overlooked, plain radiographs of the spine can provide an initial interpretation of the spinal column stability and should always be included in the workup. Obvious vertebral collapse with a kyphotic deformity, for example, can be easily noted on a plain lateral radiograph. CT scan of the spine can further elucidate bony involvement of the lesion in all three columns of the spine (Fig. 59–1I). MRI is required to identify the severity of the SCC and to distinguish between neural compression secondary to soft tumor extension and retropulsed pathologic bone into the spinal canal. Spinal MRI can also further define the extent of tumor extension within the spinal canal and the paraspinal region (Fig. 59–1C,G,H). Bone scans are utilized to help determine if a spinal lesion is a result of multiple metastatic lesions and to identify alternate biopsy sites. It must remembered that bone scans detect bone turnover and formation and can be negative in the presence of certain lytic lesions such as multiple myeloma (Fig. 59–1D).[4,5]

C. *Lesion Type*

Unstable Pathway

If the pathologic spinal lesion is considered "unstable," urgent spinal stabilization and decompression are planned after the patient's medical condition is optimized even if the histopathology of the spinal lesion is not known. In such a case, a definitive pathologic specimen can be obtained at the time of the spinal canal decompression and stabilization procedure.

For the "unstable" spinal lesion, if the primary malignancy is known, urgent decompression and stabilization can be accomplished with appropriate preoperative planning. If the lesion is known or suspected to be a highly vascular tumor (e.g., renal cell carcinoma), preoperative arterial embolization is imperative. If the histopathology of the lesion is not known, it is recommended that the spinal lesion be embolized preoperatively. Embolization can significantly decrease intraoperative blood loss, providing better visualization to facilitate tumor resection and spinal cord decompression. Renal cell carcinomas are the most common clinically occult cancer to present with SCC.[15] The risk of excessive blood loss associated with vascular spinal lesions and the likelihood of an unknown spinal lesion being a renal cell carcinoma support the use of preoperative embolization for unknown spinal lesions[16,48] (Fig. 59–2).

Stable Pathway

If the neurologic deficit is stable and the spine is determined to be mechanically stable, nonsurgical treatment modalities can be utilized. As mentioned, radiation therapy (RT) is the most commonly used nonsurgical treatment method for metastatic lesions. If the spinal lesion is radiosensitive (breast cancer, prostate cancer, lymphoma, myeloma) and the spine is

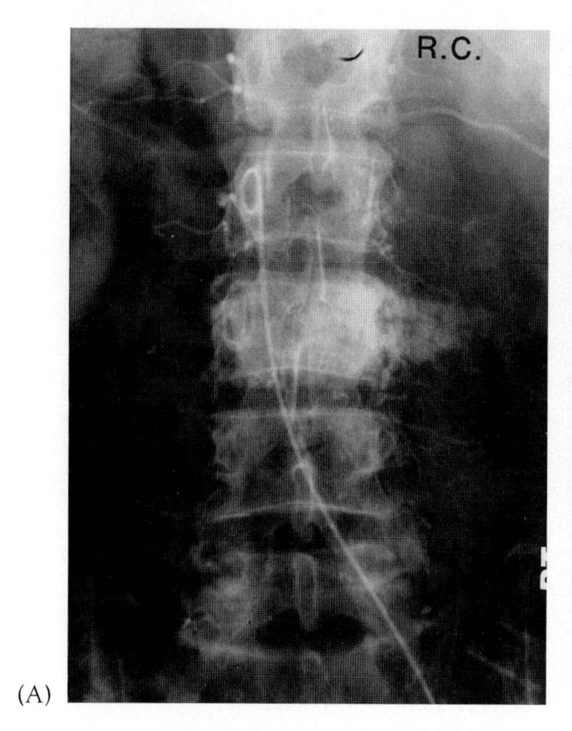

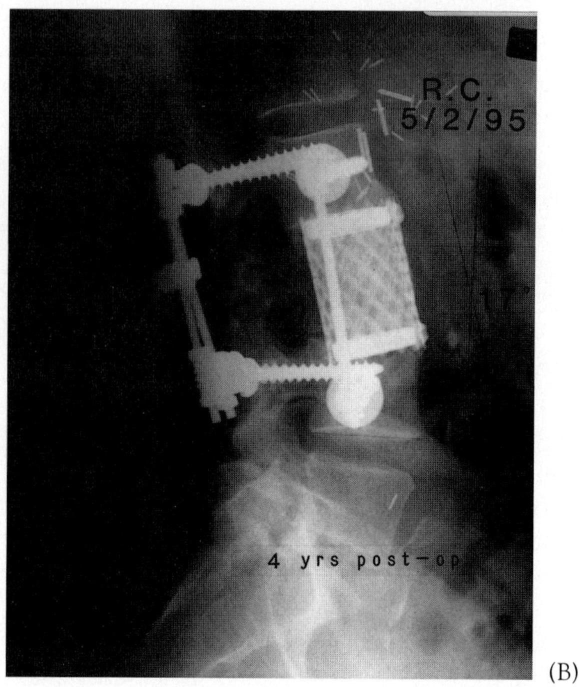

(A) (B)

FIGURE 59–2
(A) Embolization of a metastatic renal cell carcinoma involving the L3 vertebra. Note the blush of the contrast material into the vertebral body owing to the extreme vascularity of these lesions. (B) Postoperative radiograph of the anterior titanium mesh cage used to support the anterior column after anterior decompression and vertebral corpectomy. Posterior instrumentation was utilized because of the posterior column involvement of the metastatic tumor.

considered stable, RT is an appropriate treatment. The spine can be braced for additional support during the radiation treatments to help prevent pathologic collapse. The radiation dose and dose intervals vary from hospital to hospital, but typically 2500–4500 cGy (rads) is the maximum radiation the spinal cord can receive, as higher doses correlate with the development of transverse myelopathy.[5,13,50–52] Lymphoma is an excellent example of a highly radiosensitive spinal lesion that responds remarkably even in the presence of neurologic compromise. Other nonsurgical treatment modalities (i.e., chemotherapy, hormonal therapy) or surgical intervention may be indicated if the metastatic lesion is radioresistant. If a radioresistant spinal lesion exists with the potential to cause significant vertebral body involvement, pathologic collapse, and instability, surgical excision and stabilization are required.

D. *Vertebral Biopsy*

If the primary lesion is unknown, a biopsy is required to determine histology. CT-guided 22-gauge percutaneous biopsies can be done under local anesthesia in an outpatient setting. They have been shown to yield positive results for 60–95% of lytic spinal lesions.[4,5,14] Percutaneous or open Craig needle biopsy can be performed if the fine-needle biopsy was not diagnostic.

E. *Medical Condition*

The patient's overall prognosis and medical condition also determine treatment. If it is medically risky for the patient to undergo a major spinal procedure, alternative nonoperative treatments are utilized. Additional medical concerns include the patient's nutritional and immunologic status, the use of adjunctive chemotherapy, and the patient's skin condition following radiation therapy. DeWald et al.[21] found that the patient's immune status had a significant impact on the overall success of surgery. Patients with metastatic disease have often already undergone chemotherapy or radiotherapy, and may have lost a significant amount of weight. An immunoincompetent state increases surgical risk not only in terms of postoperative infection and wound dehiscence but with respect to the development of decubitus ulcers and sepsis. Poor nutrition also plays a role in wound healing and the prevention and healing of decubitus ulcers. Serum albumin and transferrin levels and a white blood cell count are required to help determine the nutritional state and immunologic state of the patient.

F. Spinal Decompression

The surgical approach for decompression is dictated by the location of the spinal lesion: an anterior approach (thoracotomy or flank) for anterior lesions and a posterior approach for lesions involving the posterior elements.[12,34,44] Two-thirds of metastatic lesions involve the vertebral body versus the posterior elements.[4,10,34,50] For this reason, most spinal decompressions are best approached anteriorly via a thoracotomy or a retroperitoneal flank approach. It is the perceived complexity of an anterior spinal procedure that has led to the incorrect assumption that posterior decompression via laminectomy alone would be sufficient to relieve pressure on the spinal cord. Anterior compression on the spinal cord due to a pathologic lesion of the vertebrae acts as a fulcrum over which the spinal cord is draped in a kyphotic position.[12,14,21] Attempted decompression posteriorly via excision of the posterior elements, including the laminae and interspinous ligaments, when the compression lies anteriorly results in an increase in the kyphotic moment and continued or increased spinal cord compression anteriorly.[5,8,21,29,30,41,42] If the metastatic lesion has resulted in an unstable spine, spinal stability must be reestablished.[21,53] Anterior corpectomy for decompression requires reconstruction of the anterior column, which is accomplished using a strut device made from methylmethacrylate, allograft bone (femur, ilium), or a metallic cage (Fig. 59–2B).

G. Posterior Element Assessment

Once the anterior column has been reconstructed after spinal canal decompression of an anterior metastatic lesion, the posterior column of the spine must be reassessed. If the lesion also involves posterior elements, such as the pedicles or facet joints, posterior spinal instrumentation augmentation may be required. This preferably done the same day as the anterior decompression/reconstruction. Posterior stabilization is accomplished using posterior rod instrumentation with multiple fixation points using either hooks or screws. The strength of the rod fixation is determined by the number of fixation points to the spine. Posterior rod constructs supplementing an anterior spinal reconstruction typically span one level above and one level below the lesion (Fig. 59–2B). Posterior adjunctive instrumentation is also required when two or more vertebral bodies have been excised anteriorly. Patients with multiple metastatic lesions of the spine are best treated with longer posterior rod stabilization with or without an anterior corpectomy.[2,12,53] Less commonly, SCC results from a metastatic lesion involving the posterior elements. In this case, as the SCC is located posteriorly, decompression can be accomplished via a posterior laminectomy and stabilized utilizing posterior instrumentation, as necessary.

H. Adjuvant Treatment

Postoperative radiation therapy, chemotherapy, or both are often utilized as adjunctive treatment following surgical decompression and excision of a metastatic lesion. Adjunctive chemotherapy or radiation should be withheld at least 2 weeks after surgery and preferably up to 6 weeks.[4,5,25] Early postoperative irradiation or chemotherapy can prohibit proper wound healing and lead to disabling, potentially life-threatening wound dehiscence with exposure of the underlying spinal hardware and neural structures.

I. Nonoperative Treatment

For patients deemed to be medically unstable, nonoperative treatments include brace support, pain management, hospice care, patient education, and additional radiation. Braces can be used to support the spine and allow the patient to be mobilized at least to an upright sitting position. Unfortunately, most braces are not tolerated well by adults. Lesions in the cervical spine require a hard cervical collar or halo-vest; lesions in the mid to upper thoracic spine require a cervical-thoracic-lumbar-sacral orthosis (CTLSO); and lumbar and lower thoracic spine require a thoracic-lumbar-sacral orthosis (TLSO). None of these braces is sufficient for a long-term solution for unstable pathologic lesions and should be reserved for terminal patients with less than 6 weeks of expected survival or when there is severe cardiopulmonary disease, where the morbidity/mortality risk is too high for a major surgical procedure.

Additionally, it is necessary to educate not only the patient but also the family about a paraparetic or paralyzed condition. The neurologically impaired patient requires a significant amount of assistance, often with extensive rehabilitation. This can be difficult, as typically the neurologic impairment has occurred at a terminal stage in the patient's life.

Conclusions

Patients with SCC due to metastatic disease of the spine must be simultaneously evaluated with regard to neurologic impairment, stability of the spine, and tumor type. A multidisciplinary approach is required for these patients including an internist, medical oncologist, radiation oncologist, and spinal surgeon. Compressive tumor extension can be treated effectively by radiotherapy for lesions that are radiosensitive, but radiotherapy cannot reverse a neurologic deficit if the SCC is a result of instability, vertebral collapse, or kyphosis. Spinal lesions with impending instability or current instability require spinal stabilization. The goals of surgery are to maintain or restore neurologic function and spinal stability, relieve pain, and maintain an independent quality of life. If the patient is medically able to undergo spinal surgery and has a life expectancy of 3 months or more, surgical intervention should be strongly considered.

References

1. Khosla A, Martin DS, Awwad EE. The solitary intraspinal vertebral osteochondroma: an unusual cause of compressive myelopathy: features and literature review. Spine 1999;24:77–81.
2. Kostuik JP, Errico TH, Gleason TF, et al. Spinal stabilization of vertebral column tumors. Spine 1988;13:250–256.
3. Weinstein JN, McLain RF. Primary tumors of the spine. Spine 1987;12: 843–851.
4. Bell GR. Surgical treatment of spinal tumors. Clin Orthop 1997;335: 54–63.
5. Asdourian PL. Metastatic disease of the spine. In: Bridwell KH, DeWald RL (eds). The Textbook of Spinal Surgery, 2nd ed. Philadelphia: Lippincott, 1997;2007–2050.
6. Cobb CA III, Leavens ME, Eckles N. Indications for non-operative treatment of spinal cord compression due to breast cancer. J Neurosurg 1977; 47:653–658.
7. Miller F, Whitehill R. Carcinoma of the breast metastatic to the skeleton. Clin Orthos 1984;184:121–127.
8. Sundaresan N, Galicich JH, Bains MS, Martini N, Beattie EJ. Vertebral body resection in the treatment of cancer involving the spine. Cancer 1984;53:1393–1396.
9. Jacobs SC. Spread of prostatic cancer to bone. Urology 1983;21:337–344.
10. Asdourian PL, Weidenbaum M, DeWald RL, Hammerberg KW, Ramsey RG. The pattern of vertebral involvement in metastatic vertebral breast cancer. Clin Orthos 1990;250:164–170.
11. Batson OV. The function of the vertebral veins and their role in the spread of metastases. Ann Surg 1940;112:138–149.
12. Hammerberg KW. Surgical treatment of metastatic spine disease. Spine 1992;17:1148–1153.
13. Lord CF, Herndon JH. Spinal cord compression secondary to kyphosis associated with radiation therapy for metastatic disease. Clin Orthos 1986;210: 120–127.
14. Mardjetko SM, DeWald CJ. Management of metastatic spinal disease. Spine 1996;10:89–105.
15. Schaberg JC, Gainor BJ. A profile of metastatic carcinoma of the spine. Spine 1985;10:19–20.
16. King GJ, Kostuik JP, McBroom RJ, et al. Surgical management of metastatic renal cell carcinoma of the spine. Spine 1991;16:265–271.
17. Barron KD, Hirano A, Araki S, Terry RD. Experiences with metastatic neoplasms involving the spinal cord. Neurology 1959;9:91–106.
18. Ushio Y, Posner R, Posner JB, Shapiro WR. Experimental spinal cord compression by epidural neoplasm. Neurology 1977;27:422–429.
19. Brihaye J, Ectors P, Lemort M, Van Houtte P. The management of spinal epidural metastases. Adv Tech Stand Neurosurg 1988;16:121–176.
20. Gilbert RW, Kim JH, Posner JB. Epidural spinal cord compression from metastatic tumor: diagnosis and treatment. Ann Neurol 1978;3: 40–51.
21. DeWald RL, Bridwell KH, Prodromas C, Rodts MF. Reconstructive spinal surgery as palliation for metastatic malignancies of the spine. Spine 1985;10:21–26.
22. Galasko CS. Spinal instability secondary to metastatic cancer. J Bone Joint Surg Br 1991;73:104–108.
23. Helwig-Larsen S. Clinical outcome in metastatic spinal cord compression: a prospective study of 153 patients. Acta Neurol Scand 1996;94: 269–275.
24. Lee CK, Rosa R, Fernand R. Surgical treatment of tumors of the spine. Spine 1986;11:201–208.
25. McAfee PC, Zdeblick TA. Tumors of the thoracic and lumbar spine: surgical treatment via the anterior approach. J Spinal Disord 1989;2:145–154.
26. Onimus M, Schraub S, Bertin D, Bosset JF, Guidet M. Surgical treatment of vertebral metastasis. Spine 1986;11:883–891.
27. McKinley WO, Conti-Wyneken AR, Vokac CW, Cifu D. Rehabilitative functional outcome of patients with neoplastic spinal cord compressions. Arch Phys Med Rehabil 1996;77:892–895.
28. O'Neil J, Gardner V, Armstrong G. Treatment of tumors of the thoracic and lumbar spinal column. Clin Orthop 1986;227:103–112.
29. Sundaresan N, Digiacinto GV, Hughes JE, Cafferty M, Vallejo A. Treatment of neoplastic spinal cord compression: results of a prospective study. Neurosurgery 1991;29:645–650.
30. Sundaresan N, Galicich JH, Lane JM, Bains MS, McCormack P. Treatment of neoplastic epidural cord compression by vertebral body resection and stabilization. J Neurosurg 1985;63:676–684.
31. Bohlman HH, Sachs BL, Carter JR, Riley L, Robinson RA. Primary neoplasms of the cervical spine: diagnosis and treatment of twenty-three patients. J Bone Joint Surg Am 1986;68:483–494.
32. Katagiri H, Takahashi M, Inagaki J, et al. Clinical results of nonsurgical treatment for spinal metastases. Int J Radiat Oncol Biol Phys 1998; 42:1127–1132.
33. Kostuik JP, Weinstein JN. Differential diagnosis and surgical treatment of metastatic spine tumors. In: Frymoyer JW (ed) The Adult Spine: Principles and Practice. New York: Raven, 1991;861–888.
34. Sundaresan N. Spinal metastasis: current status and recommended guidelines for management. Neurosurgery 1979;5:726–746.
35. Constans JP, de Divitiis E, Donzelli R, Spaziante R, Meder JF, Haye C. Spinal metastases with neurological manifestations: review of 600 cases. J Neurosurg 1983;59:111–118.
36. Dunn RC Jr, Kelly WA, Wohns RNW, Howe JF. Spinal epidural neoplasia: a 15 year review of the results of surgical therapy. J Neurosurg 1980; 52:47–51.
37. Findlay GF. Adverse effects of the management of malignant spinal cord compression. J Neurol Neurosurg Psychiatry 1984;47:761–768.
38. Martenson JA, Evans RG, Lie MR, et al. Treatment outcome and complications in patients treated for malignant epidural spinal cord compression (SCC). J Neurooncol 1985;3:77–84.
39. Raichle ME, Posner JB. The treatment of extradural spinal cord compression. Neurology 1970;20:391.
40. Young RF, Post EM, King GA. Treatment of spinal epidural metastases: randomized prospective comparison of laminectomy and radiotherapy. J Neurosurg 1980;53:741–748.
41. Harrington KD. Anterior cord decompression and spinal stabilization for patients with metastatic lesions of the spine. J Neurosurg 1984;61:107–117.
42. Harrington KD. Anterior decompression and stabilization of the spine as a treatment for vertebral collapse and spinal cord compression from metastatic malignancy. Clin Orthop 1988;233:177–197.
43. Onimus M, Papin P, Gangloff S. Results of surgical treatment of spinal thoracic and lumbar metastases. Eur Spine J 1996;5:407–411.
44. Perrin RG, McBroom RJ. Anterior versus posterior decompression for symptomatic spinal metastasis. Can J Neurol Sci 1987;14:75–80.
45. Perrin RG, McBroom RJ. Spinal fixation after anterior decompression for symptomatic spinal metastasis. Neurosurgery 1988;22:324–327.
46. Siegal T, Siegal T. Surgical decompression of anterior and posterior malignant epidural tumors compressing the spinal cord: a prospective study. Neurosurgery 1985;17:424–432.

47. Siegal T, Tiqva P, Siegal T. Vertebral body resection for epidural compression by malignant tumors: results of forty-seven consecutive operative procedures. J Bone Joint Surg Am 1985;67:375–382.
48. Nelson PK, Setton A, Berenstein A. Vertebrospinal angiography in the evaluation of vertebral and spinal cord disease. Neuroimaging Clin N Am 1996;6:589–605.
49. Cantu RC. Corticosteroids for spinal metastases. Lancet 1968;2:912.
50. Maranzano E, Latini P, Checcaglini F, et al. Radiation therapy in metastatic spinal cord compression: a prospective analysis of 105 consecutive patients. Cancer 1991;67:1311–1317.
51. Maranzano E, Latini P, Perrucci E, Beneventi S, Lupattelli M, Corgna E. Short-course radiotherapy (8 Gy × 2) in metastatic spinal cord compression: an effective and feasible treatment. Int J Radiat Oncol Biol Phys 1997;38:1037–1044.
52. Tong D, Gillick L, Hendrickson FR. The palliation of symptomatic osseous metastases: final results of the study by the Radiation Therapy Oncology Group. Cancer 1982;50:893–899.
53. Bauer HC. Posterior decompression and stabilization for spinal metastases: analysis of sixty-seven consecutive patients. J Bone J Surg Am 1997; 79:514–522.

Chapter 60

Superior Vena Cava Syndrome

Cam Nguyen
V. Amod Saxena

The superior vena cava (SVC) syndrome is an urgent medical condition that requires prompt, efficient diagnosis. Treatment is based on the histology of the underlying condition, and it is essential to recognize SVC syndrome early in its clinical course so proper therapy can be initiated as soon as possible.[1,2] The SVC is the main pathway for venous return from the head and neck, upper extremities, and upper thorax. The SVC, which drains into the right atrium, is located in the mid-mediastinum and is surrounded by the trachea, right mainstem bronchus, ascending aorta, right pulmonary artery, perihilar/paratracheal lymph nodes, thoracic vertebral bodies, and sternum. Abnormalities of any of these structures may compress the SVC,[3] producing the syndrome. The SVC syndrome is usually caused by cancer: 65% of cancer-related cases are caused by lung tumors and 35% by lymphomas or other mediastinal masses. Benign causes, which are rare, include aortic dissection, substernal goiter, tuberculosis, fungal infections, and constrictive pericarditis.

Often patients with SVC syndrome are first seen in the emergency room with a variety of symptoms produced by compression of vascular and airway structures. Early involvement of the surgeon, anesthesiologist, medical oncologist, and radiation oncologist is essential, as it brings together a team of specialists, each with a different expertise required to manage the situation promptly. Many of these patients, especially those with lymphoma, can be cured with appropriate therapy.

A. Diagnosis

The diagnosis of SVC syndrome should be suspected based on a constellation of clinical symptoms and physical findings. The common symptoms, in order of frequency, are dyspnea (62%), facial edema (50%), cough (24%), upper extremity swelling (18%), chest pain (15%), and dysphagia (9%). Physical findings are usually obvious: neck vein distension (66%), chest wall venous distension (54%), facial edema (46%), cyanosis (20%), and upper extremity edema (14%). Figure 60–1 represents a woman with SVC obstruction due to lung cancer. Note the chest wall vein distension due to chronic obstruction and the slight facial edema.

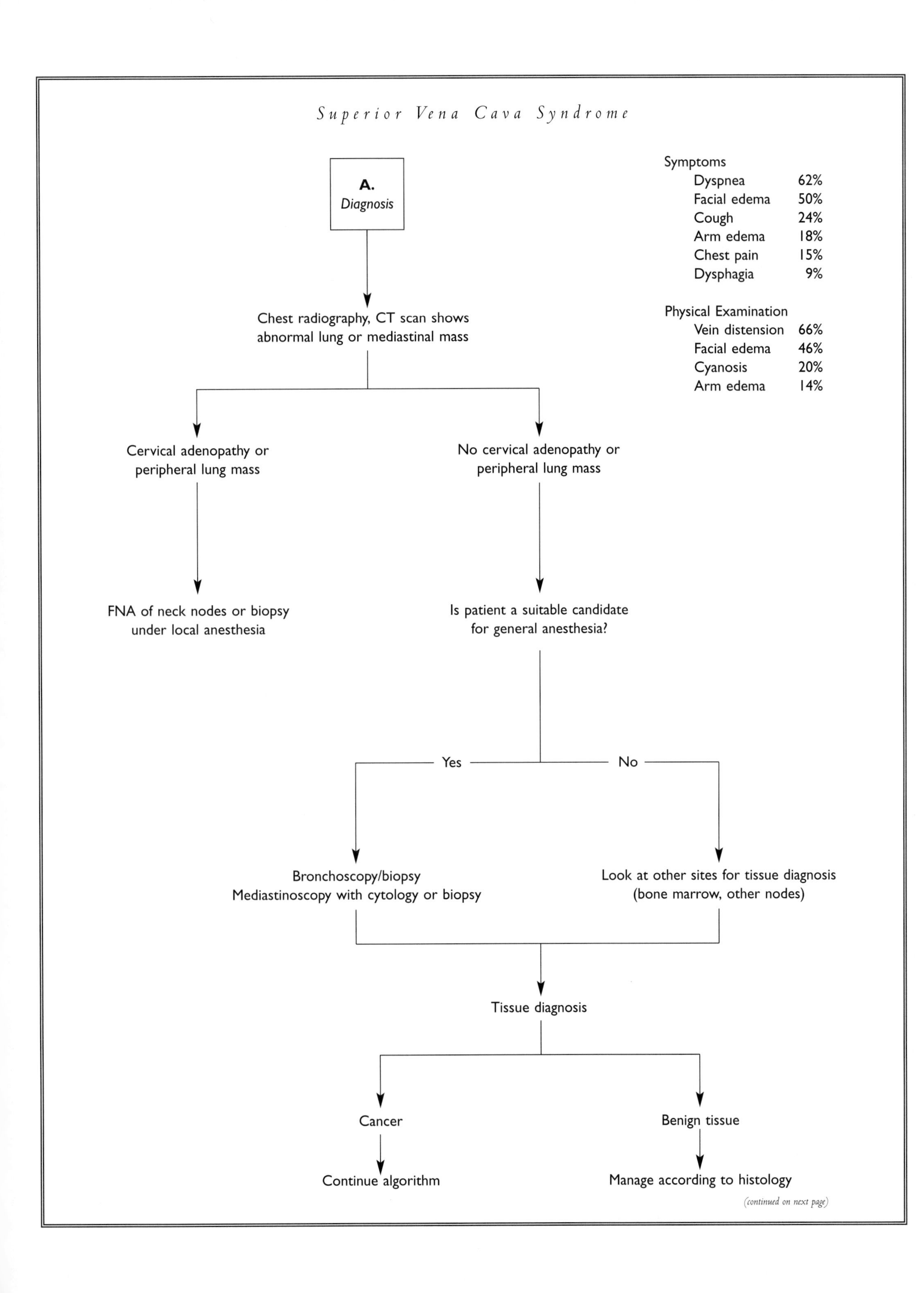

(continued on next page)

Superior Vena Cava Syndrome (continued)

B.
Treatment

Non-small cell lung carcinoma

Irradiation: total dose 6000 cGy, 30 fractions
Chemotherapy:
Cisplatin 100 mg/m^2 days 1 and 29
Vinblastine 5 mg/m^2 weekly for 5 weeks
or
Paclitaxel-based regimen

Small cell lung carcinoma

Chemotherapy:
Etoposide 100 mg/m^2 day 1–13
Cisplatin 25 mg/m^2 day 1–3
4 cycles repeated every 3 weeks
Irradiation-possible adjunct

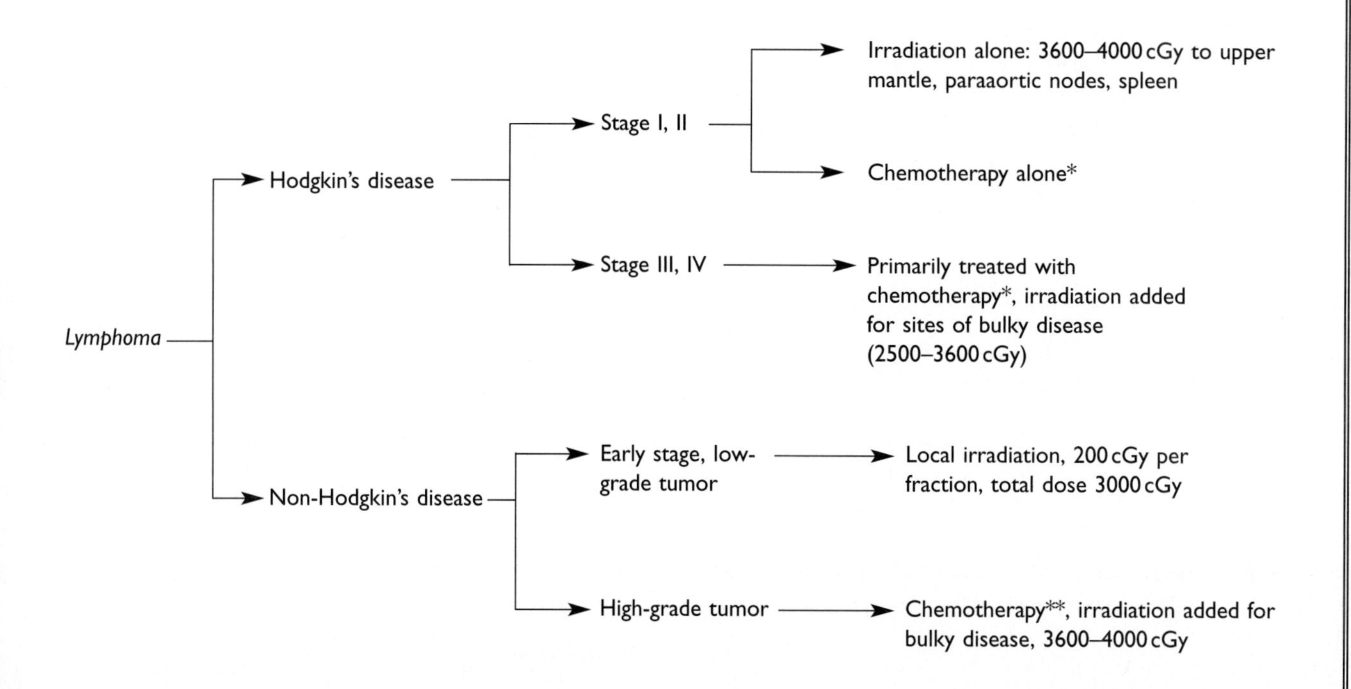

*MOPP (mustard, oncovin, procarbazine, prednisone)
ABVD (adriamycin, bleomycin, vincristine, dacarbazine)

**CHOP (cyclophosphamide, adriamycin, oncovin, prednisone)

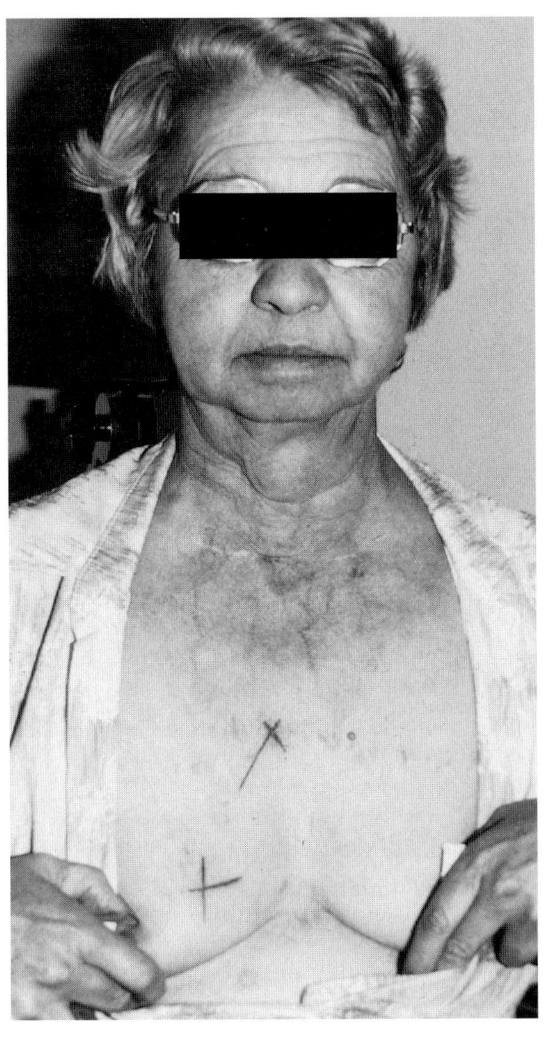

FIGURE 60–1
Patient with lung cancer causing superior vena cava (SVC) obstruction. Note the chest wall vein distension due to chronic obstruction and the slight facial edema. As the condition worsens, the facial edema becomes more pronounced.

Initial diagnostic tests include a chest radiograph and computed tomographic (CT) scan of the thorax. As findings on a radiograph can be subtle, the CT scan is an essential part of the workup: It helps delineate regional anatomy more precisely. Usually, a mediastinal or lung mass is seen in the SVC area. Histologic diagnosis should then be obtained with the easiest, least invasive route.[4]

If palpable cervical or supraclavicular nodes are present, fine-needle aspiration (FNA) should be performed. If the FNA is nondiagnostic, excisional biopsy is indicated. For patients who do not have obvious neck nodes, one should obtain tissue directly from the mediastinal/lung mass.

The patient is then assessed for general anesthesia. Some patients are hemodynamically unstable, making anesthesia risky. Furthermore, a bulky mediastinal mass may pose an airway management problem and difficulty with intubation/extubation.[5] On occasion it is necessary to consider urgent radiotherapy (RT) to shrink the mass, without having a tissue diagnosis. In actuality, this is rarely the case because with modern anesthesia techniques difficult extubation is a rare event. An accurate histologic diagnosis is essential for providing curative treatment; administering RT without a histologic diagnosis can make subsequent tissue studies difficult[6] and potentially compromise definitive treatment.

If the patient is suitable for anesthesia, bronchoscopy is performed if a lung mass is seen on the CT scan. Biopsy, cytologic examination, or both should be performed on any suspicious lesions. If the patient has a mediastinal mass, mediastinoscopy or anterior thoracotomy could be performed, the choice of procedure being based on the location of the mass.[7] Again, one should attempt the least traumatic procedure to secure a tissue diagnosis. Occasionally, a benign process is diagnosed and should be managed according to the histology.

In the rare situation that the patient cannot undergo general anesthesia, one should look at other sites for a tissue diagnosis. If lymphoma or small cell lung cancer is suspected clinically, one should obtain bone marrow aspirates and biopsy for diagnosis and staging. Non-small cell lung cancer rarely involves the bone marrow.

B. *Treatment*

Non-Small Cell Lung Carcinoma

For non-small cell lung carcinoma (NSCLC), the choice of therapy is determined by the stage of the disease. Surgical resection is chosen for early disease and combination chemotherapy/RT for advanced disease.[8–10] Unfortunately, most patients with NSCLC *and* SVC syndrome usually have advanced tumors; if there is no evidence of metastatic disease, combined RT and chemotherapy (cisplatin- or paclitaxel-based) can be given with curative intent. Because of the urgent nature of the SVC syndrome, a few large fractions of RT are given to relieve compression on the SVC quickly. Typically, a dose of 300–400 cGy (1 cGy = 1 rad) per fraction is delivered to the mediastinum including the mass. Giving large doses of radiation per fraction may cause an increased risk of late side effects; therefore only a few *large* fractions of RT are given for rapid relief of symptoms. In the potentially curative situation, a total dose of 6000 cGy is given over 30 fractions (200 cGy/fraction) with chemotherapy. The mainstay of therapy for NSCLC is RT with chemotherapy added to potentiate the effects of RT; the effects of chemotherapy on RT can be additive or synergistic.

A common chemotherapeutic regimen is cisplatin and vinblastine. Intravenous cisplatin (100 mg/m^2) is given on days 1 and 29. Intravenous vinblastine (5 mg/m^2) is given weekly for five consecutive weeks beginning on day 1. Chest RT is started on day 50 to a total dose of 6000 cGy, as mentioned earlier.

If the patient with NSCLC *and* SVC syndrome is found to have distant metastatic disease, palliative RT alone is given. The most common regimen of RT is 3000 cGy in 10 fractions (300 cGy/fraction) delivered to the mediastinum including the mass. Chemotherapy can be withheld during this phase of palliative RT because of the poor prognosis of metastatic lung cancer and the potential for side effects with combined therapy. The general principle of palliation is quick relief of symptoms with minimal side effects. Chemotherapy given concurrently with chest RT can cause significant side effects; it may be used later, however, to control metastatic disease.

Small Cell Lung Carcinoma

Patients with small cell lung carcinoma (SCLC) are treated according to stage. The mainstay of treatment is chemotherapy[11] for both metastatic and limited/localized disease. Limited-stage SCLC is potentially curable and is treated primarily with chemotherapy, with RT to the mediastinum added as consolidative therapy. The most commonly used regimen is etoposide (100 mg/m^2 days 1–3) and cisplatin (25 mg/m^2 days 1–3) for a total of four cycles, repeated every 3 weeks. It was previously believed that RT was more effective than chemotherapy for relieving SVC compression in SCLC patients. However, this concept was challenged by data from Spiro et al.,[12] who showed that chemotherapy alone is highly effective in relieving SVC syndrome caused by SCLC.

Lymphoma

Mediastinal lymphoma causing SVC syndrome represents a challenging situation. Many of these cases are potentially curable, and every attempt should be made to minimize late side effects due to therapy. Again, close collaboration between the medical and radiation oncologists is essential to achieve a high cure rate with the lowest risk of pulmonary or cardiac toxicity. For example, adriamycin-based chemotherapy followed by mediastinal RT can cause cardiac damage. Various chemotherapy regimens are available,[13,14] and one must choose a regimen capable of giving acceptable cure rates with minimal risk of complications when combined with RT. For Hodgkin's disease (HD) common chemotherapy regimens are MOPP (nitrogen mustard/ Oncovin (vincristine) / procarbazine / prednisone) and ABVD (adriamycin / bleomycin / vincristine / dacarbazine). For non-Hodgkin's lymphoma (NHL) a common regimen is CHOP (cyclophosphamide/adriamycin/Oncovin (vincristine)/prednisone); alternatively, second- or third-generation regimens are available. The details of chemotherapy doses for HD and NHL are rather complex and beyond the scope of this chapter. For further details, Armitage's review of this subject is excellent.[13]

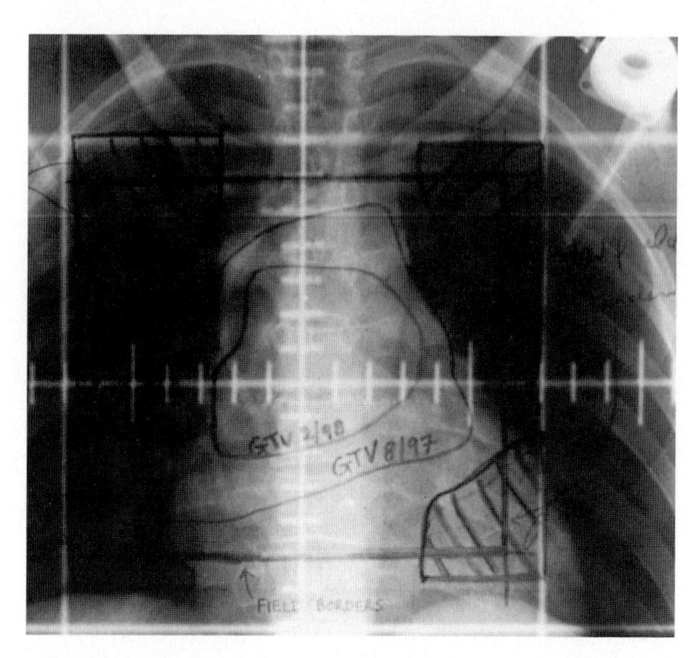

FIGURE 60–2
Radiotherapy (RT) planning film of a 38-year-old woman with mediastinal lymphoma causing SVC compression. Note the gross tumor volume at presentation (GTV 08/97). The second gross tumor volume (GTV 02/98) represents the residual tumor after RT (600 cGy in three fractions) and chemotherapy. This patient was treated with further RT and was in remission. The RT fields are square (12 × 12 cm), and the hatched area represents the blocks to shape the RT field. The portacath (used for chemotherapy) can be seen in the upper right-hand corner of the film.

Figure 60–2 shows an RT planning film of a 38-year-old woman with a mediastinal lymphoma causing SVC compression. Note the gross tumor volume at presentation (GTV 08/97). The second gross tumor volume (GTV 02/98) represents residual tumor after RT (600 cGy in three fractions) and chemotherapy. This patient was treated with further RT, and the treatment induced remission. It was believed that RT was more effective than chemotherapy in relieving SVC compression caused by lymphoma, but data have now shown that chemotherapy alone is as effective as RT in relieving the SVC syndrome.[15] In general, local RT is used for early-stage low-grade NHL with curative intent. High-grade NHL is treated primarily by chemotherapy, with local RT added for sites of bulky disease. Stages I and II of HD can be cured with RT alone or chemotherapy alone. More advanced disease (stages III and IV) is treated by chemotherapy primarily, with RT added for sites of bulky disease.

Because NHLs are generally radioresponsive, conventional fractionation of RT is used. Typically, a dose of 200 cGy is given per fraction. For low-grade lymphomas, a total dose of 3000 cGy is sufficient. For high-grade lymphomas a higher dose is necessary, typically 3600–4400 cGy if used alone and lower (3600–4000 cGy) if used as consolidative therapy following administration of chemotherapy. The treated volume is called "involved-field," referring to the involved lymph node and its next draining nodal echelon.

If RT is used alone as definitive treatment for HD, 3600–4000 cGy is delivered to the upper mantle area (whole neck and supraclavicular, axillary, and mediastinal regions) followed by prophylactic RT to the paraaortic nodes and spleen. If chemotherapy is used as the primary treatment and RT as consolidative therapy, a lower dose (2500–3600 cGy) is delivered, usually to the involved region.

Mediastinal RT can cause acute and long-term side effects. Acute side effects include skin erythema and esophagitis. Long-term side effects include pericarditis, cardiomyopathy (especially in patients receiving adriamycin), pulmonary fibrosis, and myelitis. These side effects are unusual with modern RT techniques, which deliver high quality RT, taking into account the normal tissue tolerances. For example, if the spinal cord dose is kept at 4500 cGy, the risk of radiation-induced myelitis is virtually zero.

In the rare situation that the SVC syndrome fails to respond to nonsurgical therapy (chemotherapy, RT), the patient should be assessed for surgery. Experience with bypass grafting for SVC compression is limited. It is generally recommended that autologous grafts of the same caliber as the SVC be used. Some investigators use saphenous vein,[16,17] and at our institution Piccione et al.[18] used autologous pericardium to reconstruct the SVC after resection of a malignant tumor. Again, this is a rare situation; and the bypass procedure should be considered only by a vascular surgeon experienced with this technique.

With prompt diagnosis and management, a patient with SVC syndrome does not necessarily carry a worse prognosis than a patient with the same histology and stage but without SVC syndrome. In fact, some investigators think that patients with cancer and SVC syndrome have a better prognosis because the cancer is discovered earlier, but this point is debatable.[19] van Houtte et al.[19] showed that the 2-year survival was 15% both for patients with SVC syndrome and for those without SVC syndrome. In this series, SVC syndrome was found not to be a negative prognostic factor.

Conclusions

The SVC syndrome can be caused by a benign condition (aortic dissection, substernal goiter, tuberculosis or fungal infections, constrictive pericarditis), in which case the prognosis is generally good, or more commonly by a malignancy, in which case prompt diagnosis and therapy is essential for good outcome with the least late side effects. It cannot be overemphasized that a close collaboration between the internist, surgeon, medical oncologist, and radiation oncologist is necessary for a successful outcome.

References

1. Armstrong BA, Perez CA, Simpson JR, et al. Role of irradiation in the management of superior vena cava syndrome. Int J Radiat Oncol Biol Phys 1987;13:531–539.
2. Bell DR, Woods RL, Levi JA. Superior vena cava obstruction: a 10-year experience. Med J Aust 1986;145:566–568.
3. Schechter MM. The superior vena cava syndrome. Am J Med Sci 1954;227:46.
4. Painter TD, Karf M. Superior vena cava syndrome: diagnostic procedures. Am J Med Sci 1983;285:2–6.
5. Jeffrey GM, Mead GM, Whitehouse JMA. Life-threatening airway obstruction at the presentation of Hodgkin's disease. Cancer 1991;67:506–510.
6. Loeffler JS, Leopold KA, Recht A, et al. Emergency prebiopsy radiation for mediastinal masses: impact on subsequent pathologic diagnosis and outcome. J Clin Oncol 1986;4:716–721.
7. Jahangiri M, Goldstraw P. The role of mediastinoscopy in superior vena caval obstruction. Ann Thorac Surg 1995;59:453–455.
8. Dillman RO, Seagren SL, Propert KJ, et al. A randomized trial of induction chemotherapy plus high-dose radiation versus radiation alone in stage III non-small cell lung cancer. N Eng J Med 1990;323:940–945.
9. Byhardt RW. The evolution of Radiation Therapy Oncology Group (RTOG) protocols for non-small cell lung cancer. Int J Radiat Oncol Biol Phys 1995;32:1513–1525.
10. Sause WT, Scott C, Taylor S, et al. Radiation Therapy Oncology Group (RTOG) 88-08 and Eastern Cooperative Oncology Group (ECOG) 4588: preliminary results of a phase III trial in regionally advanced, unresectable non-small-cell lung cancer. J Natl Cancer Inst 1995;87:198–205.
11. Perry MC, Herdon JE II, Eaton WL, et al. Thoracic radiation therapy added to chemotherapy in limited small cell lung cancer: an update of Cancer & Leukemia Group B (CALGB) study 8083. Proc Am Soc Clin Oncol 1996;15:A1150.
12. Spiro SG, Shah S, Harper PG, et al. Treatment of obstruction of the superior vena cava by combination chemotherapy with and without irradiation in small cell carcinoma of the bronchus. Thorax 1983;38:501–505.
13. Armitage JO. Therapy of non-Hodgkin's lymphoma. N Engl J Med 1993;328:1023–1030.
14. Fisher RI, Gaynor ER, Dahlberg S, et al. Comparison of a standard regimen (CHOP) with three intensive chemotherapy regimens for advanced non-Hodgkin's lymphoma. N Engl J Med 1993;328:1002–1006.
15. Perez-Soler R, McLaughlin P, Velasquez WS, et al. Clinical features and results of management of superior vena cava syndrome secondary to lymphoma. J Clin Oncol 1984;2:260–266.
16. Scherck JP, Kerstein MD, Stansel HC. The current status of vena caval replacement. Surgery 1974;76:209–233.
17. Doty DB, Doty JR, Jones KW. Bypass of superior vena cava: fifteen years experience with spiral vein graft for obstruction of superior vena caused by benign disease. J Thorac Cardiovasc Surg 1990;99:889–895.
18. Piccione W Jr, Faber LP, Warren WH. Superior vena cava reconstruction using autologous pericardium. Ann Thorac Surg 1990;50:417–419.
19. Van Houtte P, De Jager R, Lustman-Marechal J, et al. Prognostic value of the superior vena cava syndrome as the presenting sign of small-cell anaplastic carcinoma of the lung. Eur J Cancer 1980;16:1447–1450.

Chapter 61

Cardiac Tamponade

David Esposito
Keith W. Millikan

A. Mechanism

Cardiac tamponade occurs as a result of fluid accumulating in the pericardial sac, which may in turn cause hemodynamic compromise. In the cancer patient it can occur as a result of obstruction of pericardial lymphatics by a primary cardiac malignancy or, more commonly, by metastatic disease to the pericardium. Primary cancers most commonly associated with metastases to the pericardium are lung and breast cancers, melanoma, lymphoma, and leukemia. Radiation to the chest used to treat various cancers can also cause pericardial effusions.[1] Overall, 15–40% of effusions are due to neoplastic processes and 4–7% to radiation.[2]

B. Pathophysiology

The pericardial sac normally contains 15–50 ml of fluid. The pressure of this fluid is usually at atmospheric levels; it changes with respiration and is less than the right and left ventricular end-diastolic pressures (EDPs). As the fluid in the pericardial sac increases, pressure increases until the intrapericardial pressure is greater than the ventricular EDP. At this point, diastolic filling is impaired and cardiac output decreases. The body compensates with systemic arteriolar vasoconstriction, increased blood volume, venoconstriction, and tachycardia. The severity of the symptoms depends on the rate of fluid accumulation, the volume of fluid, and the compliance of the pericardium. In the acute setting or if the pericardium is stiffened because of malignant infiltration or radiation fibrosis, as little as 150 ml of fluid can cause tamponade. With gradual accumulation of fluid, the pericardium can accommodate 1–2 liters before compressive symptoms arise.[1]

C. Diagnosis

The symptoms of pericardial tamponade are vague and are usually first attributed to other causes. Symptoms include chest pain or discomfort, anxiety, and dyspnea. Clinical signs range from mild tachycardia to circulatory collapse. *Pulsus paradoxus* is characterized by a systolic blood pressure decrease

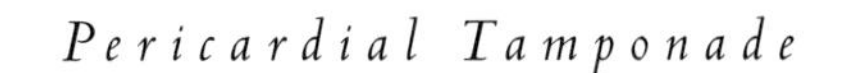

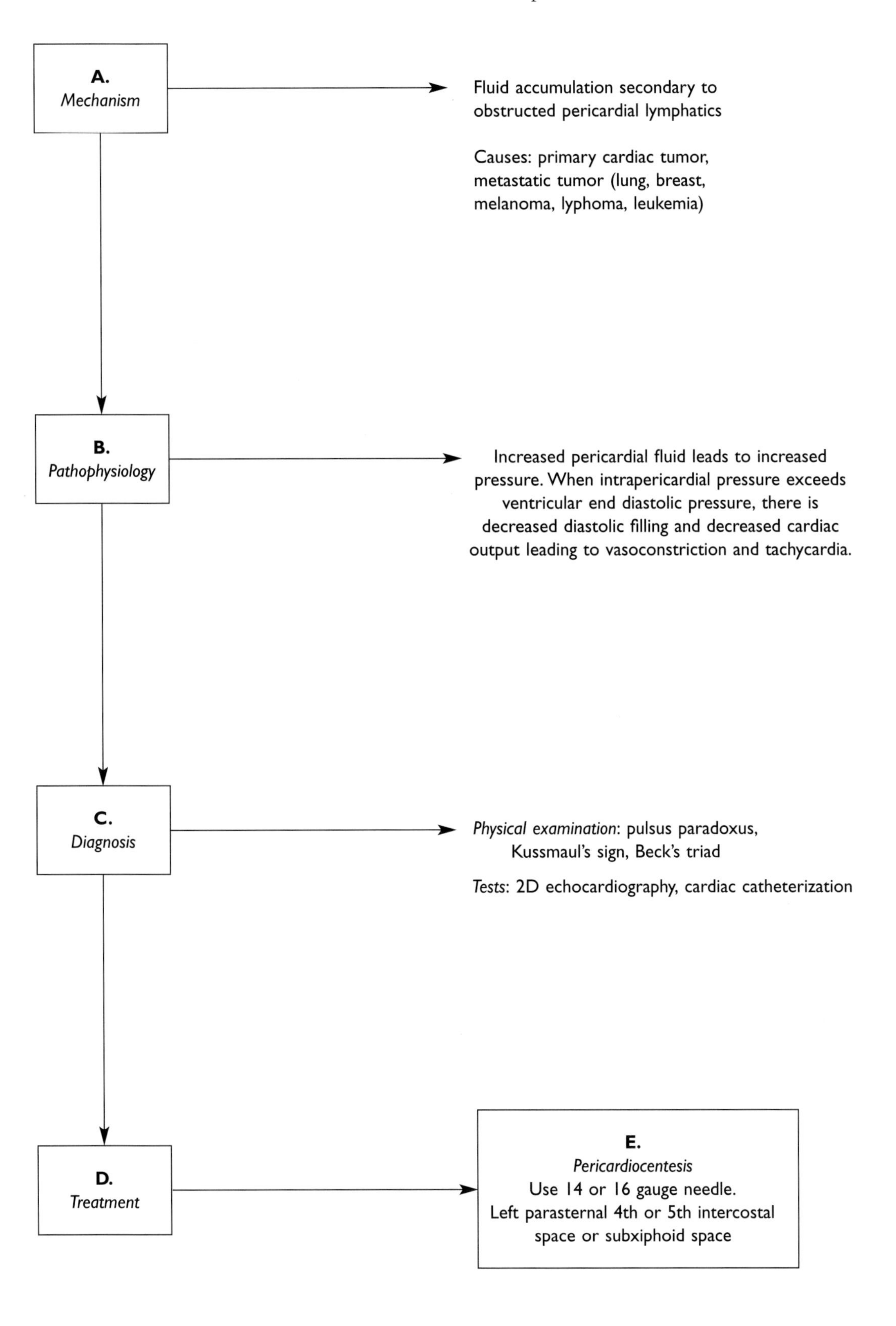

(continued on next page)

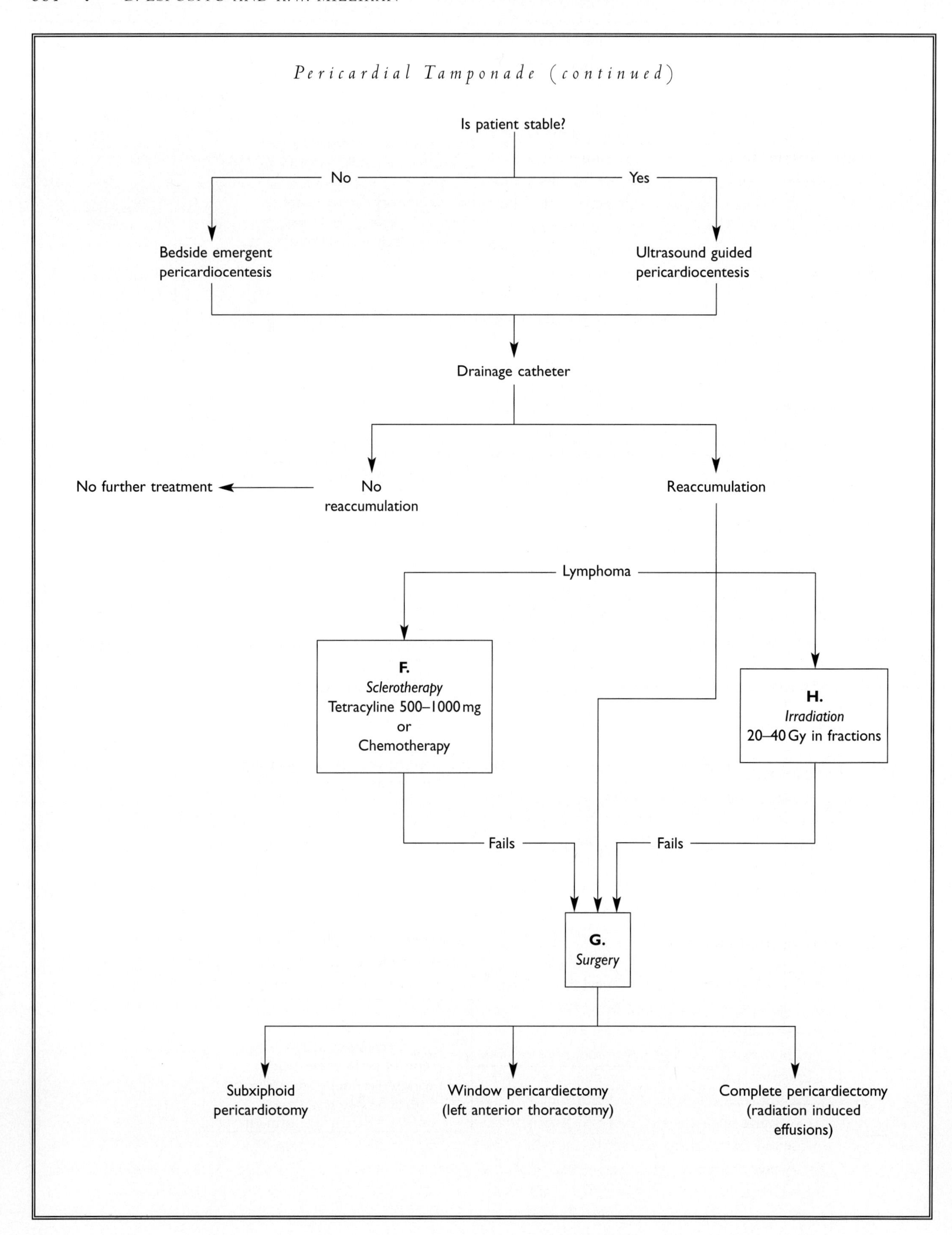
Pericardial Tamponade (continued)
Is patient stable?
No
Yes
Bedside emergent pericardiocentesis
Ultrasound guided pericardiocentesis
Drainage catheter
No further treatment
No reaccumulation
Reaccumulation
Lymphoma
F.
Sclerotherapy
Tetracyline 500–1000 mg
or
Chemotherapy
H.
Irradiation
20–40 Gy in fractions
Fails
Fails
G.
Surgery
Subxiphoid pericardiotomy
Window pericardiectomy (left anterior thoracotomy)
Complete pericardiectomy (radiation induced effusions)

systolic of more than 20 mm Hg with inspiration. Usually both pulsus paradoxus and Kussmaul's signs are seen and occur by the same mechanism; that is, they are an exaggeration of the normal inspiratory decline of left ventricular stroke volume and arterial pressure. This occurs because of the transmission of the negative intrathoracic pressure to the pericardium during inspiration. *Kussmaul's sign* is an increase in venous pressure with inspiration. *Beck's triad* consists of jugular venous distension, muffled heart sounds, and hypotension. These signs are pathognomonic and should alert the clinician to the diagnosis of tamponade immediately. Electrocardiography shows decreased voltage in all leads and sinus tachycardia. Two-dimensional echocardiography is the best tool to confirm the diagnosis, as it has the ability to detect pericardial fluid and collapse of the ventricles during diastole. This should be the test of choice for stable patients with suspected tamponade. Cardiac catheterization demonstrates that all chamber pressures are elevated and equal. It is thought that any patient who is not in extremis would benefit from cardiac catheterization to help establish the hemodynamic significance of the effusion and help determine the cause. Measurement of right-sided heart pressure and pericardial pressures simultaneous with pericardiocentesis: (1) confirm tamponade; (2) determine the degree of hemodynamic compromise; (3) document improvement in hemodynamic function during fluid withdrawal; and (4) diagnose coexisting abnormalities such as left ventricular failure, constrictive pericarditis, and pulmonary hypertension. Unstable patients suspected of having tamponade should be treated as such until proven otherwise, and diagnostic tests only delay treatment and jeopardize the patient.[3]

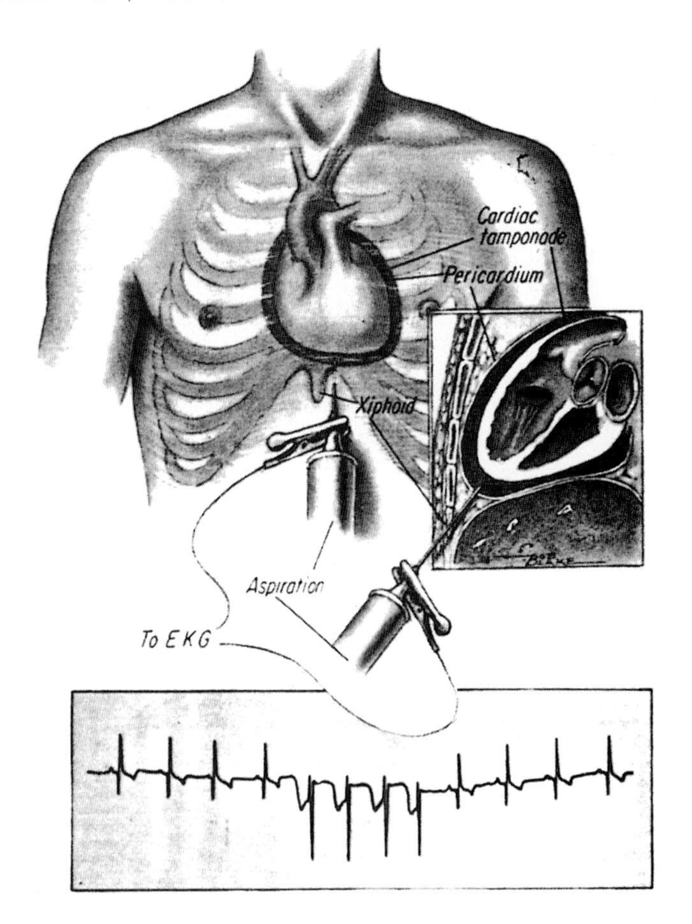

FIGURE 61–1
Technique of pericardiocentesis. (Reproduced with permission from Ebert P.: The pericardium. In Sabiston DC, and Speneer FC (eds): Gibbon's Surgery of the Chest, 4th ed. Philadelphia WB, Saunders 1983.)

D. *Treatment*

Appropriate systemic therapy aimed at the underlying neoplasm may provide long-term palliation. Pericardiocentesis with or without instillation of chemotherapeutic or sclerosing agents, surgery, and radiation therapy are also important in the management of this process.[4]

E. Pericardiocentesis

The treatment for cardiac tamponade is removal of the pericardial fluid. In the emergency setting this can be done at the bedside by inserting a needle via a left parasternal approach into the fourth or fifth interspace or via the subxiphoid route under local anesthesia. The patient's head and thorax are tilted upward, enhancing the accumulation of fluid anteriorly and inferiorly. A 14- or 16-gauge needle is attached to a stopcock and syringe and is inserted just underneath and to the left of the xiphoid process. A precordial electrocardiogram (ECG) lead is attached to the needle as it is inserted at a 30°–45° angle posteriorly, aimed at a point between the scapulae. The needle is advanced until fluid is encountered or the ECG indicates contact with the heart in the form of a negative deflection of the QRS complex (Fig. 61–1). Blood aspirated from the pericardium does not clot owing to rapid defibrination from cardiac motion. Aspiration of clotting blood indicates that it was obtained from a cardiac chamber.

Removal of even a small amount of fluid produces rapid, dramatic improvement of a patient in extremis. Once decompression is accomplished, a drainage catheter can be inserted over a guidewire to drain and monitor the rate of subsequent reaccumulation. This is especially important for malignant effusions. If the patient is stable, needle pericardiocentesis under ultrasound guidance can help avoid potential complications such as laceration of the heart, internal mammary or coronary arteries, or lung. The complication rate is approximately 5% with this procedure.[3]

Without further treatment, malignant effusions recur in more than 50% of patients. This figure can be decreased to less than 25% if a drainage catheter is used. Options for management of persistent malignant effusions include sclerotherapy, surgery, and radiation therapy.[5]

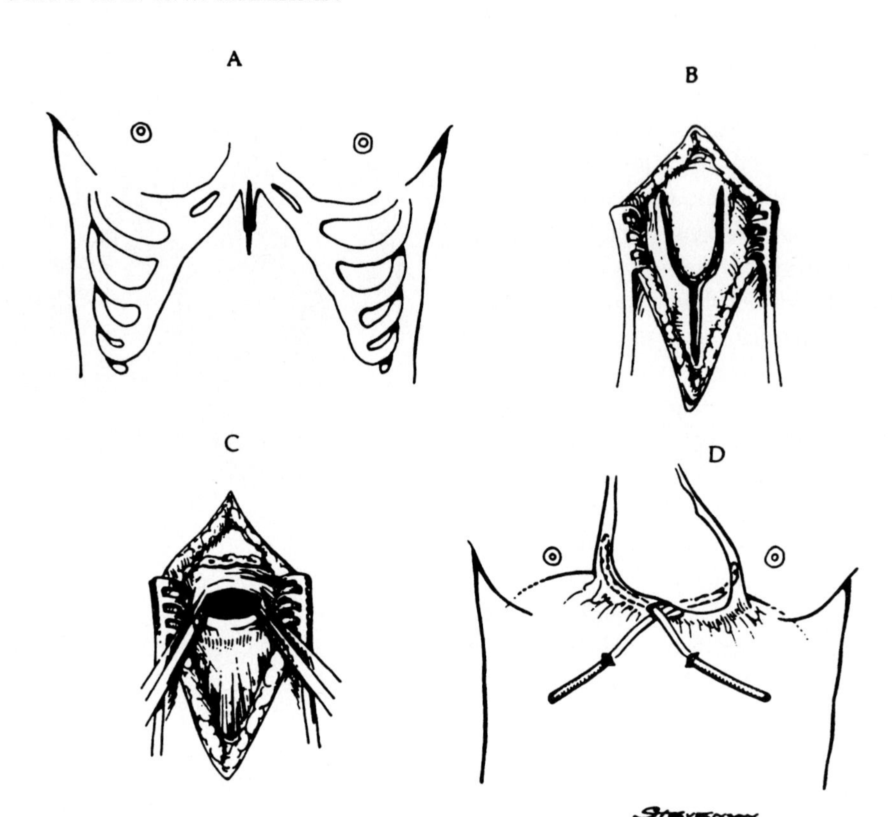

FIGURE 61–2
Technique of subxiphoid pericardial window. (Reproduced with permission from Hankins JR, Satterfield JR, Aisner J, et al. Pericardial window for malignant pericardial effuision. Ann Thorac Surg. 1980. Nov; 30(5):465–471.)

F. Sclerotherapy

Sclerosis is accomplished by instilling 500–1000 mg of tetracycline into the pericardial space. Bleomycin and nitrogen mustard have also been used successfully when instilled into the pericardial space for lung cancer and lymphoma. These agents generate an inflammatory response that leads to fibrosis and obliteration of the space. Multiple instillations are usually necessary and should be repeated until less than 25 ml drains over a 24-hour period. Sclerosis is successful in 86% of cases.[4]

G. Surgery

Subxiphoid Pericardiotomy Subxiphoid pericardiotomy avoids thoracotomy and can be done under local anesthesia. An incision is made to the left of the xiphoid down to the rectus muscle. Dissection is done cephalad, superior to the transversus abdominis muscle, to expose the pericardium. The pericardium is then incised, and a drainage catheter is placed (Fig. 61–2). The catheter is left in place until less than 25 ml drains over 24 hours. Recurrence with this procedure is 7%.[3]

Window Pericardiectomy Window pericardiectomy is done through a left anterior thoracotomy. A portion of pericardium is excised, allowing drainage of fluid into the left pleural space. The fluid is first evacuated from a thoracostomy tube and later, after the tube has been removed, is absorbed via the pleural space. Success rates approach 80%.

Complete Pericardiectomy Complete pericardiectomy is reserved for radiation-induced pericardial effusions. It can be done through a left anterior thoracotomy, bilateral thoracotomies, or median sternotomy. With this procedure the entire pericardium is decorticated from around the right and left ventricles. It is associated with an operative mortality of 4–15% and a long-term success rate of 75%.[1]

H. Irradiation

Radiation therapy is useful for treating the stable patient with symptoms of tamponade due to infiltration with lymphoma. Directed doses of radiation are given in 2- to 3-Gy fractions to a total dose of 20–40 Gy.[1]

Survival

Once a malignant pericardial effusion is detected, survival is related to the tumor type; it ranges from 3.5 months for lung cancer to 18.5 months for breast cancer.[1] Thus the presence of a pericardial effusion does not preclude meaningful survival, underlining the importance of prompt detection.

References

1. Bergen DH, Feig BW, Fuhrman GM (eds). The MD Anderson Surgical Oncology Handbook, 2nd ed. Boston: Little Brown, 1995.
2. Ball JB, Morrison JB. Cardiac tamponade. Postgrad Med J 1997;73:141–145.
3. Sabiston DC. Textbook of Surgery, 15th ed. Philadelphia: Saunders, 1997; 1946–1949.
4. Smith FE. Cardrovascular complications of malignancy. In Smith FE, Lane M (eds). Medical Complications of Malignancy. New York: John Wiley, 1984; 1–11.
5. Hancock EW. Cardiac tamponade. Heart Disease Stroke 1994; May/June; (3):155–158.

Chapter 62

Adrenal Insufficiency

William B. Inabnet III

A. Introduction

Adrenal insufficiency (AI) is caused by dysfunction of the hypothalamus-pituitary-adrenal (HPA) axis that leads to inadequate secretion of adrenocortical hormones. With *primary AI*, commonly referred to as Addison's disease, the adrenal cortex is compromised resulting in decreased adrenocortical function. During the 1930s tuberculosis was the most common cause of primary AI, but currently autoimmune adrenalitis accounts for more than 75% of cases.[1,2] Conditions that disrupt the hypothalamus-pituitary axis lead to *secondary AI* by impairing secretion of adrenocorticotropin hormone (ACTH) from the anterior pituitary gland. Although the level of disruption of the HPA axis is different for primary and secondary AI, the endpoint is the same: decreased ACTH release and function.

Essential to appreciating the pathophysiology, diagnosis, and treatment of AI is an understanding of the biosynthesis and regulation of adrenocortical hormones. The hypothalamus synthesizes and releases corticotropin-releasing hormone (CRH) in response to a variety of stimuli from the central nervous system. CRH reaches the pituitary gland via the portal circulation, stimulating secretion of ACTH by the anterior pituitary gland. ACTH is released into the systemic circulation, where it stimulates the zona fasciculata and zona reticularis of the adrenal cortex to release glucocorticoids and androgens, respectively.[3] The zona glomerulosa, the outer layer of the adrenal cortex, which secretes aldosterone, is regulated by the renin-angiotensin system and to a much lesser extent by ACTH.[4] For this reason, aldosterone deficiency is *not* a component of secondary AI, as ACTH plays a negligible role in the biosynthesis of aldosterone. ACTH secretion is regulated by multiple factors, including cortisol, the circadian rhythm, CRH, and stress. Cortisol exerts a negative feedback on CRH, thereby regulating ACTH synthesis and release.

The biologic activity of cortisol is complex, playing a key role in carbohydrate and protein metabolism and regulation of the immune system. Cortisol secretion is under the influence of the circadian rhythm, with levels peaking at 8:00 a.m. and reaching a trough between 10:00 p.m. and 2:00 a.m. Events that cause stress, such as surgery, sepsis, or trauma, disrupt the normal diurnal variation of cortisol, leading to increased synthesis and secretion of glucocorticoids. With AI, the adrenal response to stressful stimuli

Adrenal Insufficiency

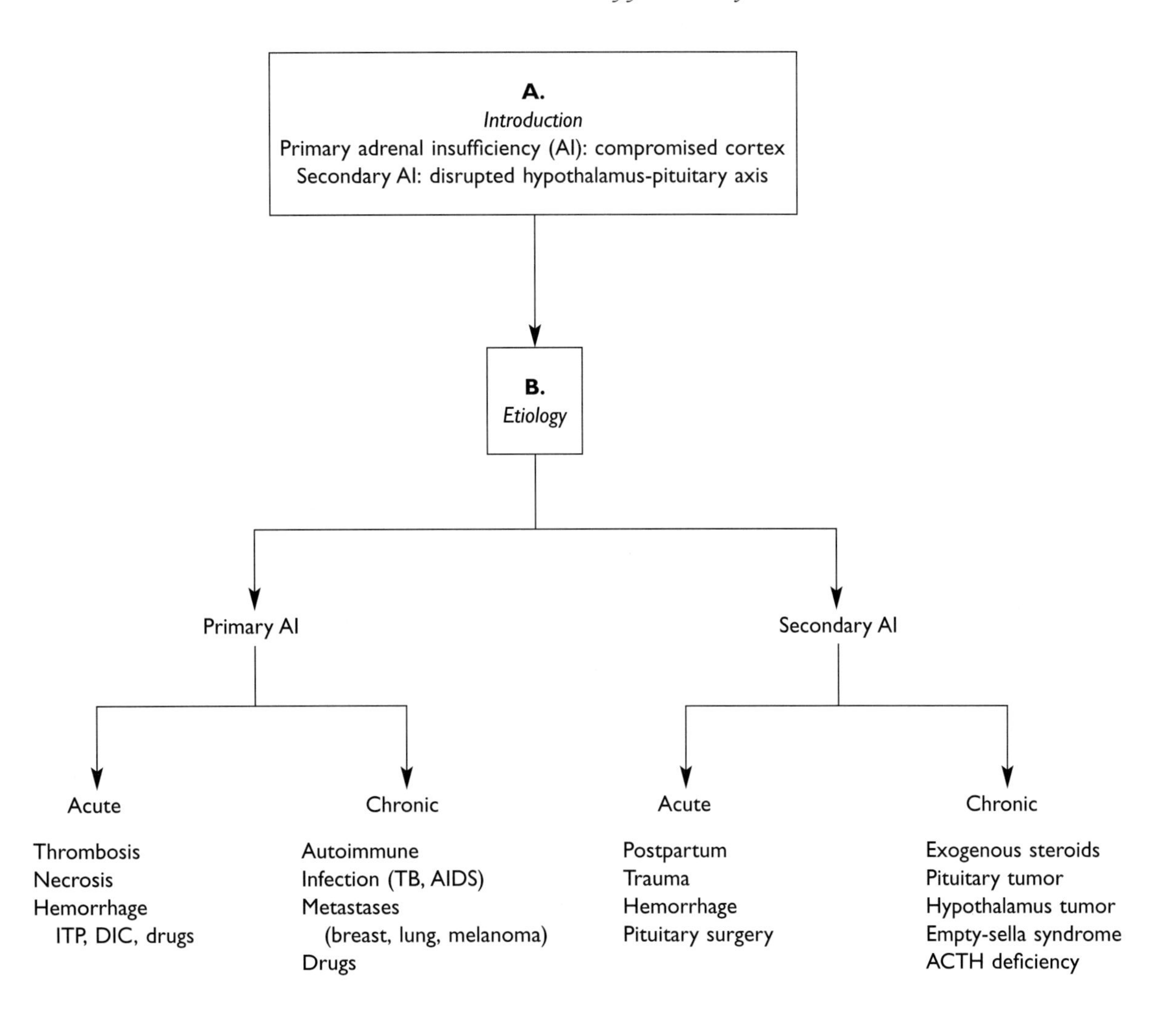

C.
Clinical Manifestations

General
Hemodynamic
Hyperpigmentation (primary AI)
Gastrointestinal
Psychiatric
Endocrine
Laboratory findings

(continued on next page)

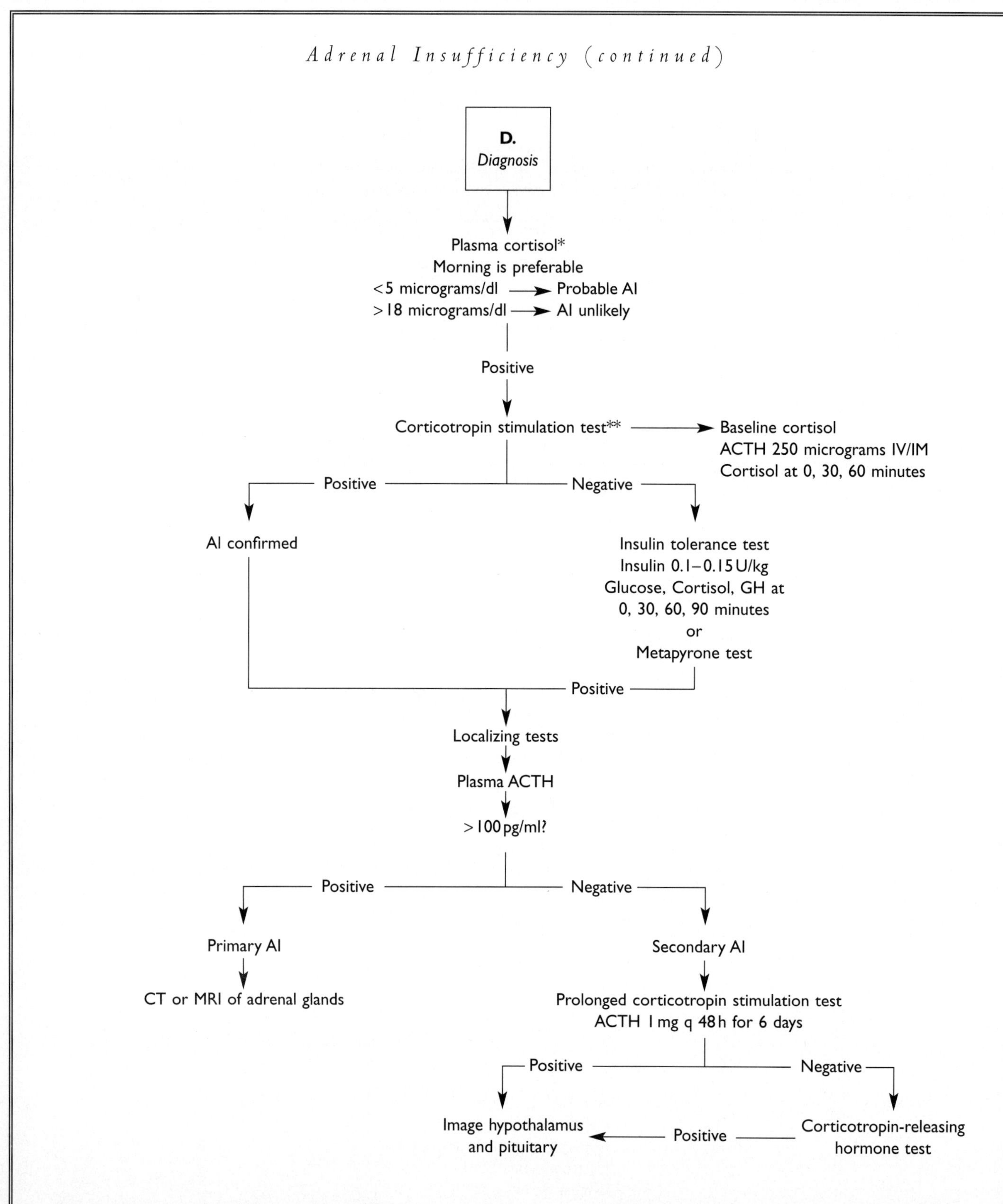

Adrenal Insufficiency (continued)
D.
Diagnosis
Plasma cortisol*
Morning is preferable
<5 micrograms/dl → Probable AI
>18 micrograms/dl → AI unlikely
Positive
Corticotropin stimulation test** → Baseline cortisol
ACTH 250 micrograms IV/IM
Cortisol at 0, 30, 60 minutes
Positive
Negative
AI confirmed
Insulin tolerance test
Insulin 0.1–0.15 U/kg
Glucose, Cortisol, GH at
0, 30, 60, 90 minutes
or
Metapyrone test
Positive
Localizing tests
Plasma ACTH
>100 pg/ml?
Positive
Negative
Primary AI
CT or MRI of adrenal glands
Secondary AI
Prolonged corticotropin stimulation test
ACTH 1 mg q 48 h for 6 days
Positive
Negative
Image hypothalamus
and pituitary
Positive
Corticotropin-releasing
hormone test
*Normal plasma cortisol does not rule out AI.
**Useful for primary and chronic secondary AI; of little benefit for acute secondary AI.

Adrenal Insufficiency (continued)

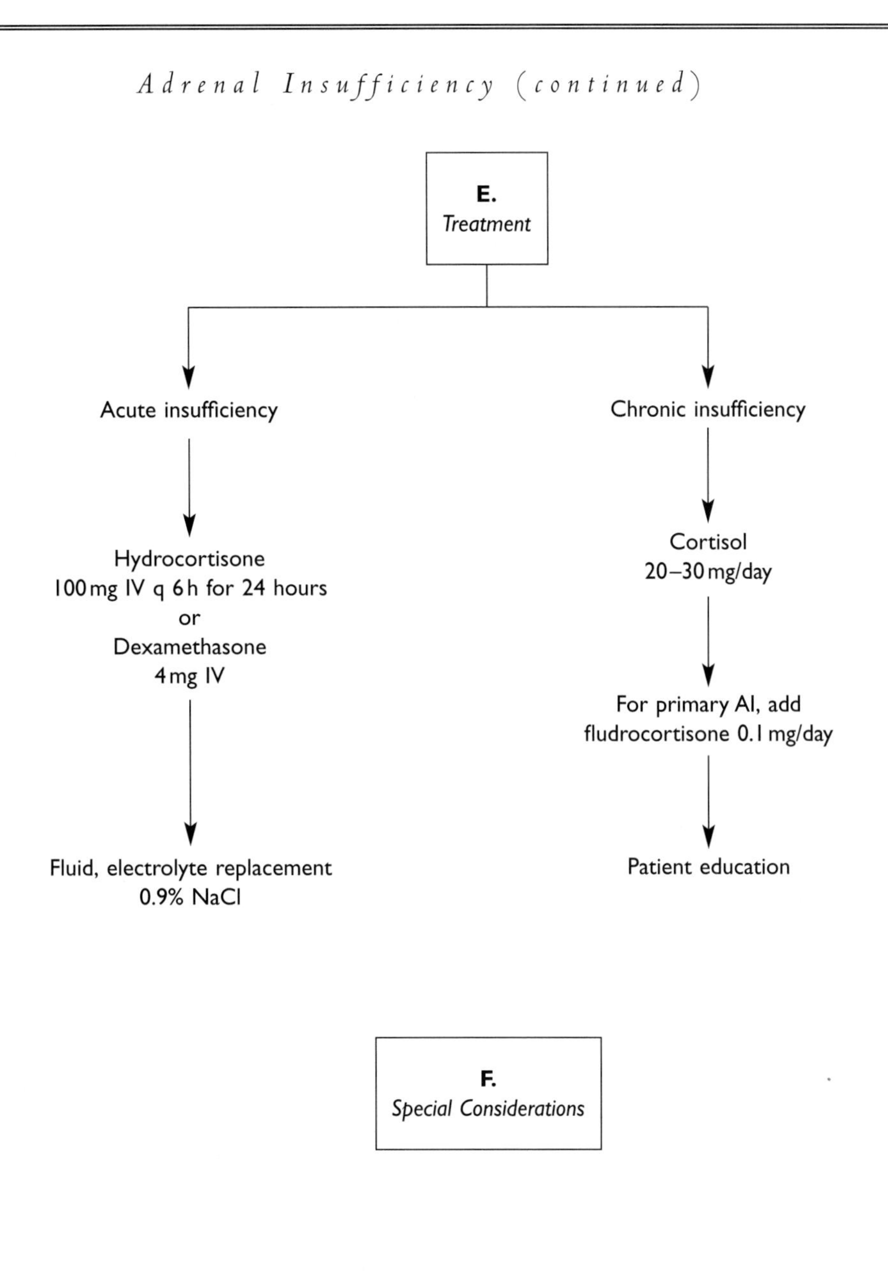

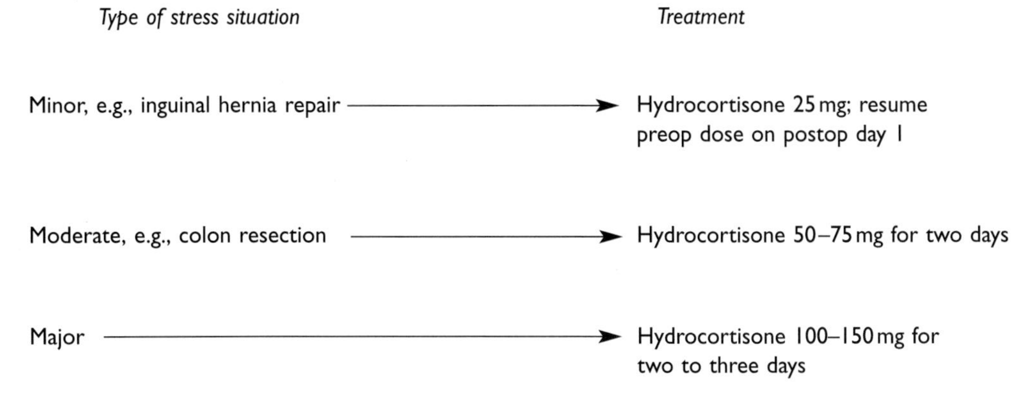

is inadequate, leading to a wide array of nonspecific symptoms. Early recognition and treatment of adrenal failure are essential because AI is usually fatal if not diagnosed and treated in a timely manner.

B. *Etiology*

The clinical manifestations of primary AI result from deficiencies of aldosterone, cortisol, and androgens (all three layers of the cortex). Although the adrenal medulla is typically spared, epinephrine synthesis is dependent on high local concentrations of cortisol,[4] the deficiency of which may blunt normal synthesis of epinephrine, further compromising the adrenal response to stress.

Secondary AI occurs as a result of dysfunction of the hypothalamus or pituitary glands, the end result of which is decreased release of ACTH. Differentiating between primary and secondary AI is essential for the management of these patients, as the clinical manifestations, workup, and treatment vary.

Primary Adrenal Insufficiency

Acute-onset primary AI is a truly life-threatening emergency. Events that acutely compromise adrenal perfusion (e.g., adrenal hemorrhage, thrombosis, necrosis) can lead to acute adrenal failure. The adrenal gland has a rich arterial blood supply derived from the inferior phrenic artery, aorta, and adrenal artery. Fifty to sixty small arterioles converge to form a subcapsular plexus that communicates with a vascular plexus at the corticomedullary junction. The medullary sinusoids, in turn, drain into the thick-walled, muscular adrenal vein. The left adrenal vein empties into the left renal vein, whereas the right adrenal vein drains directly into the vena cava.

The pathogenesis of adrenal hemorrhage is in part related to the unique circulatory anatomy of the adrenal gland. Because the corticomedullary junction is the farthest removed from the adrenal arterial supply, this region has a disproportionally high oxygen demand and is particularly vulnerable to ischemic changes. Disease states that cause hypotension, such as sepsis or hemorrhagic shock, can acutely compromise adrenal perfusion, leading first to ischemia and then necrosis and hemorrhage at the corticomedullary junction. In contrast, sudden increases in adrenal perfusion may contribute to the pathogenesis of adrenal thrombosis by exceeding the limited venous drainage of the adrenal gland, thereby promoting venous stasis and platelet aggregation. This sequence of events can result in thrombosis, necrosis, and central hemorrhage, the end result of which is compromised adrenal function.[3]

Although adrenal hemorrhage is often associated with anticoagulation therapy, it is unclear if excessive anticoagulation is the underlying event.[3,5,6] In many cases hemorrhage occurs even though the prothrombin time is within normal limits.[5] Other causes of coagulopathy that may lead to adrenal hemorrhage include the presence of the lupus anticoagulant, idiopathic thrombocytopenic purpura (ITP), disseminated intravascular coagulation (DIC), uremia, and drug-induced coagulopathy (e.g., cephalosporins).[5]

The *Waterhouse-Friderichsen syndrome*, a rare disease that occurs in children, is characterized by bilateral adrenal hemorrhage, meningococcal septicemia, purpura, and vascular collapse.[3] Acute AI should be suspected, diagnosed, and treated in patients with meningococcal septicemia, shock, and the characteristic skin purpura. If untreated, the Waterhouse-Friderichsen syndrome has a poor prognosis.

Adrenal vein thrombosis is a well recognized complication of adrenal venography.[2] Iatrogenic adrenal vein thrombosis is typically a unilateral process and theoretically should not cause AI. However, some patients have a functioning adrenal adenoma that causes suppression of the contralateral adrenal gland.[7] In this setting, adrenal vein thrombosis of the gland with the adenoma could lead to acute-onset primary AI.

Several diseases may cause a slow, insidious onset of primary AI, the most common of which is *autoimmune adrenalitis* (65–90% of all cases of primary adrenal failure).[1–3] The adrenal glands experience diffuse bilateral infiltration of cytotoxic lymphocytes that cause uniform destruction of the adrenal cortex, a process that spares the adrenal medulla. Autoimmune adrenalitis is often associated with other autoimmune diseases, which has allowed classification of this disease into two types: polyglandular autoimmune (PGA) syndrome types I and II. PGA syndrome types I and II share several common features, including primary AI, hypothyroidism, vitiligo, alopecia, and pernicious anemia.[2] Features unique to the PGA syndrome type I include early age of onset, hypoparathyroidism, chronic mucocutaneous candidiasis, and no HLA association. Patients with PGA syndrome type II usually present during adulthood and have a high frequency of insulin-dependent diabetes mellitus, thyroid autoimmunity, and HLA association.

A variety of infections can cause primary AI. *Tuberculosis* was once the most common cause of primary adrenal destruction but now accounts for only 10% of cases in developed countries.[2] Tuberculous AI should be suspected in patients with slow-onset adrenal failure and a positive tuberculin skin test. Most patients have radiographic evidence of pulmonary involvement.[1] In acute cases the adrenal glands are enlarged bilaterally, whereas in chronic cases the adrenal glands appear diffusely calcified. There has been a recent increase in the incidence of tuberculosis in the United States, particularly in the inner cities; accordingly, the incidence of tuberculous AI may also increase.[8]

There is a clear association between fungal infections and primary AI.[1–3] Disseminated *histoplasmosis*, which is endemic in certain parts of the United States, is the most common fungal cause of adrenal failure, leading to AI in more than 50% of infected patients.[3] Other, less common fungal etiologies include blastomycosis, cryptococcosis, and coccidiomycosis.

The *acquired immunodeficiency syndrome* (AIDS) results in adrenocortical destruction in 5–10% of patients during the late stages of the disease.[3,8] Opportunistic pathogens, such as cytomegalovirus (CMV), *Mycobacterium avium*, and *Cryptococcus*, infiltrate the adrenal gland; the human immunodeficiency virus (HIV) can also directly infiltrate the adrenal gland, as can Kaposi's sarcoma. Drugs commonly used to treat patients with AIDS, including rifampin and ketoconazole, can contribute to adrenal failure. Adrenal involvement should be suspected in patients with unexplained hypotension and generalized decompensation.

Several drugs used to treat Cushing's disease inhibit adrenal steroidogenesis, including *o,p'*-DDD (mitotane), metyrapone, ketoconazole, and aminoglutethimide.[1] Other, more commonly used drugs, such as rifampin, phenytoin, and phenobarbital, can lead to AI by accelerating cortisol catabolism.[3]

Metastases to the adrenal gland are common, occurring in approximately 22% of all patients with adenocarcinoma.[9] Primary tumors with a high propensity to metastasize to the adrenal gland include breast and lung cancers and melanoma. Despite the high incidence of adrenal gland involvement, AI due to malignant disease is rare, occurring in fewer than 5% of patients[10]; extensive destruction of bilateral adrenal tissue is necessary before AI becomes clinically apparent.[9,10] In this setting, cure is rarely possible, although steroid replacement therapy may greatly improve the quality of life.

Secondary Adrenal Insufficiency

Secondary AI results from impaired synthesis and release of ACTH from the anterior pituitary gland or from compromised secretion of CRH from the hypothalamus. Diseases that disrupt pituitary perfusion can lead to abrupt onset of secondary AI. Postpartum pituitary necrosis (Sheehan syndrome) may occur in patients with postpartum hemorrhage and hypotension, leading to deficient production of ACTH, gonadotropins, and thyroid-stimulating hormone (TSH).[11] Other causes of acute-onset secondary AI include necrosis or bleeding into a pituitary macroadenoma, head trauma, and pituitary surgery for Cushing's disease.[4]

Administration of exogenous steroids is the most common cause of AI, resulting in a slow, insidious onset of symptoms in the unstressed patient.[8,12] Exogenous steroids cause negative feedback inhibition of the HPA axis primarily by suppressing the synthesis and release of CRH by the hypothalamus. The use of exogenous steroids is commonplace, playing an important role in the immunosuppression of transplant patients and in the management of a variety of common diseases such as asthma, arthritis, and inflammatory bowel disease. These patients have an increased risk of developing postoperative AI if perioperative glucocorticoid coverage is not provided.[12] Even a short 1-week course of corticosteroid therapy can lead to secondary AI.[8] Other, less common causes of slow-onset secondary AI include primary or metastatic pituitary tumors, tumors of the hypothalamus, the empty-sella syndrome, and isolated ACTH deficiency.[4]

C. Clinical Manifestations

The clinical manifestations of AI range from a gradual onset of symptoms in the unstressed patient to sudden vascular collapse during events that cause stress. Many of the symptoms are nonspecific and vague in nature, often resulting in a missed or delayed diagnosis. The diagnosis of AI requires a high index of suspicion and familiarity with the clinical manifestations of adrenocortical deficiency. There is also considerable overlap of the symptomatology of AI and that of other disease processes. This is particularly true in oncologic patients, who often experience anorexia, weight loss, and vomiting due to the underlying neoplastic process or the administration of adjuvant therapy.

Generalized symptoms of AI include fatigue, muscle weakness, asthenia, arthralgia, and anorexia.[3] Vague abdominal complaints such as abdominal pain, cramps, or diarrhea are common. A low-grade fever and tachycardia often precede more serious manifestations such as hypotension and shock.[9] Other nonspecific presenting features include postural dizziness, weight loss, and decreased libido.[4]

The hemodynamic manifestations of AI range from orthostatic hypotension in patients with chronic adrenal failure to catecholamine-resistant shock in the acute setting.[3,8] Postural hypotension is more pronounced in patients with primary AI than in those with secondary AI due to the hypovolemic effects of aldosterone insufficiency. Decreased aldosterone production leads to sodium wasting, volume depletion, and impaired excretion of potassium.[1] In addition, patients often experience a craving for salt.[4] In the stressed patient with untreated adrenal failure, the hemodynamic instability closely resembles that of sepsis, characterized by profound hypotension, high cardiac output, normal pulmonary capillary wedge pressure, and low systemic vascular resistance.[1] Cardiac contractility and work are also decreased. In addition, decreased local cortisol levels impair the synthesis and release of catecholamines from the adrenal medulla, which also contributes to the pathogenesis of shock in these patients. Many of the hemodynamic manifestations resolve shortly after administration of glucocorticoids.[3]

Hyperpigmentation is one of the most specific findings in primary AI, occurring in up to 90% of patients.[3] Because hyperpigmentation results from elevated levels of ACTH, this

and any delay in such improvement should raise the question of an incorrect diagnosis. After initiating therapy, the underlying cause of the adrenal crisis must be identified and appropriately treated.

The goal of long-term therapy is to maintain the patient on the lowest possible dose of oral glucocorticoid replacement therapy. Numerous glucocorticoid preparations are available with varying potencies, including cortisol, cortisone, prednisone, and dexamethasone.[3] Even though in normal states the adrenal glands produce 15–20mg of cortisol per day, most patients with AI require 20–30mg of cortisol (or an equivalent dose) per day.[2] The dose is usually divided into two or three daily doses. Attempting to mimic the normal pulsatile secretion of endogenous cortisol by dose staggering is of little benefit. Certain drugs (e.g., rifampin, phenytoin, barbiturates) increase the metabolism of steroids in the liver, often necessitating higher doses of replacement therapy. In patients with primary AI, a mineralocorticoid must also be administered as a substitute for aldosterone. Fludrocortisone (Florinef) 0.1 mg per day is the drug of choice, the adequacy of which can be monitored by checking for postural hypotension and by following plasma sodium levels.

Whereas secondary AI due to exogenous steroid use is usually reversible, most primary AIs lead to permanent adrenal failure. Patient education is of utmost importance for long-term management of chronic primary AI. Patients must always wear a Medic-Alert bracelet or necklace listing their medical condition, medications, and appropriate emergency contact numbers. Preloaded syringes of dexamethasone should always be in close proximity to the patient. For minor febrile illnesses, patients can double or triple their maintenance dose without consulting a physician. All major sources of stress (e.g., trauma, myocardial infarction, sepsis) require increased dosing of steroid therapy.

F. Special Considerations

Providing adequate perioperative glucocorticoid coverage for patients with AI is critical to a successful surgical outcome. When preparing a patient for major surgery, the traditional approach has been to administer perioperative stress-dose steroids consisting of 300mg of hydrocortisone in divided doses over the 24 hours surrounding surgery. Studies have shown, however, that the current recommended dose of perioperative glucocorticoids is excessive.[12,19] Glucocorticoid administration should be adjusted to the magnitude of the stress and the known glucocorticoid production associated with it. Using this approach, Salem et al. revised the recommendations for perioperative glucocorticoid coverage.[12]

Whereas the traditional perioperative glucocorticoid coverage is based on anecdotal information from the 1950s, these new recommendations are based on accumulated experimental data of the adrenal response to stress.[12] The degree of surgical stress can be divided into mild, moderate, and severe categories, each requiring differing amounts of glucocorticoid coverage. For *minor surgical stress*, such as an inguinal hernia repair, the perioperative glucocorticoid target is a bout 25 mg of hydrocortisone equivalent.[12] If the operation is uneventful, the preoperative maintenance dose can be resumed on the first postoperative day. Surgical procedures associated with *moderate surgical stress* include open cholecystectomy, colon resection, and lower extremity revascularization. The glucocorticoid target for these procedures is approximately 50–75 mg of hydrocortisone equivalent for 1–2 days. For patients experiencing *major surgical stress*, the steroid target should be 100–150mg of hydrocortisone per day for 2–3 days. With each category of surgical stress, the exact steroid dosing should be adjusted to the overall medical condition of the patient and to the occurrence of any perioperative complications.

References

1. Burke CW. Adrenocortical insufficiency. Clin Endocrinol Metab 1985; 14:947–976.
2. Burke CW. Primary adrenocortical failure. In: Grossman A (ed) Clinical Endocrinology. Oxford: Blackwell Scientific, 1992:393–404.
3. Werbel SS, Ober KP. Acute adrenal insufficiency. Endocrinol Metab Clin North Am 1993;22:303–328.
4. Oeklers W. Adrenal insufficiency. N Engl J Med 1996;335:1206–1212.
5. Dahlberg PJ, Goellner MH, Pehling GB. Adrenal insufficiency secondary to adrenal hemorrhage: two case reports and a review of cases confirmed by computed tomography. Arch Intern Med 1990;150:905–909.
6. Siu SC, Kitzman DW, Sheedy PF, Northcut RC. Adrenal insufficiency from bilateral adrenal hemorrhage. Mayo Clin Proc 1990;65: 664–670.
7. Huiras CM, Pehling GB, Caplan RH. Adrenal insufficiency after operative removal of apparently nonfunctioning adrenal adenomas. JAMA 1989; 261:894–898.
8. Numann PJ. Addison's disease and acute adrenal hemorrhage. In: Clark OH, Duh Q-Y (eds) Textbook of Endocrine Surgery. Philadelphia: Saunders, 1997:523–528.
9. Ihde JK, Turnbull AD, Bajorunas DR. Adrenal insufficiency in the cancer patient: implications for the surgeon. Br J Surg 1990;77:1335–1337.
10. Kung AW, Pun KK, Lam KL, et al. Addison crisis as presenting feature in malignancies. Cancer 1990;65:177–179.
11. Prager D, Braunstein PD. Pituitary disorders during pregnancy. Endocrinol Metab Clin North Am 1995;24:1–14.
12. Salem M, Tainsh RE, Bromberg J, et al. Perioperative glucocorticoid coverage: a reassessment 42 years after emergence of a problem. Ann Surg 1994;219:416–425.
13. Grinspoon SK, Biller BM. Clinical review 62: laboratory assessment of adrenal insufficiency. J Clin Endocrinol Metab 1994;79:923–931.
14. Schulte HM, Chrousos BP, Avgerinos P, et al. The corticotropin-releasing hormone stimulation test: a possible aid in the evaluation of patients with adrenal insufficiency. J Clin Endocrinol Metab 1984;58:1064–1067.

15. Baker DE, Glazer GM, Francis IR. Adrenal magnetic resonance imaging in Addison's disease. Urol Radiol 1988;9:199–203.
16. Gilfeather M, Woodward PJ. MR imaging of the adrenal glands and kidneys. Semin Ultrasound CT MR 1988;19:53–66.
17. Glazer GM, Francis IR, Quint LE. Imaging of the adrenal glands. Invest Radiol 1988;23:3–11.
18. Buxi TB, Vohra RB, Sujathay. CT in adrenal enlargement due to tuberculosis: a review of literature with five new cases. Clin Imaging 1992; 16:102–108.
19. Glowniak JV, Loriaux DL. A double blind study of perioperative steroid requirements in secondary adrenal insufficiency. Surgery 1997;121:123–129.

CHAPTER 63

Hypercalcemic Crisis

RODERICH E. SCHWARZ

A. Introduction

Calcium, ubiquitous in the body, is the most common mineral element. The normal adult body contains 1000 g of calcium, more than 98% of which is localized in bones.[1] Under normal conditions tightly controlled homeostasis of body calcium leads to a constant calcium level in the extracellular fluid (ECF) compartment. The serum calcium level relates directly to this ECF calcium concentration; and factors that regulate it include calcium itself by means of a calcium receptor,[2] parathyroid hormone (PTH), and 1,25-dihydroxyvitamin D_3 [$1,25(OH)_2D_3$].[3]

In the ECF calcium exists in three forms: 50% is ionized calcium, which represents the biologically active calcium fraction; 10% is complexed to anions including bicarbonate, phosphate, and sulfate; and 40% is protein-bound, primarily to albumin. It has been established that 1 g of albumin can bind 0.8 mg of calcium per deciliter. To correct for hypoalbuminemia, this amount should be added to the measured serum calcium level for each gram of albumin below 4 g/dl. For those readers who prefer formulas, it translates into:

$$\text{Corrected calcium (mg/dl)} = \text{measured calcium} + \{[4 - \text{albumin (g/dl)}] \times 0.8\}$$

Ionized serum calcium is dependent on the pH of the ECF. Acidemia decreases protein binding of calcium and increases ionized calcium (hypocalcemic symptoms can be temporized with respiratory acidosis through rebreathing). For each 0.1 incremental decrease in pH, the ionized calcium level rises 0.2 mg/dl (0.05 mmol/L). A calcium level of 1 mg/dl equals 0.25 mmol/L (SI unit) or 0.5 mEq/L; a level of 1 mmol/L equals 4 mg/dl. The normal range of total serum calcium is 8.5–10.5 mg/dl (2.1–2.6 mmol/L), and that of ionized serum calcium is 4.48–4.92 mg/dl (1.12–1.23 mmol/L). Although better suited for clinical decision-making, ionized calcium levels are still not widely measured. The guidelines in this chapter therefore continue to refer to total serum calcium values in both conventional and SI units.

Hypercalcemic Crisis

A.

Introduction

Calcium regulated by parathyroid hormone, vitamin D^3

Corrected calcium = measured calcium + {[4 − albumin(g/dl)] × 0.8}

For each 0.1 fall in pH, ionized calcium rises 0.2 mg/dl

B.

Clinical Presentation

Mild hypercalcemia: frequently asymptomatic, found incidentally on electrolyte panels

Moderate or severe hypercalcemia: neuromuscular signs, polyuria, reduction in extracellular volume, kidney stones, gastrointestinal symptoms, bradycardia, bone pain

C.

Differential Diagnosis

Primary hyperparathyroidism: rarely causes hypercalcemic crisis, diagnosed by elevated PTH

Hypercalcemia of malignancy: elevated PTH not generally seen, caused usually by breast or lung cancer

Drug induced: rarely leads to severe symptoms

Granulomatous disease

Metabolic disorders

D.

Diagnosis

Tests needed:
- Serum calcium
- Serum phosphate
- Serum chloride
- Intact PTH
- PTH-related peptide

Imaging studies to assess extent of cancer:
- Bone scan
- Plain film radiography

(continued on next page)

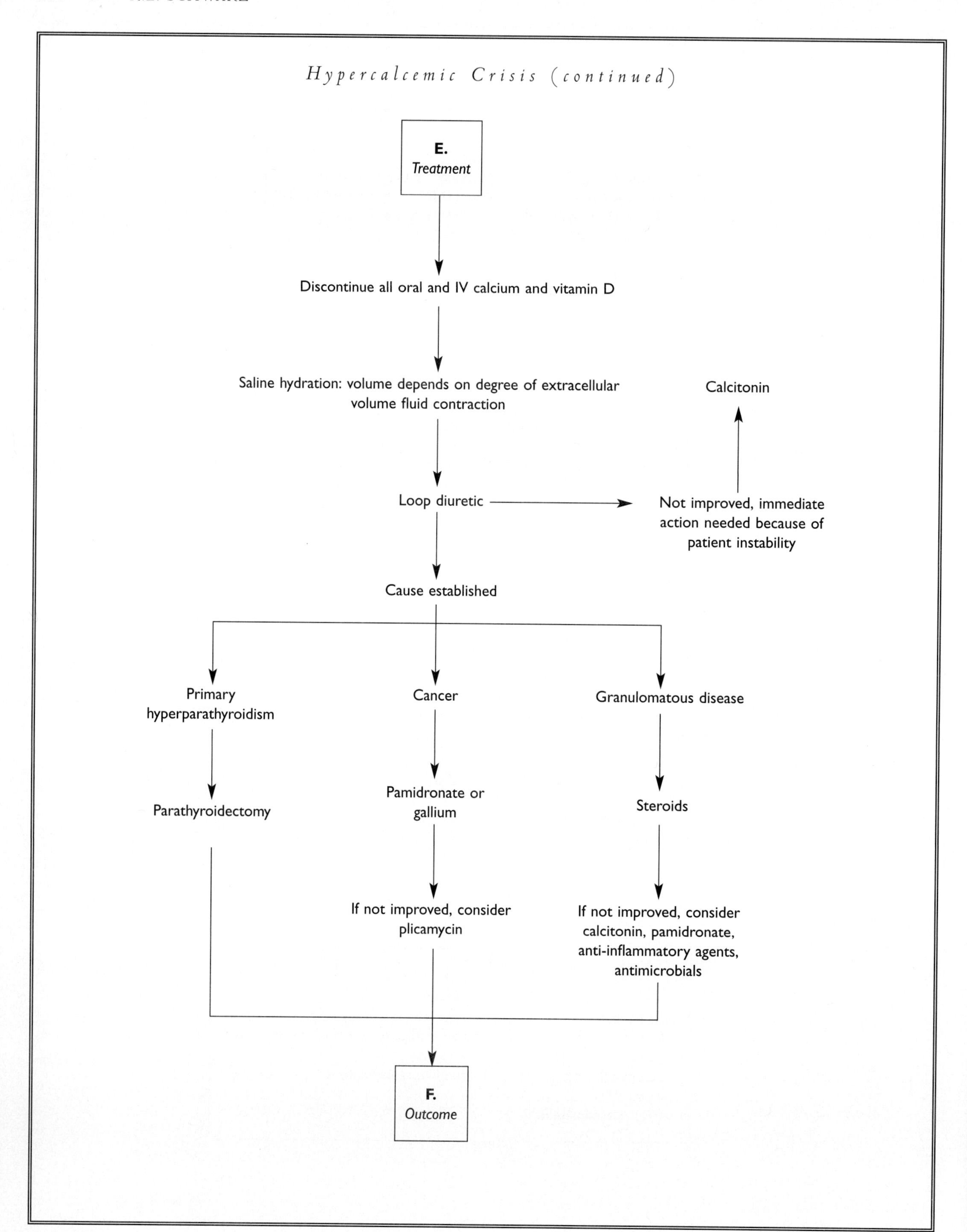
Hypercalcemic Crisis (continued)
E.
Treatment
Discontinue all oral and IV calcium and vitamin D
Saline hydration: volume depends on degree of extracellular volume fluid contraction
Calcitonin
Loop diuretic
Not improved, immediate action needed because of patient instability
Cause established
Primary hyperparathyroidism
Cancer
Granulomatous disease
Parathyroidectomy
Pamidronate or gallium
Steroids
If not improved, consider plicamycin
If not improved, consider calcitonin, pamidronate, anti-inflammatory agents, antimicrobials
F.
Outcome

B. Clinical Presentation

Hypercalcemia results from a relative increase of calcium influx from bone or intestine compared to the efflux into or through kidney, bone, or intestine. This imbalance may be caused by acute or chronic mechanisms. The rate of increase of the calcium concentration can determine whether symptoms occur and how quickly treatment measures should be instituted, as compensation mechanisms to chronic hypercalcemia exist. Accordingly, the rate of calcium elevation may be more important than the actual level. For clinical purposes it appears useful to categorize hypercalcemia into mild, moderate, and severe forms; although "hypercalcemic crisis" implies the presence of severe (>14 mg/dl; >3.5 mmol/L), symptomatic, or potentially life-threatening hypercalcemia,[4] moderate hypercalcemia may lead to an unstable presentation requiring emergent therapeutic intervention as well. The treatment of symptomatic moderate or severe hypercalcemia is presented in this chapter, and some general guidelines for the workup and management of mild hypercalcemia (10.5–12.0 mg/dl; <3.0 mmol/L) are discussed.

Mild hypercalcemia frequently remains asymptomatic, is usually detected on routine laboratory electrolyte panel screens, and is most commonly associated with hyperparathyroidism. *Moderate or severe hypercalcemia* may present with complex symptom presentations of variable degree. Neuromuscular manifestations can include mental status changes, drowsiness, lethargy, proximal muscle weakness, stupor, and coma. Renal problems involve a hypercalciuria-related tubular defect mimicking diabetes insipidus, which may lead to polyuria, a decrease in glomerular filtration, and ECF volume reduction. Nephrolithiasis or nephrocalcinosis can result from hypercalcemia. Gastrointestinal manifestations may be vague, ranging from anorexia to constipation, nausea, vomiting, peptic ulcer development, and pancreatitis. The cardiovascular effects of hypercalcemia reflect changes in neurotransmission: bradycardia and shortened systole with acute hypercalcemia; shortened QT interval with moderate elevation; and QT interval elongation with severe hypercalcemia. These conditions may lead to symptomatic arrhythmias. In addition, an elevated calcium level may potentiate digitalis toxicity. Bone pain is a common result of active skeletal turnover processes. Hypercalcemia may aggravate pruritus and weight loss.

C. Differential Diagnosis

The more common causes of hypercalcemia are shown in Table 63–1. Primary hyperparathyroidism is by far the most common cause and leads to hypercalcemia in more than 50% of cases. However, both patient and surgeon should be considered fortunate if this cause is identified in a surgical oncology practice setting, as hypercalcemia secondary to malignancy is the much more likely scenario.[5] The increased PTH secretion of hyperparathyroidism leads to increased renal calcium reabsorption, increased bone turnover, and an increase in serum 1,25-$(OH)_2D_3$, which causes enhanced intestinal absorption. An intact PTH (iPTH) elevation is diagnostic, although inappropriate low urine excretion due to familial hypercalcemic hypocalciuria should be ruled out. Many patients have no or mild symptoms. Hypercalcemic crisis due to primary hyperparathyroidism is rare; it is most often is due to a parathyroid adenoma, although it can occur with parathyroid cancer or mediastinal parathyroid cysts.[6]

TABLE 63–1.
Causes of hypercalcemia

Primary hyperparathyroidism
Malignancy
Metastatic bone involvement
No bone metastases
Drugs
Thiazide diuretics
Vitamin D
Calcium carbonate
Lithium
Tamoxifen
Granulomatous diseases
Sarcoid
Wegener's granulomatosis
Others (tuberculosis, leprosy)
Metabolic disorders
Renal failure
1, 25-Dihydroxyvitamin D_3 replacement therapy for dialysis patients
Aluminum intoxication in dialysis patients
Secondary hyperparathyroidism
Osteoporosis
Paget's disease
Familial hypercalcemic hypocalciuria
Hyperthyroidism
Milk-alkali syndrome
Immobilization

The hypercalcemia of malignancy, in contradistinction, does not manifest through an elevated iPTH. The causes are direct bone destruction with osteoclast activation (osteoclast-activating factor, lymphotoxin, other cytokines) or paraneoplastic secretion of a PTH-related peptide (PTH-rP) that binds to PTH receptors but is not identified on iPTH assays.[7] The constellation of tumor-derived PTH-rP secretion is also termed humoral hypercalcemia of malignancy.[4] If iPTH is elevated in the setting of an advanced malignancy, two separate disease mechanisms should be suspected. The underlying malignancy is most often known and is the obvious cause of the hypercalcemia. The most common cancers to cause hypercalcemia are lung and breast

TABLE 63-2.
Pharmacologic therapy for hypercalcemia

Drug	Mechanism of action	Side effects
Biophosphonates	Stabilize bone mineral	Renal dysfunction
Etidronate		
Pamidronate		
Zoledronic acid		
Alendronate		
Calcitonin	Counteracts bone resorption by osteoclasts; increases renal calcium excretion	Tachyphylaxis not useful as a single agent
Plicamycin	Inhibits osteoclast-mediated resorption	Nephrotoxicity, hepatotoxicity, thrombocytopenia, coagulopathy
Gallium nitrate	Stabilizes bone material	Nephrotoxicity, hypophosphatemia, anemia

cancer (25–30% each), multiple myeloma, squamous cell cancer of the head and neck, renal cell cancer, and T cell lymphoma.[3,8] Occasionally, parathyroid cancer presents with a severely elevated calcium level due to PTH hypersecretion. Up to 10.9% of all patients with hematologic neoplasms and 5.6% of patients with solid tumors have been found to develop hypercalcemia.[9] The rate of calcium elevation secondary to malignancy can be rapid, and patients are frequently symptomatic. In general, malignancy is the most common cause for severe hypercalcemia and hypercalcemic crisis.

Drug-induced hypercalcemia rarely leads to severe symptoms, and usually symptoms disappear after discontinuation of the drug. In the presence of granulomatous processes, tissue conversion of $25(OH)D_3$ to $1,25(OH)_2D_3$ can be increased; this is particularly amenable to glucocorticosteroid treatment. Hypercalcemia in the setting of renal failure is uncommon and usually a result of treatment factors in patients undergoing dialysis.

D. Diagnosis

Laboratory tests suggested for the workup of suspected or proven hypercalcemia include assays for serum calcium (or ionized serum calcium, see above), phosphate, chloride, iPTH, and possibly PTH-rP. A phosphate level of <3.5 mg/dl (causing an elevated chloride/phosphate ratio) is commonly associated with hyperparathyroidism; the reverse can be expected in malignancy-associated hypercalcemia. Elevated serum alkaline phosphatase and urinary hydroxyproline levels may indicate increased bone turnover. Imaging studies are rarely necessary or helpful: Bone scans, plain film radiography, or magnetic resonance imaging (MRI) may aid in the diagnosis and determining the extent of cancer metastatic to bone; preoperative computed tomography (CT) scans of the neck and chest are suggested for the rare case of suspected parathyroid cancer. During hypercalcemic crises the PTH level determination is crucial, even when an advanced malignancy is known or suspected, as the proper treatment of the underlying condition may differ greatly.[10]

E. Treatment

Pharmacologic Options

The general pharmacologic treatment options for hypercalcemia are listed in Tables 63–2 and 63–3. *Rehydration*, whether accomplished intravenously or, for mild cases, orally, is generally helpful for expanding the ECF and increasing renal perfusion and secretion; it usually suffices to decrease an elevated calcium level. Intravenous fluid administration is the recommended immediate treatment for symptomatic hypercalcemia. *Diuresis* may allow more aggressive hydration with larger amounts of intravenous saline solution, especially in patients with congestive heart failure. Intravenous furosemide or other loop diuretics should be used only in the well hydrated patient, as they may compromise the ECF and thus increase serum calcium in the absence of adequate hydration; thiazide diuretics are always contraindicated in hypercalcemic patients. Intravenous phosphorus should be avoided because of the risk of inducing metastatic calcification or nephrocalcinosis.

Biphosphonates are effective agents for treating hypercalcemia secondary to enhanced osteoclastic bone destruction. They stabilize bone mineral through direct binding and by inhibiting enzymes specific for phosphate-containing substrates[12]; they also have a long half-life. Etidronate (7.5 mg/kg IV over 4 hours for 3–7 days) and pamidronate (60–90 mg once over 12–24 hours, single dose) are approved for treating hypercal-

TABLE 63–3.
Pharmacologic treatment options for hypercalcemia, time to effect, and estimated cost

Substance	Suggested dose	Time to effect (hours)	Amount for cost calculation	Estimated cost ($)
Normal saline	200–400 ml/hr IV	6–12	4 L	13.50
Furosemide	40–80 mg/hr IV q2–4 h	6–12	1200 mg	55.00
Pamidronate	60–90 mg once over 2–4 hours; sometimes slower; single dose	24–48	90 mg	540.00
Zoledronic acid	4–8 mg once over 15 minutes	12	(no standard price yet)	
Calcitonin	2–8 U/kg SC or IM q6–12 h	1–4	16 U/kg, 70 kg	127.35
Plicamycin	10–50 μg/kg IV; brief infusion	24–48	25 μg/kg, 70 kg	78.35
Gallium nitrate	100–200 mg/m^2/day continuous infusion, up to 5 days	24–48	200 mg/m^2, 1.72 m^2 5 days	415.50
Prednisone	40–100 mg/day	~72	80 mg	6.70

Dose recommendations according to Warrell.[11]

cemia; alendronate is available for the treatment of osteoporosis but has calcium-lowering side effects. Multiple other biphosphonates are under clinical investigation. Pamidronate is more effective than etidronate (efficacy rate of 60–80% versus 30–40%) and has fewer side effects with regard to renal dysfunction.[13] A single dose frequently normalizes the calcium level within 1 week. Biphosphonates play an important role in the continued management of patients with bone metastases, even if hypercalcemia is no longer present. They can slow progression of the disease and alleviate bone pain.[14] Pamidronate administered once monthly can reduce subsequent morbidity from the skeletal metastases of breast cancer.[15] Recently, zoledronic acid was found to be superior to pamidronate in the treatment of hypercalcemia of malignancy; its other advantages include the ability for more rapid infusion (15 minutes) and its longer duration of action.[15a]

Salmon calcitonin (2–8 U/kg SC or IM q6–12 h) counteracts bone resorption by osteoclasts and increases renal calcium excretion. Although the effect is weak and tachyphylaxis is common, calcitonin acts within hours and can be considered an additional agent for patients with severe hypercalcemia aside from biphosphonates or plicamycin, as the latter take longer to show effect. Calcitonin is rarely useful as a single agent for treating hypercalcemia.

Plicamycin (mithramycin 10–50 μg/kg IV, brief infusion) inhibits osteoclast-mediated bone resorption through RNA blockade. It is highly effective in lowering serum calcium quickly but has potentially serious side effects, including nephrotoxicity, hepatotoxicity, thrombocytopenia, and coagulopathy with hemorrhagic complications. However, single doses are usually tolerated well. Its use is limited to situations where serum calcium must be reduced rapidly.

Gallium nitrate (100–200 mg/m^2/day, continuous infusion up to 5 days) stabilizes bone minerals through direct binding and decreases their solubility.[16] Although its relative efficacy is high (up to 80%), the onset of action takes several days; the effect lasts approximately a week. There are significant, frequent side effects, including nephrotoxicity, hypophosphatemia, and anemia; and gallium nitrate is expensive.

Glucocorticosteroids (e.g., prednisone 40–100 mg/day or an equivalent) are useful in situations where hypercalcemia is caused by tissue macrophage-induced excessive formation of $1,25(OH)_2D_3$ (e.g., granulomatous disorders, hematologic malignancies, vitamin D toxicity). They are inexpensive and well tolerated, but their efficacy is lower than that of the agents listed above. Oral availability facilitates their use in the outpatient setting. Steroids are also of benefit in delaying tachyphylaxis after calcitonin treatment initiation. Hypercalcemia refractory to steroid therapy in sarcoidosis patients can be treated with chloroquine, hydrochloroquine, or ketoconazole.[17]

Prostaglandin inhibition (e.g., by indomethacin, 75–150 mg/day) has been useful for cases of hypercalcemia of malignancy with direct bone invasion and destruction where prostaglandins may have a causative role. Although there appears to be no role for first-line treatment with nonsteroidal antiinflammatory medications, they should be considered for patients whose hypercalcemia remains refractory to other treatment. It should be noted that acetaminophen given before pamidronate infusion can ameliorate its side effects.[18]

Hemodialysis is a rarely necessary but highly effective therapy for the unstable patient with therapy-refractory hypercalcemia.

Oral *phosphorus* (1–3 g/day PO) can be considered for treatment of hypercalcemia, but it is not largely effective, has frequent gastrointestinal side effects, and can cause extraosseous calcification. It is not widely used.

Treatment of the underlying condition is frequently the only therapy required for mild hypercalcemia (10.5–12.0 mg/dl; <3.0 mmol/L). For patients with primary hyperparathyroidism, surgical resection of oversecreting tissue (usually one parathyroid adenoma) is curative. Urgent surgical intervention is rarely necessary but may be indicated for acutely symptomatic cases of hyperparathyroidism due to benign or malignant parathyroid processes after aggressive hydration has been initiated.

Therapeutic Decisions

Hypercalcemia per se does not necessarily require treatment. Of the several treatment options available, a specific approach must be chosen depending on the clinical setting. Generally, treatment decisions are based on the degree of hypercalcemia, the severity of symptoms, their resolution, the underlying cause of hypercalcemia, and cost-benefit considerations. Therefore treatment suggestions for individual patients may vary considerably. The key questions are as follows: How urgent is the therapeutic intervention (is there a true crisis)? How likely is it to succeed based on the underlying condition? Does treatment require hospital admission? Is expensive treatment justified? Can the patient tolerate potential side effects?

Mild, Asymptomatic Hypercalcemia Mild, asymptomatic hypercalcemia (10.5–12.0 mg/dl; <3.0 mmol/L) usually requires no immediate calcium-lowering treatment, although therapy of the underlying condition should be considered, such as parathyroidectomy. Stopping oral calcium intake, increasing oral hydration, and adjusting medications are additional measures. Outpatient treatment is adequate; diuretics should not be prescribed. When osteoporosis is the primary disease process, hormonal replacement or manipulation (raloxifene) should be considered.

Mild, Symptomatic Hypercalcemia For symptomatic mild hypercalcemia (10.5–12.0 mg/dl; <3.0 mmol/L), outpatient treatment appears feasible when renal function is normal, mentation is intact, and no arrhythmias are present. The patient should be able to take oral fluids and medication, and access to medical care should not be limited; these criteria are likely to be satisfied with appropriate family support.

Asymptomatic, Moderate Hypercalcemia Asymptomatic moderate hypercalcemia (12–14 mg/dl; 3.0–3.5 mmol/L) does not always require hospital admission, but it is probably treated most safely in the hospital setting. The search for the underlying condition should be initiated in a timely manner, and additional treatment should be considered based on the known or suspected etiology. Repeat calcium testing and clinical assessment are recommended on a short-term basis to not miss worsening hypercalcemia or the development of symptoms.

Symptomatic, Moderate/Severe Hypercalcemia For symptomatic, moderate (12–14 mg/dl; 3.0–3.5 mmol/L) or severe (>14 mg/dl; >3.5 mmol/L) hypercalcemia, irrespective of symptoms, inpatient treatment and monitoring are mandatory. The basic treatment goals include restoring adequate hydration, facilitating urinary calcium excretion, inhibiting osteoclast activity, and treating the underlying condition if possible.[10] Aggressive intravenous hydration with saline solution (4–10 L/day) is the initial treatment step. The effect of this treatment is only temporary, but it is extremely helpful, immediate, inexpensive, and easily administered. Diuresis is induced if the urine output remains inadequate or to allow high-volume intravenous hydration without the resulting congestive heart failure.[1] Close monitoring of electrolytes, creatinine, blood urea nitrogen (BUN), and calcium is suggested. In addition to hydration, calcium-directed treatment is virtually always necessary under these circumstances. Pamidronate (or zoledronic acid) or gallium nitrate, but not both, should be administered after hydration has been initiated successfully. If hypercalcemic complications demand immediate lowering of the calcium level, calcitonin should be considered. If severe hypercalcemia persists and requires additional therapy, plicamycin is an option. In case of renal failure, dialysis may resolve the hypercalcemia without the need for expensive calcium-lowering drugs. For patients with cancer-associated severe hypercalcemia, there may be no realistic treatment options for the underlying condition. It is suggested that the patient's or relatives' advanced directives be reviewed carefully and that one consider limiting the management to supportive care or comfort care if indicated.

F. *Outcome*

Information on the results after treatment of significant or symptomatic hypercalcemia is surprisingly sparse. Depending on the underlying condition, most patients can expect outcomes ranging from complete resolution after successful treatment of the underlying condition (hyperparathyroidism) to some temporary or intermediate-term relief with short-term survival (hypercalcemia of malignancy). Hypercalcemic crisis, although a life-threatening emergency, today rarely results in the patient's death so long as appropriate treatment is administered. The relative efficacy of hypercalcemia therapy, defined as the percentage of patients with serum calcium of >12 mg/dl (>3 mmol/L) who achieve normalization of serum calcium levels after a single course of therapy, has been listed as follows: gallium nitrate (75–80%), pamidronate (60–77%), plicamycin (50%), etidronate (30–40%), calcitonin (30%), oral phosphorus (30%), normal saline (20%), corticosteroids (0–40%, depending on the disease process).[11]

Survival of patients with hypercalcemia of malignancy is generally poor, with the median survival ranging from several days to a few months.[19,20] The degree of elevation of the calcium level does not appear to carry prognostic significance.[21] The response to hypercalcemia-oriented treatment, however, with a decrease in the serum calcium level to less than 12 mg/dl was found to improve the median survival from 9 to 35 days.[22] The critical determinant of prolonged survival appears to be whether specific antineoplastic therapy is available and can be instituted after initial control of the hypercalcemia. In one series antineoplastic treatment of patients with hypercalcemia allowed a median survival of 135 days compared to 30 days without it.[23] This may explain the poor outcome of hypercalcemic patients with gastrointestinal cancer, where effective systemic treatment generally does not exist (mean survival 33 days).[24] In light of these poor results, the question of whether aggressive treatment for severe hypercalcemia of advanced malignancy should be considered in the absence of available effective systemic treatment options appears generally justified and should be answered based on the patient's individual clinical circumstances.

References

1. Chan FK, Koberle LM, Thys-Jacobs S, Bilezikian JP. Differential diagnosis, causes, and management of hypercalcemia. Curr Probl Surg 1997;34: 445–523.
2. Brown EM, Pollak M, Seidman CE, et al. Calcium-ion-sensing cell-surface receptors. N Engl J Med 1995;333:234–240.
3. Bushinsky DA, Monk RD. Calcium. Lancet 1998;352:306–311.
4. Edelson GW, Kleerekoper M. Hypercalcemic crisis. Med Clin North Am 1995;79:79–92.
5. Walls J, Ratcliffe WA, Howell A, Bundred NJ. Parathyroid hormone and parathyroid hormone-related protein in the investigation of hypercalcaemia in two hospital populations. Clin Endocrinol (Oxf) 1994;41:407–413.
6. Gurbuz AT, Peetz ME. Giant mediastinal parathyroid cyst: an unusual cause of hypercalcemic crisis—case report and review of the literature. Surgery 1996;120:795–800.
7. Potts J Jr. Hyperparathyroidism and other hypercalcemic disorders. Adv Intern Med 1996;41:165–212.
8. Mundy GR, Guise TA. Hypercalcemia of malignancy. Am J Med 1997; 103:134–145.
9. Burt ME, Brennan MF. Incidence of hypercalcemia and malignant neoplasm. Arch Surg 1980;115:704–707.
10. Bilezikian JP. Clinical review 51: management of hypercalcemia. J Clin Endocrinol Metab 1993;77:1445–1449.
11. Warrell RP. Metabolic emergencies. In: DeVita VT, Hellman S, Rosenberg SA (eds) Cancer: Principles and Practice of Oncology, 5th ed. Philadelphia: Lippincott-Raven, 1997:2486–2500.
12. Rogers MJ, Watts DJ, Russell RG. Overview of bisphosphonates. Cancer 1997;80:1652–1660.
13. Gucalp R, Ritch P, Wiernik PH, et al. Comparative study of pamidronate disodium and etidronate disodium in the treatment of cancer-related hypercalcemia. J Clin Oncol 1992;10:134–142.
14. Fulfaro F, Casuccio A, Ticozzi C, Ripamonti C. The role of bisphosphonates in the treatment of painful metastatic bone disease: a review of phase III trials. Pain 1998;78:157–169.
15. Theriault RL, Lipton A, Hortobagyi GN, et al. Pamidronate reduces skeletal morbidity in women with advanced breast cancer and lytic bone lesions: a randomized, placebo-controlled trial: protocol 18 Aredia Breast Cancer Study Group. J Clin Oncol 1999;17:846–854.

15a. Major P, Lortholary A, Hon J, et al. Zoledronic acid is superior to pamidronate in the treatment of hypercalcemia of malignancy: a pooled analysis of two randomized, controlled clinical trials. 7 Clin Oncol 2001;19:558–567.

16. Warrell R Jr. Gallium nitrate for the treatment of bone metastases. Cancer 1997;80:1680–1685.
17. Sharma OP. Vitamin D, calcium, and sarcoidosis. Chest 1996;109:535–539.
18. Reasner CA, Isley WL. Endocrine emergencies: recognizing clues to classic problems. Postgrad Med 1997;101:231–234. Erratum. Postgrad Med 1997;102:28.
19. Blomqvist CP. Malignant hypercalcemia—a hospital survey. Acta Med Scand 1986;220:455–463.
20. Takai E, Yano T, Iguchi H, et al. Tumor-induced hypercalcemia and parathyroid hormone-related protein in lung carcinoma. Cancer 1996;78: 1384–1387.
21. De Wit S, Cleton FJ. Hypercalcemia in patients with breast cancer: a survival study. J Cancer Res Clin Oncol 1994;120:610–614.
22. Kimura S, Sato Y, Matsubara H, et al. A retrospective evaluation of the medical treatment of malignancy-associated hypercalcemia. Jpn J Cancer Res 1986;77:85–91.
23. Ralston SH, Gallacher SJ, Patel U, et al. Cancer-associated hypercalcemia: morbidity and mortality: clinical experience in 126 treated patients. Ann Intern Med 1990;112:499–504.
24. Monno S, Nagata A, Furuta S. Hypercalcemia of cancer in the digestive tract. J Clin Gastroenterol 1987;9:78–82.

CHAPTER 64

Hypoglycemia

DAVID BALDWIN, JR.

In humans, plasma glucose is closely regulated between 50 and 100 mg/dl. Studies by Merimee and Tyson have shown that after 72 hours of fasting the plasma glucose level stabilizes at 55–75 mg/dl in normal men and at 35–60 mg/dl in normal premenopausal women.[1] Thus fasting values less than 55 mg/dl in men or less than 35 mg/dl in women are diagnostic of hypoglycemia. Occasionally, patients who have undergone total gastrectomy experience postprandial or reactive hypoglycemia as part of the constellation of symptoms that occur with the "dumping syndrome." Rarely patients develop autoimmune insulin antibodies, which have been implicated in postprandial hypoglycemia.[2] Reactive hypoglycemia does not appear to be an early manifestation of type II diabetes mellitus.

Plasma glucose is maintained in the normal range during fasting by activating hepatic gluconeogenesis through the four counterinsulin hormones (epinephrine, glucagon, growth hormone, cortisol) and by suppressing insulin secretion. The signs and symptoms of hypoglycemia can be divided into two categories: *adrenergic* and *neuroglycopenic* (Table 64–1). During hypoglycemia, a hierarchical sequence of counterinsulin hormone release is triggered. As plasma glucose drops below 70 mg/dl, epinephrine and glucagon are released, producing adrenergic symptoms. Growth hormone release is triggered when glucose drops below 60 mg/dl and cortisol release below 50 mg/dl. As the plasma glucose level drops below the minimum needed for cerebral metabolism, the patient exhibits progressive neuroglycopenic symptoms, from mild confusion to seizures and coma.

A. Diagnosis

In 1938 Whipple established the classic triad necessary to diagnose hypoglycemia: (1) symptoms of neuroglycopenia must be present; (2) synchronous plasma glucose must be less than 40–50 mg/dl; and (3) symptoms must be promptly relieved by administration of glucose. It is mandatory that Whipple's triad be met before hypoglycemia is diagnosed.

Whereas the symptoms of neuroglycopenia are somewhat specific for hypoglycemia, the adrenergic symptoms are nonspecific and are commonly experienced in the postprandial state. For many years it was widely held by patients and physicians alike that reactive or postprandial hypoglycemia was a

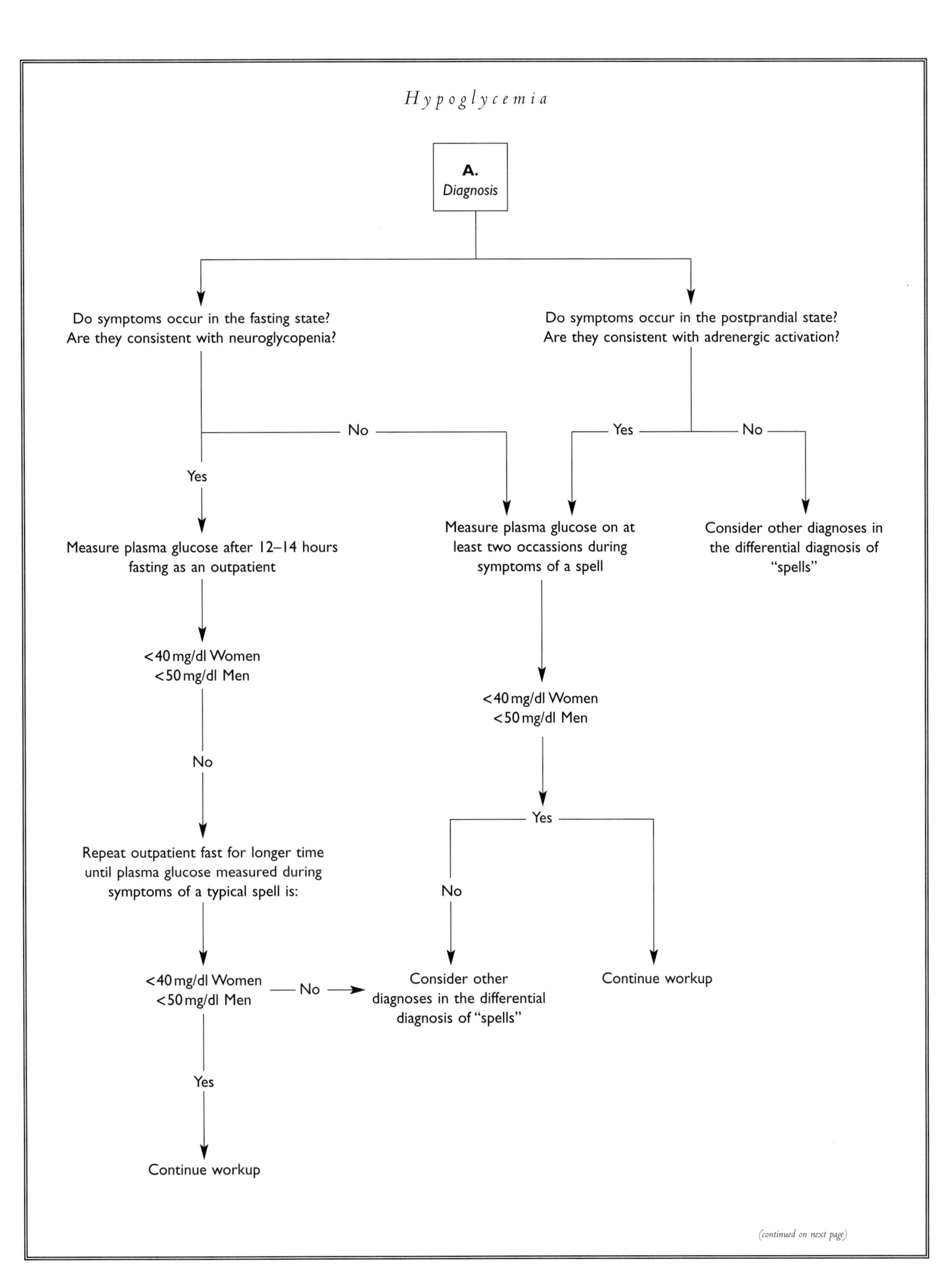

(continued on next page)

Hypoglycemia (continued)

B.
Definitive Diagnosis and Treatment

Admit to hospital for supervised 72 hour fast. Establish IV access. Free access to oral water; measure blood glucose by bedside reflectance meter every 6 hours until level less than 60 mg/dl is noted and then every 2–3 hours until it is less than 50 mg/dl; then change to plasma glucose measurement every 1–2 hours. Frequent examination of the patient for signs and symptoms of neuroglycopenia is critical. When the patient has a plasma glucose level less than 40 mg/dl and is exhibiting signs of neuroglycopenia, obtain the following studies:

Serum insulin
Plasma C-peptide
Serum sulfonylureas
Serum cortisol

Provide the patient with 25 g of IV or PO glucose and observe for rapid reversal of all signs of neuroglycopenia. Was Whipple's triad fulfilled? If yes, continue the fast, checking plasma glucose every 1–2 hours until once again the patient is neuroglycopenic and has a plasma glucose level less than 40 mg/dl; then obtain a second set of the above studies, provide glucose, and terminate the fast.

common phenomenon and that it could be diagnosed by performing a 5-hour oral glucose tolerance test (OGTT). More recently, evidence suggests that reactive hypoglycemia is a nonentity. First, it is common for plasma glucose values to dip into the hypoglycemic range after ingestion of 100 g of glucose by normal individuals. Second, there is a poor correlation between symptoms and plasma glucose levels during the OGTT. Third, and most important, only 5% of patients complaining of reactive hypoglycemic symptoms have a blood glucose level less than 50 mg/dl while experiencing these symptoms.[3] Thus Whipple's triad is not present in these patients, and hypoglycemia cannot be diagnosed. The OGTT no longer has any role in evaluating patients with symptoms suggestive of hypoglycemia.[4] The exact etiology for these commonly experienced postprandial symptoms is not known, but one study suggested that when caffeine is ingested with the meal sympathoadrenal activation occurs with a marked increase in reactive adrenergic symptoms at normal plasma glucose levels.[5]

It cannot be overemphasized that investigation of the precise cause of hypoglycemia can be undertaken only when Whipple's triad is present. Patients with symptomatic spells who do not satisfy the criteria for Whipple's triad often have an alternate diagnosis (Table 64–2) that is established only after further study.

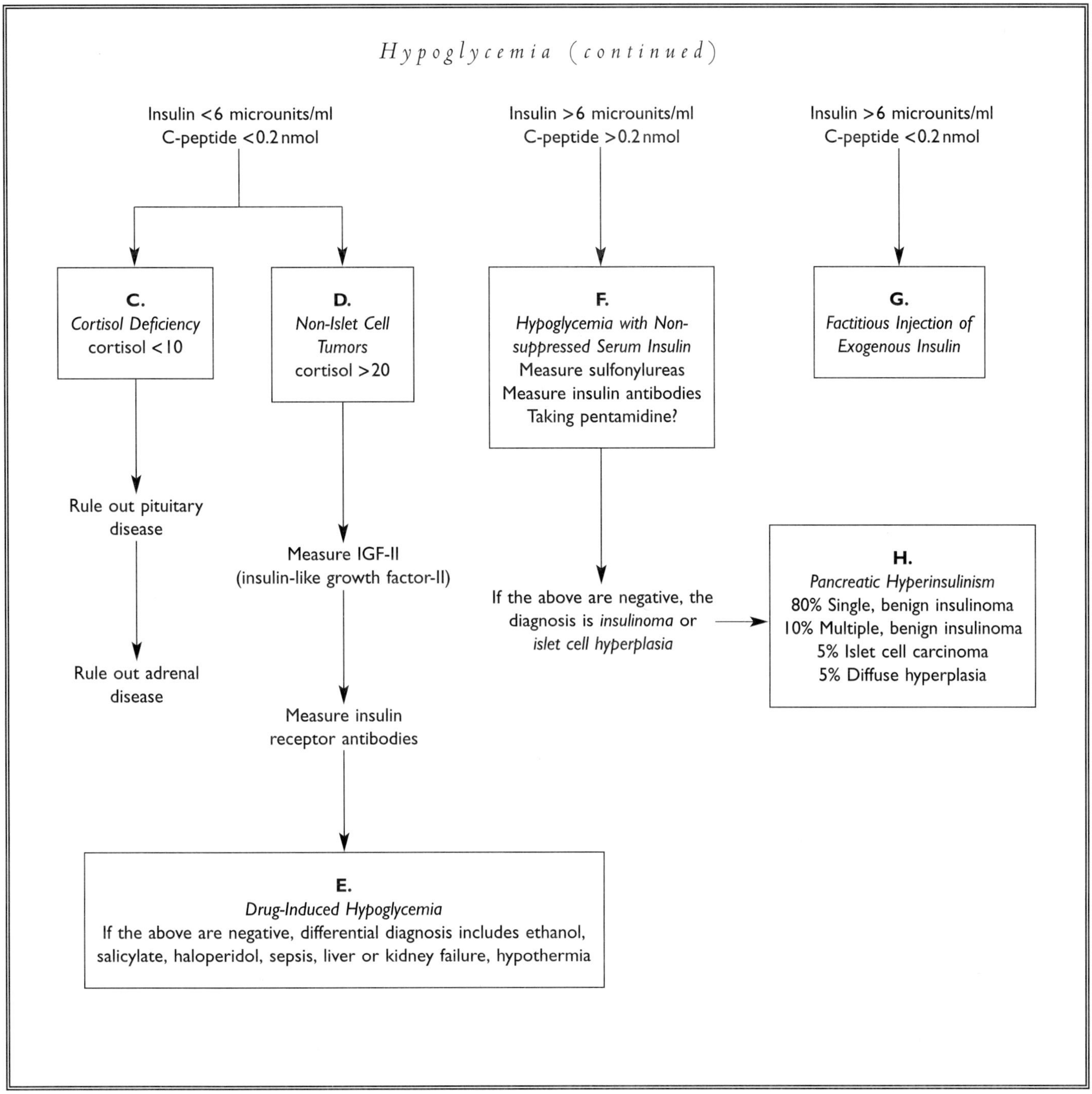

Hypoglycemia (continued)

Insulin <6 microunits/ml
C-peptide <0.2 nmol

C.
Cortisol Deficiency
cortisol <10

Rule out pituitary disease

Rule out adrenal disease

D.
Non-Islet Cell Tumors
cortisol >20

Measure IGF-II (insulin-like growth factor-II)

Measure insulin receptor antibodies

E.
Drug-Induced Hypoglycemia
If the above are negative, differential diagnosis includes ethanol, salicylate, haloperidol, sepsis, liver or kidney failure, hypothermia

Insulin >6 microunits/ml
C-peptide >0.2 nmol

F.
Hypoglycemia with Non-suppressed Serum Insulin
Measure sulfonylureas
Measure insulin antibodies
Taking pentamidine?

If the above are negative, the diagnosis is *insulinoma* or *islet cell hyperplasia* →

H.
Pancreatic Hyperinsulinism
80% Single, benign insulinoma
10% Multiple, benign insulinoma
5% Islet cell carcinoma
5% Diffuse hyperplasia

Insulin >6 microunits/ml
C-peptide <0.2 nmol

G.
Factitious Injection of Exogenous Insulin

B. Definitive Diagnosis and Treatment

Once true hypoglycemia has been diagnosed, serum insulin, C-peptide, cortisol, and sulfonylurea levels can direct the classification into one of two pathophysiologic groups. Patients with suppressed insulin (<6 μU/ml) and C-peptide (<0.2 nmol) levels due to negative feedback regulation of the beta cells by hypoglycemia have one of the diagnoses listed in Table 64–3. Patients whose insulin levels are not suppressed by hypoglycemia have one of the diagnoses listed in Table 64–4.

C. Cortisol Deficiency

Patients with primary adrenal insufficiency (Addison's disease) or isolated ACTH deficiency may have hypoglycemia. Patients with panhypopituitarism lose growth hormone in addition to

TABLE 64–1.
Symptoms of hypoglycemia

Adrenergic symptoms (epinephrine)
Anxiety
Tremor
Sweating
Palpitations
Neuroglycopenic symptoms
Headache
Lethargy
Confusion
Seizures
Coma

cortisol secretion and thus are more likely to experience hypoglycemia. Typically, these patients provide many other diagnostic clues, such as fatigue, weight loss, orthostatic hypotension, and hyponatremia.[6]

Cortisol secretion is the dominant counterregulatory response to hypoglycemia. Indeed, an insulin-induced hypoglycemic challenge is the gold standard for evaluating the hypothalamic-pituitary-adrenal (HPA) axis. All patients in whom the HPA axis is intact have an elevated serum cortisol level (>20 μg/dl) in response to hypoglycemia; determining whether this response is intact can shed light on the underlying diagnosis. Thus finding *low* insulin and *low* cortisol levels at the time of Whipple's triad establishes that cortisol deficiency is the cause of the hypoglycemia.

TABLE 64–2.
Differential diagnosis of paroxysmal spells

Endocrine causes
Hypoglycemia
Thyrotoxicosis
Pheochromocytoma
Menopause
Carcinoid
Cardiovascular causes
Angina pectoris
Arrhythmia
Orthostatic hypotension
Orthostatic tachycardia
Psychological causes
Anxiety/panic
Hyperventilation
Neurologic causes
Atypical seizures
Atypical migraine

TABLE 64–3.
Hypoglycemia with suppressed serum insulin levels

Hypopituitarism
Isolated corticotropin deficiency
Primary adrenal insufficiency
Mesenchymal tumors producing insulin-like growth factor-II
Autoimmune insulin receptor antibodies
Drugs
Ethanol
Salicylates
Haloperidol
Sepsis
End-stage renal failure
End-stage liver failure
Starvation

D. Non-Islet Cell Tumors

It has been known for years that certain non-islet cell tumors are associated with hypoglycemia. Included are large retroperitoneal mesenchymal tumors such as sarcomas and hepatomas. Studies have shown that these tumors secrete excess *insulin-like growth factor II (IGF-II)*.[7,8] IGF-binding protein-3 levels and growth hormone levels are both lowered by the excess of IGF-II. Thus high levels of unbound IGF-II are available to stimulate insulin receptors, thereby causing hypoglycemia. The hypoglycemia is exacerbated by concomitant suppression of growth hormone secretion. This syndrome should be suspected in patients who have a low insulin level but a high cortisol level at the time of Whipple's triad; it can be confirmed by measuring serum IGF-II levels and by obtaining a computed tomography (CT) scan of the abdomen.

The development of anti-insulin receptor antibodies is a rare autoimmune phenomenon. These antibodies often develop in association with other autoimmune diseases, such as systemic lupus erythematosus, and block the insulin receptor, causing a diabetic state that is highly resistant to insulin. These antibodies may rarely stimulate the insulin receptor, mimicking insulin, and produce profound hypoglycemia. This phenomenon has been described in patients with lupus and with Hodgkin's

TABLE 64–4.
Hypoglycemia with nonsuppressed serum insulin levels

Insulinoma
Exogenous insulin injection
Beta cell stimulation by sulfonylureas
Autoimmune insulin antibodies
Beta cell destruction by pentamidine

disease.[9,10] The condition is easily diagnosed by a serum assay for insulin receptor antibodies.

E. *Drug-Induced Hypoglycemia*

Most patients with drug-induced hypoglycemia have taken insulin or a sulfonylurea. The next most common drug capable of causing hypoglycemia is ethanol.[11] When hypothermia complicates alcoholism, the risk of hypoglycemia is increased.[12] Other drugs implicated in hypoglycemia include salicylates and haloperidol.

Patients with sepsis, end-stage renal failure, and end-stage liver failure may have hypoglycemia secondary to primary failure of hepatic gluconeogenesis.[13–15] Patients with starvation can experience hypoglycemia as a late complication secondary to lack of amino acid substrate for gluconeogenesis. Hypoglycemia in these patient groups should be readily identifiable by the typical clinical characteristics.

F. *Hypoglycemia with Nonsuppressed Serum Insulin*

If serum insulin levels are not suppressed (i.e., >6 μU/ml) when Whipple's triad occurs, a diagnosis from Table 64–4 is likely. As mentioned above, patients may develop autoimmune insulin antibodies, especially after exposure to methimazole.[2] These rare patients usually experience postprandial hypoglycemia. Because serum insulin is measured by immunoassay, the presence of insulin antibodies in the patient's serum introduces significant artifact. In the usual double-antibody immunoassay, insulin levels appear to be extremely high (>200 μU/ml). Such extremely high values are not seen in any other situation except proximate exogenous injection of insulin. When such elevated values are encountered, serum should be assayed for the presence of insulin antibodies.

Because pentamidine has been widely used to treat *Pneumocystis* pneumonia, complications involving the pancreatic beta cells have been described. Hypoglycemia occurs in 14% of pentamidine-treated patients,[16] and it may occur after any treatment duration. Its risk is increased by azotemia. It is caused by direct cytotoxic damage to the beta cells with inappropriate release of insulin. Eventually, if the damage is prolonged, permanent beta cell destruction and insulin-dependent diabetes mellitus may ensue.

G. *Factitious Injection of Exogenous Insulin*

Two of the most challenging etiologies of hypoglycemia to diagnose are factitious ingestion of sulfonylurea and factitious injection of insulin. These patients are usually women, usually have a medical background, and are familiar with diabetes mellitus. Many of these patients have significant depression, and suicides have resulted from factitious hypoglycemia. Many have features of Munchausen syndrome, and one-third of patients described in the literature have undergone inappropriate pancreatic operations in a fruitless search for an insulinoma.

Factitious injection of insulin is recognized by an **elevated** insulin level at the time of Whipple's triad coupled with a synchronous **suppressed** C-peptide level (<0.2 nmol).[17] Because insulin and C-peptide are co-secreted on an equimolar basis from their common beta cell precursor proinsulin, this inverse ratio indicates an exogenous source of insulin. Other tests such as insulin high-performance liquid chromatography (HPLC) or an assay for insulin antibodies are unlikely to be helpful now that most available insulin is of the human structure. The need for concordant insulin and C-peptide assays for correctly diagnosing insulinoma cannot be overemphasized. However, because stimulation of beta cell secretion by a sulfonylurea also produces concordant elevation of insulin and C-peptide at the time of hypoglycemia, the diagnosis of insulinoma must always be "ruled in" by finding no sulfonylurea present in serum collected at the time of hypoglycemia.[18] Serum should be collected during at least two episodes of hypoglycemia, and the results of the above-described testing must have no ambiguity if mistaken diagnoses are to be avoided.

H. *Pancreatic Hyperinsulinism*

Once a patient is found to have serum insulin levels higher than 6 μU/ml, plasma C-peptide levels higher than 0.2 nmol, serum cortisol levels higher than 20 μg/dl, and a negative assay for sulfonylureas at the time of Whipple's triad on more than one occasion, the diagnosis of pancreatic hyperinsulinism is established. Most (80%) patients have a single benign insulinoma, 5% have an islet cell carcinoma producing insulin, 5% have diffuse islet cell hyperplasia (nesidioblastosis), and 10% have multiple benign insulinomas, especially in association with multiple endocrine neoplasia (MEN) type I. Seven percent of insulinomas occur in patients with MEN-I. Most insulinomas occur in patients 20–60 years of age.

All patients with insulinoma have preprandial hypoglycemia, and exacerbation of symptoms by exercise is common. The onset of symptoms is typically insidious, with the median interval from the onset of symptoms to the diagnosis of hypoglycemia reported to be 2 years in several series.[19,20] Only 50% of patients brought to emergency rooms with neuroglycopenic symptoms were correctly diagnosed with hypoglycemia, so a high degree of suspicion is needed for prompt diagnosis. A common mistake is to give patients intravenous glucose to correct severe hypoglycemia before blood samples are obtained for insulin, C-peptide, cortisol, and sulfonylurea assays. All patients with a

TABLE 64–5.
Localization of insulinoma

Test	Sensitivity (%)	References
Ultrasomography (US)	38	21–24
Computed tomography (CT)	24	21–25
Angiography	40	21–26
Portal venous sampling (PVS)	79	21, 24, 25
Intraarterial calcium stimulation (IACS)	88	24
Endoscopic US (EUS)	75	26, 27
Intraoperative US (IOUS)	92	21–24, 28
Surgical palpation	75	21, 22, 28

suspected insulinoma should be admitted to the hospital for a 72-hour fast. One-third develop Whipple's triad within 12 hours, one-third within 24 hours, and the remainder between 24 and 72 hours.

Once the insulinoma is diagnosed, most patients are referred for definitive surgical resection. Diazoxide may be useful in patients who are not surgical candidates (e.g., those with metastatic islet cell carcinoma). The role of preoperative localization studies is controversial, but many endocrine surgeons prefer such a study if the expertise is available. Table 64–5 lists the sensitivity of various localization procedures.

Ultrasonography, CT, and angiography are widely available, but they are difficult to justify as cost-effective or useful given their low sensitivity compared to that of intraoperative ultrasonography. Portal venous sampling (PVS) requires transhepatic puncture and blood sampling for insulin assays in multiple pancreatic venous loci. Its sensitivity of 70–90% is likely not attainable except in the few centers with considerable experience.[21,24,25] Endoscopic ultrasonography is noninvasive, but few centers have the experience.[26,27] Doppman et al. have described a novel approach in which a sampling catheter is placed in the right hepatic vein.[24] Calcium gluconate is injected sequentially into the superior mesenteric, gastroduodenal, and splenic arteries. Insulin is measured at 30 seconds and 2.0 minutes after each injection. Intraarterial calcium stimulation (IACS) is less invasive than PVS and in initial studies is 90% sensitive for localizing the adenoma to the pancreatic head or to the body and tail. IACS is not technically demanding and thus should have good success in most larger centers.

Intraoperative ultrasound (IOUS) have become the gold standard of localization techniques.[21–24,28] It is widely available in most large centers; and when performed by an experienced endocrine surgeon, close to 100% of single insulinomas can be successfully resected by enucleation or distal pancreatectomy. Thus it has been suggested that preoperative localization studies are neither necessary nor cost-effective.[29,30] However, given the ease and accuracy of IACS, it is likely to continue to be widely utilized. Perhaps preoperative localization can facilitate laparoscopic resection of insulinomas aided by laparoscopic ultrasonography.[31,32]

Patients with MEN-I usually have multiple adenomas, and current surgical strategy usually includes distal pancreatectomy and enucleation of all tumors localized in the pancreatic head by IOUS.[33,34] The risk of recurrence is 20% at 10 years, compared with a 5% recurrence rate at 10 years for sporadic insulinoma.[35] Pancreatic nesidioblastosis is treated with diazoxide or by subtotal pancreatectomy.

References

1. Merimee T, Tyson J. Stabilization of plasma glucose during fasting: normal variations in two separate studies. N Engl J Med 1974;291:1275–1278.
2. Burch H, Clement S, Sokol M, Landry F. Reactive hypoglycemic coma due to insulin autoimmune syndrome: case report and literature review. Am J Med 1992;92:681–685.
3. Palardy J, Havranknova J, Lepage R, et al. Blood glucose measurements during symptomatic episodes in patients with suspected postprandial hypoglycemia. N Engl J Med 1989;321:1421–1425.
4. Johnson D, Dorr K, Swenson W, Service J. Reactive hypoglycemia. JAMA 1980;243:1151–1155.
5. Kerr D, Sherwin R, Pavalkis F, et al. Effect of caffeine on the recognition of and responses to hypoglycemia in humans. Ann Intern Med 1993;119: 799–804.
6. Oelkers W. Adrenal insufficiency. N Engl J Med 1996;335:1206–1212.
7. Le Roith D. Insulin-like growth factors. N Engl J Med 1997;336:633–640.
8. Daughaday W, Emanuele M, Brooks M, Barrato A, Kapadia M, Rotwein P. Synthesis and secretion of insulin-like growth factors II by a leiomyosarcoma with associated hypoglycemia. N Engl J Med 1988;319:1434–1440.
9. Braund W, Naylor B, Williamson D, et al. Autoimmunity to insulin receptor and hypoglycemia in patient with Hodgkin's disease. Lancet 1987;1: 237–240.
10. Moller D, Ratner R, Borenstein D, Taylor S. Autoantibodies to the insulin receptor as a cause of autoimmune hypoglycemia in systemic lupus erythematosus. Am J Med 1988;84:334–338.
11. Malouf R, Brust J. Hypoglycemia: causes, neurological manifestations, and outcome. Ann Neurol 1985;17:421–430.
12. Fitzgerald FJ. Hypoglycemia and accidental hypothermia in an alcoholic population. West J Med 1980;133:105–107.
13. Arem R. Hypoglycemia associated with renal failure. Endocrinol Metab Clin North Am 1989;18:103–121.
14. Service F. Hypoglycemic disorders. N Engl J Med 1995;332:1144–1151.
15. Fischer K, Lees J, Newman J. Hypoglycemia in hospitalized patients: causes and outcomes. N Engl J Med 1986;315:1245–1250.
16. Waskin H, Stehr-Green J, Helmick C, Sattler F. Risk factors for hypoglycemia associated with pentamidine therapy for Pneumocystis pneumonia. JAMA 1988;260:345–347.
17. Grunberger G, Weiner J, Silverman R, Taylor S, Gorden P. Factitious hypoglycemia due to surreptitious administration of insulin: diagnosis, treatment, and long-term follow-up. Ann Intern Med 1988;108:252–257.
18. Klonoff D, Barrett B, Nolte M, Cohen R, Wyderski R. Hypoglycemia following inadvertent and factitious sulfonylurea overdosages. Diabetes Care 1995;18:563–567.
19. Service FJ, Dale A, Elveback L, Jiang N-S. Insulinoma: clinical and diagnostic features of 60 consecutive cases. Mayo Clin Proc 1976;51:417–429.

20. Fajans S, Vinik A. Insulin-producing islet cell tumors. Endocrinol Metab Clin North Am 1989;18:45–75.
21. Doherty G, Doppman J, Shawker T, et al. Results of a prospective strategy to diagnose, localize, and resect insulinomas. Surgery 1991;110:989–997.
22. Galiber A, Reading C, Charboneau J, et al. Localization of pancreatic insulinoma: comparison of pre- and intraoperative US with CT and angiography. Radiology 1988;166:405–408.
23. Grant C, van Heerden J, Charboneau W, James M, Reading C. Insulinoma: the value of intraoperative ultrasonography. Arch Surg 1988;123:843–848.
24. Doppman J, Chang R, Fraker D, et al. Localization of insulinomas to regions of the pancreas by intra-arterial stimulation with calcium. Ann Intern Med 1995;123:269–273.
25. Pasieka J, McLeod M, Thompson N, Burney R. Surgical approach to insulinomas: assessing the need for preoperative localization. Arch Surg 1992;127:442–447.
26. Rosch T, Lightdale C, Botet J, et al. Localization of pancreatic endocrine tumors by endoscopic ultrasonography. N Engl Med 1992;326:1721–1726.
27. Thompson N, Czako P, Fritis L, et al. Role of endoscopic ultrasonography in the localization of insulinomas and gastrinomas. Surgery 1994;116: 1131–1138.
28. Norton J, Cromack D, Shawker T, et al. Intraoperative ultrasonographic localization of islet cell tumors: a prospective comparison to palpation. Ann Surg 1988;207:160–168.
29. Van Heerden J, Grant C, Czako P, Service J, Charboneau J. Occult functioning insulinomas: which localizing studies are indicated? Surgery 1992;112:1010–1015.
30. Alexrod L. Insulinoma: cost-effective care in patients with a rare disease. Ann Intern Med 1995;123:311–312.
31. Sussman L, Christie R, Whittle D. Laparoscopic excision of distal pancreas including insulinoma. Aust NZ J Surg 1996;66:414–416.
32. Gagner M, Pomp A, Herrara M. Early experience with laparoscopic resections of islet cell tumors. Surgery 1996;120:1051–1054.
33. Demeure M, Klonoff D, Karam J, Duh Q-Y, Clark O. Insulinomas associated with multiple endocrine neoplasia type I: the need for a different surgical approach. Surgery 1991;110:998–1004.
34. Diarmuid S, O'Riordain M, O'Brien T, van Heerden J, Service F, Grant C. Surgical management of insulinoma associated with multiple endocrine neoplasia type I. World J Surg 1994;18:488–494.
35. Service FJ, McMahon M, O'Brien P, Ballard D. Functioning insulinoma: incidence, recurrence, and long-term survival of patients: a 60-year study. May Clin Proc 1991;66:711–719.

CHAPTER 65

Tumor Lysis Syndrome

DAVID B. WILSON

Tumor lysis syndrome (TLS) has classically been associated with the treatment of rapidly dividing myeloproliferative and lymphoproliferative neoplasms. As increasingly effective chemotherapy regimens are being discovered and utilized, TLS has become a common problem with other neoplasms including solid organ tumors. TLS is an oncologic emergency that causes rapid, and severe metabolic changes and end-organ dysfunction. Characterized by *hyperuricemia*, *hyperkalemia*, *hyperphosphatemia*, and *hypocalcemia*, TLS is the result of rapid destruction of large numbers of neoplastic cells. The syndrome usually follows the initiation of chemotherapy, but it can accompany radiation therapy, surgical resection, endocrine therapy, or hyperthermia. It may even occur spontaneously. The metabolic derangements result from release of cellular potassium, phosphate, and purine degradation products into the bloodstream. Therapy is aimed first at preventing the syndrome once high risk groups are identified and then at supporting cardiac and renal function to allow clearance of the by-products.

A. Solid Organ Tumors

Tumor lysis syndrome rarely occurs during the treatment of solid organ cancers. A review of the literature revealed 27 cases of TLS that occurred during treatment of small cell lung cancer (seven cases), breast carcinoma (five cases), neuroblastoma (four cases), metastatic adenocarcinoma (two cases), thymoma, ovarian carcinoma, vulvar carcinoma, seminoma, melanoma, leiomyosarcoma, rhabdomyosarcoma, medilloblastoma, and hepatoblastoma (one case each). In these reported cases, TLS occurred with various treatment regimens including single-agent and combination chemotherapy, radiation therapy, chemoradiotherapy, hormonal therapy, biologic response modifiers including immunotherapy, and chemoimmunotherapy.[1–3]

B. Hematologic Tumors

Malignancies with a large tumor burden and high sensitivity to chemotherapy, such as Burkitt's lymphoma and acute lymphoblastic leukemia (ALL), often lead to TLS.

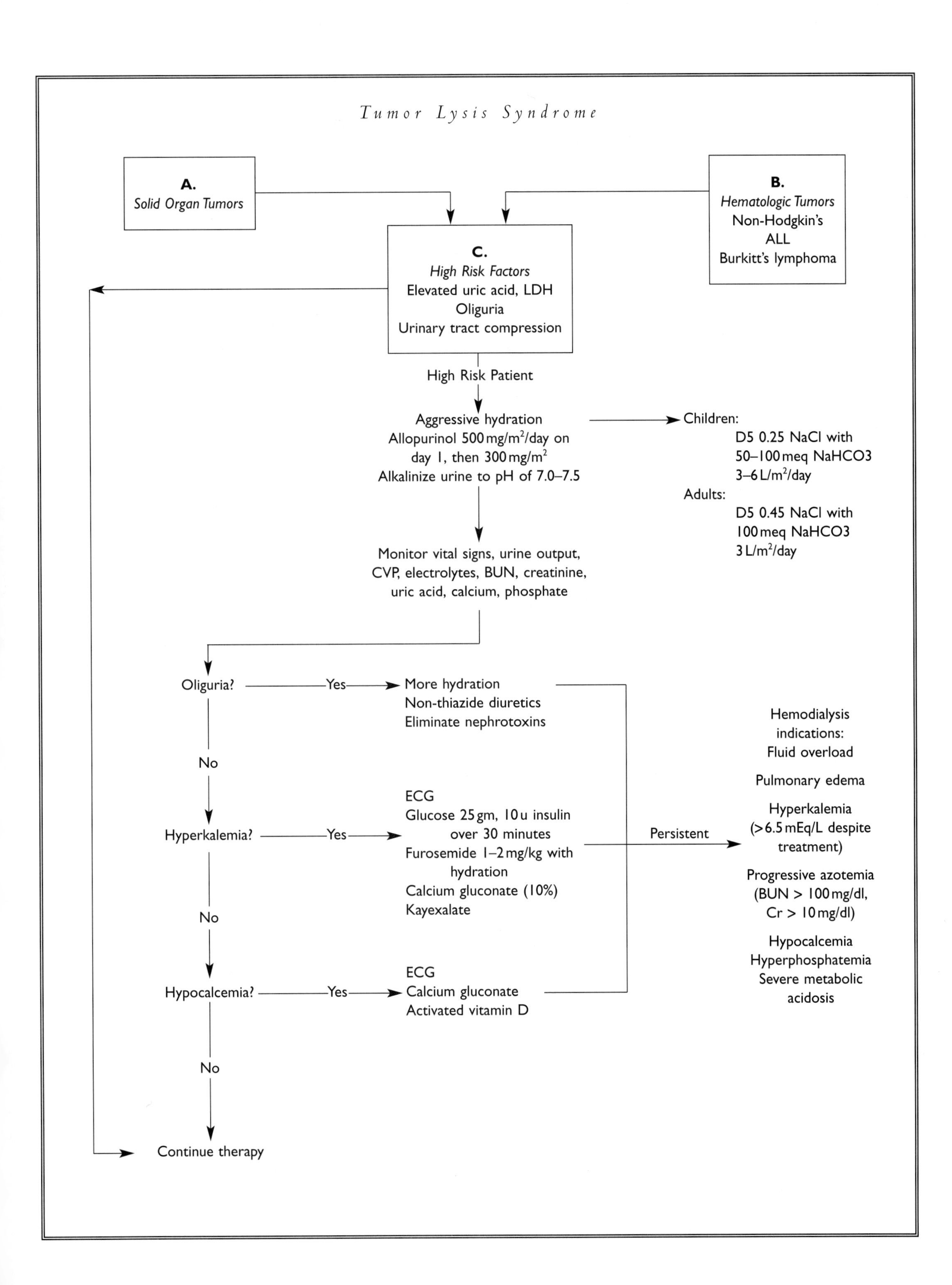

Tumor Lysis Syndrome
A.
Solid Organ Tumors
B.
Hematologic Tumors
Non-Hodgkin's
ALL
Burkitt's lymphoma
C.
High Risk Factors
Elevated uric acid, LDH
Oliguria
Urinary tract compression
High Risk Patient
Aggressive hydration
Allopurinol 500 mg/m²/day on day 1, then 300 mg/m²
Alkalinize urine to pH of 7.0–7.5
Children:
D5 0.25 NaCl with 50–100 meq NaHCO3
3–6 L/m²/day
Adults:
D5 0.45 NaCl with 100 meq NaHCO3
3 L/m²/day
Monitor vital signs, urine output, CVP, electrolytes, BUN, creatinine, uric acid, calcium, phosphate
Oliguria?
Yes
More hydration
Non-thiazide diuretics
Eliminate nephrotoxins
No
Hyperkalemia?
Yes
ECG
Glucose 25 gm, 10 u insulin over 30 minutes
Furosemide 1–2 mg/kg with hydration
Calcium gluconate (10%)
Kayexalate
No
Hypocalcemia?
Yes
ECG
Calcium gluconate
Activated vitamin D
No
Continue therapy
Persistent
Hemodialysis indications:
Fluid overload
Pulmonary edema
Hyperkalemia (>6.5 mEq/L despite treatment)
Progressive azotemia (BUN > 100 mg/dl, Cr > 10 mg/dl)
Hypocalcemia
Hyperphosphatemia
Severe metabolic acidosis

C. High Risk Patient

Patients with elevated pretreatment uric acid and lactate delydrogenase (LDH) levels are at increased risk of developing TLS. These parameters are indirect indications of cellular turnover seen in rapidly dividing neoplasms. Oliguria is the main risk factor for developing acute renal failure with TLS. Extrinsic urinary tract compression and renal lymphomatous infiltration are possible risk factors as well. All patients with non-Hodgkin's lymphoma and ALL are considered at risk because of the high response rates of these malignancies to cytotoxic therapy. Patients with bulky treatment-sensitive solid organ tumors who develop oliguria and elevated LDH or uric acid levels should also be considered at high risk for TLS.

Standard treatment includes optimizing the patient's metabolic status prior to initiating therapy. Aggressive hydration to replace volume deficits is started with 5% dextrose in 0.25% normal saline D_5 0.2% NaCl plus 50–100 mEq/L $NaHCO_3$ at 3–6 L/m^2/day in children, or D_5 0.45% NaCl + 100 mEq/L $NaHCO_3$ at 3 L/m^2/day in adults. These patients often have a total volume deficit of 5–6 liters.

Treating dehydration is one method of avoiding renal failure. Another is to decrease the precipitation of uric acid in the kidney. Alkalization of the urine to pH 7.0–7.5 (pKa of uric acid 7.4) using sodium bicarbonate increases uric acid solubility. Uric acid is 98% ionized as urate at normal serum pH. At the renal tubule's lower pH, the ionized percentage drops and urate becomes less soluble. This leads to precipitation and crystallization in the tubules and collecting ducts. Decreasing the kidney's total load of uric acid is another strategy for avoiding renal failure. Allopurinol is a renally excreted potent inhibitor of xanthine oxidase, the enzyme responsible for the liver's conversion of purine metabolites to uric acid. Treatment with allopurinol decreases uric acid excretion and increases the kidney's load of hypoxanthine and xanthine, more soluble precursors to uric acid. A dose of 500 mg/m^2 is given on day 1, followed by 300 mg/m^2 on subsequent days. The dosage is reduced in the presence of renal failure. Adenosine, also a purine breakdown product, acts directly on the renal microvasculature to decrease the glomerular filtration rate. Preglomerular vasoconstriction and postglomerular vasodilation combine to decrease glomerular perfusion, thereby further compromising renal function. Treatment is supportive (Table 65–1).

TABLE 65–1.
Etiology of acute renal failure in tumor lysis syndrome

Dehydration
Decreased glomerular filtration rate secondary to adenosine-regulated preglomerular vasoconstriction and postglomerular vasodilatation
Obstructive nephropathy secondary to uric acid crystallization in the collecting ducts
Obstructive nephropathy secondary to calcium phosphate crystallization in the tubules

Patients at high risk require close monitoring during therapy, including urine output and central venous pressure (CVP) measurements. If a patient becomes oliguric, intensive care unit (ICU) monitoring is indicated. Electrolytes, blood urea nitrogen, creatinine, uric acid, ionized calcium, and phosphate levels should be checked twice daily.

Anticipation of the common metabolic problems in TLS allows their early recognition and treatment. Oliguria should be treated with either volume or nonthiazide diuretics based on the central venous pressure. Nephrotoxic drugs should be stopped. Failure to respond should lead to early consultation with a nephrologist and preparation for hemodialysis.

Hyperkalemia results from the release of intracellular potassium, leading potentially to cardiac arrhythmias and sudden death. Standard treatment methods apply. An electrocardiogram should be obtained; and peaked T waves, widening of the QRS complexes, or atrioventricular dissociation should prompt immediate temporary measures. A 10% calcium gluconate solution, 10–30 ml is given for myocardial stabilization. Intravenous sodium bicarbonate 50–150 mEq over 5 minutes and insulin and dextrose in the form of 10 U of regular insulin in 50 ml $D_{50}W$ over 30–60 minutes provide a temporary shift of potassium into the intracellular compartment. Furosemide 1–2 mg/kg intravenously and hydration increase excretion in the presence of maintained renal function. Potassium-binding resins such as sodium polystyrene sulfonate in sorbitol can be given orally as tolerated to eliminate potassium via the gastrointestinal tract. Rectal administration should be avoided in neutropenic patients. Failure to respond to these measures is an indication for emergent hemodialysis.

The release of massive amounts of phosphate from tumor nucleoproteins into the serum leads to an inverse decrease in serum calcium. Calcium homeostasis is regulated mainly by parathyroid hormone (PTH) and vitamin D. The increase in

TABLE 65–2.
Indications for hemodialysis

Fluid overload/pulmonary edema
Hyperkalemia >6.5 mEq/L despite treatment
Progressive azotemia (BUN > 100 mg/dl, Cr > 10 mg/dL)
Hypocalcemia/hyperphosphatemia
Severe metabolic acidosis

BUN, blond urea nitrogen; Cr, creatinine.

phosphate levels overwhelms this autoregulation and leads to calcium phosphate precipitation in the kidneys. Renal interstitial inflammation and tubular atrophy ensue. Hypocalcemia caused by precipitation of calcium phosphate and lowered calcitrol levels can cause neuromuscular irritability, tetany, and obtundation. These symptoms can be resistant to calcium supplementation and respond only to 1,25-dihydroxycholecalciferol replacement.[4] Most patients require supplements of 0.01–0.05 μg/kg IV three times per week. The dose is started at 0.01 μg/kg and titrated to keep serum calcium at 9–10 μg/dl. Hemodialysis can also treat resistant symptomatic hypocalcemia by decreasing the serum phosphate level.

Hemodialysis should be considered early in TLS for several indications. Such indications are fluid overload, hyperkalemia despite treatment, progressive azotemia, symptomatic hypocalcemia, and severe metabolic acidosis (Table 65–2).

References

1. Kalemkerian GP, Darwish B, Varterasian ML. Tumor lysis syndrome in small cell carcinoma and other solid organ tumors. Am J Med 1997;103:363–367.
2. Boisseau M, Bugat R, Mahjoubi M. Rapid tumor lysis syndrome in a metastatic colorectal cancer increased by treatment. Eur J Cancer 1996;32A: 737–738.
3. Yokoi K, Miyazawa N, Kano Y, et al. Tumor lysis syndrome in invasive thymoma with peripheral blood T-cell lymphocytosis. Am J Clin Oncol 1997;20:86–89.
4. Lorigan PC, Woodings PL, Morgenstern GR. Tumour lysis syndrome, case report and review of the literature. Ann Oncol 1996;7:631–636.

CHAPTER 66

Compromised Airway

T.K. VENKATESAN
NADER SADEGHI
PETER MURPHY

A. Introduction

The approach to the compromised airway is a logical, stepwise progression. The importance of individualizing the treatment plan cannot be adequately emphasized. What follows is our philosophy on managing the adult airway in the setting of head and neck cancer.

The patient with head and neck cancer poses a challenge to optimal airway management. Any unanticipated threat to the airway creates the potential for sudden death. Airway compromise may be secondary to neuromuscular dysfunction, mass effect from tumors, or inflammatory processes.

There are many strategies for securing the airway, and the ultimate plan should be selected after consultation between the surgeon, anesthesiologist, and patient. At the time of the preoperative evaluation, all pertinent information including the rate of evolution of symptoms, the degree of respiratory compromise, and the results of laboratory and radiographic data must be reviewed. Several options should be considered and a choice made based on the clinical situation, the skill of the personnel available, and the equipment at hand. Furthermore, the plan must be flexible and should make room for modification as indicated.

The options for management are based on the urgency of the clinical situation. The use of postoperative adjunctive therapy in the form of chemotherapy and radiotherapy should also be factored in. The age of the patient and the presence of co-existing illnesses may require some alteration of the approach. Because airway intervention is usually reversible, the same team should meet at intervals to decide when respiratory independence can be tolerated and to plan for weaning from ventilatory support.

B. Assessment

A quick survey should focus on the mental status of the patient and the presence of restlessness, agitation, tachypnea, stridor, and hoarseness. Nasal flaring, cheek puffing, use of accessory muscles of respiration, intercostal retractions, and paradoxical respiration reflect the severity of airway compromise and dictate the urgency for intervention. Surprisingly, cyanosis is a late sign. Loss of consciousness is

The Compromised Airway

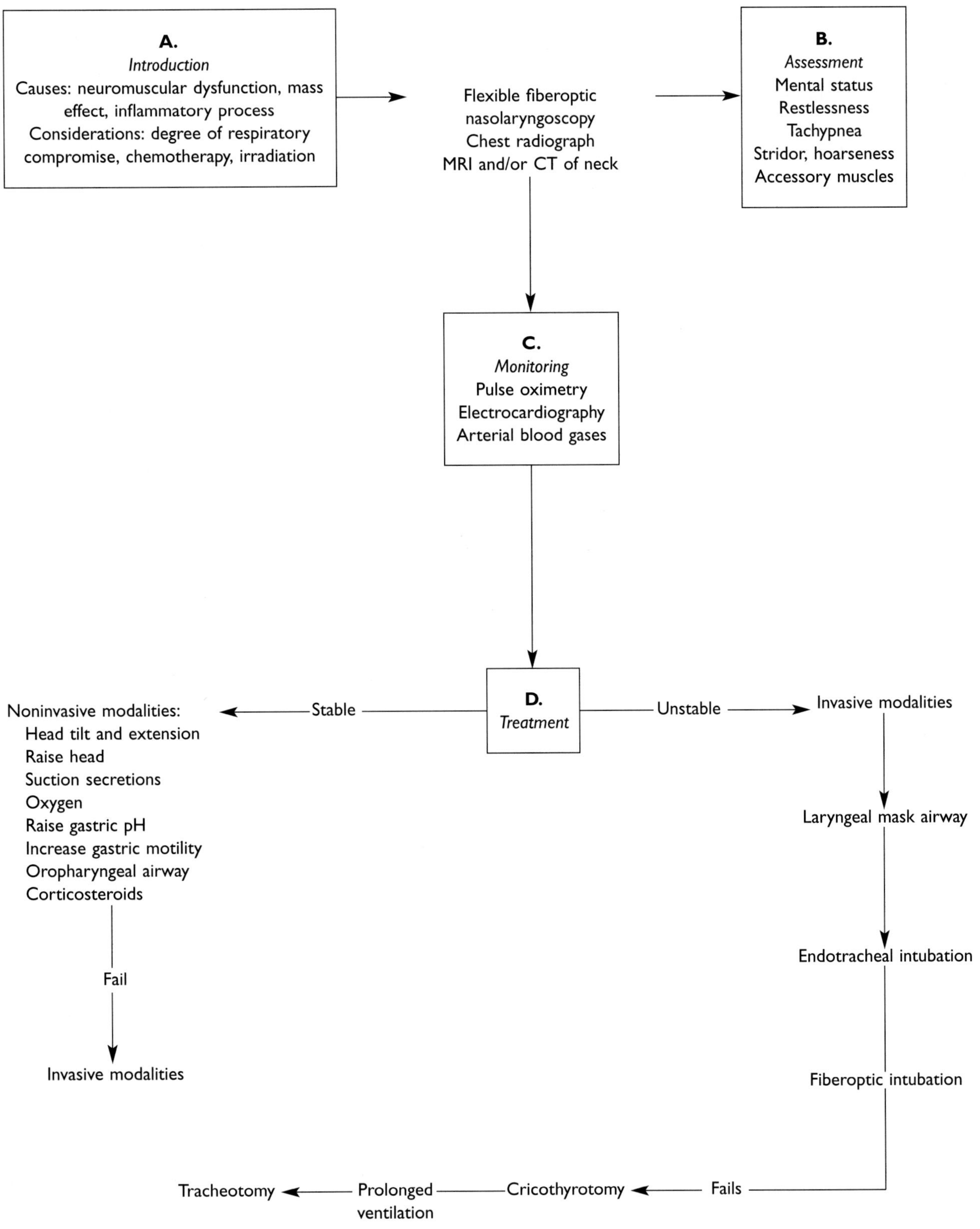

A.
Introduction
Causes: neuromuscular dysfunction, mass effect, inflammatory process
Considerations: degree of respiratory compromise, chemotherapy, irradiation

→ Flexible fiberoptic nasolaryngoscopy
Chest radiograph
MRI and/or CT of neck

→ **B.**
Assessment
Mental status
Restlessness
Tachypnea
Stridor, hoarseness
Accessory muscles

↓

C.
Monitoring
Pulse oximetry
Electrocardiography
Arterial blood gases

↓

D.
Treatment

Stable → Noninvasive modalities:
- Head tilt and extension
- Raise head
- Suction secretions
- Oxygen
- Raise gastric pH
- Increase gastric motility
- Oropharyngeal airway
- Corticosteroids

Fail → Invasive modalities

Unstable → Invasive modalities
→ Laryngeal mask airway
→ Endotracheal intubation
→ Fiberoptic intubation
→ Fails → Cricothyrotomy → Prolonged ventilation → Tracheotomy

uncommon; but if narcotics have been administered, their combined effect with hypoxia can produce sudden respiratory depression that is lethal. A history of airway compromise and its management in the past may avoid a delay in establishing an airway. Aspiration with ensuing pneumonia diminishes the pulmonary reserve and should be taken into account. A brief neurologic assessment should be part of the physical examination.

A short muscular neck, full dentition, retrognathia, trismus, and limitation of temporomandibular joint mobility are important when choosing the approach to the airway. The presence of cervical masses, contractures, and deviation of the larynx or trachea should be noted. The presence of excessive secretions or blood renders laryngoscopy technically difficult and frustrating.

Flexible fiberoptic nasolaryngoscopy has made airway assessment more objective and safe, and it allows assessment of vocal cord function. In a nonemergent setting, a chest radiograph and soft tissue lateral neck radiograph may add valuable information. In the stable patient, a computed tomography (CT) scan of the neck with infusion provides accurate data regarding the anatomy and extent of disease, and it helps plan therapy, including the approach to the airway.

Electrolyte imbalance, if present, should be corrected to avoid cardiac rhythm disturbances during airway management. An arterial blood gas analysis may enable quantification of the severity of airway compromise and the duration of the problem. It may also affect the urgency of securing the airway.

C. *Monitoring*

Pulse oximetry, electrocardiography, and arterial blood pressure monitoring at least every 5 minutes are considered standards of care by the American Society of Anesthesiology (ASA). Regular and frequent measurements and the integration of clinical judgment and experience are emphasized. With the use of endotracheal or tracheostomy tubes, capnography and peak airway pressures are useful parameters for following the adequacy and safety of artificial ventilation. Electronic monitoring does not reduce the need for clinical assessment by inspection, palpation, and auscultation.

D. *Treatment*

The modalities employed to secure the airway can conveniently be classified into two broad categories—noninvasive and invasive—each of which is applicable in both emergent and nonemergent situations.

Noninvasive Modalities

Positioning The primary cause of airway obstruction is flexion of the head at the atlantoaxial joint, and the etiology of the obstruction is the atonic tongue. Head tilt (extension) is the most effective means for maintaining the patency of the hypopharyngeal airway. Raising the head about 5.0–7.5 cm in addition to the head tilt maximizes airway patency.

Suction A functioning suction apparatus and catheters, soft and rigid (Yankauer), are imperative. With the presence of thick, viscid secretions, it may be necessary to irrigate with normal saline and then proceed with suctioning.

Prevention of Aspiration The use of drugs to increase the pH of gastric fluid and promoters of gastric emptying can diminish the impact of potential aspiration. Cricoid pressure with the Sellick maneuver is applied during induction and intubation and may mitigate the chances of regurgitation and aspiration. Paramount to decreasing the risk of aspiration is maintenance of a patent upper airway and avoidance of inflating the stomach during positive-pressure ventilation.

Artificial Airways Oropharyngeal airways keep the base of the tongue anterior and clear the pharyngeal passage. Using an incorrect size may be counterproductive and cause airway obstruction by displacing the tongue posteroinferiorly. Nasopharyngeal airways extend from the external nares to the base of tongue and are useful in situations where the obstruction is thought to be at the level of the nasopharynx or oropharynx and the patient is conscious.

Oxygen With good mask ventilation using 100% oxygen for a minimum of 3 minutes, oxygen saturation of hemoglobin and the amount of dissolved oxygen in the blood is increased. This extends the time available for securing the airway. Inspired air should be humidified to prevent the desiccating effects of high flow.

Corticosteroids Dexamethasone with a long half-life of 36–72 hours decreases the severity of aspiration-related symptoms and may reduce the need for intubation. It is thought to act by decreasing capillary endothelial permeability and mucosal edema, stabilizing the lysosomal membrane, and reducing the inflammatory reaction.

Invasive Modalities

Laryngeal Mask Airway A simple, effective solution when endotracheal intubation has failed consists of a silicone rubber tube with an angled elliptical mask that has an inflatable balloon. The device is placed without visualization by inserting it through the mouth and into the hypopharynx, where it comes to rest over the glottis. The main drawback of this laryngeal mask airway is that the cuff does not seal the glottis safely from gastric fluid reflux, and for the same reason it is not airtight enough for use with positive-pressure ventilation. Nevertheless, this simple tool can be life-saving.

Endotracheal Intubation In the setting of the compromised airway, direct laryngoscopy may not be able to achieve atraumatic intubation. Despite optimal positioning and proper equipment and technique, there is still a possibility of failed intubation. The use of a malleable stylet with the distal end bent into a hockey-stick configuration may aid intubation.

Endotracheal intubation may be continued for several days; but if it appears that prolonged ventilatory support is required, conversion to tracheostomy is indicated. This may avoid the laryngeal injury that typically occurs in the posterior commissure, with damage to the arytenoid and interarytenoid area. It is not clear how long endotracheal intubation must be in place before damage occurs, but most agree that conversion to tracheostomy should be considered after 7 days.

Fiberoptic Intubation Fiberoptic intubation provides excellent, safe, quick access to the difficult airway. Several of the factors that make conventional intubation challenging (e.g., trismus, limited neck mobility, a tortuous and distorted pharynx) are overcome by fiberoptic intubation. The ability to administer topical anesthesia, suction secretions, and insufflate oxygen during fiberoptic intubation make this technique appealing in the awake patient with airway compromise. The drawbacks are the cost of the instrument, the extreme delicacy of the glass fiber threads, the vulnerability of the small lens to secretions and blood, the limited field of view, and the need for special skills. Topical anesthesia is essential, and a drying agent should be administered beforehand. In addition, injecting local anesthetic percutaneously into the trachea provides good analgesia and suppresses the cough reflex. Fiberoptic intubation should not be considered a last resort for managing difficult intubations but the initial method adopted in special circumstances.

Cricothyrotomy In the event of failed intubation and difficult mask ventilation, placing a large-bore catheter through the cricothyroid membrane may be lifesaving. Surgical cricothyrotomy involves an incision in the cricothyroid membrane and insertion of a tracheostomy tube or endotracheal tube into the trachea. If long-term intubation is anticipated, conversion to a tracheotomy is recommended to minimize laryngeal injury.

Rigid Bronchoscopy The use of a rigid ventilating bronchoscope in the difficult airway setting is another option available. Familiarity with the equipment and technique is crucial to the success of the procedure.

Tracheostomy Standard tracheostomy is a safe, established airway access procedure that has stood the test of time. Ideally, the tracheostomy should begin *only* after the patient has been intubated, even in the emergency setting. Failing to do so can lead to a fatal outcome from bleeding that fills the bronchial tree.

Tracheostomy may be done under local anesthesia in the operating room with the neck hyperextended. Ideally, the incision is oriented transversely at the level of the second tracheal cartilage. The thyroid isthmus is retracted superiorly or inferiorly or is clamped and divided. The second and third cartilages are incised vertically, or a window created keeping the ensuing hole as small as possible. Long-term complications include infection, hemorrhage (erosion into the innominate artery), and airway obstruction (granulation, stricture).

Conclusions

The compromised airway is a clinical problem that should be anticipated and prevented through effective communication and planning. Formulation of a strategy for care that provides for modification based on data acquired through constant monitoring is crucial to the success of securing the airway. Familiarity with the equipment available and expertise in the techniques utilized dictate the outcome.

CHAPTER 67

Mental Status Changes

RICHARD W. BYRNE

A. Introduction

Neurologic symptoms that develop in patients previously treated for cancer are a common reason for hospital admission and are second only to pain control as a cause of hospitalization to an oncologic unit.[1] Mental status changes may consist of deterioration in alertness, orientation, memory, perception, or comprehension.[1] The spectrum of mental status change ranges from subtle changes of memory to deep coma. The etiologies of these changes and their likelihood of resolving or improving with treatment vary greatly.

B. History and Physical Examination

The most important tools a physician has when evaluating and treating mental status changes are the neurologic history and physical examination. During the history a detailed account of the following is critical. Which aspect of the mental status has changed? What are its time course and precipitating factors (e.g., new medications, drug interactions, recent trauma, type of cancer involved, presence of metastases)?

Whether the complaints are motor, sensory, or gait in origin is important. Cranial nerve deficits, fever, photophobia, neck stiffness, headache, nausea, vomiting, seizure activity, alcohol or illicit drug use, previous psychiatric disorder, diabetes, systemic infection, and coagulopathy are important as well. It must be remembered that the cause of mental status changes can be multifactorial. A clear example is that brain metastases may cause a seizure or cerebral hemorrhage, either of which can cause mental status changes independent of the metastasis itself.

On surgical services the neurologic and mental status examinations are often minimized or overlooked on admission. "Nonfocal" is a common documented assessment of the central nervous system; this early oversight leaves one at a disadvantage when a patient is found to have impaired mental status later in the course of his or her treatment. One of the most common scenarios is an elderly patient

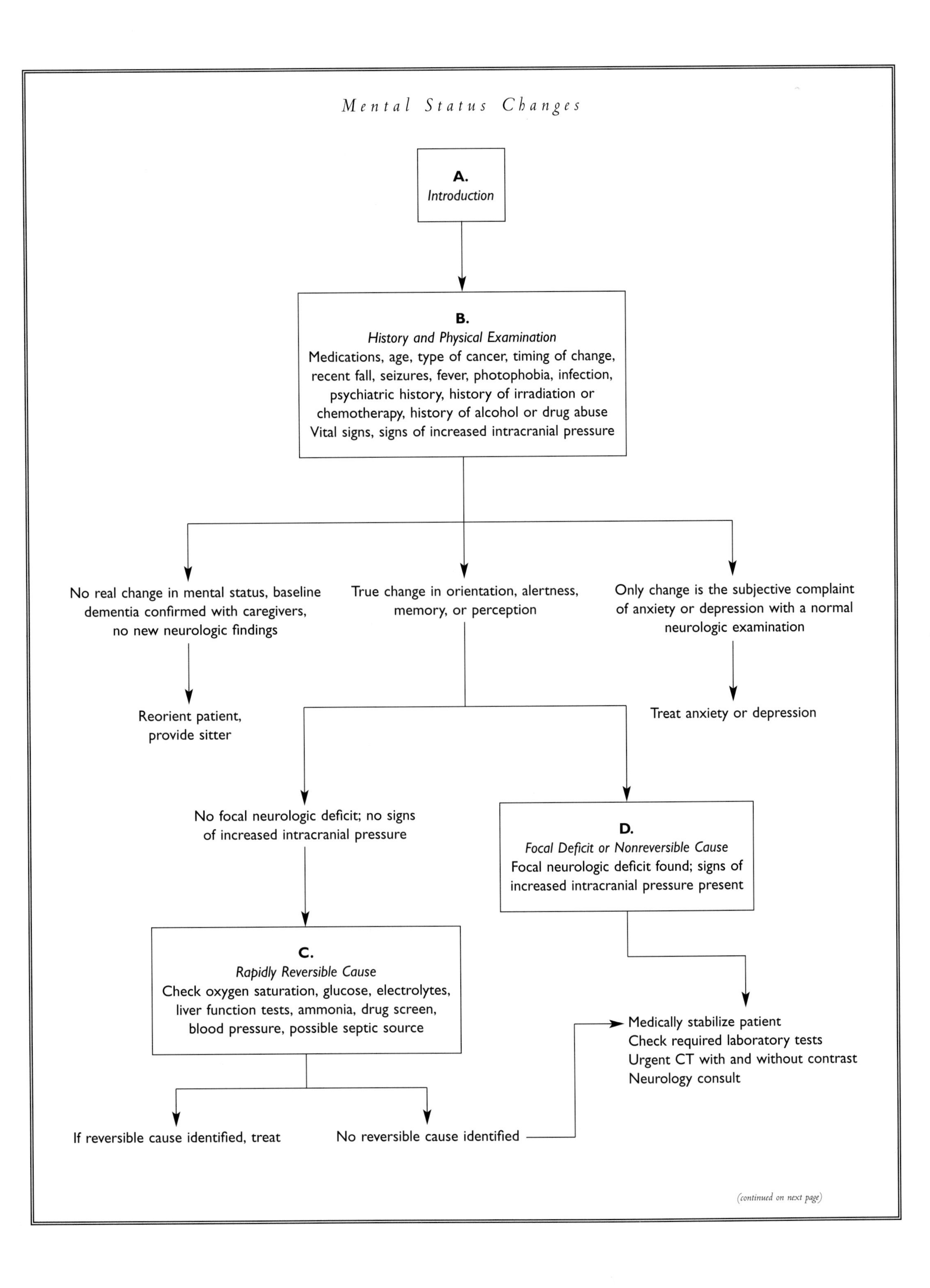

(continued on next page)

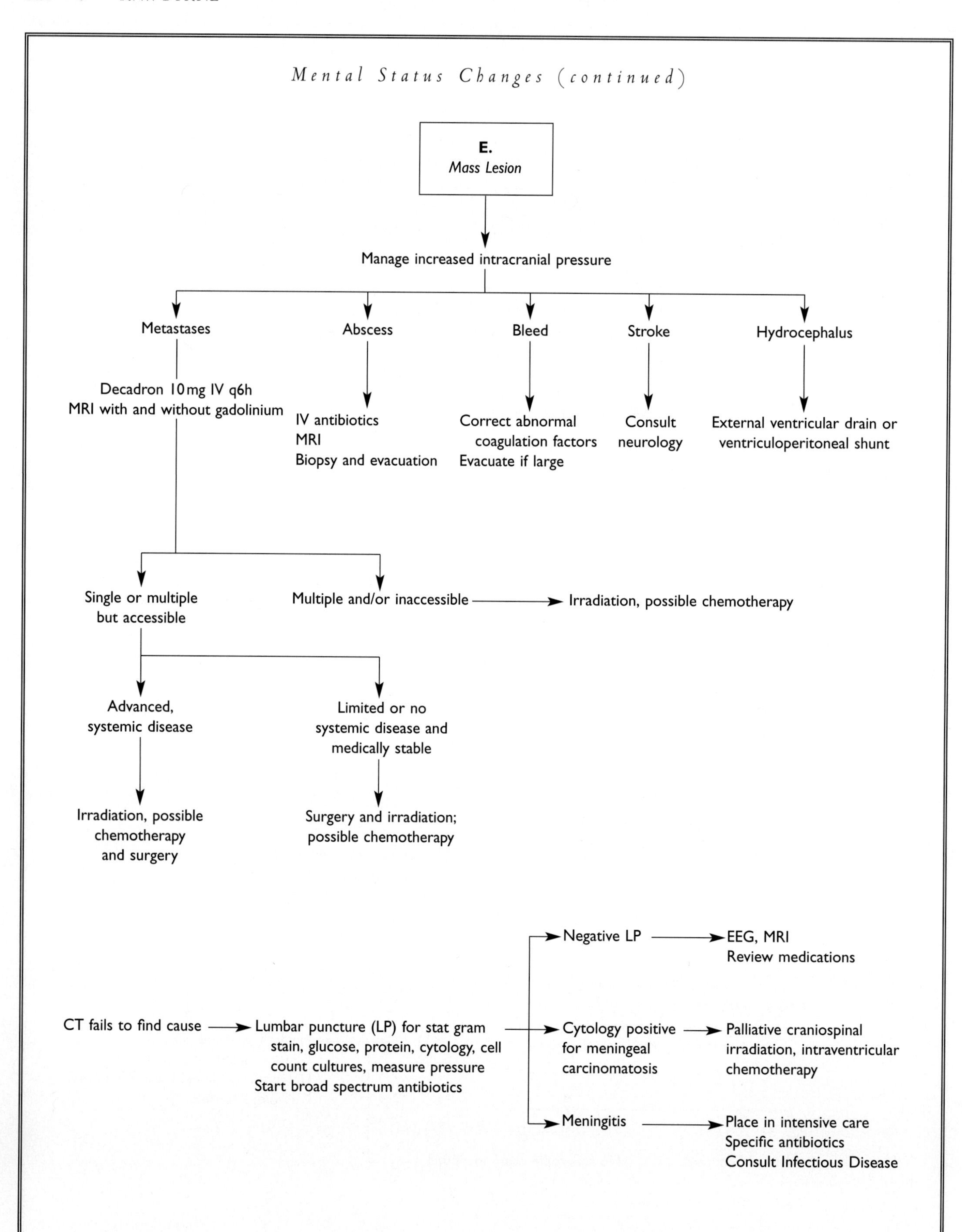
Mental Status Changes (continued)
E.
Mass Lesion
Manage increased intracranial pressure
Metastases
Abscess
Bleed
Stroke
Hydrocephalus
Decadron 10 mg IV q6h
MRI with and without gadolinium
IV antibiotics
MRI
Biopsy and evacuation
Correct abnormal coagulation factors
Evacuate if large
Consult neurology
External ventricular drain or ventriculoperitoneal shunt
Single or multiple but accessible
Multiple and/or inaccessible
Irradiation, possible chemotherapy
Advanced, systemic disease
Limited or no systemic disease and medically stable
Irradiation, possible chemotherapy and surgery
Surgery and irradiation; possible chemotherapy
CT fails to find cause
Lumbar puncture (LP) for stat gram stain, glucose, protein, cytology, cell count cultures, measure pressure
Start broad spectrum antibiotics
Negative LP
EEG, MRI
Review medications
Cytology positive for meningeal carcinomatosis
Palliative craniospinal irradiation, intraventricular chemotherapy
Meningitis
Place in intensive care
Specific antibiotics
Consult Infectious Disease

with mild dementia who becomes disoriented when sleep-deprived, on new medications in a strange environment. This scenario can be anticipated and avoided by asking the family about prior episodes. These patients are best handled with reorientation, reassurance, family help, sitters, or mild anxiolytics.

Portenoy and Krupp,[2] who studied patients with systemic cancer referred to a neurologist, noted that the referring service missed almost half of the cases of neurologic weakness, 85% of the cases of cranial nerve palsy, and 75% of the cases of sensory loss. It is clear from this study and others like it[1–4] that the best way to improve care for oncologic patients with mental status changes is to improve the neurologic history and physical examinations.

The physical examination may include the following: inspection for signs of trauma; tests of orientation, memory, intelligence, and speech; functional assessments of cranial nerves, motor, sensory (pin, touch, position), cerebellar, and deep tendon reflexes and gait. The presence of a focal neurologic deficit or signs of increased intracranial pressure (ICP) direct the evaluation. Lack of a focal deficit suggests a systemic, metabolic, or toxic cause that may be readily identifiable, treatable, and potentially reversible.

C. Rapidly Reversible Cause

Laboratory testing should first be directed at rapidly reversible causes of mental status change (e.g., hypoglycemia, hypoxia, hyponatremia, uremia). Such tests include assays for arterial blood gases and serum glucose and electrolytes; measurement of drug levels; and a toxicology screen. Blood and urine cultures should be ordered if sepsis is suspected, liver function tests checked if liver failure is suspected, and a coagulation profile evaluated if an intracranial bleed is suspected or a lumbar puncture is planned. If laboratory testing reveals any of these rapidly reversible causes of mental status changes, they should be corrected before they reach a critical stage. Rapid correction of significant hyponatremia (<120 mEq/L) can lead to central pontine myelinolysis. If the patient's mental status returns to baseline, it is unlikely that a second cause is present. However, it is important to determine the underlying reason for the metabolic or toxic derangement.

A thorough neurologic and mental status history, physical examination, and laboratory testing lead to a diagnosis in almost half of all cancer patients.[1] Gilbert and Grossman analyzed all admissions to the Johns Hopkins Oncology Center over a 3-month period and found that 46% of patients had a neurologic disorder related to their cancer. Of 162 patients, 25 had mental status changes. Twelve of these patients had metabolic derangements or drug toxicity that were readily diagnosed by history, physical examination, and laboratory testing.[1]

D. Focal Deficit or Nonreversible Cause

Patients who do not have a clear, rapidly reversible cause of their mental status change should be evaluated with computed tomography (CT) of the brain with and without contrast. Most patients who have a true mental status change or a new focal neurologic deficit and who lack a metabolic or toxic cause either have a structural lesion or require a lumbar puncture to rule out meningitis or meningeal carcinomatosis. CT scans are essential in both instances.

E. Mass Lesion

The structural lesions encountered in this scenario are the following: *metastases* (single or multiple), *abscess*, *stroke* (hemorrhagic or ischemic), *intracranial bleed*, or *hydrocephalus*. If any one of these conditions is diagnosed on CT scan, an urgent neurosurgical or neurologic consultation is recommended along with initial attempts at medical stabilization. The treatment of each of these conditions is largely dependent on the patient's prognosis from his or her systemic disease and the type of intracranial event. Patients with a significant mass lesion who are medically stable should undergo craniotomy; consideration is given to resection of a solitary metastasis, evacuation of an intra- or extraaxial hemorrhage, or drainage of an abscess. Significant hydrocephalus requires ventriculostomy or ventriculoperitoneal shunt after the etiology of the hydrocephalus is determined.

Most patients who present with cerebral metastases complain of headache or focal neurologic deficits. Approximately 40% of patients present with mental status changes.[5] Initial resuscitation includes administering Decadron 10 mg IV every 6 hours. Factors that affect the choice of treatment for patients with brain metastases include the following.

1. *Tumor type* (Table 67–1). Most metastatic tumors are best treated with gross total surgical removal, postoperative whole-brain irradiation, and chemotherapy appropriate for the type of tumor.[6–10] (Radiation therapy doses are usually 3000–4000 rad initially.) Alternatively, highly aggressive tumors, such as small cell lung cancer, usually are multiple and are best treated with whole-brain irradiation.[8]

2. *Single versus multiple metastases*. A single metastasis in a surgically accessible area in a medically stable patient is best treated with surgery. Stereotactic radiosurgery is a reasonable choice in some cases.[11–13] Some have had good results with resecting multiple brain metastases.[14] Patients with more than four metastases are almost always treated with whole-brain radiation therapy (WBRT) rather than with surgery.

3. *Tumor location*. Deep-seated brain metastases are best treated with WBRT or stereotactic radiotherapy. Fortunately,

TABLE 67–1.
Median survival of 583 patients with single brain metastasis

Primary	No. of patients	Median survival (months)	Mean survival (months)	One-year survival (%)
Lung	227	11.0	22.8	47.6
Lung (small cell)	10	18.8	22.0	60.0
Melanoma	73	6.0	16.5	33.0
Colon	63	7.0	11.8	31.7
Breast	50	13.4	22.8	54.0
Kidney	39	14.0	21.5	53.8
Miscellaneous	38	8.7	21.0	47.4
Urogenital	31	9.0	21.1	41.9
Sarcoma	25	6.3	21.6	40.0
Unknown	19	10.0	17.7	47.4
Esophageal	8	5.7	7.1	25.0
Total	583	9.4	19.7	44.4

All patients underwent craniotomy between 1974 and 1992. (Reproduced with permission from Arbit E, Wronski M. Clinical decision making in brain metastases. Neurosurg Clin N Am 1996 ful; 7(3):449.)

most metastases originate peripherally near the gray-white junction of the cortex.[15,16] These tumors are more accessible and therefore more amenable to resection, provided the patient is an acceptable candidate for surgery.

4. *General medical condition*. An uncontrolled primary tumor, the presence of multisystem metastases, advanced patient age, and advanced comorbid medical conditions are reasons to pursue nonsurgical treatment. Brain metastases usually are a manifestation of disseminated disease, with metastases involving the liver, lungs, or bone. In such cases, craniotomy is rarely if ever indicated. The brain is rarely the sole site of metastatic disease.

If no structural lesion is found and the patient is not coagulopathic, a lumbar puncture (LP) should be performed. The cerebrospinal fluid (CSF) is checked for cell count, glucose, protein, Gram stain, and culture. In addition, 5–10 ml should be sent for cytology and the CSF pressure noted in the supine lateral position. In patients strongly suspected to have meningitis, intravenous antibiotics with broad-spectrum coverage should be given immediately after the LP. Sometimes it is appropriate to give the antibiotics before the LP if the LP is delayed. A neurology and infectious disease consult may be helpful at this point.

In cases where the LP does not show infection, cytology may reveal malignant cells indicating meningeal carcinomatosis. For most cancers this is accompanied by cranial nerve deficits and a poor prognosis, even with systemic and intrathecal therapy. An LP with cytologic analysis has 100% specificity but is much less sensitive.[5]

Occasionally, no diagnosis can be reached even for the patient who presents with new mental status changes that persist and is evaluated according to this algorithm. In this case, an electroencephalogram should be obtained to rule out nonconvulsive seizures. If this test is negative, a magnetic resonance image of the brain may reveal rare problems, such as evidence of encephalitis or metastases despite a negative CT scan and LP evaluation.

References

1. Gilbert M, Grossman S. Incidence and nature of neurologic problems in patients with solid tumors. Am J Med 1986;81:951–954.
2. Portenoy R, Krupp L. Neurologic consultation in the management of patients with systemic cancer admitted to a community hospital. Cancer Invest 1986;44:293–296.
3. Silberforb P. Chemotherapy and cognitive defects in cancer patients. Annu Rev Med 1983;34:35–46.
4. Levine P, Silberforb P, Lipowski Z. Mental disorders in cancer patients: a study of 100 psychiatric referrals. Cancer 1978;42:1385–1391.
5. LeChevalier T, Smith FP, Caille P, et al. Sites of primary malignancies in patients presenting with cerebral metastases: a review of 120 cases. Cancer 1985;56:880–882.
6. Yamamoto T, Matsumura A, Fujita K, et al. Cerebral metastasis of parathyroid carcinoma. Neurol Med Chir 1996;36:96–98.
7. Hammoud MA, McCutcheon IE, Elsouki R, et al. Colorectal carcinoma and brain metastasis: distribution, treatment, and survival. Ann Surg Oncol 1996;3:453–463.
8. Andrews RJ, Gluck DS, Konchingeri RH. Surgical resection of brain metastases from lung cancer. Acta Neurochir (Wien) 1996;138:382–389.

9. Sampson JH, Carter JH Jr, Friedman AH, et al. Demographics, prognosis, and therapy in 702 patients with brain metastases from malignant melanoma. J Neurosurg 1998;88:11–20.
10. Nussbaum ES, Djalilian HR, Cho KH, et al. Brain metastases: histology, multiplicity, surgery, and survival. Cancer 1996;78:1781–1788.
11. Breneman JC, Warnick RE, Albright RE Jr, et al. Stereotactic radiosurgery for the treatment of brain metastases: results of a single institution series. Cancer 1997;79:551–557.
12. Wronski M, Maor MH, Davis BJ, et al. External radiation of brain metastases from renal carcinoma: a retrospective study of 119 patients from the M.D. Anderson Cancer Center. Int J Radiat Oncol Biol Phys 1997; 37:753–759.
13. Auchter RM, Lamond JP, Alexander E, et al. A multiinstitutional outcome and prognostic factor analysis of radiosurgery for resectable single brain metastasis. Int J Radiat Oncol Biol Phys 1996;35:27–35.
14. Bindal RK, Sawaya R, Leavens ME, et al. Reoperation for recurrent metastatic brain tumors. J Neurosurg 1995;83:600–604.
15. Nicolson GL, Menter DG, Herrmann JL, et al. Brain metastasis: role of trophic, autocrine, and paracrine factors in tumor invasion and colonization of the central nervous system. Curr Top Microbiol Immunol 1996;213(Pt 2):89–115.
16. Hwang TL, Close TP, Grego JM, et al. Predilection of brain metastasis in gray and white matter junction and vascular border zones. Cancer 1996;77:1551–1555.

CHAPTER 68

Bone Marrow-Suppressed Cancer Patient

GAIL SHIOMOTO
PINESH MONGE
NAFEEZA KHOKA

Bone marrow suppression in a cancer patient may involve one or more of the marrow compartments and may present as neutropenia, anemia, or thrombocytopenia. Each compartment is discussed separately.

Neutropenia

A. Epidemiology

Following myelosuppressive chemotherapy, neutropenia is a major risk factor for serious bacterial infection and a frequent reason for hospitalization during or following chemotherapy. About 5–10% of cancer patients still succumb to infectious complications associated with neutropenia despite appropriate interventions. The febrile neutropenic patient is therefore considered a medical emergency requiring immediate diagnostic and therapeutic intervention.[1] Neutropenia is defined as a neutrophil count less than 500/μl or less than 1000/μl with a predicted decrease to less than 500/μl. Fever is defined as a single oral temperature of 38.3°C (101°F) or ≥38.0°C (100.4°F) for at least 1 hour.[2]

B. Diagnosis

For the initial evaluation of the febrile, neutropenic patient, a thorough physical examination of the patient must include inspection of the periodontium, pharynx, larynx, esophagus, lungs, perineum, skin/bone marrow aspirate sites, vascular catheter sites, and tissue around the nail beds. Two sets of blood cultures for bacteria and fungi should be obtained for all patients. For patients with central venous catheters, blood cultures from each lumen and from a peripheral vein are needed to rule out a catheter infection. If the tissue through which the catheter is tunneled is inflamed or draining, the fluid should be Gram-stained and cultured for bacteria and fungi. Diarrheal stools should be tested for *Clostridium difficile* toxin, bacteria (*Salmonella*, *Yersinia*), viruses (rotavirus, cytomegalovirus), or protozoa (*Cryptosporidum*).

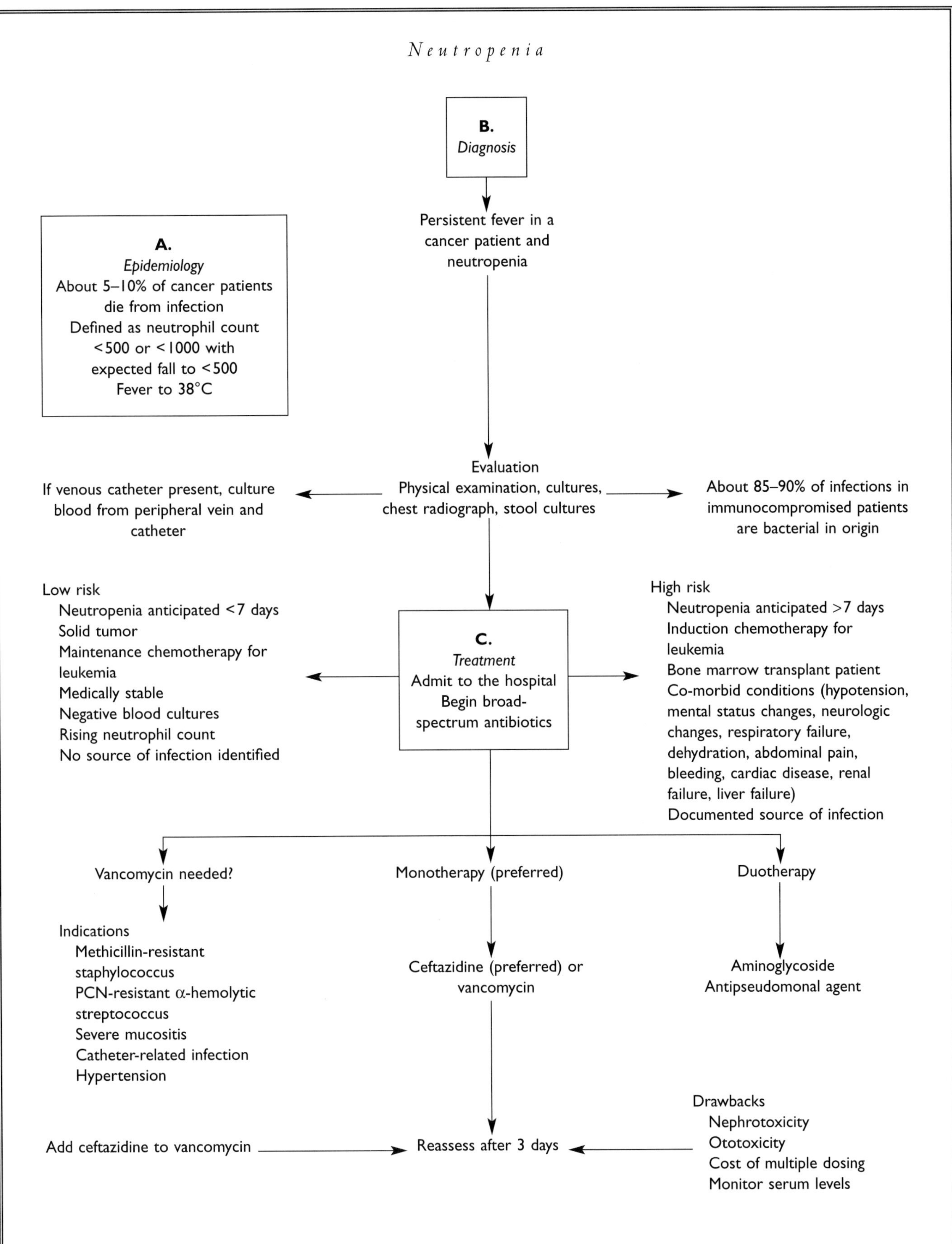

(continued on next page)

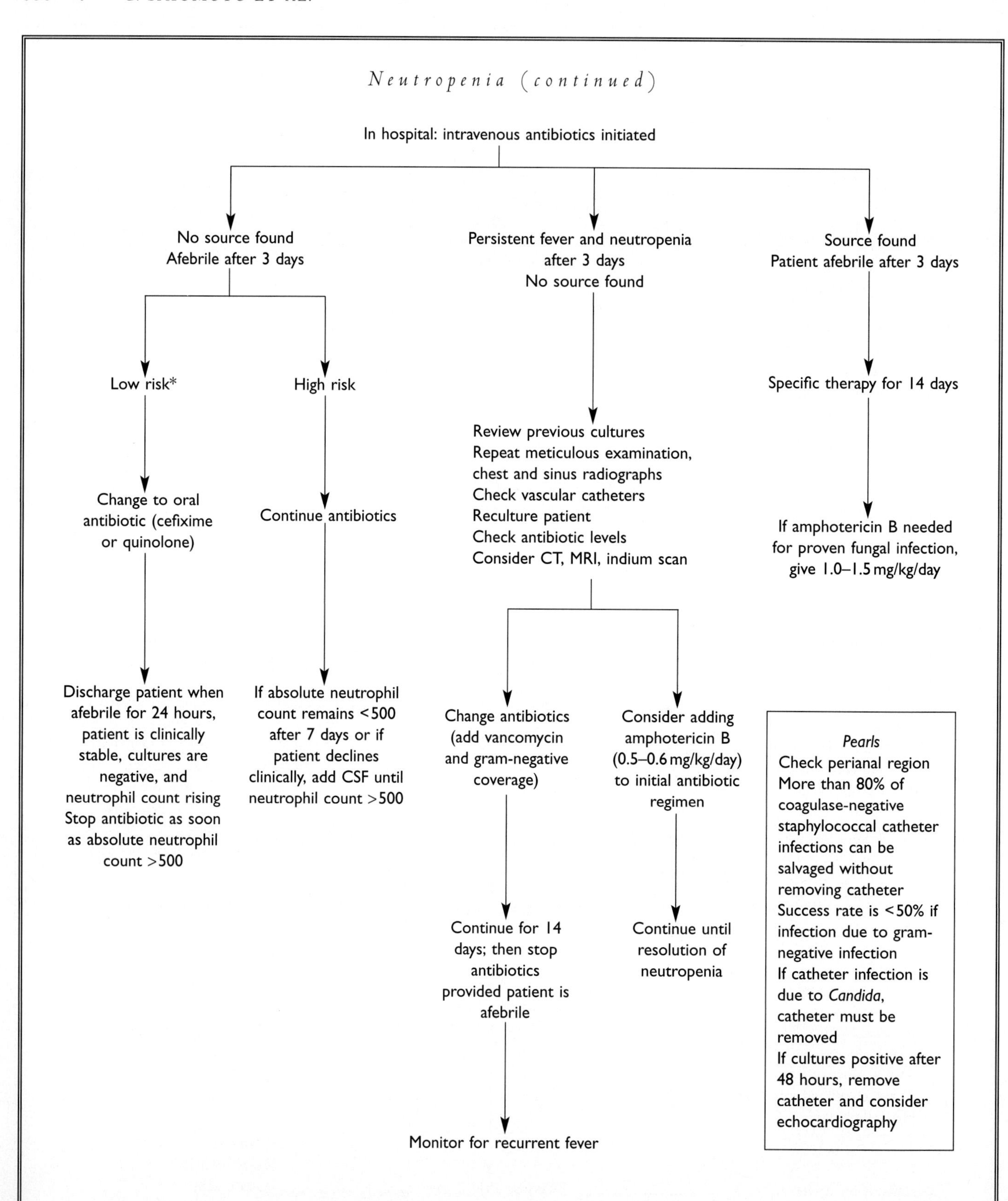

Neutropenia (continued)
In hospital: intravenous antibiotics initiated
No source found
Afebrile after 3 days
Low risk*
Change to oral antibiotic (cefixime or quinolone)
Discharge patient when afebrile for 24 hours, patient is clinically stable, cultures are negative, and neutrophil count rising
Stop antibiotic as soon as absolute neutrophil count >500
High risk
Continue antibiotics
If absolute neutrophil count remains <500 after 7 days or if patient declines clinically, add CSF until neutrophil count >500
Persistent fever and neutropenia after 3 days
No source found
Review previous cultures
Repeat meticulous examination, chest and sinus radiographs
Check vascular catheters
Reculture patient
Check antibiotic levels
Consider CT, MRI, indium scan
Change antibiotics (add vancomycin and gram-negative coverage)
Continue for 14 days; then stop antibiotics provided patient is afebrile
Monitor for recurrent fever
Consider adding amphotericin B (0.5–0.6 mg/kg/day) to initial antibiotic regimen
Continue until resolution of neutropenia
Source found
Patient afebrile after 3 days
Specific therapy for 14 days
If amphotericin B needed for proven fungal infection, give 1.0–1.5 mg/kg/day
Pearls
Check perianal region
More than 80% of coagulase-negative staphylococcal catheter infections can be salvaged without removing catheter
Success rate is <50% if infection due to gram-negative infection
If catheter infection is due to Candida, catheter must be removed
If cultures positive after 48 hours, remove catheter and consider echocardiography
*Outpatient treatment may be considered if low risk and bone marrow recovery seen.

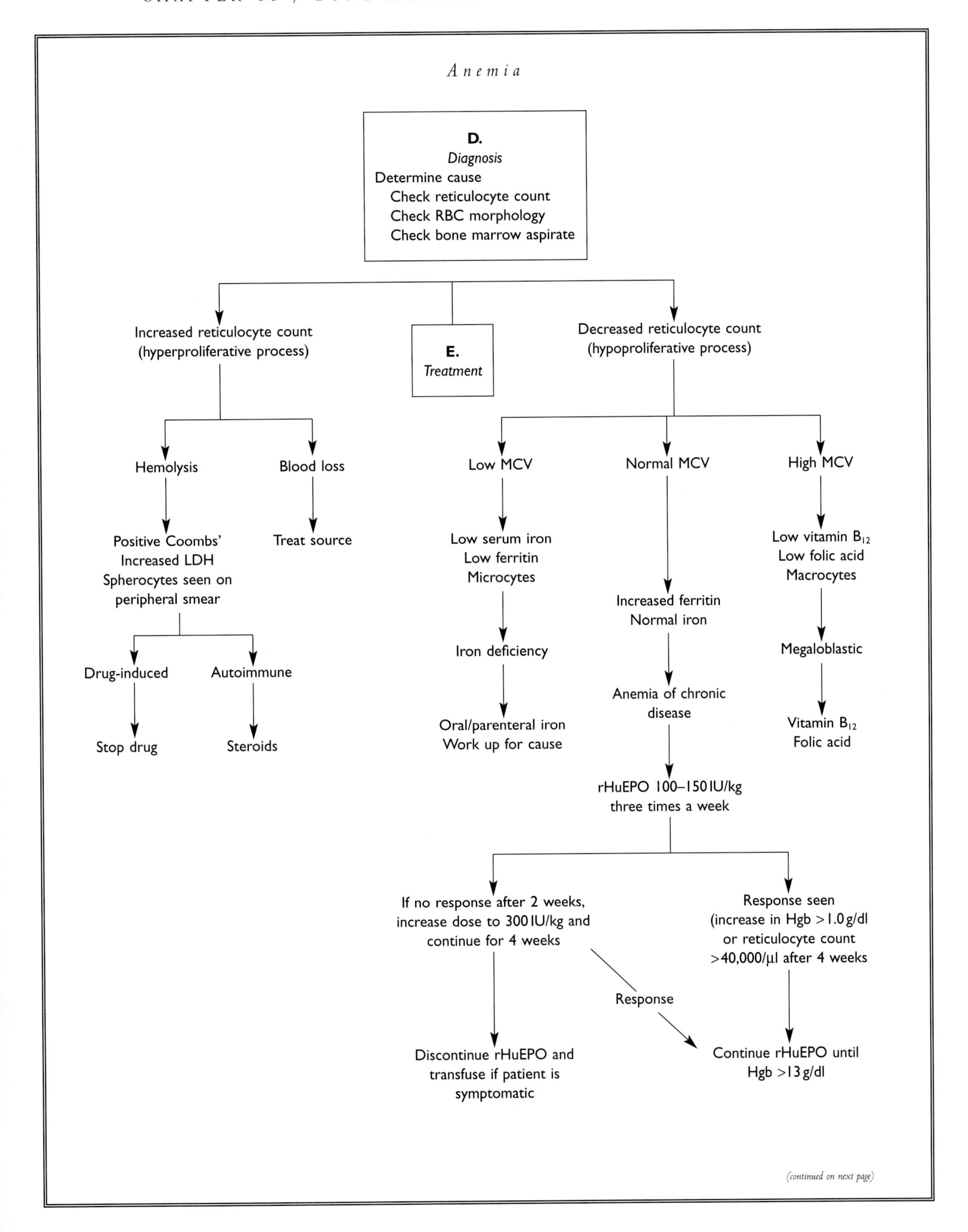

(continued on next page)

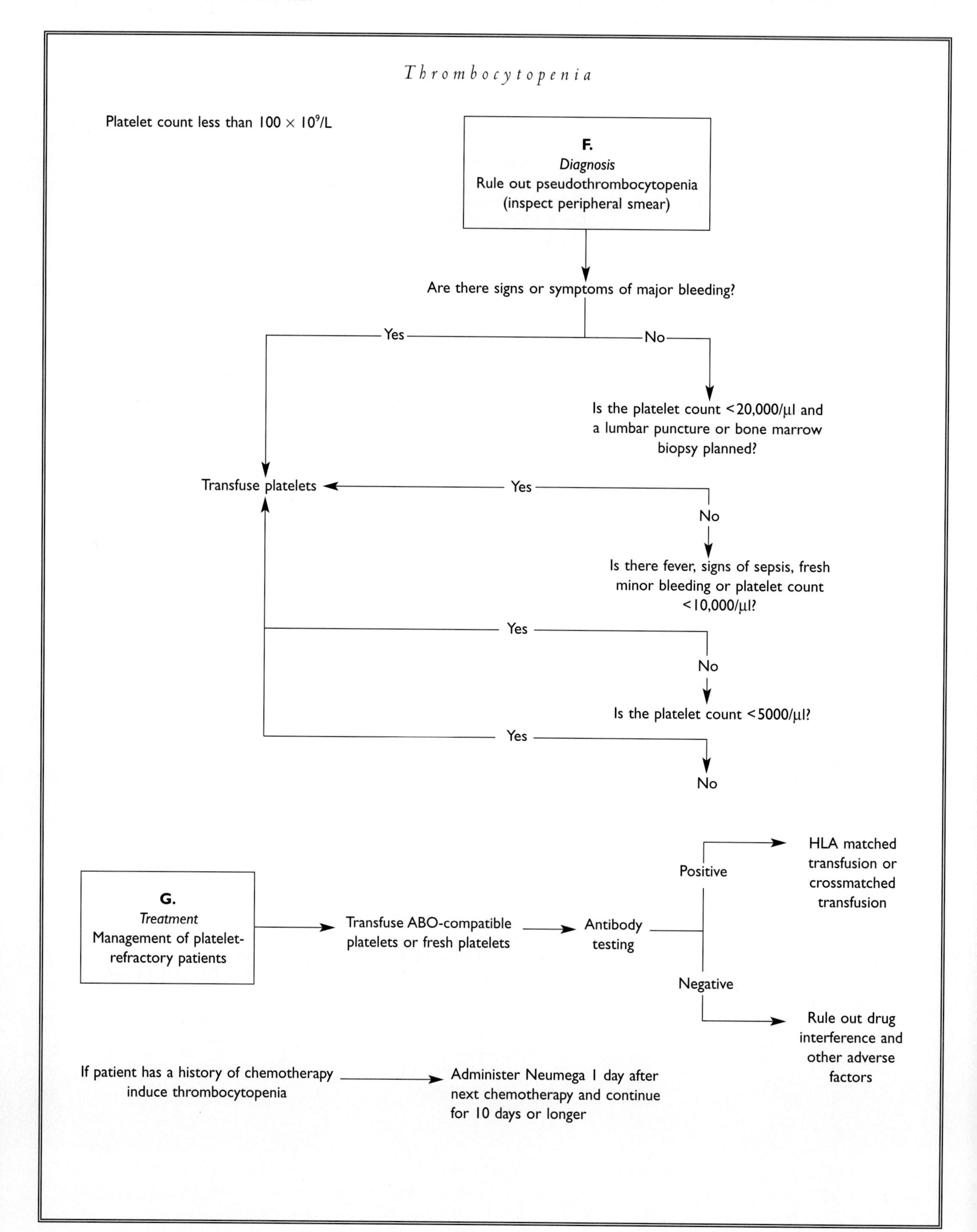

Thrombocytopenia
Platelet count less than 100 × 10⁹/L
F.
Diagnosis
Rule out pseudothrombocytopenia (inspect peripheral smear)
Are there signs or symptoms of major bleeding?
Yes
No
Is the platelet count <20,000/µl and a lumbar puncture or bone marrow biopsy planned?
Transfuse platelets
Yes
No
Is there fever, signs of sepsis, fresh minor bleeding or platelet count <10,000/µl?
Yes
No
Is the platelet count <5000/µl?
Yes
No
G.
Treatment
Management of platelet-refractory patients
Transfuse ABO-compatible platelets or fresh platelets
Antibody testing
Positive
HLA matched transfusion or crossmatched transfusion
Negative
Rule out drug interference and other adverse factors
If patient has a history of chemotherapy induce thrombocytopenia
Administer Neumega 1 day after next chemotherapy and continue for 10 days or longer

Urine cultures are indicated if there are signs or symptoms of a urinary tract infection or if a patient has a chronic indwelling bladder catheter. A baseline chest radiograph is obtained to rule out pneumonia. Skin lesions suspected of infection should be examined and be subjected to cultures, Gram stains, and cytology. Finally, specimens are collected for a complete blood count and serum transaminase, electrolyte, urea nitrogen, and creatinine assays.[3]

Approximately 60–70% of documented infections are due to gram-positive organisms, which may be methicillin-resistant and susceptible to vancomycin or teicoplanin.[4] Eighty-five percent of severe infections are due to eight pathogens, identified by the 3 + 3 + 2 rule: three gram-positive cocci (hemolytic *Streptococcus*, *Staphylococcus aureus*, *Staphylococcus epidermidis*), three gram-negative bacilli (*Escherichia coli*, *Klebsiella pneumoniae*, *Pseudomonas aeruginosa*), and two fungal infections (*Candida*, *Aspergillus*).[4] Variation can be found in the bacterial isolates from different hospitals, and it is important to know the distribution and their antimicrobial sensitivities in the center where the patient is being treated.[4]

C. Treatment

Practices vary, but febrile neutropenic cancer patients are usually admitted to the hospital for observation and initiation of antibiotic therapy. A risk analysis for potentially serious septic complications is prepared and is determined by the anticipated length of neutropenia, the type of cancer being treated, the presence of co-morbid medical conditions, and the documented presence of infection (e.g., blood cultures, catheter infection, perianal cellulitis). Low risk status is conferred by the following: anticipated neutropenia lasting less than 7 days, solid tumor, maintenance chemotherapy for leukemia (rather than for induction or bone marrow transplant), no evidence of renal or hepatic dysfunction, normal mental status, and negative cultures. Patients at greatest risk of infection are those with absolute neutrophil counts less than 500/μl lasting longer than an estimated 7 days. Low risk patients are less likely to have recurrent fever following an initial course of empiric antibiotic therapy and are less likely to be readmitted to the hospital for additional treatment.

Once the patient is admitted to the hospital and the necessary cultures have been obtained, *empiric* intravenous antibiotics are administered. If a documented source of infection and the responsible pathogen are identified, *specific* antibiotics are prescribed. Regarding empiric therapy, prompt institution is mandatory to reduce mortality and improve survival. The regimen chosen depends on institutional practices and local resistance patterns; choices include monotherapy with ceftazidine or imipenem or multiple drug combinations with an aminoglycoside, which has a risk of nephrotoxicity and ototoxicity and requires monitoring of serum levels. Ceftazidine is the preferred antibiotic; imipenem is more frequently associated with *C. difficile*-induced diarrhea, nausea, and vomiting and the emergence of resistant strains of *P. aeruginosa*.

Vancomycin is not routinely included in most empiric antibiotic regimens. Its use is dictated by individual institutional practices, but it should be given for infections with penicillin-resistant α-hemolytic streptococci and methicillin-resistant *S. aureus*. It is also indicated for cases of severe mucositis and catheter-related infections.

Following institution of empiric in-hospital therapy and estimating the risk of septic complications, a decision is made regarding whether to continue treatment on an inpatient or outpatient basis. Outpatient treatment is possible for the low risk patient provided some recovery of bone marrow function is seen (slowly rising neutrophil count); close monitoring of the patient is essential, as 20–30% of patients are readmitted with recurrent fever. There is no reliable way to identify these patients prospectively, but discharge should not be considered until the neutrophil count is higher than 500/μl, the patient has been afebrile for at least 24 hours, and cultures are negative for 48 hours. If these criteria are satisfied, the potential for readmission is lessened.

Cessation of antibiotic therapy is determined by the duration of neutropenia. For afebrile patients with neutropenia lasting less than 7 days, stopping treatment once the neutrophil count has been restored is acceptable. If the neutropenia lasts longer than 7 days, continuing antibiotics for the duration of the neutropenia is considered proper even if no source has been identified. For patients with a known source of infection, stopping the antibiotics on day 14 should be considered provided the patient has been afebrile and there is no clinical or laboratory evidence of persistent infection.

Empiric antifungal therapy should be considered for neutropenic patients who have persistent fevers despite a 7-day course of empiric antibiotic therapy. The benefit stems from the fact that fungal infection may accompany broad-spectrum antibiotic therapy, and early treatment decreases the incidence of invasive fungal infection, thereby decreasing mortality. Amphotericin B is preferred over ketoconazole. For empiric therapy a dose of 0.5–0.6 mg/kg/day is chosen and continued for the duration of the neutropenia. For patients with documented fungal infection, amphotericin B is given at a dose of 1.0–1.5 mg/kg/day.

Colony-stimulating factor (CSF) may be indicated when worsening of the course is anticipated and there is an expected long delay in recovery of the marrow. It is indicated in the presence of pneumonia, hypotensive episodes, severe cellulitis, or multisystem dysfunction secondary to sepsis and for patients who remain severely neutropenic and have documented infection that fails to respond to appropriate antimicrobial therapy.

Colony-stimulating factor may be given as an adjunct to patients receiving chemotherapy. For conventional chemotherapy doses, CSF is given to patients who have had previous neutropenic fever episodes; subsequent chemotherapy doses are attenuated. If high-dose chemotherapy without stem cell support is to be given and the risk of febrile neutropenia exceeds 40%, CSF is given. Likewise, if high-dose chemotherapy with stem cell support is prescribed, CSF is given as well. The dose of CSF is $250\,mcg/m^2/d$ and is given until the absolute neutrophil count is higher than $500/\mu l$ for 3 days.[5,6]

Anemia

Anemia, a common hematologic abnormality in cancer patients, can detract from their quality of life. A significant number of patients require transfusions during the course of their illness.[7] The causes are usually multifactorial, and often more than one mechanism is responsible. Treatment of cancer-related anemia presents a special treatment challenge. It is imperative therefore to understand the pathophysiology in each case to treat the anemia effectively. In the past, blood transfusion was the only option, but the availability of recombinant human erythropoietin (rHuEPO) now provides a safer, more cost-effective alternative.

Numerous causes of anemia have been identified in cancer patients (Table 68–1). Hemolysis may be secondary to certain chemotherapeutic agents (cisplatin, fludarabine) or can be autoimmune in origin, as occurs in 20% of patients with chronic lymphocytic leukemia, lymphoma, and rarely solid tumors such as gastric adenocarcinoma and ovarian carcinoma.[8] Iatrogenic or intrinsic tumor factors can cause significant blood loss. Other causes of anemia are nutritional deficiencies (iron, vitamin B_{12}, folic acid) and bone marrow suppression due to tumor invasion, myelofibrosis, or infection. Anemia of chronic disease (ACD) is the most common cause of anemia in cancer patients, but this is a diagnosis of exclusion. ACD in cancer is usually mild (hemoglobin 8–10 g/dl), and it has an insidious onset. The serum erythropoietin level is inappropriately low in patients with cancer, as the normal linear relation between the degree of anemia and the serum erythropoietin level is lost.[9] The severity of anemia is not influenced by the stage of malignancy or whether the patient is receiving cytotoxic treatment.

D. Diagnosis

One must first try to determine the cause of the anemia. The history regarding previous blood counts and cytotoxic treatment

TABLE 68–1.
Mechanism, causes, and characteristics of anemia in cancer patients

Mechanism	Characteristics
Hemolysis	Coombs' positive; increased reticulocytes, increased LDH, spherocytes on peripheral smear
Autoimmune: CLL, lymphoma, gastric adenocarcinoma, ovarian carcinoma	
Drug-induced: cisplatin, fludarabine	
Microangiopathy	Fragmented cells on peripheral smear, increased LDH
Tumor: gastric adenocarcinoma	
Drug-induced: mitomycin C, cyclosporine	
Hemorrhage	
Iatrogenic: surgery, phlebotomy	Increased/normal reticulocyte count; increased/normal mean corpuscular volume
Intrinsic tumor factor: tumor invasion of blood vessel, or mucosal bleeding (e.g., gastric, head and neck and cervical carcinoma, intratumoral bleeding)	
Nutritional deficiency	
Iron deficiency	Peripheral smear: microcytic hypochromic, low serum iron, low ferritin, increased TIBC
Inadequate intake	
Vitamain B_{12}/folic acid	Macrocytic cells on peripheral smear, low serum levels of vitamin B_{12}/folic acid
Increase requirement	
Bone marrow suppression	Neoplastic cells on bone marrow biopsy
Tumor invasion	Hypocellular marrow
Myeloablative treatment	Fibrosis on bone marrow biopsy
Myelofibrosis	Decreased EPO; normocytic normochromic cells on peripheral smear; increased ferritin; decreased serum iron; decreased reticulocytes
Anemia of chronic disease	

CLL, chronic lymphocytic leukemia; LDH, lactose dehydrogenase; TIBC, total iron-binding capacity; EPO, erythropoietin.

must be reviewed, which helps determine the duration and rapidity with which the anemia developed. The reticulocyte count is one of the most important parameters that must be checked. If it is increased, it indicates a hyperproliferative process (i.e., hemolysis or acute blood loss), whereas a low reticulocyte count is diagnostic of a hypoproliferative process (i.e., bone marrow suppression or vitamin B_{12} deficiency). A normal reticulocyte count is seen with iron deficiency and ACD.

The morphology of red blood cells on a peripheral blood smear helps differentiate between iron deficiency (microcytic hypochromic), vitamin B_{12} and folic acid deficiency (macrocytic), and hemolysis (spherocytes, or fragmented red blood cells). A bone marrow aspirate and biopsy are necessary in some cases to document iron deficiency or tumor invasion as the cause of anemia.

E. Treatment

Next, the anemia must be treated (i.e., nutritional supplements for vitamin B_{12}, folic acid, and iron deficiency anemia, and steroids for autoimmune hemolytic anemia). If it is determined that a low erythropoietin level is the cause of the anemia, it is treated with rHuEPO or blood transfusion. Many randomized trials have shown the efficacy and safety of rHuEPO in cancer patients; ACD associated with cancer can be corrected in approximately 50% of patients so treated.[10,11] The exact dose and schedule are controversial, although most recommend a starting dose of 100–150 IU/kg SC three times a week. If no response is noted by 4 weeks, the dose is increased to 300 IU/kg. Response is defined by an increase in the hemoglobin level of more than 1 g/dl or a reticulocyte count higher than 40,000/μl after 4 weeks of therapy. There is no benefit in escalating the dose further in a nonresponding patient. RHuEPO is available as an intravenous preparation, although the subcutaneous route is just as effective. Oral or parenteral iron supplementation is needed during the first 4–6 weeks of treatment with rHuEPO, as partial iron deficiency can cause unresponsiveness to rHuEPO.[12]

The advantages of rHuEPO are that it decreases the need for blood transfusion and therefore avoids the risk of transmitting serious infection or causing alloimmunization, a nonhemolytic transfusion reaction, and iron overload. There is evidence that allogeneic transfusion can increase the recurrence and metastasis of cancer.[13,14] Quality of life is improved, with a significant increase in energy level, ability to perform daily activities, and overall sense of well-being.[15] There is no evidence that rHuEPO enhances malignancy.[12] It is more cost-effective than blood transfusion, and it can be given concomitantly with other myelosuppressive treatment.

Factors that predict a favorable response to treatment with rHuEPO include a serum erythropoietin level less than 100 mU/ml and a hemoglobin concentration increased by more than 0.5 g/dl after 2 weeks of treatment or a serum ferritin level less than 400 ng/ml after 2 weeks of treatment.[16] An increase in baseline reticulocyte count of more than 40,000/μl after 4 weeks of treatment also predicts a favorable response.[17] Pretreatment serum erythropoietin levels are not consistently useful for predicting response. Side effects include occasional facial flushing, headache, hypertension, and deep vein thrombosis, but the risks of these complications are not significantly higher than in controls.

Thrombocytopenia

Thrombocytopenia is common and may be due to the disease itself or its treatment (i.e., irradiation or chemotherapeutic agents). When thrombocytopenia is sufficiently severe, the patient may experience extensive bleeding. Intracranial bleeding is a common cause of death. Timely intervention with platelet transfusion may prevent fatal complications.

The causes of thrombocytopenia are outlined in Table 68–2. Thrombocytopenia may result from impaired production, increased utilization, accelerated destruction of platelets, or sequestration by the spleen.[18,19] Bone marrow suppression by chemotherapy and irradiation causes decreased production of platelets. Other causes of impaired production include tumor involvement of the marrow, vitamin deficiencies, and fibrosis. Immune or nonimmune mechanisms may cause increased peripheral destruction of platelets; immune mechanisms are seen more frequently with hematologic malignancies than with solid neoplasms.

TABLE 68–2.
Etiology of thrombocytopenia[a] in cancer patients

Mechanism	Causes
Increased destruction	
Immune	Autoimmune hemolytic anemia, infections, collagen vascular disease, transfusion reactions, idiopathic
Nonimmune	Disseminated intravascular coagulopathy, thrombotic thrombocytopenia, hemolytic uremic syndrome, prosthetic heart valves, sepsis
Sequestration	Hypersplenism
Decreased production	
Abnormal marrow	Infiltration: fibrosis or tumor
	Suppression: treatment-related
	Vitamin deficiency
	Inherited disorder

[a] Platelet count less than 100×10^9/L.

F. Diagnosis

The peripheral smear should be inspected for clumps of platelets, which can be seen in cases of pseudothrombocytopenia. The decision to transfuse platelets is determined by clinical events, associated co-morbid conditions, and the platelet count. In 1962 Gaydos et al. reported a quantitative relation between the platelet count and the frequency of hemorrhage in patients with acute leukemia.[20] Based on this report a platelet count of 20,000/μl has been adapted as a target for prophylactic platelet transfusion, although many clinicians, in the absence of active bleeding or other co-morbid conditions (i.e., infections), may opt to observe patients closely. Platelets should be transfused if there is (1) any *major* bleeding irrespective of platelet count; (2) a *minor* bleed or a fever and a platelet count less than 10,000/μl; (3) a planned minor invasive procedure, (i.e., lumbar puncture) with a count less than 20,000/μl; or (4) a platelet count less than 5000/μl. Any causative agent including chemotherapy should be withheld if surgery is planned. The platelet count should be maintained at ≥50,000/μl during the intraoperative and immediate postoperative period. Immediate posttransfusion platelet counts should be obtained to be certain the desired platelet count has been reached before proceeding to surgery.[21] Appropriateness of response can be influenced by body surface area.[22] The initial therapy for thrombocytopenic patients remains a pooled random donor platelet concentrate. In a 70kg adult, 1 unit of random donor platelet concentrate increases the recipient platelet count by 5000–10,000/μl. Transfusion of 6–10 units is needed on each occasion.

G. Treatment

If platelet transfusion fails to restore normal counts, the following are important guidelines: (1) Transfuse ABO compatible blood. ABO incompatibility decreases the posttransfusion platelet increment by 10–20%.[23] (2) Fresh platelet transfusion can be used to overcome refractoriness, but this may not be easy to obtain as viral disease testing requires a minimum of 48 hours. (3) If there is no response to transfusion, perform antibody testing to rule out alloimmunization. If antibodies are present, transfuse with cross-matched or HLA-matched platelets. (4) Leukoreduction filters should be used in patients who are to receive multiple transfusions to decrease the risk of alloimmunization.

Neumega (oprelvekin) is a recombinant form of platelet growth factor, human interleukin-11, that promotes production of the body's platelet supply in cancer patients with solid tumors or lymphoma who are undergoing chemotherapy. If given to patients who have previously received platelets, Neumega (50μg/kg) significantly decreases the likelihood of platelet transfusion during a subsequent cycle of chemotherapy. Adverse effects of Neumega are fluid retention, peripheral edema, dyspnea, tachycardia, conjunctival redness, and atrial arrhythmia (10%).[24]

References

1. Chanock SJ, Pizzo PA. Fever in the neutropenic host. Infect Dis Clin North Am 1996;10:777–796.
2. Hughes WT, Armstrong D, Bodey GP, et al. 1997 Guidelines for the use of antimicrobial agents in neutropenic patients with unexplained fever: Infectious Diseases Society of America. Clin Infect Dis 1997;25:551–573.
3. Freifield A, Walsh T, Pizzo P. Infections in cancer. In: DeVita V (ed) Principles and Practice of Oncology. New York: Lippincott, 1997.
4. Huang AK. Infections in the patient with cancer. In: Djulbegovis B (ed) Decision Making in Oncology. New York: Churchill Livingstone, 1997.
5. Fleming D. Use of growth factors. In: Djulbegovis B (ed) Decision Making in Oncology. New York: Churchill Livingstone, 1997.
6. Pizzo P. Infectious complications of chemotherapy and supportive therapy for patients with hematologic malignancies. In: Bone R (ed) Current Practice of Medicine. New York: Churchill Livingstone, 1996.
7. Skillings JR, Sridhar FG, Wong C, Paddock L. The frequency of red cell transfusion for anemia in patients receiving chemotherapy: a retrospective cohort study. Am J Clin Oncol 1993;16:22–25.
8. Moliterno AR, Spivak JL. Anemia of cancer. Hematol Oncol Clin North Am 1996;10:345–363.
9. Miller CB, Jones RJ, Piantadosi S, Abeloff MD, Spivak JL. Decreased erythropoietin response in patients with the anemia of cancer. N Engl J Med 1990;322:1689–1692.
10. Kasper C, Terhaar A, Fossa A, Welt A, Seeber S, Nowrousian MR. Recombinant human erythropoietin in the treatment of cancer related anemia. Eur J Haematol 1997;58:251–256.
11. Ludwig H, Fritz E, Kotzmann H, Hocker P, Gisslinger H, Barnas U. Erythropoietin treatment of anemia associated with multiple myeloma. N Engl J Med 1990;332:1693–1699.
12. Cazzola M, Mercuriali F, Brugnara C. Use of recombinant human erythropoietin outside the setting of uremia. Blood 1997;89:4248–4267.
13. Mohandas K, Aledort L. Transfusion requirements, risks, and costs for patients with malignancy. Transfusion 1995;35:427–430.
14. Klein HG. Immunologic aspects of blood transfusion. Semin Oncol 1994;21(suppl 3):16–20.
15. Glaspy J, Bukowski R, Steinberg D, Taylor C, Tchekmedyian S, Vadhan-Raj S. Impact of therapy with epoietin alfa on clinical outcomes in patients with nonmyeloid malignancies during cancer chemotherapy in community oncology practice: Procrit Study Group. J Clin Oncol 1997;15:1218–1234.
16. Ludwig H, Fritz E, Leitgeb C, Pecherstorfer M, Samonigg H, Schuster J. Prediction of response to erythropoietin treatment in chronic anemia of cancer. Blood 1994;84:1056–1063.
17. Henry DH. Clinical application of recombinant erythropoietin in anemic cancer patients. Hematol Oncol Clin North Am 1994;8:961–973.
18. Goldsmith GH Jr. Hemostatic disorders associated with neoplasia. In: Ratnoff OD, Forbes (eds) Disorders of Hemostasis. Orlando: Grune & Stratton, 1984:351–366.
19. Hasegawa DK, Bloomfield CD. Thrombotic and hemorrhagic manifestations of malignancy. In: Yarbow JW, Bornstein RS (eds) Oncologic Emergencies. Orlando: Grune & Stratton, 1981:141–196.
20. Gaydos LA, Freireich E, Mantel N. The quantitative relation between count and hemorrhage in patients with acute leukemia. N Engl J Med 1962; 266:905–909.

21. Bishop JF, Schiffer CA, Aisner J, Matthew SJP, Wiernik PH. Surgery in acute leukemia: a review of 167 operations in thrombocytopenic patients. Am J Hematol 1987;26:147–155.
22. Slichter S. Principles of platelet transfusion therapy. In: Hoffman R, Benz EJ, Shattil SJ, Furie B, Cohen HJ, Silbenstein LE (eds) Hematology: Basic Principles and Practice, 2nd ed. New York: Churchill Livingstone, 1995:1987.
23. Yankee RA, Grumet FC, Rogentine GN. Platelet transfusion: the selection of compatible platelet donors for refractory patients by lymphocyte HLA typing. N Engl J Med 1969;281:1208–1212.
24. Isaacs C, Robert NJ, Bailey FA, et al. Randomized placebo-controlled study of recombinant human interleuken-11 to prevent chemotherapy-induced thrombocytopenia in patients with breast cancer receiving dose-intensive cyclophosphamide and doxorubicin. J Clin Oncol 1997;15:3368–3377.

Section 14

Diagnostic and Therapeutic Challenges

CHAPTER 69

Occult Axillary Metastases

SETH P. HARLOW

A. Epidemiology

Axillary metastasis from an occult primary malignancy is an uncommon first presentation for cancer. The incidence of axillary metastasis from breast cancer (the most common malignancy to present this way) is 0.3–0.8% of operable patients.[1–3] Approximately 2.2% of patients with melanoma present initially with axillary metastases without a known primary location.[4] Other malignancies that present with an axillary metastasis less frequently include other skin cancers (squamous cell, Merkel's cell, and skin adnexal tumors), lung cancer, gastrointestinal cancers (esophagus, stomach, pancreas, gallbladder, and colon), thyroid cancer, undifferentiated carcinomas, and rarely sarcomas. Primary lymphomas may also present with isolated axillary lymphadenopathy and should be included in the differential diagnosis.

B. Patient Evaluation

A careful detailed history and physical examination are important when evaluating the patient with axillary adenopathy. The historian should inquire about any skin lesions that may have been previously removed or were noted to have regressed spontaneously, regardless of how much time may have elapsed. A history of breast lumps or prior biopsies, chronic cough, hemoptysis, hoarseness, dysphagia, abdominal pains, bowel habit changes, blood per rectum, fevers, night sweats, and weight loss should also be elicited. The patient should also be asked about prior trauma, infections, cat scratches, or recent viral illness. A social history including smoking and alcohol use is needed.

Although most causes of axillary adenopathy are not malignant, the physical examination should focus on evaluating possible primary tumor locations, most importantly the breasts and skin. An evaluation of additional metastatic sites, such as other lymph node basins, liver enlargement, or pleural effusions should be performed. The number of enlarged lymph nodes, their size, and whether they are fixed to one another or other structures should be noted.

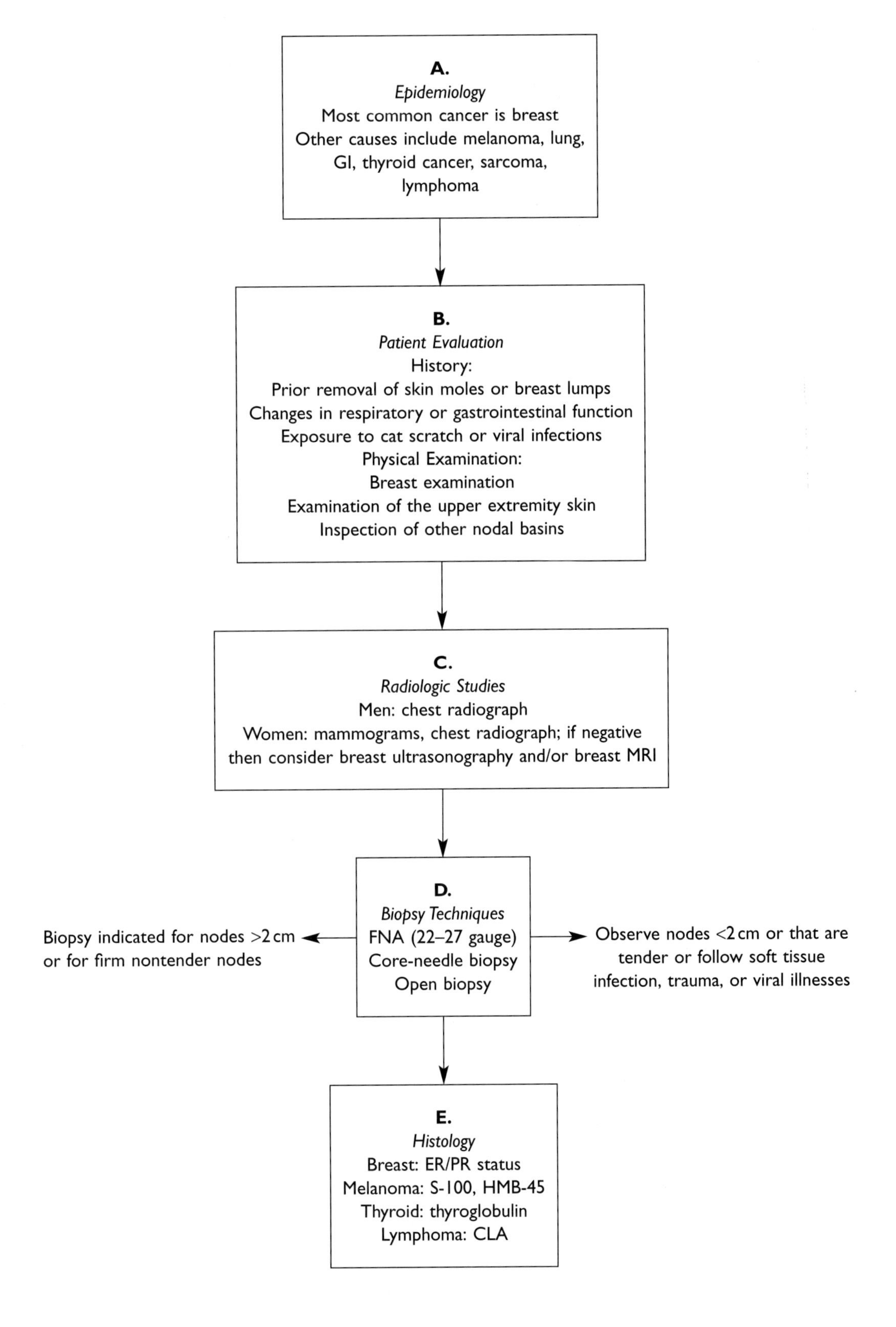

(continued on next page)

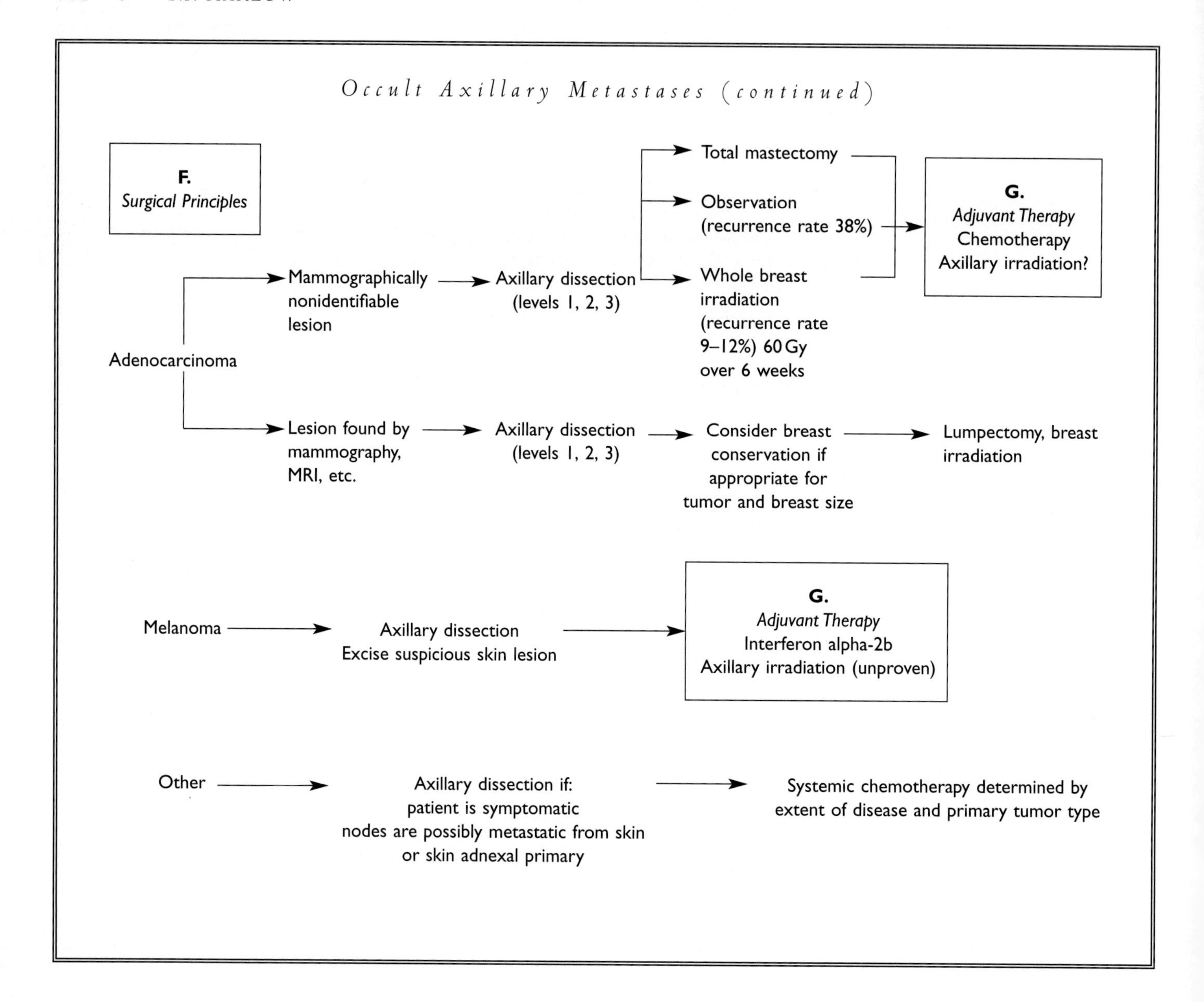

C. *Radiologic Studies*

Radiologic studies are indicated for all patients presenting with suspicious axillary lymphadenopathy, including a chest radiograph and bilateral mammography in women. High quality mammography may reveal findings suggestive of cancer (mass, calcifications), and chest radiographs may reveal a solitary lung nodule or multiple lesions consistent with metastatic disease. In women with metastatic adenocarcinoma to the axillary lymph nodes, an occult ipsilateral breast primary is the most likely source. If the lesion is not detected using mammography or physical examination, it is appropriate to perform whole-breast ultrasonography to search for an occult primary. The surgeon should be aware of the possibility of a contralateral breast cancer as well. Breast magnetic resonance imaging (MRI) has been evaluated as an imaging tool for breast cancer especially when looking for occult primary lesions. Using MRI, Tilanus-Linthorst et al.[5] were able to identify the primary tumor location in four women with mammographic and clinically occult breast cancers, leading them to recommend the use of breast MRI in this patient population.

For patients with metastatic melanoma, a careful skin search should be performed. Any suspicious lesion should be biopsied. Melanomas may be amelanotic; therefore, any nonpigmented nodular lesion should be considered a possible primary tumor. A history of a pigmented skin lesion removed in the past or that regressed spontaneously should alert the treating physician that this may be the primary site.

For patients in whom a primary tumor site cannot be identified after physical examination, chest radiography, and mammography, further testing is warranted. It may include bone scans and computed tomography (CT) scans of the chest and abdomen. The likelihood of identifying the primary tumor location is small, but other metastatic disease may be identified, which can influence clinical decision making. Extensive testing to evaluate the aerodigestive tract for primary tumors in asymptomatic patients is rarely fruitful and is unlikely to influence patient survival.

D. Biopsy Techniques

Generally, an axillary lymph node 2 cm or larger that is firm and nontender should be considered suspicious for harboring cancer and certainly should be biopsied. Findings that favor simple observation include small or painful nodes recently palpable following soft tissue infection, trauma, or a viral illness. In these patients follow-up at 2–3 months, with biopsy if they are still palpable, is a reasonable strategy. The available biopsy techniques include the following.

1. *Fine-needle aspiration* (FNA). This technique uses a 22- to 27-gauge needle, is readily suitable for use in the outpatient clinic, and is quite reliable for identifying metastatic disease. Identifying and typing lymphomas may be difficult by FNA alone.

2. *Core-needle biopsy*. This technique uses a 14- to 18-gauge core-needle and allows large samples to be taken for histopathologic evaluation while retaining the ability to be performed in the outpatient setting. This technique is slightly more invasive than FNA, and care should be taken to avoid puncturing the axillary vessels and creating a pneumothorax by the thrust of the needle.

3. *Open biopsy*. Open biopsy of enlarged axillary lymph nodes provides enough tissue to reach a definitive diagnosis using hematoxylin and eosin stains, immunohistochemical stains, and even electon microscopy. This technique is more costly and more invasive than other biopsy techniques.

E. Histology

Special stains may be helpful for identifying the likely origin of metastatic disease in axillary lymph nodes. Positive immunohistochemical stains for estrogen and progesterone receptors indicate a breast primary. S-100 and HMB-45 staining are suitable for malignant melanoma; thyroglobulin can indicate a thyroid primary; and common leukocyte antigen (CLA) is used to detect lymphoma. With this knowledge, surgeons can then focus their evaluation on those specific areas in an attempt to locate the primary tumor.

F. Surgical Principles

The surgical management of these patients depends largely on the primary tumor location. Although a tumor that expresses estrogen (ER) or progesterone (PR) receptors is highly suggestive of a breast primary, at least half of the breast cancers that present as an axillary mass are ER/PR-negative. Therefore occult axillary adenocarcinoma in a women without a known primary site is generally treated as breast cancer. In men adenocarcinomas most likely arise from lung or gastrointestinal tract primaries.

Surgical management of metastatic *adenocarcinoma* in women should include an axillary dissection (levels I, II, and III) to stage and control regional disease. The breast has been managed quite variably in different centers. If chest radiography and a CT scan of the chest are negative and mammography does *not* reveal a lesion, most still advocate total mastectomy on the ipsilateral side. Sectioning the specimen discloses a primary breast lesion in approximately 60–70% of cases.[6] Local recurrence rates after mastectomy are similar to those found in patients with detectable tumors and range from 2% to 9% in most series. Some centers have adopted an observation-only management program for the breast after lymph node dissection; the local recurrence rates in these patients is approximately 38%, with recurrence seen at 5–60 months.[6] Patients have been managed by whole-breast irradiation alone (60 Gy over 6 weeks) and have been found to have local recurrence rates of 9–12%,[6] which are not dissimilar to recurrence rates for detectable breast cancer treated with breast conservation. Two retrospective studies from M.D. Anderson Cancer Center[7] and Memorial Sloan-Kettering Cancer Center[1] have shown equivalent survival rates when comparing mastectomy and whole-breast irradiation. Therefore breast conservation may be safely considered an option in these patients. If radiologic studies reveal a lesion, consideration can be given to breast conservation, as the primary tumor is usually small in such instances.

In the case of occult malignant *melanoma*, when there is no evidence of systemic metastases, appropriate surgical treatment of the axillae should be a full axillary lymph node dissection. Additionally, any suspicious skin lesion should be excised to determine if it is the primary site. Survival rates of patients with metastatic melanoma from an unknown primary site are similar to those for whom the primary site is known, supporting the use of similar surgical procedures for managing axillary nodes.[4]

The surgical treatment of *axillary metastases* from non-breast/nonmelanoma primaries is not as clear-cut. For most of these patients the nodal metastases are simply a manifestation of systemic disease, and surgical removal is unlikely to influence survival. Palliative resection of large masses is indicated if the patient is symptomatic. Complete axillary dissection is warranted if there is a possibility that the nodes represent regional disease from a skin or skin adnexal primary. Surgeons should also be aware that some breast cancers show squamous differentiation histologically, a fact that must be considered in women presenting with metastatic squamous cell carcinoma to the axillae. Cancers with poor differentiation should be further evaluated by immunohistochemistry studies to be certain the tumor is not a lymphoma or an amelanotic melanoma.

G. Adjuvant Therapy

Breast Primary Lesion

Occult breast primaries are considered stage II lesions by the American Joint Committee on Cancer (AJCC) criteria.[8] As for patients with detectable breast primaries, the number of metastatic nodes is of major prognostic significance, with four or more positive nodes having high systemic recurrence rates. Commonly used chemotherapy regimens that have been found to improve survival significantly after breast cancer include CMF [cytoxan/methotrexate 5-fluorouracil (5-FU) for six cycles], AC (adriamycin/cyclophosphamide for four cycles), and CAF (cyclophosphamide/adriamycin/5-FU for six cycles);[9] newer agents such as the taxanes (docetaxel or paclitaxel) have significant antitumor effects on breast cancer, and their use in adjuvant trials is presently under study. In an overview analysis, standard-dose systemic chemotherapy has been found to reduce the systemic recurrence rates of breast cancer by approximately 30%.[10] The efficacy of higher-dose chemotherapy, with or without bone marrow/stem cell rescue, in high risk patients (four or more positive nodes) is the subject of ongoing studies, and its use should be limited to such trials. In regard to the use of combined chemoendocrine therapies, the combination of 5 years of tamoxifen plus chemotherapy for ER-positive patients is superior to either alone with respect to disease-free survival. For premenopausal patients the benefit is derived chiefly from the chemotherapy, with tamoxifen added after chemotherapy has been completed. For postmenopausal patients, the major benefit is derived from tamoxifen; however, there is a definite improvement in disease-free survival with combined chemotherapy and tamoxifen compared to tamoxifen alone, although this improvement may only be about 3–5%.

Following axillary dissection of clinically palpable nodes, patients are at higher risk of regional recurrence than those with clinically negative nodes. Whereas complete axillary dissection is quite good at controlling regional disease, adjuvant irradiation of the axillae and supraclavicular and internal mammary nodes may be used postoperatively for high risk patients (four or more positive nodes, extracapsular extension of tumor) to minimize this risk.[11]

Melanoma

A study by the Eastern Cooperative Oncology Group (ECOG), utilizing adjuvant interferon alfa-2b, given over 1 year in high risk melanoma patients (node-positive or tumor depth ≥4.0 mm), has demonstrated a significant improvement in survival for patients receiving adjuvant therapy compared to observation alone.[12] Patients with nodal metastases of an unknown primary would fall into the category of high risk (stage III) patients and would be candidates for this treatment. Patients on the ECOG study who received interferon had improved 5-year overall survival rates (47% vs. 36%) and 5-year relapse-free survival rates (37% vs. 26%), compared to those with observation alone. These patients may also be eligible for newer trials comparing tumor vaccines or other immunotherapies to interferon alfa-2b.

Axillary recurrence of melanoma following dissection is a potential problem in this group of patients. At present there are no randomized studies that demonstrate lower recurrence rates with nodal irradiation following axillary dissection. A single-arm study by Ang et al.,[13] evaluating the effectiveness of postoperative irradiation (30 Gy in five fractions over 2.5 weeks) in previously untreated patients, showed a regional control rate of 92% at 5 years. This treatment is currently being studied in a prospective randomized trial by the Radiation Therapy Oncology Group (RTOG) to see if it offers improvement over surgery alone.

Other Primaries

Currently there are no standardized adjuvant protocols for patients with metastatic disease thought not to be from a breast or melanoma primary. Patients thought to have metastatic differentiated thyroid cancer may benefit from radioactive iodine. Consideration should be given to adjuvant radiation to the axillae and supraclavicular nodes, as this may well improve regional control. Adjuvant chemotherapy may be considered, with the most commonly used drugs being 5-FU and cisplatin.

Conclusions

Occult axillary metastases in women usually arise from a primary breast cancer. Axillary dissection and either breast irradiation or mastectomy may be performed if radiologic tests fail to reveal a breast tumor. If mammography reveals a nonpalpable malignant lesion, breast conservation is an option, but axillary dissection and irradiation of the remaining breast should be performed. Consideration should be given to systemic chemotherapy and possible regional radiotherapy in selected patients. Such cases in men are usually due to metastatic melanoma or tumors arising in the lungs or gastrointestinal tract. Axillary dissection is indicated for melanoma, but in other instances it should be performed only if the patient is symptomatic from bulky disease.

References

1. Baron PL, Moore MP, Kinne DW, et al. Occult breast cancer presenting with axillary metastases: updated management. Arch Surg 1990;125:210–214.

2. Fitts WT, Streiner GC, Enterline HT. Prognosis of occult carcinoma of the breast. Am J Surg 1963;106:460–463.
3. Owen HW, Dockerty MD, Gray HK. Occult carcinoma of the breast. Surg Gynecol Obstet 1954;98:302–308.
4. Wong JH, Cagle LA, Morton DL. Surgical treatment of lymph nodes with metastatic melanoma from unknown primary site. Arch Surg 1987; 122:1380–1383.
5. Tilanus-Linthorst MM, Obdeijn AI, Bontenbal M, et al. MRI in patients with axillary metastases of occult breast carcinoma. Breast Cancer Res Treat 1997;44:179–182.
6. Forquet A, DeLaRochefordiere A, Campana F. Occult primary cancer with axillary metastases. In: Harris JR, Lippman ME, Morrow M, Hellman S (eds) Diseases of the Breast. Philadelphia: Lippincott-Raven, 1996;892–896.
7. Ellerbroek N, Holmes F, Singletary E. Treatment of isolated axillary metastases in patients with an occult primary consistent with breast [abstract]. Int J Radiat Oncol Biol Phys 1989;17(suppl 1):178.
8. Beahrs OH, Henson DE, Hutter RVP, et al (eds). Handbook for Staging of Cancer. Manual for Staging of Cancer, 4th ed. Philadelphia: Lippincott, 1993;161–167.
9. Osborne CK, Clark GM, Ravdin PM. Adjuvant systemic therapy of primary breast cancer. In: Harris JR, Lippman ME, Morrow M, Hellman S (eds) Diseases of the Breast. Philadelphia: Lippincott-Raven, 1996;548–578.
10. Early Breast Cancer Trialists Collaborative Group. Systemic treatment of early breast cancer by hormonal, cytotoxic or immune therapy. Lancet 1992;39:71–85.
11. Early Breast Cancer Trialists Collaborative Group. Effects of radiotherapy and surgery in early breast cancer: an overview of the randomized trials. N Engl J Med 1995;333:1444–1455.
12. Kirkwood JM, Strawderman MH, Ernstoff MS, et al. Interferon alpha-2b adjuvant therapy of high risk resected cutaneous melanoma: the Eastern Cooperative Oncology Group trial EST 1684. J Clin Oncol 1996;14:7–17.
13. Ang KK, Byers RM, Peters LJ, et al. Regional radiotherapy as adjuvant treatment for head and neck malignant melanoma. Arch Otol Head Neck Surg 1990;116:169.

CHAPTER 70

Cervical Lymph Node

JACQUELINE HARRISON
CONSTANTINE V. GODELLAS

A. Epidemiology and Etiology

An isolated cervical mass in an adult should be considered malignant until proven otherwise. This maxim is derived from the "rule of 80s," which states that of adult patients with a nonthyroidal neck mass approximately 80% have a neoplasm, 80% of these are malignant, 80% of these malignancies are metastatic, and 80% of the primaries are located above the clavicles. This rule is a simplification of data collected over 19 years by Gray et al.[1]

One of the most important aspects of the patient's history is his or her *age*. Congenital and benign lesions are more common in the pediatric population, whereas metastatic cancer is the most common cause of the isolated nonthyroidal neck mass in patients over 40 years of age. The *time course* of the lesion is also important. Masses that enlarge rapidly over a matter of days and are of less than 2 weeks' duration are usually infectious, although some neoplasms (e.g., lymphoma) may increase in size at an alarming rate.[2] The presence or absence of *pain* is also an important distinguishing characteristic; most malignant lesions are painless. The presence of tenderness usually signifies an infectious origin, although necrosis or hemorrhage into a malignant lesion causing rapid capsular expansion can lead to pain and swelling.[3] Risk factors for *infections* with the human immunodeficiency virus (HIV), mononucleosis, and tuberculosis should be assessed, including a history of exposure, intravenous drug abuse, and risky sexual practices. These diagnoses can be established by serologic or skin testing. A history of head and neck *malignancy* or lung or gastrointestinal cancer should be sought. Risk factors for upper aerodigestive tract cancers should be assessed, particularly a history of *alcohol and tobacco use*. In addition, other symptoms indicative of upper aerodigestive tract cancers should be sought, including dysphagia, hoarseness, epistaxis or nasal discharge, hemoptysis, shortness of breath, and otalgia.

B. Physical Examination

Evaluation of the mass itself includes an accurate assessment of its location, size, and consistency. Thorough knowledge of the lymphatic drainage of the salivary glands, thyroid gland, oral cavity, and nasopharynx is invaluable for directing attention to those organs if there is metastatic nodal disease

Cervical Mass

In adults, 80% of non-thyroid masses are neoplastic
Of these, 80% are malignant
Of these, 80% are metastatic
Of these, 80% have a head and neck primary

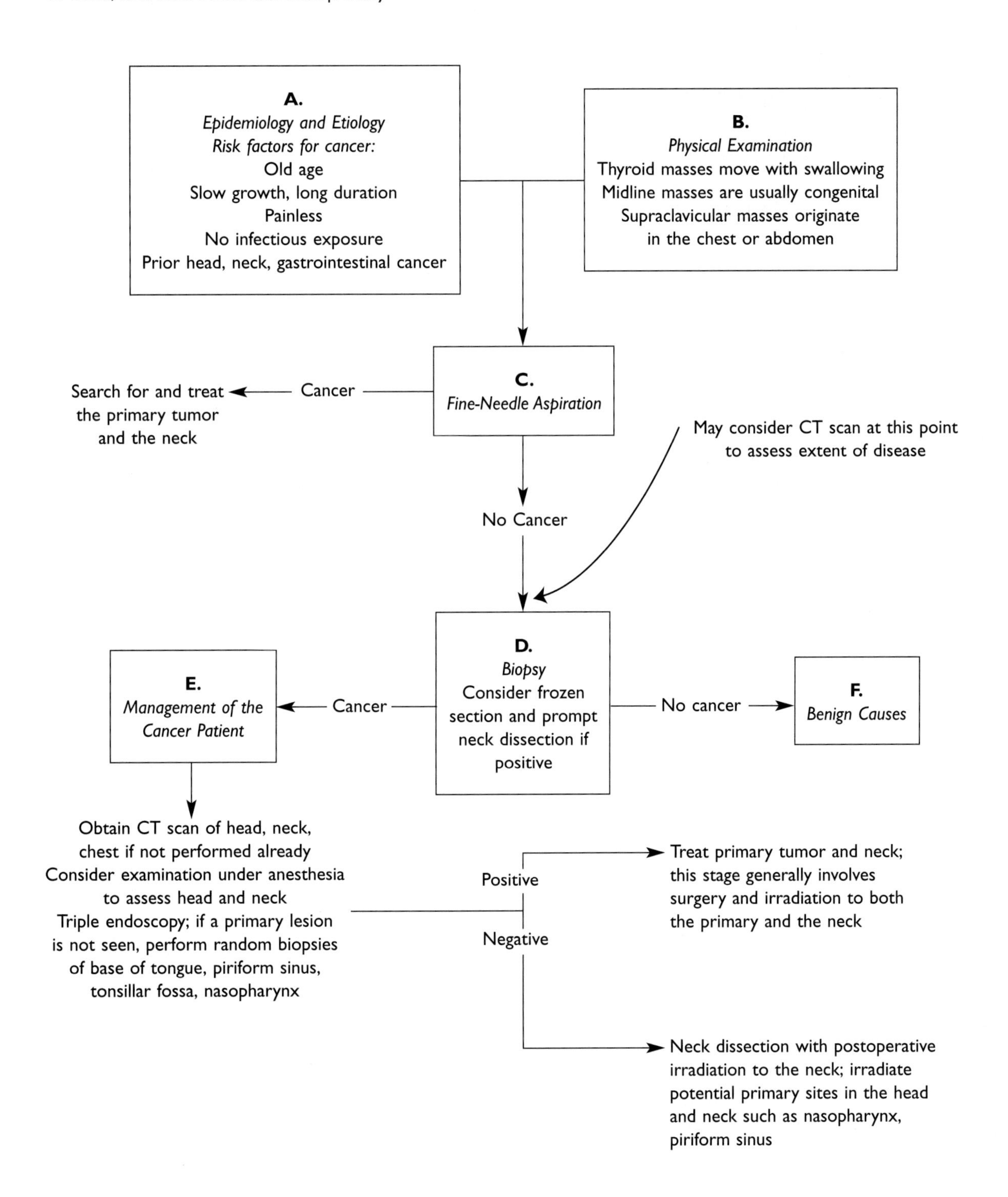

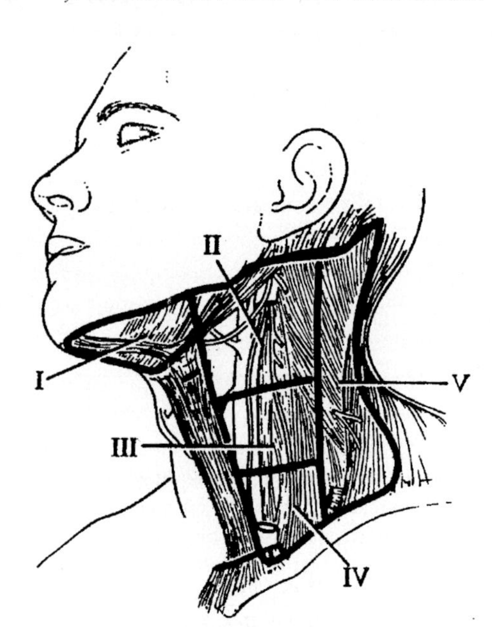

FIGURE 70–1
Memorial Sloan-Kettering cervical lymph node levels.

in specific areas of the neck. The regional head and neck lymphatics, as grouped by the Memorial Sloan-Kettering Cancer Center leveling system, are depicted in Figure 70–1 and detailed in Table 70–1. Parotid, suboccipital, and preauricular nodes are not included in the Memorial Sloan-Kettering leveling system.

The mass should be palpated while the patient swallows. The thyroid's association with the pretracheal fascia binds it to the trachea and larynx so thyroidal masses move with swallowing, helping to differentiate these lesions from other masses. Nonthryoidal midline masses are more often congenital than neoplastic. Among them, the most common is the thyroglossal duct cyst, a remnant of the duct connecting the foramen cecum to the thyroid isthmus. Supraclavicular masses (e.g., Virchow's node) are more likely to originate from a source in the thorax or abdomen.

In addition to examining the mass, a careful search for possible primary sites of cancer should be undertaken. The scalp should be thoroughly examined, as should the face and neck, for melanomas and squamous cell cancers. The oral cavity should be carefully inspected and palpated, with special attention to the base of the tongue, a common site for occult carcinomas. Palpation is extremely important, as many of these tumors have no visible mucosal abnormality but feel indurated on palpation. The nasopharynx should be examined using a nasal speculum to examine the anterior nares, and the larynx should be examined via indirect laryngoscopy. The latter is performed using a warmed dentist's mirror. With the patient and examiner both seated and the examiner wearing a head lamp, the patient's tongue is held forward so the oropharyngeal structures can be seen better. The mirror is introduced into the patient's mouth, with special care to avoid touching the base of the tongue with the mirror. By angling the mirror, the oropharynx, larynx, and hypopharynx can be visualized. Instructing the patient to say "e" allows assessment of vocal cord mobility and improved visualization of the piriform sinuses, postcricoid hypopharynx, and the laryngeal portion of the epiglottis. Depressing the tongue with a tongue blade and placing the mirror behind the soft palate allows visualization of this part of the nasopharynx.[4]

Complete physical examination of these patients, especially those with level IV or V nodes, includes an examination of the chest, abdomen, pelvis, and extremities, including inspection of other lymph node chains (axillary and inguinal basins). A digital rectal examination in patients of both genders, as well as a bimanual pelvic examination in women, should also be performed.

C. *Fine-Needle Aspiration*

If after a complete history and physical examination a neoplasm is suspected, fine-needle aspiration (FNA) should be undertaken for confirmation. FNA is an office procedure requiring only a 10-cc syringe and a 22-gauge needle. The patient lies supine so the surgeon can stabilize the mass with the nondominant hand. Anesthesia is usually unnecessary. The 22-gauge needle with attached syringe is passed into the mass. About 2 cc of air should be in the barrel of the syringe prior to aspirating the mass. Once in the mass, suction is applied to the syringe and multiple passes are made through the mass. Suction is released prior to removing the needle, and the 2 cc of air in the syringe is used to express the aspirate out of the needle onto a glass slide, which is then placed in alcohol or sprayed with fixative. If cystic fluid or blood is aspirated, multiple passes are not performed. Cystic lesions can include thyroglossal duct cysts, cystic hygroma, branchial cleft cysts, parathyroid cysts, and cystic degeneration of papillary carcinoma of the thyroid. If cystic fluid is aspirated, it is sub-

TABLE 70–1.
Drainage patterns of the cervical lymph nodes

Lymph node basin[a]	Primary site
Level I	Lip, facial skin, oral cavity
Level II	Oral cavity, oropharynx, nasopharynx, hypopharynx, larynx
Level III	Thyroid, oral cavity, oropharynx, hypopharynx, larynx
Level IV	Oropharynx, hypopharynx, larynx, thyroid, cervical esophagus
Level V	Posterior scalp and pinna, nasopharynx, thyroid, lung, GI tract, breast, GU tract

GI, gastrointestinal; GU, genitourinary.
[a] See Figure 70–1.

mitted for cytologic evaluation. FNA is particularly good for establishing a diagnosis of squamous cell carcinoma, thyroid carcinoma, melanoma, and well differentiated adenocarcinoma. FNA is not accurate for diagnosing lymphomas, sarcomas, neuroendocrine tumors, or poorly differentiated adenocarcinomas. FNA is not able to establish a diagnosis in about 10% of aspirated lesions owing to insufficient material, sampling error, or the presence of certain pathologies that cannot be adequately diagnosed by FNA alone (e.g., lymphoma). In these instances an open biopsy is necessary.[5] Negative reports do not rule out carcinoma, as the false-negative rate of FNA in experienced hands is about 7%.[6]

D. Biopsy

Open biopsy is indicated when FNA was unsuccessful. It should not be undertaken lightly, as the morbidity can be significant. Particularly, the incidence of infection and tumor recurrence at open biopsy sites is considerable, and incisional biopsy is associated with higher infection rates and tumor fungation than excisional biopsy. A 1984 study by Gooder and Palmer found an infection rate of 23% associated with incisional biopsy versus 9% with excisional biopsy. The incidence of fungation was 21% in the incisional biopsy group compared to 11% in the excisional group and 7% in the nonbiopsied group.[7] It is unclear whether distant metastasis is affected by biopsy of cancerous nodes. A 1978 review by McGuirt and McCabe showed a significant increase in distant metastasis with incisional lymph node biopsy (39%) compared to patients without biopsy or biopsy only at the time of neck dissection,[8] in contrast to the Gooder and Palmer review, which found no difference in the distant metastatic rate between these two groups.[7] Clearly, if open biopsy is necessary, complete excision of the node is preferable if feasible. Large nodes or groups of matted nodes may make complete excision technically impossible. In addition, special attention and forethought should be directed to the placement of the surgical incision so it can be excised easily if neck dissection is required. An ideal approach is to prepare the patient for formal neck dissection at the time of frozen section node biopsy and then proceed with definitive surgical therapy based on results of the frozen section rather than closing the wound and subjecting the patient to a two-stage procedure.

E. Management of the Cancer Patient

If on FNA a diagnosis of squamous cell carcinoma is obtained and no primary lesion has been found by physical examination, indirect laryngoscopy, or plain radiography, computed tomography (CT) scans of the head, neck, and chest are indicated. If FNA suggests adenocarcinoma, neuroendocrine carcinoma, or poorly differentiated cancer, CT scans of the neck, chest, abdomen, and pelvis are indicated provided the history, physical examination, and plain films have not suggested a primary tumor. In addition to detecting the primary lesion, the extent of lymphadenopathy can be evaluated by CT or magnetic resonance imaging (MRI).

The most established means of imaging neck masses are MRI and CT. CT is the more commonly used modality, mainly because of its lesser expense and faster acquisition time. The use of ultrasonography is limited to its occasional use in guiding FNA and evaluating thyroid lesions. Advantages of MRI include its ability to image multiple planes, better soft tissue contrast, no radiation exposure, and no need for intravenous contrast material. With the development of lymph node-delineating contrast agents and spectroscopy, MRI may supplant the role of CT in imaging neck masses and head and neck cancer.

Benign neoplasms appear homogeneous with both CT and MRI. On CT solid tumors are similar in attenuation to muscle, and cystic tumors are similar in attenuation to cerebrospinal fluid. On both CT and MRI, benign tumors have preserved fascial planes and are encapsulated. In contrast, malignant tumors are poorly circumscribed, heterogeneous in appearance, and have poorly defined fascial planes. Cystic or necrotic areas in the tumor are of low attenuation on CT. Infectious processes are evaluated equally well with either CT or MRI, which are useful for delineating the extent of the process. In addition, cellulitis can be differentiated from an abscess with either modality. Imaging should be carried down to the level of the superior mediastinum, as infectious processes in the neck can extend along fascial planes down to this level. The CT scan is more sensitive than MRI for detecting calcifications in granulomatous lymphadenopathy (i.e., tuberculosis, sarcoidosis).

If a thorough head and neck examination reveals a primary tumor in a patient with palpable neck disease, imaging (e.g., CT scan) is performed to determine the extent of the disease. The primary tumor and the cervical metastases are the treated, usually with surgery and irradiation. Patients with metastatic neck disease and no known primary tumor, despite a thorough history, physical examination, chest radiography, or CT scan of the head, neck, and chest, should undergo triple endoscopy (panendoscopy). Panendoscopy consists of direct laryngoscopy, esophagoscopy, and bronchoscopy. If no tumor is found, random biopsy specimens should be obtained from the base of the tongue, piriform sinus, ipsilateral tonsillar fossa, and nasopharynx. These areas are the most likely statistically to harbor an occult carcinoma.[9] If these biopsies are positive, the treatment plan for the primary tumor and neck metastases can be established. If the biopsies are negative, the node is excised, with frozen section assessment followed by neck dissection. Even though random biopsies were negative, the areas most likely to harbor an occult cancer are irradiated.

Whether all patients with diagnosed head and neck carcinomas should undergo triple endoscopy remains controversial. The incidence of synchronous upper aerodigestive tract cancers in patients with a diagnosed head and neck carcinoma is considerable, documented at 5–16%.[10–12] Proponents of routine triple endoscopy in head and neck tumor patients point out that early, treatable carcinomas can be detected. Additionally, if an advanced synchronous tumor is found, it may alter the treatment of the head and neck tumor. Opponents of routine triple endoscopy point out that in most of the patients with synchronous cancers, a careful history and physical examination along with chest radiography and esophagography detected the synchronous tumors. Routine triple endoscopy is not cost-effective.[13]

F. Benign Causes

Infectious and inflammatory causes of a neck mass must be included in the differential diagnosis for patients of all ages, especially pediatric patients. Dental caries is not an uncommon cause of cervical lymphadenopathy and can be seen on oral examination. A history of exposure to cats may raise suspicion of cat scratch disease. Splenomegaly, a pharyngeal exudate, and a history of exposure may lead one to suspect mononucleosis.

Acute Lymphadenitis

One of the most common causes of neck masses in children is acute lymphadenitis. This infection is characterized by tenderness and erythema of the overlying skin. The pathogen is usually *Staphylococcus* or *Streptococcus*, with the portal of entry being the throat. Treatment is gram-positive antibiotic coverage, such as amoxicillin/clavulanic acid or erythromycin. Organized abscesses should be incised and drained.[14]

Mononucleosis

Mononucleosis, caused by the Epstein-Barr virus, is a common cause of a neck mass in adolescents. Usually the lymphadenopathy is accompanied by an exudative pharyngitis, splenomegaly, and systemic symptoms such as malaise and fever. Diagnosis is by examination of the peripheral blood smear, with findings of increased numbers of mononucleocytes (10–20% of the white blood cells) and atypical mononucleocytes. The Monospot test, a serologic test, confirms the diagnosis. Treatment is supportive with rest and hydration.

Actinomycosis

Actinomycosis is caused by *Actinomyces israelii*, a fastidious gram-positive anaerobe that forms part of the normal oral flora. Most common in young healthy adults, this disease is usually preceded by trauma to the oral cavity, often dental manipulation. The infection coalesces into suppurative lumps that can form sinuses that drain the characteristic "sulfur granules," which are composed of bacterial colonies. The diagnosis can be suspected by a history of preceding trauma and confirmed with anaerobic culture of FNA material. Because these organisms are easily killed by aerobic conditions, culturing the offending organism can be difficult. Histopathology, with a finding of sulfur granules, can also confirm the diagnosis. Treatment is with intravenous penicillin until the lesions subside, then a long course of oral penicillin.[15]

Cat Scratch Disease

Cat scratch disease is a zoonotic infection with an incidence of 24,000 cases per year in the United States. It is caused by *Bartonella henselae*, a gram-negative coccobacillus isolated within the last 10 years. The victim usually has a history of being bitten or scratched by a kitten about 2 weeks before the onset of cervical lymphadenopathy. Eighty percent of victims are children, and this disease has a seasonal pattern, peaking in late fall and winter. The diagnosis is established by the presence of three of the following: a typical history, onset of lymphadenopathy about 2 weeks after the exposure, a positive cat scratch disease skin test, or a positive culture for *Bartonella* from FNA material from the lymph node. Treatment is expectant, as this disease is self-limited and the lymphadenopathy resolves within 2–6 months.[16]

Toxoplasmosis

Toxoplasmosis is a zoonotic infection caused by exposure to cat feces or ingestion of uncooked meat. The causative organism is *Toxoplasma gondii*, a complex parasite. This infection can be devastating in immunocompromised patients and infants, involving the central nervous system. The disease usually mimics mononucleosis, with systemic manifestations of malaise and fever. Diagnosis by serologic testing for immunopobulin M antibodies to the parasite. Treatment is supportive for isolated lymphadenopathy in immunocompetent patients, and with pyrimethamine, sulfadiazine, and leucovorin in immunosuppressed patients or those with central nervous system involvement.[16]

Scrofula

A granulomatous infection, scrofula is usually caused by atypical mycobacterial infection (*Mycobacterium avium intracellulare*, *Mycobacterium kansasii*). It primarily affects children, usually with the development of high cervical lymphadenopathy (levels I and II). Diagnosis is by FNA, demonstrating the acid-fast bacilli or yielding positive mycobacterial cultures, positive skin testing, or caseating granulomas on open biopsy.[17]

References

1. Gray SW, Skandalakis JE, Androulakis JA. Non-thryoid tumors of the neck. Contemp Surg 1985;26:13–24.
2. Pangalis GA, Vassilakopoulos TP, Boussiotis VA, et al. Clinical approach to lymphadenopathy. Semin Oncol 1993;20:570–582.
3. Kubota TT. The evaluation of peripheral lymphadenopathy. Prim Care 1980;7:461–471.
4. Beenken SW, Maddox WA, Lerist MM. Workup of a patient with a mass in the neck. Adv Surg 1995;28:371–383.
5. Lefebvre JL, Coche-Dequeant B, Van JT, et al. Cervical lymph nodes from an unknown primary tumor. Am J Surg 1990;160:443–446.
6. Zakowski MF. Fine-needle aspiration cytology of tumors: diagnostic accuracy and potential pitfalls. Cancer Invest 1994;12:505–516.
7. Gooder P, Palmer M, Cervical lymph node biopsy: a study of its morbidity. Laryngol Otol 1984;98:1031–1040.
8. McGuirt WF, McCabe BF. Significance of node biopsy before definitive treatment of cervical metastatic carcinoma. Laryngoscope 1978;88: 594–597.
9. Jakobsen J, Aschenfeldt P, Johansen J, et al. Lymph node metastases in the neck from unknown primary tumour. Acta Oncol 1992;31:653–655.
10. Weaver A, Fleming SM, Knechtges TC, et al. Triple endoscopy: a neglected essential in head and neck cancer. Surgery 1979;86:493–496.
11. Cahan WG, Castro EB, Rosen PP, et al. Separate primary carcinomas of the esophagus and head and neck region in the same patient. Cancer 1976;37:85–89.
12. Shapshay SM, Hong WK, Fired MP, et al. Simultaneous carcinomas of the esophagus and upper aerodigestive tract. Otolaryngol Head Neck Surg 1980;88:373–377.
13. Benninger MS, Enruque RR, Nichols RD, et al. Symptom-directed selective endoscopy and cost containment for evaluation of head and neck cancer. Head Neck 1993;15:532–536.
14. Reibel JF. The patient with a neck mass. Comp Ther 1997;23:737–741.
15. Miller M, Haddad AJ. Cervicofacial actinomycosis. Oral Surg Oral Med Oral Pathol Oral Radiol Endosc 1998;85:496–508.
16. Midani S, Ayoub EM, Anderson B. Cat-scratch disease. Adv Pediatr 1996;43:397–418.
17. Davenport M. Lumps and swellings of the head and neck. BMJ 1996; 312:368–371.

CHAPTER 71

Mediastinal Masses

DAVID ESPOSITO
KEITH W. MILLIKAN

A. Anatomy

The boundaries of the mediastinum are the thoracic inlet superiorly, the diaphragm inferiorly, the sternum anteriorly, the vertebral column posteriorly, and the right and left parietal pleura laterally. The mediastinum is artificially divided into three regions for convenience in localizing lesions: the anterosuperior, middle, and posterior compartments (Fig. 71–1).

The *anterosuperior* mediastinum, also referred to as simply the anterior mediastinum, is that portion anterior to the pericardium and pericardial reflection. The *middle mediastinum* is bordered anteriorly by the anterior pericardial reflection and posteriorly by the posterior pericardial reflection. The *posterior mediastinum* extends from the posterior pericardial reflection to the vertebral column. The anterosuperior mediastinum contains the thymus, aortic arch and its branches, great veins, lymphatics, and fatty areolar tissue. The middle mediastinum contains the heart, pericardium, phrenic nerves, tracheal bifurcation and main bronchi, hila of the lungs, and their lymph nodes. In the posterior mediastinum lies the esophagus, vagus nerves, sympathetic nervous chain, thoracic duct, descending aorta, azygos system, paravertebral lymph nodes, and fatty areolar tissue. Based on the contents of each mediastinal division, the physician can tailor his or her workup of a lesion based on its location.[1]

Of mediastinal masses, 54% are located in the anterosuperior compartment, 26% in the middle compartment, and 20% in the posterior compartment. The most common anterior mediastinal masses are thymoma (31%), lymphoma (23%), and germ cell tumors (17%). Other masses include thyroid tissue, cysts, and carcinoma. Middle mediastinal masses are likely cysts (61%) or lymphoma (21%). Posterior masses represent neurogenic tumors (52%) or cysts (32%) (Table 71–1). Approximately 25–42% of mediastinal masses are malignant. The rate of malignancy is influenced by the location of the tumor and the age of the patient. For instance, 59% of anterior, 29% of middle, and 16% of posterior masses are malignant. Patients in their second to fourth decade of life have the highest likelihood of harboring a malignancy, as this age group corresponds to the peak incidence of lymphoma and germ cell tumors, two common mediastinal tumors. Most (73%) of the masses in children are benign.[2]

Mediastinal Masses

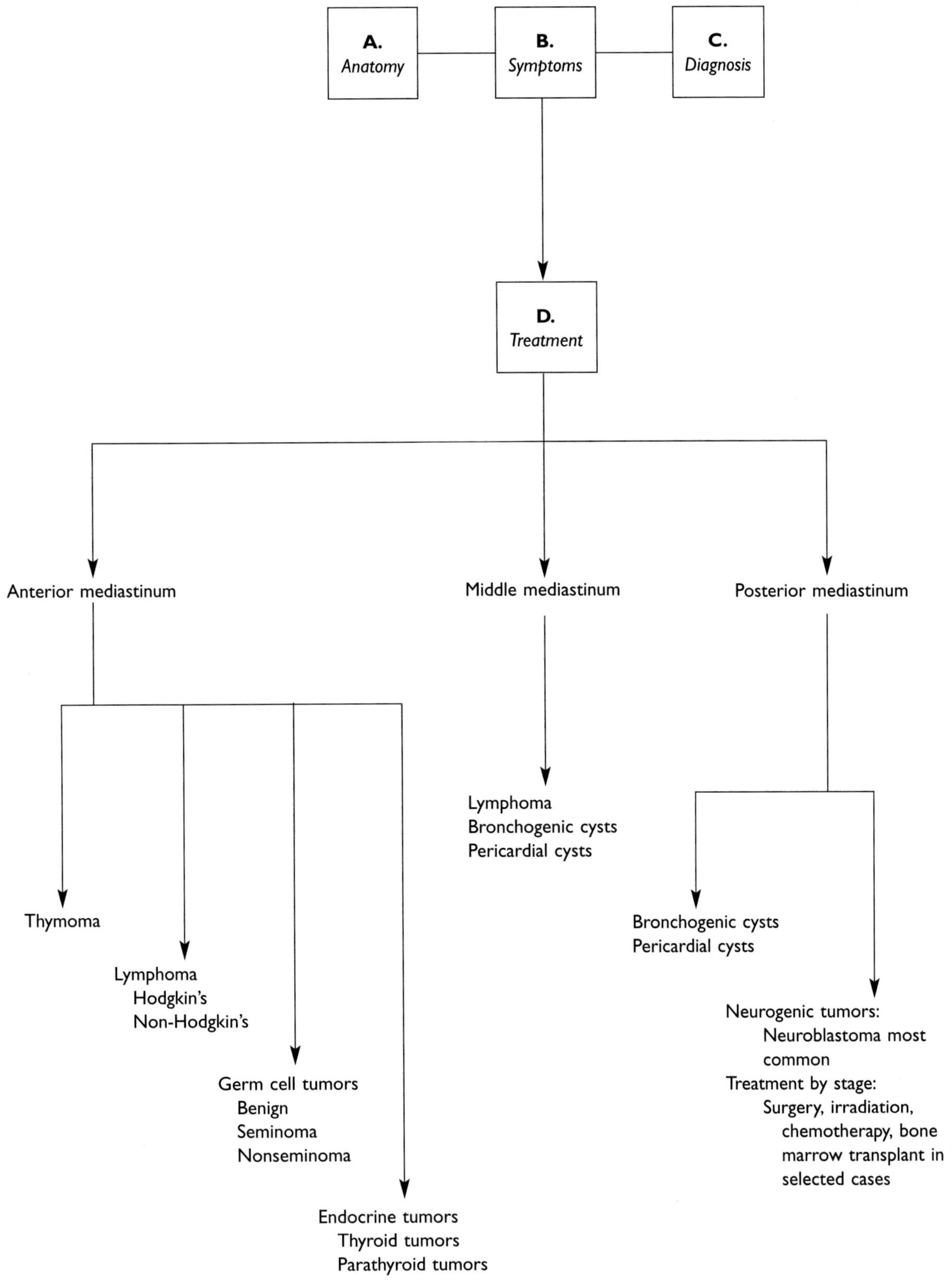

A. *Anatomy* — **B.** *Symptoms* — **C.** *Diagnosis*

↓

D. *Treatment*

↓

Anterior mediastinum

- Thymoma
- Lymphoma
  - Hodgkin's
  - Non-Hodgkin's
- Germ cell tumors
  - Benign
  - Seminoma
  - Nonseminoma
- Endocrine tumors
  - Thyroid tumors
  - Parathyroid tumors

Middle mediastinum

- Lymphoma
- Bronchogenic cysts
- Pericardial cysts

Posterior mediastinum

- Bronchogenic cysts
- Pericardial cysts
- Neurogenic tumors:
  - Neuroblastoma most common
- Treatment by stage:
  - Surgery, irradiation, chemotherapy, bone marrow transplant in selected cases

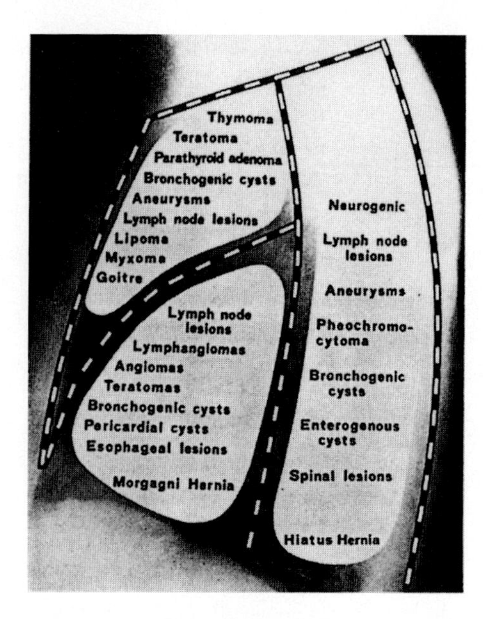

FIGURE 71–1
Three mediastinal compartments (anterior, middle, posterior) and the masses commonly found in each compartment. (Reproduced with permission from Burkell CC, Cross JM. Mass lesions of the mediastinum. In: MM Ravitch (ed.) Current Problems in Surgery, Chicago: Year Book Medical Publishers, 1969)

B. Symptoms

Most patients (56–65%) are asymptomatic and present with an incidental chest radiographic finding. Symptomatic patients experience local effects due to invasion or to compression or systemic effects from tumor products. Benign tumors are more often asymptomatic than malignant ones (54% vs. 15%). Likewise, in a 20-year review of 441 patients at Duke University, 76% of asymptomatic patients had benign tumors, and 62% of symptomatic patients had malignant tumors.[1] Children are more likely (78%) to have symptoms due to the limited space in their mediastinum. Anterior, middle, and posterior masses have a 75%, 45%, and 50% incidence of symptoms, respectively. Symptoms include chest pain, dyspnea, cough, fever, weight loss, and superior vena cava syndrome. Some mediastinal tumors produce hormones or antibodies that may produce a systemic syndrome. Examples include thyroid goiter (thyrotoxicosis), pheochromocytoma (hypertension), germ cell tumors (hypoglycemia due to secretion of an insulin-like substance), and thymoma (myasthenia gravis). Each specific tumor has its own set of associated symptoms, discussed later in the chapter.

C. Diagnosis

The goals of the workup of a mediastinal mass are to: (1) differentiate a primary mediastinal mass from other types of lesion; (2) recognize associated systemic manifestations that may affect perioperative care; (3) evaluate for compressive symptoms; (4) assess resectability; and (5) identify co-morbidities to optimize the patient's overall medical condition. This is done differently depending on the location of the tumor and the differential diagnosis.

All patients should undergo a careful history and physical examination to detect conditions that can help make the diagnosis and decrease the risk of perioperative complications. Posteroanterior and lateral chest radiographs show the location and size of the tumor, the displacement of adjacent structures, the density (cystic versus solid), and the calcifications.[3]

Computed tomography (CT) or magnetic resonance (MRI) should be employed next, as it offers more accurate anatomic detail of the lesion and its relation to the surrounding structures. CT may help differentiate tumors from vascular or other abnormalities that may present as a mediastinal lesion and may also be diagnostic for some lesions (i.e., cysts) based on a characteristic appearance, location, or density. Overall, however, the CT scan accurately diagnoses only 68% of mediastinal lesions. Once the chest radiograph and CT scan have been done, there are still many patients for whom the diagnosis is uncertain.[3]

Other techniques can be used based on the clinician's index of suspicion. Echocardiography can be useful for middle medi-

TABLE 71–1.
Anatomic location of primary tumors and cysts of the mediastinum

Tumor or cyst	%
Anterosuperior mediastinum (n = 245)	
Thymic neoplasms	31
Lymphomas	23
Germ cell tumors	17
Benign	9
Malignant	8
Carcinoma	13
Cysts	6
Mesenchymal tumors	4
Endocrine tumors	5
Other	1
Middle mediastinum (n = 83)	
Cysts	61
Lymphomas	20
Mesenchymal tumors	8
Carcinoma	6
Other	5
Posterior mediastinum (n = 113)	
Neurogenic tumors	52
Benign	40
Malignant	12
Cysts	32
Mesenchymal tumors	10
Endocrine tumors	2
Other	4

SOURCE: Davis and Sabiston.[2]

astinal masses. Serologic tests may be useful in some patients, such as young males in whom serum β-human chorionic gonadotropin (β-hCG) or α-fetoprotein (AFP) may diagnose nonseminomas. Fine-needle aspiration (FNA) should be considered for any patient whose diagnosis is uncertain. It can be done safely in any mediastinal region guided by CT, ultrasonography, fluoroscopy, or endoscopic ultrasonography; and it is accurate in 80–90% of cases. The most errors in diagnosis are encountered with lymphoma. FNA is not required for all anterior masses. Cutting needle techniques have increased the sensitivity of needle biopsy. Complications occur with 20–25% of FNAs and include pneumothorax and hemoptysis. Because the optimal treatment of some tumors (i.e., lymphomas) requires precise histologic subclassification, surgeons are often asked to provide tissue specimens for this purpose. The anterior mediastinum is best approached via a limited upper median sternotomy, the middle mediastinum via mediastinoscopy, and the posterior mediastinum via a limited posterior thoracotomy.[1]

D. Treatment

Treatment of specific lesions is discussed in detail later in the chapter, but for patients undergoing surgical resection there are a few caveats to remember. Anterior masses are best approached through a median sternotomy or anterolateral thoracotomy, whereas middle and posterior lesions are best approached via a posterolateral thoracotomy. Thoracoscopy is useful for the diagnosis and treatment of mediastinal masses and is safe, especially for lesions in the middle and posterior mediastinum. Benign lesions can be removed thorascopically, but this approach is considered inadequate for removing malignant lesions. Most patients undergo surgical excision successfully, although some have severe cardiopulmonary complications during general anesthesia.

Anterosuperior Masses (Anterior Mediastinum)

Once an anterior mass is diagnosed by chest radiography and defined by CT scan, the workup proceeds based on the entity that seems to be the most likely diagnosis. Thymoma, lymphoma, germ cell tumors, and endocrine tumors are the most common causes of masses in this location.

THYMOMA Thymoma is the most common anterior mediastinal mass, usually presenting during the third to fifth decade of life. It occurs with equal frequency in men and women but is extremely rare in children.[3] Patients with thymomas usually present with symptoms, either from a local mass effect or systemic syndromes associated with the immunologic function of the gland (myasthenia gravis, red blood cell aplasia, hypogammaglobulinemia).

Myasthenia gravis (MG) is seen in 10–50% of patients with thymoma; conversely 8–40% of patients with MG have a thymoma.[1] MG is an acquired autoimmune disorder characterized by circulating antibodies to the acetylcholine receptor, leading to a deficiency of acetylcholine receptors at the motor end-plate. Symptoms of MG are due to weakness and fatigue of skeletal muscles (most commonly muscles innervated by the cranial nerves). Patients experience diplopia, ptosis, difficulty swallowing, slurred speech, loss of facial expression, and easy fatigability of the limbs (proximal muscles more so than distal muscles). As the disease progresses, universal muscle weakness is encountered, leading to dyspnea and respiratory failure. Rapid progression usually occurs during the first year after diagnosis, and most deaths occur within the first 3 years. MG is diagnosed using the anticholinesterase test, in which edrophonium administration results in rapid yet transient alleviation of symptoms. Electromyography studies show progressive decreases in the amplitude of the muscle response from the first to the fifth stimulus. Serologic tests for the acetylcholine receptor antibody can also be diagnostic. Because of the high incidence of thymoma in MG patients, all those diagnosed with MG should undergo CT scans or MRI.[1]

Red blood cell aplasia is seen in 5–10% of patients with thymoma and is characterized by the absence of red blood cell precursors. The etiology of this syndrome is unknown, but an autoimmune cause is suspected.

Hypogammaglobulinemia is seen with about 5% of thymomas. Patients exhibit a decrease in both cellular and humoral immunity.[3]

Surgical Treatment The primary treatment for patients with thymoma is surgical resection whenever possible. An extended thymectomy, with removal of the entire thymus and the surrounding fatty-areolar tissue, is recommended to ensure excision of all glandular tissue.[4] The best exposure is obtained via a median sternotomy, and the surgeon should remember to outline the extent of disease with surgical clips to plan postoperative radiation portals should they become necessary. In patients with MG, perioperative management is vital for preventing complications. Anticholinesterase inhibitors should be discontinued, as it can help decrease the amount of pulmonary secretions and avoid inadvertent cholinergic weakness. Plasmapheresis should be undertaken within 72 hours of the operation to improve the patient's muscle strength.[1] Postoperatively, aggressive pulmonary toilet is of the utmost importance.

Prognosis depends on the stage of the tumor. Stage I is a well encapsulated thymoma without invasion and is associated with 85–100% 5-year survival. Stage II exhibits pericapsular growth into the adjacent fat, pleura, or mediastinum and is associated with 60–80% 5-year survival. Stage III disease has invasion of the adjacent organs or intrathoracic metastases, with a 5-year survival of 40–70%. Stage IV tumors are those with extrathoracic metastases, and the 5-year survival approaches 50%.[1] Patients with MG who undergo extended thymectomy can expect alleviation of their symptoms in 85–96% of cases and drug-free remission 46–63% of the time. About 30% of patients with red blood cell aplasia improve after thymectomy, but the hypogammaglobulinemia remits only occasionally.[2]

Radiation Therapy Radiation therapy is indicated after thymectomy in patients with stage II and III disease. Studies have shown surgery and irradiation to be far superior to surgery alone in these patients.[1] In fact, patients with stage III disease can expect close to 100% survival at 5 years and 95% survival 10–15 years after surgery and radiation therapy. A dose of 3500–5000 cGy should be used in these circumstances. Preoperative radiation therapy can be useful in patients with superior vena caval obstruction or extensive disease. Unresectable or incompletely resected disease should be treated with 40–50 Gy postoperatively.[3]

Chemotherapy Chemotherapy is only moderately active against thymic tumors and therefore should be reserved for recurrent or widely metastatic disease. Cisplatin-based regimens have provided response rates up to 75% and 3-year survival rates in the range of 30%.[1]

LYMPHOMA Although the mediastinum is frequently involved in patients with systemic lymphoma (40–70%), it is the sole site of disease in only 5–10% of cases. CT and MRI are useful for delineating the extent of the disease to differentiate it from cardiovascular structures, selecting radiation portals, following the response, and diagnosing relapse.[1] Lymphomas are diagnosed by biopsy; and because treatment is vastly different depending on the histologic subclassification, a large quantity of tissue is needed. Mediastinoscopy or thoracotomy is often necessary to obtain this tissue for diagnosis, as needle biopsy is usually inadequate. Complete staging must be done in all patients, which includes a detailed physical examination and history looking for constitutional ("B") symptoms (right sweats and weight loss), complete laboratory tests, chest radiography, CT scan of the chest and abdomen, and bone marrow biopsy in all patients. Liver biopsy, staging laparotomy, gallium scan, bone scan, and lymphangiography are reserved for specific indications.[5] The Ann Arbor staging system is used for both Hodgkin's and non-Hodgkin's lymphomas, although its usefulness for non-Hodgkin's lymphoma is limited. Stage I has involvement of a single lymph node basin or a single extralymphatic site. Stage II has involvement of two or more lymph node regions on the same side of the diaphragm. Stage III has involvement on both sides of the diaphragm. Stage IV indicates disseminated disease. The suffix B indicates the presence of "B" symptoms.[5]

Hodgkin's Lymphoma Hodgkin's lymphoma is most commonly seen in the anterior mediastinum, and 50% of all patients with the disease have mediastinal involvement. There are four types of Hodgkin's disease based on the predominant cell type: nodular sclerosing, lymphocyte-predominant, mixed cellularity, and lymphocyte-depleted. The nodular sclerosing (55–75%) and lymphocyte-predominant (40%) cell types are the most common ones to occur in the mediastinum. Symptoms include chest pain, dyspnea, hoarseness, and constitutional symptoms (e.g., fever, weight loss, sweats). The CT scan is used to gauge the extent of the tumor and lung involvement and to plan radiation portals. The diagnosis can be made by sampling involving cervical lymph nodes or, in the absence of this involvement, the mediastinal tumor itself. Treatment depends on the stage and volume of disease and focuses on irradiation and chemotherapy. The role of surgery is only to obtain tissue for diagnosis and to assist in pathologic staging of the disease (i.e., staging laparotomy for patients with clinical stage I or IIA disease).[3]

Radiation Therapy Radiation therapy is the mainstay of treatment for Hodgkin's lymphoma. In patients with stage I and IIA nonbulky disease, radiation therapy is the sole treatment. Patients with bulky disease or an advanced stage require chemotherapy in addition. Because Hodgkin's disease spreads via lymphatic contiguity, three radiation fields were designed to cover likely sites of disease. The mantle field covers the submandibular, cervical, supraclavicular, infraclavicular, axillary, mediastinal, and hilar nodes. The paraaortic field covers the transverse processes of the abdominal vertebral bodies and the spleen. The pelvic field includes the common iliac, hypogastric, external iliac, and inguinal nodes. Most patients receive mantle and paraaortic irradiation but rarely pelvic irradiation. A total dose of 4000 cGy is given. Patients with stage I and IIA have a higher than 80% long-term disease-free survival beyond 10 years, with less than 10% mortality from the Hodgkin's disease. Relapses can usually be successfully treated with combination chemotherapy.[5]

Chemotherapy Patients with stage IIB, III, and IV disease should receive combination chemotherapy in addition to radiation. The regimen of mechlorethamine/vincristine (Oncovin)/procarbazine/prednisone (MOPP) has a complete response rate of 80–90%. CHOP (cyclophosphamide/doxorubicin/vincristine [Oncovin]/prednisone) and ABVD (doxorubicin/bleomycin/vinblastine/dacarbazine) have also been used, especially for MOPP-resistant tumors. Long-term survival depends on a variety of prognostic indicators, but even the group with the worst prognosis has 5-year survival rates higher than 50%. Relapse can be treated with irradiation, chemotherapy, bone marrow transplant, or a combination of modalities.[5]

Non-Hodgkin's Lymphoma Non-Hodgkin's mediastinal lymphoma is either a manifestation of generalized disease or an isolated large, bulky anterior mass. Constitutional symptoms are present in 50% of patients and signal a poorer prognosis. Complete staging, as in Hodgkin's disease, is essential, as other organs are frequently involved. The two most common subtypes are lymphoblastic (60%) and diffuse large cell lymphomas (40%).[3]

Lymphoblastic Lymphoma The lymphoblastic lymphoma is a distinct entity that presents as a mediastinal mass in older children and young adults, males more commonly than females. The tumor cells express T cell antigens, and the disease is usually at an advanced stage at diagnosis (91% stage III or IV). There is early bone marrow involvement, early central nervous system (CNS) metastases, and frequently associated leukemia. Radiation therapy produces an initial response, but there is uniform recurrence; therefore chemotherapy is the treatment of choice.

Diffuse Large Cell Lymphoma The diffuse large cell lymphoma is a predominantly B cell tumor, most commonly seen in young females. Treatment consists of chemotherapy, with irradiation reserved for relapses.

Chemotherapy Lymphoblastic lymphoma is treated similarly to lymphoid leukemia, with either C-MOPP (cyclophosphamide-MOPP) or CHOP. Early intrathecal prophylaxis is recommended because of the propensity for CNS involvement. Complete response rates approach 100% with minimal relapses.

Large cell lymphoma is treated with CHOP, C-MOPP, M-BACOD (methotrexate/bleomycin/doxorubicin [Adriamycin]/cyclophosphamide/vincristine [Oncovin]/dexamethasone) or MACOP-B (methotrexate/doxorubicin (Adriamycin)/ cyclophosphamide/vincristine [Oncovin]/prednisone/bleomycin). The 5-year survival is 50%.[1]

GERM CELL TUMORS Germ cell tumors are benign or malignant tumors that originate from primordial germ cells that fail to complete their migration from the urogenital ridge and thus come to rest in the mediastinum. They have no relation to gonadal tumors, and no workup of the testes is warranted other than a careful physical examination. Malignant tumors are seen predominantly in men, but benign tumors are seen equally in men and women. They are diagnosed with chest radiography followed by CT scans of the chest and abdomen to assess the extent of disease and to check for metastases to the liver and retroperitoneum. Serum β-human chorionic gonadotropin (β-hCG) and α-fetoprotein (AFP) are useful for differentiating seminomas from nonseminomas.[6]

Benign Tumors Teratoma, the most common mediastinal germ cell tumor, consists of tissue elements from all three primitive embryologic layers. It is usually asymptomatic until it grows large enough to cause compressive symptoms. CT scans show a predominantly fatty mass with a cystic component, often containing calcifications, teeth, or bone. Treatment is exclusively with surgical excision. No additional therapy is needed.

Seminoma Seminomas represent 50% of all malignant germ cell neoplasms; and unlike most germ cell tumors, they usually remain intrathoracic with only local extension. When metastases do occur, they spread first via the lymphatics, then the blood. Bone and lungs are the most common sites of metastatic disease. Seminomas rarely produce β-hCG ($<7\%$) and never produce AFP. Complete excision is the treatment of choice; if excision is not possible, the treatment is controversial. Radiation therapy to the mediastinum and adjacent lymph node basins with a dose of 4500–5000 rad over 6 weeks, with salvage chemotherapy for residual disease, is advocated by some. Both of these techniques offer excellent long-term survival. It is agreed that for bulky or extramediastinal disease chemotherapy is superior to irradiation.[2] Others support initial cisplatin-based chemotherapy (VBP); [vincristine/bleomycin/prednisione vincristine/Adriamycin/bteomycin (VAB)]; and salvage surgery for residual disease.

Nonseminoma Malignant nonseminomatous tumors include choriocarcinoma, embryonal cell carcinoma, malignant teratoma, and yolk sac tumors. These tumors differ from seminomatous tumors in that they are much more aggressive, frequently present with disseminated disease, are rarely radiosensitive, and produce either β-hCG or AFP in more than 90% of cases. The local invasiveness and frequent metastases usually preclude the use of surgery to resect the disease. Surgery is used only to obtain tissue for diagnosis in patients whose tumors do not produce AFP or β-hCG. Treatment is with multiagent cisplatin-based chemotherapy. The serum AFP and β-hCG levels are monitored for response. When these levels normalize, surgical exploration and removal of residual disease are undertaken. If the serum markers fail to normalize, a second dose of different chemotherapeutic agents is needed. Patients who have a complete response to chemotherapy without residual disease in the surgical specimen can expect 35–40% long-term survival. The presence of residual disease or of relapse signals an extremely poor prognosis, with a mean survival of about 6 months.[2]

ENDOCRINE TUMORS

Thyroid Tumors Thyroid tissue is sometimes found in the chest and therefore may present as a mediastinal mass. Although thyroid extension into the substernal region is common, totally intrathoracic thyroid tumors are rare, representing only 1% of all mediastinal masses. These tumors arise from heterotopic thyroid tissue, most commonly in the anterior mediastinum, but they can also arise in the middle and posterior compartments. Chest radiography shows a sharply circumscribed dense mass, and the CT scan shows a contrast-enhancing lesion. The ^{131}I scan "lights up" functioning thyroid tissue; but because most thyroid malignancies are nonfunctioning they are not seen. Once a thyroid tumor is suspected, the ^{131}I scan should be done to document the presence of thyroid tissue outside the thorax. Fine-needle aspiration (FNA) can be done to document malignancy. All symptomatic and malignant tumors should be excised. Patients without symptoms but with normal functioning thyroid tissue in the neck should also undergo excision, as these tumors (adenomas) tend to enlarge and eventually become symptomatic. Asymptomatic patients whose sole thyroid tissue rests in the thorax should be observed and followed with serial CT scans. If the tumor enlarge, they are excised. The tumors should be approached via median sternotomy or anterolateral thoracotomy because the blood supply is from thoracic vessels.[1]

Parathyroid Tumors Parathyroid adenomas are found in the mediastinum in 10% of hyperparathyroid patients, but most are accessible via the traditional cervical incision. Sternotomy is needed in only 2.5% of cases. The inferior gland is most commonly located in the anterior mediastinum near the thymus, as they both arise from the third branchial cleft. The superior glands arise from the fourth branchial cleft and therefore are most commonly found in the posterior mediastinum. Symptoms are those of hyperparathyroidism, as the small size of these tumors precludes local mass effects. Diagnosis is by CT scan, MRI, ultrasonography, thallium scan, or venous sampling. They are too small to be seen on chest radiography. If no glands are found during neck exploration, sternotomy should be performed.[1]

Middle Mediastinal Masses

Middle mediastinal masses are most commonly cysts, although lymphoma and other tumors are occasionally present in this area as well. More than 75% of these cysts are asymptomatic, and they rarely cause any morbidity. As they increase in size, however, they may cause compressive-type symptoms and should be differentiated from malignancies.

Bronchogenic Cysts Bronchogenic cysts represent 6% of all primary mediastinal masses and 34% of all cysts. They originate as a sequestration of the ventral foregut, and the wall consists of cartilage, mucous glands, smooth muscle, and fibrous tissue with an inner layer of ciliated respiratory epithelium. They are found proximal to the trachea and posterior to the carina. Two-thirds are asymptomatic, but children often exhibit compressive symptoms. Surgical excision is recommended to obtain a definitive histologic diagnosis, alleviate symptoms, and prevent complications and because malignant degeneration has been described.[1]

Pericardial Cysts Pericardial cysts represent 6% of all primary mediastinal masses and 33% of all cysts. They classically occur at the right (70%) or left (22%) pericardiophrenic angle; 8% occur at other sites on the pericardium. They may or may not have communication with the pericardial sac. They are seen on chest radiography, and the CT scan classically reveals a pericardiophrenic location, near-water attenuation, and smooth borders. When this classic appearance is encountered, simple needle aspiration can be done and the patient followed with serial CT scans. Surgical excision is reserved for patients in whom the diagnosis is in doubt or in whom a malignancy is suspected.[1]

Posterior Mediastinal Masses

Posterior masses are most commonly neurogenic tumors or cysts. Occasionally lymphomas or other tumors are seen in this region as well. Neuroblastoma is the most common neurogenic tumor, although ganglioneuroblastoma, ganglioneuroma, neurilemoma, neurofibroma, and paraganglioma are seen as well.

Neurogenic Tumors Neurogenic tumors may arise from the sympathetic ganglia, intercostal nerves, or paraganglia cells. They are seen in a greater proportion in children, although their peak incidence is during adulthood. Tumors in children are more likely to be malignant. They may present as an asymptomatic posterior mediastinal mass on chest radiography or with symptoms due to mechanical factors. Chest and back pain arise when compression or invasion occurs into the bone, chest wall, or associated nerves. Compression of the tracheobronchial tree leads to cough or dyspnea. Pancoast syndrome and Horner syndrome can occur with invasion of the brachial or cervical sympathetic chains, respectively. About 10% of tumors extend into the spinal column and are called "dumbbell tumors" because of their shape, exhibiting large paraspinal and intraspinal portions connected by an isthmus of tissue traversing the intervertebral foramen. Sixty percent of dumbbell tumors produce symptoms of spinal cord compression. CT scans, MRI, or CT myelograms should be done to evaluate the presence of an intraspinal component. There may also be systemic symptoms due to production of neurohormonal elements (i.e., catecholamines, vasoactive intestinal peptide).

Neuroblastoma, the most common neurogenic tumor, arises from cells of the sympathetic nervous system. It is most commonly seen in the retroperitoneum, but 10–20% are primarily located in the mediastinum. Neuroblastomas are highly invasive, with most having already metastasized to the liver, lungs, bone, brain, or lymph nodes at the time of diagnosis. They are usually symptomatic, with cough, dyspnea, or back and chest pain. Spinal cord compression and paraplegia occur in 33% of children with this disease. Neuroblastomas have a unique immunobiology in that spontaneous regression and mutation is well documented, and T cells are capable of suppressing tumor growth.[1]

Treatment of neuroblastoma depends on the stage of the disease. Stage I represents a well circumscribed, noninvasive tumor. Stage II has local invasiveness without crossing the midline. Stage III has tumor crossing the midline, and stage IV indicates metastatic disease.

The treatment for stage I disease is surgical excision alone. Stage II disease is treated with surgical excision and adjuvant radiation therapy. Stages III and IV are treated using a multimodality approach that consists of an initial debulking surgical excision followed by irradiation and multiagent chemotherapy; finally, a second-look operation is undertaken to assess for and resect residual disease. Chemotherapeutic agents in use against neuroblastoma are cisplatin, doxorubicin, cyclophosphamide, and etoposide. Some success with relapses or refractory disease has been seen with ablative chemotherapy followed by an autologous bone marrow transplant.

Patients less than 1 year of age have an excellent prognosis, even if widespread disease is present. As age and extent of involvement increase, the prognosis worsens. Expression of the N-*myc* gene and particularly of the N-myc protein are associated with an unfavorable prognosis.[1]

References

1. Davis RD, Oldham HN, Sabiston DC. The mediastinum. In: Sabiston DC, Spencer FC (eds) Surgery of the Chest, 6th ed. Philadelphia: Saunders, 1995;576–611.
2. Davis RD, Sabiston DC. The mediastinum. In: Sabiston DC (ed) Textbook of Surgery: The Biological Basis of Modern Surgical Practice, 15th ed. Philadelphia: Saunders, 1997;1906–1932.
3. Aisnev J, Antman KH, Belanic P. Pleura and Mediastinan. In: Abeloff MD et al. (eds) Clinical Oncology. New York: Churchill Livingstone, 1995; 1166–1180.
4. Bulkley GB, Bass KN, Stephenson GR, et al. Extended cervicomediastinal thymectomy in the integrated management of myasthenia gravis. Ann Surg 1997;226:324–335.
5. Freedman AS, Nadler LM. Malignancies of lymphoid cells. In: Harrison's Principles of Internal Medicine, 14th ed. New York: McGraw-Hill, 1998;695–711.

Suggested Reading

Blossom GB, Steiger Z, Stephenson LW. Neoplasms of the mediastinum. In: Cancer: Principles and Practice of Oncology, 5th ed. Philadelphia: Lippincott-Raven, 1997;951–969.

Fraser RS, Pare JAP, Fraser RG, Pare PD. Disease of the mediastinum. In: Synopsis of Diseases of the Chest, 2nd ed. Philadelphia: Saunders, 1994;905–939.

Martini N, McCormack PM, Rusch VW, Bains MS, Burt ME. Tumors of the mediastinum. In: Moossa AR, Schimpff SC, Robson MC. et al. (eds) Comprehensive Textbook of Oncology, 2nd ed. Baltimore: Williams & Wilkins, 1990;711–731.

Chapter 72

Liver Masses

ISAAC SAMUEL
GREGORY S. FOSTER
KEITH W. MILLIKAN

Liver mass lesions (Table 72–1) may or may not cause symptoms. *Asymptomatic masses* are usually discovered incidentally during clinical examination or following imaging studies performed to evaluate other conditions. *Symptomatic masses* may present with pain, fever, jaundice, or weight loss; occasionally, they present as an abdominal emergency due to hemorrhage or rupture. Approximately 50% of patients with hepatocellular adenomas present with abdominal pain. Larger masses may be associated with jaundice when they cause mechanical obstruction of the biliary tract. Right upper quadrant pain, fever, and weight loss may be associated with infectious or neoplastic processes.

A history of alcoholic cirrhosis, chronic hepatitis, or other forms of cirrhosis increases the risk for hepatocellular carcinoma. A history of estrogen or androgen use is associated with hepatocellular adenoma. Neoplasms of the liver may also be caused by exposure to chemical carcinogens such as thorium dioxide (Thorotrast), aflatoxin, vinyl chloride, and arsenic. Patients infected with the human immunodeficiency virus (HIV) are at increased risk for developing primary hepatic lymphoma or liver abscesses.

Laboratory abnormalities of liver function are inconsistently seen and may even be normal in the presence of liver masses. For patients with abnormal liver function tests, serologic studies for hepatitis should be obtained. The tumor markers α-fetoprotein and carcinoembryonic antigen are useful in the diagnosis and postoperative follow-up of hepatocellular carcinoma, cholangiocarcinoma, and metastatic colon carcinoma.

Imaging studies are utilized not only to detect hepatic masses but also to determine their number, size, and location; assess vascular invasion; and detect the presence of extrahepatic disease. The results of imaging studies are used to determine and plan tumor resection. Multiple imaging modalities, including ultrasonography, computed tomography (CT), CT angiography, magnetic resonance imaging (MRI), magnetic resonance angiography (MRA), conventional angiography, CT-enhanced arteriography, CT-enhanced portography, radionuclide scans, and intraoperative ultrasonography (IOUS) are currently available to the clinician. These imaging techniques are often complementary, rather than competitive, when evaluating the diverse pathologic features of liver masses. The choice of imaging modalities used

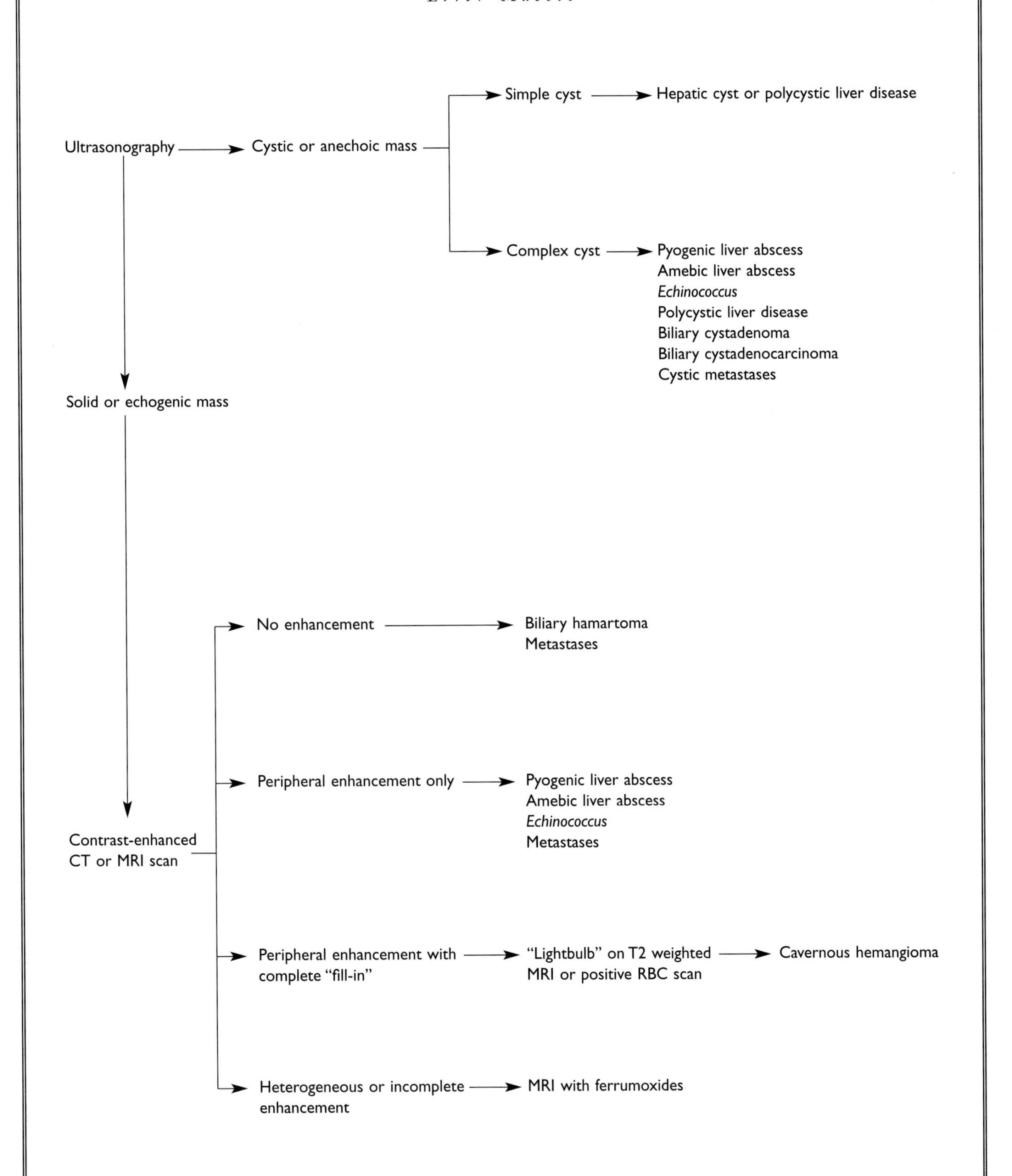

(continued on next page)

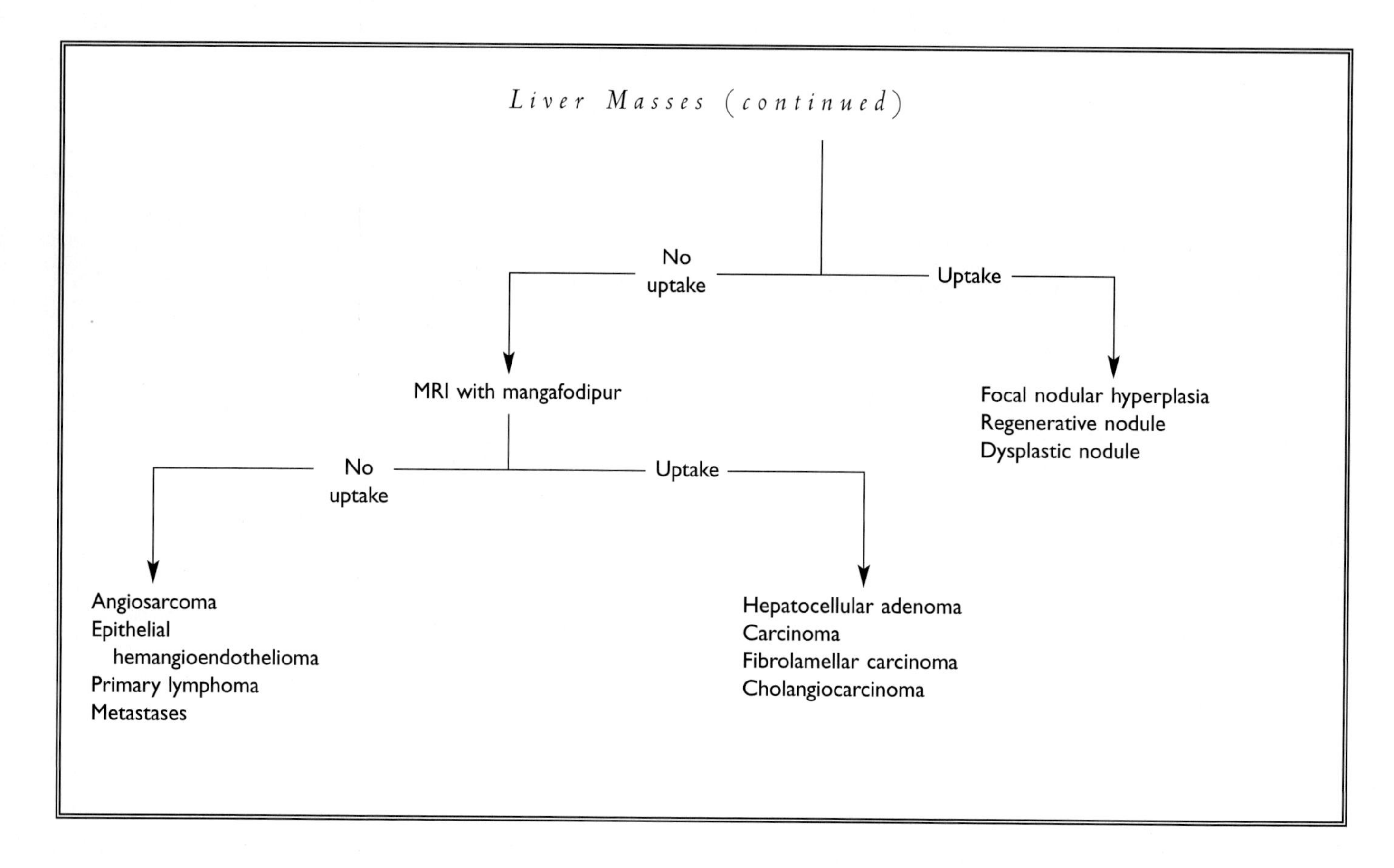

in a given case depends on multiple factors, including patient history, laboratory finding, prior imaging studies, and institutional preferences. Although preoperative imaging is routinely performed, IOUS is the most sensitive *in vivo* method, including physical inspection and palpation of the liver, for detecting liver neoplasms. The results of IOUS may alter surgical management.

The radiologic algorithm summarizes the use of imaging studies for evaluating the most common liver masses. Ultrasonography is often the initial imaging modality, as it is relatively inexpensive and convenient to perform. Most lesions determined to be cystic using ultrasound criteria do not require further evaluation. Solid or indeterminate liver masses usually require additional evaluation with contrast-enhanced CT scans or MRI for lesion characterization. Conventional angiography or noninvasive angiographic studies using CT or MRI are usually reserved for preoperative vascular mapping or evaluation of vessel patency.

Cavernous Hemangioma

Cavernous hemangioma, the most common benign tumor of the liver detected by imaging studies, is found during about 7% of autopsies. These lesions are congenital benign hamartomas characterized histologically by dilated vascular spaces lined with vascular endothelium. Most patients with cavernous hemangioma are asymptomatic. Patients with large (5 cm) hemangiomas may present with vague right upper quadrant pain, early satiety, nausea, vomiting, and fever. Rarely, patients develop obstructive jaundice or gastric outlet obstruction. Although bleeding and rupture are rare, acute thrombosis of a large cavernous hemangioma may progress to consumption coagulopathy. Abdominal examination may reveal hepatomegaly or a right upper quadrant bruit.

Cavernous hemangioma may be diagnosed by the characteristic pattern seen on contrast-enhanced CT. On precontrast images there is a well defined mass that is isodense to the aortic blood pool. Dynamic CT scans obtained following intravenous contrast demonstrate globular peripheral enhancement beginning in the portal venous phase with progressive, complete centripetal filling. The lesions become isodense to liver on images obtained after delays of 5–60 minutes following contrast administration. Similar enhancement patterns may also be demonstrated with MRI scans performed with intravenous gadolinium chelates (Fig. 72–1). However, this classic pattern of lesion enhancement is demonstrated in only approximately half of all cavernous hemangiomas. When the enhancement pattern is not typical, cavernous hemangioma may be diagnosed if the lesion has features suggestive of hemangioma using a complementary imaging technique, such as T2-weighted MRI or radionuclide scans. Typically, cavernous hemangiomas are markedly bright

TABLE 72–1.
Classification of liver masses

- Solid, nonmalignant
  - Cavernous hemangioma
  - Hepatocellular adenoma
  - Focal nodular hyperplasia
  - Biliary hamartoma
  - Confluent hepatic fibrosis
  - Inflammatory pseudotumor of the liver
- Cystic, nonmalignant
  - Hepatic cyst
  - Polycystic liver disease
  - Biliary cystadenoma
- Cystic, infectious
  - Pyogenic liver abscess
  - Amebic liver abscess
  - Echinococcal cyst
  - Hepatic microabscess
- Cystic, malignant
  - Biliary cystadenocarcinoma
  - Metastatic disease
- Solid, malignant
  - Hepatocellular carcinoma
  - Fibrolamellar carcinoma
  - Cholangiocarcinoma
  - Gallbladder carcinoma
  - Angiosarcoma
  - Epithelioid hemangioepithelioma
  - Primary hepatic lymphoma
  - Metastatic disease

lesions on heavily T2-weighted images (obtained with an echo time of more than 120 ms), a feature uncommon to solid liver lesions. A technetium-99 m-tagged red blood cell radionuclide scan may confirm the diagnosis as a "hot spot" if the lesion is >2 cm in diameter. Cavernous hemangiomas are often lobulated and have fine internal septations. Angiography is no longer commonly used to diagnose hemangiomas. Ultrasound images display the cavernous hemangioma as a hyperechoic homogeneous lesion; however, ultrasonography is not reliable as a sole imaging modality for this diagnosis.

Needle biopsy of cavernous hemangiomas is relatively contraindicated owing to the risk of substantial hemorrhage. Cavernous hemangiomas are resected only if symptomatic and if it is surgically feasible without undue risk. Resection involves enucleation and ligation of the feeding arteries.

Hepatocellular Adenoma

Hepatocellular adenoma is the most common benign liver tumor in young women. More than 90% of hepatocellular adenomas occur in women of childbearing age. Long-term oral contraceptive use is the most commonly identified predisposing factor. Estrogens stimulate activity of mitogenic factors such as hepatocyte growth factor. Up to 25% of men with hepatocellular adenoma give a history of androgen use. The histology of hepatocellular adenoma is characterized by the presence of hyperplastic hepatocytes with a lack of biliary architecture.

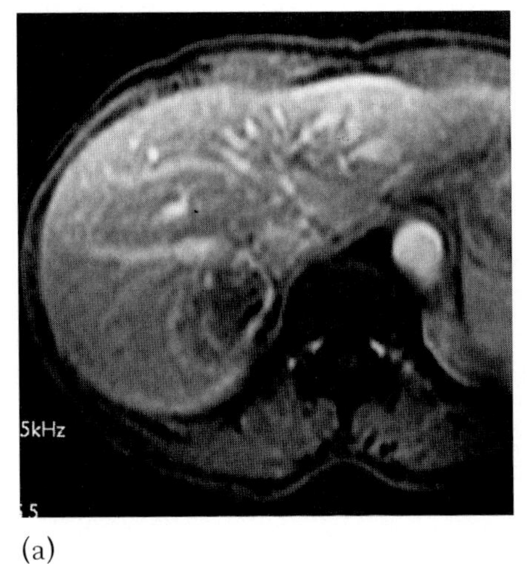

(a)

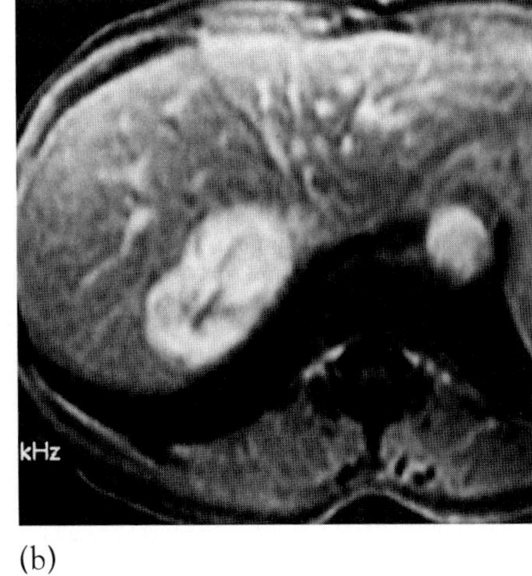

(b)

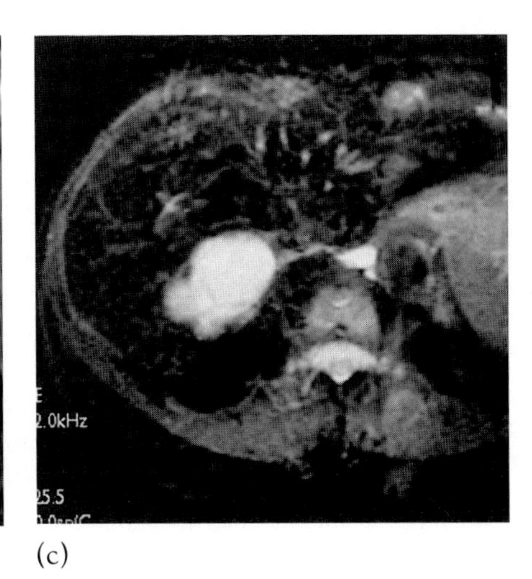
(c)

FIGURE 72–1
Cavernous hemangioma in a 66-year-old woman. (a) Portal venous phase gadolinium-enhanced magnetic resonanc (MR) image shows typical nodular peripheral enhancement. (b) Delayed phase-enhanced MR image obtained 5 minutes after injection shows complete lesion enhancement. (c) T2-weighted MR image shows typical bright appearance. Lobulated margins and internal septations are also common features.

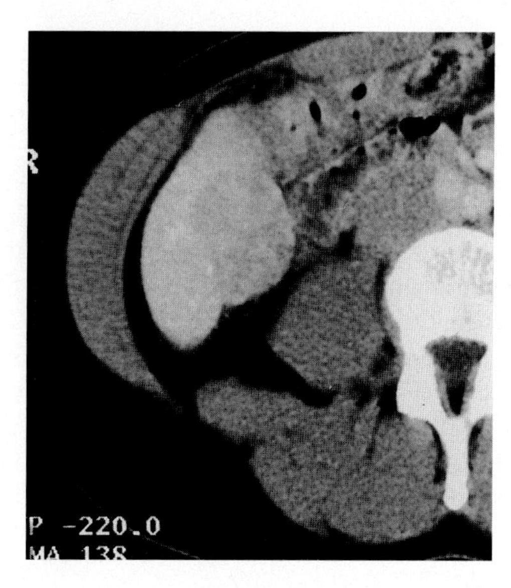

FIGURE 72–2
Hepatocellular adenoma in a 41-year-old woman. Contrast-enhanced computed tomography (CT) scan shows a heterogeneously enhancing mass arising from the inferior margin of the right lobe of the liver.

Most patients are symptomatic at presentation, with abdominal pain occurring in up to 50% of patients. Hepatomegaly or a palpable right upper quadrant mass may be elicited. Up to 30% of patients with hepatocellular adenoma present as surgical emergencies related to intralesional hemorrhage or intraperitoneal rupture with hypovolemic shock. Liver function tests are often abnormal, but α-fetoprotein is not elevated.

The imaging features are those of a hypervascular mass, often with internal hemorrhage or necrosis. These features are best demonstrated with dynamic enhanced CT or MRI enhanced with gadolinium chelates (Fig. 72–2). Ultrasonography is usually less specific but typically shows a heterogeneous hyperechoic lesion. The presence of functional hepatocytes in the lesion may be confirmed by either MRI with mangafodipir contrast or a radionuclide hepatobiliary scan. Hepatocellullar adenoma may be differentiated from focal nodular hyperplasia histologically by its paucity of reticuloendothelial (Kupffer) cells. Hepatocellular adenoma usually appears "cold" on technetium-99 sulfur colloid radionuclide scans or MRI scans performed with intravenous ferrumoxides. Angiographic studies demonstrate a hypervascular tumor with arteriovenous shunting. These imaging features are indistinguishable from those of malignant hepatocellular neoplasms.

A needle biopsy may be indicated to confirm the diagnosis, but the risk of malignant seeding or tumor rupture discourages its use. Asymptomatic hepatocellular adenomas <6 cm may be observed. Pregnancy and estrogen use are associated with tumor growth and increased risk of rupture. Spontaneous regression of hepatocellular adenomas has been reported following cessation of estrogen therapy. Women who are considering using birth control pills should practice alternative methods of contraception.

Hepatocellular adenomas ≥6 cm have an appreciable risk of malignant transformation or rupture. Resection is indicated if the mass is symptomatic, >6 cm, progressing in size with serial studies, or associated with elevated serum α-fetoprotein levels. Rupture of a hepatocellular adenoma is a surgical emergency, and immediate resection is indicated. Preoperative angiography with hepatic artery embolization has been used to stabilize the patient and minimize intraoperative blood loss.

Focal Nodular Hyperplasia

Focal nodular hyperplasia occurs in both genders and all age groups. Although the incidence is highest in young women, there is no association with oral contraceptive use. Focal nodular hyperplasia is thought to arise from a hyperplastic response around a vascular malformation. The lesions are usually asymptomatic and are often detected incidentally by imaging procedures. Bleeding complications and malignant transformation are rare. Symptomatic patients complain of abdominal discomfort or have right upper quadrant tenderness.

Focal nodular hyperplasia lesions are lobulated, and there is usually a central stellate scar. Peripheral lesions may show umbilication of the liver surface. Abnormal liver function tests are seen in fewer than 20% of patients. Internal hemorrhage or necrosis is rarely present in focal nodular hyperplasia. The lesions brightly enhance, and the central scar is commonly seen in contrast-enhanced CT or MRI images (Fig. 72–3). The presence of Kupffer cells in the lesion on histologic examination confirms the diagnosis. A technetium-99 sulfur colloid radionuclide scan or MRI scan performed with intravenous ferrumoxides can confirm the diagnosis. Increased Kupffer cell uptake of the radionuclide in the area of focal nodular hyperplasia appears as either a "hot spot" or a normal area, in contrast to other liver masses that demonstrate reduced uptake ("cold spot"). The lesions appear isointense or hypointense relative to liver on T2-weighted MR images obtained following administration of ferrumoxides.

The histopathology of focal nodular hyperplasia is that of normal-appearing hepatocytes with the presence of bile ducts and Kupffer cells. Asymptomatic focal nodular hyperplasia should be observed, whereas lesions that demonstrate growth or cause substantial symptoms are resected.

Biliary Cystadenoma

Biliary cystadenoma is a rare cystic tumor, most commonly seen in women. The lesions are typically septated and multiloculated

(a)

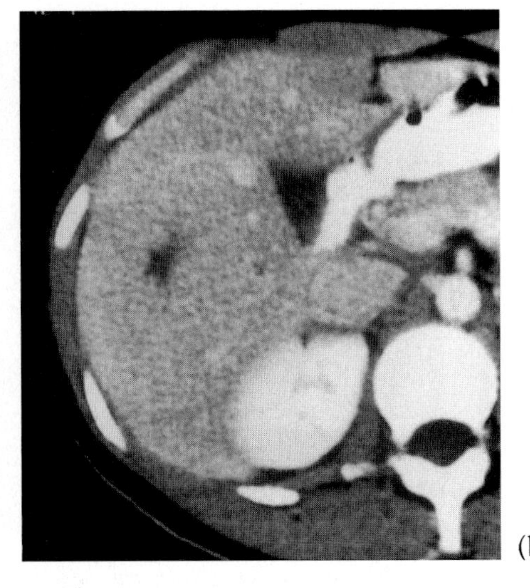

(b)

FIGURE 72–3
Focal nodular hyperplasia in a 27-year-old woman. (a) CT scan obtained without intravenous contrast demonstrates a large, low-density mass within the right lobe of the liver. (b) Following intravenous contrast, the mass brightly enhances. A nonenhancing central scar is present.

(Fig. 72–4). The presence of papillary projections or calcification may indicate transformation to cystadenocarcinoma (see below). Lesions may be initially confused with echinococcal cysts or pyogenic abscesses. Lesions with benign cytology and negative cultures may be aspirated and observed, but definitive treatment is surgical excision.

Biliary Hamartoma

Biliary hamartomas, also called von Meyenburg complexes, are benign biliary malformations consisting of ductal components with fibrous stroma. They are seen in up to 15% of autopsies and are often detected as incidental lesions on imaging studies. Biliary hamartomas are frequently multiple and usually present as hypodense solid lesions measuring <5 mm. The lesions usually do not enhance with contrast agents. Because of their small size, they often cannot be accurately characterized using imaging studies and may be confused with small cysts or metastases (Fig. 72–5). Biopsy may be required to make the diagnosis in patients with a history of malignancy.

Confluent Hepatic Fibrosis

Confluent hepatic fibrosis is a lesion that commonly occurs with advanced cirrhosis. Lesions are usually wedged-shaped and consist of retraction of portions of the right lobe of the liver. There is usually associated hypertrophy of the left and caudate lobes. Lesions typically appear hypervascular relative to the adjacent cirrhotic liver on portal venous and parenchymal phase CT and MR scans. As the lesions consist entirely of fibrous tissue, there is no lesionsal uptake of the MR contrast agents ferrumoxides or mangafodipir.

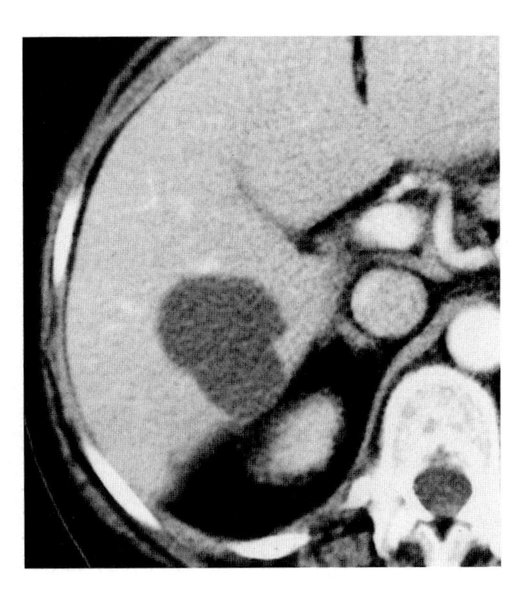

FIGURE 72–4
Biliary cystadenoma in a 73-year-old woman. Contrast-enhanced CT scan shows a cyst with faint septation.

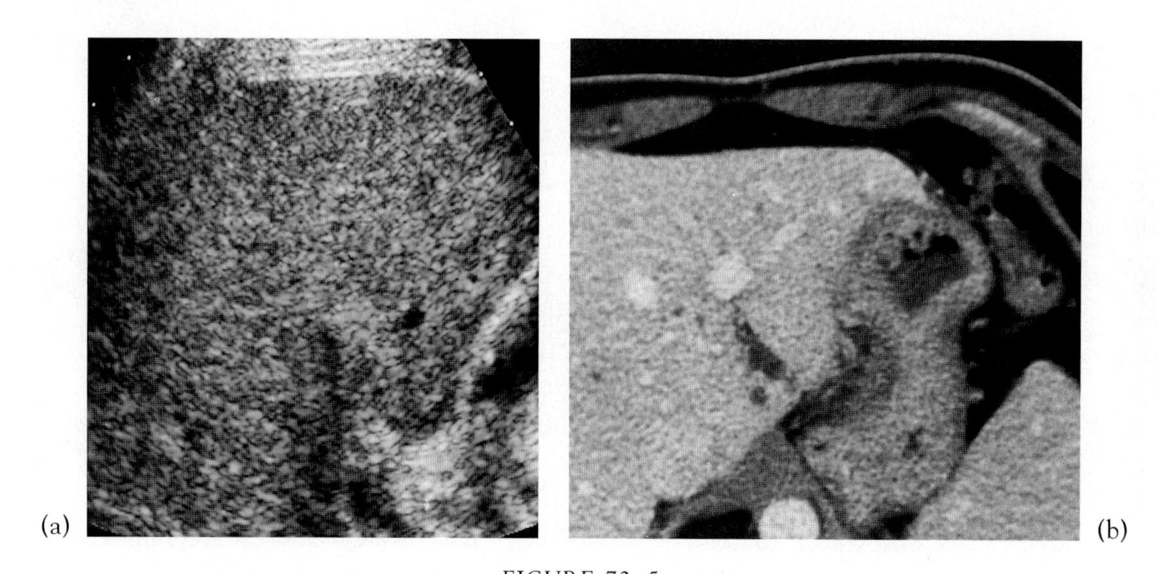

FIGURE 72–5
Biliary hamartomas in a 24-year-old woman. (a) Ultrasonography demonstrates multiple hypoechoic nodules. (b) Contrast-enhanced CT scan shows multiple 2- to 3-mm low-density lesions.

Inflammatory Pseudotumor of the Liver

Inflammatory pseudotumor of the liver is a rare lesion with features suggestive of liver malignancy. The lesions are typically multifocal and consist of focal polyclonal proliferation of plasma cells, lymphocytes, histiocytes, and eosinophils combined with a fibrous stroma. Lesions demonstrate variable, inhomogeneous enhancement with features suggestive of malignancy (Fig. 72–6). The diagnosis may be difficult to obtain with biopsy techniques, and resection may be required.

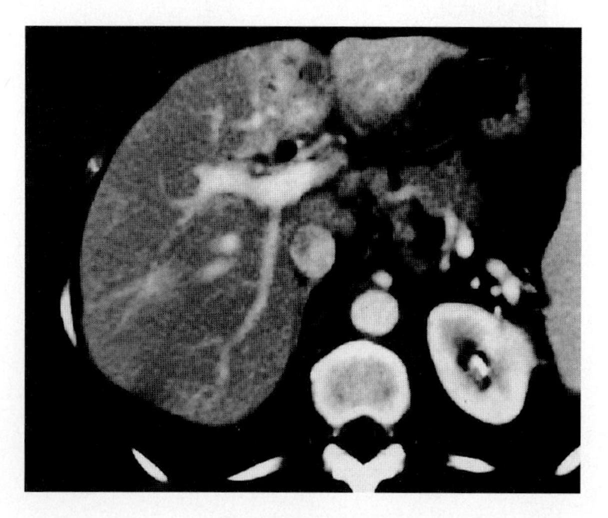

FIGURE 72–6
Inflammatory pseudotumor in a 67-year-old woman. The contrast-enhanced CT scan shows poorly defined lesions with irregular rim enhancement.

Hepatic Cyst

Hepatic cysts are common and are usually asymptomatic. If the cyst is symptomatic, patients may describe pain, vague discomfort, or early satiety. Compression of adjacent structures may cause obstructive jaundice or gastric outlet obstruction. Acquired liver cysts may be traumatic or neoplastic. Traumatic cysts have no epithelial lining, are associated with a history of trauma, and contain hemosiderin in their fibrotic walls. They are treated in a fashion similar to that for congenital liver cysts. Malignant liver cysts are uncommon but may be due to malignant degeneration of a primary hepatic tumor, may arise as a primary biliary cystadenoma or cystadenocarcinoma, or may be secondary deposits arising from cystic carcinomas of the pancreas or ovary. Hydatid cysts are described below.

Ultrasound images of simple cysts show a smoothly bordered anechoic mass with posterior acoustic enhancement (Fig. 72–7). The presence of internal echoes on ultrasonography raises suspicion of infection or malignancy and is an indication for ultrasound-guided aspiration of the fluid for culture and cytology. Simple cysts do not demonstrate internal or mural enhancement following contrast enhancement on CT or MRI scans. The fluid in uncomplicated cysts has an attenuation of 0–30 Hounsfield units and has a uniformly high signal on T2-weighted MR images.

Asymptomatic patients do not require surgery, but such patients should be followed for any sign of cyst enlargement. Aspiration of cyst fluid is usually not an effective treatment for symptomatic cysts, as reaccumulation of fluid is common. Laparoscopic unroofing of large hepatic cysts is a successful mode of surgical treatment. The lesions may also be

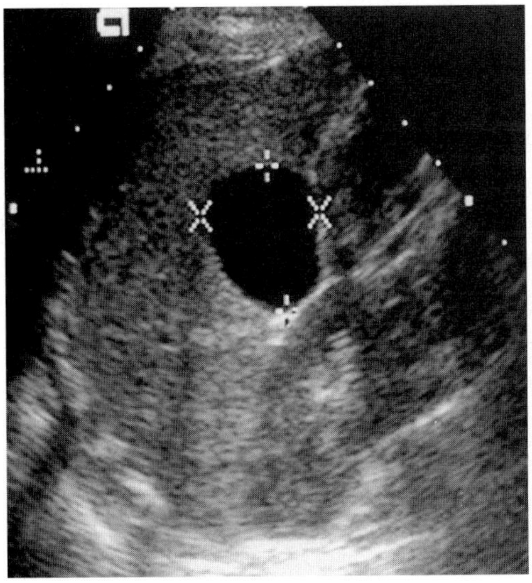

FIGURE 72–7
Hepatic cyst in a 32-year-old woman. Ultrasonography shows an anechoic lesion with posterior acoustic enhancement.

ablated by image-guided percutaneous injection of sclerosing agents.

Polycystic Liver Disease

Congenital polycystic disease can affect the kidney, liver, spleen, and pancreas and is associated with intracranial aneurysms. Adult polycystic liver disease is usually asymptomatic and is diagnosed during the routine investigation of patients with polycystic kidney disease. Imaging studies demonstrate multiple hepatic cysts of various sizes, ranging from several millimeters to several centimeters. Cysts may have internal septations or hemorrhage. Multiple renal cysts almost always coexist (Fig. 72–8). Venous compression or sepsis can lead to ascites and liver failure. Symptomatic cysts are treated with techniques similar to those used with simple cysts. Combined liver and kidney transplantation is required in some individuals with advanced disease.

Pyogenic Liver Abscess

Pyogenic liver abscesses arise as a consequence of infection, such as cholangitis, gastrointestinal sepsis, trauma, prior surgery, or subacute bacterial endocarditis. Alcoholic cirrhosis, diabetes mellitus, HIV infection, and hepatic metastases predispose to the development of pyogenic liver abscesses. The typical presentation includes right upper quadrant pain, fever, chills, and weight loss. Chest radiographs may show elevation of the right hemidiaphragm and radiopacities in the right lower lung field. The most common organisms cultured are *Escherichia coli*, *Klebsiella*, *Proteus*, *Bacteroides*, and *Peptostreptococcus*. Ultrasonography and CT are useful for identifying liver abscesses, demonstrating biliary tract obstruction, evaluating associated extrahepatic conditions, and guiding placement of a catheter for external drainage. Debris in the abscess appears hyperechoic on ultrasound images, which may lead to an incorrect diagnosis of a solid mass lesion. Contrast-enhanced CT is useful for demonstrating the enhancing abscess wall and the nonenhancing abscess cavity (Fig. 72–9).

Image-guided external drainage and intravenous antibiotics for 2 weeks followed by oral antibiotics for 4 weeks is adequate treatment in most cases. Laparotomy is required when percutaneous drainage fails, such as in cases in which there is multiloculation, inspissated thick pus, or excessive solid debris.

Amebic Liver Abscess

Amebic liver abscess is caused by *Entamoeba histolytica*. The clinical presentation is similar to that of pyogenic liver abscess. A single, large abscess in the dome of the right lobe of the liver is the typical presentation. A history of travel to an endemic area and a history of alcoholism are important predisposing factors. Serologic tests, such as the enzyme-linked immunosorbent assay (ELISA) and immunofluorescence tests, are available to confirm the diagnosis. Ultrasonography and CT are the initial imaging tests most frequently performed (Fig. 72–10).

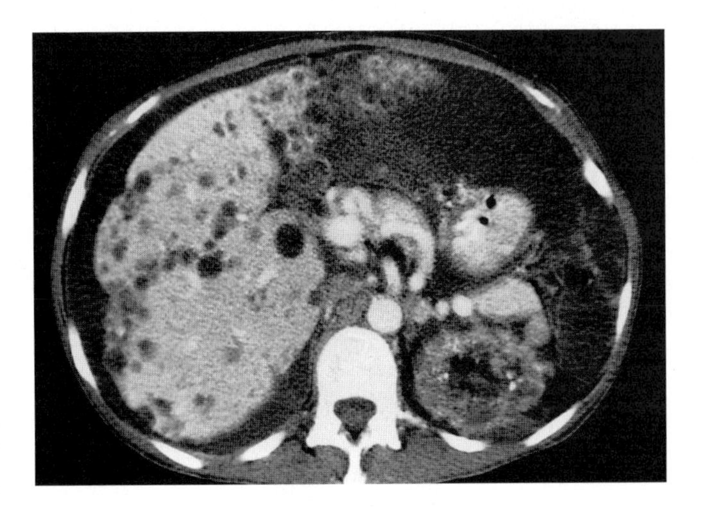

FIGURE 72–8
Polycystic disease of liver and kidney in a 61-year-old woman. Contrast-enhanced CT sean shows multiple hepatic and renal cysts.

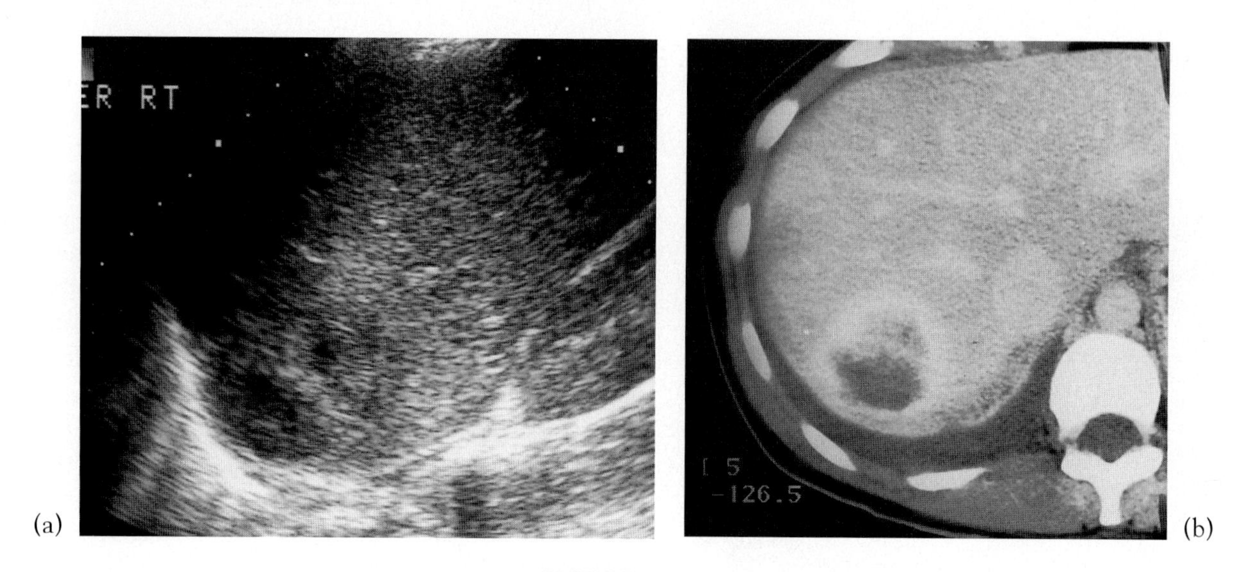

(a) (b)

FIGURE 72–9
Pyogenic liver abscess in a 42-year-old woman. (a) Ultrasonography shows an apparently solid liver lesion. (b) Contrast-enhanced CT scan shows nonenhancing central necrosis with enhancement of the abscess wall.

Most amebic liver abscesses resolve without drainage when treated with metronidazole 750 mg three times daily; chloroquine is added for acutely ill patients. Patients who do not respond to treatment with metronidazole and chloroquine require therapeutic aspiration and drainage. Aspiration occasionally reveals an unsuspected pyogenic abscess. Large left liver lobe amebic abscesses are also an indication for therapeutic drainage due to the imminent danger of fatal intrapericardial rupture.

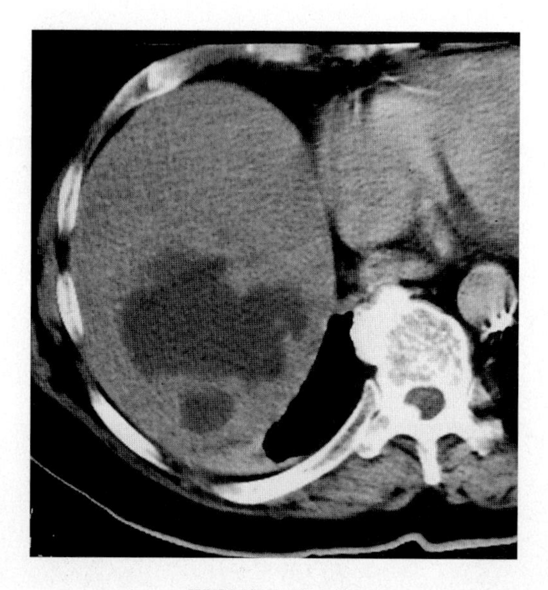

FIGURE 72–10
Amebic liver abscess in a 77-year-old woman. CT scan shows a loculated fluid density mass near the dome of the liver.

Hydatid Cyst of the Liver

Echinococcal (hydatid) cysts of the liver arise from infestation by the tapeworm *Echinococcus granulosus*. The dog is the primary host, which spreads the disease by the fecal-oral route to intermediate hosts such as sheep, cattle, and humans. Echinococcosis occurs when the swallowed egg develops into an embryo in the intermediate host gut, enters the portal circulation, and lodges in the liver to develop a hydatid cyst. Less often the organ involved is the brain, lung, spleen, or bone. When dogs consume the viscera of animals with echinococcosis, they are infested with the tapeworm and the life cycle is thus propagated.

Symptomaic patients experience abdominal pain or jaundice. A mass may be palpable. A plain radiograph of the abdomen may show an "egg-shell calcification" of the hydatid cyst. Serologic tests are positive in approximately 80% of cases. Ultrasonography and CT are the most commonly used diagnostic imaging tests (Fig. 72–11).

Surgery is used to excise the cysts under controlled circumstances. Inadvertent spillage of cyst contents may result in spread of disease and is associated with an increased risk for anaphylaxis. Mebendazole 200 mg/kg/day is given before and after surgery to minimize recurrence. Image-guided percutaneous treatment with intracystic administration of scolicidal

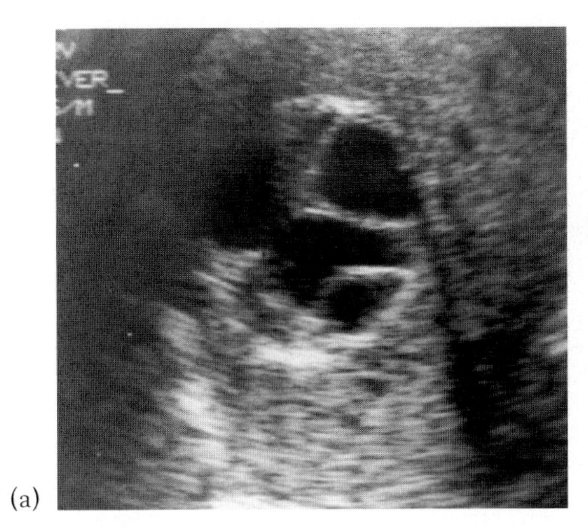

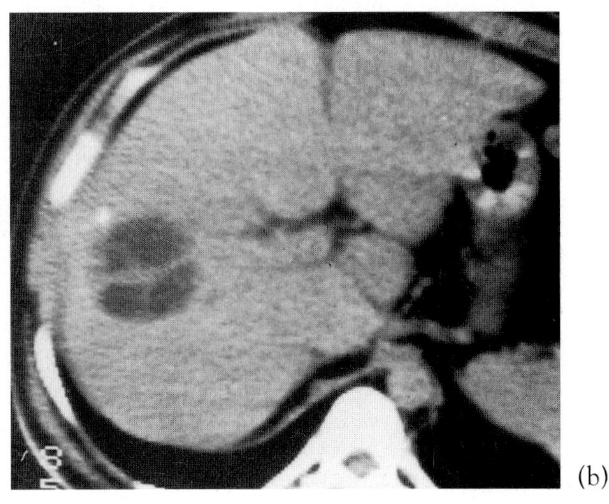

(a) (b)

FIGURE 72–11
Echinococcal cyst of the liver in a 46-year-old man. (a) Ultrasonography shows a septated cystic mass. (b) CT scan shows characteristic peripheral calcification.

agents has also been performed in some centers as primary treatment.

Hepatic Microabscess

Hepatic microabscess occur as a result of diffusely disseminated infectious processes, such as fungal infection and mycobacterial disease. Similar findings may be seen in acute granulomatous processes, such as sarcoidosis and disseminated *Pneumocystis carinii*. The lesions appear as multiple 2- to 10-mm poorly enhancing lesions scattered throughout the liver (Fig. 72–12). The differential diagnosis includes metastatic disease and biliary hamartoma. The diagnosis may be facilitated by percutaneous aspiration.

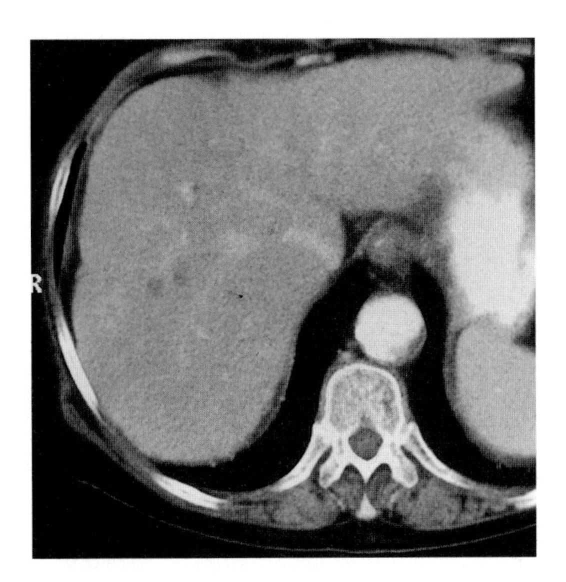

FIGURE 72–12
Candida microabscesses in a 69-year-old woman. Contrast-enhanced CT scan shows small, low-density, poorly enhancing hepatic lesions.

Liver Malignancies

Most hepatic neoplastic disease in North America is the result of metastatic disease, whereas in Asian countries such as Japan primary hepatic malignancies constitute most of the hepatic neoplasms. Hepatocellular carcinoma (hepatoma) and intrahepatic cholangiocarcinoma are the most common primary malignancies of the liver. Other, rarer primary cancers of the liver include biliary cystadenocarcinoma, sarcoma, epithelioid hemangioendothelioma, and primary hepatic lymphoma.

Hepatocellular Carcinoma

Predisposing factors for hepatocellular carcinoma include hepatitis B and C, cirrhosis from any cause, and exposure to hepatotoxins. The duration of hepatitis virus infection correlates with an increased risk of hepatocellular carcinoma. Patients with macronodular cirrhosis have a greater risk of developing hepatocellular carcinoma than those with micronodular cirrhosis. Hepatotoxins predisposing to the development of hepatocellular carcinoma include aflatoxin (from the fungus *Aspergillus flavus*), thorium dioxide, vinyl chloride, and arsenic.

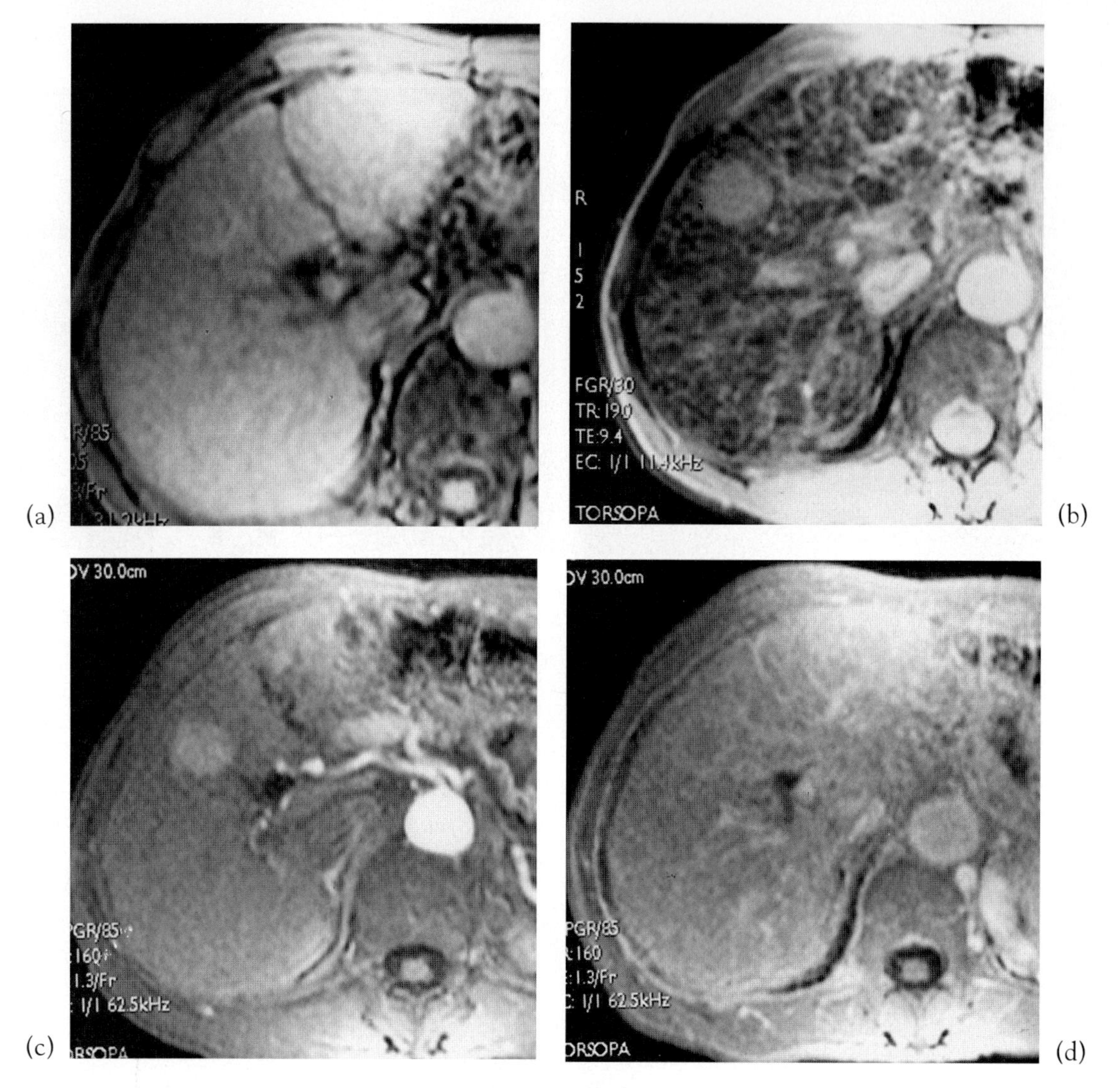

FIGURE 72–13
Hepatocellular carcinoma in a 66-year-old man with chronic hepatitis B infection and elevated serum α-fetoprotein. (a) T1-weighted MR image shows a vague lesion in segment 4. (b) Ferrumoxides-enhanced T2-weighted image shows micronodular cirrhosis and lack of contrast uptake in the nodule. (c) Gadolinium-enhanced arterial phase image demonstrates bright enhancement, which shows central "washout" on the parenchymal phase image (d).

Hepatocellular carcinoma afflicts men three times more commonly than women. Many patients are asymptomatic, and the lesions are commonly discovered on imaging studies. When hepatocellular carcinoma is symptomatic, there is painful hepatomegaly associated with anorexia and weight loss. Hemorrhage into the mass causes sudden, severe pain; and hemorrhage into the free intraperitoneal cavity may produce shock and hypovolemia. Abnormalities of liver enzymes may be present but are a nonspecific finding. α-Fetoprotein levels are elevated in more than 70% of patients and correlate with tumor size. α-Fetoprotein levels are elevated not only in patients with hepatocellular carcinoma but also in those with hepatitis, cirrhosis, massive hepatic necrosis, pregnancy, and yolk sac tumors. The clinical triad of a liver mass, positive hepatitis serology, and high α-fetoprotein levels is diagnostic of hepatocellular carcinoma.

Ultrasonography and CT are most often the first radiologic investigations performed. Ultrasonography is a useful screening test in high risk patients and is a sensitive, noninvasive test for tumors ≥2 cm. Multiphase contrast-enhanced CT or MRI is more sensitive than ultrasomography for detecting smaller lesions. Hepatocellular carcinoma is typically hypervascular on contrast-enhanced CT or MR scans (Fig. 72–13). Color doppler sonography is commonly used to evaluate the portal

(a) 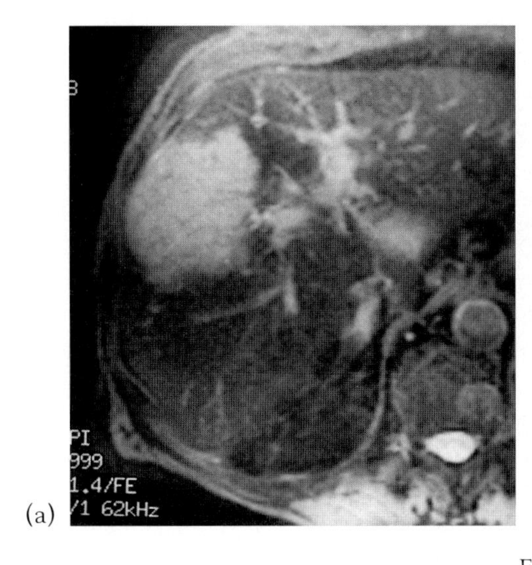

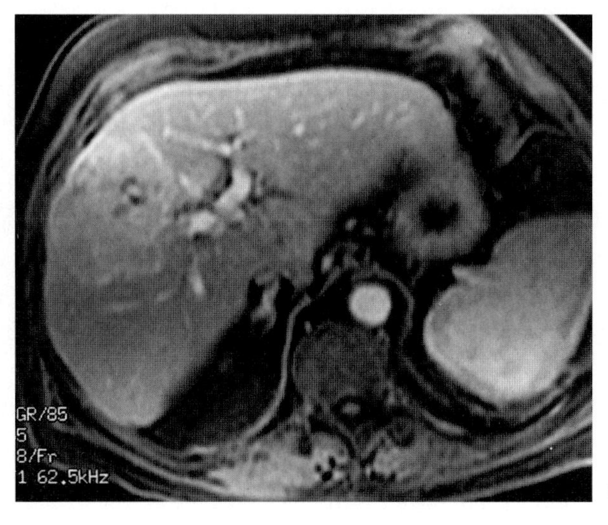 (b)

FIGURE 72–14
Fibrolamellar carcinoma in a 52-year-old woman. (a) Ferrumoxides-enhanced T2-weighted MR image shows a lobulated high-signal lesion in the right lobe of the liver. (b) Gadolinium-enhanced MR images shows enhancement of the tumor capsule. A low-intensity central scar is present.

vein, hepatic veins, and inferior vena cava and may detect vascular invasion. Tumor thrombus in large veins may exhibit an arterial Doppler waveform. MRI with MR angiography or CT with CT angiography can provide preoperative vascular maps, demonstrate hepatic arterial variants, and evaluate for extrahepatic disease. Conventional angiography, CT-enhanced arteriography, or CT-enhanced portography are also used by various institutions as part of the routine preoperative assessment. IOUS provides further information about vascular involvement and helps determine the extent of surgical resection.

Treatment depends on whether the patient has coexistent cirrhosis, as these patients do not tolerate major hepatic resections. Limited wedge resections may be feasible in patients with compensated cirrhosis and peripherally located hepatocellular carcinoma. Cryotherapy is an option for lesions <5 cm. Intraarterial chemoembolization or percutaneous intralesional ethanol injection may be effective ablative therapy for hepatocellular carcinoma in patients who are poor surgical candidates. Intravenous chemotherapy is indicated for lesions >5 cm and for multicentric lesions; however, chemotherapy alone is associated with a poor prognosis.

Curative liver resections should be performed whenever possible in noncirrhotic patients, although local recurrence is common despite successful resection. Secondary lesions are rarely amenable to repeat resection. Surgical resection is associated with an operative mortality of 5–10% and a 5-year survival rate of about 25%. Liver transplantation has been attempted for treatment of unresectable primary and metastatic liver cancers, but the recurrence rate is high (>65%). Factors influencing tumor-free survival following transplantation for hepatocellular carcinoma are lesion size <5 cm and fewer than three lesions.

Fibrolamellar Carcinoma

Fibrolamellar carcinoma, previously considered a variant of hepatocellular carcinoma, is now described as a separate entity. It duffers from hepatocellular carcinoma in that it occurs in younger patients, is not associated with predisposing factors such as cirrhosis or hepatitis, is usually not associated with elevated α-fetoprotein levels, and has a more favorable prognosis. Fibrotic bands in a laminar pattern in the tumor produce the "fibrolamellar" characteristics of this tumor. Fibrolamellar carcinoma presents as a large solitary mass with a lobulated contour. The presence of a central fibrous scar with a preponderance of calcification is another characteristic of this tumor.

Ultrasonography and CT help detect the tumor, and MRI with ferrumoxides may help differentiate if from focal nodular hyperplasia, which also has central scarring (Fig. 72–14). Histologic examination is required for final confirmation of the diagnosis. Resectable lesions have a 5-year survival rate of about 60%.

Cholangiocarcinoma

Cholangiocarcinomas may be intrahepatic or extrahepatic. Intrahepatic cholangiocarcinomas are rare and are classified into three groups: (1) peripheral cholangiocarcinoma arising in the small peripheral ducts; (2) major hepatic duct cholangiocarcinoma arising from the right of left hepatic duct near the hilum: and (3) hilar cholangiocarcinoma arising at the junction of the common hepatic duct with the left and right hepatic ducts (Klatskin tumor). Predisposing factors include ulcerative colitis, choledochal cysts, Caroli's disease, sclerosing cholangitis, chronic cholangitis, intrahepatic biliary calculi, congenital biliary atresia, and *Clonorchis* or *Opisthorchis* infestation. Cholangiocarcinoma arises from the bile duct epithelium and has a poor prognosis. Klatskin tumors present early owing to biliary tract obstruction, whereas peripheral cholangiocarcinomas usually present at an advanced stage. Regardless of presentation, the 3-year survival is 3%. In patients with cholangiocarcinoma, serum α-fetoprotein levels are normal, and serum carcinoembryonic antigen levels are often elevated.

Biliary obstruction is the most common imaging finding, and the lesions are well demonstrated by most imaging modalities (Fig. 72–15). Preoperative angiography or noninvasive angiographic imaging studies are required to ascertain portal vein involvement and invasion of the contralateral lobar hepatic artery. Further evaluation and treatment of intrahepatic cholangiocarcinomas are similar to that for hepatocellular carcinomas.

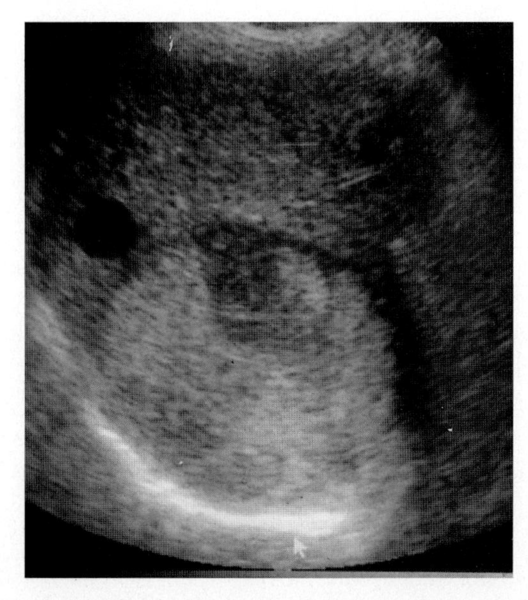

FIGURE 72–15
Intrahepatic cholangiocarcinoma in a 69-year-old man. Ultrasonography shows a hyperechoic, encapsulated mass in the right lobe. An adjacent simple cyst is present.

Biliary Cystadenocarcinoma

Biliary cystadenocarcinoma is a rare malignant tumor of the biliary tract. Most originate in the intrahepatic biliary ducts and the remainder in the extrahepatic biliary ducts or the gallbladder. Biliary cystadenocarcinomas are large, nodular, multiloculated tumors that have excrescences from the septal walls that are seen on ultrasonogophy, CT, or MRI. CT and MRI show a water-density tumor with contrast enhancement of the wall and internal elements (Fig. 72–16). Based on the radiologic appearance of these tumors, the differential diagnosis includes biliary cystadenoma, liver abscess, and echinococcal cyst. The malignancy may be diagnosed by image-guided percutaneous aspiration. In view of their malignant ptoential, biliary cystadenomas should be surgically resected in the same manner as localized biliary cystadenocarcinomas.

Gallbladder Carcinoma

Carcinoma of the gallbladder may invade the liver and present as a right upper quadrant mass. Cholelithiasis is usually present in patients with gallbladder carcinoma. If carcinoma of the gallbladder is found incidentally at cholecystectomy and does not transgress the submucosa, cholecystectomy alone is considered adequate treatment. When deeper layers of the gallbladder wall are involved, cholecystectomy with segmental liver resection is recommended (Fig. 72–17).

Angiosarcoma

Angiosarcoma is a rare tumor, with an incidence of 0.14 per million; but it is the most common primary hepatic sarcoma. Chemical carcinogens such as vinyl chloride, arsenic, and thorium dioxide are strongly implicated in its pathogenesis, and therapeutic irradiation and hemochromatosis have also been identified as predisposing factors. Angiosarcoma is a nonencapsulated lesion that is frequently multifocal and prone to intralesional hemorrhage. Fatal hemoperitoneum can also occur.

On ultrasound examination, the lesions are typically heterogenous in terms of echogenicity (Fig. 72–18). Contrast-enhanced CT scans show a hypervascular tumor with a centripetal enhancement pattern similar to that of cavernous hemangioma. The presence of residual intrahepatic Thorotrast and a hypervascular hepatic tumor is virtually diagnostic of angiosarcoma. Angiographic imaging with vascular mapping is required to ascertain resectability. Percutaneous needle biopsy for a tissue diagnosis followed by chemotherapy is the treatment for nonresectable lesions. Angiosarcoma is a highly aggressive

(a) 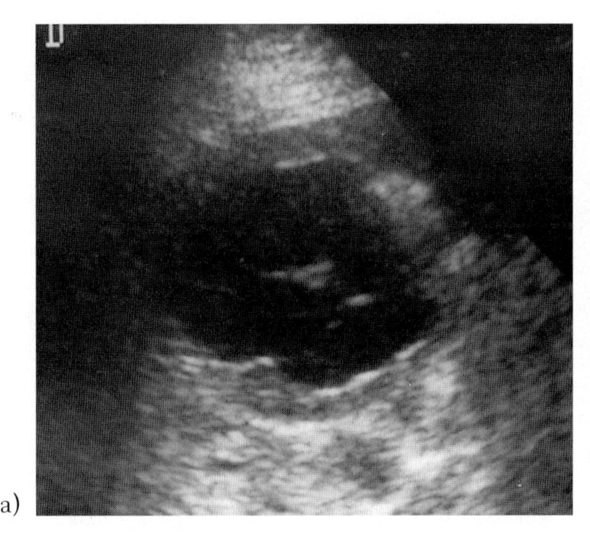 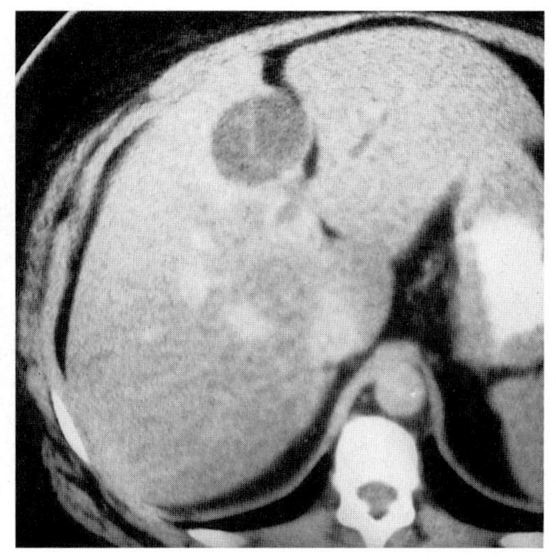 (b)

FIGURE 72–16
Biliary cystadenocarcinoma in a 49-year-old woman. (a) Ultrasonography shows a multiseptated cyst. (b) CT scan shows irregular enhancement of internal septations.

malignancy with a marked degree of local invasion and metastases leading to early death.

Epithelioid Hemangioendothelioma

Hepatic epithelioid hemangioendothelioma is a rare malignant tumor of vascular origin composed primarily of epithelioid cells with myxoid and fibrous stroma. Female/male occurrence is 2:1. No definite predisposing risk factors have been identified. The tumor usually presents as multifocal infiltrative masses scattered throughout the liver that may coalesce as the tumor progresses (Fig. 72–19).

Primary Hepatic Lymphoma

Primary hepatic lymphoma is rare compared to secondary hepatic involvement in cases of extrahepatic lymphoma. Primary hepatic lymphoma is usually of B cell origin and may

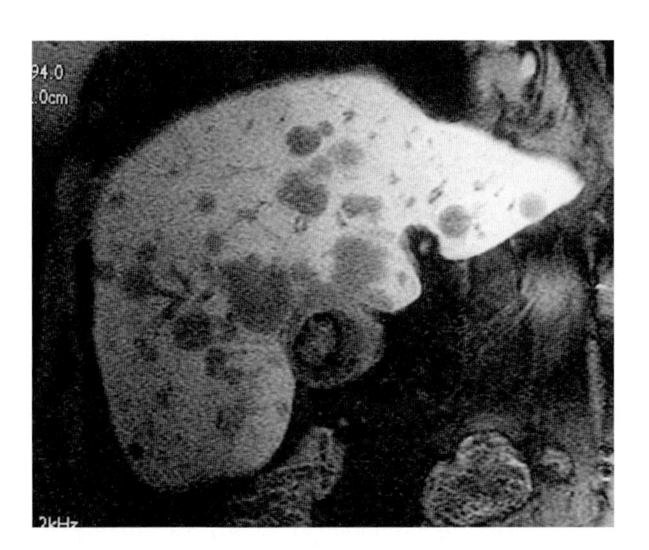

FIGURE 72–17
Gallbladder carcinoma in a 71-year-old man. Mangafodipir-enhanced coronal MR image shows concentric thickening of the gallbladder wall. Tumor extends from the gallbladder into the adjacent liver. Cholelithiasis is present.

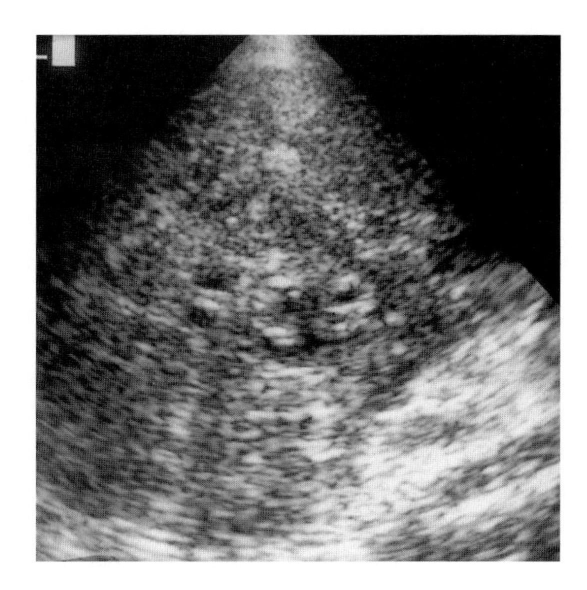

FIGURE 72–18
Angiosarcoma in a 72-year-old man. Ultrasonography shows a heterogeneous solid mass.

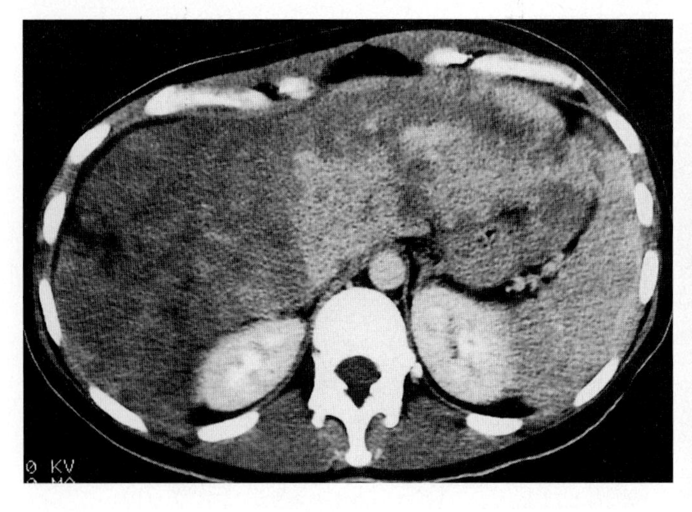

FIGURE 72–19
Epithelioid hemangioendothelioma in a 34-year-old woman. Contrast-enhanced CT scan shows diffusely infiltrative masses in both hepatic lobes.

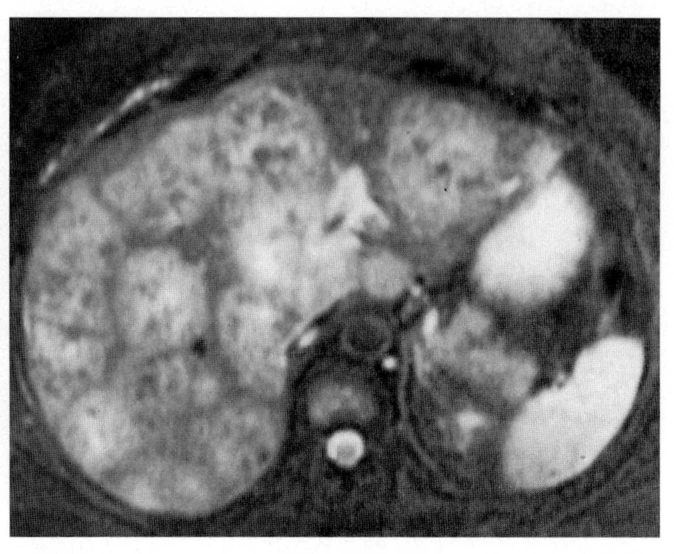

FIGURE 72–21
Metastatic colon carcinoma in a 63-year-old woman. T2-weighted MR images show multiple liver lesions with a "target" appearance.

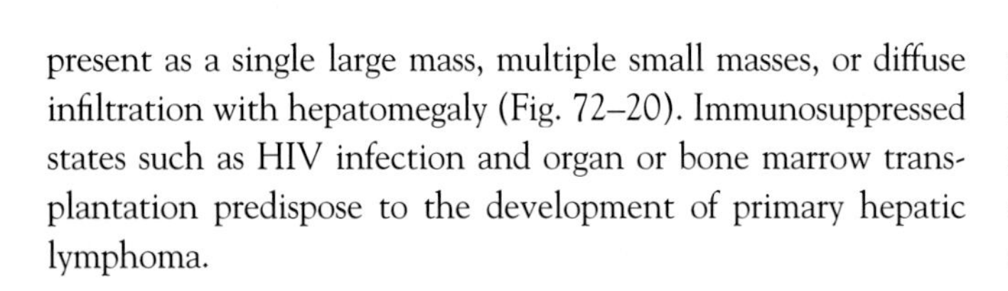

present as a single large mass, multiple small masses, or diffuse infiltration with hepatomegaly (Fig. 72–20). Immunosuppressed states such as HIV infection and organ or bone marrow transplantation predispose to the development of primary hepatic lymphoma.

Secondary Liver Malignancies

Metastatic cancers of the liver are more common in North America than primary hepatic cancers. Metastatic lesions may

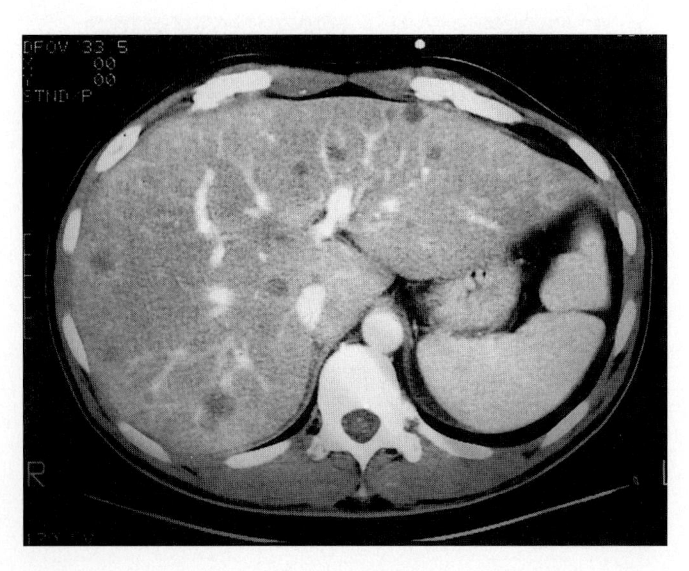

FIGURE 72–20
Large cell B cell lymphoma in a 42-year-old man with human immunodeficiency virus (HIV) infection. Contrast-enhanced CT scan shows multiple low attenuation lesions in the liver.

present as solitary lesions and may be detected prior to identification of the primary tumor. The main primary malignancies associated with liver metastases are colorectal carcinoma, breast carcinoma, lung carcinoma, melanoma, lymphoma, renal cell carcinoma, pancreatic carcinoma, and neuroendocrine tumors, such as carcinoid. Most metastatic lesions appear solid on imaging studies (Fig. 72–21). Cystic metastases are common with ovarian carcinoma and breast carcinoma.

Percutaneous biopsy is used to confirm staging or to determine the origin of the primary cancer. Although metastatic disease is usually treated with chemotherapy, resection of metastatic lesions may improve survival in patients with primary colonic carcinoma, carcinoid syndrome, or renal cell carcinoma.

Suggested Reading

Cameron JL (ed). Current surgical Therapy, 5th ed. St. Louis: Mosby, 1995; 258–280.

Fernandez MP, Redvanly RD. Primary hepatic malignant neoplasms. Radiol Clin North Am 1998;36:333–348.

Fukuya T, Honda H, Matsumata T, et al. Diagnosis of inflammatory pseudotumor of the liver. AJR Am J Roentgenol 1994;163:1087–1091.

Greenfield LJ, Mulholland MW, Oldham KT, Zelenock GB (eds). Surgery—Scientific Principles and Practice. Philadelphia: Lippincott, 1993;843–923.

Karhunen PJ. Benign hepatic tumours and tumour-like conditions in men. J Clin Pathol 1986;39:183–188.

Millikan KW. Liver mass. In: Millikan KW, Saclarides TJ (eds) Common Surgical Diseases—An Algorithmic Approach to Problem Solving. New York: Springer, 1997;246–250.

Millikan KW, Staren ED, Doolas A. Invasive therapy of metastatic colorectal cancer to the liver. Surg Clin North Am 1997;77:27–48.

Patricia JM, Pablo RR. Benign lesions of the liver. Radiol Clin North Am 1998;36:319–332.

Semelka RC, Hussain SM, Marcos HB, Woosley JT. Biliary hamartomas. J Magn Reson Imaging 1999;10:196–201.

Staren ED, Gambla M, Deziel DJ, et al. Intraoperative ultrasound in the management of liver neoplasms. Am Surg 1997;63:591–596.

Üstünsöz B, Akhan O, Kamiloglu MA, Somuncu I, Ugurel MS, Cetiner S. Percutaneous treatment of hydatid cysts of the liver: long-term results. AJR Am J Roeutgenol 1999;172:91–96.

Van Beers BE, Gallez B, Pringot J. Contrast-enhanced MR imaging of the liver. Radiology 1997;203:297–306.

Vauthey JN. Liver imaging: a surgeon's perspective. Radiol Clin North Am 1998;36:445–457.

Way LW (ed). Current Surgical Diagnosis and Treatment, 10th ed., Norwalk CT: Appleton & Lange, 1994;505–519.

CHAPTER 73

The Jaundiced Cancer Patient

JAMES A. MADURA II
DANIEL J. DEZIEL

Jaundice in a cancer patient may be a manifestation of a number of disease processes. Primary upper abdominal malignancies may present with biliary tract obstruction treatable with curative or palliative means. Although jaundice in a patient with preexisting malignancy may signal incurability, substantial symptomatic benefit and longevity can be achieved with appropriate treatment. A spectrum of benign conditions can result in hyperbilirubinemia in the cancer patient and should not be mistaken for irreversible disease.

Advancements in technology over the past two decades have improved our ability to diagnose and treat both benign and malignant biliary obstruction. A number of laboratory investigations, imaging techniques, and interventional modalities are now available for diagnostic and therapeutic use. Specifically, developments in radiologic imaging, endoscopic diagnostic and percutaneous interventions, and minimally invasive surgery have had an important impact on the management of the jaundiced patient. Unfortunately, jaundice often remains a sign of advanced malignancy. The patient's overall prognosis and physical comfort must therefore be the foremost considerations as various diagnostic and therapeutic maneuvers are entertained.

A. Diagnosis

History and Physical Examination

A thorough history at the time of presentation can provide substantial information to guide the subsequent course of the evaluation. In addition to a comprehensive interrogation regarding the onset of jaundice and any other present complaints, the history should include a detailed analysis of any prior malignancy and its treatment; other medical conditions that may be associated with jaundice (e.g., cholelithiasis, hepatitis, cirrhosis, inflammatory bowel disease, prior operations); past and present medications including chemotherapy; alcohol and drug use; and family history (especially regarding malignancy). The review of symptoms should be extensive, as subtle complaints may reveal important diagnostic and prognostic information not volunteered. Obvious examples include constipation or

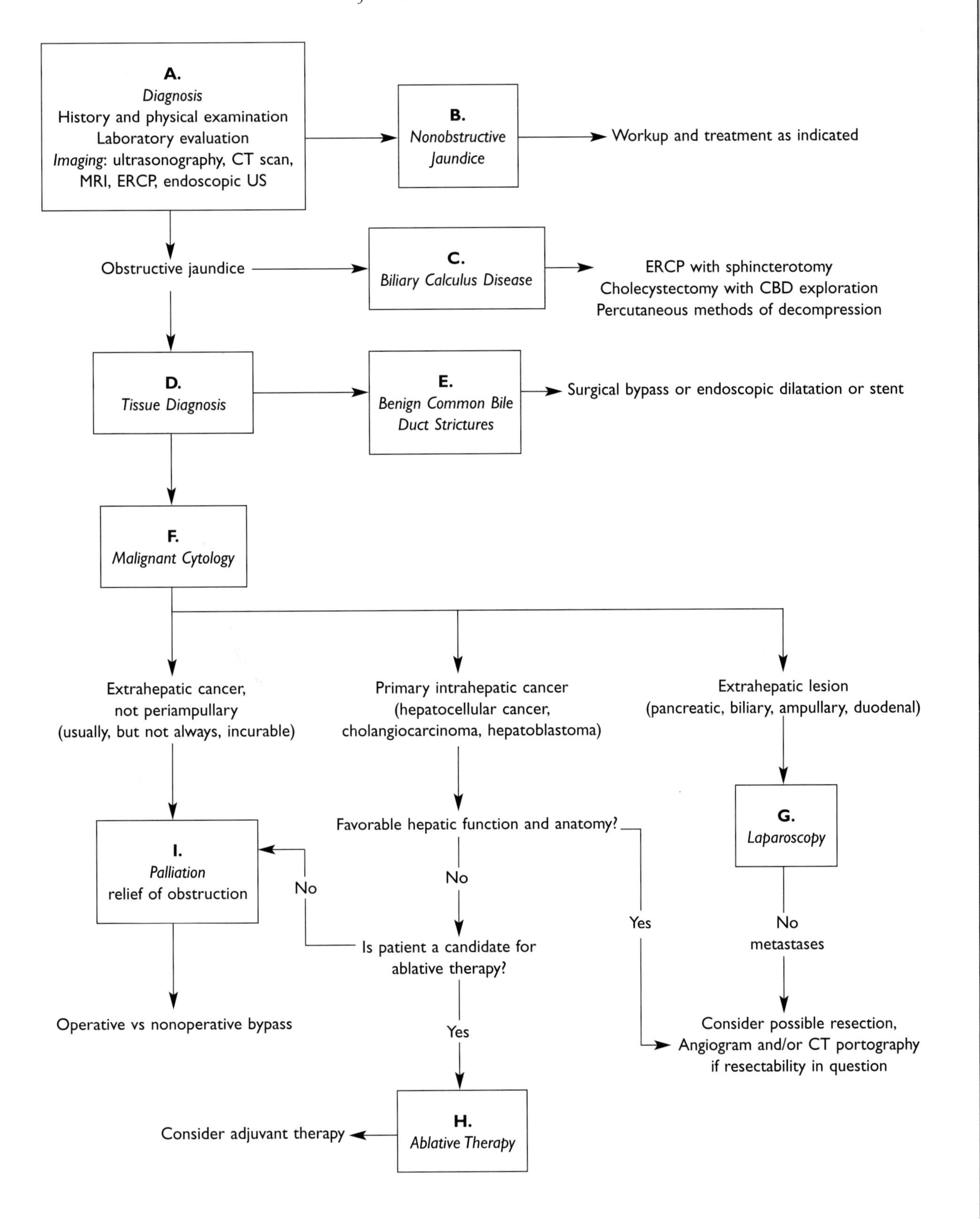

The Jaundiced Cancer Patient
A.
Diagnosis
History and physical examination
Laboratory evaluation
Imaging: ultrasonography, CT scan, MRI, ERCP, endoscopic US
B.
Nonobstructive Jaundice
Workup and treatment as indicated
Obstructive jaundice
C.
Biliary Calculus Disease
ERCP with sphincterotomy
Cholecystectomy with CBD exploration
Percutaneous methods of decompression
D.
Tissue Diagnosis
E.
Benign Common Bile Duct Strictures
Surgical bypass or endoscopic dilatation or stent
F.
Malignant Cytology
Extrahepatic cancer, not periampullary (usually, but not always, incurable)
Primary intrahepatic cancer (hepatocellular cancer, cholangiocarcinoma, hepatoblastoma)
Extrahepatic lesion (pancreatic, biliary, ampullary, duodenal)
Favorable hepatic function and anatomy?
No
Yes
I.
Palliation
relief of obstruction
No
Is patient a candidate for ablative therapy?
Yes
Operative vs nonoperative bypass
G.
Laparoscopy
No metastases
Consider possible resection, Angiogram and/or CT portography if resectability in question
H.
Ablative Therapy
Consider adjuvant therapy

changes in bowel habits that suggest a colon neoplasm or back pain due to pancreatic cancer. Weight loss is a frequent presenting complaint that accompanies the jaundice of malignant biliary obstruction. An unintended 10–15% reduction in the patient's body weight suggests malignancy until proven otherwise.

A properly and thoroughly performed physical examination may reveal important findings, either obvious or subtle. Abdominal masses and enlarged lymph nodes should be sought as well as ascites and cutaneous manifestations of liver disease (e.g., cutaneous venous collaterals, spider hemangiomas). An assessment of the patient's overall nutritional and physiologic status is important. Cholangitis is not a common initial presentation of malignant biliary obstruction. However, localized or intense abdominal pain, fever, or hemodynamic instability may signal biliary sepsis requiring urgent evaluation and treatment.

Laboratory Studies

Jaundice is defined as abnormal yellow discoloration of the skin, sclera, and mucous membranes resulting from hyperbilirubinemia. For jaundice to be detected clinically, a serum bilirubin concentration of more than 3 mg/dl must usually be present. The perceived intensity of clinical jaundice does not correlate with the serum bilirubin concentration, although a deeply jaundiced patient typically has pronounced hyperbilirubinemia. Subclinical hyperbilirubinemia in a cancer patient must also be investigated even if the patient is asymptomatic.

Laboratory studies are often revealing in jaundiced patients. A minimum battery of laboratory evaluations is shown in Table 73–1. These basic studies help discriminate between cholestatic, hemolytic, and hepatocellular jaundice. Additional studies, such as a reticulocyte count and peripheral blood smear, may help confirm a suspicion of hemolysis; and hepatitis panels, blood alcohol content, serum drug levels, and sickle cell preparations are appropriate in select patients.

Most cancer patients present with cholestatic jaundice characterized by conjugated hyperbilirubinemia. Elevated serum alkaline phosphatase levels, which are typical of cholestatic jaundice, result from increased synthesis and release of the enzyme primarily at the canalicular membrane of the hepatocyte. Liver transaminase elevations result from the hepatocellular injury that can occur with cholestasis; extreme or isolated transaminase elevations suggest causes other than obstructive biliary tract disease. Albumin and coagulation studies are quick, inexpensive measures of hepatic synthetic function.

TABLE 73–1.
Minimum laboratory evaluation of the jaundiced cancer patient

Complete blood count
Liver enzyme profile
Fractionated bilirubin
Alkaline phosphatase
Transaminases (AST/ALT)
Total protein
Albumin
Prothrombin and partial thromboplastin times

Myriad serum chemistries and tumor markers are available to investigate biliary, hepatic, and pancreatic diseases in the jaundiced cancer patient; some are practical [serum amylase, carcinoembryonic antigen (CEA), CA 19-9], and some are rather esoteric (anti-mitochondrial antibodies for primary biliary cirrhosis). However, most jaundiced cancer patients manifest a cholestatic picture of conjugated hyperbilirubinemia with variable degrees of elevation of serum alkaline phosphatase, γ-glutamyl transferase (GGT), and serum leucine aminopeptidase (SLAP). The minimal laboratory evaluation identifying these findings is usually sufficient evidence to proceed to imaging studies.

Imaging

Transabdominal ultrasonography (US) should be the initial imaging study in most jaundiced patients. US is highly accurate for evaluating cholestatic jaundice and specifically for detecting the presence and level of biliary obstruction.[1] The gallbladder, intrahepatic and extrahepatic bile ducts, liver, and usually the pancreas can be evaluated. US is excellent for documenting cholelithiasis and hepatic masses. Transabdominal US is not particularly reliable for visualizing the intrapancreatic common bile duct, and technical factors sometimes limit sonographic imaging of the pancreas. US is often the only imaging study required for benign conditions and usually provides useful information regarding malignant diseases. Accurate imaging, patient tolerance, the absence of radiation exposure, and low cost make US the preferred initial imaging test for obstructive jaundice.

Computed tomography (CT) is as reliable as US for identifying the level of biliary obstruction but provides a more comprehensive evaluation of the liver, biliary tree, pancreas, portal and retroperitoneal lymph nodes, vascular structures, and the rest of the abdominal viscera and retroperitoneum.[2] CT is the screening test of choice for evaluating the liver in patients with a history of cancer; it has a sensitivity approaching 85% for detecting the presence of metastatic lesions.[3] Primary liver tumors are perfused through the hepatic arterial system and may therefore be delineated more effectively with CT arterial portography. By administering contrast via the superior mesenteric or splenic artery during dynamic CT scanning, the liver supplied by the portal vein is preferentially enhanced. The sensitivity for detecting individual liver lesions is therefore improved.[4] In general, CT portography and angiography should be reserved for cases in which vascular involvement would change therapy and is suspected but cannot be excluded by conventional CT alone.

The role of magnetic resonance imaging (MRI) continues to evolve in the area of hepatobiliary and pancreatic imaging. Both CT and US have lower sensitivities in patients with fatty infiltration of the liver. Therefore in this group of patients and in the case of iodinated contrast allergy, MRI should be considered for diagnostic and screening examinations. With the addition of gadolinium and ferritin enhancement, MRI provides additional sensitivity and specificity for atypical liver lesions. MR cholangiopancreatography (MRCP) holds great promise for imaging neoplastic pancreaticobiliary obstruction. The initial experience with single-shot fast spin-echo MRCP has been encouragingly accurate for identifying the level of obstruction as well as the site and extent of underlying tumor while avoiding the potential complications of traditional cholangiography[5] (sepsis, bleeding, bile leak, death).[6,7] Sensitivity and specificity rates of 90% and 100%, respectively, have been demonstrated for MRCP in the detection of benign biliary obstruction (choledocholithiasis) as well.[8] With further refinements and increased availability in the future, MRCP may become the imaging modality of choice in the jaundiced patient.

The evolution of endoscopy of the pancreaticobiliary system has had a major impact on the evaluation and management of the jaundiced patient. Endoscopic retrograde cholangiopancreatography (ERCP) is now widely available and successful in more than 96% of patients in whom it is attempted. Although ERCP is an invasive procedure, major complications are rare (1% or less) and are fewer than those seen with percutaneous transhepatic cholangiography (PTC). More recently, the development of endoscopic ultrasonography (EUS) probes has enhanced the ability to assess the distal bile duct, pancreas, and peripancreatic and periportal areas. EUS has been particularly useful for detecting small pancreatic tumors not seen by other modalities and as an adjunct to CT for assessing vascular invasion.

Diagnostic and therapeutic options available at the time of ERCP include endoscopic sphincterotomy (ERCP/ES), clearance of common bile duct (CBD) stones, retrieval of brush cytology specimens, needle biopsy for the pathology diagnosis, and stenting of obstructing lesions. ERCP/ES and endobiliary stenting has proved invaluable in the management of benign bile duct obstruction and for palliation of unresectable malignant disease. Endoscopic stenting for patients with potentially resectable malignancies is a much debated issue.

B. *Nonobstructive Jaundice*

Nonobstructive jaundice in the cancer patient is usually the result of diffuse infiltration of the liver with tumor or therapy-related liver failure. Cytotoxic agents often affect liver function, as do nutritional deficiencies and occasionally parenteral nutrition. Offending agents should obviously be removed and supportive treatment instituted, but few interventions reverse the jaundice of this late-stage liver failure.

C. *Biliary Calculus Disease*

Cholelithiasis is at least as common in cancer patients as in the general population and may be more frequent owing to the lithogenic effects of blood transfusions, therapy-related hemolysis, and cholestasis due to limited oral intake, parenteral nutrition, or drugs. The approach to the cancer patient with symptomatic calculus disease should be no different than the approach to any other patient based on their physiologic status. Definitive treatment requires cholecystectomy and evaluation of the CBD for clearance. Preoperative ERCP is appropriate for jaundiced patients and is important for identifying whether obstruction is related to stones or malignancy, as the management may be quite different. Laparoscopic cholecystectomy is the standard treatment, although it is not possible in some patients with extensive prior upper abdominal surgery. For patients with jaundice due to choledocholithiasis who are not fit for surgery or whose life expectancy from cancer is limited, endoscopic therapy alone suffices. Alternatively, percutaneous methods of decompressing the bile duct may be considered.

D. *Tissue Diagnosis*

Although sometimes helpful, tissue diagnosis is not a prerequisite to further intervention in the evaluation of jaundiced cancer patients. Several techniques are available to obtain specimens, including percutaneous fine-needle aspiration (FNA) or biopsy (CT- or US-guided), endoscopic biopsy or brushing, bile sampling (percutaneously or endoscopically), laparoscopic biopsy, and open biopsy. The need for tissue diagnosis is best discussed in terms of the location of the suspect lesion.

Liver Lesions

The resectability of hepatocellular malignancies and some metastatic tumors in the liver is determined by the location, size, and multiplicity of lesions and by underlying hepatic function. Biopsy is important for newly diagnosed liver masses if their benign nature cannot be established by imaging characteristics. Most of these lesions are accessible by the percutaneous route aided by CT or US guidance. Occasionally, laparoscopic or open biopsy is indicated. For patients with known or previously treated malignancy, the appearance of new liver lesions consistent with metastasis does not necessarily require biopsy prior to intervention. Rather, these patients require assessment for the presence of any extrahepatic disease prior to planning therapy.

Bile Duct Lesions

Differentiating benign from malignant bile duct strictures is often a challenging task. It is in this arena that excessive effort is sometimes applied. Endobiliary sampling is technically difficult, with sensitivities in the rage of 35–43% for cytology and biopsy.[9] Combining cytology and biopsy improves diagnostic sensitivity, but bleeding, perforation, and tumor seeding are significant concerns. Biopsy, whether percutaneous or endoscopic, should not be condoned for suspicious lesions that are amenable to surgical extirpation in good risk patients. However, for patients with indeterminate lesions of the bile ducts, at high risk for surgical complications, or with unresectable lesions, tissue diagnosis utilizing endoscopic, percutaneous, or (rarely) surgical biopsy may be appropriate for guiding other nonsurgical therapy.

Pancreatic Lesions

Tissue diagnosis is rarely indicated prior to surgical intervention for pancreatic tumors. When history and imaging studies suggest resectable pancreatic cancer in a good risk patient, preoperative tissue sampling should not be performed. Regardless of its accuracy, it is unnecessary and does not alter the operative plan. Moreover, occasional complications or tumor seeding as the result of unnecessary percutaneous biopsy can prohibit potentially curative resection.

Rarely, the clinical setting and imaging studies suggest pancreatic lymphoma or metastatic disease to the pancreas. In these cases and in the case of obvious unresectable lesions or surgically unfit patients, attempts at tissue diagnosis may be appropriate. However, even for unresectable pancreatic cancer, percutaneous biopsy is not indicated if the patient is best treated by surgical bypass of the biliary or duodenal obstruction.

Metastatic Lesions

In the case of prior malignancy and suspected metastatic lesions presenting as jaundice, it is advisable to obtain tissue to confirm the diagnosis if it is the only known site of the patient's disease. In the rare case of resectable metastatic disease presenting as jaundice, lack of tissue diagnosis should not preclude a potentially curable resection.

E. Benign Common Bile Duct Strictures

Malignant bile duct obstruction should never be excluded based on negative cytology or tissue biopsy. The diagnosis of a benign biliary stricture is based on the patient's clinical course, which should include a logical explanation for benign rather than malignant disease, and on imaging features. The most common cause of benign stricture is previous operative injury. Other etiologies include chronic pancreatitis, stone disease with cholangitis, sclerosing cholangitis, irradiation, and hepatic arterial chemotherapy. Endoscopic methods to deal with benign CBD strictures include dilatation and endobiliary stent placement. Although quite successful at initial decompression, endobiliary stents have a finite patency rate requiring replacement every few months and a higher likelihood of recurrent cholangitis and stricture recurrence. Surgical bypass has been shown to be a more durable means of decompression. Therefore in patients who are able to tolerate an abdominal operation and who have a proposed survival of more than 1 year, surgical bypass should be considered in favor of endoscopic stenting.

F. Malignant Cytology

Extrahepatic Metastatic Lesions

As a rule, extrahepatic metastatic disease is not amenable to resection or cure. These patients generally have a limited life expectancy and should therefore undergo palliation with this in mind.

Intrahepatic Metastatic Lesions

The approach to intrahepatic metastatic lesions depends on the primary cancer, the location and size of the hepatic lesions, the presence or absence of metastatic disease outside the liver, and underlying hepatic function. Most cancer patients with jaundice have hepatocellular dysfunction, extensive metastases throughout the liver, or simultaneous extrahepatic disease, in contrast to isolated obstructing lesions. However, several tumors are amenable to resection or ablative procedures when the extent of involvement is limited. Refer to chapters on specific malignancies for further information.

Primary Intrahepatic Malignancy

Primary intrahepatic malignancies include hepatocellular carcinoma (HCC), cholangiocarcinoma, hepatoblastoma, and rarely sarcoma or mesenchymoma. The only curative therapy is complete surgical resection. In most cases this requires an anatomic resection in the form of lobectomy, extended lobectomy, or various segmentectomies. Partial resection, re-resection, and cytoreductive procedures have shown some benefit in terms of survival.[10] Criteria for resection are becoming more liberal.[11] Unfortunately, HCC most often occurs in the presence of cirrhosis, which precludes a complete, safe resection. Transplantation may be appropriate for selected patients with small HCCs and decompensated liver function.[12] A combination of chemotherapy and irradiation has been effective in reducing tumor size, improving survival, and making some lesions amenable to resection.

Primary Extrahepatic Malignancy

Periampullary tumors may be of pancreatic, biliary, ampullary, or duodenal origin. Refer to chapters on these tumors for additional information.

TABLE 73–2.
Metastatic liver lesions amenable to resection or ablation

Colon adenocarcinoma
Neuroendocrine malignancies
Desmoid tumors
Sarcomas
Melanoma
Ovarian carcinoma
Renal cell carcinoma

G. Laparoscopy

For malignant biliary obstruction considered resectable based on preoperative imaging, laparoscopy has decreased the rate of nontherapeutic laparotomy by detecting unresectable disease in 20–40% of cases.[13,14] If patients are candidates for endoscopic stenting and do not have duodenal obstruction, laparoscopic staging may avoid laparotomy. On the other hand, if one believes that surgical bypass of a biliary or duodenal obstruction provides the best palliation for a patient with unresectable cancer, there is little rationale for performing laparoscopy prior to laparotomy. Skilled laparoscopic surgeons can perform laparoscopic biliary and duodenal bypass procedures in this situation.[15,16]

H. Ablative Therapy

Most patients with intrahepatic malignant disease have unresectable tumors. Several ablative therapies have shown promise for eradicating or palliating unresectable liver malignancies. A major theoretical advantage of all of the ablative methods is the possibility of rendering patients tumor-free while sparing uninvolved hepatic parenchyma. A number of liver tumors have been treated by ablative approaches.

Cryotherapy has attracted much interest owing to the improved methods of delivering ablative hypothermia. The largest experience with this technique is for the treatment of colorectal hepatic metastases. There are anecdotal reports of other tumor types treated with this technology as well (Table 73–2). Improved survival compared to nonablative therapy and destruction of lesions not amenable to surgical resection has been demonstrated with only a 10% local failure rate at 5 years.[17] Cryosurgery is usually performed during laparotomy, but laparoscopic applications are being developed. Long-term data are needed to confirm the role of cryotherapy in the treatment of selected patients with unresectable liver tumors.

Thermal ablation using low power lasers or radiofrequency energy sources has shown promise in experimental models of solid organ tumors and is being actively investigated clinically.[18] High-intensity focused ultrasound can ablate selected tissue targets in the liver without requiring surgical exposure.[19] This technique is now being applied to human models but is still experimental.

Percutaneous ethanol injection yields survival results comparable to those in matched patients who underwent partial hepatectomy for small HCCs but has produced far less encouraging results in the treatment of hepatic metastases.[20] It therefore has a limited role in managing patients with hepatic tumors.

I. Palliation

A large proportion of cancer patients who present with jaundice have incurable disease and limited life expectancy at presentation. Additionally, many potentially curable lesions require complex operations that may be prohibitive to elderly or debilitated patients. A number of interventions are available to provide relief of biliary obstruction, improve the quality of life, and even extend survival in some instances. Relief of biliary obstruction is advisable in most if not all scenarios, as decompression can relieve the symptoms of jaundice, notably pruritus, anorexia, and malaise. The route of decompression (percutaneous, endoscopic, surgical) must be chosen on an individual basis with regard to the site of obstruction, the patient's condition, and expected survival. In general, the disadvantages of surgical intervention are related to the perioperative mortality and morbidity. Most series of palliative operations for obstructive jaundice report mortality rates near 10%, but these operations have fewer subsequent hospitalizations for cholangitis and recurrent jaundice than after percutaneous or endoscopic procedures, which may require stent or catheter changes.

Operative versus Nonoperative Biliary Bypass

Several factors influence the decision to perform nonoperative or surgical bypass for unresectable pancreatic cancer causing biliary obstruction. Patient-related factors include overall health status, co-morbid conditions, and expected survival; procedure-related factors include mortality and morbidity.[21] It has been shown that surgical bypass is superior to endoscopic or percutaneous biliary drainage with regard to the success and durability of the biliary decompression with a trend toward improved survival.[22] Simultaneous duodenal bypass can be performed for concomitant or impending duodenal obstruction in selected patients, negating the need for additional procedures later in the course of the disease. In cases of limited life expectancy and patient factors prohibiting major surgery, endoscopic and percutaneous routes of biliary drainage are acceptably effective and continue to evolve with the introduction of new stent technology.[23] Cost advantages have been proposed in favor of endoscopic decompression but tend to favor surgery when patient survival is extended and when more expensive stent materials are used.[24]

Biliary obstruction from unresectable bile duct carcinoma can be relieved by both surgical and nonoperative methods. The variety of presentations with regard to the location of the obstruction make it important to individualize the approach to these patients. Intrahepatic segment III biliary-enteric bypass has been demonstrated to provide excellent palliation with relatively few late complications and minimal morbidity and mortality in patients with hilar lesions.[25] However, limited life expectancy and diffuse disease at presentation in most patients with cholangiocarcinoma favor less invasive procedures. Internal biliary drainage utilizing endoscopic or combined endoscopic-radiologic techniques can provide effective palliation without the hindrance of external drainage devices.[26]

Endoscopic versus Percutaneous Biliary Drainage

In general, the rates of successful biliary drainage for malignant obstructive jaundice are similar for both endoscopic and percutaneous interventions. An endoscopic approach is preferred for distal bile duct obstruction but has a lower success rate for proximal obstruction. Procedural complication rates may be lower for endoscopic interventions.

Special Considerations

Routine *preoperative biliary drainage* does not decrease the risk of subsequent surgery for patients with malignant biliary obstruction. In fact, endoscopic stent decompression of malignant biliary obstruction has been associated with an increase in postoperative infectious complications in patients with periampullary cancer.[27,28] Biliary stenting should therefore be considered a palliative procedure in this group of patients, limited to those who are not operative candidates due to the extent of the disease, the inability to tolerate a major operation, or in the case of obstructive cholangitis.

References

1. Weltman DI, Zeman RK. Acute diseases of the gallbladder and bile ducts. Radiol Clin North Am 1994;32:933–950.
2. Gulliver DJ, Baker ME, Cheng CA, Meyers WC, Pappas TN. Malignant biliary obstruction: efficacy of thin section dynamic CT in determining resectability. AJR Am J Roentgenol 1992;159:503–507.
3. Baker ME, Pelley R. Hepatic metastases: basic principles and implications for radiologists. Radiology 1995;197:329–337.
4. Nelson RC, Chezmar JL, Sugarbaker PH, Bernardino ME. Hepatic tumors: comparison of CT during arterial portography, delayed CT, and MR imaging for preoperative evaluation. Radiology 1989;172:27–34.
5. Schwartz LH, Coakley FV, Sun Y, Blimgart LH, Fong Y, Panicek DM. Neoplastic pancreaticobiliary duct obstruction: evaluation with breathhold MR cholangiopancreatography. AJR Am J Roentgenol 1998;170:1491–1495.
6. Bilboa MK, Dotter CT, Lee TG, Katon RM. Complications of retrograde cholangiography (ERCP): a study of 10,000 cases. Gastroenterology 1976; 70:314–320.
7. Harbin WP, Mueller P, Ferrucci JT. Transhepatic cholangiography: complications and use pattern of the fine needle technique. Radiology 1980; 135:15–22.
8. Reinhold C, Bret PM. Current status of MR cholangiography. AJR Am J Roentgenol 1996;166:1285–1295.
9. Ponchon T, Gagnon P, Berger F, et al. Value of endobiliary brush cytology and biopsies for the diagnosis of malignant bile duct stenosis: results of a prospective study. Gastrointest Endosc 1995;42:565–572.
10. Tang ZY. Treatment of hepatocellular carcinoma. Digestion 1998;59: 556–562.
11. Nagasue N. Liver resection for hepatocellular carcinoma: indications, techniques, complications, and prognostic factors. J Hepatobiliary Pancreat Surg 1998;5:7–13.
12. Olthof KM. Surgical options for hepatocellular carcinoma: resection and transplantation. Liver Transpl Surg 1998;4(suppl 1):S98–S104.
13. Cushieri A. Laparoscopy for pancreatic cancer: does it benefit the patient? Eur J Surg Oncol 1988;14:41–44.
14. Warshaw AL, Tepper JE, Shipley WU. Laparoscopy in the staging and planning of therapy for pancreatic cancer. Am J Surg 1986;151:76–80.
15. Targarona EM, Pera M, Martinez J, et al. Laparoscopic treatment of pancreatic disorders: diagnosis and staging, palliation of cancer and treatment of pancreatic pseudocysts. Int Surg 1996;81:1–5.
16. Raj PK, Mahoney P, Linderman C. Laparoscopic cholecystojejunostomy: a technical application in unresectable biliary obstruction. J Laparoendosc Adv Surg Tech A 1997;7:47–52.
17. Ravikumar TS, Cane R, Cady B, et al. A 5-year study of cryosurgery in the treatment of liver tumors. Arch Surg 1991;126:1520–1524.
18. Krasner N. Palliative laser therapy for tumors of the gastrointestinal tract. Baillieres Clin Gastroenterol 1991;5:37–59.
19. Yang R, Sanghvi NT, Rescorla FJ, Kopecky KK, Grosfeld JL. Liver cancer ablation with extracorporeal high-intensity focused ultrasound. Eur Urol 1993;23(suppl 1):17–22.
20. Bartolozzi C, Lencioni R. Ethanol injection for the treatment of hepatic tumors. Eur Radiol 1996;6:682–696.
21. Shumate CR, Baron TH. Palliative procedures for pancreatic cancer: when and which one? South Med J 1996;89:27–32.
22. Deziel DJ, Wilhelmi B, Staren ED, Doolas A. Surgical palliation for ductal adenocarcinoma of the pancreas. Am Surg 1996;62:582–588.
23. Lichtenstein DR, Carr-Locke DL. Endoscopic palliation for unresectable pancreatic carcinoma. Surg Clin North Am 1995;75:969–988.
24. Raikar GV, Melin MM, Ress A, Lettieri SZ. Cost-effective analysis of surgical palliation versus endoscopic stenting in the management of unresectable pancreatic cancer. Ann Surg Oncol 1996;3:470–475.

25. Jarnagin WR, Burk E, Powers C, Fong Y, Blumgart LH. Intrahepatic biliary enteric bypass provides effective palliation in selected patients with malignant obstruction at the hepatic duct confluence. Am J Surg 1998;175: 453–460.
26. Kuvshinoff BW, Armstrong JG, Fong Y, et al. Palliation of irresectable hilar cholangiocarcinoma with biliary drainage and radiotherapy. Br J Surg 1995;82:1522–1525.
27. Pitt HA, Gomes AS, Lois JF, et al. Does preoperative percutaneous biliary drainage reduce operative risk or increase hospital cost? Ann Surg 1985; 201:545–552.
28. McPherson GAD, Benjamin IS, Hodgson HJF, et al. Preoperative percutaneous transhepatic biliary drainage: the results of a controlled trial. Br J Surg 1984;71:371–375.

CHAPTER 74

Adnexal Masses

MARIE WELSHINGER

A. Epidemiology

Every female at birth has a 5–7% lifetime risk of developing an ovarian neoplasm and a 1.4% lifetime risk of developing a malignant ovarian tumor. The ovary can produce a diversity of tumors with respect to both histologic structure and biologic behavior. Evaluation of an adnexal mass represents a significant clinical challenge when one considers both gynecologic and nongynecologic possibilities (Table 74–1).

B. Histology

The classification of ovarian neoplasms is based on the presumed cell of origin, and these lesions are therefore categorized histologically into three major categories (Table 74–2). Tumors arising from the *coelomic epithelium* (or mesothelium) covering the ovary account for 60–70% of all ovarian neoplasms. The epithelial ovarian carcinomas comprise 90% of all ovarian cancers. Tumors arising from the specialized gonadal stroma (*sex cord-stromal tumors*) include the theca and granulosa cells, the Sertoli-Leydig cells, and their precursors. Some include the lipoid cell tumors in this category. The sex cord-stromal groups each account for 5–10% of ovarian neoplasms and comprise about 7% of all ovarian malignancies. Tumors arising from *germ cells* arise from unfertilized ovum and are composed of tissue representing the cell of origin (dysgerminoma), extraembryonic tissue (yolk sac, trophoblast), embryonic tissue (polyembryoma, immature teratoma), or adult tissue (dermoid cyst, monodermal teratoma). Gonadoblastomas can also be included in this category. Although 20–25% of ovarian neoplasms are germ cell in origin, they comprise only 5% of ovarian malignancies.

C. Diagnosis

In a female patient with an adnexal mass, the goals of preoperative evaluation and diagnostic workup are aimed at excluding nongynecologic causes, determining one's level of suspicion of ovarian malignancy, and preparing the patient for exploratory surgery. Although there are usually no early symptoms

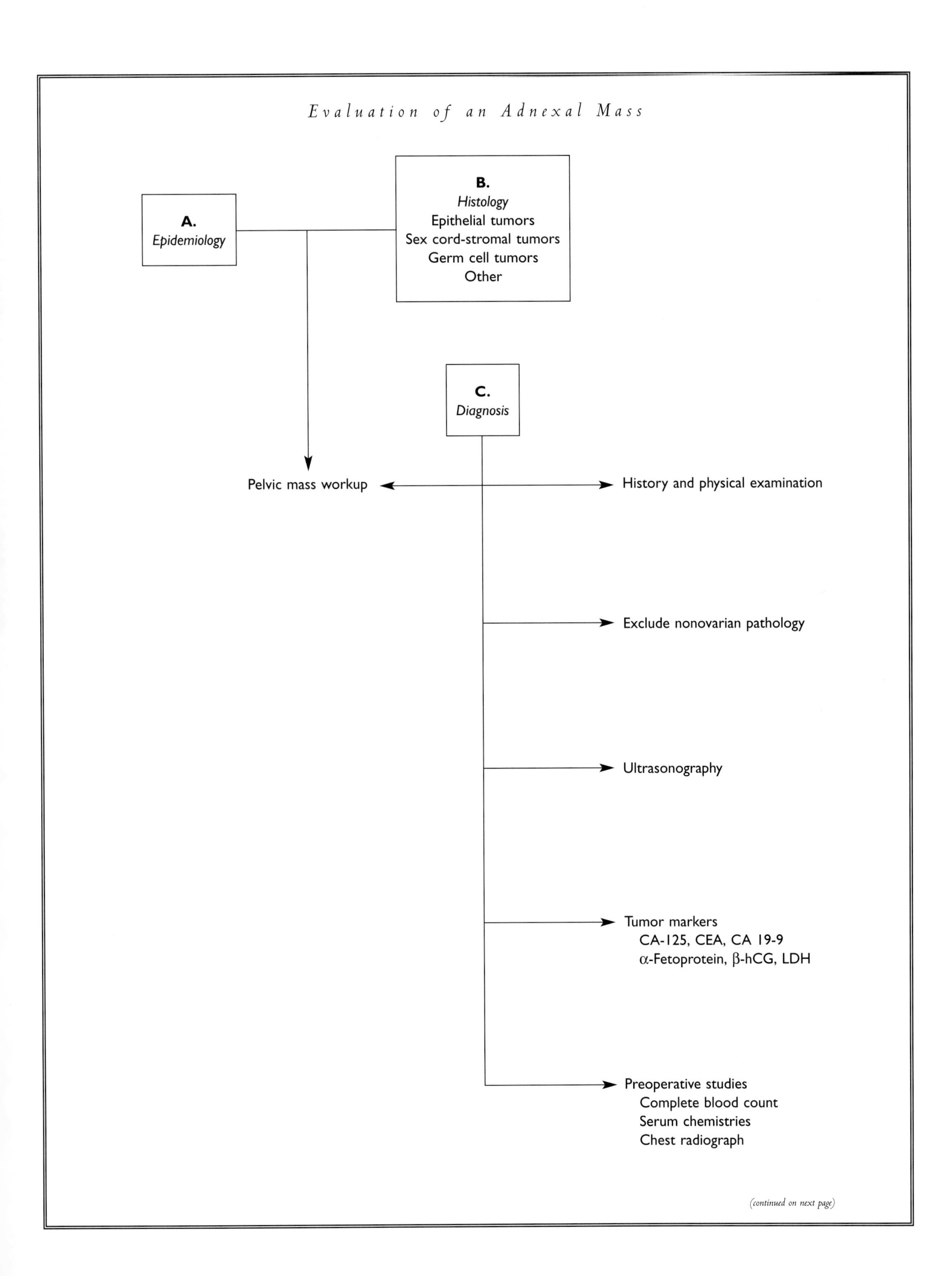

(continued on next page)

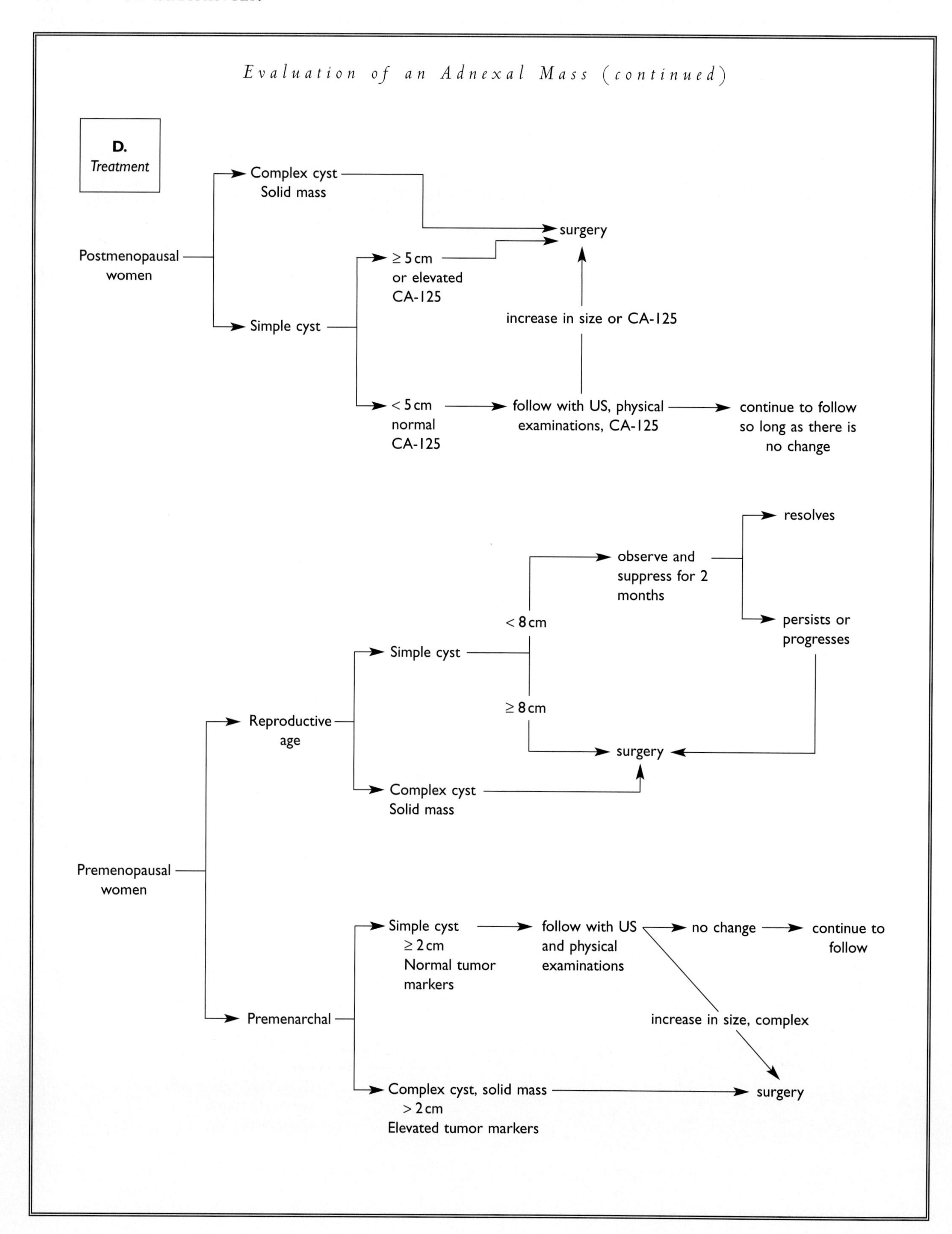
Evaluation of an Adnexal Mass (continued)
D.
Treatment
Postmenopausal women
Complex cyst
Solid mass
surgery
≥ 5 cm
or elevated
CA-125
Simple cyst
increase in size or CA-125
< 5 cm
normal
CA-125
follow with US, physical examinations, CA-125
continue to follow so long as there is no change
resolves
observe and suppress for 2 months
< 8 cm
persists or progresses
Simple cyst
Reproductive age
≥ 8 cm
surgery
Complex cyst
Solid mass
Premenopausal women
Simple cyst
≥ 2 cm
Normal tumor markers
follow with US and physical examinations
no change
continue to follow
Premenarchal
increase in size, complex
Complex cyst, solid mass
> 2 cm
Elevated tumor markers
surgery

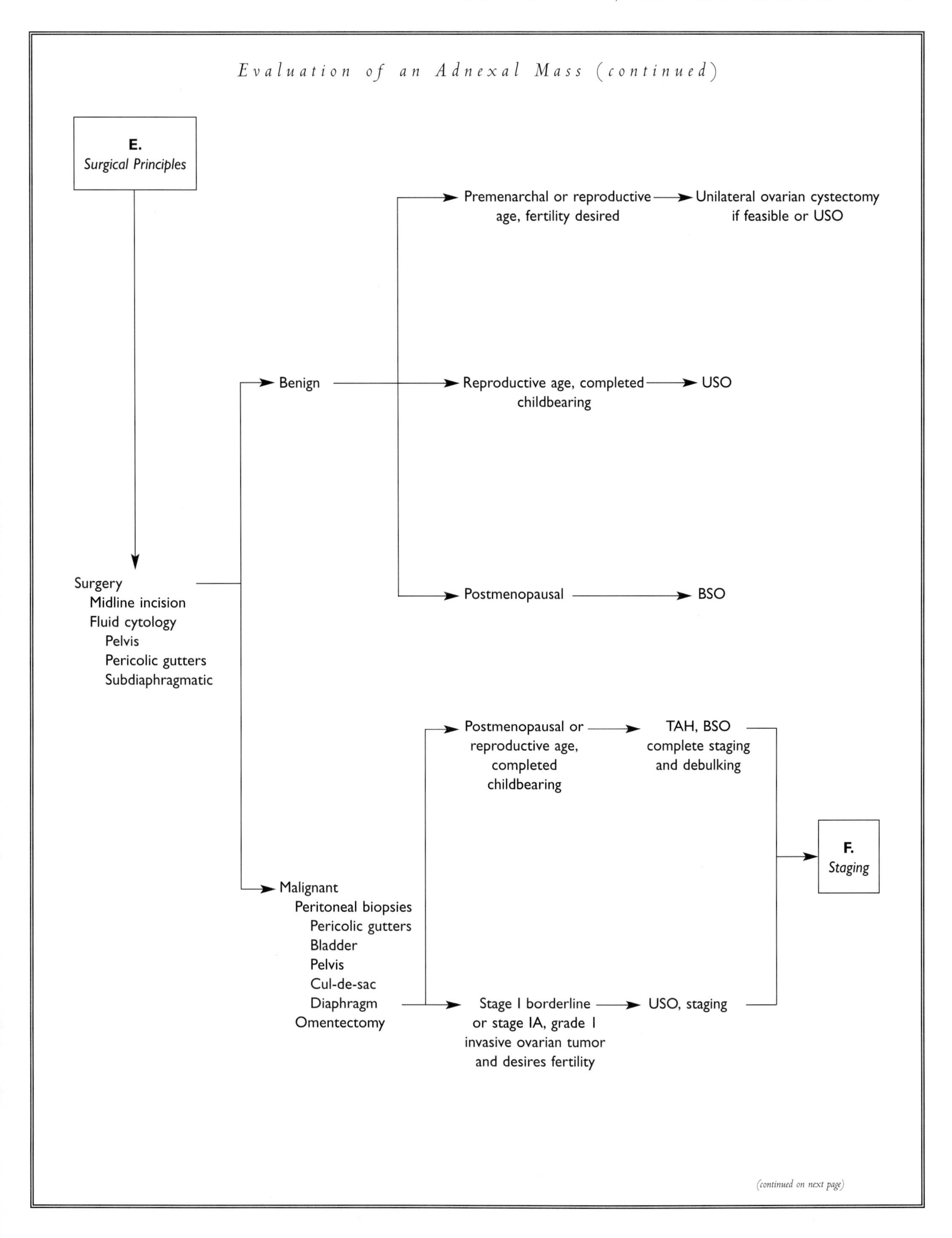

(continued on next page)

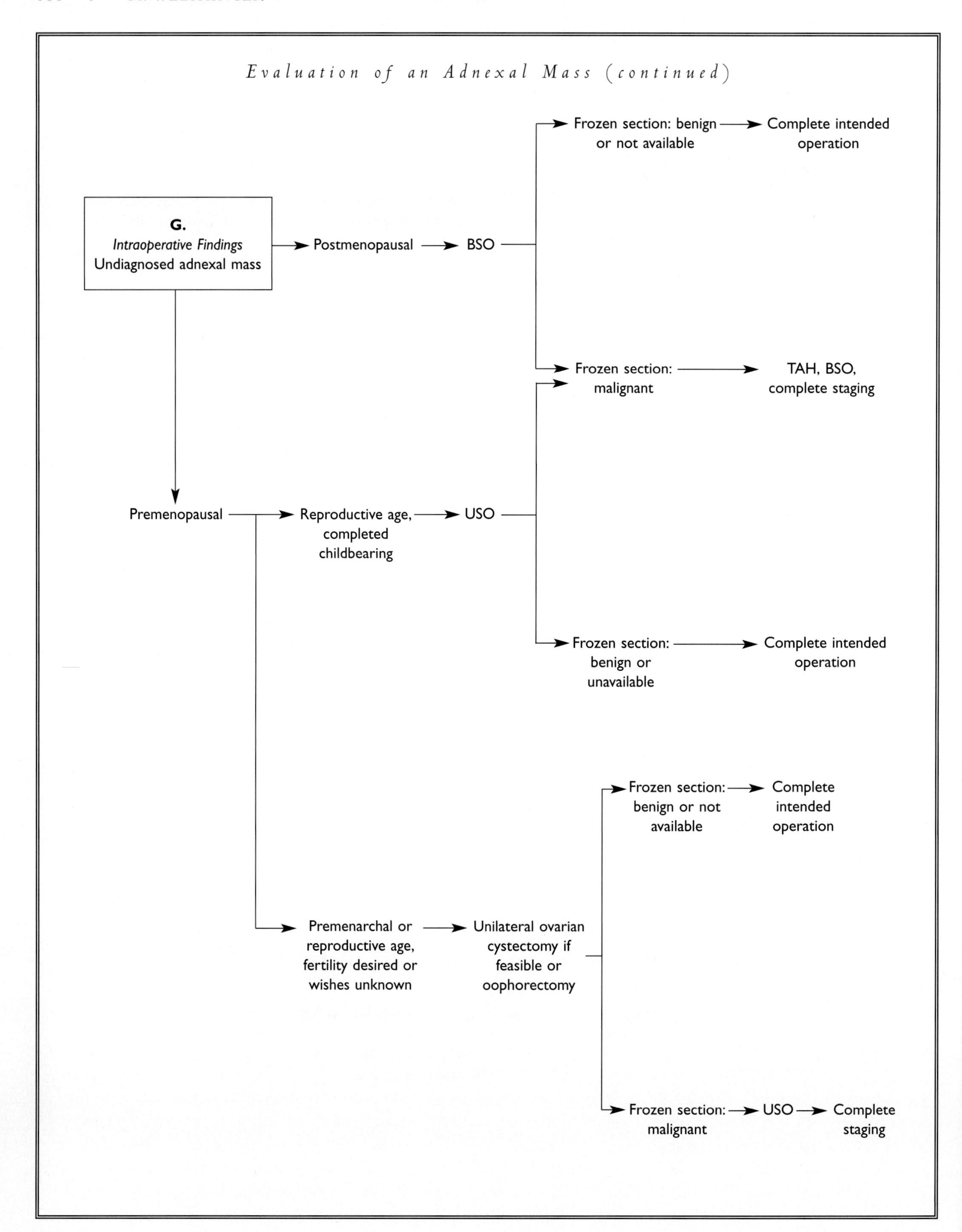
Evaluation of an Adnexal Mass (continued)
G.
Intraoperative Findings
Undiagnosed adnexal mass
Postmenopausal
BSO
Frozen section: benign or not available
Complete intended operation
Frozen section: malignant
TAH, BSO, complete staging
Premenopausal
Reproductive age, completed childbearing
USO
Frozen section: benign or unavailable
Complete intended operation
Premenarchal or reproductive age, fertility desired or wishes unknown
Unilateral ovarian cystectomy if feasible or oophorectomy
Frozen section: benign or not available
Complete intended operation
Frozen section: malignant
USO
Complete staging

TABLE 74–1.
Differential diagnosis of an adnexal mass

Etiology	Neoplastic	Nonneoplastic
Ovary	Primary ovarian neoplasm (benign or malignant)	Endometriosis
Fallopian tube	Primary tubal neoplasm	Tuboovarian abscess Hydrosalpinx Paraovarian cyst Ectopic pregnancy
Uterus	Pedunculated or interligamentous myoma	Intrauterine pregnancy in a bicornuate uterus
Bowel	Primary appendiceal or colon neoplasm Primary small bowel neoplasm	Appendiceal abscess Crohn's disease Diverticular abscess
Miscellaneous	Lymphoma	Abdominal wall hematoma or abscess
	Mesothelial tumor Retroperitoneal neoplasm Urachal cyst	Anterior sacral meningocele Distended bladder Pelvic kidney

of ovarian cancer, a thorough history may reveal symptoms associated with increasing tumor mass, peritoneal or bowel serosal spread of tumor, ascites, or a pleural effusion. It is important to consider the patient's age, as the risk of ovarian cancer is significantly higher in premenarchal and postmenopausal women with an adnexal mass than in women of reproductive age.

The *physical examination* must include both bimanual (pelvic) and rectovaginal examinations. Findings such as bilaterality, irregular contours, immobility, or solid consistency are suggestive of malignancy, as are ascites and nodularity in the posterior cul-de-sac.

Other primary cancers metastatic to the ovary should be excluded. A barium enema or colonoscopy is indicated in symptomatic patients and perhaps in asymptomatic patients over the age of 45 to exclude a primary colonic lesion with ovarian involvement. These tests may also be useful for determining the likelihood that a large bowel resection with or without colostomy or ileostomy (or both) will be needed. Any patient with occult blood in the stool or symptoms of intestinal obstruction should also have her colon examined. Evaluation of the upper gastrointestinal tract should be considered on the basis of symptoms or the presence of bilateral solid ovarian tumors such as might occur with metastatic gastric carcinoma.[2,3] Chest radiography should be undertaken preoperatively to detect pleural effusions or metastatic disease. Intravenous urography may be indicated to define the course of the ureters or exclude the rare pelvic kidney. If the patient has not been previously screened, mammography is indicated. A palpable breast mass must be evaluated, as breast cancer can metastasize to the ovaries. Cervical cytology should be obtained, although its value for detecting ovarian cancer is limited. Patients with irregular menses or postmenopausal bleeding should have an endometrial biopsy and endocervical curettage.

Ultrasonography (US) can distinguish ovarian masses as being solid or cystic and can further evaluate cystic masses according to the absence (simple) or presence (complex) of mural nodularity, septations, and internal echoes. Transvaginal imaging has been proposed as a more specific alternative to abdominal sonography.[4,5] Additional information with respect to lymph node or liver metastases may be obtained from computed tomography (CT) with oral and intravenous contrast or magnetic resonance imaging (MRI). However, imaging studies cannot replace exploratory surgery, pathologic evaluation of the mass, or thorough surgical staging. Clinically, a solid tumor is always considered neoplastic, and the etiology of a simple cystic tumor can range from a physiologic follicle or corpus luteum cyst to an early borderline or frankly invasive ovarian carcinoma. The solid or complex composition of teratomas and epithelial ovarian tumors suggests malignancy, although both can present as a simple cyst, and both have benign and malignant counterparts. Thus gross features may be important to the clinician during the process of making

TABLE 74–2.
Modified World Health Organization comprehensive classification of ovarian tumors

- I. Common "epithelial tumors"
  - Serous, Mucinous, Endometrioid, Clear cell, Brenner, Mixed epithelial — *benign, borderline, or malignant*
  - Undifferentiated
  - Mixed mesodermal tumors
  - Unclassified
- II. Sex cord-stromal tumors
  - A. Granulosa stromal cell
    - 1. Granulosa cell
    - 2. Thecoma-fibroma
  - B. Androblastomas; Sertoli-Leydig cell tumors
    - 1. Well differentiated
    - 2. Intermediate differentiation
    - 3. Poorly differentiated
    - 4. With heterologous elements
  - C. Lipid cell tumors
  - D. Gynandroblastoma
  - E. Unclassified
- III. Germ cell tumors
  - A. Dysgerminoma
  - B. Endodermal sinus tumor
  - C. Embryonal cell carcinoma
  - E. Choriocarcinoma
  - F. Teratomas
    - 1. Immature
    - 2. Mature (dermoid cyst)
    - 3. Monodermal (struma ovarii, carcinoid)
  - G. Mixed forms
  - H. Gonadoblastoma
- IV. Soft tissue tumors not specific to the ovary
- V. Unclassified tumors
- VI. Secondary (metastatic) tumors
- VII. Tumor-like conditions (e.g., pregnancy luteoma)

From: Morrow et al.,[1] with permission.

management decisions, but they do not provide the basis for definitive treatment.

Tumor markers may prove useful in the diagnosis and management of several types of ovarian tumor and should be assayed in patients suspected or known to have ovarian cancer (Table 74–3). CA-125 levels are elevated (>35 U/ml) in more than 80% of patients with nonmucinous epithelial ovarian carcinomas but only 1% of the normal population. Approximately half the patients with early-stage (I–II) ovarian cancer have elevated levels. In postmenopausal patients with a pelvic mass, CA-125 levels higher than 65 U/ml are predictive of malignancy in 75% of cases.[7] In premenopausal women, CA-125 can be confounding because of the many benign conditions associated with an elevated level. Endometriosis, leiomyomas, pelvic inflammatory disease, hepatitis or cirrhosis, and nonovarian malignancies can produce a high CA-125 level. *Serum CA 19-9* is potentially useful in patients with mucinous ovarian carcinomas, is often elevated in patients with malignant (immature) teratomas, and may be elevated in patients with mucinous tumors of the gastrointestinal tract.

Carcinoembryonic antigen (CEA) levels, although not specific for ovarian cancer, may be elevated in patients with ovarian cancer or alert the clinician to rule out colon, pancreatic, or breast cancer. During the workup of a patient with a confirmed adnexal mass, serum CA-125 and CEA assays are routinely recommended, and a CA 19-9 assay is occasionally helpful.

α-Fetoprotein (AFP), *β-human chorionic gonadotropin* (β-hCG), and *lactate dehydrogenase* (LDH) levels should be measured preoperatively in *young* patients with a cystic-solid or solid adnexal mass. Many germ cell tumors produce biologic markers, which may aid in the diagnosis of these tumors (Table 74–4). More importantly, elevated markers may be used to

TABLE 74–3.
Tumor markers in the management of ovarian neoplasms

Tumor marker	Types of tumor identified
CA-125	Nonmucinous epithelial ovarian carcinoma Can be elevated in malignant germ cell tumors
CA 19-9	Mucinous epithelial ovarian carcinoma Immature teratoma
Carcinoembryonic antigen	Mucinous epithelial ovarian carcinoma
α-Fetoprotein	Endodermal sinus tumor Embryonal cell carcinoma Mixed germ cell tumors
Human chorionic gonadotropin	Ovarian choriocarcinoma Embryonal cell carcinoma Mixed germ cell tumors
Lactate dehydrogenase	Dysgerminoma
Neuron-specific enolase	Dysgerminoma
Inhibin	Granulosa cell tumor

TABLE 74–4.
Serum tumor markers in malignant germ cell ovarian tumors

Histology	α-FP	β-hcg
Dysgerminoma	–	–
Embryonal carcinoma	+	+
Endodermal sinus tumor	+	–
Choriocarcinoma	–	+
Immature teratoma	–	–
Polyembryoma	+/–	+

monitor response to treatment or detect subclinical disease recurrence. Table 74–3 summarizes the various tumor markers and the neoplasms with which they are most likely to be associated.

D. Treatment

Once the diagnosis of an adnexal mass is confirmed the recommended course of action depends on the age and menopausal status of the patient and the physical and ultrasonographic findings. All postmenopausal women with an adnexal mass should undergo surgical exploration.

The one exception may be the patient with a normal CA-125 level and an asymptomatic unilocular cyst < 5 cm in diameter detected on US. In 1989 Goldstein et al. reported on 28 consecutive surgical specimens in postmenopausal patients, all with unilocular, unilateral ovarian cysts < 5 cm in maximum diameter, with no excrescences, septations, or ascites detected by transabdominal US. All were benign, and the authors concluded that serial US follow-up may be justified in the management of such patients.[8] Serial CA-125 determination is also recommended for following these patients.

Premenopausal patients are divided into two categories: premenarchal and reproductive age patients. For asymptomatic patients of reproductive age, simple, mobile, smooth-contoured, unilateral adnexal cysts < 8 cm can be followed for two cycles and reevaluated.[9] Hormonal suppression with a monophasic oral contraceptive may be used. A nonneoplastic lesion should regress, as measured by pelvic examination and US. If the mass is persistent, increases in size, or becomes complex in nature, it is presumed neoplastic and must be removed surgically. In women of reproductive age, any mass that is complex or has other findings consistent with malignancy (Table 74–5) should be surgically evaluated.

A premenarchal female with an adnexal mass measuring ≥2 cm usually requires surgical exploration.[10] Serum β-hCG and AFP titers, a complete blood count (CBC), and liver enzyme assays are necessary in young patients. A chest radiograph is important because germ cell tumors can metastasize to the lung or mediastinum. A karyotype should be obtained preoperatively on all premenarchal females because of the propensity of these tumors to arise in dysgenetic gonads. At the time of surgery, consideration must be given to the preservation of fertility whenever possible.

TABLE 74–5.
Frequent gross features favoring a diagnosis of benign versus malignant ovarian tumors

Benign	Malignant
Preoperative information	
Unilateral	Bilateral
Smooth surface	Excrescences on surface
Freely mobile	Fixed/adherent to adjacent structures
Ascites absent	Ascites present
Simple cystic	Complex cystic, solid, or partly solid, mural nodularity or thickening
Normal CA-125	Elevated CA-125 (postmenopausal patients)
Intraoperative and pathologic information	
Capsule intact	Capsule ruptured
Uniform appearance	Variegated
Entire tumor viable	Areas of hemorrhage and necrosis
Smooth cystic lining	Intracystic papillations or intramural nodules
Smooth peritoneal surface	Peritoneal implants

Once surgical removal is indicated, the type of approach (laparoscopy versus laparotomy) must be addressed. The role of laparoscopic surgery for adnexal masses is controversial, and the following guidelines should be followed. Preoperative clinical or US findings suspicious of malignancy (Table 74–4) should be managed by laparotomy. If laparoscopy is undertaken, a potentially neoplastic cyst should be removed intact, not biopsied or drained and left in situ. No cyst should intentionally be drained into the peritoneal cavity. Inspection of the entire abdomen and pelvis is obligatory. Visual or pathologic evidence of malignancy is an indication to convert to laparotomy.

E. Surgical Principles

For patients whose preoperative evaluation suggests malignancy, consultation with a gynecologic oncologist is recommended. To perform truly comprehensive staging, a midline abdominal incision is utilized to allow adequate access to the upper abdomen. Aspiration of ascites or peritoneal lavage is performed to obtain fluid for cytologic examination. Separate specimens are submitted from the pelvis, right and left pericolic gutters, and undersurfaces of the right and left hemidiaphragms. An encapsulated adnexal mass should be removed intact if possible. Rupture and spillage of malignant cells in the peritoneal cavity increases the stage of disease and may adversely affect prognosis. A 2-cm margin of infundibulopelvic ligament (ovarian vessel pedicle) is taken with the specimen.

If frozen section diagnosis indicates the presence of ovarian cancer, a complete staging procedure is indicated. Exploration in every case requires a systematic visual and palpatory examination of all intraabdominal surfaces and viscera, proceeding clockwise from the pelvic cul-de-sac to the cecum, cephalad along the right pericolic gutter to the right hemidiaphragm, liver surface, and gallbladder, followed by palpation of the transverse colon, omentum, lesser sac, and stomach. From the left hemidiaphragm, this essential evaluation proceeds caudad along the descending colon to the rectosigmoid colon. Retroperitoneal pelvic and aortic lymph nodes are palpated, and the small intestine and its mesentery are inspected from the ligament of Treitz to the ileocecal valve. Suspicious areas and any adhesions are biopsied. If there is no evidence of disease outside the ovary, multiple peritoneal biopsies are performed for staging and prognostic purposes. They include biopsies of both paracolic gutters, the peritoneum overlying the bladder, the pelvic side walls and cul-de-sac, and the diaphragm, which alternatively can be sampled by scraping it with a tongue depressor and making a cytologic smear. An infracolic omentectomy is performed, and the lesser sac is entered, allowing ligation of the gastroepiploic vessels along with all small branches to the infracolic omentum. However, for patients with inflammatory adhesions due to prior surgery or omental tumor, whether microscopic metastases or a bulky "omental cake," dissection may be difficult and care must be taken to avoid injury to the mesenteric vessels. The exploration of the retroperitoneal space and dissection of the pelvic and paraaortic lymph nodes is performed by incising the peritoneum overlying the psoas muscles. Any enlarged lymph nodes are removed. Complete sampling includes bilateral external and internal iliac and obturator lymph nodes in the pelvis and right and left common iliac and paraaortic lymph nodes outside the pelvis.

F. Staging

The entire staging evaluation, including biopsies, can be performed with the uterus and contralateral ovary intact. The fate of these organs depends on the menopausal status of the patient and her future childbearing wishes, as well as the pathology and stage of disease at diagnosis. For postmenopausal patients or premenopausal patients who have completed their childbearing, hysterectomy and contralateral oophorectomy is recommended and can be performed following removal of the ovarian mass.

G. Intraoperative Findings

A sterilization procedure is contraindicated in children or young women of reproductive age. Conservative surgical management is a consideration when a Stage I low malignant potential (borderline) tumor or Stage IA well differentiated (grade 1) tumor is present (Table 74–6). The opposite ovary is evaluated, and any suspicious cyst or nodule is biopsied. Wedge biopsy of a normal-appearing contralateral ovary is discouraged, as it may affect future fertility. With borderline tumors, ovarian cystectomy is appropriate management, even if both ovaries are abnormal. Completion of the more standard operation [total abdominal hysterectomy/bilateral salpingo-orphorectomy (TAH /BSO)] is recommended after completion of childbearing for patients with a history of early-stage disease or at the time of staging for patients with borderline tumors and spread outside the ovary (Stage II and above). Standard surgery is advised for patients with invasive epithelial ovarian carcinomas other than Stage IA grade I. Note that in light of new reproductive techniques, a patient with bilateral invasive disease confined to the ovaries (Stage IB) may undergo preservation of the uterus for potential reproduction with a donor egg, an option that should be discussed preoperatively with patients wishing to preserve fertility.

For most human solid tumors, aggressive surgical resection is justified only if all known tumor can be removed. For patients with epithelial ovarian cancer, however, there is theoretical and

TABLE 74–6.
FIGO (1986) staging system for carcinoma of the ovary

Stage	Criteria
I	Growth limited to the ovaries
IA	Growth limited to one ovary; no malignant ascites present or washings containing malignant cells; no tumor on the external surface; capsule intact
IB	Growth limited to both ovaries; no malignant ascites present or washings containing malignant cells; no tumor on the external surfaces; capsule(s) intact
IC[a]	Tumor classified as stage IA or IB but with malignant ascites present or washings containing malignant cells, or tumor on the external surface of one or both ovaries, or with capsule(s) ruptured
II	Growth involving one or both ovaries with pelvic extension
IIA	Extension and/or metastases to the uterus and/or tubes; no malignant ascites present or washings containing malignant cells; no tumor on the external surface(s); capsule(s) intact
IIB	Extension to other pelvic tissues; no malignant ascites present or washings containing malignant cells; no tumor on the external surface(s); capsule(s) intact
IIC[a]	Tumor classified as either stage IIA or IIB but with malignant ascites present or washings containing malignant cells, or tumor on the external surface of one or both ovaries, or with capsule(s) ruptured
III	Tumor involving one or both ovaries with peritoneal implants outside the pelvis and/or positive retroperitoneal or inguinal nodes. Superficial liver metastasis equals stage III; tumor limited to the true pelvis but with histologically proven malignant extension to small bowel or omentum
IIIA	Tumor grossly limited to the true pelvis with negative nodes but with histologically confirmed microscopic seeding of abdominal peritoneal surfaces
IIIB	Tumor involving one or both ovaries with negative nodes but with histologically confirmed implants of abdominal peritoneal surfaces, none exceeding 2 cm in diameter
IIIC	Implants of abdominal peritoneal surfaces exceeding 2 cm in diameter and/or positive retroperitoneal or inguinal lymph nodes
IV	Tumor involving one or both ovaries with distant metastasis; if pleural effusion present, there must be positive cytology; parenchymal liver metastasis indicates stage IV

Staging of ovarian carcinoma is based on findings at clinical examination and by surgical exploration. The histologic findings are considered in the staging, as are the cytologic findings as far as effusions are concerned.

[a] Notes about staging: To evaluate the impact on the prognosis of the various criteria for allotting cases to stage IC or IIC, it would be of value to know whether rupture of the capsule was spontaneous or caused by the surgeon and if the source of the malignant cells detected was peritoneal washings or ascites.

From FIGO,[6] with permission.

clinical support for the concept that debulking of large tumor masses is beneficial for the patient, even if complete tumor removal is not possible. Patients with other than Stage I disease documented at initial exploratory laparotomy should undergo cytoreductive surgery to remove as much of the tumor and its metastases as possible. This includes TAH/BSO, omentectomy, and resection of any metastatic lesions from the peritoneal surface or from the intestines. Hoskins et al.[11] reported on the effect of residual disease diameter on survival following primary cytoreductive surgery. Only patients whose tumors were suboptimally debulked (residual nodules > 1 cm in diameter) were included. A statistically significant improvement in survival was noted when patients with 1–2 cm diameter residual nodules were compared to those having nodules > 2 cm. Aggressive primary cytoreductive surgery is associated with acceptable morbidity and mortality when performed by experienced surgeons.[12] The National Institutes of Health Consensus Development Conference on Ovarian Cancer held in 1994 concluded that "aggressive attempts at cytoreductive surgery as the primary management of ovarian cancer will improve the patient's opportunity for long-term survival."[13] Optimal cytoreduction is difficult to achieve in the presence of extensive disease on the diaphragm, in the parenchyma of the liver, along the base of the small bowel mesentery, in the lesser omentum, or in the porta hepatis. Stage IV ovarian cancer patients require special consideration with respect to cytoreduction. One small study failed to demonstrate a survival benefit for stage IV patients whose lesions were optimally cytoreduced.[14] In the absence of definitive information, it seems reasonable to attempt cytoreduction in patients whose tumors are stage IV only by virtue of a malignant pleural effusion but to be less aggressive in the face of multiple parenchymal liver lesions.[15]

Although the previous paragraphs are dedicated to the workup and management of known adnexal masses, adnexal masses are often found incidentally at the time of laparotomy for emergent or elective nongynecologic procedures. The management is similar, although decisions are sometimes rendered more difficult as fertility desires are seldom known preoperatively.

Postmenopausal patients or reproductive age patients who have completed childbearing can undergo bilateral (BSO) or unilateral (USO) salpingo-oophorectomy, respectively. Frozen section results dictate further management.

Premenarchal patients and patients desiring fertility should be treated conservatively, with ovarian cystectomy if feasible or USO if necessary to remove the mass. Frozen section results and surgical stage, if malignant, dictate further management. If the frozen section results are equivocal or unavailable, conservative management (cystectomy or USO) is appropriate; and restaging can be performed if the final pathology is consistent with malignancy.

The majority of ovarian cancers are epithelial in origin; therefore the management of germ cell and sex cord-stromal tumors is only briefly summarized. Ovarian germ cell tumors account for 20–25% of ovarian neoplasms but only 5% of ovarian malignancies, and these occur predominantly in young women (mean and median age 19 years). The possibility of a germ cell malignancy should be included in the differential diagnosis of any young woman with an ovarian mass, especially if the mass is solid, if other signs of malignancy are present (Table 74–4), or if tumor markers are elevated (Table 74–3). Although generally regarded as highly malignant, 60–75% of malignant ovarian germ cell tumors are stage I at diagnosis, and conservative surgery (consisting of unilateral oophorectomy, staging biopsies, sampling lymph nodes, and omentectomy) is appropriate. A cystic lesion of the contralateral ovary should be enucleated. Biopsy of a normal-appearing ovary is indicated only in the case of dysgerminoma, 15% of which can be covertly bilateral. Current data indicate that the most active adjuvant chemotherapy for germ cell cancers of the ovary is the combination of bleomycin, etoposide, and cis-platinum.

Sex cord-stromal cancers are rare and are characterized by somewhat unpredictable biologic behavior. Most are unilateral and can be treated with oophorectomy and staging. In women who have completed childbearing, hysterectomy with bilateral adnexectomy with surgical staging is recommended. Because estrogen stimulation can occur with functioning granulosa cell and theca cell tumors, 50% of patients have endometrial hyperplasia or polyps and up to 15% have endometrial carcinoma. As previously noted, abnormal bleeding must be evaluated preoperatively. Preservation of the uterus cannot be recommended in the presence of endometrial cancer. Adjuvant therapy depends on the surgical stage, histologic subtype, patient's desire for fertility, and various prognostic factors. Surgery alone is sufficient for several sex cord-stromal tumors, and adjunctive therapy should be considered for patients with advanced disease or other poor-prognostic features. Optimal adjuvant chemotherapeutic regimens for sex cord-stromal tumors have not yet been determined.

Conclusions

The primary workup of a patient with an undiagnosed pelvic mass includes a history and physical examination, ultrasonography, serum CA-125 or other appropriate tumor markers in selected patients, chest radiography, and serum liver chemistries. Additional studies such as CT, colonoscopy, or upper gastrointestinal imaging may be performed when clinically warranted. If the operative evaluation of a pelvic mass reveals an ovarian carcinoma, comprehensive staging and TAH/BSO is recommended. Young patients who want to retain childbearing capacity and have low grade, low stage tumors can undergo unilateral salpingo-oophorectomy with comprehensive staging. If the patient clinically has Stage III or IV disease, cytoreductive surgery is recommended. Chemotherapy is based on tumor histology, stage, and grade.

References

1. Morrow CP, Curtin JP, Townsend DE. Tumors of the ovary: the adnexal mass. In: Morrow CP, Curtin JP, Townsend DE (eds) Synopsis of Gynecologic Oncology, 4th ed. New York: Churchill Livingstone, 1993; 215–232.
2. American College of Obstetricians and Gynecologists. Cancer of the Ovary. Technical Bulletin 141. Washington, DC: ACOG, 1990.
3. DePriest PD, Puls LE, Schwartz RW, et al. Metastatic gastric cancer presenting as a pelvic mass. J Ky Med Assoc 1993;91:193–194.
4. DePriest PD, Gallion HH, Pavlik EJ, et al. Transvaginal sonography as a screening method for the detection of early ovarian cancer. Gynecol Oncol 1997;65:408–414.
5. DePriest PD, van Nagell JR, Gallion HH, et al. Ovarian cancer screening in asymptomatic postmenopausal women. Gynecol Oncol 1993;51:205–209.
6. FIGO. Staging announcement: FIGO Cancer Committee. Gynecol Oncol 1986;25:383.
7. Malkasian GD, Knapp RC, Lavin PT, et al. Preoperative evaluation of serum CA 125 levels in premenopausal and postmenopausal patients with pelvic masses: discrimination of benign from malignant disease. Am J Obstet Gynecol 1988;159:341–346.
8. Goldstein SR, Subramanyam B, Snyder JR, et al. The postmenopausal cystic adnexal mass: the potential role of ultrasound in conservative management. Obstet Gynecol 1989;38:8–10.
9. American College of Obstetricians and Gynecologists. Ovarian Cystectomy. Criteria Set 24. Washington, DC: ACOG, 1996.
10. Berek JS, Hacker NF. Nonepithelial ovarian and fallopian tube cancers. In: Berek JS, Hacker NF (eds) Practical Gynecologic Oncology, 2nd ed. Baltimore: Williams & Wilkins, 1994;377–402.
11. Hoskins WJ, McGuire WP, Brady MF, et al. The effect of diameter of largest residual disease on survival after primary cytoreductive surgery in patients

with suboptimal residual epithelial ovarian carcinoma. Am J Obstet Gynecol 1994;170:974–979.
12. Venesmaa P, Ylikorkala O. Morbidity and mortality associated with primary and repeat operations for ovarian cancer. Obstet Gynecol 1992;79:162–172.
13. NIH Consensus Development Conference on Ovarian Cancer: Screening, treatment, and follow-up. Gynecol Oncol 1994;55:S173.
14. Goodman HM, Harlow BL, Sheets EE, et al. The role of cytoreductive surgery in the management of stage IV epithelial ovarian carcinoma. Gynecol Oncol 1992;46:367–371.
15. Ozols RF, Rubin SC, Thomas G, et al. Epithelial ovarian cancer. In: Hoskins WJ, Perez CA, Young RC (eds) Principles and Practice of Gynecologic Oncology, 2nd ed. Philadelphia: Lippincott-Raven, 1997;919–986.

CHAPTER 75

Malignant Pleural Effusion

ROBERTO V. BARRESI
KEITH W. MILLIKAN

A. Introduction

Malignant pleural effusion (MPE) refers to the accumulation of fluid in the pleural space due to neoplastic involvement of the pleura by direct tumor extension or metastatic dissemination. The diagnosis is made when exfoliated malignant cells are recovered from pleural fluid or are identified in pleural tissue obtained by percutaneous biopsy, or thoracoscopy, or thoracotomy or at autopsy.[1,2] MPE may be the presenting sign of malignancy or, more commonly, manifest after a cancer diagnosis has been established.[3,4]

Patients who develop MPE are usually symptomatic, and the severity of the symptoms depends more on the rate of fluid accumulation than on the absolute amount of fluid. Symptoms typically include dyspnea, cough, and pleuritic chest pain, leading to reduced ability to perform routine daily activities and an overall diminished quality of life. Other systemic complaints, such as fatigue, anorexia, weight loss, and generalized malaise are often related to the underlying malignancy.

Although the underlying malignancy is most often the cause of effusion, some patients with proven malignancy have cytology-negative effusions and no evidence of tumor directly involving the pleural surface. Pleural effusions developing in these patients may result from "benign" etiologies (e.g., congestive heart failure or nonobstructive pneumonia). If none of these other causative factors can be identified, these effusions are referred to as "paramalignant." Lymphatic obstruction is a notable cause of paramalignant effusion and is likely essential for the accumulation of large volumes of fluid in patients with cancer. Other causes of paramalignant effusion include bronchial obstruction, leading to atelectasis and a resultant transudative effusion, or pneumonia with an associated parapneumonic exudative effusion. Finally, pleural effusions may arise because of the systemic effects of malignancy or the adverse effects of cancer therapy.

The diagnosis of MPE heralds a poor prognosis,[5] as it indicates an advanced disease stage. The median survival time of patients presenting with MPE ranges from 4 to 12 months. At the time of diagnosis, approximately 75% of patients with MPE have thoracic symptoms. The major objective of MPE therapy is therefore cost-effective symptom palliation.

Malignant Pleural Effusion

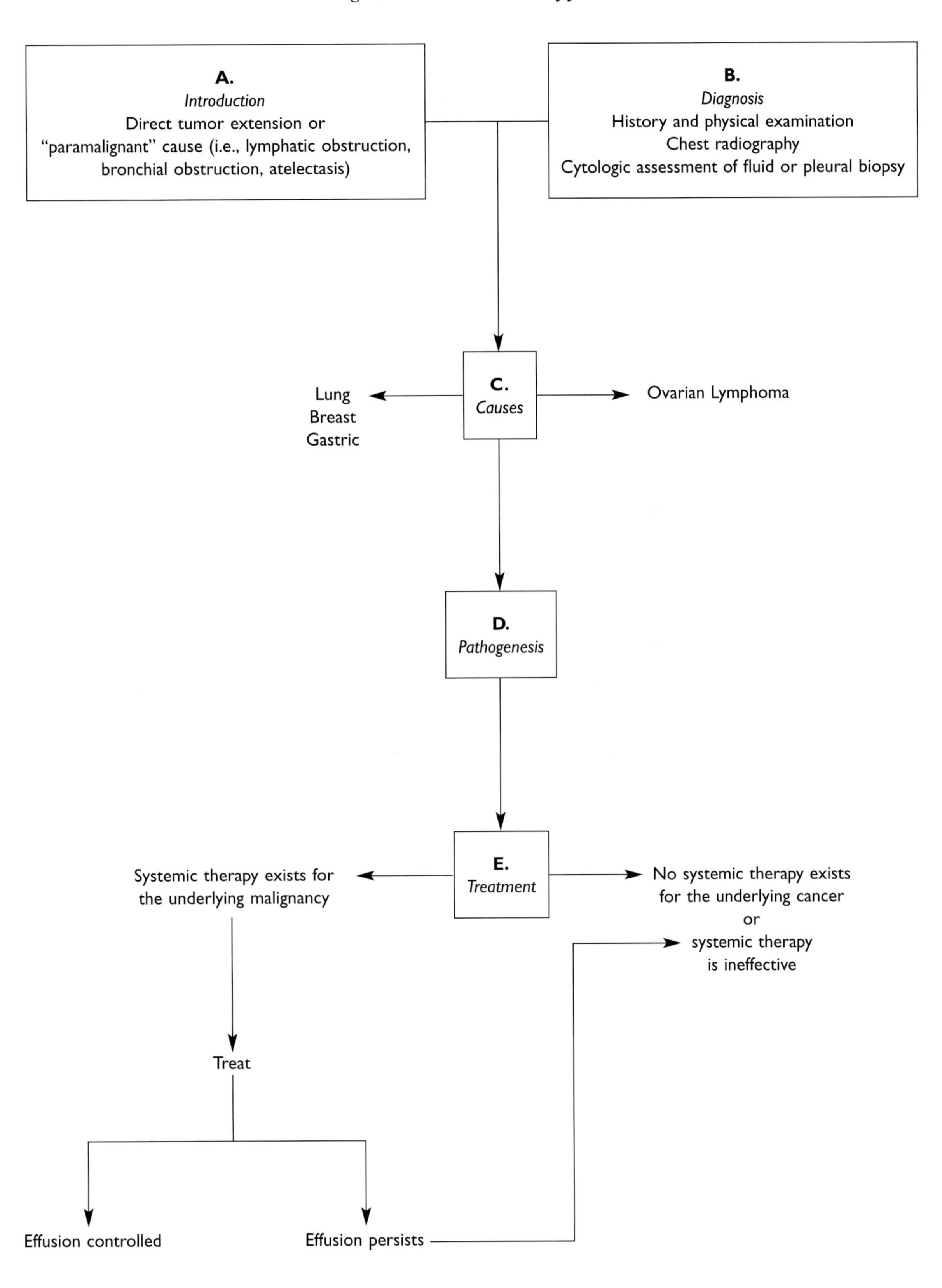

(continued on next page)

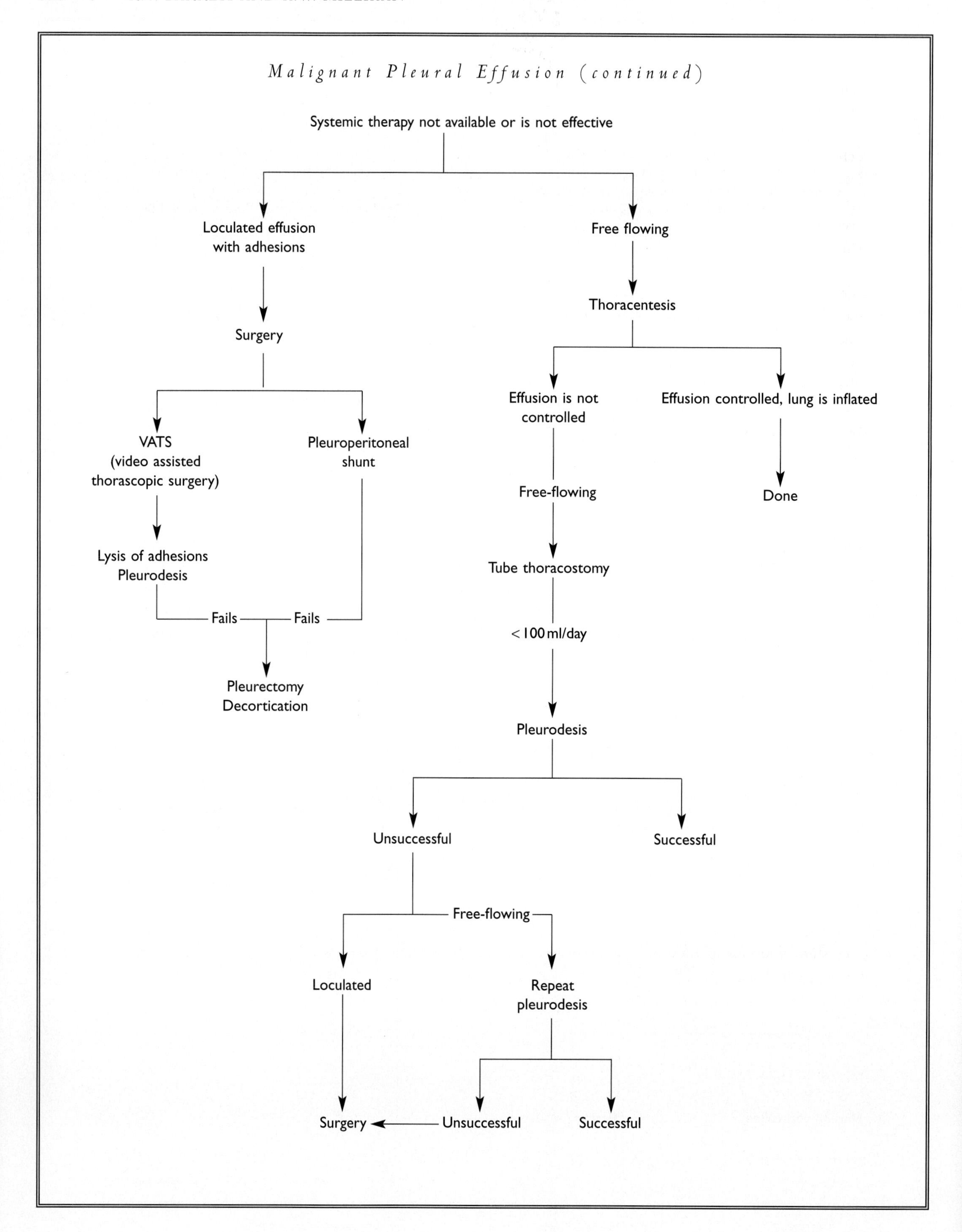
Malignant Pleural Effusion (continued)
Systemic therapy not available or is not effective
Loculated effusion with adhesions
Free flowing
Thoracentesis
Surgery
Effusion is not controlled
Effusion controlled, lung is inflated
VATS (video assisted thoracoscopic surgery)
Pleuroperitoneal shunt
Free-flowing
Done
Lysis of adhesions
Pleurodesis
Tube thoracostomy
Fails
Fails
< 100 ml/day
Pleurectomy
Decortication
Pleurodesis
Unsuccessful
Successful
Free-flowing
Loculated
Repeat pleurodesis
Surgery
Unsuccessful
Successful

B. Diagnosis

As with any medical illness, the approach to MPE begins with obtaining a complete medical history and performing a detailed physical examination. The typical symptoms (dyspnea, cough, pleuritic chest pain) in association with generalized fatigue and weight loss suggest malignancy. Physical findings may include percussion dullness, vocal fremitus, and diminished breath sounds over the affected area of effusion. Occasionally, massive pleural effusions are noted to cause bulging of the intercostal spaces, deviation of the trachea away from the affected hemithorax, and decreased diaphragmatic excursion.

Chest radiography remains a low cost means of confirming the presence of a pleural effusion. As little as 175 ml of pleural fluid may be detected on an upright chest radiograph as a ground-glass shadow obscuring the diaphragm, costophrenic angle, and a variable quantity of the pleural space. Lateral decubitus views are even more sensitive, with the ability to detect as little as 100 ml of fluid. Computed tomography, though not routinely needed for confirmation, can detect yet smaller amounts of fluid in the pleural space. Effusion ipsilateral to the primary lesion is commonplace with carcinoma of the lung. When the primary malignancy is extrapulmonary, with the possible exception of carcinoma of the breast, there appears to be no ipsilateral propensity, and bilateral effusions are not uncommon.

The pleural effusion is generally large (500–2000 ml) in most patients who present with carcinomatous involvement of the pleura. Approximately 10% of these patients present with effusions of less than 500 ml, whereas 10% present with massive MPEs, obliterating virtually an entire hemithorax. About 70% of patients who present with a massive pleural effusion have an underlying malignancy.[6]

Bilateral effusions, in the presence of a normal cardiac silhouette, suggest malignancy. Nearly 50% of patients with such radiographic findings have MPE or paramalignant effusions. In such cases, however, other nonmalignant etiologies should be considered, such as cirrhosis, asbestosis, lupus pleuritis, rheumatoid pleurisy, hypoalbuminemia, and constrictive pericarditis.

In general, large pleural effusions lead to a contralateral mediastinal shift. Effusions of 1500 ml or more *without* a concomitant mediastinal shift usually result from malignancy. In such cases one must consider: (1) malignant mediastinal lymphadenopathy leading to a fixed mediastinum; (2) malignant mesothelioma (the radiodensity represents tumor, whereas the effusion may be minimal); (3) carcinoma of the ipsilateral mainstem bronchus (leading to atelectasis); and (4) extensive ipsilateral pulmonary malignant infiltration (mimicking a large effusion).

Once it has been determined that an abnormal fluid collection exists, establishing a diagnosis of cancer is rather straightforward. Cytologic examination is the best means of diagnosing MPE and is easily accomplished with thoracentesis. At least 250 ml of fluid is necessary for an adequate sample, as volumes less than this often contain too few cells for accurate analysis.[7] This procedure can be performed safely at the bedside using local anesthesia; it has a high diagnostic yield and may provide temporary relief of pulmonary symptoms. Complications of thoracentesis include pneumothorax, lung parenchymal laceration, and pleural shock (an exaggerated vagal response); moreover, if a large volume of fluid is removed rapidly from the pleural space, reexpansion pulmonary edema may ensue. Approximately 50% of MPEs are diagnosed by cytologic examination using this method, and the yield increases by 10% with repeat cytology.[8]

A pitfall in the cytologic assessment of MPEs is that a paucity of identifiable cancer cells may lead to a false-negative report. Additionally, mesothelial cell abnormalities and macrophages collected in the sedimented specimen may lead to a false-positive report. For these reasons, flow cytometry provides a useful adjunct to routine cytopathologic examination. Flow cytometry identifies chromosomal abnormalities (irrespective of the state of cancer cell proliferation) in samples containing malignant cells. The results are expressed as a DNA index, with aneuploidy (DNA index outside the normal range) shown to correlate significantly with the presence of malignant cells in the specimen. Although this technique is fast and accurate, it adds considerable cost to the diagnostic evaluation and should be reserved for cases in which routine cytology is indeterminate.

Pleural biopsy using a Cobe-Abrans needle is another means by which pleural malignancy can be demonstrated. This percutaneous technique, however, is associated with a low yield, particularly if used alone.[9] Aside from the potential complications of lung injury and pneumothorax, this approach is "blind" and may fail to demonstrate cancer in localized lesions due to sampling error. Over time, the role of thoracoscopy with directed pleural biopsy has gained favor. The technique is associated with less morbidity than thoracotomy and has a diagnostic yield of 93–96%.[10]

Cytologic examination of effusions from a mesothelioma or lymphoma has a low diagnostic yield. These neoplasms generally require large tissue samples (via thoracoscopy or thoracotomy) to confirm the diagnosis.

Despite the techniques outlined here, the cause of nearly 25% of pleural effusions remains unclear; either thoracoscopic biopsy or limited thoracotomy is required to establish a definitive diagnosis. With the advances in video-assisted thoracoscopic equipment and the associated reductions in patient discomfort, overall cost of hospitalization, length of stay, and morbidity, thoracoscopy is increasingly replacing open biopsy in the diagnostic armamentarium of pleural disease.

C. Causes

The most common causes of exudative pleural effusions are cancer and pneumonia.[11] Numerous reviews have verified that the major causes of MPE are primary lung, breast, ovarian, and gastric carcinomas and lymphoma. Together, breast cancer, lung cancer, and lymphoma account for more than 75% of all MPEs.

Carcinoma of any organ has the ability to metastasize to the pleura. Lung cancer, however, is the most common malignancy to invade the pleura and produce MPE and paramalignant effusion. Cancerous pleural involvement is apparent in 5–15% of patients with pulmonary carcinoma at the time of presentation, and up to 50% of patients with disseminated disease develop this complication. Between 7% and 15% of patients with lung cancer eventually exhibit MPE. Second in incidence is breast cancer, with ovarian and gastric cancer representing 5% or fewer of the cases. Hodgkin's and non-Hodgkin's lymphomas are responsible for nearly 10% of all MPEs. Finally, no primary cancer has been identified in approximately 7% of patients with malignant effusion.

D. Pathogenesis

The visceral and parietal pleurae are each composed of a single layer of mesothelial cells. These layers, in close apposition in the normal state, give rise to a potential space, through which 5–10 liters of pleural fluid pass each day. The parietal pleura is perfused by the high-pressure systemic circulation, whereas the visceral pleura is perfused primarily by the pulmonary circulation. This gives rise to a net pressure gradient that, in accordance with Starling's law, normally tends to drive a low-protein-containing fluid from the parietal pleura to the visceral pleura. The small amount of protein entering the pleural space is readily cleared by lymphatics underlying the pleural surfaces and transported to the systemic circulation by way of the thoracic duct. Approximately 80–90% of the fluid is absorbed by the pulmonary venous capillaries, and the remainder is reabsorbed by the pleural lymphatics.

An important characteristic of the parietal pleura is the existence of lymphatic stomas, which are small openings situated randomly among the parietal pleural mesothelial cells. These stomas empty into the lymphatic lacunae, which coalesce into collecting lymphatics and join the intercostal trunk lymphatics. The flow of lymph is thus directed predominantly in the direction of the mediastinal lymph nodes.

Malignant pleural effusion results when there is an interruption in the delicate balance of the normal fluid dynamics as it traverses the pleural space. Thus events leading to increased secretion or decreased reabsorption result in an accumulation of fluid. In patients with MPE (despite preserved hydrostatic and oncotic pressures) fluid accumulates owing to inflammation or disruption of the pulmonary venous capillary endothelium or impaired lymphatic drainage due to direct obstruction by tumor infiltrates. Bloody MPEs are the result of direct invasion of tumor into blood vessels, occlusion of venules, tumor-induced angiogenesis, or increases in capillary dilatation due to vasoactive substances.

Paramalignant effusions, on the other hand, may be either directly or indirectly caused by tumors but are not associated with pleural metastases. Paramalignant effusion develops secondary to mediastinal lymph node metastases, obstructing bronchial tumors giving rise to atelectasis or pneumonia, and obstruction of the thoracic duct. The effusions associated with chemotherapy and radiation therapy are thus paramalignant effusions as well. Paramalignant effusions differ from MPEs by their negative cytology, lower cell count, higher platelet count, and higher glucose level.

E. Treatment

The management of MPE depends on several factors. First and foremost, one must consider the treatment potential of the primary malignancy and the patient's overall prognosis. Systemic therapy, aimed at treating oat-cell carcinoma of the lung or lymphoma, may adequately control the MPE. For such treatment regimens, thoracentesis may be employed to palliate symptoms but is not considered the primary treatment modality per se.

When the pleural effusion is malignant or paramalignant and no specific systemic therapy is adequate to control the effusion, the primary aim of therapy should be optimal palliation. Inherently, one should attempt to avoid unnecessary hospitalization, excessive cost, and treatments with increased risk of complications. The major therapies designed to manage MPE are (1) thoracentesis; (2) tube thoracostomy and drainage (3); tube thoracostomy and drainage with instillation of a sclerosing agent; (4) talc poudrage (5); pleuroperitoneal shunt; and (6) pleurectomy.

Thoracentesis

For patients with advanced disease and short life expectancy, adequate palliation can be achieved by intermittent thoracentesis.[12] Comfort measures, including adequate analgesia and oxygen supplementation, may be combined with intermittent placement of a small-bore catheter into the pleural space to evacuate the effusion. The benefit of this therapy is generally short-lived, and effusions with symptoms are expected to recur in virtually all patients. Repeated thoracentesis predisposes to the formation of adhesions, loculated effusions, and empyema, making overall management more difficult.

Tube Thoracostomy and Drainage

Placement of a chest tube with evacuation of the pleural fluid gives nearly immediate relief of symptoms, provided the lung has the capacity to reexpand. As with repeated thoracentesis, however, MPE and symptoms are likely to recur soon after the tube is withdrawn. Generally speaking, this technique is not recommended for long-term therapy.

Tube Thoracostomy and Drainage with Instillation of a Sclerosing Agent

By far the most commonly used therapy for managing MPE, tube thoracostomy and drainage with instillation of a sclerosing agent are offered by most institutions. A chest tube is placed in the pleural space in the sixth or seventh interspace at the midaxillary line under aseptic conditions and local anesthesia; it is then connected to a drainage collection system with 15–20 cmH_2O suction applied. Drainage is allowed to continue until less than 100 ml/day is evacuated, the lung is reexpanded, and the pleural surfaces are apposed to one another. The sclerosing agent is then delivered into the pleural space through the drainage tube, after which the tube is clamped. The patient is instructed to change position every 20 minutes for 2 hours to ensure even distribution of the sclerosant. The clamp is then released, and the fluid is again allowed to drain for 24 hours prior to removing the chest tube. Success is determined by assessing symptoms and by follow-up radiographs to evaluate for any evidence of MPE recurrence.

A number of sclerosing agents have been utilized, some with better success than others.[13] The primary role of these agents is to induce chemical pleuritis, causing adhesions to form between the pleural surfaces, thereby reducing the propensity for recurrent pleural fluid collection. The "optimal" sclerosant is sterile; is of high molecular weight; has high chemical polarity, low regional clearance, and high systemic clearance; and is well tolerated by the patient.

Talc Talc was introduced for pleural poudrage in 1935 and remains one of the most effective sclerosing agents in current use. The mechanism by which this agent works is inducing an intense reactive pleuritis. It can be administered as a slurry (5–10 g of talc in 0.9% NaCl) through the chest tube or insufflated into the pleural space during thoracoscopic procedures. Talc pleurodesis is highly effective, with nearly a 100% success rate after a single application. The most common adverse effects noted are fever and pain. Occasional episodes of acute respiratory distress syndrome (ARDS) have been reported following the procedure.

Tetracycline Until recently tetracycline was commercially available in the United States in an injectable form. After instillation of 1 g in 30–50 ml 0.9% NaCl into a well drained pleural space, it had a reported success rate of 59–94% for controlling MPE. The mechanism of tetracycline's action on inducing pleurodesis is thought to be via stimulation of mesothelial cell release of fibroblast growth factor-like substances. Currently, it is of only historic interest.

Doxycycline Administered as a 500 mg dose in 30–100 ml 0.9% NaCl, the success rate of doxycycline for controlling MPE is reported to be 60–72%. Although similar to the mechanism proposed for tetracycline, doxycycline seems to require repeated instillation to achieve maximal benefit. Side effects associated with its utilization include fever and chest discomfort.

Minocycline A single study tested the efficacy of minocycline in seven patients with MPE. Six patients (86%) responded completely, and no significant untoward effects were noted.

Quinacrine Quinacrine is an antimalarial agent that has proved to be as effective as tetracycline in controlling MPE. However, fever, hallucinations, severe pleuritic chest pain, and convulsions following its administration have hampered its further use in clinical practice.

Antineoplastic Agents and Biologic Therapies

Antineoplastic Agents In contrast to sclerosants, chemotherapeutic agents were introduced with the aim of providing not only chemical pleurodesis but treatment of the underlying malignancy locally and systemically. Several chemotherapeutic agents have been used to control MPE, including bleomycin, doxorubicin, mitoxantrone, cisplatin, and cytarabine.

Bleomycin, with a success rate of 63–85%, is delivered intrapleurally as 60 U in 50 ml of 5% dextrose solution. Although absorbed systemically, toxicity has rarely been reported. Pain and fever, the most frequently reported side effects, can be minimized with prophylactic therapy. Its reported mechanism of action is mainly by induction of chemical pleurodesis.

Doxorubicin (10–40 mg) has a reported response rate of 39–80%, and adverse reactions include nausea, vomiting, pain, and fever. *Mitoxantrone*, in preliminary studies, has mild toxicity and a response rate similar to that of tetracycline and bleomycin.

The combination of *cisplatin* (1200 mg) and *cytarabine* (100 mg/m^2) has demonstrated a complete response rate in only 49% of participants. However, with its minimal toxicity and prolonged duration of MPE control (9 months), this combination of chemotherapeutic agents deserves further investigation.

BIOLOGIC RESPONSE MODIFIERS The biologic response modifiers include the interferons and interleukin-2 (IL-2). *Interferons* up-regulate major histocompatibility complex (MHC) expression, increase natural killer cell function, and improve macrophage cytotoxic function. Intrapleural interferon-β (IFNβ) has been administered to patients with MPE (without pleural drainage), with an overall response rate of 38%. Moreover, local instillation of recombinant interferon alfa-2b has an observed response rate of 70%.[14] Observed adverse reactions included flu-like symptoms. Overall, it appears that neither of these agents is more effective at controlling MPE than bleomycin. *Interleukin-2* (recombinant), given intrapleurally, has caused the disappearance of cancer cells in the pleural fluid and resolution of the effusion. Its only untoward effect thus far has been fever.[15]

Corynebacterium parvum, a gram-positive anaerobe, though not widely available, has been studied in the management of MPE. Extracts from this bacterium, given weekly at doses of 5–10 mg, have been reported to control 90–100% of MPEs at 1 month. The presumed mode of action is via induction of an inflammatory response against the lipopolysaccharide bacterial cell wall. In several studies the effectiveness of *C. parvum* is comparable to that of tetracycline and bleomycin. Adverse effects include pain and fever.[16]

Picibanil, a streptococcal preparation, has been shown to be effective for patients with MPE. It is thought that it increases expression of intercellular adhesion molecule-1 (ICAM-1) and is reported to be 70–73% effective.

SURGICAL OPTIONS

When other means of controlling the symptoms associated with MPE have failed, one may consider operative therapy. Using *video-assisted thoracoscopic surgery* (VATS), patients can undergo pleurectomy and decortication with relatively low morbidity and mortality. In the past this procedure was done without video assistance and required a formal thoracotomy with its attendant risks. As experience with minimally invasive techniques grows, we can expect a further reduction in operative and perioperative complications.

Patients with intractable MPE who are not candidates for conventional sclerotherapy (e.g., trapped lung) have another option. A high-flow, pressure-activated manual *pleuroperitoneal pump reservoir* can be surgically implanted between the pleural and peritoneal cavities under local or general anesthesia. This device is designed to allow free egress of the MPE into the peritoneal cavity if such pressure gradients are reached, and it provides the ability to decompress the pleural space manually. Once implanted, patients may be managed on an outpatient basis with considerable improvement in their quality of life. Drawbacks include potential clogging of the one-way valves with cellular debris and infection of the implanted device.

Conclusions

Malignant pleural effusion, a common complication of advanced malignancy, is associated with significant morbidity and mortality. The symptoms of MPE (dyspnea, cough, pleuritic pain) can be debilitating and can result in prolonged hospitalization at a considerable cost. Several therapeutic regimens have been designed to improve such patients' quality of life by palliating these symptoms. Although controversy still exists as to which therapy is optimal for individual patients, a critical review of the existing management options allows patients and physicians to have open discussions on the utility of the currently available treatment strategies.

References

1. Sahn SA. Malignancy metastatic to the pleura. Clin Chest Med 1998; 19:351–361.
2. Hsu C. Cytologic detection of malignancy in pleural effusion: a review of 5255 samples from 3811 patients. Diagn Cytopathol 1987;3:8.
3. Belani CP, Pajeau TS, Bennett CL. Treating malignant pleural effusions cost consciously. Chest 1998;113:78S–85S.
4. Tattersall M. Management of malignant pleural effusion. Aust NZ J Med 1998;28:394–396.
5. Chernow B, Sahn SA. Carcinomatous involvement of the pleura: an analysis of 96 patients. Am J Med 1977;63:695.
6. Maher GG, Berger HW. Massive pleural effusion: malignant and nonmalignant causes in 46 patients. Am Rev Respir Dis 1972;105:458.
7. Fiocco M, Krasna MJ. The management of malignant pleural and pericardial effusions. Hematol Oncol Clin North Am 1997;11:253–265.
8. Fraser RS, Colman N, Müller NL, Paré PD. Pleural effusion. In: *Diagnosis of Diseases of the Chest, 4th ed.* Philadelphia: Saunders, 1999;2739–2778.
9. Winkelmann M, Pfitzer P. Blind pleural biopsy in combination with cytology of pleural effusions. Acta Cytol 1981;25:373–376.
10. Weisberg D, Daufman M. Diagnostic and therapeutic pleuroscopy: experience with 127 patients. Chest 1980;78:732.
11. Fraser RS, Coleman N, Müller NL, Paré PD. The pleura. In: *Synopsis of Diseases of the Chest, 2nd ed.* Philadelphia: Saunders, 1994;868–895.

12. Colice GL, Rubins JB. Practical management of pleural effusions: when and how should fluid accumulations be drained? Postgrad Med 1999;105:67–77.
13. Belani CP, Ziskind AA, Dhawan M, Lemmon CC. Management of malignant pleural and pericardial effusions. In: Aisner J, Green, Perry, Arriagada, Martini (eds). *Comprehensive Textbook of Thoracic Oncology*. Baltimore: Williams & Wilkins, 1996;880–905.
14. Rosso R, Rimoldi R, Salvati F, et al. Intrapleural natural beta interferon in the treatment of malignant pleural effusion. Oncology 1998;45:253–256.
15. Yasumoto K, Ogura T. Intrapleural application of recombinant interleukin-2 patients with malignant pleurisy due to lung cancer: a multi-institutional cooperative study. Biotherapy 1991;3:345–349.
16. Grossi F, Pennucci MC, Tixi L, Cafferata MA, Ardizzoni A. Management of malignant pleural effusions. Drugs 1998;55:47–58.

CHAPTER 76

Malignant Ascites

H. DREXEL DOBSON III

Ascites is often a manifestation of advanced cancer, and its presence denotes a worsening prognosis. Overall, cancer is responsible for 10% of all cases of ascites,[1] and approximately half of these patients have ascites as the presenting feature of their disease.[1] Intraperitoneal causes of malignant ascites include cancers of the ovary, pancreas, stomach, uterus, and colon; extraperitoneal tumors capable of causing malignant ascites originate in breast, lung, and lymphomatous tissue.[2] Overall, these lesions collectively account for more than 80% of cases of malignant ascites; in approximately 20% of all cases ascites is due to tumors of unknown origin. Survival, albeit dismal, is dependent on the site of origin; lymphomas have a mean survival of 58–78 weeks, ovarian cancer 30–35 weeks, and cancers of the gastrointestinal tract 12–20 weeks. Ascites from tumors of unknown origin have the worst prognosis, and survival varies between 7 days and 12 weeks at best.[3]

A. Diagnosis

Ascites may be due to a variety of causes (Table 76–1), and the underlying diagnosis is usually made based on the history and physical examination assisted by radiographic studies, cytologic examination, serum tumor markers, and ultimately surgical exploration. Symptomatic patients present with various findings including swollen lower extremities, dyspnea, increasing abdominal girth, abdominal pain, and nausea. Anorexia is common and may be accompanied by vomiting.[4] Physical limitations include decreased mobility and fatigue. Patients can either gain or lose weight depending on their balance between retention of ascitic fluid and nutritional status, which may be severely compromised. Physical signs include abdominal distension, bulging flanks, shifting dullness to percussion, and a marked fluid wave. The presence of a fluid wave has a diagnostic specificity of 90% and a sensitivity of 62%.[1]

Imaging studies may help identify ascites but are infrequently helpful for determining the cause. Plain abdominal films are unreliable for detecting ascites, although if a significant amount of fluid is present the abdomen has a "ground-glass" appearance and the borders of the psoas muscles are not discernible. Ultrasonography is useful for identifying as little as 100 ml of intraabdominal fluid and can be

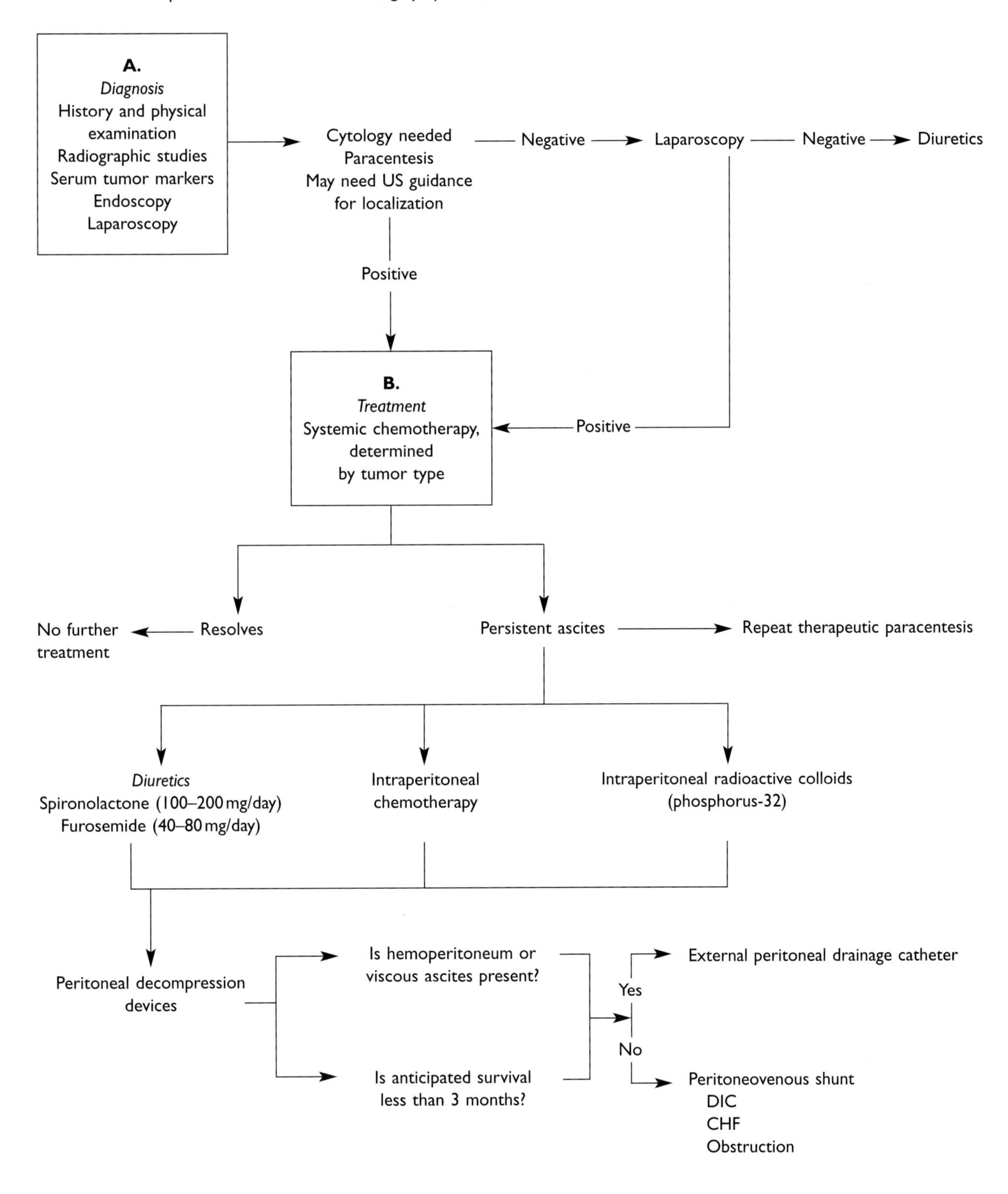
Malignant Ascites
Intraperitoneal cancers: ovary, pancreas, stomach, uterus, colon
Extraperitoneal cancers: breast, lung, lymphoma, melanoma
A.
Diagnosis
History and physical examination
Radiographic studies
Serum tumor markers
Endoscopy
Laparoscopy
Cytology needed
Paracentesis
May need US guidance for localization
Negative
Laparoscopy
Negative
Diuretics
Positive
B.
Treatment
Systemic chemotherapy, determined by tumor type
Positive
No further treatment
Resolves
Persistent ascites
Repeat therapeutic paracentesis
Diuretics
Spironolactone (100–200 mg/day)
Furosemide (40–80 mg/day)
Intraperitoneal chemotherapy
Intraperitoneal radioactive colloids (phosphorus-32)
Peritoneal decompression devices
Is hemoperitoneum or viscous ascites present?
Is anticipated survival less than 3 months?
Yes
No
External peritoneal drainage catheter
Peritoneovenous shunt
DIC
CHF
Obstruction

TABLE 76–1.
Pathophysiologic classification of ascites

Osmotic ascites
Hepatic dysfunction/insufficiency
Malnutrition
Protein-losing states (i.e., nephrotic syndrome, enteropathies)
Hydrostatic ascites (hepatic congestion)
Congestive heart failure
Cirrhosis/advanced liver disease
Constrictive pericarditis
Hepatic vein occlusion
Portal vein occlusion
Exogenous sources
Neoplastic (primary, secondary, mesothelial)
Infectious (bacterial, tuberculous, fungal, parasitic)
Pancreatic
Biliary
Chylous

useful for targeting fluid for cytology. Alternative techniques that can identify ascites include computed tomography (CT) and magnetic resonance imaging (MRI). CT findings suggestive of peritoneal carcinomatosis or tumor implantation throughout the peritoneum may include ascites or enhancement of thickened peritoneum (or both) on contrast-enhanced scans. The ascites may or may not be loculated. A stellate mesenteric appearance suggests an infiltrative process that may be benign or malignant.[5] Cytologic examination should be performed to rule out an infectious process, especially if a primary tumor is not identified on CT or endoscopic examination(s).

Ascitic fluid should be sampled and submitted for laboratory tests and cytologic examination. Cytology has a specificity of 100% but is only 60% sensitive for diagnosing malignancy.[1,2] If the initial cytologic assessment failed to diagnose cancer, repeat cytologic aspiration should be performed if warranted because of suspicious clinical or radiologic findings. Studies have shown that patients with peritoneal carcinomatosis *and* ascites have positive or suspicious cytology in 87% of cases. Biochemical assays may be helpful for distinguishing between malignant and nonmalignant ascites; but to date, no one test or group of tests is routinely or consistently useful in this regard. Measurement of fibronectin in the ascitic fluid is a promising indicator of an underlying cancer but is currently not diagnostic.[1] A serum albumin concentration higher than 32 g/L has been associated with improved survival in patients with nonovarian cancer.[4]

Abdominal paracentesis is valuable for the diagnosis and treatment of malignant ascites and may provide symptomatic relief for about 90% of patients.[1] Patients with previous abdominal surgery, a history of intraabdominal chemotherapy, or loculated collections should undergo ultrasound-guided paracentesis to minimize the risk of visceral injury. Up to 10 liters of ascites can be drained safely using an indwelling trocar over a 24- to 48-hour period. Too rapid removal of ascites can precipitate intravascular volume depletion and oliguria; therefore large-volume paracentesis should be accompanied with colloid infusion to prevent cardiovascular collapse.[2] Repeated paracentesis of protein-rich ascites may cause plasma protein depletion.[1] Complications include cardiovascular collapse, secondary bacterial peritonitis, pulmonary emboli, and nutritional depletion; careful attention to detail can prevent these complications. Paracentesis remains the therapy by which all others are judged in the treatment of malignant ascites.

Laparoscopic exploration is rapidly gaining favor for patients whose initial workup was indeterminate. Several studies have used laparoscopy and biopsy for diagnosis, which was achieved in roughly 90% of patients. Laparoscopy has a morbidity of 6%. Prolonged ascitic leakage from a port site is the most common complication and has caused two deaths from peritonitis among a cohort of 227 cases. Port-site recurrence has a low incidence probably because of the limited long-term survival after the procedure.[1]

B. *Treatment*

Various treatment modalities have been proposed, most of which are palliative in nature and serve to ameliorate symptoms. The first line of treatment is *systemic therapy* specific for the particular class or type of tumor. In this regard, good results have been noted primarily for ovarian cancer. Secondary treatment strategies should focus on providing relief of symptoms and preventing recurrence of ascites.

Diuretics

Diuretics are beneficial, especially aldosterone antagonists, as they interrupt renin-angiotensin activation. Intravascular depletion is thought to be a result of increased accumulation of fluid in the abdominal cavity by impaired lymphatic drainage and increased fluid secretion from both normal peritoneal cells and tumor cells. Spironolactone 100–200 mg/day may be used alone initially or in combination with a loop-acting diuretic, such as furosemide 40–80 mg/day to help control ascites.[3]

Intraperitoneal Chemotherapy

Chemosensitive tumors that cause malignant ascites may respond to systemic therapy or local administration of chemotherapeutic agents. As medications are absorbed into the portal circulation, they are usually metabolized to their inactive metabolites during their first pass through the liver; this produces less systemic toxicity. Intraperitoneal chemotherapy has produced variable results,[3] and there are few reports in the literature describing its use. Loggie and colleagues reported 34 patients with disseminated intraperitoneal gastrointestinal cancers treated with cytoreductive surgery and intraperitoneal hyperthermic chemotherapy (mitomycin C). Ascites was controlled in 75% of cases and prevented in all patients with positive intraperitoneal cytology. The 1-year survival was 39%; patients without ascites had a 1-year survival of 89% using this approach.[6]

Other studies have used bleomycin, cisplatin, and 5-fluorouracil (5-FU) with promising results. Most notably, Alberts and colleagues conducted a phase 3 trial of intraperitoneal cisplatin therapy for ovarian cancer. After staging laparotomy and tumor debulking, 546 patients were randomized to receive six courses of intravenous cyclophosphamide (600 mg/m^2 body surface area per course) plus either intraperitoneal cisplatin (100 mg/m^2) or intravenous cisplatin (100 mg/m^2); each was administered at 3-week intervals. The median survival was found to be significantly longer for the intraperitoneal cisplatin group than for the group given intravenous medication (49 vs. 41 months). A decreased incidence of toxic effects was noted as well.[7] Recio and colleagues found that salvage platinum-based intraperitoneal chemotherapy produced a significantly longer progression-free survival and 5-year survival in selected patients with small-volume ovarian cancer.[8] Romensch et al. found that bismuth-212 delivers high linear energy transfer, which is densely ionizing and does not require the presence of cellular oxygen in in vitro or in vivo animal models of ovarian cancer cell lines. The extrapolated human dose would be about 270 mCi of activity, which should be well tolerated by human subjects. Further trials are under way.[9]

Scheithauer and colleagues have shown that a regimen of intraperitoneal and intravenous 5-FU (200 mg/m^2) and leucovorin (200 mg/m^2) was effective in reducing colorectal locoregional tumor recurrences with or without liver or other organ site involvement compared to standard therapy with 5-FU and levamisole in stage III colon cancer patients.[10] The investigational combination therapy was given intravenously on days 1–4 and intraperitoneally on days 1 and 3 every 4 weeks for six courses. Improved disease-free survival and a survival advantage was found for the intraperitoneal/intravenous group, with a 43% reduction in mortality. No difference in survival was found in patients with stage II disease.

Intraperitoneal Radiocolloids

Intraperitoneal radiocolloids have been used since the 1940s to treat malignant ascites and are particularly useful for ovarian cancer. Traditionally instilled at the time of surgery, intraperitoneal phosphorus has also been given at intervals after debulking surgery. Phosphorus-32 (^{32}P) is most useful, as it penetrates tissues to a depth of 8 mm and has a half-life of about 14 days. Response rates of 40–54% have been noted.[1,3] Side effects include bowel necrosis and bowel obstruction. Currently, no randomized study has confirmed any survival advantage with this treatment modality. Young and colleagues conducted a prospective randomized national cooperative trial of adjuvant therapy in patients with localized ovarian carcinoma.[11] A total of 141 patients with poorly differentiated stage I tumors or stage II tumors confined to the pelvis were randomly assigned to treatment with melphalan or a single intraperitoneal dose of ^{32}P (15 mCi) at surgical staging. The two groups had similar 5-year disease-free survivals (80% for both groups) and overall survivals (81% vs. 78%). Others reported promising results in patients with disseminated ovarian carcinoma treated with intravenous cisplatin therapy coupled with concomitant intraperitoneal instillation of 5 mCi of ^{32}P at each monthly cycle for up to eight cycles. The overall 3-year survival was 63%, thought to be due to an enhanced and possibly supraadditive effect of cisplatin on the cytotoxicity from ^{32}P irradiation.

Peritoneal Decompression Devices

Peritoneal decompression devices have been used as adjuncts to relieve malignant ascites. There are two categories: peritoneovenous shunts and external drainage catheter devices. The Le Veen shunt was introduced in 1974 for decompressing ascites secondary to liver failure. The Denver shunt was subsequently introduced for the same purpose (Fig. 76–1). They have since been used for malignant ascites and provide palliation in up to 70% of patients.[1–3] Straus and colleagues reviewed the experience with LeVeen shunts in 37 cancer patients and found that 73% had long-term function (mean 10.6 weeks) or functioned until the death of the patient (mean 11.6 weeks).[12]

The most common reason for shunt failure is occlusion, which can be prevented by avoiding shunts in patients with hemoperitoneum or viscous ascites.[2,12] Another complication is activation of the coagulation cascade due to systemic introduction of ascitic fluid; this is seen more commonly in cirrhotic patients. Although this complication is rare in those with malignant ascites, its presence should be sought; in fact, certain protocols suggest that elevated fibrinogen split products is an indicator of adequate shunt function.[1] LeVeen and LeVeen believed that disseminated intravascular coagulopathy (DIC) is due to excessive tissue plasminogen activator and can be treated with ε-aminocaproic acid.[13] Tempero and colleagues believed that activated clotting factors and platelet aggregation are responsible.[14] Bracci and colleagues advocated interruption of shunting when DIC is observed.[15] Tumor dissemination to the insertion sites and the systemic circulation has not been

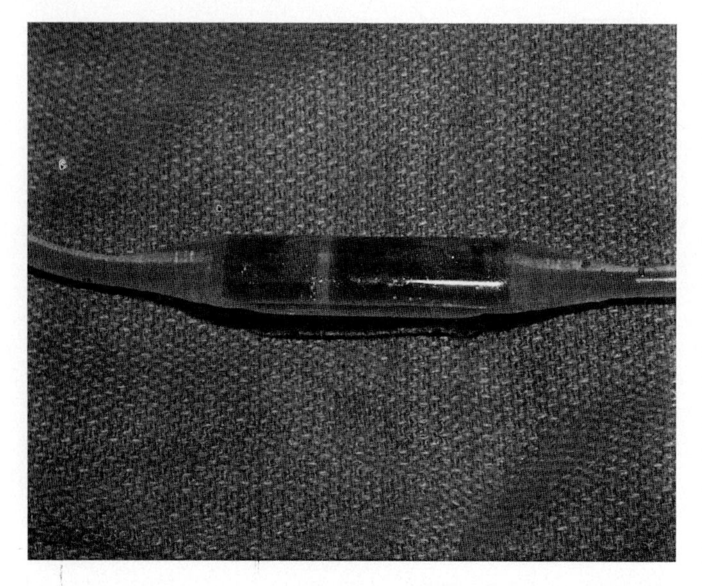

FIGURE 76–1
Denver peritoneovenous shunt.

observed commonly in vivo, although intuitively it should occur.[1,2] Congestive heart failure has been observed after shunt insertion secondary to massive fluid shifts; hence patients should be closely monitored postoperatively, perhaps in an intensive care unit, and may require diuretic therapy. Schumacher and colleagues reviewed the Straus et al. experience as well as an additional 52 patients and found that only 31% of 89 patients maintained a patent shunt and lived for more than 2 months.[16] Twelve patients (13%) died within 30 days of surgery as a result of complications of shunt placement; most notably, cardiorespiratory failure (4), peritonitis (2), small bowel obstruction (2), pneumonia (1), subdural hematoma (1), massive gastrointestinal bleed (1), and pulmonary embolism (1). Subclinical DIC and temperature elevations were observed and appeared to serve as an indicator of shunt function. Schumacher and colleagues believed the high morbidity and mortality and fair (at best) symptomatic relief limit the usefulness of shunt devices and suggested the use of external peritoneal drainage catheters. Anecdotal mention of 17 patients treated in this manner indicated ease of placement, with immediate and reproducible relief of symptoms, no perioperative mortality, and only one complication (catheter leakage).[16]

There are no prospective trials comparing the use of peritoneovenous shunts and external peritoneal drainage catheters. Malignant ascites of gastrointestinal origin may preclude shunt insertion, as the prognosis is poor and the inherent risk of this procedure is not justified. Generally, only patients who are expected to survive longer than 3 months with adequate cardiac function and nonviscous ascites should be considered for shunt placement. The decision regarding whether an external catheter is preferable must take into consideration the potential for shunt-related complications, the patient's ability to tolerate them, and whether an already dismal prognosis should be compromised by a more invasive, potentially morbid procedure.

Future modalities for the therapy of malignant ascites include immunotherapy with intraabdominal immunostimulants and matrix metalloproteinase inhibitors. OK-432 has shown promising results in a Japanese study, conferring a response rate of 62% and increased survivals of 3–10 months.[1,3] Early studies of metalloproteinase inhibitors in other cell lines have shown regression of tumor cells by interfering with angiogenesis.[1] These treatments are currently in their experimental stages and must be validated before they are applied clinically.

Malignant ascites is a complication of disseminated tumor burden in the peritoneal cavity. The therapy should be aimed at identifying the primary neoplasm and instituting appropriate therapeutic modalities. Relief of malignant ascites is paramount, and palliation of symptoms should be considered the most important priority in these patients with dismal prognoses.

References

1. Parsons SL, Watson SA, Steele RJ. Malignant ascites. Br J Surg 1996;83: 6–14.
2. Smith IC, Heys SD, Eremin O. Surgical management of patients with advanced cancer. Eur J Surg Oncol 1997;23:178–182.
3. Sharma S, Walsh D. Management of symptomatic malignant ascites with diuretics: two case reports and a review of the literature. J Pain Symptom Manage 1995;10:237–242.
4. Parsons SL, Lang MW, Steele RJ. Malignant ascites: a 2-year review from a teaching hospital. Eur J Surg Oncol 1996;22:237–239.
5. Kim Y, Cho O, Song S. Peritoneal lymphomatosis: CT findings. Abdom Imaging 1998;23:87–90.
6. Loggie BW, Perini M, Fleming RA. Treatment and prevention of malignant ascites associated with disseminated intraperitoneal malignancies by aggressive combined modality therapy. Am Surg 1997;63:137–143.
7. Alberts DS, Liu PY, Hannigan EV, et al. Intraperitoneal cisplatin plus intravenous cyclophosphamide versus intravenous cisplatin plus intravenous cyclophosphamide for stage III ovarian cancer. N Engl J Med 1996;335: 1950–1955.
8. Recio FO, Piver MS, Hempling RE, Driscoll DL. Five year survival after second-line cisplatin-based intraperitoneal chemotherapy for advanced ovarian cancer. Gynecol Oncol 1998;68:267–273.
9. Romensch J, Whitock J, Schwartz J, Hines J, Reba R, Harper P. In vitro and in vivo studies on the development of the alpha-emitting radionuclide bismuth 212 for intraperitoneal use against microscopic ovarian carcinoma. Am J Obstet Gynecol 1997;176:833–840.
10. Scheithauer W, Kornek GV, Marczell A, et al. Combined intravenous and intraperitoneal chemotherapy with fluorouracil + leucovorin vs fluorouracil + levamisole for adjuvant therapy of resected colon carcinoma. Br J Cancer 1998;77:1349–1354.
11. Young RC, Walton LA, Ellenberg SS, et al. Adjuvant therapy in stage I and stage II epithelial ovarian cancer: results of two prospective randomized trials. N Engl J Med 1990;322:1021–1027.

12. Straus AK, Roseman DL, Shapiro TM. Peritoneovenous shunting in the management of malignant ascites. Arch Surg 1979;114:489–491.
13. LeVeen EG, LeVeen HH. The place of peritoneovenous shunt in the treatment of ascites. ASAIO Trans 1989;35:165–168.
14. Tempero MA, Davis RB, Reed E, Edney J. Thrombocytopenia and laboratory evidence of disseminated intravascular coagulation after shunts for ascites in malignant disease. Cancer 1985;55:2718–2721.
15. Bracci F, Bracaglia C, Zampino MA, Farina F, Cucchiarra G. The Denver peritoneojugular shunt: current indications. Minerva Med 1989;80:363–366.
16. Schumacher DL, Saclarides TJ, Staren ED. Peritoneovenous shunts for the palliation of the patient with malignant ascites. Ann Surg Oncol 1994;1: 378–381.

Section 15

Surgical Adjuncts

CHAPTER 77

Management of the Patient with Pain

JUDITH A. PAICE

Cancer pain is often undertreated owing to knowledge deficits, misconceptions regarding addiction and tolerance, inadequate assessment, and regulatory concerns.[1] To provide optimal control, surgeons treating patients with cancer-related pain must overcome these barriers and become informed about pain assessment techniques and appropriate use of analgesics. Pain can be minimized, and in many cases prevented, during diagnostic and surgical interventions.[2] After surgery good pain relief provided by skillful surgeons allows adequate inspiration, earlier ambulation, and improved range of motion,[2,3] which can enhance recovery. Furthermore, several studies have suggested that adequate delivery of analgesics, with resultant control of pain, favorably affects immune competence.[4] This is of particular concern to the individual with cancer.

The Agency for Healthcare Research and Quality, formerly the Agency for Health Care Policy and Research, developed clinical practice guidelines for acute pain management in 1992.[2] Included in these guidelines are algorithms for surgical pain treatment, differentiating the preoperative and intraoperative phases from the postoperative care. These algorithms also serve as a framework for the treatment of patients undergoing surgery for cancer. In 1994 the Agency released *Management of Cancer Pain*, describing the treatment of pain associated with malignancy throughout the disease continuum.[1]

Preoperative and Intraoperative Care

Pain management should begin before the surgical procedure or postoperative period. Prior to surgery it is essential to assess carefully the patient's pain and pain experiences. One should obtain a complete pain history, perform a thorough assessment, and conduct any indicated diagnostic studies. A treatment plan is generated based on this information, and patients and family members are made aware of this plan prior to surgery. During surgery analgesic and anesthetic techniques are incorporated to prevent pain to the greatest degree possible.

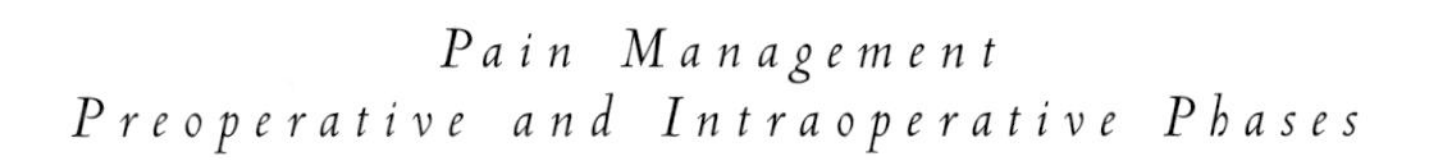

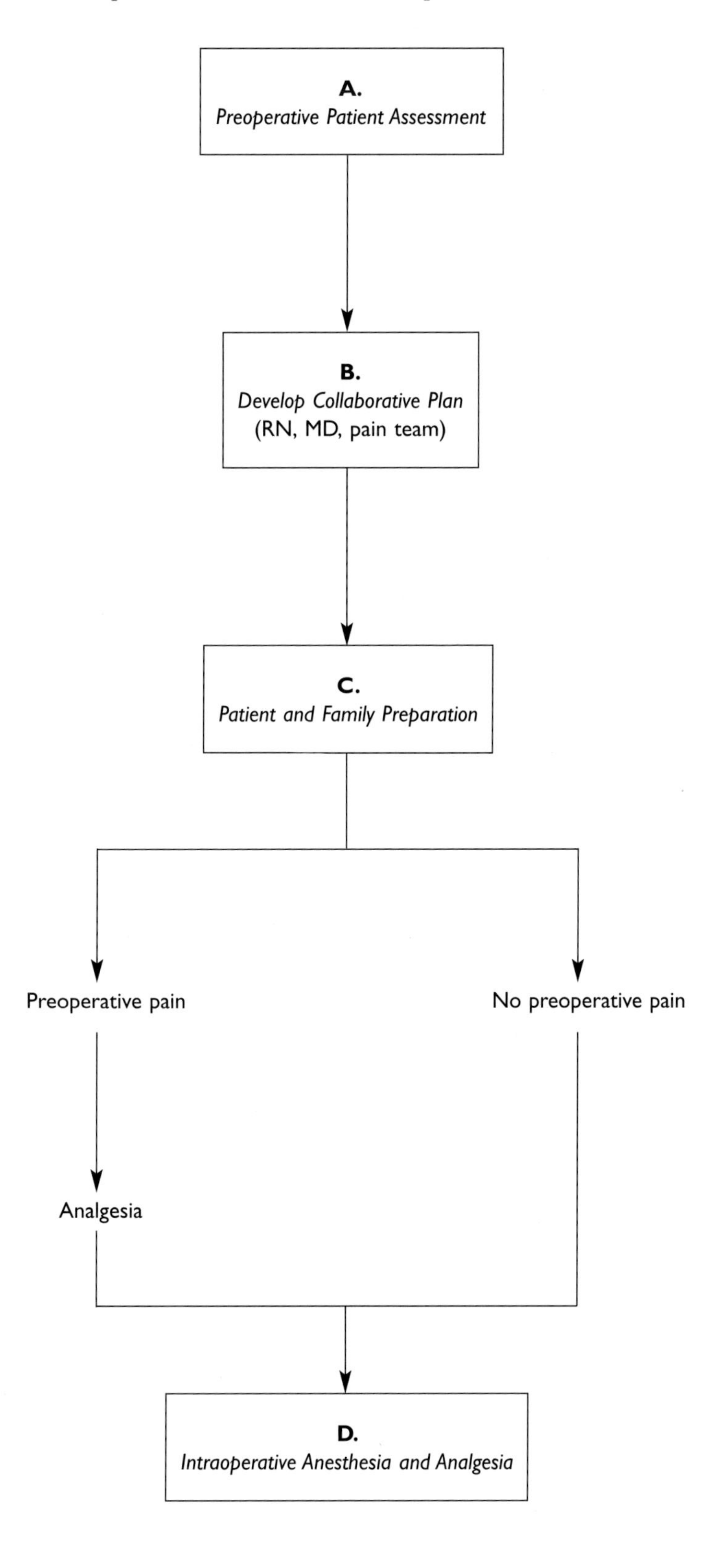

(continued on next page)

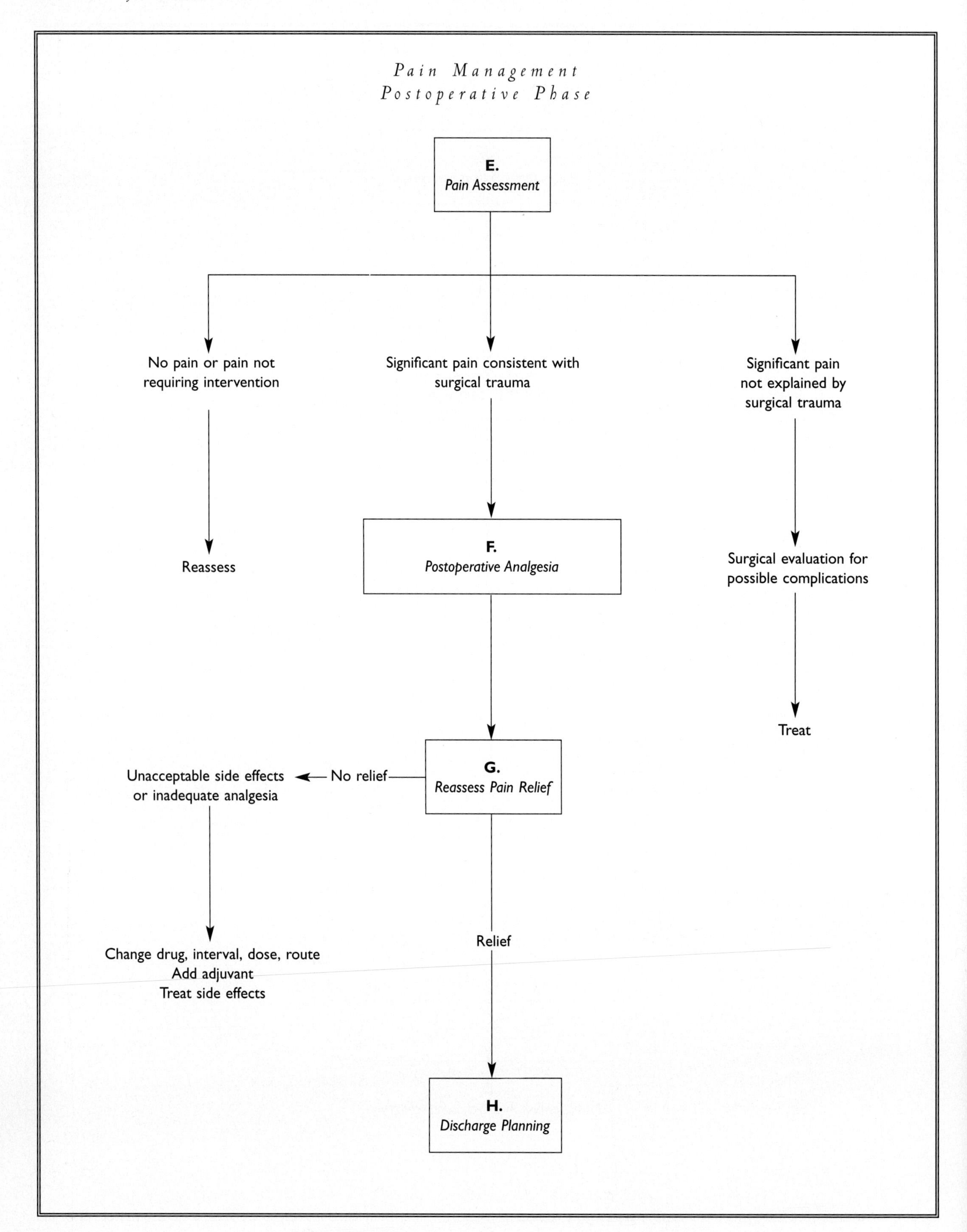
Pain Management
Postoperative Phase
E.
Pain Assessment
No pain or pain not requiring intervention
Significant pain consistent with surgical trauma
Significant pain not explained by surgical trauma
Reassess
F.
Postoperative Analgesia
Surgical evaluation for possible complications
Treat
Unacceptable side effects or inadequate analgesia
No relief
G.
Reassess Pain Relief
Change drug, interval, dose, route
Add adjuvant
Treat side effects
Relief
H.
Discharge Planning

A. *Preoperative Patient Assessment*

HISTORY Self-report is the most reliable indicator of an individual's pain. A pain history is critical and should include questions regarding the locations of pain, the present complaint, and any other chronic painful conditions preexisting the cancer diagnosis.[1,2] Intensity can be quantified using a simple 0 to 10 scale, where 0 indicates "no pain," and 10 signifies the "worst pain imaginable." For the few patients unable to use a numeric scale, descriptors such as none, mild, moderate, or severe can be used.

The quality of the pain, derived from the adjectives used by patients to describe the sensation, can suggest etiology and treatment.[5,6] Nociceptive pain, described as "aching" or "throbbing," is frequently associated with bone or soft tissue damage. Visceral pain, a subtype of nociceptive pain, is described as "squeezing" or "cramping." This pain is often generated by tumor involvement of the gastrointestinal or genitourinary systems. Neuropathic pain, associated with damage to the peripheral or central nervous system, is characterized using terms such as "burning," "tingling," or "shooting." Examples of neuropathic pain syndromes common with malignancy are listed in Table 77–1.

A thorough medication history is essential, and this information has direct implications for postoperative pain management. Patients should be asked about current analgesic medication use [including nonsteroidal antiinflammatory drugs (NSAIDs), opioids, and adjuvants], previous analgesic use, and any adverse effects noted with these drugs. Because of the effect of NSAIDs on platelet function, these agents should be discontinued prior to an invasive procedure.[7] Furthermore, the patient currently taking opioids for cancer pain requires significantly higher postoperative opioid doses than opioid-naive patients.[1] Patients may report past allergic responses to opioids when in fact they experienced nausea or vomiting. Clarify true allergy (e.g., bronchospasm) from common, and treatable, adverse effects. This is also an important time to query patients about fears of addiction or tolerance and dispel these concerns.

PHYSICAL EXAMINATION

The diagnostic evaluation includes a meticulous physical examination with particular attention to the neurologic examination. These data assist in identifying the etiology of the pain and any preexisting sensory changes. Laboratory values may reflect renal or liver abnormalities, which preclude the use of certain analgesics, such as meperidine and acetaminophen, respectively.[1,2] Despite the importance of physiologic data, an absence of obvious pathology does not preclude the reality of the patient's pain complaint.

B. *Develop Collaborative Plan*

A plan for pain management is developed by incorporating the data obtained from the pain history and physical examination. This may include a discussion with the anesthesiologist regarding intraoperative blocks or infusions to preempt pain (see below). Postoperative management may include parenteral administration of opioids, with or without patient-controlled analgesia (PCA).[8] Other options include spinal (usually epidural) delivery of an opioid alone or in combination with local anesthetics or clonidine.[2] This plan is based on the patient's previous response to analgesics, the type of surgery planned, and the patient's ability to participate in therapy.

TABLE 77–1.
Neuropathic pain states common with malignancy

Neuropathic pain states
Neuropathic pain originating from injury of the central nervous system
Brachial, cervical, or lumbosacral plexopathy due to tumor or radiation fibrosis
Spinal cord compression
Neuropathies originating from peripheral nerve injury
Acute and postherpetic neuropathies
Chemotherapy-induced peripheral neuropathies
Cranial neuropathies due to leptomeningeal disease or metastases to the base of the skull
Postlimb amputation/stump pain and phantom limb pain
Postmastectomy syndrome
Postnephrectomy pain
Postradical neck dissection
Postthoracotomy syndrome
Radiation-induced peripheral nerve tumors
Tumor infiltration of peripheral nerves

C. Patient and Family Preparation

Patients who are given procedural information and coping strategies are likely to have less pain and shorter lengths of stay.[9] Patients and their family members or caregivers should be assured that pain will be treated and should be informed about their responsibilities related to pain control. Patients should be advised and encouraged to report pain to the medical staff. Optimally, patients are educated regarding related technology, such as PCA, prior to surgery. Include families or caregivers in these discussions to help reinforce the material or identify fears and misconceptions they may have regarding pain and its management.

Many patients with cancer present with pain prior to surgery. This pain should be managed aggressively while planning for surgery. The patient with adequate relief is better prepared to tolerate the stress of surgery and less likely to experience complications associated with unrelieved pain.

D. Intraoperative Anesthesia and Analgesia

A complete discussion of intraoperative anesthetic techniques can be found in numerous textbooks.[10,11] Recent information suggests that additional techniques may actually prevent pain, which may inhibit central nervous system sensitization.[12] Once sensitized, nonpainful stimulation may be perceived as painful. This is one hypothesis for the origin of postsurgical pain states.[13] Studies of preemptive analgesia have employed intravenous opioids or NSAIDs, epidural infusions of opioids and local anesthetics, nerve blocks, infiltration of the wound with local anesthetics, or combinations of these techniques.[14,15] The benefits of these techniques can be profound. For example, preoperative epidural analgesia for elective limb amputation reduced phantom limb pain, a potentially debilitating complication of surgery.[16] A randomized, controlled study of preemptive epidural analgesia started prior to induction for radical prostatectomy demonstrated a 33% reduction in pain when comparing subjects who received either fentanyl or bupivacaine versus saline.[17] This relief resulted in improved activity 3.5 weeks after surgery. Furthermore, there was no difference in postoperative complications among the three groups, providing evidence of the safety of these preemptive techniques.

Postoperative Management

Postoperative analgesia begins long before termination of the intraoperative anesthetic. Optimizing postoperative management is critical and depends on an ongoing assessment, knowledge of the available pharmacologic agents, the routes of administration of these drugs, and the principles that guide the use of these medications.

E. Pain Assessment

The assessment of postoperative pain depends on the data derived from the pain history conducted preoperatively. Immediately upon termination of the operative anesthesia and frequently during the postoperative period patients are queried regarding the presence of pain.[2] Should the patient report no pain, reassessment continues on an ongoing basis. Moderate to severe pain that is not consistent with the typical postoperative course demands surgical evaluation for complications, which should then be treated. Pain that is consistent with the surgical trauma should be treated with analgesics.

F. Postoperative Analgesia

There are three primary categories of medications used to treat pain, including NSAIDs, opioids, and adjuvant medications. Most cancer patients with postoperative pain can obtain relief using these agents, either singly or in combination. The dosing schedule is critical and depends on the relative duration of action of the drug and the patient's response. Attention also must be paid to preventing and treating the adverse effects of these drugs. Various routes of administration are available, particularly when the oral route is not feasible.

Nonopioids Nonsteroidal antiinflammatory drugs or acetaminophen can be used alone to relieve mild pain or in combination with an opioid for moderate to severe pain. Both agents have analgesic and antipyretic effects. NSAIDs can be effective when treating bone pain or pain associated with inflammation.[1,2] The potent NSAID ketorolac can be given intramuscularly or intravenously, although the enhanced potency is associated with an increased prevalence of adverse effects.[18] Adverse effects of all NSAIDs include gastrointestinal bleeding, bleeding from other sites including the operative site, and nephrotoxicity; these drugs should therefore be avoided in patients with a current or prior history of gastrointestinal ulcers, thrombocytopenia, or renal dysfunction.[7,18,19]

Acetaminophen doses higher than 4000 mg/day may lead to liver failure.[20] This is of particular concern when using admixtures of weak opioids, such as hydrocodone and acetaminophen. These formulations often contain 500 mg of acetaminophen per tablet. Therefore a typical postoperative order of one or two tablets every 4 hours could lead to a daily dose of 6000 mg of acetaminophen, 50% more than the recommended dose.

OPIOIDS Opioids are the mainstay of postoperative pain management. The pure agonist opioids (morphine, hydromorphone, codeine, oxycodone, fentanyl) are preferred over mixed agonist-antagonists.[1] Mixed agonist-antagonist opioids (butorphanol, pentazocine, dezocine) are more likely to cause cognitive changes, and their long-term use is complicated by the lack of oral preparations. Furthermore, it is of particular concern in surgical oncology that these agents can precipitate withdrawal symptoms when given to patients currently taking pure agonist opioids. Thus the cancer patient on a regimen of morphine for preexisting pain can experience the abstinence syndrome when given a mixed agonist-antagonist.

Meperidine (Demerol) is to be avoided in the treatment of cancer-related pain.[1,2,21–23] Meperidine is often underdosed; typically, 75 mg IM is given every 4 hours. The morphine equivalence is approximately 10 mg, an inadequate postoperative dose for many adults. In addition, the duration of action of meperidine is usually 2–3 hours, so every-4-hour administration is inadequate. Likewise, oral meperidine has poor oral availability, with 50 mg PO approximately equivalent to two aspirin tablets.[21] Most important, meperidine's metabolite normeperidine accumulates during renal dysfunction. Elevated plasma levels of normeperidine are toxic to the central nervous system, leading to irritability, tremors, seizures, and death.[22,23]

A common problem in the management of postoperative cancer pain is lack of recognition of tolerance to opioids. Usual postoperative opioid doses are applied to patients already receiving significant amounts of morphine prior to surgery, leading to severe pain after surgery. Equianalgesic conversions should be conducted to provide the patient's usual opioid dose along with additional amounts of drug to treat the postoperative pain. For example, oral morphine doses must be approximately three times the parenteral dose to provide equal analgesia.[1] Thus a patient receiving 150 mg of oral morphine per day (approximately equal to 50 mg parenterally) prior to surgery requires an intravenous morphine infusion of 2.0 mg/h to merely meet the preoperative opioid requirements. The infusion of morphine should be increased and bolus doses made available to treat the postoperative pain.

Traditionally, intramuscular routes are used to deliver opioids after surgery, yet this route results in great variability in absorption of the drug.[2] Furthermore, intramuscular injections are painful and can cause local tissue trauma, particularly in the cachectic cancer patient.[1] Therefore the oral route should be taken when patients are able to use their gastrointestinal tracts. When not able to swallow or ingest medications, the intravenous, subcutaneous, or rectal routes can be used.[24–26] Although useful for chronic pain, transdermal administration of fentanyl is not indicated for postoperative pain owing to the long interval to the onset of therapeutic plasma levels after applying the patch (approximately 17 hours).[27]

ADJUVANTS Adjuvant medications include tricyclic antidepressants, anticonvulsants, corticosteroids, local anesthetics, clonidine, and others.[1] Many patients with chronic pain associated with malignancy receive tricyclic antidepressants, anticonvulsants, or corticosteroids. The use of these agents for postoperative pain has not been well documented. However, to prevent return of the chronic painful condition, these agents should be resumed after surgery as soon as the patient is able to tolerate oral medications.

Of particular benefit during the postoperative period is the use of local anesthetics.[5] These agents are traditionally given epidurally or intrathecally, although interpleural administration has been shown to provide relief.[28,29] Bupivacaine is often combined with fentanyl or other opioids when given epidurally in doses that provide analgesia without motor blockade.[30] Continuous infusions and patient-controlled epidural analgesia (PCEA) are the standard methods of delivery.[31] Another adjuvant, clonidine, is a noradrenergic agonist known to relieve pain associated with surgery, cancer, and labor when given epidurally.[32] Commercial preparations are currently available in concentrations of 100 μg/ml.

G. *Reassess Pain Relief*

UNACCEPTABLE SIDE EFFECTS The side effects of opioids are easily managed in most patients.[1,2] Tolerance to these effects also develops rapidly, usually within 24–48 hours. Nausea and vomiting can be treated with antiemetics or switching the opioid. Urinary catheterization alleviates retention, seen frequently in men with prostatism. Pruritus responds to diphenhydramine to some degree. A change in opioid may also be required. Respiratory depression, although feared, is rare and easily reversed with naloxone.[33] Furthermore, because sedation always precedes respiratory depression, there is a warning period that allows the clinician time to act if indicated. Constipation can be prevented through the prophylactic use of stool softeners and laxatives.

INADEQUATE ANALGESIA Inadequate analgesia is generally treated by changing the dose, the drug, the interval, or the route.[2] Inadequate relief in the absence of adverse effects can usually be treated by dose escalation. Changing the opioid may be required if inadequate relief is coupled with adverse effects not responding to treatment. As-needed (PRN) dosing of analgesics has been shown to lead to inadequate analgesia. Stable and continued plasma levels of the analgesic lead to consistent pain relief, thereby avoiding periods of over- and undermedication. Analgesics should be administered on a schedule based on the pharmacokinetics of a particular drug, with titration based on the patient's response, as large individual variability in dose and duration exists.[1] The oral route is preferred when patients are able to take medicines by mouth. Intravenous administration is preferred when the patient cannot take anything by mouth. Epidural delivery of an opioid with local anesthetic or clonidine is an alternative when relief is ineffective.[28,32]

H. Discharge Planning

Discharge planning should include a simple, convenient, noninvasive pain treatment regimen for use after hospitalization.[1,2,34] Patients are given written instructions regarding their treatment plan, including the drug, dosage, adverse effects, and the name of a professional to contact should pain be uncontrolled.[2]

Conclusions

Surgeons treating patients with cancer must overcome numerous barriers to provide optimal pain control. Preoperative assessments and patient and family preparation reduce complications and enhance recovery. Intraoperative measures, including preemptive analgesia, can limit postoperative pain and potentially prevent chronic painful conditions. After surgery, good pain relief allows adequate inspiration, earlier ambulation, improved range of motion, enhanced immune function, and ultimately improved care for the patient.

References

1. Jacox A, Carr DB, Payne R, et al. Management of Cancer Pain. Clinical Practice Guideline No. 9. AHCPR Publication 94-0592. Rockville, MD: Agency for Health Care Policy and Research, Public Health Service, US Department of Health and Human Services, 1994.
2. Acute Pain Management Guideline Panel. Acute Pain Management: Operative or Medical Procedures and Trauma. Clinical Practice Guideline. AHCPR Publication 92-0032. Rockville, MD: Agency for Health Care Policy and Research, Public Health Service, US Department of Health and Human Services, 1992.
3. Egbert AM, Parks LH, Short LM, et al. Randomized trial of postoperative patient-controlled analgesia vs intramuscular narcotics in frail elderly men. Arch Intern Med 1990;150:1897–1903.
4. Page GG, Ben-Eliyahu S. The immune-suppressive nature of pain. Semin Oncol Nurs 1997;13:10–15.
5. Cousins M, Power I. Acute and postoperative pain. In: Wall PD, Melzak R (eds) Textbook of Pain (4th Ed.). Edinburgh: Churchill Livingstone, 1999:447–491.
6. Coda BA, Bonica JJ. General considerations of acute pain. In: Loeser JD, Butler SH, Chapman CR, Turk DC (eds) Bonica's management of pain, 3rd ed. Philadelphia: Lippincott Williams & Wilkins, 2001:222–240.
7. Schafer AI. Effects of nonsteroidal antiinflammatory drugs on platelet function and systemic hemostasis. J Clin Pharmacol 1995;35:209–219.
8. Ripamonti C, Bruera E. Current status of patient-controlled analgesia in cancer patients. Oncology 1997;11:373–384.
9. Reading AE. The effects of psychological preparation on pain and recovery after minor gynecological surgery: a preliminary report. J Clin Psychol 1982;38:504–512.
10. Barash PG, Cullen BF, Stoelting RK. Clinical Anesthesia, 3rd ed. Philadelphia: Lippincott-Raven, 1997.
11. Longnecker DE, Tinker JH, Morgan GE. Principles and Practices of Anesthesiology, 2rd ed. St. Louis: Mosby, 1997.
12. Woolf CJ. Evidence for a central component of post-injury pain hypersensitivity. Nature 1983;306:686–688.
13. Woolf CJ, Chong MS. Preemptive analgesia: treating postoperative pain by preventing the establishment of central sensitization. Anesth Analg 1993;77:362–379.
14. Hannibal K, Galatius H, Hansen A, et al. Preoperative wound infiltration with bupivacaine reduces early and late opioid requirements after hysterectomy. Anesth Analg 1996;83:376–381.
15. Dahl JB, Kehlet H. Preoperative epidural fentanyl, neuroplasticity, and postoperative pain. Anesthesiology 1993;78:801–803.
16. Bach S, Noreng MF, Tjellden NU. Phantom limb pain in amputees during the first 12 months following limb amputation, after preoperative lumbar epidural blockade. Pain 1988;33:297–301.
17. Gottschalk A, Smith DS, Jobes DR, et al. Preemptive epidural analgesia and recovery from radical prostatectomy. JAMA 1998;279:1076–1082.
18. Allison MC, Howatson AG, Torrance CJ, et al. Gastrointestinal damage associated with the use of nonsteroidal antiinflammatory drugs. N Engl J Med 1992;327:749–754.
19. Souter AJ, Fredman B, White PF. Controversies in the perioperative use of nonsteroidal antiinflammatory drugs. Anesth Analg 1994;79:1178–1190.
20. McGoldrick MD, Bailie GR. Nonnarcotic analgesics: prevalence and estimated economic impact of toxicities. Ann Pharmacother 1997;31:221–227.
21. Principles of analgesic use in the treatment of acute pain and cancer pain, 4th ed. Glenview, IL, American Pain Society, 1999.
22. Kaiko RF, Foley KM, Grabinski PY, et al. Central nervous system excitatory effects of meperidine in cancer patients. Ann Neurol 1983;13:180–185.
23. Szeto HH, Inturrisi C, Houde R, et al. Accumulation of normeperidine, an active metabolite of meperidine, in patients with renal failure or cancer. Ann Intern Med 1977;86:738–741.
24. Nelson KA, Glare PA, Walsh D, et al. A prospective, within-patient, crossover study of continuous intravenous and subcutaneous morphine for chronic cancer pain. J Pain Symptom Manage 1997;13:262–267.
25. SempleTJ, Upton RN, Macintyre PE, et al. Morphine blood concentrations in elderly postoperative patients following administration via an indwelling subcutaneous cannula. Anaesthesia 1997;52:318–323.
26. Cole L, Hanning CD. Review of the rectal use of opioids. J Pain Symptom Manage 1990;5:118–126.
27. Calis KA, Kohler DR, Corso DM. Transdermally administered fentanyl for pain management. Clin Pharm 1992;11:22–36.
28. Liu S, Carpenter RL, Neal JM. Epidural anesthesia and analgesia: their role in postoperative outcome. Anesthesiology 1995;82:1474–1506.
29. Raffin L, Fletcher D, Sperandio M, et al. Interpleural infusion of 2% lidocaine with 1:200,000 epinephrine for postthoracotomy analgesia. Anesth Analg 1994;79:328–334.
30. De Leon-Casasola OA, Parker B, Lema MJ, et al. Postoperative epidural bupivacaine-morphine therapy. Anesthesiology 1994;81:368–375.
31. Rockemann MG, Seeling W, Duschek S, et al. Epidural bolus clonidine/morphine versus epidural patient-controlled bupivacaine/sufen-

tanil: quality of postoperative analgesia and cost-identification analysis. Anesth Analg 1997;85:864–869.
32. Eisenach JC, DuPen S, Dubois M, et al. Epidural clonidine analgesia for intractable cancer pain. Pain 1995;61:391–399.
33. Ballantyne JC, Carr DB, Diferante S, et al. The comparative effects of postoperative analgesic therapies upon pulmonary outcome: cumulative meta-analyses of randomized, controlled trials. Anesth Analg 1998;86: 598–612.
34. Paice JA, Stanton-Hicks M. Extension of pain treatment: Home care. In: Raj PP (ed) Practical management of pain, 93rd ed. St. Louis: Mosby, 2000:961–967.

CHAPTER 78

Nutritional Support

JANET MILLIKAN
KEITH W. MILLIKAN

A. Initial Nutritional Considerations

Approximately 40–80% of cancer patients experience some degree of malnutrition[1] leading to increased morbidity and mortality rates, decreased tolerance of cancer treatment, and decreased quality of life.[2,3] The degree of malnutrition varies depending on disease type and stage. Malnutrition develops because of: (1) the cancer process itself (e.g., tumor obstructing the gastrointestinal tract); (2) side effects of cancer treatment (i.e., radiation enteritis); (3) cancer cachexia.

Cancer cachexia is a devastating burden to the host and is present with both advanced and early malignant disease. It is a tumor-derived, progressive wasting syndrome characterized by anorexia, weight loss, asthenia, anemia, and nutrient metabolism abnormalities distinct from those observed with simple starvation. Although its symptoms are easy to identify, its cause is unknown, making it difficult to treat. Causative factors include: (1) humorally mediated factors affecting the hypothalamus and ultimately decreasing appetite and intake; (2) malabsorption; (3) changes in energy expenditure; (4) humoral factors secreted by tumor cells or produced elsewhere in the body in response to the presence of the tumor; (5) response to antineoplastic therapy; and (6) deranged nutrient/substrate metabolism. Research has focused on the role of cytokines [tumor necrosis factor-α (TNFα), interleukins 1 and 6 (IL-1, IL-6), interferon-γ (INFγ), and leukemia-inhibiting factor] as factors responsible for the cachexia syndrome. It is generally thought that the syndrome is due to a combination of these factors.[4–9]

Anorexia and weight loss are common components of malnutrition, experienced by approximately 50% of cancer patients.[3,10] Some clinicians speculate that anorexia and the resulting decrease in oral intake are the result of a cytokine-induced increase in hypothalmic, serotonergic activity.[11,12] Weight loss by a cancer patient does not parallel that seen with simple starvation.[13] Increased catabolism of whole-body protein, decreased protein synthesis, and insulin action due to increased circulating glucose levels prevents lipolysis, resulting in weight loss of equal amounts of fat and protein.[6,14,15] The incidence of weight loss in patients with gastrointestinal cancers tends to be higher than in patients with breast cancer, sarcomas, acute nonlymphocytic leukemia, and favorable non-Hodgkin's lymphoma. Patients with advanced cancers have the highest degree of body mass depletion. The positive correlation between

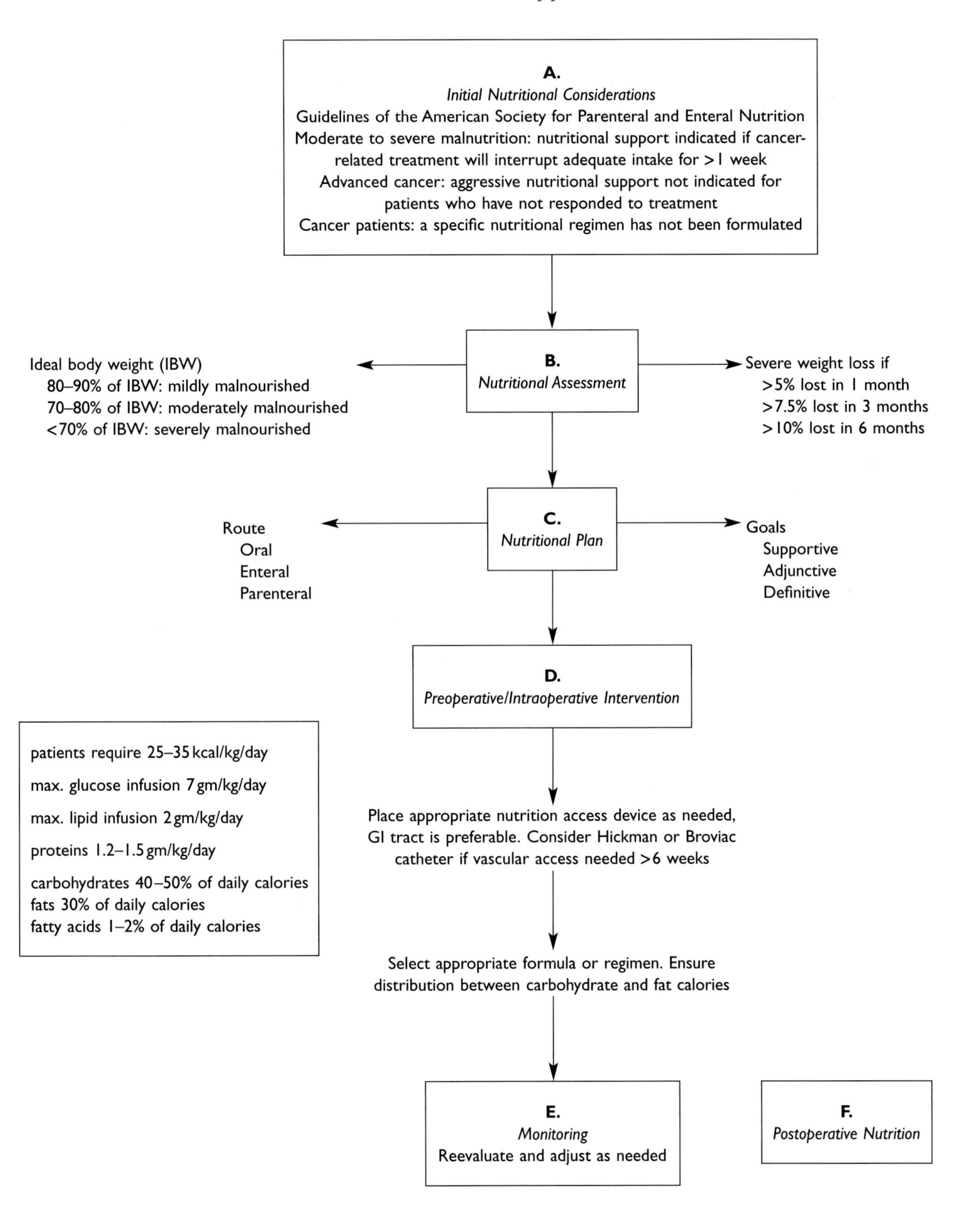

Nutritional Support
A.
Initial Nutritional Considerations
Guidelines of the American Society for Parenteral and Enteral Nutrition
Moderate to severe malnutrition: nutritional support indicated if cancer-related treatment will interrupt adequate intake for >1 week
Advanced cancer: aggressive nutritional support not indicated for patients who have not responded to treatment
Cancer patients: a specific nutritional regimen has not been formulated
B.
Nutritional Assessment
Ideal body weight (IBW)
80–90% of IBW: mildly malnourished
70–80% of IBW: moderately malnourished
<70% of IBW: severely malnourished
Severe weight loss if
>5% lost in 1 month
>7.5% lost in 3 months
>10% lost in 6 months
C.
Nutritional Plan
Route
Oral
Enteral
Parenteral
Goals
Supportive
Adjunctive
Definitive
D.
Preoperative/Intraoperative Intervention
patients require 25–35 kcal/kg/day
max. glucose infusion 7 gm/kg/day
max. lipid infusion 2 gm/kg/day
proteins 1.2–1.5 gm/kg/day
carbohydrates 40–50% of daily calories
fats 30% of daily calories
fatty acids 1–2% of daily calories
Place appropriate nutrition access device as needed, GI tract is preferable. Consider Hickman or Broviac catheter if vascular access needed >6 weeks
Select appropriate formula or regimen. Ensure distribution between carbohydrate and fat calories
E.
Monitoring
Reevaluate and adjust as needed
F.
Postoperative Nutrition

Determining the Best Feeding Method

Function of the gastrointestinal tract

Nonfunctional

Consider preoperative parenteral nutrition prior to surgery as indicated by nutritional status and continue as needed after surgery

Functional

Support nutritional requirements orally, as tolerated, to meet at least 90% of the patient's nutritional needs with regular food and/or nutritional supplements

Patient unable to meet nutritional needs with regular foods and/or supplements before or after surgical intervention

Tube feedings not a safe or viable option

Tube feedings possible

Tube feeding expected to be needed for <6 weeks

Long term enteral access needed (>6 weeks)

Nasoenteric tube

Tube enterostomy

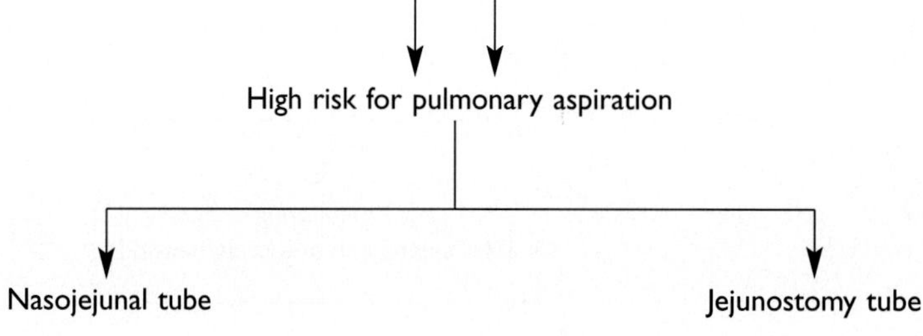

a cancer patient's weight loss and decreased survival, decreased quality of life, and decreased performance and productivity explains the emphasis on trying to reverse this problem.[3,16,17] Host depletion is a major concern in the surgical patient, as it correlates with an increased incidence of postoperative complications including sepsis, wound dehiscence, ileus, immune compromise, impaired pulmonary function, and death.[18–21]

Logically, it seems simple that if supplemental nutrition is provided the host can be repleted, or depletion can be prevented. However, studies have not conclusively supported "universal" nutritional therapy for most cancer patients. Klein and Koretz reviewed more than 70 prospective, randomized, controlled studies of nutritional support; results failed to show a positive benefit in terms of improved morbidity, mortality, or length of stay for most cancer populations. Of note, however, is that most of the studies reviewed had problems with study design and sample size, limiting their value.[22] Current studies are showing promise as to the positive benefits of using nutritional support for malnourished patients.[23–26] One such study of patients undergoing gastrointestinal surgery showed that there were fewer wound complications, fewer infections, and decreased length of hospital stay when patients were fed an arginine/omega-3 fatty acid/RNA-supplemented enteral formula compared with patients supported with standard enteral formulas.[24] Studies evaluating the use of glutamine supplementation in many patient populations continue to show the positive effects of this amino acid on gut immune function, nitrogen balance, and decreased bacterial translocation. A thorough review was presented by Herskowitz and Souba.[26]

Researchers have yet to put to rest several ongoing issues, such as whether the patient can actualize protein accrual and improve lean body mass[27–29] and whether tumor growth is stimulated by nutritional support.[30,31] With these issues in mind, guidelines for nutritional support of cancer patients provided by the American Society for Parenteral and Enteral Nutrition (ASPEN) Board of Directors are as follows: (1) individuals diagnosed with moderate or severe malnutrition who are expected to undergo cancer treatment that will inhibit or prolong adequate intake for more than 1 week should have nutritional intervention; (2) patients with mild malnutrition or advanced-stage cancer who have a documented nonresponse to cancer treatment are not likely to benefit from total parenteral nutrition (TPN) and should not be considered candidates for aggressive nutritional support; (3) no specialized nutritional support exists for cancer patients despite many efforts to formulate a cancer-specific nutrition regimen.[32] Despite conflicting findings, use of nutritional support (TPN) continues to rise.[33] Current thinking and practice by some clinicians indicates that death by starvation for patients with curable, treatable, or stable cancers is inappropriate; and nutritional intervention is warranted when cancer treatments are to be continued for the purpose of saving the patient.[33,34]

B. *Nutritional Assessment*

Nutritional support must be considered when the malnourished cancer patient undergoes surgery. Determining nutritional status (degree of malnutrition) is accomplished by reviewing the patient's: (1) dietary history; (2) weight and metabolic status; (3) physical assessment; (4) laboratory data; (5) medical history, including gastrointestinal symptoms and the treatment plan.[35–38] An in-depth description of a nutritional screening process called the Scored Patient-Generated Global Assessment (PG-SGA) can be found elsewhere.[38–41] This type of assessment may detect problems earlier in the patient's course and allows quantification of the overall nutritional status.

Despite new techniques for evaluating malnutrition, historical methods continue to be used and have included assessment of proteins, measuring body weight, and determining the degree of weight loss. If the weight is 80–90% of ideal body weight (IBW), the patient is mildly malnourished; 70–80% of IBW constitutes moderate malnourishment; and less than 70% of IBW is categorized as severe body mass depletion. Weight loss is considered *significant* if: (1) 5% weight loss occurred in 1 month; (2) 7.5% of the patient's weight was lost in 3 months; or (3) 10% of body weight was lost in 6 months. A patient's weight loss is considered *severe* if: (1) more than 5% of body weight is lost in 1 month, (2) more than 7.5% of body weight is lost in 3 months; or (3) more than 10% of body weight is lost in 6 months. Serum albumin levels are often used to assess visceral protein stores; however, thyroxine-binding prealbumin is becoming a more popular indicator given its short half-life of 2–3 days compared to albumin's half-life of 21 days.[42] *Mild* visceral protein loss is reflected by an albumin level of 2.8–3.5 g/dl or a prealbumin reading of 10–15 mg/dl. *Moderate* depletion is an albumin level of 2.1–2.7 g/dl or a prealbumin reading of 5–10 mg/dl. *Severe* visceral protein store depletion is <2.1 g/dl of albumin or a prealbumin level of <5 mg/dl.[35,43]

Questions about the predictive power of anthropometrics and plasma proteins have arisen given the variations that are due to factors other than malnutrition (i.e., fluid status and surgery). Baker et al. and Detsky et al. have shown clinical judgment to be a useful predictor of malnutrition.[44,45] The PG-SGA may be the best way to evaluate nutritional status given that this method allows patient scoring on the following features: (1) weight change; (2) dietary intake or lack thereof; (3) gastrointestinal symptoms; (4) functional capacity; (5) stress; and (6) physical signs.[46,47]

C. *Nutritional Plan*

Once the presence or potential for moderate to severe malnutrition has been identified, an individualized plan for nutritional support can be established. All cancer patients and, perhaps most importantly, the surgical patient can benefit from a thorough evaluation of the overall treatment plan (surgery, chemotherapy, irradiation) and its possible side effects. Anticipating treatment side effects can help the surgeon plan for postoperative nutrition. Such forethought can prevent (1) additional postoperative procedures (i.e., placement of a jejunostomy tube at a later time instead of simultaneously with the planned cancer surgery) and (2) replacement of inappropriate equipment (i.e., replacing single-lumen catheters with a catheter with multiple lumens for chemotherapy and TPN). Identifying the postoperative need for nutritional support preoperatively can help reduce potential postoperative complications.[16] Table 78–1 lists possible nutrition-related side effects of cancer therapies.[48]

Determining a patient's nutrient requirements is based on an overall assessment. Studies have shown that cancer patients have abnormal resting energy expenditures (REE) that can be unpredictable and not necessarily hypermetabolic depending on the tumor type and cancer stage.[49,50] For example, Dempsey et al. studied REEs in gastrointestinal cancer patients and found that those with gastric cancers were predominantly hypermetabolic and patients with pancreatic or hepatobiliary tumors were predominantly hypometabolic.[49] Fredrix et al. demonstrated elevated REEs in lung cancer patients but normal REEs in gastric and colorectal cancer patients.[50] In addition, patients undergoing major abdominal surgery increase their energy expenditure by approximately 10% during the first few postoperative days; it returns to baseline after 5 days.[51] One must also consider that tumor removal tends to normalize the REE.[42] Obtaining serial REEs to evaluate changes in an individual patient's nutritional requirements is ideal. Once the REE is established, the clinician may provide the patient with a nutrition prescription at 115–130% of REE for maintenance and 150% of REE for nutritional repletion.

TABLE 78–1.
Cancer treatments and their nutritional side effects

Surgical procedures
- Oropharyngeal resection: chewing and swallowing problems
- Esophagectomy: early satiety, achlorhydria, gastric stasis, diarrhea, steatorrhea secondary to vagotomy
- Gastrectomy (total or high subtotal): dumping syndrome, malabsorption, early satiety
- Jejunectomy: malabsorption of nutrients
- Ileal resection: bile salt losses, steatorrhea, diarrhea, fat and fat-soluble vitamin malabsorption, calcium and magnesium depletion, hyperoxaluria, renal stones
- Massive bowel resection: malabsorption, dehydration, malnutrition with vitamin B_{12} malabsorption, blind loop syndromes, metabolic acidosis, salt and water imbalance with ostomies
- Pancreatectomy: malabsorption, diabetes mellitus

Radiation therapy
- Head and neck: loss of teeth, loss of taste, odynophagia, esophagitis, dysphagia, nausea, stenosis, fibrosis with esophageal strictures, fistulas
- Abdomen and pelvis: erosion of mucosal lining and loss of intestinal villa, resulting in bowel damage with diarrhea, malabsorption, stenosis, or obstruction; possible ulceration with bleeding, vomiting, and resulting weight loss

Chemotherapy
- Toxic effects vary with the drugs. Possible side effects: mucositis, oral ulcerations, stomatitis, glossitis, nausea, vomiting, diarrhea, constipation, hepatotoxicity, electrolyte imbalance, nephrotoxicity

Ongoing evaluation of the patient's status to allow appropriate nutritional provisions is always prudent. For maintenance, cancer patients require 25–35 kcal/kg/day with additional requirements for weight gain.[52] When determining TPN composition, a mixed fuel system of amino acids, carbohydrates, and fat is ideal; this regimen prevents excess glucose use (the maximal glucose infusion rate is 7 g/kg/day)[53] and promotes appropriate lipid provisions (maximal lipid infusion rate is 2 g/kg/day). Carbohydrates are typically provided to the patient at 40–50% of their calorie needs, and fat makes up 30% of the calories, with essential fatty acids providing 1–2% of calories to prevent essential fatty acid deficiency. Protein needs range from 1.2 to 1.5 g/kg/day with increased requirements for those with large intestinal losses or severe stress.[52]

Providing specific nutrient prescriptions is determined by the ability of the patient to handle the necessary fluid loads. Review of the patient's volume status and cardiovascular, renal, hepatic, and pulmonary systems helps determine the patient's reaction to added volume via the feeding regimen. Average fluid requirements for adult patients are 30 ml/kg or 1400 ml/m^2.[54] If the patient is meeting the estimated nutritional requirements, no nutritional intervention may be necessary. However, many oncologic operations prevent nutritional intake or change the way the patient can receive nutrients.

Once it has been determined that the patient requires aggressive nutritional support, three routes can be used: oral, enteral, or parenteral. Determining the best route is based on the patient's overall assessment and expected tolerance. Oral or enteral feedings are preferred to the parenteral route if the gut is functional and nutritional needs can be met.[39] When deciding between enteral or parenteral feeding, refer to the algorithm.[55] Oral feedings may not be an option for the malnourished cancer patient who has difficulty eating average quantities of food and drink. Nutritional supplements, such as Ensure, are nutrient-dense but require that a significant volume be consumed, which may not be tolerated by patients with nausea. Enteral feeding provides liquid nutrients via a feeding tube, typically a nasoenteric or tube enterostomy. TPN is provision of a hyperosmolar dextrose/amino acid/lipid-based solution via a central vein.

Nutrition is provided to prevent progression of malnutrition, to improve nutritional status, and to maintain patient body composition, functional status, and quality of life. In the outcome/results-based health care system it is important to focus on the objective of nutritional therapy. As described by Shils, these objectives are categorized as follows: (1) definitive—sustains life in those who cannot receive nutrition by any other means; (2) supportive—allows future or additional treatments by supporting the patient's nutritional needs; and (3) adjunctive—uses nutritional therapy as part of the treatment plan.[56] Nutritional support is not a cancer treatment but can help improve/maintain the patient's status to tolerate invasive, rigorous cancer treatments.

D. Preoperative/Intraoperative Intervention

Once the goals and best route of nutritional support have been established, patients with treatable cancers who have moderate to severe malnutrition may benefit from 7–10 days of preoperative nutritional support if surgery can be delayed without harm.[57] A review by Daley et al. revealed a trend toward improved nutritional status in the severely malnourished patient who received preoperative nutrition.[2] This benefit may not outweigh the cost of intervention, as clinical outcomes remain less well defined.[22] If surgery is undertaken without preoperatively addressing nutritional derangements, one must still consider what the postoperative nutritional needs may be. If surgery is performed emergently, the procedure should include providing access for a postoperative feeding regimen. This may involve placing an enterostomy tube or central venous catheter.

Access to the gastrointestinal tract or a central vein is necessary for provision of nutrients. For oral supplementation the patient must be able to chew/swallow solid food and liquids without a gastrointestinal obstruction preventing its passage. A patient should not undergo oral dietary manipulation if vomiting or diarrhea prevent adequate digestion and absorption. The enteral route is preferred if the gastrointestinal tract is functioning and adequate oral intake is not possible. Tubes can be placed in the stomach, jejunum, or duodenum via laparotomy, laparoscopy, fluoroscopy, or endoscopy.[58] Creative tube placement may be necessary for the head and neck cancer patient, as nasogastric and nasojejunal tubes are contraindicated for patients with extensive neck involvement or thrombocytopenia. Thrombocytopenia may pose a problem when placing central venous lines. Also, a patient who has previously had multiple lines may have thrombosis of the commonly used veins. The standard approach for central venous access is percutaneous, infraclavicular subclavian vein catheterization. Long-lasting Hickman or Broviac Silastic catheters are typically used if one anticipates needing central access for longer than 6 weeks. Multiple-lumen catheters allow administration of various fluids (i.e., antibiotics or chemotherapy) at the same time as TPN infusion.

Selecting the most appropriate oral supplements, enteral formula, or TPN formulation permits one to meet estimated nutritional requirements. Many tube-feeding formulas are available for use. Given that no specialized formulas have been recommended for the oncology patient, selection should be based on (1) the patient's macronutrient requirements; (2) patient-specific, disease-specific nutrient requirements/restrictions; and (3) formula availability. Formulas exist that vary in water, protein, carbohydrate, and fat content. There are also, formulas available with fiber, partially hydrolyzed nutrients, or disease-specific nutrients.[59] Typically, the hospital formulary dictates what is available during the patient's hospital stay. Once the formula has been selected, the clinician must determine the appropriate delivery system and length of administration. Enteral formulas can be administered by bolus, intermittently, or by electronic pump methods. The length of time for feeding delivery typically depends on the volume necessary to meet the patient's nutrient needs and the patient's expected tolerance.

The macronutrient components (water, carbohydrate, protein, fat) and micronutrient requirements (vitamins, minerals, electrolytes, trace elements) for TPN solutions should be determined carefully. A guide on how to formulate patient-specific TPN has been described by Maillet.[60] Carbohydrates in TPN solutions supply 3.4 kcal/g, and fat in TPN solutions supplies 9 kcal/g. Typical electrolyte additives for TPN solutions are sodium 60–120 mEq, potassium 60–100 mEq, chloride 60–120 mEq, calcium 200–400 mg, phosphorus 300–400 mg, and magnesium 8–10 mEq. Lipids can be included in the TPN solutions or "piggybacked" into the standard parenteral solution. It is important to ensure proper distribution between carbohydrate calories and fat calories to prevent excess administration of either substrate. Hyperglycemia and hepatic steatosis are unwanted side effects of excess glucose infusion and can further compromise the oncology patient with specific metabolic derangements (described later in the chapter). Excess lipid administration can create an impaired immune response and elevated liver function tests, which are unwelcome side effects. The typical initiation of TPN is 1 liter of the patient's goal solution. Lipids can be added once a normal triglyceride level has been established (triglyceride level must be within normal limits prior to use of total nutrient admixtures). Advancement to the patient's goal TPN occurs when the initial liter of TPN is tolerated.

E. Monitoring

Monitoring guidelines for all TPN patients include daily intake and output; chemistry panels that include electrolytes, minerals, triglycerides, protein stores, blood glucose, and liver function tests; coagulation factors; daily weights, and nitrogen balance. Monitoring the tolerance to oral and enteral feedings varies but typically includes laboratory values, body weight, fluid status, and abdominal side effects.

The surgeon must also be aware of metabolic derangements that may affect the patient's ability to tolerate nutritional support. Carbohydrate derangements included increased glucose production and increased resistance and tolerance to insulin. Protein metabolism changes include increased whole-body protein turnover and decreased muscle protein synthesis. Abnormalities in fat metabolism include depletion of fat stores with increased lipid turnover and hyperlipidemia.[12] These metabolic derangements likely contribute to ineffective utilization of absorbed or infused nutrients, thereby preventing host repletion. It is important to be aware of these potential abnormalities when prescribing and monitoring nutritional supplementation. Adjustments may be necessary to help control a patient's abnormal response to nutritional therapy (i.e., decrease the amount of glucose calories in the feeding regimen of patients with elevated blood glucose or try to correct it with insulin).

F. *Postoperative Nutrition*

Feedings are discontinued prior to surgery. Starting nutritional support for the malnourished patient can begin almost immediately after operation. Postsurgical goals for nutritional support will likely differ from the patient's preoperative goals. Early in the postoperative period a patient's REE can be elevated by 10%, and the protein requirement likely has increased secondary to the stress of surgical intervention. The macronutrients supplied to the patient must often be adjusted. Patients who may have been given oral supplements preoperatively may require enteral or parenteral nutrition for a time. If the patient's gastrointestinal tract is functioning and capable of tolerating volume, enteral feeding is a viable modality. Otherwise, TPN followed by a gradual transition from TPN to enteral feedings is an option.

Nutrition for the terminally ill cancer patient is another complex area in which the surgeon is often involved. Certainly quality of life issues are important considerations for this group of patients. Such issues were thoughtfully addressed by Bozzetti et al.[33] A committee of experts developed a three-step process to meet needs and expectations of the terminally ill cancer patient. Step 1 involved using eight parameters to reach a decision regarding feeding: (1) oncologic/clinical condition; (2) symptoms; (3) expected length of survival; (4) nutritional and hydration status; (5) oral intake; (6) psychological profile; (7) gut function and available routes of nutrient administration; and (8) the need for specialized services required for the prescribed nutrition support method. Step 2 was to make the decision to feed or hydrate the patient based on the pros and cons of step 1 and a well defined endpoint (i.e., quality of life improved, maintain survival). Step 3 entailed periodic reevaluation of the patient to determine whether the goals have been reached or have become unattainable because of new developments.

The clear benefit from nutritional support of the cancer setting is preventing death by starvation. Further well controlled studies are needed to narrow or broaden the scope of nutritional support for the cancer patient. Currently, the clinician must evaluate patient specifics when determining the appropriateness of aggressive nutritional support, including: (1) the expected response rate to anticancer therapy; (2) the question of whether risks outweigh benefits of the intervention or vice versa; (3) whether the gastrointestinal tract can support nutritional needs. The "best" way to support malnourished cancer patients nutritionally remains elusive; but to be able to determine and implement appropriate nutritional regimens is important in this patient population.

References

1. Chute CG, Greenberg ER, Baron J, Korson R, Baker J, Yates J. Presenting conditions of 1539 population-based cancer patients in New Hampshire and Vermont. Cancer 1985;56:2107–2111.
2. Daly JM, Redmond HP, Gallagher H. Perioperative nutrition in cancer patients. J Parent Ent Nutr 1992;16(suppl):100S–105S.
3. DeWys WD, Begg D, Lavin PT, et al. Prognostic effects of weight loss prior to chemotherapy in cancer patients. Am J Med 1980;69:491–497.
4. Kern KA, Norton JA. Cancer cachexia. J Parent Ent Nutr 1988;12:286–298.
5. Langstein HN, Norton JA. Mechanisms of cancer cachexia. Hematol Oncol Clin North Am 1991;5:103–123.
6. Ng E, Lowry SF. Nutritional support and cancer cachexia: evolving concepts of mechanisms and adjunctive therapies. Hematol Oncol Clin North Am 1991;5:161–184.
7. Holroyde GP, Reichard GA. General metabolic abnormalities in cancer patients: anorexia and cachexia. Surg Clin North Am 1986;66:947–956.
8. Fearon KCH, Carter DC. Cancer cachexia. Ann Surg 1988;208:1–5.
9. Tisdale MJ. Cancer cachexia: metabolic alterations and clinical manifestations. Nutrition 1997;13:1–7.
10. Grosvenor M, Bulcavage L, Chlebowski RT. Symptoms potentially influencing weight loss in a cancer population. Cancer 1989;63:330–334.
11. Laviano A, Renvyle T, Yang Z-J. From laboratory to bedside: new strategies in the treatment of malnutrition in cancer patients. Nutrition 1996;12: 112–122.
12. Laviano A, Meguid MM, Yang Z-J, et al. Cracking the riddle of cancer anorexia. Nutrition 1996;12:706–710.
13. Brennan MF. Uncomplicated starvation vs. cancer cachexia. Cancer Res 1977;58:1867–1873.
14. Cohn SH, Gartenhaus W, Sawitsky A, et al. Compartmental body composition of cancer patients with measurement of total body nitrogen, potassium and water. Metabolism 1981;30:222–227.
15. Heymsfield SB, McManus CB. Tissue components of weight loss in cancer patients. Cancer 1985;55:238–249.
16. Meguid MM, Meguid V. Preoperative identification of the surgical cancer patient in need of post-operative supportive total parenteral nutrition. Cancer 1985;55:258–272.
17. Warren S. The immediate cause of death in cancer. Am J Med Sci 1933; 84:610–615.

18. Bozetti F, Migliavacca S, Gallus G, et al. Nutritional markers as prognostic indicators of post-operative sepsis in cancer patients. J Parent Ent Nutr 1985;9:464–470.
19. Rumley TO, Copeland EM. Value of nutritional support in adult cancer patients. Surg Clin North Am 1986;66:1177–1198.
20. DeWys WD. Management of cancer cachexia. Semin Oncol 1985;12: 452–460.
21. Inagaki J, Rodriguez V, Bodey GP. Causes of death in cancer patients. Cancer 1974;33:568–573.
22. Klein S, Koretz R. Nutrition support in patients with cancer: what do the data really show? Nutr Clin Pract 1994;9:91–100.
23. Ziegler TR, Young LS, Benfell K, et al. Clinical and metabolic efficacy of glutamine-supplemented parenteral nutrition after bone marrow transplant. Ann Intern Med 1992;116:821–828.
24. Daly JM, Liberman MD, Goldfine J, et al. Enteral nutrition with supplemented arginine, RNA, and omega-3 fatty acids in patients after operation: immunologic, metabolic, and clinical outcome. Surgery 1992;112: 56–67.
25. Zogbaum AT, Farkas S, Pease CR, Fitz FA, Duffy VB. Enteral feedings are associated with improved adherence to radiation treatment, prescription and weight maintenance in head and neck cancer patients [abstract]. J Am Diet Assoc 1996;96(suppl):A-35.
26. Herskowitz K, Souba WW. Intestinal glutamine metabolism during critical illness: a surgical perspective. Nutrition 1990;6:199–206.
27. Warnold I, Eden E, Lundholm K. The inefficiency of total parenteral nutrition to stimulate protein synthesis in moderately malnourished patients. Ann Surg 1988;207:143–149.
28. Moller-Loswick AC, Zack-Risson H, Bennegard K, Sandrom R, Lundholm K. Insufficient effect of total parenteral nutrition to improve protein balance in peripheral tissues of surgical patients. J Parent Ent Nutr 1991;15:669–675.
29. Streat SJ, Beddoe AH, Hill GL. Aggressive nutritional support does not prevent protein loss despite fat gain in septic intensive care patients. J Trauma 1987;27:262–266.
30. Torosian M. Stimulation of tumor growth by nutritional support. J Parent Ent Nutr 1992;16:72S–75S.
31. Mullen JL, Buzby GP, Gertner MH, et al. Protein synthesis dynamics in human gastrointestinal malignancies. Surgery 1980;87:331–338.
32. ASPEN. Board of Directors. Guidelines of the use of parenteral and enteral nutrition in adult and pediatric patients. J Parent Ent Nutr 1993;17: 1SA–52SA.
33. Bozzetti F, Amadori D, Bruera E, et al. Guidelines on artificial nutrition versus hydration in terminal cancer patients. Nutrition 1996;12:163–167.
34. Bloch A. Feeding the cancer patient: where have we come from, where are we going? Nutr Clin Pract 1994;9:87–89.
35. Hopkins B. Assessment of nutritional status. In: Gottschlic M, Matalese L, Shronts E (eds) Nutrition Support Dietetics: Core Curriculum. Silver Spring, MD: American Society for Parenteral and Enteral Nutrition, 1993:15–70.
36. Charney P. Nutritional assessment in the 1990's: where are we now? Nutr Clin Pract 1995;10:131–139.
37. Hammond K. Physical assessment: a nutritional perspective. Nurs Clin North Am 1997;32:779–790.
38. Buzby KM. Overview: screening, assessing, and monitoring. In: Bloch AS (ed) Nutrition Management of the Cancer Patient. Gaithersburg, MD: Aspen, 1990:15–23.
39. Ottery FD. Supportive nutrition to prevent cancer cachexia and improve quality of life. Semin Oncol 1995;3:98–111.
40. Jeejeebhoy KN, Meguid MM. Assessment of nutritional status in the oncologic patient. Surg Clin North Am 1986;66:1077–1090.
41. Bloch AS. Cancer. In: Gottschlich M, Matatese L, Shronts E (eds) Nutrition Support Dietetics: Core Curriculum. Silver Spring, MD: American Society for Parenteral and Enteral Nutrition, 1993:213–227.
42. Church JM, Hill GL. Assessing the efficacy of intravenous nutrition in general surgical patients: dynamic nutritional assessment with plasma proteins. J Parent Ent Nutr 1987;11:135–139.
43. Blackburn GL, Bistrian BR, Maini BS, et al. Nutritional and metabolic assessment of the hospitalized patient. J Parent Ent Nutr 1977;1:15–25.
44. Baker JP, Detsky AS, Wesson DE, et al. Nutritional assessment: a comparison of clinical judgement and objective measures. N Engl J Med 1982; 306:969–972.
45. Detsky AS, Baker JP, Mendelson RA, et al. Evaluation of accuracy of nutritional assessment techniques applied to hospitalized patients: methodology and comparisons. J Parent Ent Nutr 1984;8:153–159.
46. Desky AS, McLaughlin JR, Baker JP, et al. What is subjective global assessment of nutritional status? J Parent Ent Nutr 1987;11:8–13.
47. Jeejeebhoy KN, Detsky AS, Baker JP. Assessment of nutritional status. J Parent Ent Nutr 1990;14:193S–196S.
48. Shils ME. Nutrition and diet in cancer. In: Shils ME, Young VR (eds) Modern Nutrition in Health and Disease. Philadelphia: Lea & Febiger, 1988:1408.
49. Dempsy DT, Feurer EK, Knox LS, Crosby LO, Buzby GP, Mullen JL. Energy expenditure in malnourished gastrointestinal cancer patients. Cancer 1984;53:1265–1273.
50. Fredrix EW, Soeters PB, Wonters EF, Deerenberg IM, von Meyenfeldt MF, Savis WM. Effects of different tumor types on resting energy expenditure. Cancer Res 1991;51:6138–6141.
51. Elwyn DH, Kinney JM, Askanazi K. Energy expenditure in surgical patients. Surg Clin North Am 1981;61:545–556.
52. Herrmann VM, Fuhrman MP, Borum PR. Wasting diseases. In: Merrit RJ, Klein S, Souba WW, et al. (eds) The ASPEN Nutrition Support Practice Manual. Silver Spring, MD: American Society for Parenteral and Enteral Nutrition, 1998:11(1)–11(15).
53. Wolfe RB, O'Donnell TF, Stone MD, et al. Investigation of factors determining the optimal glucose infusion rate in total parenteral nutrition. Metabolism 1980;29:892–899.
54. Dempsey DT, Mullen JL. Macronutrient requirements in the malnourished cancer patient: how much of what and why? Cancer 1985;55:290–294.
55. Ideno KT. Cancer. In: Gottschlich ME, Matatese LE, Shronts EP (eds) Nutrition Support Dietetics: Core Curriculum. Silver Spring, MD: American Society for Parenteral and Enteral Nutrition, 1993:83.
56. Shils ME. Principles of nutritional therapy. Cancer 1979;43(suppl): 2093–2102.
57. Veterans Affairs Total Parenteral Nutrition Cooperative Study Group. Perioperative total parenteral nutrition in surgical patients. N Engl J Med 1991;8:525–532.
58. Minard G. Enteral access. Nutr in Clin Pract 1994;10:172–182.
59. Weinstein DS, Furman J. Enteral formulas. Nurs Clin North Am 1997; 32:669–682.
60. Maillet JO. Calculating parenteral feedings: a programmed instruction. J Am Diet Assoc 1984;84:1312–1323.

CHAPTER 79

Genetic Testing for Cancer Susceptibility

TINA J. HIEKEN

A. Introduction

There has been a recent rapid increase in discoveries related to the molecular genetic events underlying the development of human cancers. Many germline mutations predisposing to cancer susceptibility now have been identified, which has led to increased efforts to apply such information clinically, such as with the use of genetic testing to assess an individual's likelihood of developing certain cancers. This chapter presents a general overview of the steps required for genetic testing to assess cancer risk.

A number of genes have been implicated in the familial forms of some cancers, and these are summarized in Table 79–1.[1–19] As a caution to the reader, this list and the recommendations for testing are constantly and rapidly evolving as new information emerges. At present, commercial testing is available for several germline mutations, including those in *BRCA1*, *BRCA2*, *APC*, *hMSH2*, *hMLH1*, and *CDKN2A*. However, routine testing of high risk individuals is recommended as the accepted standard of care only for familial adenomatous polyposis coli (*APC*), retinoblastoma (*RB1*), von Hippel-Lindau disease (*VHL*), and familial medullary thyroid cancer and multiple endocrine neoplasia (MEN) type II (*RET*).[5,20,21] There is a presumed, but as yet unproven, benefit for some individuals in genetic testing for other familial cancer syndromes, including familial breast and ovarian cancer (*BRCA1*, *BRCA2*), hereditary nonpolyposis colon cancer (*hMSH2*, *hMLH1*, *hPMS1*, *hPMS2*, *hMSH6*), and Li-Fraumeni syndrome (*p53*).[22] Although commercial testing is now available for germline mutations in other cancer predisposition genes such as *CDKN2A* (implicated in some cases of hereditary malignant melanoma), such testing is indicated only in the context of a research study.

Practice guidelines for predisposition genetic testing for cancer in adults are rapidly evolving but remain incomplete. Although technologic advances are rapid and the number of commercially available tests is increasing, how to use such information to benefit patients remains unclear. A limited number of position papers and protocols have appeared during the past few years.[21–30] The guidelines in the following pages include a synthesis of these recommendations from the American Society of Clinical Oncology, the American Society of Human Genetics, the National Advisory Council for Human Genome Research, the National Society of Genetic Counselors, and other organizations. Many of these

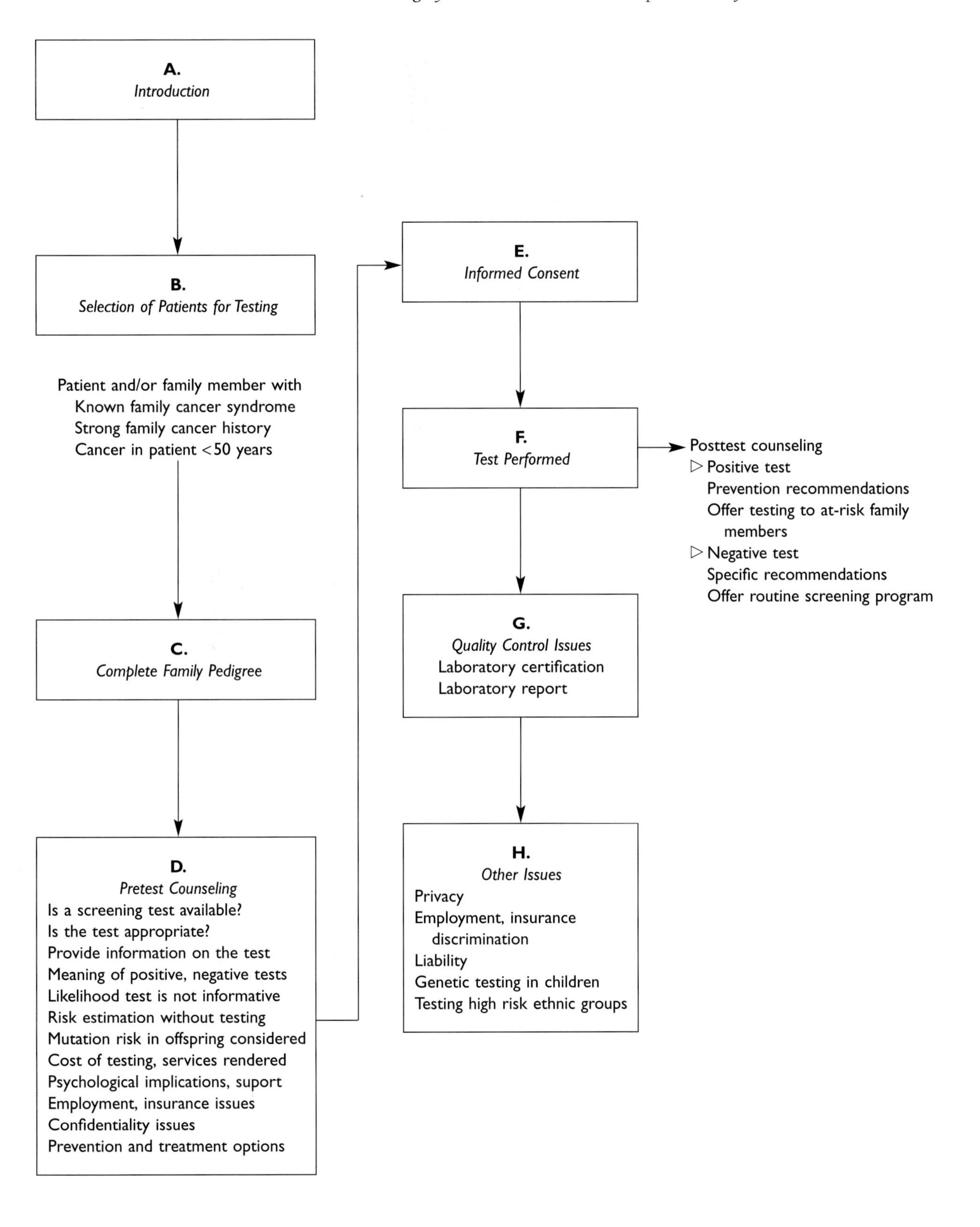

Genetic Testing for Cancer Susceptibility
A.
Introduction
B.
Selection of Patients for Testing
Patient and/or family member with
Known family cancer syndrome
Strong family cancer history
Cancer in patient <50 years
C.
Complete Family Pedigree
D.
Pretest Counseling
Is a screening test available?
Is the test appropriate?
Provide information on the test
Meaning of positive, negative tests
Likelihood test is not informative
Risk estimation without testing
Mutation risk in offspring considered
Cost of testing, services rendered
Psychological implications, suport
Employment, insurance issues
Confidentiality issues
Prevention and treatment options
E.
Informed Consent
F.
Test Performed
Posttest counseling
▷ Positive test
Prevention recommendations
Offer testing to at-risk family members
▷ Negative test
Specific recommendations
Offer routine screening program
G.
Quality Control Issues
Laboratory certification
Laboratory report
H.
Other Issues
Privacy
Employment, insurance discrimination
Liability
Genetic testing in children
Testing high risk ethnic groups

TABLE 79–1.
Genes implicated in familial forms of some cancers

Malignancy	Syndrome	Implicated gene	Chromosome	Refs.
Basal cell skin cancer	Gorlin syndrome (basal cell carcinoma and nevi)	*NBCCS*	9q	1
Breast cancer	Hereditary breast-ovarian cancer	*BRCA1*	17q21	2
		BRCA2	13q12-13	3
Colon cancer	Familial adenomatous polyposis	*APC*	5q21	4,5
	Hereditary nonpolyposis colon cancer (also endometrial, ovarian, stomach, small bowel cancers)	*hMSH2*	2p16	6–11
		hMLH1	3p21	
		hPMS1	2q31-33	
		hPMS2	7q11.2	
		hMSH6	2p15-16	
Melanoma	Familial melanoma (also glioblastoma)	*CDKN2A*	9p21	12,13
Renal cell carcinoma	Von Hippel-Lindau (also pheochromocytoma, hemangioblastoma)	*VHL*	3p25-26	14
Retinoblastoma	Retinoblastoma (also osteosarcoma, soft tissue sarcoma)	*RB1*	13q14	15
Soft tissue sarcoma	Li-Fraumeni syndrome (also leukemia, osteosarcoma; brain, breast, adrenocortical carcinoma)	*p53*	17p13	16,17
Thyroid cancer	Familial medullary thyroid cancer	*RET*	10q11.2	18,19
	Multiple endocrine neoplasia (MEN) type IIA (medullary thyroid cancer, pheochromocytoma) and MEN-IIB	*RET*	10q11.2	

organizations have presented conflicting policy directives.[31] Therefore, the focus of this chapter is on the complexity of genetic testing for cancer risk assessment and on the importance of appropriate patient selection, education, counseling, and informed consent to the decision-making process leading to testing.

B. Selection of Patients for Testing

At this time, genetic testing for cancer predisposition is not indicated for unselected patients in the general population. In general, individuals who seek or are offered testing are those who themselves or their family members have a known family cancer syndrome or a strong family cancer history or who have cancers that develop before age 50. Genetic testing may be offered to clarify the diagnosis of a suspected familial cancer syndrome. The first step is to create a written record of the family medical history. A targeted physical examination of the individual requesting testing is probably appropriate to see if there is any evidence of the cancer in question. If such evidence exists, further diagnostic workup takes precedence over predisposition testing.

C. Complete Family Pedigree

Because most information provided to an individual family member is orally transmitted, confirmation of the diagnoses of affected family members and the precise age of onset is critical. Information should be sought for three generations on both maternal and paternal sides. Every effort should be made to create an accurate family pedigree. This requires that pathology report-confirmation of the patient's or family member's diagnoses be obtained prior to instituting testing.[32]

D. Pretest Counseling

Pretest counseling is ideally provided in a multidisciplinary setting and includes specialist physicians, psychologists, nurses, social workers, and genetic counselors. When assessing cancer risk for a known hereditary cancer syndrome, it is helpful to invite all interested family members to this informational pretest session. Although the major potential benefit of genetic testing for cancer risk is to reduce cancer mortality through prevention or timely screening and early detection in predisposed individuals, other, less apparent psychological and social benefits of testing may be important to individuals. The likelihood that such benefits will accrue to an individual seeking testing depends on a number of factors.

First, is the proper test available? Second, is the test an appropriate one for the disease in question? Information on the specific test to be performed should be provided at this stage. The nature of the test proposed, either direct DNA sequencing or indirect analysis, should be disclosed. The tests that may be appropriately utilized include linkage analyses, protein truncation analyses, single-strand conformational polymorphism testing, allele-specific oligonucleotide assays, and tumor microsatellite instability (replication error) testing as well as direct DNA sequencing of various portions of the candidate gene. Information on how often the test in question gives an informative result should be provided. The meaning of positive and negative test results should be explained to the individual in a comprehensible fashion free of medical jargon. It is important to stress that while an inherited predisposition to certain common cancers may be due most frequently to mutations in better-known genes, rare genetic syndromes do account for some familial cancers. For example, familial breast cancer, while most often associated with mutations in *BRCA1* or *BRCA2*, can be due to Cowden's disease (*PTEN*), Peutz-jeghers syndrome (*STK11/LKB1*), Muir-Torre syndrome (*MSH2/MLH1*) or ataxia telangiectasia (*ATM*).[33] Also, patients need to be informed of possible increased risk of other malignancies, other than the one that initiated testing, associated with germline mutations in some genes. While it may be well-known that *BRCA1* and *BRCA2* mutations confer an increased risk of ovarian cancer, as well as breast cancer, and that female HNPCC mutation carriers have an increased risk of endometrial cancer as well as colon cancer, other associations may be less well-known and new information is continually becoming available as greater numbers of patients are tested and followed for the development of disease. For example, *CDKN2A* mutations (which may be detected in melanoma-prone families) confer a four-fold increased risk for the development of breast cancer and a 30-fold increased risk of pancreatic cancer.[34]

The likelihood of developing the cancer in question if a specific genetic alteration is identified should be addressed. This process is becoming quite challenging as more genetic tests are applied to familial cancer syndromes with lower (or unestablished) penetrance, and accurate estimation of risk may be difficult. Also, whenever a new mutation in a gene is discovered its functional significance is uncertain, as it may represent a polymorphism rather than a true mutation. An explanation of other factors, genetic and environmental, that may influence the onset of disease should be offered. It is important to stress that predisposition testing is usually probabilistic rather than deterministic. The implication of a negative test result must be clarified so the individual understands that he or she may still develop the cancer in question.[30] There is no currently available genetic test that permits identification of more than 95% of all mutation carriers. Even with complete sequencing of the entire coding region of the suspect gene, false negatives can occur such as in the case of a mutation in the promoter or other region that affects gene expression. The sensitivity of other assays is lower. For hereditary cancer syndromes associated with abnormalities in multiple genes, the picture may be even more complicated. For example, for hereditary nonpolyposis colon cancer, which is associated with mutations in multiple genes in the DNA mismatch repair pathway, a germline mutation is detected in fewer than 75% of kindreds with tumor microsatellite instability, suggesting that as-yet undiscovered genes may be involved.[35]

After information on the specific test has been provided, the options for risk estimation without genetic testing must be reviewed (e.g., the use of the Gail or Claus models for estimating breast cancer risk). Models for estimating the likelihood of finding mutations in various cancer-associated genes for an individual with a family history of the disease are being proposed.[5,36–39] The rapidly changing nature of this field and the possibility of storing DNA specimens for future use may be discussed.

The risk of passing the mutation on to children must be addressed for the specific hereditary syndrome. Other issues that should be covered during the pretest counseling phase include the cost of testing, the psychological risks of testing or declining testing,[40] the risks of employment and insurance discrimination, and confidentiality issues. The medicolegal and privacy issues are addressed in greater detail later in the chapter.

The prevention and intervention options (i.e., proposed follow-up care plan after testing) must be addressed. Such recommendations vary greatly depending on the specific cancer in question and need to be presented in a factual manner by the appropriately informed physician specialist. For example, for patients found to have a *BRCA1* or *BRCA2* mutation, information on penetrance is evolving and is probably lower than originally estimated; that is, not all patients with the mutation develop breast cancer.[41–43] In addition, prophylactic mastectomy (or oophorectomy) does not entirely ablate the risk for the development of cancer in the future, and the benefit of such measures remains unproven.[44,45] While a recent study suggests that prophylactic mastectomy for *BRCA1* and *BRCA2* carriers is efficacious, at least in the short-term, the effect of concomitant prophylactic oophorectomy, selection bias, and other confounding factors limit the conclusions that can be drawn from these data.[46] Also, studies examining the efficacy of prophylactic intervention to decrease cancer risk have looked at the development of cancer as an endpoint, rather than for a survival benefit. These issues remain to be resolved. Therefore careful consideration by an informed individual is mandatory before an irrevocable decision is made to have prophylactic surgery. In addition to available treatment and surveillance plans, the medical, behavioral, and social implications of test results should be discussed. The possibility of guilt, anxiety, depression, changes in family relationships, and so forth needs to be explored.[47] The motives for requesting testing should be discussed. Common reasons for seeking testing include anxiety about passing the risk on to children and concern about surveillance and prevention options.[48] The potential life-altering effects of testing on the individual must be acknowledged.[49]

All information should be presented in a balanced, nonjudgmental, nondirective fashion. Patients may weigh the risks and benefits of testing in a manner differently from health care professionals, as there are many complicated social, family, and personal issues involved. Individuals who seek testing should be encouraged to bring a support person to their educational and counseling sessions. Supplemental written materials, summarizing the information discussed, allow the patient to refer back to accurate information at a later date and share the information with other people should he or she desire.

E. Informed Consent

Issues involved in obtaining informed consent include a full understanding of the items outlined above. A recent analysis of laboratories performing molecular genetic testing showed that informed consent was required by only 34% for predisposition testing and by 44% for presymptomatic testing.[50] Clearly, responsible physicians and centers providing genetic testing for cancer risk must always obtain written informed consent. In addition, whether the patient is participating in a research protocol or in clinically based testing should be disclosed. Because there is an absence of data on the appropriate medical management of mutation carriers for all but a few familial cancer syndromes, patients should be encouraged to participate in research protocols or central data registries to provide long-term outcome data whenever possible.

In summary, the hazards and benefits of testing must be defined. The counseling team must also ensure that the individual is psychologically equipped to deal with the results of testing. Awareness of the potential problems of testing, including disclosure, insurance, and employment issues, is extremely important.[51] The goal of this process of education and counseling is to facilitate true voluntary, informed decision-making on the part of the individual requesting testing. The informed consent document should enumerate each of these issues and be written in clearly understood language in a manner that protects both the individual who seeks testing and the health care provider.[29]

F. Test Performed

The logistics of testing should be reviewed ahead of time. The usual source for genetic testing is DNA obtained from peripheral blood leukocytes. DNA retrieved from tumor blocks may be utilized if an affected relative is deceased. Issues regarding payment, collection, and disposition of specimens, as well as the time frame and manner in which the test results are disclosed, should be clearly stated in advance.

Posttest Counseling

Test results are best given in person by a medical professional with or without a trained genetic counselor. Survey data suggest that a cancer specialist is preferred to a primary care provider by most patients.[52] Results are best given in a comfortable setting with sufficient time permitted to explain the implication of the results and answer questions on pertinent issues. Follow-up medical and psychological care should be available and offered. Telephone numbers are provided so patients can call with future questions and concerns. Recommendations for screening guidelines, regardless of testing results, are provided, and referrals are made to appropriate medical specialists for long-term care.

Positive Test

Conferring information to an individual about a positive test result—that the patient is indeed a likely mutation carrier—must be done in a compassionate as well as factually accurate manner. Intervention, prevention, and screening recommendations necessarily depend on the specific cancer in question. Such recommendations are also rapidly evolving as more knowledge on penetrance and the natural history of the carrier state accrues.[43,53] Testing should also be offered to at-risk family members. Helping affected individuals to develop positive coping strategies and to adhere to medical recommendations for prevention or screening regimens is extremely important. There is evidence that compliance with screening and prevention recommendations may be low even among newly diagnosed gene mutation carriers, such as in an ongoing study of *BRCA1* testing participants.[54] Reiteration of the importance of these measures by the physician and genetic counselor can improve compliance.

Negative Test

It is important for individuals who are not gene carriers to know that they still need screening. Depending on the disease entity being evaluated, the individual may still require intensive screening measures (i.e., not those offered to the general population). The known sensitivity of the test in question should be disclosed. For example, whereas *RET* mutation analysis including exons 10, 11, and 14 has a sensitivity of 95%, exclusion of exon 14 analysis decreases the sensitivity of the test to about 80%.[55] Routine cancer screening recommendations, such as those promulgated by the American Cancer Society, should be reiterated for other individuals. If the proband has not been shown to have the mutation being evaluated, the individual tested needs to know that a negative test result may not confer any protection, and the individual may well remain at high risk for the future development of the particular cancer. It is important to discuss the uncertainty and continued evolution of knowledge associated with the molecular biology of genetic testing for cancer risk assessment.

G. *Quality Control Issues*

Genetic testing for clinical use must be done in a laboratory in compliance with the Clinical Laboratories Improvement Act (CLIA) regulations.[30] Studies performed in a research laboratory must be validated by a CLIA-certified laboratory before being used for clinical purposes. Accreditation from the College of American Pathologists/American College of Medical Genetics' Molecular Pathology program is desirable but not required by any federal law. Some states have special certification programs for laboratories providing clinical molecular genetic testing. The sensitivity and specificity of genetic testing depends not only on the test provided but the laboratory providing the test. At present, it appears that a great deal of reliance is placed on the ordering physician as the present regulatory system governing genetic testing is minimal, and such tests are not subject to Food and Drug Administration (FDA) regulation.[56] Physicians offering genetic testing must be aware of these issues.

Interpretation of the results of genetic predisposition tests is not as straightforward as the interpretation of other laboratory tests routinely evaluated by clinical practitioners. The commercial laboratory report must include information on the accuracy of the test performed, the nature and predictive value of the mutation identified (or not identified), and whether such a mutation has been previously reported. An ambiguous or uninformative result must be clearly stated and any recommendations for further testing appended to the report. Ideally, references to the current medical literature should be provided with the test result.

H. *Other Issues*

Privacy

Prior to testing patients should be informed of who will receive the test results and where such information will be stored. In some centers, patients undergoing genetic testing are identified by a code number, and such information is stored separately from the general medical records. At-risk individuals must be informed prospectively that even with such safeguards in place confidentiality cannot be guaranteed.[57] In addition, although sequestering medical information may restrict access by insurers and employers, it may be detrimental in terms of medical care and providing information for future generations. In addition, the physician's fiduciary duty to warn in order to prevent harm to a third party may conflict with patient confidentiality when an individual is found to be a mutation carrier and does not inform other family members of their possible risk status.[58,59] The current status of the law appears to favor duty to the patient rather than to family members unless unusual circumstances exist.[60]

Employment and Insurance Discrimination

As alluded to earlier, some of the gravest concerns of both high risk individuals and physicians surrounding genetic testing for cancer susceptibility involve the potential for "genetic discrimination." Cases of such employment or insurance discrimination have been documented.[61,62] The usual scenario in which insurability problems arise is when an individual tries to alter an existing policy or obtain new insurance coverage. Until federal legislation that prohibits discrimination based on genetic testing is enacted, the fear of loss of insurance or employment is the single most significant factor keeping individuals from pursuing genetic testing.[63] To this end, 12 states have enacted legislation restricting the use of genetic testing in the context of insurance practice, and at least 15 other states have such legislation pending.[64] In this regard, it is important to remember that carriers of a defined germline mutation associated with increased cancer risk are not ill and do not invariably develop cancer.

Liability Issues

Another issue concerns the legal liability assumed by genetic counselors, whose disclosures may influence decisions about childbearing, for example, and expose individuals to various forms of socioeconomic discrimination as alluded to above.[58,59] Additional legal questions will be raised as genetic testing for heritable cancer becomes more accepted and available. Will physicians have a duty to offer genetic testing to a patient with a personal and family history suggestive of a heritable cancer syndrome? Will physicians caring for an individual with a known mutation have a de facto responsibility to inform third parties such as at-risk relatives? These questions remain to be answered.

Genetic Testing in Children

A few studies have suggested that many parents believe they should be able to provide informed consent for genetic testing for cancer susceptibility to their minor children.[65] However, the long-term consequences, both physical and psychological, are unknown, and the potential for significant psychological damage to children is a real concern.[66] Although the primary focus should be on what is in the best medical interest of the child, debate remains on the appropriateness of genetic testing of children, especially for adult-onset disorders and those where there is no known intervention to change the outcome. Hereditary cancer syndromes associated with the onset of tumors during childhood, such as familial medullary thyroid carcinoma, familial adenomatous polyposis, and retinoblastoma, warrant genetic testing of children, as interventions are available and appear to be of benefit in reducing morbidity and mortality from the disease.[5,20,21,67]

Genetic Testing of Certain Ethnic Groups

Although there is currently almost uniform agreement that genetic testing for cancer risk is not indicated as a population screening tool, there have been suggestions that certain ethnic groups may benefit from testing for certain cancer syndromes. One example is screening Ashkenazi Jewish women for breast cancer. Since the discovery of the high prevalence of specific mutations in *BRCA1* and *BRCA2* among Ashkenazi Jewish women, one study of unselected patients found that all identified carriers in their study reported at least one first- or second-degree relative with a history of breast or ovarian cancer.[68] Thus they concluded that testing is probably not indicated unless there is also a family or personal history of breast cancer. No benefit to genetic testing as screening for any racial or ethnic group has been shown at this time.

References

1. Reis A, Kuster W, Linss G, et al. Localization of the gene for the nevoid basal cell carcinoma syndrome. Lancet 1992;339:617–619.
2. Futreal PA, Liu Q, Shattuck-Eidens D, et al. BRCA1 mutations in primary breast and ovarian carcinomas. Science 1994;266:120–122.
3. Tavtigian S, Simard J, Romens J, et al. The complete BRCA2 gene and mutations in chromosome 13q-linked kindreds. Nat Genet 1996; 12:333–337.
4. Kinzler KW, Nilbert MC, Su L, et al. Identification of FAP locus genes from chromosome 5q21. Science 1991;253:661–664.
5. Giardello FM, Brensinger JD, Peersen GM, et al. The use and interpretation of commercial APC gene testing for familial adenomatous polyposis. N Engl J Med 1997;336:823–827.
6. Leach FS, Nicolaides N, Papadopoulos N, et al. Mutations of a MutS homolog in hereditary non-polyposis colorectal cancer. Cell 1993;75: 1215–1225.
7. Lynch HT, Smyrk TC, Watson P, et al. Genetics, natural history, tumor spectrum and pathology of hereditary nonpolyposis colorectal cancer: an updated review. Gastroenterology 1993;104:1535–1549.
8. Papadopoulos N, Nicolaides NC, Wei Y, et al. Mutation of a mutL homolog in hereditary nonpolyposis colon cancer. Science 1994;263:1625–1629.
9. Nicolaides NC, Papadopoulos N, Liu B, et al. Mutations of two PMS homologues in hereditary nonpolyposis colon cancer. Nature 1994;371:75–80.
10. Akiyama Y, Sato H, Yamada T, et al. Germ-line mutation of the hMSH6/GTBP gene in an atypical hereditary nonpolyposis colorectal cancer kindred. Cancer Res 1997;57:3920–3923.
11. Miyaki M, Konishi M, Tanaka K, et al. Germline mutation of MSH6 as the cause of hereditary nonpolyposis colorectal cancer [letter]. Nat Genet 1997;17:271–272.
12. Kamb A, Shattuck-Eidens D, Eeles R, et al. Analysis of the p1 gene (CDKN2) as a candidate for the chromosome 9p melanoma susceptibility locus. Nat Genet 1994;8:23–26.
13. Monzon J, Liu L, Brill H, et al. CDKN2A mutations in multiple primary melanomas. N Engl J Med 1998;338:879–887.
14. Latif F, Tory K, Gnarra J, et al. Identification of the von Hippel-Lindau disease tumor suppressor gene. Science 1993;260:1317–1320.
15. Lee WH, Bookstein R, Hong F, et al. Human retinoblastoma susceptibility gene: cloning, identification, and sequence. Science 1994;235:1987–1990.
16. Malkin D, Li FP, Strong LC, et al. Germ line p53 mutations in a familial syndrome of breast cancer, sarcomas, and other neoplasms. Science 1990;250:1233–1238.
17. Birch JM, Hartley AL, Tricker KJ, et al. Prevalence and diversity of constitutional mutations in the p53 gene among 21 Li-Fraumeni families. Cancer Res 1994;54:1298–1304.
18. Mulligan LM, Kowk JBJ, Healey CS, et al. Germ-line mutations of the RET proto-oncogene in multiple endocrine neoplasia type 2A. Nature 1993; 363:458–461.
19. Hofstra RM, Landsvater RM, Cecherini I, et al. A mutation in the RET proto-oncogene associated with multiple endocrine neoplasia type 2B and sporadic medullary thyroid carcinoma. Nature 1994;267:375–379.
20. Lips CJM, Landsvater RM, Hoppener JWM, et al. Clinical screening as compared with DNA analysis in families with multiple endocrine neoplasia type 2A. N Engl J Med 1994;331:828–835.
21. Petersen GM, Cordori A-M. Genetic testing for familial cancer. In: Vogelstein B, Kinzler KW (eds) The Genetic Basis of Human Cancer. New York: McGraw-Hill, 1998;591–599.
22. Statement of the American Society of Clinical Oncology: genetic testing for cancer susceptibility. J Clin Oncol 1996;14:1730–1736.
23. Li FP, Garber JE, Friend SH, et al. Recommendations on predictive testing for germ line p53 mutations among cancer-prone individuals. J Natl Cancer Inst 1992;84:1156–1160.
24. Biesecker BB, Boehnke M, Calzone K, et al. Genetic counseling for families with inherited susceptibility to breast and ovarian cancer. JAMA 1993;269:1970–1974.
25. Bowcock AM, Biesecker BB, Collins F, et al. Statement of the American Society of Human Genetics on genetic testing for breast and ovarian cancer predisposition. Am J Hum Genet 1994;55:i–iv.
26. National Advisory Council for Human Genome Research. Statement on use of DNA testing for presymptomatic identification of cancer risk. JAMA 1994;271:785.
27. Petersen GM. Genetic counseling and predictive testing for colorectal cancer risk. Int J Cancer 1996;69:53–54.
28. Baty BJ, Venne VL, McDonald J, et al. BRCA1 testing: genetic counseling protocol development and counseling issues. J Genet Couns 1997;6: 223–244.
29. Geller G, Botkin JR, Green MJ, et al. Genetic testing for susceptibility to adult-onset cancer: the process and content of informed consent. JAMA 1997;277:1467–1474.
30. McKinnon WC, Baty BJ, Bennett RL, et al. Predisposition genetic testing for late-onset disorders in adults: a position paper of the National Society of Genetic Counselors. JAMA 1997;278:1217–1220.
31. Kodish E, Wiesner GL, Mehlman M, et al. Genetic testing for cancer risk: how to reconcile the conflicts. JAMA 1998;279:179–181.
32. Parent ME, Ghadirian P, Lacroix A, et al. The reliability of recollections of family history: implications for the medical provider. J Cancer Educ 1997;12:114–120.
33. Domchek SM, Garber JE. Genetic testing for breast cancer. Principles and Practice of Oncology, supplement, volume 15, number 7, 2001.
34. Borg A, Sandberg T, Nilsson K, et al. High frequency of multiple melanomas and breast and pancreatic carcinomas in *CDKN2A* mutation-positive melanoma families. J Natl Cancer Inst 2000;92:1260–1266.
35. Liu B, Parsons R, Papadopoulos N, et al. Analysis of mismatch repair genes in hereditary nonpolyposis colorectal cancer patients. Nat Med 1996;2: 169–174.
36. Couch FJ, DeShano ML, Blackwood A, et al. BRCA1 mutations in women attending clinics that evaluate the risk of breast cancer. N Engl J Med 1997;336:1409–1415.
37. Shattuck-Eidens D, Oliphant A, McClure M, et al. BRCA1 sequence analysis in women at high risk for susceptibility mutations: risk factor analysis and implications for genetic testing. JAMA 1997;278:1242–1250.

38. Wijnen JT, Vasen FHA, Khan PM, et al. Clinical findings with implications for genetic testing in families with clustering of colorectal cancer. N Engl J Med 1998;339:511–518.
39. Aaltonen LA, Salovaara R, Kristo P, et al. Incidence of hereditary nonpolyposis colorectal cancer and the feasibility of molecular screening for the disease. N Engl J Med 1998;338:1481–1487.
40. Lerman C, Hughes C, Lemon SJ, et al. What you don't know can hurt you: adverse psychologic effects in members of BRCA1-linked and BRCA2-linked families who decline genetic testing. J Clin Oncol 1998;16:1650–1654.
41. Easton DF, Ford D, Bishop DT. Breast Cancer Linkage Consortium: breast and ovarian cancer incidence in BRCA1 mutation carriers. Am J Hum Genet 1994;56:265–271.
42. Struewing JP, Hartge P, Wacholder S, et al. The risk of cancer associated with specific mutations of BRCA1 and BRC2 among Ashkenazi Jews. N Engl J Med 1997;336:1401–1408.
43. Ford D, Easton DF, Stratton M, et al. Genetic heterogeneity and penetrance analysis of the BRCA1 and BRCA2 genes in breast cancer families. Am J Hum Genet 1998;62:676–689.
44. Burke W, Daly M, Garber J, et al. Recommendations for follow-up care of individuals with an inherited predisposition to cancer. II. BRCA1 and BRCA2. JAMA 1997;277:997–1003.
45. Schrag D, Kuntz KM, Garber JE, et al. Decision analysis: effect of prophylactic mastectomy and oophorectomy on life expectancy among women with BRCA1 or BRCA2 mutations. N Engl J Med 1997;33:1465–1471.
46. Meijers-Heijboer H, van Geel B, van Putten WLJ, et al. Breast cancer after prophylactic bilateral mastectomy in women with a *BRCA1* or *BRCA2* mutation. New Engl J Med 2001;345:159–164.
47. MacDonald DJ. Genetic predisposition testing for cancer: effects on families' lives. Holist Nurs Pract 1998;12:9–19.
48. Lynch HT. A descriptive study of BRCA1 testing and reactions to disclosure of test results. Cancer 1997;79:2219–2228.
49. Lerman C, Croyle R. Emotional and behavioral responses to genetic testing for susceptibility to cancer. Oncology 1996;10:191–195.
50. McGovern M, Benach MO, Wallenstein S, Desnick RJ, Keenlyside R. Quality asurance in molecular genetic testing laboratories. J Am Med Assoc 1999;281:835–840.
51. Kash M. Psychosocial and ethical implications of defining genetic risk for cancers. Ann NY Acad Sci 1995;768:41–52.
52. Audrain J, Rimer B, Cella D, et al. Genetic counseling and testing for breast-ovarian cancer susceptibility: what do women want? J Clin Oncol 1998;16:133–138.
53. Frank TS, Manley SA, Olopade OI, et al. Sequence analysis of BRCA1 and BRCA2: correlation of mutations with family history and ovarian cancer risk. J Clin Oncol 1998;16:2417–2425.
54. Few BRCA1 carriers take recommended precautions. Oncol New Int 1998;7:1.
55. Decker RA, Peacock ML. Update on the profile of multiple endocrine neoplasia type 2a RET mutations. Cancer 1997;80:557–568.
56. Malinowski MJ, Blatt RJR. Commercialization of genetic testing services: the FDA, market forces and biological tarot cards. Tulane Law Rev 1997;1211.
57. Mehlman MJ, Kodish ED, Whitehouse P, et al. The need for anonymous genetic counseling and testing. Am J Hum Genet 1996;58:393–397.
58. Dickens BM, Pei N, Taylor KM. Legal and ethical issues in genetic testing and counseling for susceptibility to breast, ovarian and colon cancer. Can Med Assoc J 1996;154:813–818.
59. Deftos LJ. Genomic torts: the law of the future—the duty of physicians to disclose the presence of a genetic disease to the relatives of their patients with the disease. Univ San Francisco Law Rev 1997;32: USFL Rev 105.
60. Anderlik MR, Lisko EA. Medicolegal and ethical issues in genetic cancer syndromes. Sem Surg Oncol 2000;18:339–346.
61. Lapham EV, Kozma C, Weiss JO. Genetic discrimination: perspectives of consumers. Science 1996;274:621–624.
62. Jacobs LA. At-risk for cancer: genetic discrimination in the workplace. Oncol Nurs Forum 1998;25:475–480.
63. Kinney A, DeVellis B, Skrzynia C, Millikan R. Genetic testing for colorectal carcinoma susceptibility: Focus group responses of individuals with colorectal carcinoma and first-degree relatives. Cancer 2001;91:57–65.
64. Bornstein RA. Genetic discrimination, insurability and legislation: a closing of the legal loopholes. J Law Policy 1996;551.
65. Benkendorf JL, Reutenauer JE, Hughes CA, et al. Patients' attitudes about autonomy and confidentiality in genetic testing for breast-ovarian cancer susceptibility. Am J Med Genet 1997;73:296–303.
66. Grosfeld FJ, Lips CJ, Beemer FA, et al. Psychological risks of genetically testing children for a hereditary cancer syndrome. Patient Educ Couns 1997;32:63–67.
67. Skinner MA, DeBenedetti MK, Moley JR, et al. Medullary thyroid carcinoma in children with multiple endocrine neoplasia types 2A and 2B. J Pediatr Surg 1996;31:177–181.
68. Richards CS, Ward PA, Roa BB, et al. Screening for 185delAG in the Ashkenazim. Am J Hum Genet 1997;60:1085–1098.

Chapter 80

When You May Legally Withdraw Treatment

MARK C. MANTOOTH

The question of when a physician may legally withdraw therapy is pertinent whenever the physician is no longer legally obligated to treat or continue treating a patient. In this analysis, we assume that treatment has already begun to avoid the need to discuss the legal and philosophic distinctions between withholding and withdrawing medical treatment. For our purposes, we attempt here to focus on the general circumstances when a physician may legally withdraw medical treatment.[1] We concentrate on a single state, Illinois, which has the two typical advanced directive statutes (the living will and the durable power of attorney) and a health care surrogate statute, while exploring the overlay of federal requirements. Note, however, that the distinctions between the various states' laws remain vast and subtle.

A physician's obligation to treat a patient generally arises out of a contractual arrangement between the physician and the patient, by which each party has certain responsibilities and rights. With this arrangement, the physician obligates him- or herself to treat the patient in accordance with the medical standard for that specialty in that geographic region. As medical specialties develop, however, courts are increasingly looking to national standards to determine the proper standard of conduct to apply for each medical specialty.

The patient's primary obligation under this contractual arrangement is to compensate the physician for the services rendered. Among his or her rights, the patient retains authority to consent to receive medical services, exercised by providing "informed consent."[2] For the patient's consent to be "informed," the physician must first inform the patient of the foreseeable risks and consequences associated with the treatment and any reasonably acceptable alternative therapies.[3] When consenting to the therapy, the patient must simultaneously be legally competent, clinically capable of understanding the information, free of coercion, and acting voluntarily.

During a course of treatment, the physician's duty to treat may be terminated in one of several ways. The physician may, *with adequate and proper notice to the patient*, terminate the patient—physician relationship. What the courts consider to be "adequate and proper notice" varies widely based on the circumstances of the particular patient—physician relationship and the governing state law. Courts have looked at such factors as the parties' subjective views whether their relationship had terminated, the

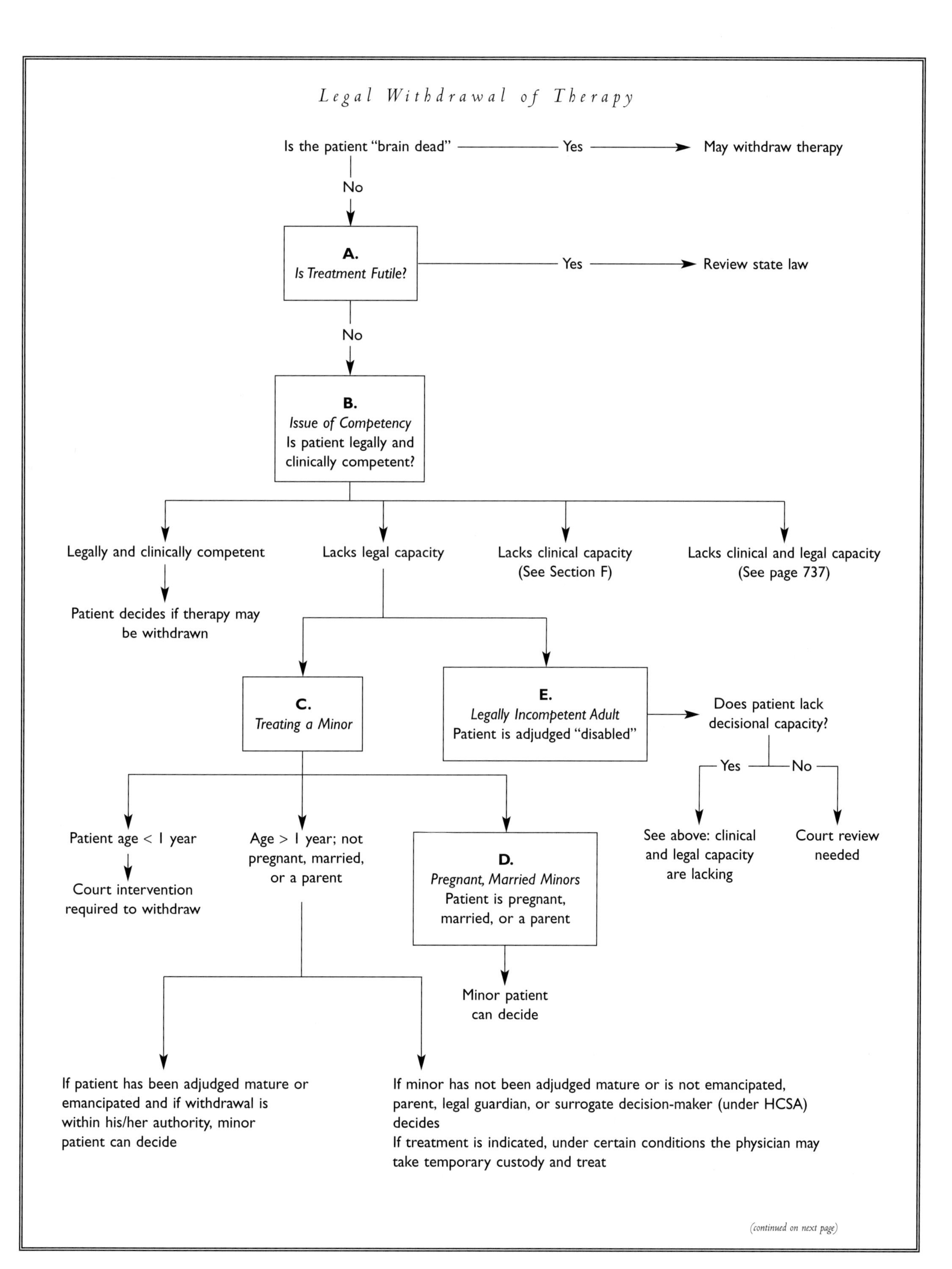

(continued on next page)

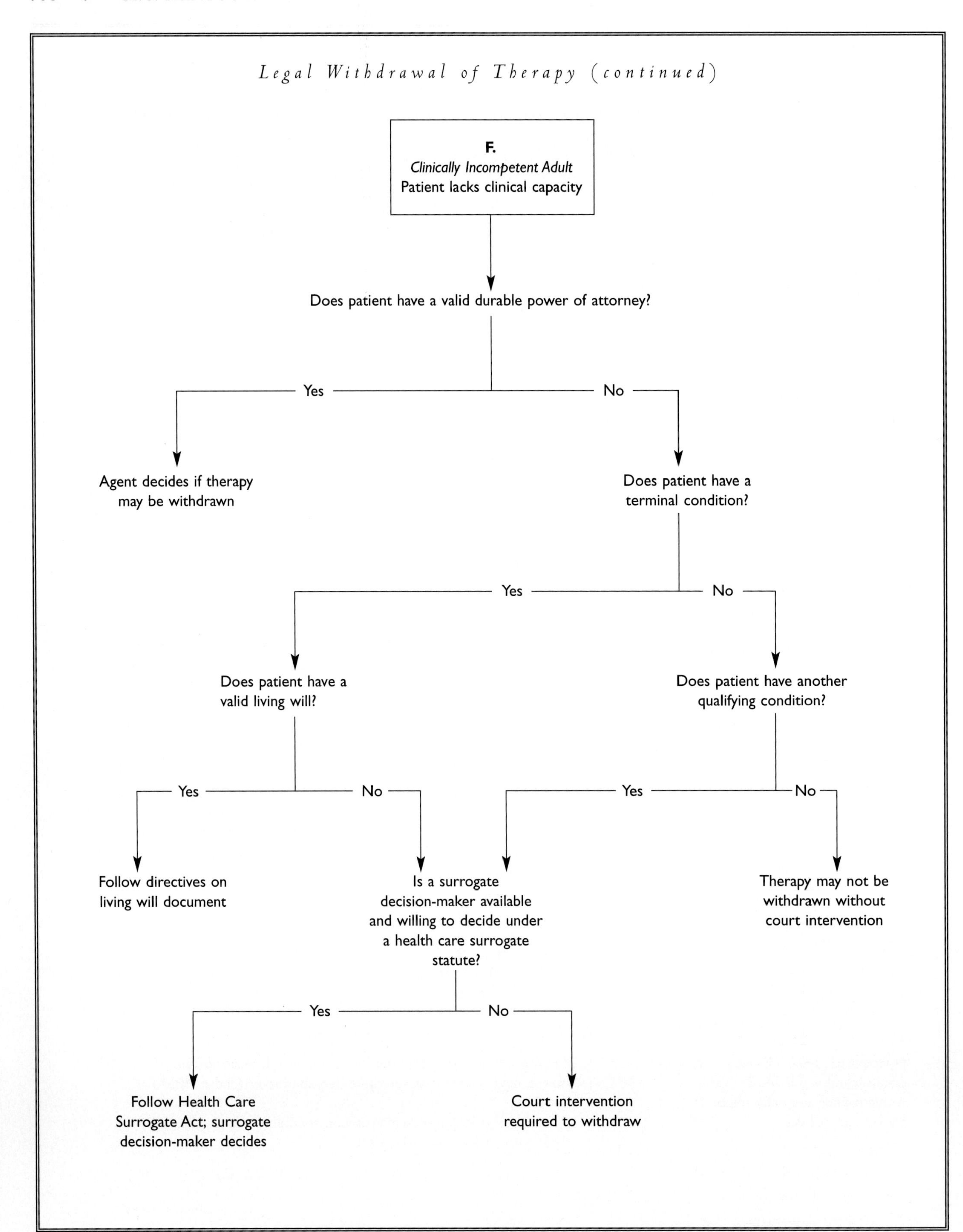
Legal Withdrawal of Therapy (continued)
F.
Clinically Incompetent Adult
Patient lacks clinical capacity
Does patient have a valid durable power of attorney?
Yes
No
Agent decides if therapy may be withdrawn
Does patient have a terminal condition?
Yes
No
Does patient have a valid living will?
Does patient have another qualifying condition?
Yes
No
Yes
No
Follow directives on living will document
Is a surrogate decision-maker available and willing to decide under a health care surrogate statute?
Therapy may not be withdrawn without court intervention
Yes
No
Follow Health Care Surrogate Act; surrogate decision-maker decides
Court intervention required to withdraw

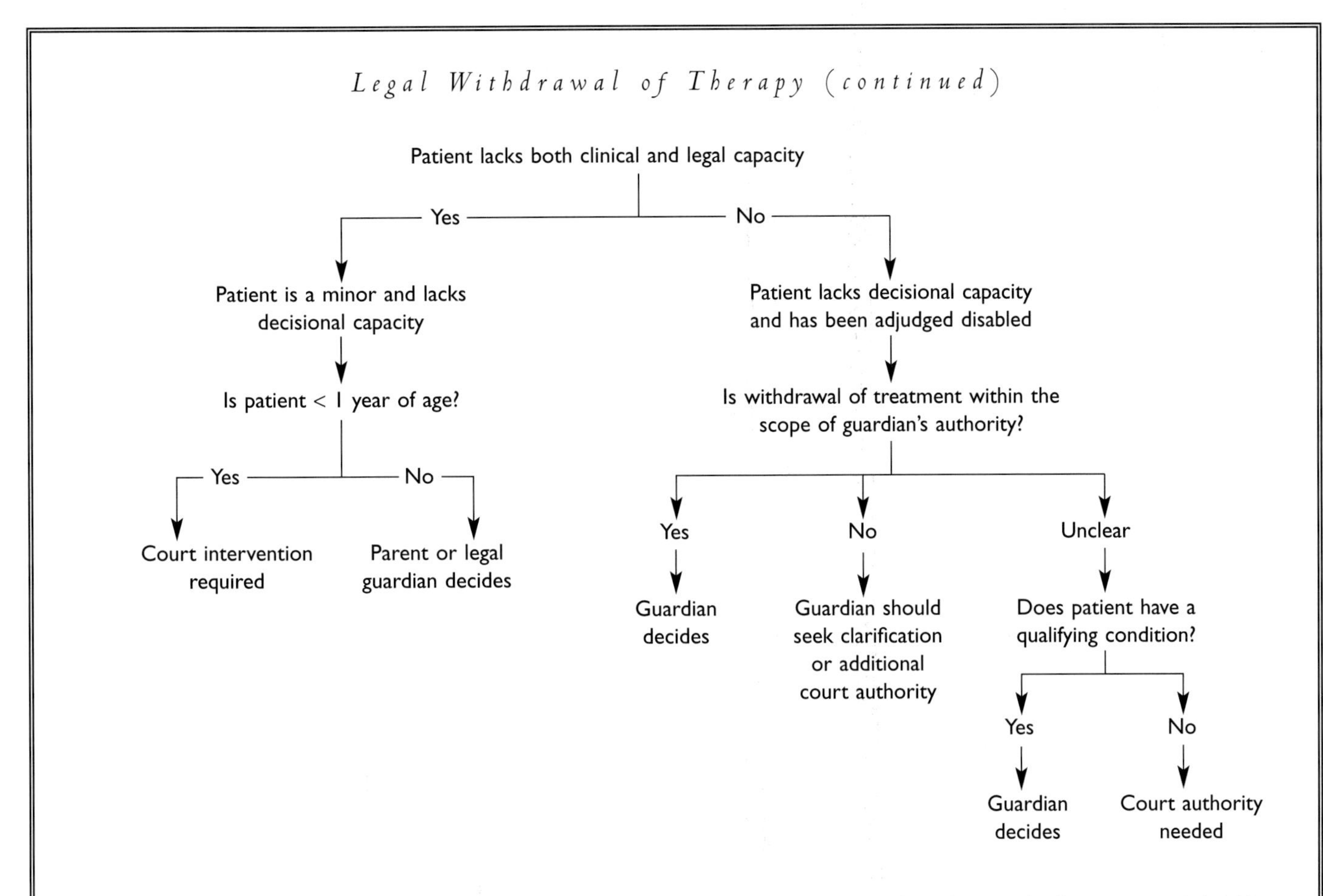

length of the relationship, the frequency of their interactions, whether the physician was still monitoring the patient's condition, whether the patient was still relying on the physician's advice, and whether the patient had begun to consult with another physician concerning the same problems.[5] One court concluded for instance that once the patient moved out of the geographic area and stopped seeing the physician, the relationship had terminated, notwithstanding an isolated, single doctor visit more than a decade after the patient moved.[6]

Under managed care scenarios, the physician's obligation may also be affected by the terms and conditions of his or her provider agreement with the managed care organization as well as the terms of the plan's arrangement with its enrollees. A physician's legal duty to treat a patient also ends upon the death of the patient—with death typically being defined as the irreversible cessation of total brain function, including the brain stem, according to the usual and customary standards of medical practice.[7] When the patient meets these criteria, the patient is referred to as being "brain dead."

A. Is Treatment Futile?

Over the years, the law has struggled to determine whether a physician has a legal duty to treat or continue to treat a patient when the proposed treatment would be "futile." Moreover, the courts have yet to articulate clearly when treatment may be deemed "futile," although when defining the term in the context of the Emergency Medical Treatment and Active Labor Act (EMTALA) the Fourth Circuit Court of Appeals in *In Re Baby K*[8] considered as *not* being futile, treatment that could alleviate the conditions that were making a condition *acute*. In that case, the parents of a 2-month old anencephalic child brought the child to their community hospital's emergency unit when the child was suffering respiratory distress. Following the second admission, the hospital sought a court injunction to allow it to refuse treatment for the child because in light of the child's anencephaly the physicians considered the treatment "futile." The federal district and appellate courts disagreed, however, finding that the plain language of EMTALA requires "stabilizing treatment for any individual who comes to a participating hospital, is diagnosed as having an *emergency* condition, and cannot be transferred."[9]

A physician's duty to treat may also be eradicated by the patient terminating the patient–physician relationship or by simply refusing to consent to a specified course of treatment.[10] Just as a patient has a right to accept treatment, a patient also enjoys a right to refuse treatment. The patient's refusal, however, must be an informed refusal. The physician is obligated to inform the patient of the risks and consequences associated with his or her refusal. The patient–physician discussion and the patient's refusal should be documented in the patient's medical record.

B. Issue of Competency

What if the patient is incapable of exercising this right? When can a patient refuse treatment, and when can the physician rely on the patient's refusal? For a person to be capable of giving legally binding consent or refuse to consent, the person must simultaneously have *legal competency* (also known as "legal capacity") and *clinical competency* (frequently referred to as "decisional capacity"). A person has *legal competency* if he or she is of majority age, which is 18 years of age in Illinois, and a court has not determined that he or she is "incompetent" or "disabled" as defined under the applicable probate or mental health statute. A person is *clinically competent*, or has decisional capacity, if he or she can understand the nature and consequences of the proposed course of treatment and can communicate an informed decision as determined by the attending physician.[11]

C. Treating a Minor

If the patient lacks legal capacity because he or she is a minor, the general rule is that the parent or legal guardian must provide consent on behalf of the patient.[12] In Illinois the following are exceptions to this rule. If the parents refuse to consent but the treatment is medically indicated and the treatment itself does not involve a similar, substantial risk, the physician may—while following certain procedures—still treat the patient. In Illinois the physician could take temporary protective custody of the child, treat the child, notify the child's parents or guardian, and report the case to the Department of Children and Family Services.[13] If the parents refuse to consent and the treatment itself poses significant risk to the child, the physician would have to assume protective custody of the child and immediately petition the court for the authority to treat the child. Regarding terminating care, unless the conditions of the Illinois Health Care Surrogate Act are met the physician would be obligated to continue treating the child according to the standard of care. If the minor is protected under the federal Child Abuse Amendments of 1984 and the accompanying regulations, a physician would be required to treat or continue treating that minor patient unless a court order authorized removal of the medically indicated treatment.[14]

D. Pregnant, Married Minors

Illinois law recognizes several exceptions when a minor may consent for treatment and a few scenarios when the minor may consent to have treatment withdrawn. The Illinois Consent by Minors to Medical Procedures Act permits pregnant or married minors, or a minor who is a parent, to consent or refuse to consent to medical treatment.[15] Under the Emancipation of Mature Minors Act, a court may declare a person 16 years of age or older emancipated if the person is of sound mind and has the capacity and maturity to manage his or her own affairs, including financial matters, and the court determines that emancipation is in the minor's and minor's family's best interests.[16] Typically, this statute would be used if the minor wished to consent or refused to consent to medical treatment and his or her parents objected. When deciding an emancipation case, the court would articulate in its written order the specific rights and responsibilities the minor would have upon emancipation.

Under Illinois common law, some Illinois state courts have recognized a right to consent or refuse consent to treatment for minors who can understand the nature and consequences of a proposed medical therapy. In *In re E.G.*,[17] an Illinois trial court found that a 17-year-old who had leukemia and refused to consent to blood transfusions on religious grounds was mature enough to exercise adult judgment and refuse treatment. In reviewing the trial court's decision, the Illinois Supreme Court confirmed that the testimony of the patient, a psychiatrist, and a hospital attorney supported the court's finding that E.G. was mature.[18] The Illinois Supreme Court under these circumstances extended to E.G. the right that adults enjoy to refuse medical care.[19]

The Illinois Health Care Surrogate Act (HCSA) also enables surrogate decision-makers to consent to the withdrawal of medical treatment for minor patients under certain circumstances, as discussed below.

E. Legally Incompetent Adult

An adult patient may also lack legal competence if a court determines that the patient is a "disabled person" or lacks entirely the mental or physical capability to manage his or her personal affairs or for some other specified reason.[20] During the court's investigation of the person's mental capacity, the court typically receives extensive testimony from a physician that confirms for the court that the person also lacks clinical competence. Upon finding that the person lacks sufficient understanding or lacks the capacity to make or communicate responsible decisions concerning his or her own care, the court can declare that the person is a "disabled person" under the state's probate act or similar statute, and that person thereby loses the legal capacity to enter into contracts or engage in certain legally binding transactions, including consenting to or refusing medical treatment.[21] During the process of adjudicating a person disabled, the court designates a relative, friend, or interested party to function as that person's legal guardian. The scope of the guardian's authority varies depending on the petition and the court order, but the court generally articulates the scope of the guardian's authority, including the ability to consent to medical treatment on behalf of the patient.[22]

The Illinois Probate Act requires the guardian to make responsible decisions for the disabled person that protect and promote his or her well-being, including providing informed consent for medically indicated treatment.[23] If continued treatment is not medically indicated, the guardian may similarly consent to the withdrawal of treatment, but only as authorized by the court.[24] Conflicts arise when treatment is medically indicated, but the guardian requests that the therapy be stopped. Most states have enacted advance directive and health care proxy or surrogacy statutes to govern many of these scenarios.

F. *Clinically Incompetent Adult*

In the absence of an applicable advance directive or a health care surrogacy statute, the U.S. Supreme Court in *Cruzan v. Missouri Dept. of Health*[25] implicitly found a constitutional right for a person in a persistent vegetative state to refuse life-sustaining medical treatment.[26] Nancy Cruzan, a 25-year-old woman, was involved in an automobile accident when driving down a country road and was later found lying face down on the ground in standing water, suffering from anoxia and severe brain damage. The emergency medical response team successfully restored her breathing and heartbeat, but she never regained consciousness or apparently an awareness of her environment; she was determined to be in a persistent vegetative state. Approximately 3 weeks after the accident, Nancy Cruzan's parents consented to having a feeding tube surgically inserted in Nancy's stomach but soon requested that it be withdrawn. Ultimately, the U.S. Supreme Court decided that the state where Nancy Cruzan was being treated, Missouri, could require clear and convincing evidence of Nancy Cruzan's wishes before a court appointed guardian could consent to the withdrawal of artificial nutrition and hydration.[27]

In Illinois the Supreme Court in *In Re Estate of Longeway*[28] decided that a terminally ill, incompetent patient could refuse or have withdrawn life-sustaining medical treatment, including artificial nutrition and hydration.[29] This right would be exercised by the court-appointed surrogate decision-maker deciding on behalf of the patient, consistent with the patient's previously expressed intent and desires.[30] The Court further stated that although the judiciary was ill-suited to resolve situations involving complex medical procedures, the intervention of a judge remained proper to guard against improper decisions, to protect the estate and the patient, and to ensure that proof of the patient's desires are demonstrated by clear and convincing evidence.[31]

In a case decided soon after *Longeway*, the Illinois Supreme Court in *In Re Estate of Greenspan*[32] reaffirmed the *Longeway* holding, but modified and expanded its application.[33] In *Greenspan*, the patient, an 82-year-old man, had organic brain syndrome, had suffered a stroke, and for approximately 5 years had been in a chronic vegetative state. When the Illinois Supreme Court was presented with the argument that because Mr. Greenspan did not have a terminal condition the *Longeway* holding did not apply, the Court in a tortured line of reasoning concluded that Mr. Greenspan's chronic condition was also "terminal." It reasoned that an illness is terminal when (1) death is imminent, and (2) death-delaying procedures would serve only to prolong the dying process.[34] Because artificial nutrition and hydration have been defined statutorily as part of "death delaying procedures," the Court decided it would judge whether Mr. Greenspan's condition was "terminal" if the patient's death was "near at hand" after the feeding tube was withdrawn.[35]

When an Advance Directive Exists

The Patient Self-Determination Act of 1990 (PSDA)[36] remains one of the few federal statutes that address the withdrawal of medical treatment, and then it does so only indirectly. The PSDA requires that all Medicare and Medicaid provider organizations, including hospitals, home health agencies, nursing facilities, hospices, and prepaid health care organizations, maintain written policies and procedures regarding advance directives. These organizations must also educate their own staffs about advance directives, provide patients upon admission with written information about advance directives, inquire whether the person has executed an advance directive, document within the person's medical record pertinent information, and comply with state laws concerning advance directives.[37]

Generally, two types of advance directives exist: living wills and appointment directives, also referred to as durable powers of attorney for health care. Most states currently have statutes for some form of one or both of these advance directives; Illinois has both. The Illinois Living Will Act (LWA)[38] provides that an adult or emancipated minor of sound mind may execute a document directing health care providers to withdraw life-sustaining treatment if they lose decisional capacity, develop a terminal condition, and death is imminent. Consequently, for a physician to rely on a properly executed living will and withdraw life-sustaining treatment, the patient must be incapable of understanding and communicating an informed decision about the treatment, and the physician must have examined the patient and determined that the patient has a terminal condition and that death is imminent.

The other applicable Illinois advance directive, the Illinois Powers of Attorney for Health Care Law,[39] permits a person (the principal) to execute a written document that, unlike the LWA, appoints another person (the agent) to make health care decisions for the principal only if the principal loses decisional capacity. This statute, as intended by the legislature, grants the agent broad authority in making treatment decisions for the principal.[40] Upon a good faith determination by the health care provider that the patient lacks the capacity to give informed consent, the provider shall consult with and obtain consent from the agent.[41] By statute, the agent is authorized to consent to, refuse consent for, or authorize the withdrawal of any health care for the principal, with "health care" being defined as "any care, treatment, service or procedure to maintain, diagnose, treat or provide for the patient's physical or mental health or personal care."[42] The agent is directed to act on the principal's benefit and in accordance with any limitations indicated on the executed document.

When a Properly Executed Advance Directive Does Not Exist

In Illinois, if a person has failed to execute properly either a living will or a durable power of attorney or is a minor, the Illinois Health Care Surrogate Act (HCSA) may still apply. The HCSA was promulgated to establish a private decision-making process for patients who had not executed an advance directive and who lacked decisional capacity. If the patient lacked decisional capacity and did not have a properly executed durable power of attorney, the HCSA would statutorily identify potential surrogate decision-makers to provide informed consent for the patient. If the surrogate's decision required the withholding or withdrawal of life-sustaining treatment, the patient would also have to have a qualifying condition; and if that qualifying condition was a terminal condition, he or she could not have an applicable living will. In other words, the HCSA would not apply to a medical condition for which an advance directive could be implemented.

As defined in the HCSA, a qualifying condition means one of three medical conditions to which a patient's attending physician and at least one other qualified physician have certified the patient has. The conditions include: a terminal condition, permanent unconsciousness, and an irreversible or incurable condition.[43] It is important to note that not all of these conditions require the patient's condition to be terminal. "Permanent unconsciousness" is depicted by a chronic condition, sometimes identified as a "persistent vegetative state."

Once the attending physician and another qualified physician have certified and documented in the patient's chart that the patient has a qualifying condition, the attending physician has to identify the appropriate surrogate decision-maker from a prioritized list, which includes next of kin.[44] After the attending physician has identified the person who has the highest priority on the surrogate list, that person would have the same rights as the patient in terms of receiving the patient's medical information and, within the parameters of the HCSA, consenting to treatment or to the withdrawal of treatment. The HCSA, however, explicitly states that the surrogate decision-maker must make health care decisions, "conforming as closely as possible to what the patient would have done or intended under the circumstances, taking into account evidence that includes, but is not limited to, the patient's personal, philosophical, religious and moral beliefs and ethical values relative to the purpose of life, sickness, medical procedures, suffering, and death."[45] If the patient's wishes are unknown, the surrogate would have to decide according to the patient's best interests as determined by the surrogate decision-maker.[46]

Despite the diversity of the state statutes and the vagaries of the various statutory terms, reviewing the laws of Illinois with the federal law overlay should provide a basic understanding of the legal issues and concepts in play. Because of the legal import of factual distinctions, the physician should consult an attorney who is familiar with the applicable state law when confronted with a clinical scenario involving the withdrawal of medical treatment.

References and Notes

1. This article does not address the peculiarities concerning consenting and refusing to consent to mental health treatment. During the discussion of advance directives, be aware of the potential interplay of mental health declarations, which grant to designated agents legal authority to consent to mental health treatment. See Mental Health Treatment Preference Declaration Act, 755 Ill. Comp. Stat. Ann. 43/1–43/115 (West 2001).
2. In addition to viewing the right to consent as a contractual right, the courts have also viewed consent as a common law right of "every individual to the possession and control of his own person," [*Union Pacific Ry. Co. v. Botsford*, 141 U.S. 250, 251, 11 S.Ct. 1000, 1001 (1891)], as a right found in the First Amendment free exercise of religion clause [See *In Re Estate of Brooks*, 32 Ill.2d361, 205 N.E.2d 435 (1965)], and as a restricted constitutional right to privacy [*Cruzan v. Missouri Dept. of Health*, 497 U.S. 261 (1990)]. Some states, such as Illinois, also require statutorily that health care providers obtain informed consent prior to treating any patient who has a nonemergent condition. Medical Patient Rights Act, 410 Ill. Comp. Stat. Ann. 50/3(a)(West 2001).
3. *Weekly v. Solomon*, 156 Ill. App. 3d 1011, 1016, 510 N.E.2d 152 (1987); *Hansbrough v. Kosyak*, 141 Ill. App. 3d 538, 551, 490 N.E.2d 181 (1986) (same duty); *see also Whittaker v. Honegger*, 284 Ill. App. 3d 739, 742, 674 N.E.2d 1274 (1996).
4. Uniform Anatomical Gift Act, 755 Ill. Comp. Stat. Ann. 50/2 (West 2001). See *In Re Haymer*, 115 Ill. App. 3d 349 (1983) (when determining the time of death, court focuses on cessation of brain activity).

5. *Blanchette v. Barrett*, 229 Conn. 256, cited in *Wit v. St. Vincent's Medical Center*, 52 Conn. App. 699, 727 A.2d 802 (1999). See also *Kahaner v. Berkley*, 1999 Conn. Super. LEXIS 897 (Conn. Supp. Ct. Mar. 24, 1999), (when determining whether the patient-physician relationship had been terminated, this Connecticut court looked at whether the doctor and his office considered the person to be the physician's patient still, whether the physician's office retained the patient's records, whether the physician was still medically supervising the use of certain prescription medications, whether the patient's medical records showed some indication that the physician considered himself to be engaged in an ongoing course of treatment, and whether the physician had discussed termination of his relationship with the patient).
6. *Aznel v. Gasso*, 154 Ill. App. 3d, 507 N.E.2d 83 (1st Dist., 1987).
7. Uniform Anatomical Gift Act, 755 Ill. Comp. Stat. Ann. 50/2 (West 2001). See *In re Haymer*, 115 Ill. App. 3d 349 (1983) (when determining the time of death, court focuses on cessation of brain activity). See also *In Re Estate of Sewart*, 236 Ill. App. 3d 1, 602 N.E.2d 1277 (1991) (an Illinois appellate court articulated two standards by which to determine death: the irreversible cessation of total brain function and an "irreversible cessation of circulatory respiratory functions according to usual and customary standards of practice." 236 Ill. App. 3d at 14–15, 602 N.E.2d at 1277).
8. 16 F.3d 590 (4th Cir. 1994).
9. *Id.*
10. Health Care Surrogate Act, 755 Ill. Comp. Stat. Ann. 40/20(a) (West 2001).
11. 755 Ill. Comp. Stat. Ann. 40/10 (West 2001).
12. Consent by Minors to Medical Procedures Act, 410 Ill. Comp. Stat. Ann. 210/2 (West 2001).
13. Abused and Neglected Child Reporting Act, 325 Ill. Comp. Stat. Ann. 5/5 (West 2001).
14. Volunteers for Children Act, 42 U.S.C. §5101 et seq., as amended by section 121(3) of the Child Abuse Amendments of 1984. In the applicable regulations, the term "infant" means "an infant less than one year of age. . . ." 45 C.F.R. §1340.15 (2001).
15. Consent by Minors to Medical Procedures Act, 410 Ill. Comp. Stat. Ann. 210/2 (West 2001).
16. Emancipation of Mature Minors Act, 750 Ill. Comp. Stat. Ann. 30/1 et seq. (West 2001).
17. 133 Ill. 2d 98, 549 N.E.2d 322 (1989).
18. 133 Ill. 2d at 107, 549 N.E.2d at 326.
19. In *In Re* E.G., the Illinois Supreme Court considered whether E.G. exercised the judgment of an adult, whether the evidence of E.G.'s wishes was clear and convincing, and the views of E.G.'s parents. *See* W. Brewster *In Re* E.G., *A Minor: Death Over Life: A Judicial Trend Continues as the Illinois Supreme Court Grants Minors the Right to Refuse Life-Saving Medical Treatment*, 23 J. Marshall L. Rev. 771 (1990).
20. The Illinois Probate Act defines "disabled person" as a "person 18 years or older who (a) because of mental deterioration or physical incapacity is not fully able to manage his person or estate; or (b) is a person with mental illness or a person with a developmental disability and who because of his mental illness or developmental disability is not fully able to manage his person or estate, or (c) because of gambling, idleness, debauchery or excessive use of intoxicants or drugs, so spends or wastes his estate as to expose himself or his family to want or suffering." Probate Act, 755 Ill. Comp. Stat. Ann. 5/11a-2 (West 2001).
21. To protect patients' right to consent to treatment, Illinois courts have found that persons adjudged "disabled" may not always lack capacity to make health care decisions. See *In Re* Guardianship of Austin, 615 N.E.2d 411, 418 (Ill. App. Ct. 4th Dist. 1993), and In re Austwick, 656 N.E.2d 773 (Ill. App. Ct., 1st Dist. 1995) (adjudication of disability does not automatically overcome presumption that the person has decisional capacity under the Health Care Surrogate Act).
22. Probate Act, 755 Ill. Comp. Stat. Ann. 5/11a-3(a) (West 2001).
23. 755 Ill. Comp. Stat. Ann. 5/11a-3(b) (West 2001).
24. In *In re Austwick*, the court ruled that a court-appointed guardian could not authorize a "do not resuscitate" order being entered for his or her elderly ward unless the patient had a qualifying condition under the Health Care Surrogate Act or without further court approval. 275 Ill. App. 3d 665, 656 N.E.2d 773 (1st Dist. 1995).
25. 497 U.S. 261 (1990).
26. 497 U.S. at 280.
27. *Id.* at 261. Under the Illinois Living Will Act and Health Care Surrogate Act, life-sustaining treatment and death-delaying procedures have been defined as including not only any medical treatment or procedure but also artificial nutrition and hydration.
28. 133 Ill.2d 33, 549 N.E.2d 292 (1989).
29. 549 N.E.2d at 298.
30. 549 N.E.2d at 299.
31. 549 N.E.2d at 300–01.
32. 137 Ill.2d 1, 558 N.E.2d 1194, 1204 (1990).
33. 558 N.E.2d at 1204.
34. *Id.* at 1203 [citing the Illinois Living Will Act (Ill. Rev. Stat., ch. 110 1/2, par. 702(d)(1987)].
35. 558 N.E.2d at 1205.
36. Patient Self-Determination Act, Omnibus Budget Reconciliation Act of 1990, Pub. L. No. 101–508, 4206 and 4751, 104 Stat. 1388–115 & 1388–204 (1991) [codified in sections of 42 U.S.C., particularly 1395cc(f) & 1396a(w) (1995)].
37. *Id.*
38. 755 Ill. Comp. Stat. Ann. 35/1 to 35/10 (West 2001).
39. 755 Ill. Comp. Stat. Ann. 45/1–1 to 45/4–12 (West 2001).
40. 755 Ill. Comp. Stat. Ann. 45/4–10 (West 2001).
41. 755 Ill. Comp. Stat. Ann. 45/4–7 (West 2001).
42. 755 Ill. Comp. Stat. Ann. 45/4–4 (West 2001).
43. The qualifying conditions are defined as follows: (1) "'terminal condition,' meaning an illness or injury for which there is no reasonable prospect of cure or recovery, death is imminent, and the application of life-sustaining treatment would only prolong the dying process; (2) 'permanent unconsciousness,' meaning a condition that, to a high degree of medical certainty, (i) will last permanently, without improvement, (ii) in which thought, sensation, purposeful action, social interaction, and awareness of self and environment are absent, and (iii) for which initiating or continuing life-sustaining treatment, in light of the patient's medical condition, provides only minimal medical benefit, and (3) 'irreversible or incurable condition,' meaning an illness or injury (i) for which there is no reasonable prospect of cure or recovery, (ii) that ultimately will cause the patient's death even if life-sustaining treatment is initiated or continued, (iii) that imposes severe pain or otherwise imposes an inhumane burden on the patient, and (iv) for which initiating or continuing life-sustaining treatment, in light of the patient's medical condition, provides only minimal medical benefit." Health Care Surrogate Act, 755 Ill. Comp. Stat. Ann. 40/10 (West 2001).
44. As provided in the statute, the priority list, with those having the highest priority at the beginning, reads as follows: (1) patient's guardian of the person; (2) patient's spouse; (3) any adult son or daughter of the patient; (4) either parent of the patient; (5) any adult brother or sister of the patient; (6) any adult grandchild of the patient; (7) close friend of the patient; (8) patient's guardian of the estate. 755 Ill. Comp. Stat. Ann. 40/25 (West 2001).
45. 755 Ill. Comp. Stat. Ann. 40/20(b-5)(1) (West 2001).
46. 755 Ill. Comp. Stat. Ann. 40/20 (West 2001).

Appendix

Commonly Used Chemotherapeutic Agents

THEODORE J. SACLARIDES

Drug	Mechanism of action	Metabolism	Indications	Route	Toxicity
Altretamine (Hexalen)	DNA alkylating agent; inhibits DNA, RNA synthesis	Liver	Ovarian, lymphoma, lung	PO	Myelosuppression, nausea, depression
Aminoglutethimide	Inhibits steroid synthesis	Liver, kidney	Breast	PO	Rash, leukopenia, adrenal insufficiency, hypothyroidism
Anastrozole (Arimidex)	Nonsteroidal aromatase inhibitor; lowers estradiol levels; no replacement therapy needed	Liver (85%), kidney (11%)	Breast	PO	Anemia, anorexia, cough, insomnia, hypertension, thrombophlebitis, fetal harm
Asparaginase	Inhibits protein synthesis dependent on asparagine	Renal, biliary	ALL, CLL, AML	IV	Bone marrow suppresion, acute renal failure, tremors, anaphylaxis, mutagenic
Bleomycin	Inhibits DNA synthesis	Liver, kidneys	Testicular, lymphoma, squamous cell	IV, IM, SQ	Nausea, pulmonary, CVA, hyperpigmentation, anaphylaxis, mutagenic
Busulfan	Interferes with DNA function	Liver	CML	PO	Bone marrow suppression, adrenal insufficiency, endocardial fibrosis, mutagenic

Drug	Mechanism of action	Metabolism	Indications	Route	Toxicity
Carboplatin	Interferes with DNA function	Kidney	Ovarian, endometrial, lung, seminoma	IV	Myelosuppression, nausea, vomiting, hematuria, pneumonitis, CVA, mutagenic, ototoxicity
Carmustine (BCNU)	Interferes with DNA, RNA synthesis	Kidney	Brain, myeloma, Hodgkin's, melanoma	IV	Myelosuppression, renal failure, pulmonary fibrosis, mutagenic
Chlorambucil (Leukeran)	Causes breaks in DNA; prevents DNA, RNA, protein synthesis	Metabolized in liver, excreted in urine	Leukemia, lymphoma, ovary, breast	PO	Myelosuppression, nausea, vomiting, pulmonary fibrosis, seizures, amenorrhea
Cisplatin (Platinol)	Binds to DNA; prevents DNA, RNA, protein synthesis	Not understood	Head and neck, testis, ovary, cervical, bladder, lung	IV	Ototoxicity, renal toxicity, myelosuppression, nausea, vomiting, pulmonary fibrosis, neuropathies, impotence, sterility
Cyclophosphamide (Cytoxan)	Alkylating agent; crosslinks DNA	Metabolized in liver, excreted in urine	Lymphoma, myeloma, leukemia, Wilms', sarcoma, rhabdomyosarcoma	PO, IV	Leukopenia, nausea, vomiting, cystitis, cardiac, mutagenesis, oligospermia, sterility
Dacarbazine (DTIC)	Alkylating agent that is cell-cycle-nonspecific; inhibits DNA, RNA synthesis	Liver	Melanoma, sarcoma, Hodgkin's, neuroblastoma	IV	Myelosuppression, nausea, vomiting, confusion, headache, mutagenic
Dactinomycin D (actinomycin)	Antibiotic; intercalates between DNA basepairs; inhibits DNA replication	Minimal metabolism, excreted in urine	Wilms', rhabdomyoscarcoma, testicular, uterine	IV	Myelosuppression, nausea, vomiting, anaphylaxis, hypocalcemia, mutagenic
Docetaxel (Taxotere)	Blocks disassembly of microtubules; prevents cell division	Liver	Breast	IV	Bone marrow suppression, elevated liver function tests, fluid retention, bronchospasm, hypersensitivity reactions, fetotoxic
Doxorubicin HCl (Adriamycin)	Anthracycline antibiotic; interferes with DNA synthesis	Hepatobiliary excretion	Leukemia, Wilms', neuroblastoma, sarcoma, breast, ovarian	IV	Bone marrow suppression, nausea, vomiting, cardiotoxicity, anaphylaxis, teratogenic, mutagenic, hyperpigmentation
Estramustine (Estracyte)	Estrogenic effect on hormone-dependent tissue	Liver	Prostate, breast	PO	Nausea, vomiting, diarrhea, elevated liver function tests, gynecomastia
Etoposide (VP-16)	Inhibits DNA topoisomerase II	Excreted in urine	Testicular, small cell lung, lymphoma, leukemia	IV, PO	Myelosuppression, mucositis, bronchospasm, fever, potentially mutagenic
Floxuridine (FUDR)	Pyrimidine antimetabolite; inhibits thymidylate synthesis, interferes with DNA synthesis	Liver	Colon metastases, primary liver, pancreatic, breast	Intraarterial	Myelosuppression, gastritis, duodenitis, duodenal ulcer, cholecystitis, renal failure, mutagenic

Drug	Mechanism of action	Metabolism	Indications	Route	Toxicity
5-Fluorouracil (5-FU)	Cell cycle-specific; inhibits thymidine synthetase	Liver	Colorectal, gastric, breast, pancreas, head and neck, renal cell, esophagus, prostate	IV	Myelosuppression, nausea, vomiting, renal failure, arrhythmias, headache, mutagenic, teratogenic
Flutamide (Eulexin)	Nonsteroidal antiandrogen; inhibits DNA synthesis in the prostate	Excreted in urine	Prostate	PO	Nausea, vomiting, diarrhea, impotence, gynecomastia, elevated liver function tests
Gemcitabine (Gemzar)	Antimetabolite; inhibits DNA synthesis, specific for S phase	Excreted in urine	Pancreatic, non-small cell lung, colon	IV	Myelosuppression, nausea, vomiting, elevated liver function tests, pulmonary toxicity, fever, renal failure
Hydroxyurea (Hydrea)	Inhibits DNA synthesis	Metabolized in liver	Head and neck, CML, ovarian, brain, melanoma	PO	Bone marrow depression, nausea, vomiting, convulsions, elevated liver function tests, elevated creatinine and BUN
Ifosfamide	Alkylating agent; destroys DNA, inhibits DNA synthesis	Liver	Germ cell testicular, sarcomas, Ewing's, lymphoma, lung, pancreas sarcoma	IV	Myelosuppression, nausea, vomiting, hemorrhagic cystitis, neurologic, infertility, mutagenic
Irinotecan (Camptosar)	Inhibits topoisomerase I, an enzyme essential for DNA replication	Liver	Colorectal	IV	Myelosuppression, diarrhea, nausea, vomiting, edema, elevated liver function tests
Levamisole	Enhances function of T lymphocytes, inhibits function of tyrosine phosphatase	Liver	Colorectal (used with 5-FU)	PO	Leukopenia, thrombocytopenia, agranulocytosis, nausea, vomiting, diarrhea, renal failure, neurologic
Lomustine (CCNU)	Alkylating agent; cell cycle-nonspecific; inhibits DNA and RNA synthesis	Urinary excretion	Brain, Hodgkin's, myeloma, gastrointestinal, non-small cell lung	PO	Myelosuppression, nausea, vomiting, nephrotoxic, pulmonary fibrosis, impairs fertility, ocular damage
Megestrol (Megace)	Antiestrogen; decreases number of estrogen receptors, inhibits release of LH receptors	Renal and fecal excretion	Endometrial, breast, cachexia, renal	PO	Leukopenia, fluid retention, weight gain, pulmonary embolism, elevated liver function tests, amenorrhea, hypercalcemia
Melphalan (Alkeran)	Cell cycle-nonspecific alkylating agent; crosslinks DNA strands	Plasma	Myeloma, breast, ovarian, testicular, sarcoma	PO, IV	Bone marrow depression, pulmonary fibrosis, anaphylaxis, bronchospasm, fetal harm, secondary neoplasms

Drug	Mechanism of action	Metabolism	Indications	Route	Toxicity
Methotrexate	S phase-specific antimetabolite; inhibits conversion of folic acid to tetrahydrofolic acid, thereby arresting DNA, RNA synthesis	Liver	Breast, head and neck, gastrointestinal non-small cell lung, osteosarcomas, ALL, trophoblastic	PO, IV, IM	Myelosuppression, nausea, vomiting, acute tubular necrosis, pulmonary infiltrates, neurologic, hypersensitivity, oligospermia, menstrual irregularities
Mitomycin C	Antitumor antibiotic; inhibits DNA synthesis	Liver	Stomach, pancreas, colon, anus, breast, uterine	IV	Myelosuppression, elevated BUN and creatinine, interstitial pneumonia, neurologic, shortness of breath, carcinogenic
Mitotane	Affects mitochondria of adrenocortical cells	Liver	Adrenal cortex, Cushing's disease, Leydig cell testis	PO	Adrenocortical insufficiency, nausea, vomiting, hemorrhagic cystitis, hypertension, hyperpigmentation, visual disturbances
Mitoxantrone HCl	Antineoplastic antibiotic; intercalates with DNA; inhibits topoisomerase II	Excreted through hepatobiliary tract	Leukemia, advanced breast, ovarian, prostate	IV	Myelosuppression, mucositis, arrhythmias, seizures, mutagenic, fever
Paclitaxel	Promotes microtubule formation and stability	Hepatobiliary	Metastatic ovarian, breast, non-small cell lung, melanoma, gastric, leukemia	IV	Bone marrow suppression, neutropenia, diarrhea, dyspnea, ECG changes, peripheral neuropathy, alopecia, facial flushing, hypersensitivity
Plicamycin, mithramycin	Binds to DNA molecules; interrupts DNA-directed RNA synthesis; inhibits osteoclasts and PTH	Liver	Testicular, hypercalcemia, hypercalciuria	IV	Thrombocytopenia, bleeding syndromes, nausea, lethargy, akathisia, elevated BUN and creatinine, elevated liver chemistries
Streptozocin	Alkylating agent; inhibits DNA synthesis; cell cycle-nonspecific	Renal	Pancreatic islet cell, carcinoid, non-small cell lung, oral	IV	Nausea, vomiting, diarrhea, hepatic, renal, proteinuria, hypersensitivity, secondary cancers
Tamoxifen	Mixed estrogen antagonist/agonist; at high concentrations blocks the G_1 cell cycle phase	Liver	Breast, endometrial, melanoma, prostate	PO	Nausea, vomiting, menopausal symptoms, dizziness, headaches, deep vein thrombosis, increased incidence of endometrial cancer
Thiotepa	Alkylating agent; reacts with DNA phosphate groups, forming crosslinkages; blocks nucleoprotein synthesis	Liver	Breast, ovary, bladder, Hodgkin's, bronchogenic	IV, intravesical	Myelosuppression, nausea, vomiting, dizziness, allergic reactions, amenorrhea, azoospermia, mutagenic, teratogenic, carcinogenic

Drug	Mechanism of action	Metabolism	Indications	Route	Toxicity
Topotecan HCl	Inhibits topoisomerase I, an enzyme essential for DNA replication	Urine, liver	Metastatic ovarian, small cell lung	IV	Bone marrow suppression, neutropenia, nausea, vomiting, dyspnea, alopecia, arthralgia, hypersensitivity
Vinblastine	Vinca alkaloid; inhibits microtubule formation in the mitotic spindle, arrests cell division in metaphase	Liver	Lymphoma, testicular, breast, bladder, renal lung	IV	Bone marrow suppression, ileus, GI bleeding, SIADH, bronchospasm, paresthesias, MI, amenorrhea, azoospermia
Vincristine	Vinca alkaloid; inhibits microtubule assembly, arrests cell division in metaphase, specific at the M and S phase	Liver	Acute leukemia, lymphoma, rhabdomyosarcoma, neuroblastoma, Wilms', myeloma, breast	IV	Bone marrow suppression, intestinal necrosis, SIADH, bronchospasm, cranial nerve dysfunction, optic atrophy, alopecia, azoospermia, amenorrhea
Vinorelbine tartrate	Vinca alkaloid (see above)	Plasma, liver	Lung, non-small cell breast, Hogdkin's, ovarian	IV	Granulocytopenia, ileus, elevated liver chemistries, SIADH, hemorrhagic cystitis, bronchospasm, peripheral neuropathy, alopecia, hypersensitivity

ALL, acute lymphocytic, leukemia; CLL, chronic lymphocytic leukemia; AML, acute myelocytic leukemia; CML, chronic myelocytic leukemia; CVA, cerebrovascular accident; BUN, blood urea nitrogen; LH, luteinizing hormone; PTH, parathyroid hormone; ECG, electrocardiogrem; GI, gastrointestinal; SIADH, syndrome of inappropriate secretion of antidiuretic hormone; MI, myocardial infarction; 5-FU, 5-fluorouracil.

Index

A

E

H

N